MYASTHENIA GRAVIS AND RELATED DISEASES

DISORDERS OF THE NEUROMUSCULAR JUNCTION

Edited by David P. Richman

The New York Academy of Sciences
New York, New York
1998

Library of Congress Cataloging-in-Publication Data

Myasthenia gravis and related diseases: disorders of the
neuromuscular junction/edited by David P. Richman.
    p. cm. — (Annals of the New York Academy of Sciences, ISSN
0077-8923; v. 841).
    Proceedings of the Ninth International Conference on Myasthenia
Gravis and Related Disorders, sponsored by the New York Academy of
Sciences and the Myasthenia Gravis Foundation of America, Inc.
(California Chapter) and held on May 7–10, 1997, in Santa Monica,
Calif.
    Includes bibliographical references and index.
    ISBN 1-57331-119-7 (cloth: alk. paper). — ISBN 1-57331-120-0
(pbk.: alk. paper).
    1. Myasthenia gravis—Congresses. 2. Myoneural junction—
Diseases—Congresses. I. Richman, David P. II. Myasthenia Gravis
Foundation (U.S.). California Chapter. III. New York Academy of
Sciences. IV. International Conference on Myasthenia Gravis and
Related Disorders (9th: 1997: Santa Monica, Calif.). V. Series.
    [DNLM: 1. Myasthenia Gravis congresses. 2. Neuromuscular
Junction—physiopathology congresses. W1 AN626YL v. 841 1998/WE
555 M9942 1998]
Q11.N5 vol. 841
[RC935.M8]
500 s—dc21
[616.7'442]
DNLM/DLC
for Library of Congress   97-52826
                                                    CIP

&/RRD
Printed in the United States of America
ISBN 1-57331-119-7 (cloth)
ISBN 1-57331-120-0 (paper)
ISSN 0077-8923

MYASTHENIA GRAVIS AND RELATED DISEASES

DISORDERS OF THE NEUROMUSCULAR JUNCTION

ANNALS OF THE NEW YORK ACADEMY OF SCIENCES

Volume 841
May 13, 1998

MYASTHENIA GRAVIS AND RELATED DISEASES

DISORDERS OF THE NEUROMUSCULAR JUNCTION[a]

Editor and Conference Organizer
DAVID P. RICHMAN

CONTENTS

---

[a]This volume is the result of the Ninth International Conference on Myasthenia Gravis and Related Disorders, which was sponsored jointly by the New York Academy of Sciences and the Myasthenia Gravis Foundation of America, Inc. (Host-California Chapter), and held on May 7–10, 1997, in Santa Monica, California.

Part II. Nonimmune Disorders of the Neuromuscular Junction

Part III. Immune Regulation and Autoimmunity

Part IV. Autoimmune (Acquired) Myasthenia Gravis

Part VII. Current Diagnosis and Treatment of Lambert-Eaton Myasthenic Syndrome

Financial assistance was received from:

Cosponsor
- MYASTHENIA GRAVIS FOUNDATION OF AMERICA, INC. (HOST-CALIFORNIA CHAPTER)

Major Funders
- NATIONAL INSTITUTE OF NEUROLOGICAL DISORDERS AND STROKE
- JACK AND JEAN CRAEMER

Supporters
- JOHN W. ALLEN, CLU, CHFC
- BAYER CORPORATION—PHARMACEUTICAL DIVISION

Introduction

DAVID P. RICHMAN

Department of Neurology
University of California, Davis
Davis, California 95616

This volume addresses the progress made in our understanding of diseases of the neuromuscular junction over the last five years. It is the product of the Ninth International Conference on Myasthenia Gravis held in Santa Monica, California, on May 7–10, 1997. The conference was the most recent in a series of international meetings jointly sponsored by the New York Academy of Sciences and the National Myasthenia Gravis Foundation, held at approximately five-year intervals.

Since 1957, when the first of these conferences was held, there has been an explosion in our understanding of the pathogenesis of the two major diseases of this synapse, myasthenia gravis and Lambert-Eaton myasthenic syndrome. Treatment of both diseases has *pari passu* improved as well. Two factors make the neuromuscular junction an extremely attractive model synapse to study: (1) its location isolated from other synapses; (2) the existence of electric organs of various fish species that consist almost solely of neuromuscular junctions.[1] The components of the synapse are, therefore, readily purified. Because of these factors, the physiology, pharmacology, biochemistry, and cellular and molecular biology of the neuromuscular junction are better understood than of any other synapse in the nervous system. For example, the three-dimensional structure of the nicotinic acetylcholine receptor is known to 9 Å resolution, and the structural transition that the channel undergoes during activation has recently been reported.[2,3]

In only a few anatomic structures other than the neuromuscular junction has there been so strong an interplay between basic biological advances and the study of the diseases affecting that structure. The pathogenesis of the major disease of the neuromuscular junction, myasthenia gravis, was serendipitously determined, during the purification and biochemical analysis of the acetylcholine receptor from eel electric organ, to involve autoimmune attack on the neuromuscular junction.[4] In turn, the autoantibodies in myasthenia gravis have provided useful probes of the structure and pharmacology of the acetylcholine receptor, and histologic study of the neuromuscular junction in myasthenia gravis has provided information on the subcellular mechanisms normally involved at the postsynaptic membrane. Moreover, the immune mechanisms involved in myasthenia gravis have provided insight into the nature of autoimmunity in general. In fact, just as it appeared that the diseases of the neuromuscular junction were nearly completely understood, the field has exploded again. This volume attempts to document those recent major advances.

During this period, the theme of interplay and cross-fertilization between study of normal functioning of the neuromuscular junction and study of the diseases of this synapse has continued full force. The most rapid advances have occurred in our understanding of the biochemical processes involved in neurotransmitter release from the motor nerve terminal. Botulism, and study of the causative neurotoxins secreted by the *Clostridium botulinum* organism, has led to the identification of a number of crucial nerve terminal proteins, which are targets of the toxins, involved in the binding cascade that results in cholinergic vesicle docking, fusion, and neurotransmitter release.[5–8] Similar advances have been made in our understanding of the formation and maintenance of the overall structure of the synapse.[5–7] Work presented here provides a view of a scaffold upon which the entire synaptic apparatus develops and is maintained. It extends from the cytoskeleton of the muscle fiber, through the end plate membrane, to the basal lamina of the synaptic cleft, through the motor nerve terminal plasma membrane, to the cytoskeleton of the terminal and its associated synaptic vesicles.

As basic knowledge of this type concerning the neuromuscular junction has advanced, the ability to determine the pathogenesis of a series of congenital (nonimmune) forms of myasthenia gravis has become a reality. The identification of those diseases, and in some cases the identification of the genes involved, has been another area of major progress during these last five years.

Considerable progress also has been made in determining the role of T cells in the autoimmune response in myasthenia gravis. A number of dominant epitopes of the acetylcholine receptor have been identified, providing the basis for new treatments directed against these cells that control the autoimmune response. In addition, the antibody response appears to involve other end plate proteins identified to play a role in synapse organization and muscle contraction.

As a result of basic work on the structure and function of this synapse, as well as laboratory and clinical studies of the immune and nonimmune diseases of this structure reported here, a number of clinical advances are presented that have provided improved treatment of patients with these diseases.

All of this information will likely provide the platform upon which the observations of the next five years will be made.

REFERENCES

1. RICHMAN, D. P. & M. A. AGIUS. 1994. Acquired myasthenia gravis: immunopathology. Neurol. Clin. North Am. **12:** 273–284.
2. UNWIN, N. 1995. Acetylcholine receptor channel imaged in the open state. Nature **373:** 37–42.
3. FAIRCLOUGH, R. H., E. GUDIPATI, M. Y. LIN, G. M. TWADDLE, D. P. RICHMAN, D. A. BURKWALL & R. JOSEPHS. 1998. A role for α(187–199) in the conversion of agonist binding energy to the opening of the acetylcholine receptor ion channel. This volume.
4. PATRICK, J. & J. LINDSTROM. 1973. Autoimmune response to acetylcholine receptor. Science **180:** 871–872.
5. FROEHNER, S. C. 1993. Regulation of ion channel distribution at synapses. Annu. Rev. Neurosci. **10:** 347–368.
6. HALL, Z. W. & J. R. SANES. 1993. Synaptic structure and development: the neuromuscular junction. Cell **72**/Neurology (Suppl.) **10:** 99–121.
7. NASTUK, M. A. & J. R. FALLON. 1993. Agrin and the molecular choreography of synapse formation. TINS **16:** 72–76.
8. BENNETT, M. A. & R. H. SCHELLER. 1994. Molecular correlates of synaptic vesicle docking and fusion. Curr. Opin. Neurobiol. **4:** 324–329.

Agrin Receptors at the Skeletal Neuromuscular Junction

JOSHUA R. SANES,[a] ELIZABETH D. APEL,[a] MEDHA GAUTAM,[b]
DAVID GLASS,[c] R. MARK GRADY,[a] PAUL T. MARTIN,[a] MIA C. NICHOL,[a]
AND GEORGE D. YANCOPOULOS[c]

[a]Department of Anatomy and Neurobiology
[b]Department of Molecular Biology and Pharmacology
Washington University School of Medicine
St. Louis, Missouri 63110

[c]Regeneron Pharmaceuticals
Tarrytown, New York

INTRODUCTION

A key step in formation of the neuromuscular junction is the accumulation of acetylcholine receptors (AChRs) in the postsynaptic membrane. AChR subunit genes are activated soon after myoblasts fuse to form myotubes, and newly synthesized AChRs accumulate in the plasma membrane to a uniform density of $\sim 10^3/\mu m^2$. In adult muscle, in contrast, AChRs are highly concentrated directly beneath the nerve terminal ($\sim 10^4/\mu m^2$) and nearly absent from extrasynaptic membrane ($\sim 10/\mu m^2$).[1,2] This precise apposition between presynaptic and postsynaptic specializations might occur in either of two ways. First, AChR clusters might form spontaneously and be associated with some molecule that attracts innervation. Alternatively, the nerve might release some signal that acts locally to induce AChR accumulation. The finding that myotubes cultured in the complete absence of neurons form "hot spots" of dense AChRs favored the first possibility. However, experiments by Anderson and Cohen[3] and by Frank and Fischbach[4] showed that in fact innervation of these cultured myotubes led to the dissolution of the "spontaneous" hot spots and to formation of new AChR clusters directly beneath the nerve. Thus, it became clear by the late 1970s that nerves induce postsynaptic specializations. Based on these studies, several groups began searching for nerve-derived synaptic organizing factors. Several candidates have been isolated in the intervening years, any of which may play physiological roles.[1,2,5] At present, however, the factor for which the best evidence has been obtained *in vivo* is agrin.

AGRIN

Agrin was isolated from *Torpedo* electric organ (a plentiful source of neuromuscular junction–like synaptic components) by McMahan and colleagues on the basis of its ability to promote formation of AChR clusters. Purified native or recombinant agrin proved competent to induce aggregation of AChRs, as well as a variety of cy-toskeletal, membrane, and matrix components that are concentrated at synaptic sites *in vivo*. Immunochemical techniques revealed that agrin was synthesized by mo-toneurons, transported down motor axons, and released into the synaptic cleft, where it bound to basal lamina. Based on these findings, McMahan proposed that agrin is a critical, nerve-derived synaptic organizing molecule.[6]

Four subsequent sets of studies have provided strong support for this "agrin hy-pothesis." First, in chimeric nerve-muscle cocultures (chick neurons innervating rat muscle), antibodies that recognize chick agrin, but not rat agrin, block formation of AChR clusters at points of nerve-muscle apposition.[7] Second, although muscles as well as nerves make agrin, only the latter make alternatively spliced isoforms (called here z^+ because they contain exons at a position called z; FIGURE 1, top) that are 1000–10,000-fold more active than the z^- isoforms made by muscle.[8–10] Third, forced expression of z^+ agrin in denervated muscle leads to formation of a postsynaptic ap-paratus that is remarkably complete, yet unopposed by any neural element.[11,12] These elegant experiments show that agrin alone is (nearly) sufficient to account for the synaptic organizing abilities of the nerve. Finally, neuromuscular development is se-verely perturbed in mutant mice from which agrin's z exons have been deleted.[13] AChR clusters are fewer in number, smaller, and less dense in mutant muscle than in wild-type littermates, and only a few are localized to nerve-muscle contacts. These mice are severe hypomorphs for all agrin isoforms, as well as lacking z^+ agrin com-pletely, so it is not clear whether their phenotype is attributable to loss of z^+ agrin alone or to agrin generally. Moreover, the mice display presynaptic as well as postsy-naptic defects, discussion of which is beyond the scope of this chapter. Nonetheless, analysis of these mice has demonstrated that agrin is necessary for synaptic differen-tiation *in vivo*.

AGRIN RECEPTORS

In view of the mounting evidence that agrin plays a critical role in neuromuscular development, it is important to identify its receptors. Over the past few years, several components of the muscle cell surface have been identified with which agrin inter-acts. They are depicted in FIGURE 1 and enumerated here:

(a) The first protein to which agrin was shown to bind was α-dystroglycan, a pe-ripheral membrane protein that is part of a complex of dystrophin-associated glyco-proteins.[14–17] The specificity and high affinity of this binding, along with the anti-body blocking experiment discussed below, led to the suggestion that dystroglycan was agrin's signaling receptor.[14–16]

(b) The neural cell adhesion molecule, N-CAM, is coregulated with AChRs in muscle: it is abundant on embryonic myotubes, becomes concentrated in the postsy-naptic membrane in adult muscle, and reappears extrasynaptically following dener-vation.[18] Moreover, agrin was isolated from brain as a major and specific het-erophilic ligand of N-CAM.[19] Thus, this molecule has a distribution and binding site consistent with the possibility that it mediates some of agrin's effects.

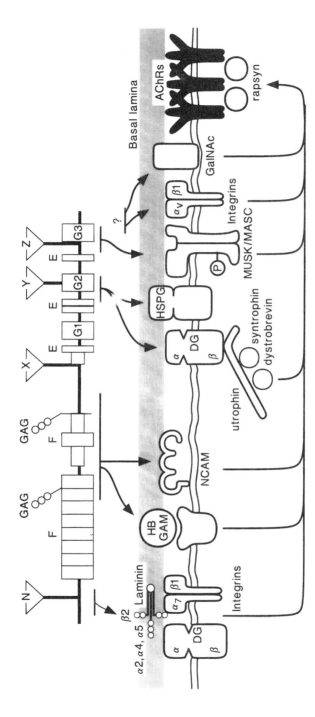

FIGURE 1. Components of the myotube surface with which agrin interacts. Schematic model of agrin is shown above the membrane. N, X, Y, and Z indicate sites of alternative splicing. Terms: E, EGF-like repeats; G, laminin-like G domains; F, follistatin-like repeats; GAG, glycosaminoglycan; HB-GAM, heparin-binding growth-associated molecule; NCAM, neural cell adhesion molecule; DG, dystroglycan; HSPG, heparan sulfate proteoglycan; MUSK, muscle-specific kinase; MASC, muscle-associated specificity component; GalNAc, β-N-acetylgalactosaminyl-terminated glycoconjugates.

(c) A growth factor called the heparin-binding growth-associated molecule (HB-GAM), or pleiotrophin, is present on muscle cell surfaces *in vivo* and at AChR-rich clusters on cultured myotubes. It binds directly to agrin, can induce clustering when presented to cultured muscle, and potentiates the effects of agrin when the two are presented together.[20]

(d) Agrin binds directly to laminins, which are major components of the muscle fiber basal lamina.[21] Laminins, in turn, play critical roles in neuromuscular development.[22] Interestingly, alternative splicing at the "N" site (FIGURE 1) may modulate binding to laminin, and agrin may bind preferentially to β2 laminins, which are themselves selectively concentrated at synaptic sites.[21,22]

(e) Integrins are present on the surface of developing muscles, serve as receptors for numerous basal lamina components (for example, laminins, collagens, fibronectin, and entactin), and have been implicated in numerous aspects of nerve and muscle development. Integrins are heterodimers of α and β subunits, both of which span the membrane. Of the 16 α and 8 β subunits that have been identified to date, developing muscles express at least 11 (α1, α3–7, α9, αv, β1, β3, and β5). At least 4 of these subunits (α3, α7, αv, and β1) are present in the postsynaptic membrane at the neuromuscular junction, presumably forming α3β1, α7β1, and αvβ1 dimers.[23] Recently, we tested the possibility that some of these subunits might be involved in agrin signaling. We found that antibodies to the integrin αv and β1 subunits inhibit the ability of agrin to induce AChR clustering. Moreover, integrins αvβ1 and αvβ3 can mediate adhesion of some nonmuscle cells to immobilized agrin.[24] Thus, integrins may mediate or modulate some of agrin's effects.

(f) Agrin binds tightly to heparin,[25–28] which resembles the heparan sulfate glycosaminoglycan moiety on many proteoglycans. Heparan sulfate proteoglycans have been implicated as receptors or coreceptors for numerous growth factors, and several such proteoglycans are present on muscle cell surfaces. Muscle cell line variants with reduced levels of cell surface heparan sulfate are also deficient in their ability to respond to agrin.[8,29] Interestingly, isoforms of agrin that contain a four-amino-acid sequence encoded by the "y" exon (FIGURE 1) bind far more avidly to heparin than do y⁻ isoforms. This exon is conserved among species (chick, human, rat, and mouse) and subject to developmental and tissue-specific regulation, suggesting that modulation of agrin's ability to bind proteoglycans may affect its function. On the other hand, inclusion of the "y" exon is not required for agrin-induced AChR clustering in vitro, indicating that the major signaling receptors are unlikely to be heparan sulfates.

(g) Glycoconjugates terminated in a β-linked N-acetylgalactosamine (βGalNAc) residue are concentrated at the neuromuscular junction, but present at very low levels extrasynaptically.[30] Lectins that bind βGalNAc potentiate the effects of agrin, indicating that a βGalNAc-terminated molecule is part of agrin's signaling pathway. Moreover, enzymatic removal of cell surface βGalNAc inhibits the effects of agrin, and exposure of additional βGalNAc on the cell surface leads to agrin-independent clustering, suggesting that the sugar itself, and not only the molecule to which it is attached, plays a role in agrin signaling.[31] The molecules to which the bioactive βGalNAc is attached have not yet been identified. Heparan sulfate glycosaminoglycans, mentioned above, do not contain GalNAc and are not recognized by GalNAc-specific lectins. On the other hand, the closely related chondroitin glycosaminoglycans do contain GalNAc and have been implicated in AChR clustering.[32] Also, the glycosylation of dystrogly-can is heterogeneous, and some forms contain GalNAc-terminated sugars that are recognized by the same lectins that affect AChR clustering.[33] It is possible that synaptic dystroglycan is GalNAc-positive and that this glycosylation enables it to interact with agrin in a way that differs from that of the bulk of muscle dystroglycan, which is GalNAc-negative.

(h) A muscle-specific receptor tyrosine kinase, MuSK, is concentrated in the postsynaptic membrane of *Torpedo* electric organ and mammalian skeletal muscle.[34,35] The facts that such tyrosine kinases are receptors for many growth factors and that tyrosine phosphorylation has been implicated in agrin's signal transduction pathway[36,37] raised the possibility that MuSK might be an agrin receptor.

Any or all of these cell surface components might be involved in agrin signaling. To date, however, the dystrophin-associated glycoproteins and MuSK have been studied in greatest detail. Moreover, genetic data are available to help evaluate their roles *in vivo*. Therefore, the following sections will focus on these two candidate receptors.

DYSTROPHIN-ASSOCIATED GLYCOPROTEINS

Dystroglycan was isolated as part of a large complex of proteins that copurifies with dystrophin, the protein mutated in Duchenne and Becker muscular dystrophies. Campbell and colleagues showed that α- and β-dystroglycan are translated as a single protein, and then proteolytically cleaved to form the α and β polypeptide.[38] α-Dystroglycan is an extracellular, peripheral membrane protein that binds to laminin-2 (merosin) in the basal lamina. β-Dystroglycan spans the membrane and binds to dystrophin, which is a cytoplasmic protein. Dystrophin, in turn, binds to actin and other cytoskeletal proteins. Thus, dystroglycan is part of a complex, the dystrophin-glycoprotein complex, that links the extracellular matrix to the cytoskeleton.[38,39] Mutations in several components of this complex, in addition to dystrophin, result in muscular dystrophies.[40]

The dystrophin-glycoprotein complex is present throughout the sarcolemma, but there are important differences between complexes in extrasynaptic regions and those at synaptic sites. Extracellularly, laminin-2 (subunit composition α2β1γ1) is abundant in extrasynaptic basal lamina, whereas the major laminins of the synaptic cleft are laminins-4 (α2β2γ1), -9 (α4β2γ1), and -11 (α5β2γ1).[41] Intracellularly, dystrophin and the dystrophin-binding proteins, α1- and β1-syntrophin, are present throughout the sarcolemma, whereas their homologues, utrophin and β2-syntrophin, are specifically localized to synaptic sites.[42–46] Moreover, some of these synaptic molecules, such as laminin β2 and utrophin, as well as dystroglycan itself, are selectively associated with AChR clusters in cultured muscle cells.[47,48]

Once the binding of agrin to α-dystroglycan was discovered,[14–17] it became attractive to hypothesize that synapse-specific components of the dystrophin-glycoprotein complex, specifically utrophin, might convert an extrasynaptic laminin-binding complex essential for muscle stability into a synaptic agrin-binding complex essential for synaptic development.[14,47] However, studies in cultured cells soon provided three sets of results inconsistent with this hypothesis. First, although Gee et al.[15] reported that antibodies to dystroglycan were able to block the ability of agrin to induce AChR clustering, Campanelli et al.[14] found only a change in cluster morphology and Sugiyama et al.[17] detected no effect, even though they used the same antibody. Second, isoforms of agrin that show little or no ability to induce AChR clustering (the z^- forms discussed above) bound to dystroglycan somewhat more tightly than z^+ isoforms that are potent clustering factors.[17,25–28,49] Third, C-terminal fragments of agrin are capable of inducing AChR clustering (albeit with low potency), but show no detectable binding to dystroglycan.[25–27] Thus, it seems unlikely that α-dystroglycan is the sole agrin signaling receptor. Unfortunately, dystroglycan-deficient mutant mice die at an early stage of embryonic development,[50] so rigorous genetic tests of dystroglycan's role in vivo are not yet feasible.

On the other hand, it has been possible to test the specific hypothesis that utrophin is crucial for development or maintenance of the neuromuscular junction. We[51] and Deconinck et al.[52] generated utrophin-deficient mutant mice and found that they appeared outwardly normal and were healthy and fertile. It was therefore straightforward to analyze their neuromuscular junctions in detail. Both groups found two subtle defects: the density of AChRs in the postsynaptic membrane and the number of junctional folds that invaginate the postsynaptic membrane were both reduced by ~20–40%. Thus, utrophin-deficient mice exhibit a mild congenital myasthenia. Nonetheless, the relatively normal structure, function, and molecular architecture of neuromuscular junctions in the mutants were inconsistent with the idea that utrophin is a required part of the primary agrin receptor.

A possible explanation for the subtle phenotype of these mutants is that utrophin can be replaced by its homologue, dystrophin. The converse idea, namely, that utrophin can compensate for loss of dystrophin, has been advanced as a potential basis for therapy in Duchenne dystrophy.[53] Interestingly, a dystrophin mutant mouse, called mdx, displays a very mild dystrophy, at least as compared to humans with essentially the same mutation.[54] We[55] and Deconinck et al.[56] therefore generated dystrophin-utrophin double mutants to determine whether the mild dystrophy observed in the absence of dystrophin or the mild myasthenia observed in the absence of utrophin reflected compensation by utrophin or dystrophin, respectively. In fact, not only were dystrophin and utrophin absent from synapses in double mutants, but levels of dystroglycan, the "synaptic" β2-syntrophin, and another dystrophin-binding protein (dystrobrevin) were all markedly reduced. However, despite this dramatic loss of dystrophin-associated and -related proteins, synaptic defects were no more severe in the double mutant than in either single mutant. Likewise, neuromuscular development is qualitatively normal in mice lacking both utrophin and dystrobrevin.[57] These data greatly weaken the case that this complex is essential for agrin signaling. On the other hand, dystrophy is severe in the double mutants and its symptoms resemble those of Duchenne dystrophy in many respects. Thus, endogenous utrophin can compensate for loss of dystrophin and apparently does so more effectively in mice than in humans. These results raise the exciting possibility that a modest upregulation of utrophin in humans could significantly attenuate the symptoms of Duchenne dystrophy.

MUSK

To test the function of MuSK *in vivo*, DeChiara *et al.*[58] generated a MuSK mutant mouse. Homozygotes developed normally *in utero*, but died at birth and displayed neuromuscular defects similar to those described above for the agrin mutant. If anything, the phenotype was more severe in MuSK than in agrin mutants—muscles bore some AChR clusters in the latter, but none in the former, even though both had normal levels of AChRs on their surface. These unexpected results provided the first evidence that MuSK might be a critical part of agrin's signal transduction pathway.

Four additional results have provided further evidence for this idea.[59,60] First, myotubes cultured from MuSK mutant mice are completely unresponsive to agrin. Second, addition of agrin to myotubes leads to a rapid activation (phosphorylation) of MuSK. Third, introduction of a dominant-negative MuSK mutant into a muscle cell line inhibits agrin's ability to induce AChR clustering. Fourth, application of chemical cross-linkers to agrin-treated myotubes leads to covalent dimerization of agrin and MuSK.

All of these results imply that MuSK could be the agrin receptor itself. On the other hand, several observations cast doubt on the simple idea that MuSK is the entire agrin receptor.[59,60] First, no direct binding of agrin to MuSK has been demonstrable, despite strenuous attempts. Second, activation of a chimeric receptor (trkC kinase extracellular domain fused to MuSK intracellular domain) with a surrogate ligand (the trkC ligand, NT-3) leads to activation of MuSK, but not to AChR clustering. Third, although addition of agrin to muscle cells activates MuSK, addition of agrin to MuSK-transfected fibroblasts does not. Thus, current evidence suggests that MuSK is a critical part of the agrin receptor, but that at least one additional component exists. This hypothetical component has been termed MASC, for muscle-associated specificity component, and efforts are under way in several laboratories to identify it. Whether one of the potential agrin receptors listed above is MASC remains to be determined.

MUSK-RAPSYN INTERACTIONS

Whatever the nature of the agrin receptor(s), one of the molecules involved in the AChR clustering process itself has now been identified with certainty. Rapsyn is a cytoplasmic peripheral membrane protein that is precisely colocalized with AChRs *in vivo* from the earliest stages of synapse formation.[1] Rapsyn may bind directly to AChRs, but this has not been shown definitively. Rapsyn was long suspected to be involved in AChR clustering based on the close association of the two molecules, but direct evidence came only after rapsyn cDNAs had been cloned and recombinant rapsyn was coexpressed with AChRs in *Xenopus* oocytes[61] or fibroblasts.[62] In both cases, the AChRs were distributed diffusely on the cell surface when expressed alone, but formed high-density clusters when coexpressed with rapsyn. In fact, rapsyn is also able to cluster several other membrane proteins normally found at synapses, including dystroglycan and MuSK.[63–67] Clustering is specific, however, in that the distribution of several membrane proteins not ordinarily concentrated at neuromuscular junctions (for example, trkA, trkC, glucose transporters, and glutamate receptors) is unaffected by coexpression with rapsyn in nonmuscle cells.

Analysis of rapsyn knockout mice proved that rapsyn is not only sufficient, but also necessary for clustering AChRs.[65] Muscles form normally in homozygous mutants and they synthesize AChRs in normal numbers, but the AChRs fail to aggregate in the postsynaptic membrane. In normal muscle, there is preferential synthesis of AChRs in synaptic areas, resulting from the selective transcription of AChR subunit genes by subsynaptic nuclei,[1,2] and this transcriptional specialization is maintained in the absence of rapsyn. Thus, AChR levels are increased at synapses, but not nearly as high as at normal end plates. The levels achieved are evidently sufficient for some movement and even shallow breathing, but the homozygotes die within a few hours of birth. Moreover, no AChR clustered in muscles cultured from the mutants, even in the presence of agrin. Finally, several components of the postsynaptic membrane and cytoskeleton (for example, erbB2, erbB3, erbB4, utrophin, and dystroglycan) fail to accumulate at synaptic sites.[65,68] Thus rapsyn is critical for executing the process of postsynaptic assembly that agrin triggers.

With the knowledge that MuSK is (or is associated with) the agrin receptor and rapsyn is a key effector of clustering, we have begun to elucidate the mechanisms by which the two molecules interact. As noted above, rapsyn and MuSK cocluster in nonmuscle cells, indicating a close molecular association between the two.[66,67] Surprisingly, however, MuSK remains concentrated at synaptic sites in the absence of rapsyn, along with at least two components of the synaptic basal lamina, laminin $\beta2$ and acetylcholinesterase.[65,66] Thus, agrin may begin its work by inducing formation of a primary scaffold that contains MuSK in the plasma membrane and key synaptic components in the overlying matrix. MuSK would then use rapsyn to recruit other synaptic components, such as AChRs, utrophin, dystroglycan, and the erbB2–4 kinases, to the synapse. In this model, MuSK would play not only a signaling role, as originally envisioned, but also a structural role in synaptogenesis, as a nucleator of clustering.

Recent studies have led to the conclusion that different domains of MuSK are responsible for carrying out its structural and signaling functions. As noted above, activation of the intracellular domain of MuSK in a chimeric receptor leads to AChR phosphorylation, but not to clustering, and inhibition of MuSK kinase activity blocks the effects of agrin.[60] Thus, the cytoplasmic kinase activity of MuSK is crucial for signaling. Surprisingly, however, the kinase domain is not necessary for association with rapsyn: rapsyn is capable of clustering chimeras that contain the ectodomain of MuSK, but not the trk-MuSK chimera containing the intracellular domain of MuSK.[66] Thus, there must be an additional component, which we have called RATL (for rapsyn-associated transmembrane linker), that mediates the association of rapsyn, which is entirely intracellular, with the ectodomain of MuSK. Moreover, the ectodomain may be the key to MuSK's ability to localize AChR clustering at synaptic sites.

A model incorporating these and other results is shown in FIGURE 2. We hypothesize that agrin binds to a MuSK/MASC complex to cause dimerization and autophosphorylation of MuSK. Agrin also causes clustering of MuSK, but it remains unclear whether this is a consequence of activation or requires a separate interaction. Activated MuSK, in turn, leads to phosphorylation of AChRs, perhaps indirectly via a kinase

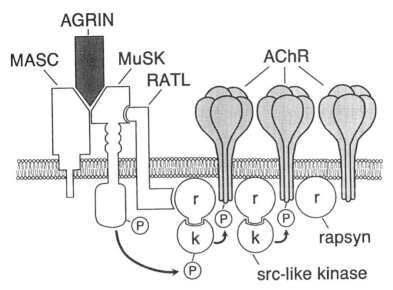

FIGURE 2. Hypothetical model of interactions between MuSK and rapsyn. See text for details. (From reference 66.)

cascade in which cytoplasmic src-like kinases are directly responsible for phosphorylating AChRs.[66,69] The phosphorylation of AChRs and other rapsyn-associated proteins[36,37,64] triggers AChR clustering. Clustering of AChRs will not occur, however, unless MuSK interacts with rapsyn, via RATL, to nucleate formation of an aggregate.

In this model, MuSK is unusual among known receptor tyrosine kinases in having a distinct role for its ectodomain. For previously studied kinases, it appears that the major role of the ectodomain is to transduce ligand binding into activation (autophosphorylation); activation of a chimera by a surrogate ligand is sufficient to mimic all the biological activities of the native receptor.[70,71] For MuSK, in contrast, we suggest that the ectodomain plays the additional role of localizing the response spatially, by forming a scaffold to which rapsyn can attach other synaptic components. A mechanism of this sort is well suited to a kinase that needs not only to initiate a response (postsynaptic differentiation), but also to localize it to a specific domain of the membrane (beneath the nerve terminal) with submicron precision.

REFERENCES

1. HALL, Z. W. & J. R. SANES. 1993. Synaptic structure and development: the neuromuscular junction. Cell **72:** 99–121.
2. DUCLERT, A. & J. P. CHANGEUX. 1995. Acetylcholine receptor gene expression at the developing neuromuscular junction. Physiol. Rev. **75:** 339–368.
3. ANDERSON, M. J. & M. W. COHEN. 1977. Nerve-induced and spontaneous redistribution of acetylcholine receptors on cultured muscle cells. J. Physiol. **268:** 757–773.

4. FRANK, E. & G. D. FISCHBACH. 1979. Early events in neuromuscular junction formation *in vitro*: induction of acetylcholine receptor clusters in the postsynaptic membrane and morphology of newly formed synapses. J. Cell Biol. **83**: 143–158.
5. FISCHBACH, G. D. & K. M. ROSEN. 1997. ARIA: a neuromuscular junction neuregulin. Annu. Rev. Neurosci. **20**: 429–458.
6. MCMAHAN, U. J. 1990. The agrin hypothesis. Cold Spring Harbor Symp. Quant. Biol. **55**: 407–418.
7. REIST, N. E., M. J. WERLE & U. J. MCMAHAN. 1992. Agrin released by motor neurons induces the aggregation of acetylcholine receptors at neuromuscular junctions. Neuron **8**: 865–868.
8. FERNS, M., W. HOCH, J. T. CAMPANELLI, F. RUPP, Z. W. HALL & R. H. SCHELLER. 1992. RNA splicing regulates agrin-mediated acetylcholine receptor clustering activity on cultured myotubes. Neuron **8**: 1079–1086.
9. RUEGG, M. A., K. W. TSIM, S. E. HORTON, S. KROGER, G. ESCHER, E. M. GENSCH & U. J. MCMAHAN. 1992. The agrin gene codes for a family of basal lamina proteins that differ in function and distribution. Neuron **8**: 691–699.
10. GESEMANN, M., A. J. DENZER & M. A. RUEGG. 1995. Acetylcholine receptor–aggregating activity of agrin isoforms and mapping of the active site, J. Cell Biol. **128**: 625–636.
11. COHEN, I., M. RIMER, T. LØMO & U. J. MCMAHAN. 1997. Agrin-induced postsynaptic-like apparatus in skeletal muscle fibers *in vivo*. Mol. Cell. Neurosci. **9**: 237–253; RIMER, M., I. MATHIESEN, T. LØMO & U. J. MCMAHAN. 1997. γ-AChR/ε-AChR switch at agrin-induced postsynaptic-like apparatus in skeletal muscle. Mol. Cell. Neurosci. **9**: 254–263.
12. JONES, G., T. MEIER, M. LICHTSTEINER, V. WITZEMANN, B. SAKMANN & H. R. BRENNER. 1997. Induction by agrin of ectopic and functional postsynaptic-like membrane in innervated muscle. Proc. Natl. Acad. Sci. U.S.A. **94**: 2654–2659.
13. GAUTAM, M., P. G. NOAKES, L. MOSCOSO, F. RUPP, R. H. SCHELLER, J. P. MERLIE & J. R. SANES. 1996. Defective neuromuscular synaptogenesis in agrin-deficient mutant mice. Cell **85**: 525–535.
14. CAMPANELLI, J. T., S. L. ROBERDS, K. P. CAMPBELL & R. H. SCHELLER. 1994. A role for dystrophin-associated glycoproteins and utrophin in agrin-induced AChR clustering. Cell **77**: 663–674.
15. GEE, S. H., F. MONTANARO, M. H. LINDENBAUM & S. CARBONETTO. 1994. Dystroglycan-α, a dystrophin-associated glycoprotein, is a functional agrin receptor. Cell **77**: 675–686.
16. BOWE, M. A., K. A. DEYST, J. D. LESZYK & J. R. FALLON. 1994. Identification and purification of an agrin receptor from *Torpedo* postsynaptic membranes: a heteromeric complex related to the dystroglycans. Neuron **12**: 1173–1180.
17. SUGIYAMA, J., D. C. BOWEN & Z. W. HALL. 1994. Dystroglycan binds nerve and muscle agrin. Neuron **13**: 103–115.
18. COVAULT, J. & J. R. SANES. 1985. Neural cell adhesion molecule (N-CAM) accumulates in denervated and paralyzed skeletal muscles. Proc. Natl. Acad. Sci. U.S.A. **82**: 4544–4548.
19. COLE, G. J. & W. HALFTER. 1996. Agrin—an extracellular matrix heparan sulfate proteoglycan involved in cell interactions and synaptogenesis. Perspect. Dev. Neurobiol. **3**: 359–371.
20. DAGGETT, D. F., M. W. COHEN, D. STONE, K. NIKOLICS, H. RAUVALA & H. B. PENG. 1996. The role of an agrin-growth factor interaction in acetylcholine receptor clustering. Mol. Cell. Neurosci. **8**: 272–285.
21. DENZER, A. J., R. BRANDENBERGER, M. GESEMANN, M. CHIQUET & M. A. RUEGG. 1997. Agrin binds to the nerve-muscle basal lamina via laminin. J. Cell Biol. **137**: 671–683.
22. NOAKES, P. G., M. GAUTAM, J. MUDD, J. R. SANES & J. P. MERLIE. 1995. Aberrant differentiation of neuromuscular junctions in mice lacking s-laminin/laminin beta 2. Nature **374**: 258–262.

23. MARTIN, P. T., S. J. KAUFMAN, R. H. KRAMER & J. R. SANES. 1996. Synaptic integrins in developing, adult, and mutant muscle: selective association of alpha1, alpha7A, and alpha7B integrins with the neuromuscular junction. Dev. Biol. **174:** 125–139.

24. MARTIN, P. T. & J. R. SANES. 1997. Integrins mediate adhesion to agrin and modulate agrin signaling. Development **124:** 3909–3917.

25. CAMPANELLI, J. T., G. G. GAYER & R. H. SCHELLER. 1996. Alternative RNA splicing that determines agrin activity regulates binding to heparin and alpha dystroglycan. Development **122:** 1663–1672.

26. HOPF, C. & W. HOCH. 1996. Agrin binding to α-dystroglycan. J. Biol. Chem. **271:** 5231–5236.

27. GESEMANN, M., V. CAVALLI, A. J. DENZER, A. BRANCACCIO, B. SCHUMACHER & M. A. RUEGG. 1996. Alternative splicing of agrin alters its binding to heparin, dystroglycan, and the putative agrin receptor. Neuron **16:** 755–767.

28. O'TOOLE, J. J., K. A. DEYST, M. A. BOWE, M. A. NASTUK, B. A. McKECHNIE & J. R. FALLON. 1996. Alternative splicing of agrin regulates its binding to heparin, α-dystroglycan, and the cell surface. Proc. Natl. Acad. Sci. U.S.A. **93:** 7369–7374.

29. GORDON, H., M. LUPA, D. BOWEN & J. HALL. 1993. A muscle cell variant defective in glycosaminoglycan biosynthesis forms nerve-induced, but not spontaneous clusters of the acetylcholine receptor and the 43-kD protein. J. Neurosci. **13:** 586–595.

30. SCOTT, L. J., F. BACOU & J. R. SANES. 1988. A synapse-specific carbohydrate at the neuromuscular junction: association with both acetylcholinesterase and a glycolipid. J. Neurosci. **8:** 932–944.

31. MARTIN, P. T. & J. R. SANES. 1995. Role for a synapse-specific carbohydrate in agrin-induced clustering of acetylcholine receptors. Neuron **14:** 743–754.

32. MOOK-JUNG, I. & H. GORDON. 1995. Acetylcholine receptor clustering in C2 muscle cells requires chondroitin sulfate. J. Neurobiol. **28:** 482–492.

33. SMALHEISER, N. R. & E. KIM. 1995. Purification of cranin, a laminin binding membrane protein. J. Biol. Chem. **270:** 15425–15433.

34. JENNINGS, C. G. B., S. M. DYER & S. J. BURDEN. 1993. Muscle-specific *trk*-related receptor with a kringle domain defines a distinct class of receptor tyrosine kinases. Proc. Natl. Acad. Sci. U.S.A. **90:** 2895–2899.

35. VALENZUELA, D. M., T. N. STITT, P. S. DiSTEFANO, E. ROJAS, K. MATTSSON, D. L. COMPTON, L. NUÑEZ, J. S. PARK, J. L. STARK, D. R. GIES, S. THOMAS, M. M. LeBEAU, A. A. FERNALD, N. G. COPELAND, N. A. JENKINS, S. J. BURDEN, D. J. GLASS & G. D. YANCOPOULOS. 1995. Receptor tyrosine kinase specific for the skeletal muscle lineage: expression in embryonic muscle, at the neuromuscular junction, and after injury. Neuron **15:** 573–584.

36. WALLACE, B. G. 1992. Mechanism of agrin-induced acetylcholine receptor aggregation. J. Neurobiol. **23:** 592–604.

37. FERNS, M., M. DEINER & Z. HALL. 1996. Agrin-induced acetylcholine receptor clustering in mammalian muscle requires tyrosine phosphorylation. J. Cell Biol. **132:** 937–944.

38. HENRY, M. D. & K. P. CAMPBELL. 1996. Dystroglycan: an extracellular matrix receptor linked to the cytoskeleton. Curr. Opin. Cell Biol. **8:** 625–631.

39. OHLENDIECK, K. 1996. Towards an understanding of the dystrophin-glycoprotein complex: linkage between the extracellular matrix and the membrane cytoskeleton in muscle fibers. Eur. J. Cell Biol. **69:** 1–10.

40. DUGGAN, D. J. & E. P. HOFFMAN. 1996. Autosomal recessive muscular dystrophy and mutations of the sarcoglycan complex. Neuromusc. Disord. **6:** 475–482.

41. PATTON, B. L., J. M. MINER, A. Y. CHIU & J. R. SANES. 1997. Distribution and function of laminins in the neuromuscular system of developing, adult, and mutant mice. Submitted.

42. OHLENDIECK, K., J. M. ERVASTI, K. MATSUMURA, S. D. KAHL, C. J. LEVEILLE & K. P. CAMP-

BELL. 1991. Dystrophin-related protein is localized to neuromuscular junctions of adult skeletal muscle. Neuron **7:** 499–508.

43. KHURANA, T. S., S. C. WATKINS, P. CHAFEY, J. CHELLY, F. TOMÉ, M. FARDEAU, J. KAPLAN & L. M. KUNKEL. 1991. Immunolocalization and development expression of dystrophin-related protein in skeletal muscle. Neuromusc. Disord. **1:** 185–194.

44. BEWICK, G. S., L. V. NICHOLSON, C. YOUNG & C. R. SLATER. 1992. Different distributions of dystrophin and related proteins at nerve-muscle junctions. Neuroreport **3:** 857–860.

45. THIMAN, N., J. M. ELLIS, D. R. LOVE, K. E. DAVIES, K. C. GATTER, G. DICKSON & G. E. MORRIS. 1991. Localization of the DMDL gene-encoded dystrophin-related protein using a panel of nineteen monoclonal antibodies: presence at neuromuscular junctions, in the sarcolemma of dystrophic skeletal muscle, in vascular and other smooth muscles, and in proliferating brain cell lines. J. Cell Biol. **115:** 1695–1700.

46. PETERS, M. F., N. R. KRAMARCY, R. SEALOCK & S. C. FROEHNER. 1994. β2-Syntrophin: localization at the neuromuscular junction in skeletal muscle. Neuroreport **5:** 1577–1580.

47. PHILLIPS, W. D., P. G. NOAKES, S. L. ROBERDS, K. P. CAMPBELL & J. P. MERLIE. 1993. Clustering and immobilization of acetylcholine receptors by the 43-kD protein: a possible role for dystrophin-related protein. J. Cell Biol. **123:** 729–740.

48. MARTIN, P. T., A. M. ETTINGER & J. R. SANES. 1995. A synaptic localization domain in the synaptic cleft protein laminin 2 (s-laminin). Science **269:** 413–416.

49. BOWEN, D. C., J. SUGIYAMA, M. FERNS & Z. W. HALL. 1996. Neural agrin activates a high-affinity receptor in C2 muscle cells that is unresponsive to muscle agrin. J. Neurosci. **16:** 3791–3797.

50. WILLIAMSON, R. A., M. D. HENRY, K. J. DANIELS, R. F. HRSTKA, J. C. LEE, Y. SUNADA, O. IBRAGHIMOV-BESKROVNAYA & K. P. CAMPBELL. 1997. Dystroglycan is essential for early embryonic development: disruption of Reichert's membrane in *Dag1*-null mice. Hum. Mol. Genet. **6:** 831–841.

51. GRADY, R. M., J. P. MERLIE & J. R. SANES. 1997. Subtle neuromuscular defects in utrophin-deficient mice. J. Cell Biol. **136:** 871–882.

52. DECONINCK, A. E., A. C. POTTER, J. M. TINSLEY, S. J. WOOD, R. VATER, C. YOUNG, L. METZINGER, A. VINCENT, C. R. SLATER & K. E. DAVIES. 1997. Postsynaptic abnormalities at the neuromuscular junctions of utrophin-deficient mice. J. Cell Biol. **136:** 883–894.

53. TINSLEY, J. M., A. C. POTTER, S. R. PHELPS, R. FISHER, J. I. TRICKETT & K. E. DAVIES. 1996. Amelioration of the dystrophic phenotype of *mdx* mice using a truncated utrophin transgene. Nature **384:** 349–353.

54. SICINSKI, P., Y. GENG, A. S. RYDER-COOK, E. A. BARNARD, M. G. DARLISON & P. J. BARNARD. 1989. The molecular basis of muscular dystrophy in the *mdx* mouse: a point mutation. Science **244:** 1578–1579.

55. GRADY, R. M., H. TENG, M. C. NICHOL, J. C. CUNNINGHAM, R. S. WILKINSON & J. R. SANES. 1997. Skeletal and cardiac myopathies in mice lacking utrophin and dystrophin: a model for Duchenne muscular dystrophy. Cell **90:** 729–738.

56. DECONINCK, A. E., J. A. RAFAEL, J. A. SKINNER, S. C. BROWN, A. C. POTTER, L. METZINGER, D. J. WATT, G. DICKSON, J. M. TINSLEY & K. E. DAVIES. 1997. Utrophin-dystrophin-deficient mice as a model for Duchenne muscular dystrophy. Cell **90:** 717–727.

57. GRADY, R. M. & J. R. SANES. 1997. In preparation.

58. DECHIARA, T. M., D. C. BOWEN, D. M. VALENZUELA, M. V. SIMMONS, W. T. POUEYMIROU, S. THOMAS, E. KINETZ, D. L. COMPTON, E. ROJAS, J. S. PARK, C. SMITH, P. S. DISTEFANO, D. J. GLASS, S. J. BURDEN & G. D. YANCOPOULOS. 1996. The receptor tyrosine kinase MuSK is required for neuromuscular junction formation *in vivo*. Cell **85:** 501–512.

59. GLASS, D. J., D. C. BOWEN, T. N. STITT, C. RADZIEJEWSKI, J. BRUNO, T. E. RYAN, D. R. GIES, S. SHAH, K. MATTSSON, S. J. BURDEN, P. S. DISTEFANO, D. M. VALENZUELA, T. M.

DeChiara & G. D. Yancopoulos. 1996. Agrin acts via a MuSK receptor complex. Cell **85:** 513–523.

60. Glass, D. J., E. D. Apel, S. Shah, D. C. Bowen, T. M. DeChiara, T. N. Stitt, J. R. Sanes & G. D. Yancopoulos. 1997. MuSK kinase domain is sufficient for phosphorylation, but not clustering of acetylcholine receptors. Proc. Natl. Acad. Sci. U.S.A. **94:** 8848–8853.

61. Froehner, S. C., C. W. Luetje, P. B. Scotland & J. Patrick. 1990. The postsynaptic 43K protein clusters muscle nicotinic acetylcholine receptors in *Xenopus* oocytes. Neuron **5:** 403–410.

62. Phillips, W. D., C. Kopta, P. Blount, P. D. Gardner, J. H. Steinbach & J. P. Merlie. 1991. Ach receptor–rich membrane domains organized in fibroblasts by recombinant 43-kilodalton protein. Science **251:** 568–570.

63. Apel, E. D., S. L. Roberds, K. P. Campbell & J. P. Merlie. 1995. Rapsyn may function as a link between the acetylcholine receptor and the agrin-binding dystrophin-associated glycoprotein complex. Neuron **15:** 115–126.

64. Qu, Z., E. D. Apel, C. A. Doherty, P. W. Hoffman, J. P. Merlie & R. L. Huganir. 1996. The synapse-associated protein rapsyn regulates tyrosine phosphorylation of proteins colocalized at nicotinic acetylcholine receptor clusters. Mol. Cell. Neurosci. **8:** 171–184.

65. Gautam, M., P. G. Noakes, J. Mudd, M. Nichol, G. C. Chu, J. R. Sanes & J. P. Merlie. 1995. Failure of postsynaptic specialization to develop at neuromuscular junctions of rapsyn-deficient mice. Nature **377:** 232–236.

66. Apel, E. D., D. J. Glass, L. M. Moscoso, G. D. Yancopoulos & J. R. Sanes. 1997. Rapsyn is required for MuSK signaling and recruits synaptic components to a MuSK-containing scaffold. Neuron **18:** 623–625.

67. Gillespie, S. K., S. Balasubramanian, E. T. Fung & R. L. Haganir. 1996. Rapsyn clusters and activates the synapse-specific receptor tyrosine kinase MuSK. Neuron **16:** 953–962.

68. Moscoso, L. M., G. C. Chu, M. Gautam, P. G. Noakes, J. P. Merlie & J. R. Sanes. 1995. Synapse-associated expression of an acetylcholine receptor–inducing protein, ARIA/heregulin, and its putative receptors, ErbB2 and ErbB3, in developing mammalian muscle. Dev. Biol. **172:** 158–169.

69. Fuhrer, C. & Z. W. Hall. 1996. Functional interaction of src family kinases with the acetylcholine receptor in C2 myotubes. J. Biol. Chem. **271:** 32474–32481.

70. Riedel, H., T. J. Dull, A. M. Honegger, J. Schlessinger & A. Ullrich. 1989. Cytoplasmic domains determine signal specificity, cellular routing characteristics and influence ligand binding of epidermal growth factor and insulin receptors. EMBO J. **8:** 2943–2954.

71. Rovelli, G., R. A. Heller, M. Canossa & E. M. Shooter. 1993. Chimeric tumor necrosis factor–TrkA receptors reveal that ligand-dependent activation of the TrkA tyrosine kinase is sufficient for differentiation and survival of PC12 cells. Proc. Natl. Acad. Sci. U.S.A. **90:** 8717–8721.

Evidence for an Association between Human Acetylcholine Receptor and Rapsyn[a]

ALEXANDRA BUCKEL, ESTHER JAMES, LESLIE JACOBSON,
JEIKE BIEWENGA, DAVID BEESON, AND ANGELA VINCENT

Neurosciences Group
Institute of Molecular Medicine
John Radcliffe Hospital
University of Oxford
Headington, Oxford OX3 9DS, United Kingdom

The acetylcholine receptor (AChR) is localized at the adult neuromuscular junction (NMJ) where it is concentrated at the crests of the postsynaptic folds. The high density of these receptors is of critical importance in synaptic transmission, and any alteration in the number of AChR or in their localization could lead to a myasthenic disorder. The cytoplasmic protein rapsyn (43-kDa protein) is thought to be responsible for anchoring the AChRs through its cytoplasmic domain, although possible sites of interaction between the AChR and rapsyn have not been defined. Mutations created within the rapsyn protein have altered AChR clustering (see also Sanes *et al.* and Hall in this volume) and have implicated a leucine zipper motif within the rapsyn structure. Utrophin is another protein that is concentrated at the neuromuscular junction, but its role in maintaining AChR clusters is not clear. β2 laminin is a component of laminins 3/4, which are neuromuscular junction–specific and concentrated extracellularly in the synaptic cleft. Here, we have used three different approaches to look for possible interactions between human rapsyn and AChRs, using utrophin and β2 laminin fragments as control proteins.[1–3]

[125]I-α-BuTx-labeled human AChR was used to overlay recombinant human rapsyn, the distal portion of utrophin, and β2 laminin recombinant fragments immobilized on nitrocellulose. FIGURE 1a shows that human AChR bound to full-length rapsyn (residues 1–412; lane 1), but not to truncated rapsyn (residues 1–151; lane 2) nor to utrophin or β2 laminin fragments (lanes 3–6).

To investigate the AChR/rapsyn interaction further, the converse approach was used in which [125]I-(recombinant)rapsyn was used to probe immobilized individual recombinant AChR subunits. FIGURE 1b shows that ^{125}I-rapsyn bound to full-length α, γ, and ε subunits (lanes 1, 4, and 5), but not to the truncated β and δ AChR subunits (lanes 2 and 3), which do not contain the cytoplasmic sequences. Rapsyn also showed very strong binding to itself (lane 6), but no binding to utrophin or β2 laminin fragments (lanes 7–10).

To determine if a coexistent association between rapsyn and AChR could be detected in muscle extracts, polyclonal antibodies directed against rapsyn and β2

[a]This work was supported by Action Research and the Muscular Dystrophy Group of Great Britain.

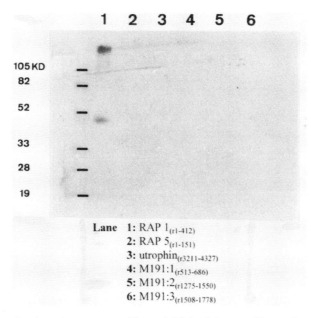

FIGURE 1a. Overlay of rapsyn, utrophin, and β2 laminin recombinants immobilized on Western blots with ¹²⁵I-BuTx-labeled AChR. Binding of AChR is observed to full-length rapsyn, but not to the shorter rapsyn recombinant nor to utrophin or β2 laminin fragments. Binding was visualized by autoradiography.

laminin were tested for immunoprecipitation of AChR. Small amounts (<10%) of ^{125}I-α-BuTx-labeled AChR could be immunoprecipitated with antirapsyn antiserum from human and mouse muscle extracts, but a similar coprecipitation was not observed when antiserum to β2 laminin was used (data not shown).

We have shown that an association between human AChR and rapsyn was evident from overlay experiments and immunoprecipitations. Similar results had previously been obtained using human AChR with mouse rapsyn (Biewenga, Beeson, and Vincent, unpublished observations, 1993). Because ^{125}I-α-BuTx–AChR binding was not seen to the shorter rapsyn polypeptide 1–151, the binding site for the AChR within rapsyn may be contained within residues 151–412; if so, the leucine zipper (residues 129–150) cannot be responsible for this interaction.

The association between rapsyn and AChR appears to be attributable, at least in part, to the binding of rapsyn to each of the α, γ, and ε subunits of the AChR; we have not yet tested binding to full-length β and δ subunits. Moreover, rapsyn appears to have a high affinity for itself, as shown by strong binding in the overlay experiments, which may account for the ability of rapsyn to cluster, even in the absence of AChR. Although the coprecipitation experiments suggest that the AChR retains some association with rapsyn after extraction, the overlay experiments indicate that this association can occur between molecules that have been denatured and separated by

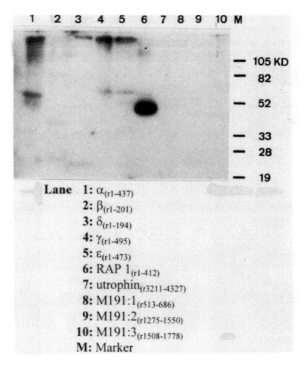

FIGURE 1b. Overlay of individual α, β, δ, γ, and ϵ recombinant AChR subunits, utrophin, $\beta2$ laminin fragments, and rapsyn itself with ^{125}I-rapsyn (full length). Binding is seen to full-length AChR subunits (α, γ, and ϵ), as well as a much greater binding to itself. Binding was visualized by autoradiography.

SDS gel electrophoresis. Therefore, the interaction does not appear to be particularly dependent on the native conformation of the molecules and it should be possible in future experiments to define more precisely the sites of interaction(s) between the proteins using shorter recombinant polypeptides and synthetic peptides.

REFERENCES

1. Philips, W. D., M. M. Maimone & J. P. Merlie. 1991. Mutagenesis of the 43 kD postsynaptic protein defines domains involved in plasma membrane targeting and AChR clustering. J. Cell Biol. **115:** 1713–1723.
2. Deconinck, A. E., A. C. Potter, J. M. Tinsley et al. 1997. Postsynaptic abnormalities at the neuromuscular junctions of utrophin-deficient mice. J. Cell Biol. **136:** 862–870.
3. Buckel, A., D. Beeson, M. James et al. 1996. Cloning of cDNA encoding human rapsyn and mapping of the RAPSN gene locus to chromosome 11p11.2–p11.1. Genomics **35:** 613–616.

Interaction between the Nicotinic Acetylcholine Receptor and Grb2

Implications for Signaling at the Neuromuscular Junction[a]

MARCIE COLLEDGE AND STANLEY C. FROEHNER[b]

Department of Physiology
University of North Carolina at Chapel Hill
Chapel Hill, North Carolina 27599-7545

INTRODUCTION

Signaling between neurons depends on a highly ordered and regulated distribution of proteins at the synapse. Neurotransmitter receptors are clustered in the postsynaptic cell in precise juxtaposition to the sites of neurotransmitter release in the presynaptic cell, ensuring rapid and efficient synaptic transmission. The bulk of our knowledge about the molecular mechanisms underlying synaptogenesis comes from studies of the neuromuscular junction (NMJ), the synapse between a motor neuron and a muscle fiber. In the end plate region of the muscle cell, nicotinic acetylcholine receptors (AChR) are amassed to a density that approaches 10,000 per μm^2. The density drops by 1000-fold just microns outside the synapse.[1,2] Disruption of this specialized postsynaptic machinery, as occurs in acquired myasthenia gravis, has serious consequences for synaptic transmission and muscle contraction. Although the signal transduction pathways underlying the initiation and maintenance of the postsynaptic specialization have not been well characterized, many lines of evidence suggest that tyrosine phosphorylation may be centrally important (see below). This chapter reviews recent experiments from our laboratory demonstrating that tyrosine phosphorylation of the AChR itself may be involved in the initiation of a signal transduction pathway through its interaction with the modular adaptor protein Grb2.[3]

TYROSINE PHOSPHORYLATION AT THE POSTSYNAPTIC MEMBRANE

The muscle nicotinic AChR is a pentameric ligand-gated ion channel, composed of four homologous subunits, in the stoichiometry $\alpha_2\beta\gamma\delta$. Each subunit is composed of a large extracellular amino-terminal domain, four transmembrane domains, and a small extracellular carboxy-terminus. A large cytoplasmic loop between the third and fourth transmembrane domains contains multiple consensus sites for phosphorylation by various kinases, including cyclic AMP–dependent protein kinase and protein

[a]This research was supported by a grant (to S. C. Froehner) from the National Institutes of Health and by a fellowship (to M. Colledge) from the Natural Sciences and Engineering Research Council of Canada.
[b]To whom all correspondence should be addressed.

kinase C (reviewed in reference 4). In addition, a single tyrosine residue in this region of the β, γ, and δ subunits of *Torpedo* AChR is the target of an unidentified tyrosine kinase (or kinases).[5] Many of the sites of phosphorylation have been mapped by sequencing phosphorylated peptide fragments of *Torpedo* AChR.[6–9] Phosphorylation sites in the β and δ subunits are conserved among species.[10] Functionally, phosphorylation of the AChR by both serine and tyrosine kinases is associated with an increased rate of receptor desensitization.[11–13]

Tyrosine phosphorylation has been postulated to play a role in the clustering of AChR in the postsynaptic membrane. AChRs isolated from *Torpedo* electric organ contain high levels of endogenous phosphotyrosine (0.5 mole phosphotyrosine per mole of subunit). This is in contrast to extremely low levels of tyrosine phosphorylation of AChRs observed in cultured myotubes[14] and BC3H1 myocytes.[15] This discrepancy suggests that innervation may regulate tyrosine phosphorylation of the AChR. Indeed, immunocytochemical experiments have identified phosphotyrosine reactivity at synaptic sites, both in *Torpedo* electric organ and at the rat NMJ.[16] At the NMJ, phosphotyrosine labeling was shown to be dependent on innervation. Phosphotyrosine immunoreactivity has also been observed at AChR clusters induced by various stimuli, including the culture substrate, electric field, and polystyrene microbeads,[17,18] as well as at clusters of AChR formed in heterologous cells by coexpression with recombinant rapsyn.[19] This labeling appears to be due not only to tyrosine phosphorylation of the AChR itself, but also to other tyrosine phosphorylated proteins present at these sites.[17] In addition, tyrosine kinase inhibitors have been shown to inhibit agrin-induced AChR clustering[20–22] as well as uncoated, bFGF (basic fibroblast growth factor)–coated, and HB-GAM (heparin-binding growth-associated molecule)–coated bead-induced clustering.[17,23,24] Moreover, the observation that agrin stimulation of cultured myotubes induces tyrosine phosphorylation of the β[21,22,25,26] and perhaps the δ[25] subunit of the AChR has led to the hypothesis that tyrosine kinase signaling may be critical in the AChR clustering pathway.

Recently, the muscle-specific receptor tyrosine kinase, MuSK, was shown to be essential for neuromuscular synapse formation.[27,28] Furthermore, agrin exerts its effects, at least in part, through activation of MuSK.[29] In addition, activation of MuSK leads to phosphorylation of the β subunit of the AChR.[29,30] These observations suggest that signaling by receptor tyrosine kinases likely plays an important role in neuromuscular synaptogenesis as it does in many other cellular processes.

Grb2-MEDIATED SIGNALING

Grb2 (*G*rowth factor *r*eceptor *b*ound protein 2) is an adaptor protein, consisting entirely of three protein binding modules: a central SH2 domain flanked by two SH3 domains.[31] In growth factor signaling, Grb2 links activated receptor tyrosine kinases to the Ras/MAP kinase signal transduction pathway (reviewed in reference 32). Ligand-driven dimerization of growth factor receptors leads to tyrosine autophosphorylation of the receptor, creating a high-affinity binding site for the SH2 domain of Grb2 (for review, see references 33–35). The Grb2/Sos (Son of sevenless) complex is then recruited from the cytoplasm to the cell membrane via the SH2 domain of Grb2. This translocation event brings Sos, a guanine-nucleotide exchange factor, to the cellular location of its substrate protein Ras, where it then activates Ras by promoting the exchange of GTP for GDP. Activated Ras initiates an MAP kinase signaling cascade, ultimately leading to changes in gene expression in the nucleus (reviewed in references 32 and 33).

Recently, Yang *et al.*[36] demonstrated a direct interaction in muscle between Grb2 and β-dystroglycan, a component of the dystrophin-glycoprotein complex. β-Dystroglycan serves as a transmembrane link between the extracellular peripheral membrane protein, α-dystroglycan, and cytoskeletal dystrophin or utrophin.[37] The identification of α-dystroglycan as a cell surface binding site for agrin[38–41] has focused much attention on the potential role of the dystrophin-associated protein complex in mediating agrin's AChR-clustering effects. The interaction between Grb2 and β-dystroglycan is mediated by the SH3 domain(s) of Grb2 and the proline-rich region of β-dystroglycan, raising the following question: what is the SH2 binding partner for Grb2 at the neuromuscular synapse? Given Grb2's role in mediating tyrosine kinase signaling in diverse cellular processes, coupled with its interaction with β-dystroglycan, we became interested in whether Grb2 might be involved in signaling at the postsynaptic membrane. As a first step, we took the approach of looking for tyrosine-phosphorylated SH2 binding partners of Grb2 in postsynaptic membranes.

IDENTIFICATION OF THE AChR δ SUBUNIT AS A Grb2 BINDING PARTNER

The electric organ of marine rays is innervated by cholinergic neurons and is highly enriched in nicotinic AChRs and other synaptic proteins whose homologues are found at the NMJ. Indeed, many synaptic proteins have been identified and characterized from postsynaptic membranes of *Torpedo* electroplax, including rapsyn, syntrophin, and agrin.[42–44] We employed a protein blot overlay approach to identify potential binding proteins of Grb2 in *Torpedo* postsynaptic membranes, using glutathione-S-transferase (GST) fusion proteins of Grb2 as a probe. GST-Grb2 fusion proteins, but not control GST proteins, consistently bound to several postsynaptic proteins of approximate molecular weights: 65 kDa, 90 kDa, 130 kDa, and 150 kDa (FIGURE 1, top; compare panels C and D, left lanes). The most prominent binding was to the 65-kDa band, which corresponds in size to the AChR δ subunit, as parallel immunoblots with Mab 88B (which recognizes both the γ and δ subunits of the AChR) labeled the same position (FIGURE 1, top, panel A). To confirm that Grb2 was indeed binding to the δ subunit and not another protein migrating to the same position, we isolated AChR by α-bungarotoxin affinity purification and repeated the overlay assays on purified AChR subunits. As anticipated, GST-Grb2, but not GST, bound to the δ subunit of the AChR (FIGURE 1, top, panels C and D, right lanes).

Grb2-AChR INTERACTION IS SH2-PHOSPHOTYROSINE-MEDIATED

Phosphotyrosine immunoblots performed on parallel samples indicated that the δ subunit was tyrosine-phosphorylated (FIGURE 1, top, panel B), suggesting that binding was mediated by the SH2 domain of Grb2. To test this, we performed protein

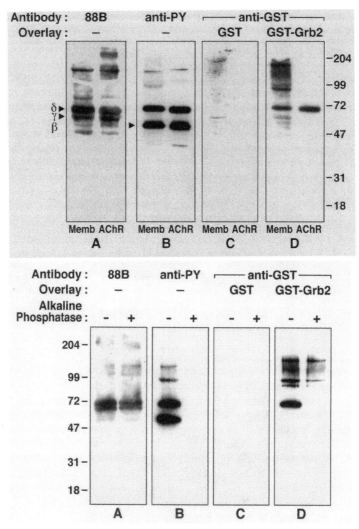

FIGURE 1. Grb2 binds to the δ subunit of the AChR. (Top) *Torpedo* postsynaptic membrane proteins and isolated AChR subunits were separated by SDS-PAGE and transferred to nitrocellulose membranes. (Panel A) Immunoblot with Mab 88B indicates the position of the γ and δ AChR subunits. Higher molecular weight bands are aggregates and dimers of the δ subunit and degradation products thereof. Minor lower molecular weight bands are degradation products of the γ and δ subunits. (Panel B) Tyrosine phosphorylation of the β and δ subunits of the AChR is shown by Western blotting using antiphosphotyrosine antibody 4G10. (Panel C) Protein overlays with control GST show no binding to membrane proteins or AChR subunits. (Panel D) Overlays with GST-Grb2 show binding to a prominent protein at 65 kDa, corresponding to the δ subunit of the AChR. Other proteins of 90, 130, and 150 kDa in membrane samples also bound Grb2. Arrows on the left indicate the position of the β, γ, and δ AChR subunits; numbers on the right indicate positions of molecular weight markers (in kDa). Reprinted from reference 3 with permission from *The Journal of Neuroscience.* (Bottom) Equivalent amounts of

overlays with fusion proteins containing each of the three individual domains of Grb2. As expected, fusion proteins that contained only the SH2 domain of Grb2 bound to the δ subunit; N- or C-terminal SH3 domain fusion proteins did not bind (data not shown). To confirm that Grb2 binding was dependent on tyrosine phosphorylation of the δ subunit, we treated *Torpedo* postsynaptic membranes with alkaline phosphatase to remove phosphotyrosine and repeated the Grb2 overlays. Although an equivalent amount of δ subunit protein was present (FIGURE 1, bottom, panel A), dephosphorylation of the δ subunit (FIGURE 1, bottom, panel B) abolished GST-Grb2 binding (FIGURE 1, bottom, panel D). Examination of the amino-acid sequence surrounding the phosphotyrosine site in the cytoplasmic domain of the δ subunit revealed a precise binding motif (pYXNX; X is any amino acid) for the SH2 domain of Grb2.[45] Indeed, a phosphopeptide corresponding to this region of the δ subunit bound to Grb2 SH2 fusion proteins with relatively high affinity (~200 nM) in surface plasmon resonance assays. A control peptide lacking phosphorylation on tyrosine exhibited no binding (data not shown). Although the β subunit of the AChR is tyrosine-phosphorylated to a similar degree as the δ subunit, specificity of the association is further supported by the observation that it does not bind to Grb2 in overlay assays (see FIGURE 1, top and bottom). This result is consistent with the fact that the tyrosine phosphorylation sites of neither the β nor the γ subunit contain appropriate Grb2 SH2 consensus sequences (FIGURE 2). Taken together, these data suggest that the AChR δ subunit and Grb2 associate, at least *in vitro*, via a specific, high-affinity phosphotyrosine–SH2 domain–mediated interaction.

GRB2 AND ACHR FORM A COMPLEX *IN VIVO*

To address whether a complex between the AChR and Grb2 exists in the cell, we asked whether Grb2 copurifies with AChR. To this end, *Torpedo* postsynaptic membranes were solubilized and AChRs were isolated using α-bungarotoxin beads. As a control for specificity of binding to the beads, solubilized membranes were preincubated with excess toxin (25 μM) before incubation with toxin beads. After extensive washing, bound proteins were eluted with SDS-sample buffer and subjected to Western blot analysis with anti-Grb2 antibodies. FIGURE 3 shows that Grb2 specifically copurifies with the AChR; Grb2 binding is dependent on the presence of AChR on the beads. Furthermore, confocal microscopy analysis indicated that Grb2 is localized in precise register with the AChR on the innervated face of the electrocyte (data

---

Torpedo membranes (5 μg) treated with (right lane) and without (left lane) alkaline phosphatase were subjected to SDS-PAGE and transferred to nitrocellulose for protein overlay analysis. (Panel A) Immunoblot with Mab 88B shows that approximately equal amounts of δ subunit protein were loaded for each condition. (Panel B) Parallel immunoblots using a cocktail of antiphosphotyrosine antibodies, 4G10 and PY20, indicate an absence of immunoreactivity in the phosphatase-treated membranes. (Panel C) Protein overlays with control GST show no binding. (Panel D) Binding of full-length GST-Grb2 to the δ subunit is abolished by phosphatase treatment of the membranes. Binding to the 90- and 150-kDa proteins is retained. Reprinted from reference 3 with permission from *The Journal of Neuroscience.*

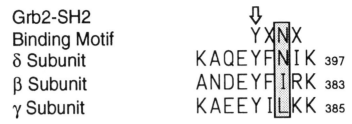

FIGURE 2. Tyrosine phosphorylation sites of *Torpedo* AChR subunits. Alignment of tyrosine phosphorylation sites in the large cytoplasmic loop of *Torpedo* β, γ, and δ subunits reveals a Grb2 SH2 consensus motif in the δ subunit, but not in the β or γ subunits. The pY+2 position is boxed and shaded. The phosphotyrosine is indicated with an arrow. Reprinted from reference 3 with permission from *The Journal of Neuroscience.*

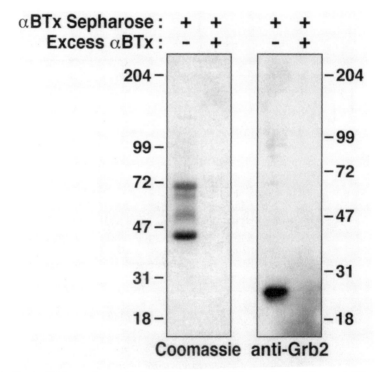

FIGURE 3. Grb2 associates with the AChR *in situ.* AChR were isolated from solubilized *Torpedo* membranes using α-bungarotoxin Sepharose, eluted in SDS buffer, and resolved by SDS-PAGE. Coomassie staining the preparation shows the four subunits of the AChR: α, ~40 kDa; β, ~50 kDa; γ, ~60 kDa; and δ, ~65 kDa. Preincubation with excess α-bungarotoxin (25 μM) prevents binding of AChR to the toxin-Sepharose (left panel). Immunoblotting the samples with anti-Grb2 antibodies reveals that Grb2 specifically copurifies with the AChR (right panel). Reprinted from reference 3 with permission from *The Journal of Neuroscience.*

not shown). These results provide evidence for a biologically relevant association between Grb2 and the nicotinic AChR at the postsynaptic membrane.

CONCLUSIONS

We have identified a previously unsuspected interaction between the tyrosine-phosphorylated δ subunit of the AChR and Grb2. To our knowledge, these data represent the first evidence of an adaptor protein binding to an ion channel. While the function of the association remains to be determined, the results raise the intriguing possi-

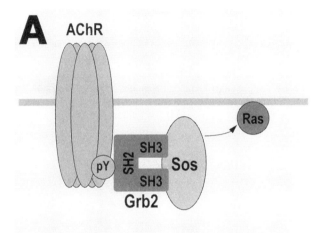

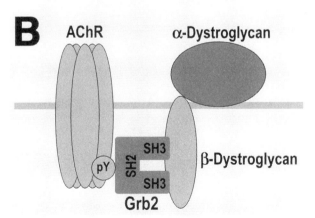

FIGURE 4. Models for downstream Grb2 interactions at the postsynaptic membrane. (A) Grb2 may mediate a signaling role by linking the AChR to the Ras signal transduction pathway through its SH3-mediated interaction with Sos. (B) Grb2 may provide a structural link between the AChR and the dystrophin-associated protein complex by binding to β-dystroglycan.

bility that tyrosine phosphorylation of the AChR may initiate a Grb2-mediated signaling cascade at the postsynaptic membrane, in a fashion analogous to activation of the Ras/MAP kinase pathway by growth factor receptor activation. Alternatively, given the observation that Grb2 can interact, via its SH3 domains, with β-dystroglycan,[36] Grb2 may provide a structural link between the AChR and the dystrophin/utrophin complex at the synapse. These two possibilities are illustrated in schematic form in FIGURE 4. Certainly, identification of SH3 binding proteins in Grb2/AChR complexes isolated from postsynaptic membranes will help to distinguish between these two possibilities.

Interestingly, we did not observe any interaction between Grb2 and β-dystroglycan in our experiments. Although Western blotting confirmed the presence of β-dystroglycan in our membrane preparations (data not shown),[38] we did not detect interaction in Grb2 overlays with a protein corresponding in size to β-dystroglycan (43 kDa). In addition, β-dystroglycan did not copurify with AChR/Grb2 complexes in affinity purification experiments. At present, aside from species or technical differences, we cannot explain the apparent discrepancy between our results and those of Yang *et al.* However, in overlay experiments using full-length Grb2 fusion proteins to probe postsynaptic membrane proteins, we consistently observed binding to proteins of 90 and 150 kDa that was not dependent on tyrosine phosphorylation (see FIGURE 1, top and bottom, panels D). Future experiments will aim to determine whether these proteins represent SH3 binding partners for Grb2 in the postsynaptic membrane.

Another important question is whether the association between the AChR and Grb2 is conserved in other species, particularly at the mammalian NMJ. While the *Torpedo* δ subunit contains a precise motif (pYXNX) for recognition by the SH2 domain of Grb2,[45] this sequence is not well conserved in mammalian δ subunits (mouse: pYFSL). This suggests that the binding affinity may be lower between Grb2 and the mammalian AChR δ subunit. One possibility is that the extremely high concentration of AChR at the NMJ might compensate for a weak interaction. In fact, a low-affinity interaction may be essential for rapid onset and termination of signaling at the mammalian end plate. We are presently pursuing answers to these questions.

ACKNOWLEDGMENTS

We are grateful to our colleagues at the University of North Carolina for helpful discussions.

REFERENCES

1. FERTUCK, N. C. & M. M. SALPETER. 1974. Localization of acetylcholine receptor by ^{125}I-labeled alpha-bungarotoxin binding at mouse motor endplates. Proc. Natl. Acad. Sci. U.S.A. **71:** 1376–1378.
2. MATTHEWS-BELLINGER, J. & M. M. SALPETER. 1978. Distribution of acetylcholine receptor at frog neuromuscular junctions with a discussion of some physiological implications. J. Physiol. **279:** 197–213.

3. COLLEDGE, M. & S. C. FROEHNER. 1997. Tyrosine phosphorylation of the nicotinic acetylcholine receptor mediates Grb2 binding. J. Neurosci. **17:** 5038–5045.

4. SWOPE, S. L., S. J. MOSS, C. D. BLACKSTONE & R. L. HUGANIR. 1992. Phosphorylation of ligand-gated ion channels: a possible mode of synaptic plasticity. FASEB J. **6:** 2514–2523.

5. HUGANIR, R. L., K. MILES & P. GREENGARD. 1984. Phosphorylation of the nicotinic acetylcholine receptor by an endogenous tyrosine-specific protein kinase. Proc. Natl. Acad. Sci. U.S.A. **81:** 6968–6972.

6. SAFRAN, A., R. SAGI-EISENBERG, D. NEUMANN & S. FUCHS. 1987. Phosphorylation of the acetylcholine receptor by protein kinase C and identification of the phosphorylation site within the receptor δ subunit. J. Biol. Chem. **262:** 10506–10510.

7. SCHROEDER, W., H. E. MEYER, K. BUCHNER, H. BAYER & F. HUCHO. 1991. Phosphorylation sites of the nicotinic acetylcholine receptor: a novel site detected in position δS362. Biochemistry **30:** 3583–3588.

8. WAGNER, K., K. EDSON, L. HEGINBOTHAM, M. POST, R. L. HUGANIR & A. J. CZERNIK. 1991. Determination of the tyrosine phosphorylation sites of the nicotinic acetylcholine receptor. J. Biol. Chem. **266:** 23784–23789.

9. YEE, G. H. & R. L. HUGANIR. 1987. Determination of the sites of cAMP-dependent phosphorylation on the nicotinic acetylcholine receptor. J. Biol. Chem. **262:** 16748–16753.

10. HUGANIR, R. L. & K. MILES. 1989. Protein phosphorylation of nicotinic acetylcholine receptors. Crit. Rev. Biochem. Mol. Biol. **24:** 183–215.

11. EUSEBI, F., M. MOLINARO & B. M. ZANI. 1985. Agents that activate protein kinase C reduce acetylcholine sensitivity in cultured myotubes. J. Cell Biol. **100:** 1339–1342.

12. HOPFIELD, J. F., D. W. TANK, P. GREENGARD & R. L. HUGANIR. 1988. Functional modulation of the nicotinic acetylcholine receptor by tyrosine phosphorylation. Nature **336:** 677–680.

13. HUGANIR, R. L., A. H. DELCOUR, P. GREENGARD & G. P. HESS. 1986. Phosphorylation of the nicotinic acetylcholine receptor regulates its rate of desensitization. Nature **321:** 774–776.

14. MILES, K., P. GREENGARD & R. L. HUGANIR. 1989. Calcitonin gene–related peptide regulates phosphorylation of the nicotinic acetylcholine receptor in rat myotubes. Neuron **2:** 1517–1524.

15. SMITH, M. M., J. P. MERLIE & J. C. J. LAWRENCE. 1987. Regulation of phosphorylation of nicotinic acetylcholine receptors in mouse BC3H1 myocytes. Proc. Natl. Acad. Sci. U.S.A. **84:** 6601–6605.

16. QU, Z., E. MORITZ & R. L. HUGANIR. 1990. Regulation of tyrosine phosphorylation of the nicotinic acetylcholine receptor at the rat neuromuscular junction. Neuron **4:** 367–378.

17. BAKER, L. & H. PENG. 1993. Tyrosine phosphorylation and acetylcholine receptor cluster formation in cultured *Xenopus* muscle cells. J. Cell Biol. **120:** 185–195.

18. PENG, H., L. BAKER & Z. DAI. 1993. A role for tyrosine phosphorylation in the formation of acetylcholine receptor clusters induced by electric fields in cultured *Xenopus* muscle cells. J. Cell Biol. **120:** 197–204.

19. DAI, Z., P. SCOTLAND, S. FROEHNER & H. PENG. 1996. Association of phosphotyrosine with rapsyn expression in *Xenopus* embryonic cells. Neuroreport **7:** 657–661.

20. DAGGETT, D. F., D. STONE, H. B. PENG & K. NIKOLICS. 1996. Full-length agrin isoform activities and binding site distributions on cultured *Xenopus* muscle cells. Mol. Cell. Neurosci. **7:** 75–88.

21. FERNS, M., M. DEINER & Z. HALL. 1996. Agrin-induced acetylcholine receptor clustering in mammalian muscle requires tyrosine phosphorylation. J. Cell Biol. **132:** 937–944.

22. WALLACE, B. G. 1994. Staurosporine inhibits agrin-induced acetylcholine receptor phosphorylation and aggregation. J. Cell Biol. **125:** 661–668.

23. BAKER, L. & H. PENG. 1995. Induction of acetylcholine receptor cluster formation by local application of growth factors in cultured *Xenopus* muscle cells. Neurosci. Lett. **185:** 135–138.
24. PENG, H. B., A. A. ALI, Z. DAI, D. F. DAGGETT, E. RAULO & H. RAUVALA. 1995. The role of heparin-binding growth-associated molecule (HB-GAM) in the postsynaptic induction in cultured muscle cells. J. Neurosci. **15:** 3027–3038.
25. QU, Z. & R. L. HUGANIR. 1994. Comparison of innervation and agrin-induced tyrosine phosphorylation of the nicotinic acetylcholine receptor. J. Neurosci. **14:** 6834–6841.
26. WALLACE, B. G., Z. QU & R. L. HUGANIR. 1991. Agrin induces phosphorylation of the nicotinic acetylcholine receptor. Neuron **6:** 869–878.
27. DECHIARA, T. M., D. C. BOWEN, D. M. VALENZUELA, M. V. SIMMONS, W. T. POUEYMIROU, S. THOMAS, E. KINETZ, D. L. COMPTON, E. ROJAS, J. S. PARK, C. SMITH, P. S. DISTEFANO, D. J. GLASS, S. J. BURDEN & G. D. YANCOPOULOS. 1996. The receptor tyrosine kinase MuSK is required for neuromuscular junction formation *in vivo*. Cell **85:** 501–512.
28. VALENZUELA, D. M., T. N. STITT, P. S. DISTEFANO, E. ROJAS, K. MATTSSON, D. L. COMPTON, L. NUNEZ, J. S. PARK, J. L. STARK, D. R. GIES, S. THOMAS, M. M. LE BEAU, A. A. FERNALD, N. G. COPELAND, N. A. JENKINS, S. J. BURDEN, D. J. GLASS & G. D. YANCOPOULOS. 1995. Receptor tyrosine kinase specific for the skeletal muscle lineage: expression in embryonic muscle, at the neuromuscular junction, and after injury. Neuron **15:** 573–584.
29. GLASS, D. J., D. C. BOWEN, T. N. STITT, C. RADZIEJEWSKI, J. BRUNO, T. E. RYAN, D. R. GIES, S. SHAH, K. MATTSSON, S. J. BURDEN, P. S. DISTEFANO, D. M. VALENZUELA, T. M. DECHIARA & G. D. YANCOPOULOS. 1996. Agrin acts via a MuSK receptor complex. Cell **85:** 513–523.
30. GILLESPIE, S. K. H., S. BALASUBRAMANIAN, E. T. FUNG & R. L. HUGANIR. 1996. Rapsyn clusters and activates the synapse-specific receptor tyrosine kinase MuSK. Neuron **16:** 953–962.
31. LOWENSTEIN, E. J., R. J. DALY, A. G. BATZER, W. LI, B. MARGOLIS, R. LAMMERS, A. ULLRICH, E. Y. SKOLNIK, D. BAR-SAGI & J. SCHLESSINGER. 1992. The SH2 and SH3 domain–containing protein Grb2 links receptor tyrosine kinases to ras signaling. Cell **70:** 431–442.
32. SCHLESSINGER, J. 1993. How receptor tyrosine kinases activate Ras. Trends Biochem. Sci. **18:** 273–275.
33. HELDIN, C-H. 1995. Dimerization of cell surface receptors in signal transduction. Cell **80:** 213–223.
34. SCHLESSINGER, J. 1994. SH2/SH3 signaling proteins. Curr. Opin. Genet. Dev. **4:** 25–30.
35. ULLRICH, A. & J. SCHLESSINGER. 1990. Signal transduction by receptors with tyrosine kinase activity. Cell **61:** 203–212.
36. YANG, B., D. JUNG, D. MOTTO, J. MEYER, G. KORETZKY & K. P. CAMPBELL. 1995. SH3 domain–mediated interaction of dystroglycan and Grb2. J. Biol. Chem. **270:** 11711–11714.
37. IBRAGHIMOV-BESKROVNAYA, O., J. M. ERVASTI, C. J. LEVEILLE, C. A. SLAUGHTER, S. W. SERNETT & K. P. CAMPBELL. 1992. Primary structure of dystrophin-associated glycoproteins linking dystrophin to the extracellular matrix. Nature **355:** 696–702.
38. BOWE, M. A., K. A. DEYST, J. D. LESZYK & J. R. FALLON. 1994. Identification and purification of an agrin receptor from *Torpedo* postsynaptic membranes: a heteromeric complex related to the dystroglycans. Neuron **12:** 1173–1180.
39. CAMPANELLI, J. T., S. L. ROBERDS, K. P. CAMPBELL & R. H. SCHELLER. 1994. A role for dystrophin-associated glycoproteins and utrophin in agrin-induced AChR clustering. Cell **77:** 663–674.
40. GEE, S. H., F. MONTANARO, M. H. LINDENBAUM & S. CARBONETTO. 1994. Dystroglycan-α, a dystrophin-associated glycoprotein, is a functional agrin receptor. Cell **77:** 675–686.

41. SUGIYAMA, J., D. C. BOWEN & Z. W. HALL. 1994. Dystroglycan binds nerve and muscle agrin. Neuron **13:** 103–115.

42. FROEHNER, S. C., A. A. MURNANE, M. TOBLER, H. B. PENG & R. SEALOCK. 1987. A postsynaptic M_r 58,000 (58K) protein at acetylcholine receptor–rich sites in *Torpedo* electroplaques and skeletal muscle. J. Cell Biol. **104:** 1633–1646.

43. GODFREY, E. W., R. M. NITKIN, B. G. WALLACE, L. L. RUBIN & U. J. MCMAHAN. 1984. Components of *Torpedo* electric organ and muscle that cause aggregation of acetylcholine receptors on cultured muscle cells. J. Cell Biol. **99:** 615–627.

44. SOBEL, A., M. WEBER & J-P. CHANGEUX. 1977. Large-scale purification of the acetylcholine receptor protein in its membrane-bound and detergent-extracted forms from *Torpedo marmorata* electric organ. Eur. J. Biochem. **80:** 215–244.

45. SONGYANG, Z., S. E. SHOELSON, J. MCGLADE, P. OLIVIER, T. PAWSON, X. R. BUSTELO, M. BARBACID, H. SABE, H. HANAFUSA, T. YI, R. REN, D. BALTIMORE, S. RATNOFSKY, R. A. FELDMAN & L. C. CANTLEY. 1994. Specific motifs recognized by the SH2 domains of Csk, 3BP2, fps/fes, GRB-2, HCP, SHC, Syk, and Vav. Mol. Cell. Biol. **14:** 2777–2785.

Fourteen Newly Recognized Proteins at the Human Neuromuscular Junctions—and Their Nonjunctional Accumulation in Inclusion-Body Myositis[a]

VALERIE ASKANAS, W. KING ENGEL, AND RENATE B. ALVAREZ

USC Neuromuscular Center
Department of Neurology
University of Southern California School of Medicine
Good Samaritan Hospital
Los Angeles, California 90017-1912

The neuromuscular junction (NMJ), the synapse between a distal axonal tip of a lower motor neuron and a muscle fiber, is a highly specialized and complicated structure. At the NMJ, the molecular composition of the muscle-fiber extracellular matrix, the plasmalemma, and the immediately postsynaptic cytoplasmic domain is distinctly different from that of the nonsynaptic regions of the same muscle fiber (reviewed in references 1–6). In general, the postsynaptic proteins may be classified as those localized to the synaptic basal lamina, the plasmalemma, or the subplasmalemmal cytoskeleton.[1–6] In virtually all species including human, the most characteristic feature of the postsynaptic plasmalemma is the high concentration of nicotinic acetylcholine receptors (AChRs). During the last two decades, considerable progress has been made in identifying mechanisms causing AChR clustering at the NMJ.[1–6] More than a dozen other proteins that either are present only at the postsynaptic domain of the NMJ or are highly concentrated there have been identified in various species (reviewed in reference 4). Remaining largely unknown are (a) the function of many of them, (b) how and why they are assembled at the NMJ, and (c) a possible pathologic role in NMJ disorders.

During the last several years, we have studied the molecular pathogenesis of sporadic inclusion-body myositis (s-IBM) and the hereditary inclusion-body myopathies (h-IBMs) (reviewed in references 7 and 8). These diseases, formerly underdiagnosed and considered infrequent syndromes, are now identified more and more often by clinicians and pathologists. Recent interest in s- and h-IBMs has been generated by the identification of abnormal accumulation within IBM muscle fibers of the group of diverse proteins previously considered characteristic of Alzheimer-disease brain and thought not to occur in diseased human muscle.[7,8]

It is particularly germane that nearly all the proteins that we have found abnormally accumulated within the IBM muscle fibers are, in normal human muscle, accumulated only at the postsynaptic domain of the NMJ (TABLE 1).

Those proteins include β-amyloid protein (Aβ),[9] two other (C- and N-terminal)

[a]Studies described in this paper were supported in part by the NIH, the Muscular Dystrophy Association, the Alzheimer Association, and the Sheldon Katz, Helen Lewis, and Ron Stever Research Funds.

TABLE 1. Comparison between IBM VMFs and NMJ[a]

	Protein Accumulated		mRNA Increased	
	NMJ, Postsynaptic	IBM, VMFs	NMJ, Postsynaptic	IBM, VMFs
Similarities				
nAChR	+	+	+	+
βAPP	+	+	+	+
prion	+	+	+	+
SOD1	+	+	0	+
43-kDa (rapsyn)	+	+		
ubiquitin	+	+		
nNOS	+	+		
iNOS	+	+		
α_1-ACT	+	+	0	0
FGF	+	+		
TGF-β1	+	+		
IL 1α	+	+		
IL 1β	+	+		
IL 6	+	+		
ApoE	+	+	0	0
Differences				
nitrotyrosine	0	+		
phosphorylated tau	0	+		
congophilia	0	+		

[a]NMJ = neuromuscular junction; IBM = inclusion-body myositis; VMFs = vacuolated muscle fibers.

epitopes of the β-amyloid precursor protein (βAPP),[10] α_1-antichymotrypsin (α_1-ACT),[13] apolipoprotein E (ApoE),[14,15] ubiquitin,[16] and cellular prion protein (PrP).[17] Those proteins were previously considered strictly neuronal and characteristic of Alzheimer's disease (AD) and prion brain diseases. The accumulation of βAPP and prion at the postsynaptic NMJ results, at least partially, from their locally increased synthesis there, evidenced by their junctionally increased mRNAs;[18,19] these same two mRNAs are also increased, along with increased SOD1-mRNA (see below), in IBM muscle fibers exhibiting increases of their corresponding proteins.

Also abnormally accumulated within IBM muscle fibers are neuronal and inducible nitric oxide synthase,[24] transforming growth factor β1,[25] fibroblast growth factor (FGF),[26] and interleukins 1α, 1β, and 6,[27] all of which are likewise accumulated at normal human NMJs. Moreover, nicotinic acetylcholine receptor (AChR) and its mRNA, and 43-kDa protein (rapsyn), which are known junctional proteins, are also abnormally accumulated within the IBM muscle.[28]

The only protein that is abnormally accumulated in the IBM muscle, but *not* accumulated at the NMJ is hyperphosphorylated tau.[11,12]

In this article, we describe examples of these 14 novel proteins accumulated at human NMJs. So far, their functions and the mechanisms controlling their expression at the NMJ are not known. Although an important contributory pathologic role of any of these proteins in disorders of the NMJ/neuromuscular transmission has not yet been identified, it can be contemplated in the various NMJ disorders, including myasthenia gravis.

We also present our hypothesis regarding a possible mechanism for the accumulation of these "junctional proteins" within nonjunctional regions of IBM muscle fibers.

β-AMYLOID PRECURSOR PROTEIN (βAPP)

Background

βAPP, a product of a chromosome-21 gene (reviewed in reference 29), exists in virtually all tissues. βAPP is a glycoprotein cell-surface component containing a large extracellular N-terminus domain, a transmembrane domain, and a short cytoplasmic carboxyl-terminus domain.[30,31] The βAPP gene produces at least three alternatively spliced transcripts encoding βAPP, containing 695, 751, or 770 amino acids; the last two contain in their extracellular region an insert of a Kunitz-type protease inhibitor.[30–35] The biological functions of βAPP are unknown, but it may play a role in mediating cell-to-cell and cell-to-matrix interaction, neurite growth, and maintenance of cell integrity and shape.[36–39] At central and peripheral synapses, its presynaptic localization was reported,[40] although at the human NMJ we find it concentrated postsynaptically (see below). β-Amyloid protein (Aβ) is a 39–42-residue polypeptide that is a part of βAPP.[29–31,41] Aβ is the major component of amyloid fibrils in blood vessels and senile plaques in the brain of patients with Alzheimer's disease, Down syndrome, Dutch hereditary cerebrovascular amyloidosis, and very advanced age (reviewed in reference 29).

NMJs

Using several well-characterized antibodies against various epitopes of βAPP including Aβ, we immunolocalized βAPP at the NMJs of normal human muscle biopsies[42] (FIGURE 1). In all biopsies, all the NMJs identified by α-BT binding had very strong immunoreactivity with antibodies to all the βAPP sequences studied (this suggests that, at normal junctions, Aβ immunoreactivity may be part of intact molecules of βAPP). The muscle nonjunctional sarcolemma was very faintly immunoreactive with all antibodies. The C-βAPP (FIGURE 1), Aβ (FIGURE 1), and N-βAPP (not shown) immunoreactivities closely colocalized with the postsynaptic cytoplasmic α-BT, desmin, and dystrophin[42] (FIGURE 1).

By gold immunoelectron-microscopy (immuno-EM), βAPP immunoreactivity was localized subjunctionally for a depth of 5–7 μm, especially between junctional nuclei and the base of the junctional folds, and also throughout the folds (FIGURES 2 and 3). Most commonly, βAPP was in amorphous patches up to 30–45 nm wide and in short filaments 5–8 nm wide. Because muscle intermediate-filament desmin is an established postsynaptic component of human NMJs[43] (FIGURE 4), we colocalized at human NMJs two βAPP epitopes and desmin by gold immuno-EM, using 5- and 15-

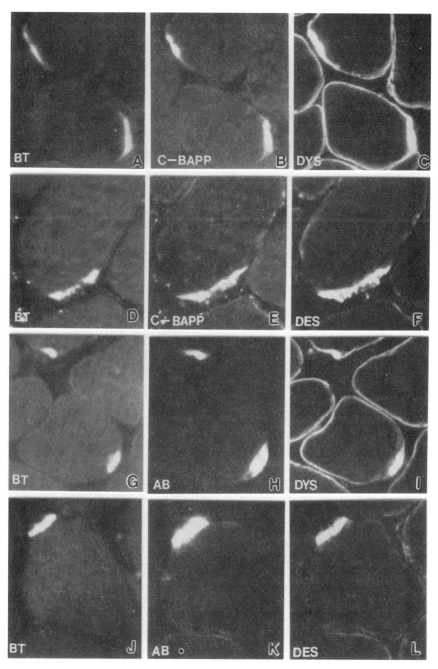

FIGURE 1. Triple-labeling of human NMJs with α-BT, C-βAPP antibody, Aβ antibody, and antibodies against desmin and dystrophin, all ×1000. (A,B,C) α-BT, C-βAPP, and dystrophin; (D,E,F) α-BT, C-βAPP, and desmin; (G,H,I) α-BT, Aβ, and dystrophin; (J,K,L) α-BT, Aβ, and desmin. There is a close colocalization of C-βAPP and Aβ with the three established postsynaptic components of the postsynaptic domain of the NMJ, namely, α-BT, desmin, and dystrophin.

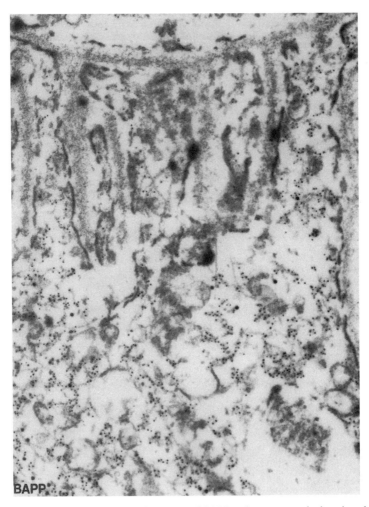

FIGURE 2. Gold immunoelectron-microscopy of βAPP at the postsynaptic domain at human NMJs (5-nm gold particles), ×48,000. βAPP is immunolocalized subjunctionally, between and below junctional folds on short filaments and small amorphous patches (dark round patches represent the labeling of AChE used to identify NMJs).

nm gold particles to simultaneously label βAPP and desmin, respectively, on the same sections. Desmin was in short filaments about 10–12 nm wide and in larger amorphous patches up to 45–90 nm wide. Therefore, similarly to desmin, βAPP appears to be an integral component of the postsynaptic cytoskeleton of human NMJs. In addition to being accumulated at the NMJ, βAPP protein appears to be locally transcribed there as evidenced by *in situ* hybridization studies demonstrating increased accumulation of βAPP-mRNA at the NMJs[18] (FIGURE 5).

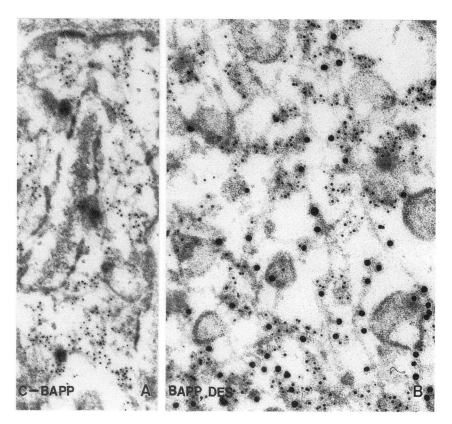

FIGURE 3. Gold immunoelectron-microscopy of βAPP and desmin at human NMJs. (A) βAPP (5-nm gold particles); (B) double-labeling of βAPP (5-nm gold particles) and desmin (15-nm gold particles). (A) ×85,000; (B) ×132,000. In A and B, βAPP is immunolocalized mainly between the junctional folds and below the folds on short filaments 5–8 nm wide; in B, βAPP is also immunolocalized on amorphous patches. Desmin is immunolocalized on short filaments 10–12 nm wide and amorphous patches 45–90 nm wide (B).

In various animal species, shown to be transcribed at the NMJ were AChRs, acetylcholinesterase, neural cell-adhesion molecule (N-CAM) (reviewed in reference 4), and utrophin.[44] Our studies of βAPP were the first to demonstrate transcription of a protein at human NMJs. Recently, using *in situ* hybridization, we have also demonstrated increased transcription at human NMJs of AChR (FIGURE 6) and prion protein (see below). The physiologic role of βAPP at the NMJ is not understood, but speculatively βAPP may be involved in the following: (a) maintaining stability and configuration of the postsynaptic membrane by associating with postsynaptic cytoskeletal components of the muscle fiber, for example, dystrophin and desmin; (b) maintaining adhesion between the postsynaptic and presynaptic components; (c) the interaction between the postsynaptic plasmalemma and basal lamina (and perhaps junction-

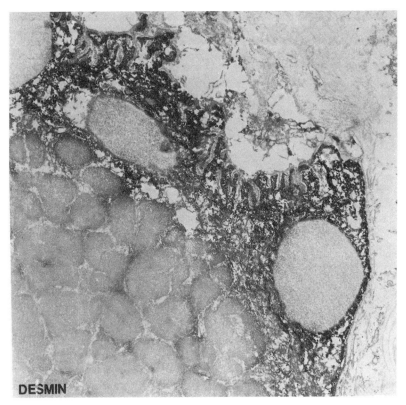

FIGURE 4. Horseradish peroxidase immunoelectron-microscopy of desmin at human NMJs, ×5600. Desmin is immunolocalized strictly postsynaptically.

al acetylcholinesterase); (d) inhibiting, by its Kunitz protease-inhibitor portion, excessive or unwanted serine proteases that may exist at the NMJ; (e) binding and internalization of synaptic substances (analogous to the demonstrated internalization of βAPP/Aβ into lysosomes); or (f) signaling, during development, from muscle fiber to the approaching motor axon, a perturbation of which may occur in βAPP-overexpressed muscle fibers (see below). The strong concentration of βAPP at human NMJs also raises the possibility that it could have a pathogenic role in some diseases affecting NMJs, such as in some patients with myasthenia gravis.

IBMs

We have reported pathologic accumulation of Aβ[9] and two other βAPP sequences[10] in nonjunctional regions of vacuolated muscle fibers of s- and h-IBMs.

Recently, we demonstrated that overexpression of βAPP in normal cultured human muscle fibers interferes with proper innervation and formation of the NMJs[47]

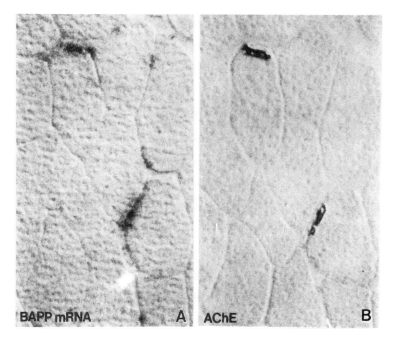

FIGURE 5. βAPP-mRNA at human NMJs. (A) *In situ* hybridization with the 751-βAPP-cRNA probe containing the KPI motif. (B) Acetylcholinesterase reaction on an adjacent section. Both ×650. βAPP-mRNA is strongly increased at two NMJs identified by the acetylcholinesterase reaction.

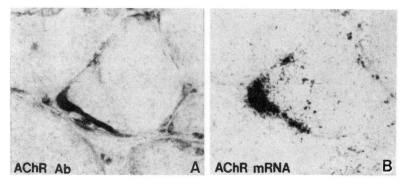

FIGURE 6. AChR immunoreactivity and AChR-mRNA at human NMJs. (A) PAP immunocytochemistry of AChR using a monoclonal antibody. (B) *In situ* hybridization with AChR-cRNA probe. Both ×1200. There is strongly concentrated AChR immunoreactivity and AChR-mRNA at the human NMJ.

(the overexpression was achieved by direct transfer into the cultured muscle fibers of the βAPP gene via a recombinant adenovirus vector[45,46]).

In our human-muscle rat-spinal-cord cocultures, the innervated human muscle fibers become fully cross-striated, are continuously and rhythmically contracting, and have acetylcholinesterase (AChE) and acetylcholine receptors (AChRs) accumulated only at the NMJs.[48,49] By contrast, βAPP-overexpressing cocultured muscle fibers apparently were not able to become properly innervated because (a) they were not cross-striated and not contracting; (b) AChE on them was in large and diffuse patches, and only 2–3% of the fibers had normal AChR clusters; and (c) axons outgrowing from the spinal cord explants had stopped when they contacted normal-control muscle fibers, but appeared to pass over the βAPP-overexpressing muscle fibers (as if not receiving a proper signal from those muscle fibers). Note that the impaired innervation was not due to an effect on spinal cord neurons of βAPP fragments released to the medium because treatment of control cultures with the conditioned medium did not alter innervation[47] (McFerrin et al., to be published). Hence, this culture system provides an excellent experimental model to study the role of βAPP and other proteins in formation and maintenance of the NMJ.

PRION PROTEIN

Background

Cellular prion protein (PrP[c]) is a normal brain constituent, 33–37 kDa, containing 253–254 amino acids. It is considered the precursor of the transmissible scrapie agent, namely, the pathologic prion protein scrapie, PrP[sc], produced by a configurational change induced in the PrP[c] by the pathologic prion molecules (reviewed in reference 20). The normal functions of PrP[c] are uncertain. PrP[c] is probably on the outer surface of the plasmalemma,[50,51] with a hypothesized role in cell-cell recognition, adhesion, or communication.[52,53]

PrP[sc] is a 33–37-kDa isoform of PrP[c] that is resistant to protease-K degradation. At least part of the brain PrP[sc] occurs as congophilic amyloid. It is found only in brains of scrapie-infected animals and in patients with Creutzfeldt-Jakob disease (CJD), Gerstmann-Sträussler-Scheinker syndrome (GSS), and kuru.[20] PrP[c] and PrP[sc] are encoded by the same gene. The amount of corresponding mRNA is the same in normal and scrapie-infected brain,[20] suggesting that PrP[sc] is derived from normal PrP[c]. Proteinase K applied to PrP[sc] from scrapie-infected brain generates a 27–30-kDa digestion-resistant fragment called PrP[27-30], whereas the PrP[c] of normal brain is completely digested by proteinase K.[20] Therefore, PrP[27-30], encoded by a normal cellular gene, is considered to be the disease-characteristic fraction of scrapie brain.[20]

NMJs

We have demonstrated that, in normal human muscle fibers, both PrP and its mRNA are localized only at the NMJs.[19,54] FIGURE 7 illustrates postsynaptic immunolocalization of PrP. By light microscopy, the topographic pattern of PrP immunoreactivity at the NMJs corresponded exactly to the localization of bound α-BT and also closely colocalized with the postsynaptically concentrated immunoreactivity of Aβ, C-βAPP, desmin, ubiquitin, and dystrophin.

By immuno-EM, prominent loci of PrP immunoreactivity were present subjunctionally within the muscle fiber to a depth of 5–7 μm; they were especially localized at the base of the junctional folds (FIGURE 8). Intense PrP immunoreactivity was also present between the folds and attached in small clusters along the muscle-fiber side of the folds. In all those locations, PrP was on 5–8-nm filaments (FIGURE 9). Thus, PrP is a part of the postsynaptic cytoskeleton, where it may help to maintain postsynaptic-fold geometry. We suggest that PrP may have an important, albeit unknown, function in normal junctional biology.

IBMs

We have demonstrated that PrP and PrP-mRNA are accumulated in nonjunctional regions of abnormal muscle fibers of s- and h-IBM.[17,19] Increased synthesis of cellular prion had not been previously reported in any human disease.[20–23]

UBIQUITIN

Background

Ubiquitin is a 76-amino-acid intracellular protein present in all eukaryocytes. It is thought to be responsible for targeting a selective breakdown of abnormal and short-lived normal proteins by an ATP-dependent pathway (reviewed in references 55 and 56). Ubiquitin also plays a role in basic cellular processes such as DNA repair and modification of cell-surface receptors.[55,56] Ubiquitin is accumulated in senile plaques of Alzheimer's disease, in Lewy bodies of Parkinson's disease, and on abnormal inclusions in lower motor neurons of patients having amyotrophic lateral sclerosis (reviewed in references 57–59).

NMJs

In normal human muscle, ubiquitin is localized postsynaptically at the NMJ where, by light microscopy, it closely colocalizes light-microscopically with bound α-BT and with desmin,[60] indicating that it is located close to the AChRs.

Ubiquitin has been shown to be covalently linked to the lymphocyte homing receptor and to the receptor for platelet-derived growth factor.[61,62] Because ubiquitination of membrane proteins appears to be highly selective, it has been proposed that a posttranslational receptor modification may play a role in signal transduction or in receptor processing.[61,63] Therefore, similar ubiquitin-related mechanisms might be important at normal NMJs.

Binding of ubiquitin to receptor proteins has been postulated to be a contributory factor to an autoimmune response against the resulting molecular complex because a

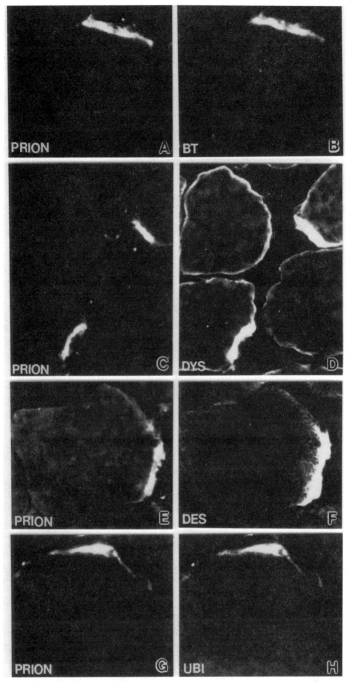

FIGURE 7. Double-labeling of human NMJs with antibodies against prion protein (PrP) and four other established junctional proteins. (A,C,E,G) PrP; (B) α-BT; (D) dystrophin; (F) desmin; (H) ubiquitin. (A,B,E,F,G,H) ×1200; (C,D) ×770. There is a close colocalization of PrP with the four other postsynaptic membrane components.

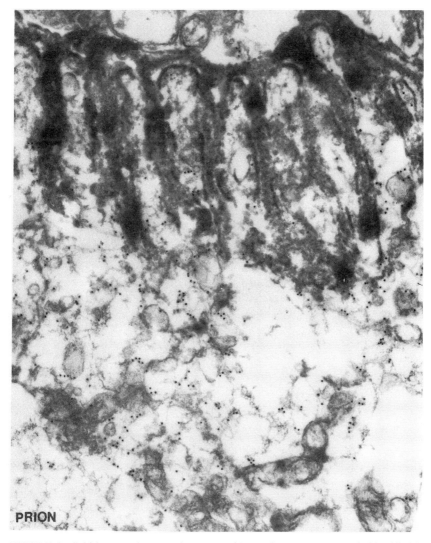

FIGURE 8. Gold immunoelectron-microscopy of PrP at human NMJs. PrP is identified by 10-nm gold particles, ×43,000. In this picture, PrP is immunolocalized subjunctionally at the base of and below the folds. The NMJ and its postsynaptic folds are identified by the dark acetylcholinesterase reaction.

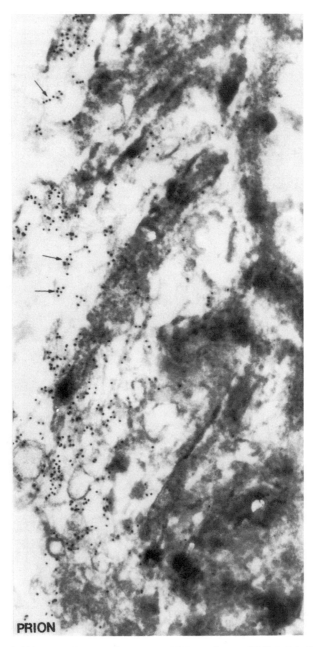

FIGURE 9. Gold immunoelectron-microscopy of PrP at a human NMJ. PrP is identified by 10-nm gold particles, ×63,000. In this particular electron micrograph illustrating a slightly obliquely cut NMJ, PrP is strongly immunolocalized between the folds and attached in small clusters (identified by arrows) along the muscle-fiber side of the folds. The NMJ and its post-synaptic folds are identified by the dark acetylcholinesterase reaction.

high percentage of patients with systemic lupus erythematosus have autoantibodies reacting with ubiquitin.[64] What role ubiquitin may play in the normal biology or pathology of the human NMJ is not yet known. Hypothetically, it may be involved in a functional posttranslational modification of the AChR or other postsynaptic proteins, or in their intracellular degradation. In myasthenia gravis, ubiquitination of the AChR could be a facilitating factor associated with the anti-AChR antibody attack. Of interest would be to determine whether patients with myasthenia gravis have circulating antibodies against ubiquitin and whether localization of ubiquitin at the NMJs is abnormal in them. Because ubiquitin is covalently bound to proteins, affinity purification of putative AChR-ubiquitin complexes should be possible.

IBMs

We have shown that ubiquitin is abnormally accumulated in nonjunctional regions of s- and h-IBM muscle fibers in several subcellular localizations, including 6–10-nm filaments and PHFs.[10,16]

α_1-ANTICHYMOTRYPSIN (α_1-ACT)

Background

α_1-Antichymotrypsin (α_1-ACT), a 68-kDa glycoprotein, is a serine protease inhibitor of the serpin superfamily (reviewed in reference 65). It preferentially inhibits cathepsin G, chymotrypsin, and mast cell chymases (reviewed in reference 66). α_1-ACT is secreted from the liver into the circulation, where it provides widespread functions to control unwanted proteolysis. α_1-ACT is an acute-phase protein because its concentration in plasma greatly increases after various types of stress.[66] α_1-ACT has been colocalized with β-amyloid protein in senile plaques of Alzheimer-disease brain.[67,68]

NMJs

α_1-ACT was strongly immunolocalized at human and rat NMJs.[69] At the NMJ, α_1-ACT closely colocalized with other postsynaptic components, including α-BT, βAPP, desmin, and dystrophin.[69] FIGURE 10 illustrates close colocalization of α_1-ACT with α-BT at human NMJs.

The function(s) of α_1-ACT at the NMJ is not known. Possibly, it plays an important role in the housekeeping of various components of the postsynaptic cytoplasm, plasmalemma, and extracellular matrix. Since cathepsin G is accumulated at the NMJ,[70] putatively α_1-ACT may, among its other functions, protect junctional proteins from cathepsin G–mediated breakdown of extracellular matrix and cellular components.[66,71,73] A proposed function of another serine protease inhibitor, nexin I (PN-I), previously localized at mouse NMJs,[72] is that it may inhibit extracellular matrix proteolysis potentially caused by plasminogen activator.[73]

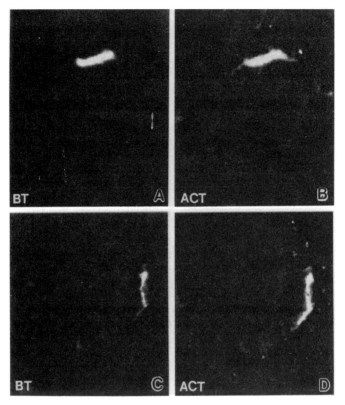

FIGURE 10. Double-labeling of human NMJs with antibodies against α_1-ACT (B,D) and α-BT (A,C), ×1200. There is a close colocalization between α_1-ACT and α-BT.

IBMs

We have reported accumulations of α_1-ACT in nonjunctional regions of abnormal muscle fibers of patients with inclusion-body myositis.[13] In those abnormal muscle fibers, as in senile plaques of Alzheimer brain, α_1-ACT colocalized with the increased accumulations of β-amyloid protein.[13,67,68]

APOLIPOPROTEIN E (ApoE) AND LOW-DENSITY LIPOPROTEIN RECEPTORS

Background

ApoE is a multifunctional apolipoprotein composed of three isoforms, E2, E3, and E4, each encoded by a different allele of a single gene on chromosome 19.[74,75]

Its role in lipid transport is well known. Newer studies demonstrated that ApoE plays a role in various cellular events unrelated to lipid transport, including immunoregulation, modulation of cell growth and differentiation,[80] and nerve regeneration.[76] In Alzheimer's disease (AD), increased ApoE immunoreactivity occurs in amyloid plaques, neurofibrillary tangles, and the cytoplasm of abnormal neurons.[77,78]

NMJs

Our original report demonstrating that ApoE is accumulated at normal human NMJs,[79] subsequently confirmed by others,[89] has been extended to emphasize its strictly postsynaptic localization there.[15]

IBMs

Our recent studies demonstrated that ApoE is accumulated in abnormal muscle fibers in sporadic and hereditary IBM.[14,15]

Low-Density Lipoprotein (LDL) Receptors

LDL receptors, which are muscle receptors for ApoE, are also immunolocalized and concentrated at the postsynaptic domain of human NMJs, according to our preliminary studies (Mirabella and Askanas, unpublished). The role of ApoE at the NMJ and the significance of increased LDL receptors there require elucidation. In s-IBM, the LDL receptors were increased in the vacuolated muscle fibers (Mirabella and Askanas, unpublished).

TRANSFORMING GROWTH FACTOR β1 (TGF-β1)

Background

TGF-β1 is a 25-kDa secretory peptide known to be a multifunctional regulator of cellular activity.[81,82] Produced by a wide variety of cells and tissues, it is both a stimulator and inhibitor of cellular replication. TGF-β1 modulates cell differentiation and extracellular matrix production in various cells and plays an important role in normal growth and development during embryogenesis and tissue repair after injury. It is a potent cytokine that possesses both proinflammatory and anti-inflammatory activities, such as suppression of T and B cell proliferation, inhibition of macrophage maturation, and activation of secretion of IgG and IgM by B cells. It has also been proposed that TGF-β1 plays a role in myogenic development in culture.[83,84]

NMJs

TGF-β1 is accumulated at normal human NMJs[25] (Mirabella *et al.*, to be published), where, by light microscopy, it colocalizes with α-BT, suggesting a postsynaptic location. Its role in the normal NMJ biology remains to be studied.

IBMs

We have demonstrated that TGF-β1 is abnormally accumulated in nonjunctional regions of IBM muscle fibers[25] (Mirabella *et al.*, to be published). Its pathogenic role is not known.

NEURONAL (n) AND INDUCIBLE (i) NITRIC OXIDE SYNTHASES (NOS), AND NITROTYROSINE

Background

Three forms of human NOS—neuronal, inducible, and endothelial—have been cloned and are encoded by different genes on chromosomes 12, 17, and 7, respectively (reviewed in references 85 and 86). Nitric oxide (NO) is a short-lived reactive gas formed by NOS directly from the guanidino nitrogen of L-arginine.[85,86] NO is considered to be both an intercellular and intracellular messenger, having many diverse functions, such as playing a role in vasodilation, mediating antimicrobial toxicity of macrophages, serving as an interneuronal messenger, and possibly influencing transcriptional and posttranscriptional regulation of gene expression.[85,86]

In contrast to many human and animal tissues in which functions of the NOS and NO have been extensively studied, their role in normal and diseased human and animal skeletal muscle is just beginning to be analyzed. Excessive production of NO is postulated to play an important role in various diseases, including neurodegenerative, inflammatory, and immunological processes.[86] The mechanisms by which NO may contribute to the pathogenesis of various diseases are not well understood, but one is thought to involve its ability to react with superoxide anion to form the highly reactive, extremely toxic molecule, peroxynitrite (reviewed in reference 87).

Peroxynitrite induces nitration of tyrosines in proteins, forming the stable component, 3-nitrotyrosine (NT).[87] Presence of NT in tissues is considered indicative of NO-induced oxidative stress.[87] NO has been reported (a) to be a messenger molecule for myoblast fusion[94] and (b) to serve as a retrograde signal, generated by muscle, for activity-dependent suppression of the presynaptic component of the developing NMJ in *Xenopus* nerve-muscle cocultures.[95]

NMJs

We have recently demonstrated in fresh-frozen sections that both nNOS and iNOS are strongly localized at the postsynaptic, but not the presynaptic, domain of normal human and rat NMJs[96] (FIGURES 11 and 12). By immuno-EM, the postsynaptic nNOS and iNOS are localized to variously sized filamentous and membranous structures.[96] nNOS, but not iNOS, is closely colocalized with intermediate-filament desmin.[96] iNOS was present in clusters not associated with desmin.[96]

The data from our studies do not agree with studies of others who reported that in various species, in fixed sections of muscle fibers, nNOS was localized exclusively at the sarcolemma, and it was either exclusively[89] or predominantly[90] present in type-II fibers. Other studies reported the following: (a) in fixed sections of frozen human and mouse muscle, nNOS is colocalized at the sarcolemma with dystrophin[91] (subsequently, in mouse skeletal muscle, the association of nNOS with the sarcolemma was postulated to be mediated by direct nNOS binding to α_1-syntrophin, a protein of the dystrophin complex containing a PDZ motif[92]) and (b) increased immunoreactivity

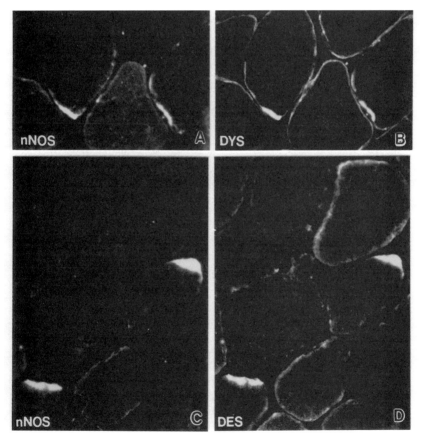

FIGURE 11. Double-immunofluorescence of human NMJs with antibodies against nNOS (A,C), dystrophin (B), and desmin (D), ×850. There is a close colocalization of nNOS with dystrophin and desmin.

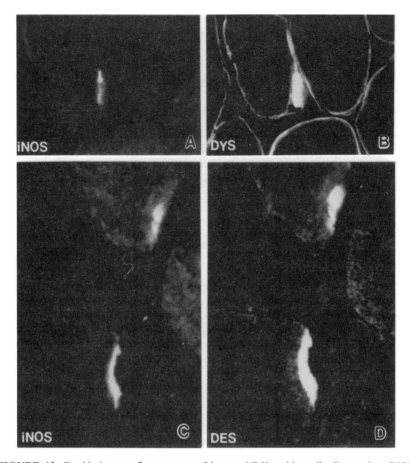

FIGURE 12. Double-immunofluorescence of human NMJs with antibodies against iNOS (A,C), dystrophin (B), and desmin (D), ×1200. iNOS colocalizes with dystrophin and desmin, but seems to occupy a smaller area than dystrophin and desmin.

of nNOS, at adult mouse NMJs, which contrary to our results was postulated to be in the presynaptic domain.[93]

The functions of the increased concentrations of nNOS and iNOS at the postsynaptic domain of the NMJ and the mechanisms of their control are not known. Recently, it was reported that NO generated by nNOS selectively enhances Ca^{2+} calmodulin-dependent phosphorylation of postsynaptic-density proteins in rat brain.[97] iNOS ultrastructurally is not closely associated with desmin[96] and its association with other junctional proteins is not known. In other situations, iNOS is mainly transcriptionally regulated and its synthesis can be stimulated by cytokines, inflammation, and other pathologic processes (reviewed in references 85, 86, and

98). In a clonal cell line of mouse muscle, induction of iNOS-mRNA by cytokines has been demonstrated.[99] Because our most recent studies demonstrate increased accumulation of interleukin 1β, 1α, and 6 postsynaptically at human NMJs,[27] it is possible that cytokines induce transcription of iNOS (and possibly of nNOS) at the NMJ. Alternatively, because a small amount of iNOS-mRNA was recently found to be constitutively present in some human tissues, including skeletal muscle,[100] it is possible that the increased iNOS at the NMJ represents its constitutive expression there.

It is not known whether the main function of the NOSs at the NMJ is to generate NO to (a) serve as a transduction signal for normal function of the NMJ, (b) provide a retrograde signal from the postsynaptic muscle fiber to the presynaptic axonal tip, or (c) help maintain a junctional or parajunctional structural component. Close colocalization of nNOS with the muscle intermediate-filament desmin suggests an important structure-function relationship. Future studies are needed to address these and other questions regarding the function of NOSs at the NMJs of normal and diseased human muscle.

Apparently, at normal human NMJs, NO, the product of the NOSs, is not generated in toxic excess to combine with superoxide to produce a very toxic peroxynitrite because no nitrotyrosine, which would reflect abnormally nitrated proteins, was detectable there.[96]

We have demonstrated by light microscopy that, at NMJs of *myasthenia gravis (MG)* patients, there is only an abnormally thin band of nNOS immunoreactivity corresponding to a similarly abnormally thin band of desmin immunoreactivity,[96] correlating with the flattening and disorganization typical of MG postsynaptic folds.[101] Lack of a similar decrease of iNOS at the myasthenic NMJs[96] suggests a different mechanism of iNOS induction and/or maintenance at the NMJ. Whether either NOS, or both, plays a role in the NMJ pathology in MG is of potential importance and should be studied.

IBMs

We have demonstrated that both nNOS and iNOS, as well as NT, are abnormally accumulated in nonjunctional regions of the vacuolated muscle fibers in sporadic IBM[88] and hereditary IBM.[103]

SUPEROXIDE DISMUTASE-1 (SOD1)

Background

Superoxide is an oxygen free-radical toxic by-product of various cellular metabolic reactions. SOD1 and other superoxide dismutases protect the cell against oxidative stress by catalyzing the dismutation of the toxic superoxide anion $O_2^{\cdot-}$, as follows: $O_2^{\cdot-} + 2H^+ \rightarrow H_2O_2 + O_2$ (and then catalase converts $H_2O_2 \rightarrow H_2O + O_2$).

NMJs

SOD1 immunoreactivity was increased at human NMJs, where by light microscopy it closely colocalized with α-BT, indicating a postsynaptic domain.[102] Accumulation of SOD1 at normal human NMJs suggests a locally increased need to diminish superoxide anion. Superoxide in excess can combine with NO, produced by the iNOS and nNOS at the NMJ, to form the very toxic peroxynitrite, which can pathologically nitrate the tyrosine groups of proteins, the result evidenced as nitrotyrosine. However, at normal human NMJs, there appears to be adequate disposal of both superoxide and NO because nitrotyrosine immunoreactivity, which indicates pathologic nitration of proteins, was not increased there[96] (in contrast to the presence of NT in nonjunctional regions of pathologic muscle fibers in inclusion-body myositis[88]). Therefore, "oxidative stress" evidenced by nitration of proteins[87] apparently does not take place at the normal human NMJ. The detailed molecular mechanisms responsible for the increased concentration of SOD1 at the NMJ require elucidation.

IBMs

Recently, we demonstrated that SOD1 and its mRNA are accumulated in nonjunctional regions of abnormal IBM muscle fibers[102] (Askanas *et al.*, to be published).

HYPOTHESIS OF "JUNCTIONALIZATION" OF NONJUNCTIONAL REGIONS OF MUSCLE FIBERS IN INCLUSION-BODY MYOSITIS

On the preceding pages, we have described 14 proteins newly recognized to be accumulated at the normal human NMJ and not elsewhere in the muscle fiber. The normal phenomena of protein and mRNA accumulation at the NMJ have been termed by us as "junctionalization" (FIGURE 13).[7,8] The postsynaptic proteins characteristic of junctionalization are induced, directly or indirectly, by the contacting motor-neuron axonal tip and presumably are governed, at least partially, by enhanced expression of the corresponding genes in muscle-fiber junctional (postsynaptic) nuclei, presumably modulated through yet-undelineated transcription factors. We have proposed a "junctionalizing master gene" whose product modulates transcription of the "junctional-protein genes". In the normal innervated mature muscle fiber, those junctional-protein genes are concurrently downregulated in the nonjunctional nuclei diffusely located in the vast nonjunctional regions of the muscle fiber (FIGURE 13). It is of particular interest that all 14 of these newly described junctional proteins, and all 3 of their studied mRNAs, have been found by us to be pathologically accumulated in the nonjunctional regions of IBM muscle fibers (e.g., βAPP,[10] prion,[17] $α_1$-ACT,[13] FGF,[26] TGFβ,[25] ubiquitin,[16] ApoE,[14,15] AChR, 43-kDa protein,[28] SOD1,[102] iNOS and nNOS,[88] and interleukins 1α, 1β, and 6[27]). Thus, these accumulated "junctional/IBM proteins" and their corresponding increased "junctional/IBM-mRNAs" are the ones normally accumulated in the muscle fiber only at the postsynaptic region of the NMJ. We have therefore proposed the concept of "pathologic junctionalization" of extrajunctional regions of the IBM muscle fiber, causing altered gene expression of the

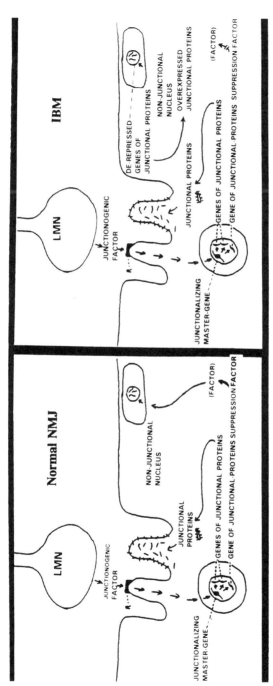

FIGURE 13. Hypothetical "junctionalization" mechanism (ectopic expression of junctional proteins) in inclusion-body myositis. In nonjunctional nuclei of IBM, there is reactivation of genes of junctional proteins or downregulation of a gene (genes?) of junctional-protein suppression-factor (by virus?, abnormal aging?, genetic factors?, others).

"IBM-junctionalized" (previously normal nonjunctional) nuclei perhaps via the proposed junctionalizing master gene[7,8] (FIGURE 13). Hypothetically, this junctionalization could be induced, directly or indirectly, by a putative virus in s-IBM or by a mutated-gene protein in h-IBM.[7,8]

ACKNOWLEDGMENTS

Our research-team colleagues who participated in various aspects of the studies described were Masako Bilak, Massimiliano Mirabella, Jesse Yang, Piraye Serdaroglu, Janis McFerrin, Eva Sarkozi, and Kazuhiro Haginoya. We are grateful to Stanley C. Froehner, Jon Lindstrom, Angela Vincent, Dennis J. Selkoe, Stanley B. Prusiner, and Steven A. Johnson, and the late George G. Glenner, for their generous gifts of antibodies and cDNA probes. Assistance in photographic processing by Maggie Baburyan and in preparation of the manuscript by Lynne Martinez is appreciated.

REFERENCES

1. BOWE, M. A. & J. R. FALLON. 1995. The role of agrin in synapse formation. Annu. Rev. Neurosci. **18:** 443–462.
2. CONNER, E. A. & M. A. SMITH. 1994. Retrograde signaling in the formation and maintenance of the neuromuscular junction. J. Neurobiol. **25:** 722–739.
3. FALLON, J. R. & Z. W. HALL. 1994. Building synapses: agrin and dystroglycan stick together. TINS **17:** 469–473.
4. HALL, Z. H. & J. R. SANES. 1993. Synaptic structure and development: the neuromuscular junction. Cell **72:** 99–121/Neuron **10:** 99–121.
5. SEALOCK, R. & S. C. FROEHNER. 1994. Dystrophin-associated proteins and synapse formation: is α-dystroglycan the agrin receptor? Cell **77:** 617–619.
6. DANIELS, M. P. 1997. Intercellular communication that mediates formation of the neuromuscular junction. Mol. Neurobiol. **14:** 143–170.
7. ASKANAS, V. & W. K. ENGEL. 1995. New advances in the understanding of sporadic inclusion-body myositis and hereditary inclusion-body myopathies. Curr. Opin. Rheumatol. **7:** 486–496.
8. ASKANAS, V. & W. K. ENGEL. 1998. Newest approaches to diagnosis and pathogenesis of sporadic inclusion-body myositis and hereditary inclusion-body myopathies, including molecular-pathologic similarities to Alzheimer disease. *In* Inclusion-Body Myositis and Myopathies. Cambridge University Press. London/New York. In press.
9. ASKANAS, V., W. K. ENGEL & R. B. ALVAREZ. 1992. Light- and electron-microscopic localization of β-amyloid protein in muscle biopsies of patients with inclusion-body myositis. Am. J. Pathol. **141:** 31–36.
10. ASKANAS, V., R. B. ALVAREZ & W. K. ENGEL. 1993. β-Amyloid precursor epitopes in muscle fibers of inclusion-body myositis. Ann. Neurol. **34:** 551–560.
11. ASKANAS, V., W. K. ENGEL, M. BILAK, R. B. ALVAREZ & D. J. SELKOE. 1994. Twisted tubulofilaments of inclusion-body myositis muscle resemble paired helical filaments of Alzheimer brain and contain hyperphosphorylated tau. Am. J. Pathol. **144:** 177–187.
12. MIRABELLA, M., R. B. ALVAREZ, M. BILAK, W. K. ENGEL & V. ASKANAS. 1996. Difference

in expression of phosphorylated tau epitopes between sporadic inclusion-body myositis and hereditary inclusion-body myopathies. J. Neuropathol. Exp. Neurol. **55:** 774–786.

13. BILAK, M., V. ASKANAS & W. K. ENGEL. 1993. Strong immunoreactivity of α_1-antichymotrypsin colocalizes with β-amyloid protein and ubiquitin in vacuolated muscle fibers of inclusion-body myositis. Acta Neuropathol. **85:** 378–382.

14. ASKANAS, V., M. MIRABELLA, W. K. ENGEL, R. B. ALVAREZ & K. WEISGRABER. 1994. Apolipoprotein E immunoreactive deposits in inclusion-body muscle diseases. Lancet **343:** 364–365.

15. MIRABELLA, M., R. B. ALVAREZ, W. K. ENGEL, K. H. WEISGRABER & V. ASKANAS. 1996. Apolipoprotein E and apolipoprotein E messenger RNA in muscle of inclusion-body myositis and myopathies. Ann. Neurol. **40:** 864–872.

16. ASKANAS, V., P. SERDAROGLU, W. K. ENGEL & R. B. ALVAREZ. 1991. Immunolocalization of ubiquitin in muscle biopsies of patients with inclusion-body myositis and oculopharyngeal muscular dystrophy. Neurosci. Lett. **130:** 73–76.

17. ASKANAS, V., M. BILAK, W. K. ENGEL, R. B. ALVAREZ, F. M. S. TOMÉ & A. LECLERC. 1993. Prion protein is abnormally accumulated in inclusion-body myositis. NeuroReport **5:** 25–28.

18. SARKOZI, E., V. ASKANAS, S. A. JOHNSON, W. K. ENGEL & R. B. ALVAREZ. 1993. β-Amyloid precursor protein mRNA is increased in inclusion-body myositis muscle. NeuroReport **4:** 815–818.

19. SARKOZI, E., V. ASKANAS & W. K. ENGEL. 1994. Abnormal accumulation of prion protein mRNA in muscle fibers of patients with sporadic inclusion-body myositis and hereditary inclusion-body myopathy. Am. J. Pathol. **145:** 1280–1284.

20. PRUSINER, S. B. 1991. Molecular biology of prion and diseases. Science **252:** 1515–1522.

21. DEARMOND, S. J. & S. B. PRUSINER. 1993. The neurochemistry of prion diseases. J. Neurochem. **61:** 1589–1601.

22. PRUSINER, S. B. & K. K. HSIAO. 1994. Human prion diseases. Ann. Neurol. **35:** 385–395.

23. OESCH, B., D. WESTAWAY, M. WALCHLI, M. P. McKINLEY, S. B. H. KENT, R. AEBERSOLD, R. A. BARRY, P. TEMPST, D. B. TEPLOW, L. HOOD, S. B. PRUSINER & C. WEISSMANN. 1985. A cellular gene encodes scrapie PrP 27–30 protein. Cell **40:** 735–746.

24. YANG, C-C., R. B. ALVAREZ, W. K. ENGEL & V. ASKANAS. 1996. Increase of nitric oxide synthases and nitrotyrosine in inclusion-body myositis. NeuroReport **8:** 153–158.

25. MIRABELLA, M., V. ASKANAS & W. K. ENGEL. 1994. Transforming growth factor-beta 1 is abnormally accumulated in vacuolated muscle fibers of sporadic inclusion-body myositis and hereditary inclusion-body myopathy [abstract]. Ann. Neurol. **36:** 320–321.

26. BILAK, M., V. ASKANAS, W. K. ENGEL & R. B. ALVAREZ. 1994. Twisted tubulofilaments (TTFs) in inclusion-body myositis (IBM) muscle contain fibroblast growth factor (FGF) and its receptor (FGF-R) [abstract]. Neurology **44:** 130.

27. HAGINOYA, K., R. B. ALVAREZ, W. K. ENGEL & V. ASKANAS. 1997. Light- and electron-microscopic immunolocalization of interleukins 1α, 1β, and 6 in vacuolated muscle fibers of sporadic inclusion-body myositis (s-IBM) [abstract]. Neurology **48:** 126.

28. ASKANAS, V., R. B. ALVAREZ, M. BILAK, S. FROEHNER & W. K. ENGEL. 1994. Muscle nicotinic acetylcholine receptor (nAChR) and its associated protein 43 Kd (43K) are highly accumulated in vacuolated muscle fibers (VMFs) of inclusion-body myositis (IBM) [abstract]. Neurology **44:** 131.

29. SELKOE, D. J. 1994. Normal and abnormal biology of the β-amyloid precursor protein. Annu. Rev. Neurosci. **17:** 489–517.

30. KANG, J., H. G. LERMAINE, A. UNTERBECK, J. M. SALBAUM, C. L. MASTERS, K. H. GRZESCHIK, G. MULTHAUP, K. BEYREUTHER & B. MULLER-HILL. 1997. The precursor

of Alzheimer's disease amyloid A4 protein resembles a cell-surface receptor. Nature **325:** 733–736.

31. ROBAKIS, N. K., N. RAMAKRISHNA, G. WOLFE & H. M. WISNIEWSKI. 1987. Molecular cloning and characterization of a cDNA encoding the cerebrovascular and neuritic plaque amyloid peptides. Proc. Natl. Acad. Sci. U.S.A. **84:** 4190–4194.

32. TANZI, R. E., J. F. GUSELLA, P. C. WATKINS, G. A. P. BRUNS, P. H. ST. GEORGE-HYSLOP, M. L. VAN KEUREN, D. PATTERSON, S. PAGAN, D. M. KURNIT & R. L. NEVE. 1987. Amyloid β protein gene: cDNA, mRNA distribution, and genetic linkage near the Alzheimer locus. Science **235:** 880–884.

33. TANZI, R. E., A. F. MCCLATCHEY, E. D. LAMERTI, L. VILLA-KAMAROFF, J. F. GUSELLA & R. L. NEVE. 1988. Protease inhibitor domain encoded by an amyloid protein precursor mRNA associated with Alzheimer's disease. Nature **331:** 528–530.

34. WIEDEMANN, A., G. KONIG, D. BUNKE, P. FISHER, N. M. SALBAUM, C. L. MASTERS & K. BEYREUTHER. 1989. Identification, biogenesis, and localization of precursors of Alzheimer's disease A4 amyloid protein. Cell **57:** 115–126.

35. PONTE, R., P. GONZALEZ-DEWHITT, J. SCHILLING, J. MILLER, D. HSU, B. GREENBERG, K. DAVIS, W. WALLACE, I. LIEBERBERG, F. FULLER & B. CORDELL. 1988. A new A4 amyloid mRNA contains a domain homologous to serine proteinase inhibitors. Nature **331:** 525–527.

36. KLIER, F. G., G. COLE, W. STALLCUP & D. SCHUBERT. 1990. Amyloid β-protein precursor is associated with extracellular matrix. Brain Res. **515:** 336–342.

37. SCHUBERT, D., L-W. JIN, T. SAITOH & G. COLE. 1989. The regulation of amyloid β protein precursor secretion and its modulatory role in cell adhesion. Neuron **3:** 689–694.

38. BREEN, K. C., M. BRUCE & B. H. ANDERTON. 1991. β-Amyloid precursor protein mediates neuronal cell-cell and cell-surface adhesion. J. Neurosci. Res. **28:** 90–100.

39. SHIVERS, B. D., C. HILBICH, G. MULTHAUP, M. SALBAUM, K. BEYREUTHER & P. H. SEEBURG. 1988. Alzheimer's disease amyloidogenic glycoprotein: expression pattern in rat brain suggests a role in cell contact. EMBO J. **7:** 1365–1370.

40. SCHUBERT, W., R. PRIOR, A. WIEDEMANN, H. DIRCKSEN, G. MULTHAUP, C. L. MASTERS & K. BEYREUTHER. 1991. Localization of Alzheimer βA4 amyloid precursor protein at central and peripheral synaptic sites. Brain Res. **563:** 184–191.

41. GLENNER, G. G. & C. W. WONG. 1984. Alzheimer's disease initial report of the purification and characteristics of a novel cerebrovascular amyloid protein. Biochem. Biophys. Res. Commun. **120:** 885–890.

42. ASKANAS, V., W. K. ENGEL & R. B. ALVAREZ. 1992. Strong immunoreactivity of β-amyloid precursor protein, including the β-amyloid protein sequence, at human neuromuscular junctions. Neurosci. Lett. **143:** 96–100.

43. ASKANAS, V., A. BORNEMANN & W. K. ENGEL. 1990. Immunocytochemical localization of desmin at human neuromuscular junctions. Neurology **40:** 949–953.

44. GRAMOLINI, A. O., C. L. DENNIS, J. M. TINSLEY, G. S. ROBERTSON, J. CARTAUD, K. E. DAVIES & B. J. JASMIN. 1997. Local transcriptional control of utrophin expression at the neuromuscular synapse. J. Biol. Chem. **272:** 8117–8120.

45. ASKANAS, V., J. MCFERRIN, S. BAQUÉ, R. B. ALVAREZ, E. SARKOZI & W. K. ENGEL. 1996. Transfer of β-amyloid precursor protein gene using adenovirus vector causes mitochondrial abnormalities in cultured normal human muscle. Proc. Natl. Acad. Sci. U.S.A. **93:** 1314–1319.

46. ASKANAS, V., J. MCFERRIN, R. B. ALVAREZ, S. BAQUÉ & W. K. ENGEL. 1997. βAPP gene transfer into cultured human muscle induces inclusion-body myositis aspects. NeuroReport **8:** 2155–2158.

47. MCFERRIN, J., S. M. PRICE, S. BAQUÉ, W. K. ENGEL & V. ASKANAS. 1997. Overexpression of β-amyloid precursor protein (βAPP) gene in cultured normal human muscle using

adenovirus vector prevents formation of neuromuscular junctions (NMJs) and functional innervation: relevance to inclusion-body myositis (s-IBM) [abstract]. Neurology **48:** 332.

48. KOBAYASHI, T., V. ASKANAS & W. K. ENGEL. 1987. Human muscle cultured in monolayer and co-cultured with fetal rat spinal cord. J. Neurosci. **7:** 3131–3141.

49. ASKANAS, V., H. KWAN, R. B. ALVAREZ, W. K. ENGEL, T. KOBAYASHI, A. MARTINUZZI & E. F. HAWKINS. 1987. *De novo* neuromuscular junction formation on human muscle fibers cultured in monolayer and innervated by fetal rat spinal cord: ultrastructural and ultrastructural-cytochemical studies. J. Neurocytol. **16:** 523–537.

50. BASLER, K., B. OESCH, M. SCOTT, D. WESTAWAY, M. WALCHLI, D. F. GROTH, M. P. McKINLEY, S. B. PRUSINER & C. WEISSMANN. 1986. Scrapie and cellular PrP isoforms are encoded by the same chromosomal gene. Cell **46:** 417–428.

51. BENDHEIM, P. E., R. A. BARRY, S. J. DEARMOND, D. P. STITES & S. B. PRUSINER. 1984. Antibodies to a scrapie prion protein. Nature **310:** 418–421.

52. BENDHEIM, P. E., A. POTEMPSKA, R. J. KASCSAK & D. C. BOLTON. 1988. Purification and partial characterization of the normal cellular homologue of the scrapie agent protein. J. Infect. Dis. **158:** 1198–1208.

53. CASHMAN, N. R., R. LOERTSCHER, J. NALBANTOGLU, I. SHAW, R. J. KASCSAK, D. C. BOLTON & P. E. BENDHEIM. 1990. Cellular isoform of the scrapie agent protein participates in lymphocyte activation. Cell **61:** 185–192.

54. ASKANAS, V., M. BILAK, W. K. ENGEL, A. LECLERC & F. M. S. TOMÉ. 1993. Prion protein is strongly immunolocalized at the postsynaptic domain of human normal neuromuscular junctions. Neurosci. Lett. **159:** 111–114.

55. FINLEY, D. & A. VARSHARSKY. 1985. The ubiquitin system: functions and mechanisms. TIBS **10:** 343–347.

56. HERSKHO, A. & A. CIECHANOVER. 1986. The ubiquitin pathway for the degradation of intracellular proteins. Prog. Nucleic Acid Res. Mol. Biol. **33:** 19–56.

57. GALLO, J. M. & B. H. ANDERTON. 1989. Ubiquitous variations in nerves. Nature **337:** 687–688.

58. MITCH, W. E. & A. L. GOLDBERG. 1996. Mechanisms of muscle wasting: the role of the ubiquitin-proteasome pathway. N. Engl. J. Med. **335:** 1897–1905.

59. LOWE, J. & R. J. MAYER. 1990. Ubiquitin, cell stress, and disease of the nervous system. Neuropathol. Appl. Neurobiol. **16:** 281–291.

60. SERDAROGLU, P., V. ASKANAS & W. K. ENGEL. 1992. Immunocytochemical localization of ubiquitin at human neuromuscular junctions. Neuropathol. Appl. Neurobiol. **18:** 232–236.

61. YARDEN, Y., J. A. ESCOBEDO, W. J. KUANG, T. YANG-FENT, T. O. DANIEL, P. TREMBLE, E. EHEN, M. ANDO, R. HARKENS, U. FRANKE, V. FRIED & L. T. WILLIAMS. 1986. Structure of the receptor for platelet-derived growth factor helps define a family of closely related growth factor receptors. Nature **323:** 226–232.

62. SIEGELMAN, M., M. W. BOND, W. GALLATIN, T. ST. JOHN, H. T. SMITH, V. FRIED & I. L. WEISSMANN. 1986. Cell surface molecule associated with lymphocyte homing is a ubiquitinated branched-chain glycoprotein. Science **231:** 823–829.

63. FRIED, V., H. T. SMITH, E. HILDEBRANDT & K. WEINER. 1987. Ubiquitin has intrinsic proteolytic activity: implications for cellular regulation. Proc. Natl. Acad. Sci. U.S.A. **84:** 3685–3689.

64. MULLER, S., J-P. BRIAND & M. H. V. VAN REGENMORTEL. 1988. Presence of antibodies to ubiquitin during the autoimmune response associated with systemic lupus erythematosus. Proc. Natl. Acad. Sci. U.S.A. **85:** 8176–8180.

65. CARREL, R. W. & J. TRAVIS. 1987. Serpins: the superfamily of plasma serine protease inhibitors. *In* Protease Inhibitors, p. 403–420. Elsevier. Amsterdam/New York.

66. Travis, J. & G. S. Salvesen. 1983. Human plasma proteinase inhibitors. Annu. Rev. Biochem. **52:** 655–709.
67. Abraham, C. R., D. J. Selkoe & H. Potter. 1988. Immunochemical identification of the serine protease inhibitor α_1-antichymotrypsin in the brain amyloid deposits of Alzheimer's disease. Cell **52:** 487–501.
68. Abraham, C. R., T. Shirahara & H. Potter. 1990. α_1-Antichymotrypsin is associated solely with amyloid deposits containing the β-protein: amyloid and cell localization of α_1-antichymotrypsin. Neurobiol. Aging **11:** 123–129.
69. Bilak, M., V. Askanas & W. K. Engel. 1994. Alpha1-antichymotrypsin is strongly immunolocalized at normal human and rat neuromuscular junctions. Synapse **16:** 280–283.
70. Bilak, M., V. Askanas & W. K. Engel. 1992. Strong immunoreactivity of serine proteinase inhibitor (serpin) alpha-1-antichymotrypsin (α_1-ACT) at the postsynaptic domain (PSD) of human and rat neuromuscular junctions (NMJs). Mol. Biol. Cell **3:** 255a.
71. Katunuma, N., N. Yasogawa, K. Kito, Y. Sanada, H. Kiwai & K. Miyoshi. 1978. Abnormal expression of a serine protease in human dystrophic muscle. J. Biochem. **83:** 625–628.
72. Festoff, B. W., J. S. Rao & D. Hantai. 1991. Plasminogen activators and inhibitors in the neuromuscular system. III. The serpin protease nexin I is synthesized by muscle and localized at neuromuscular synapses. J. Cell. Physiol. **147:** 76–86.
73. Festoff, B. W. & D. Hantai. 1987. Plasminogen activators and inhibitors: roles in muscle and neuromuscular regeneration. Prog. Brain Res. **71:** 423–431.
74. Mahley, R. W. 1988. Apolipoprotein E: cholesterol transport protein with expanding role in cell biology. Science **240:** 622–630.
75. Weisgraber, K. H. 1994. Apolipoprotein E: structure-function relationships. Adv. Protein Chem. **45:** 249–302.
76. Ignatius, M. J., P. J. Gebicke-Harter, J. H. Skene, J. W. Schilling, K. H. Weisgraber, R. W. Mahley & E. M. Shooter. 1986. Expression of apolipoprotein E during nerve degeneration and regeneration. Proc. Natl. Acad. Sci. U.S.A. **83:** 1125–1129.
77. Namba, Y., M. Tomonaga, H. Kawasaki, E. Otomo & K. Ikeda. 1991. Apolipoprotein E immunoreactivity in cerebral amyloid deposits and neurofibrillary tangles in Alzheimer's disease and kuru plaque amyloid in Creutzfeldt-Jakob disease. Brain Res. **541:** 163–166.
78. Han, S. H., G. Einstein, K. H. Weisgraber, W. J. Strittmatter, A. M. Saunders, M. Pericak-Vance, A. D. Roses & D. E. Schmechel. 1994. Apolipoprotein E is localized to the cytoplasm of human cortical neurons: a light and electron microscopic study. J. Neuropathol. Exp. Neurol. **53:** 535–544.
79. Mirabella, M., V. Askanas, W. K. Engel & K. H. Weisgraber. 1994. Immunocytochemical localization of apolipoprotein E (ApoE) in inclusion-body myositis (IBM) [abstract]. Neurology **44:** 347.
80. Akaaboune, M., M. Villanova, B. W. Festoff, M. Verdiere-Sahuque & D. Hantai. 1994. Apolipoprotein E expression at neuromuscular junctions in mouse, rat, and human skeletal muscle. FEBS Lett. **351:** 246–248.
81. Sporn, M. B., A. B. Roberts, L. M. Wakefield & R. K. Assoian. 1986. Transforming growth factor-beta: biological function and chemical structure. Science **233:** 532–534.
82. Sporn, M. B. & A. B. Roberts. 1992. Transforming growth factor beta: recent progress and new challenges. J. Cell Biol. **119:** 1017–1021.
83. Massegue, J., S. Cheifetz, T. Endo & B. Nadal-Ginard. 1986. Type beta transforming growth factor is an inhibitor of myogenic differentiation. Proc. Natl. Acad. Sci. U.S.A. **83:** 8206–8210.

84. ZENTELLA, A. & J. MASSEGUE. 1992. Transforming growth factor B induces myoblast differentiation in the presence of mitogens. Proc. Natl. Acad. Sci. U.S.A. **89:** 5176–5180.
85. DAWSON, T. M. & S. H. SYNDER. 1994. Gases as biological messengers: nitric oxide and carbon monoxide in the brain. J. Neurosci. **14:** 5147–5159.
86. NATHAN, C. & Q-W. XIE. 1994. Regulation of biosynthesis of nitric oxide. J. Biol. Chem. **269:** 13725–13728.
87. CROW, J. P. & J. S. BECKMAN. 1995. The role of peroxynitrite in nitric oxide–mediated toxicity. *In* Current Topics in Microbiology and Immunology: The Role of Nitric Oxide in Physiology and Pathophysiology. Volume 196, p. 57–73. Springer-Verlag. Berlin/New York.
88. YANG, C-C., R. B. ALVAREZ, W. K. ENGEL & V. ASKANAS. 1996. Increase of nitric oxide synthases and nitrotyrosine in inclusion-body myositis. NeuroReport **8:** 153–158.
89. KOBZIK, L., M. B. REID, D. S. BREDT & J. S. STAMIER. 1994. Nitric oxide in skeletal muscle. Nature **372:** 546–548.
90. GROZDANOVIC, Z., G. NAKOS, G. DAHRMANN, B. MAYER & R. GOSSRAU. 1995. Species-independent expression of nitric oxide synthase in the sarcolemma region of visceral and somatic striated muscle fibers. Cell Tissue Res. **281:** 493–499.
91. BRENMAN, J. E., D. S. CHAO, H. XIA, K. ALDAPE & D. S. BREDT. 1995. Nitric oxide synthase complexed with dystrophin and absent from skeletal muscle sarcolemma in Duchenne muscular dystrophy. Cell **82:** 743–752.
92. BRENMAN, J. E., D. S. CHAO, S. H. GEE, A. W. MCGEE, S. E. CRAVEN, D. R. SANTILLANO, Z. WU, F. HUANG, H. XIA, M. F. PETERS, S. C. FROEHNER & D. S. BREDT. 1996. Interaction of nitric oxide synthase with the postsynaptic density protein PSD-95 and α_1-syntrophin mediated by PDZ domains. Cell **84:** 757–767.
93. OLIVER, L., O. GOUREAU, Y. COURTOIS & M. VIGNY. 1996. Accumulation of NO synthase (type-1) at the neuromuscular junctions in adult mice. NeuroReport **7:** 924–926.
94. LEE, K. H., M. Y. BAEK, K. Y. MOON, W. K. SONG, C. H. CHUNG, D. B. HA & M-S. KANG. 1994. Nitric oxide as a messenger molecule for myoblast fusion. J. Biol. Chem. **269:** 14371–14374.
95. WANG, T., Z. XIE & B. LU. 1995. Nitric oxide mediates activity-dependent synaptic suppression at developing neuromuscular synapses. Nature **374:** 262–266.
96. YANG, C-C., R. B. ALVAREZ, W. K. ENGEL, C. K. HAUN & V. ASKANAS. 1997. Immunolocalization of nitric oxide synthases at the postsynaptic domain of human and rat neuromuscular junctions—light and electron microscopic studies. Exp. Neurol. **148:** 34–44.
97. WU, K., J-L. XU, P. C. SUEN, Y-U. HUANG & H. T. J. MOUNT. 1996. Nitric oxide increases calcium/calmodulin-dependent phosphorylation of proteins in the postsynaptic density of adult rat cerebral cortex. Mol. Brain Res. **40:** 22–26.
98. FÖRSTERMANN, U., E. I. CLOSS, J. S. POLLOCK, M. NAKANE, P. SCHWARZ, I. GATH & H. KLEINERT. 1994. Nitric oxide synthase isozymes: characterization, purification, molecular cloning, and functions. Hypertension **23:** 1121–1131.
99. WILLIAMS, G., T. BROWN, L. BECKER, M. PRAGER & B. P. GIROIR. 1994. Cytokine-induced expression of nitric oxide synthase in C2C12 skeletal muscle myocytes. Am. J. Physiol. **267:** 1020–1025.
100. PARK, C-S., R. PARK & G. KRISHNA. 1996. Constitutive expression and structural diversity of inducible isoform of nitric oxide synthase in human tissues. Life Sci. **59:** 219–225.
101. ZACKS, S. I., W. C. BAUER & J. M. BLUMBERG. 1962. The fine structure of myasthenic neuromuscular junction. J. Neuropathol. Exp. Neurol. **21:** 335–347.
102. ASKANAS, V., E. SARKOZI, R. B. ALVAREZ, J. MCFERRIN, W. K. ENGEL & T. SIDDIQUE. 1996. Superoxide-dismutase-1 (SOD1) gene and protein in vacuolated muscle fibers of spo-

radic inclusion-body myositis (s-IBM), hereditary inclusion-body myopathy (h-IBM), and cultured human muscle after β-amyloid precursor protein (βAPP) gene transfer. Neurology **46:** 487.

103. YANG, C-C., R. B. ALVAREZ, W. K. ENGEL, S. L. HELLER & V. ASKANAS. 1998. Nitric-oxide induced oxidative stress in autosomal recessive and dominant inclusion-body myopathies. Brain. In press.

Electrophysiology of Postsynaptic Activation[a]

ROBERT L. RUFF[b]

Departments of Neurology and Neuroscience
Case Western Reserve University School of Medicine
Cleveland Veterans Affairs Medical Center
University Hospitals of Cleveland
Cleveland, Ohio

INTRODUCTION

The neurotransmission defect in myasthenia gravis (MG) and some congenital disorders of neuromuscular transmission results from a failure of the postsynaptic membrane to adequately respond to acetylcholine (ACh) released from the nerve terminal.[1] Here, we examine the physiology of the postsynaptic end plate membrane and how signal transduction is disrupted in MG. The important ionic channels are the ACh receptor (AChR) and the skeletal muscle voltage-gated sodium (Na^+) channel. In this manuscript, postsynaptic membrane and end plate are used interchangeably.

NERVE TERMINAL–RELEASED ACh BINDS TO AChRs TO TRIGGER AN END PLATE POTENTIAL (EPP)

ACh is stored in vesicles within the nerve terminal.[2–6] Each synaptic vesicle releases about 10,000 ACh molecules into the synaptic cleft.[7] A nerve action potential (AP) triggers the release of 50 to 300 synaptic vesicles (i.e., the normal quantal content is between 50 and 300).[6] ACh diffuses across the synaptic cleft quickly.[8] An AChR is usually activated when two ACh molecules bind. The AChR is a large glycoprotein that contains the ACh binding domains as well as the ionic channel. When the AChR is activated, the ion channel opens, allowing cations to flow across the membrane. The influx of cations produces a depolarizing generator potential, that is, the end plate potential (EPP). Acetylcholine esterase (ChE) in the basal lamina of the postsynaptic membrane speeds the decline in concentration of ACh in the synaptic cleft.[9] Inactivation of ChE prolongs the duration of action of ACh and slows the decay of the end plate current.[5] The ChE concentration is about 3000 molecules/μm^2 of postsynaptic membrane.[9]

[a]This work was supported by the Office of Research and Development, Medical Research Service of the Department of Veterans Affairs.
[b]Address for correspondence: Neurology Service 127(W), Cleveland Veterans Affairs Medical Center, 10701 East Boulevard, Cleveland, Ohio 44106.

POSTSYNAPTIC MEMBRANE STRUCTURAL SPECIALIZATIONS

FIGURE 1 shows an electron micrograph of a rat neuromuscular junction. The branches of the nerve terminal lie in depressions of the postsynaptic membrane called primary synaptic clefts. The primary synaptic clefts are about 50 nm wide.[2] The postsynaptic membrane is folded into secondary synaptic folds that greatly increase the postsynaptic membrane area. One measure of the increased membrane at the end plate is that the membrane capacitance per unit of projected surface area (C_m) is increased at the end plate as compared to extrajunctional membrane.[10] Because the membrane is a lipid bilayer, C_m is a direct measurement of the actual amount of surface membrane. The extrajunctional and end plate membranes are not smooth, but rather are folded and contain many caveoli. Consequently, the actual membrane area is greater than the apparent or projected surface area, where the projected area is the area of a smooth cylinder with the same dimensions as the muscle fiber. A perfectly flat membrane would have a C_m normalized to projected surface area of 0.9–1 $\mu F/cm^2$.[11] The data in FIGURE 2 show that on extrajunctional membrane the capacitance is about 3–4 $\mu F/cm^2$, indicating that the extrajunctional membrane folding increases the actual membrane surface by 3–4-fold. The membrane capacitance at the end plate is higher than on extrajunctional membrane, which reflects the greater

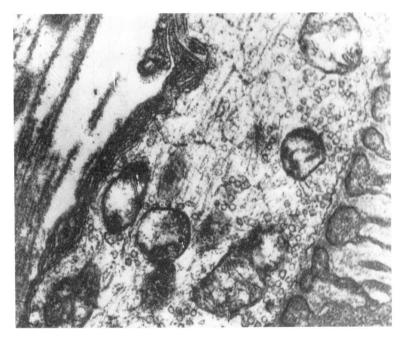

FIGURE 1. Electron micrograph of a rat neuromuscular junction from a fast-twitch skeletal muscle fiber showing junctional folds and synaptic vesicles (see text for description). Reproduced from reference 1 with permission.

membrane folding at the end plate compared with extrajunctional membrane (FIGURE 2).

The large number of AChRs on the end plate membrane makes the postsynaptic membrane very sensitive to nerve terminal–released ACh.[12] The end plate membrane AChRs are concentrated at the peaks of the secondary synaptic folds.[13] The concentration of AChRs at the end plate is about 15,000 to 20,000 receptors/μm^2.[14] The prior density measurement for AChRs was an average over the end plate; therefore, the AChR concentration is higher at the peaks of the secondary synaptic folds. Away from the end plate, the concentration of AChRs is about 1–10 receptors/μm^2.[15] The high concentration of AChRs at the end plate results in part because the nuclei near the end plate preferentially produce mRNA for AChR subunits.[16,17]

AChRs turn over by internalization and degradation of the old AChRs with replacement by new receptors. AChRs are not recycled. The half-life of AChRs, at a mature end plate, is about ten days.[18] The rates of gene transcription of AChR subunits, especially the α-subunit, are the primary controllers of the number of end plate AChRs in normal skeletal muscle. AChR degradation normally has a secondary impact on the number of AChRs at an end plate.[19–25] However, immune attack against

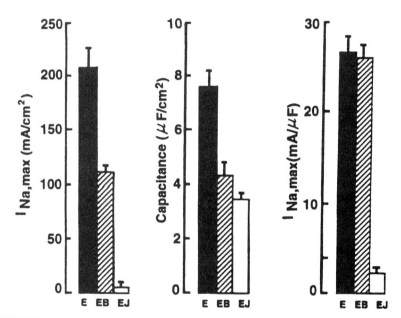

FIGURE 2. $I_{Na,max/A}$ [which is $I_{Na,max}$ normalized to projected membrane area (mA/cm²)], $I_{Na,max/C}$ [which is $I_{Na,max}$ normalized to membrane capacitance (mA/μF)], and C_m normalized to projected membrane area (μF/cm²) at the end plate (E, filled bar), end plate border (EB, hatched bar), and extrajunctional membrane > 200 μm from the end plate border (EJ, unfilled bar). Data obtained using a loose patch voltage clamp. Number of fibers studied: E = 18, EB = 20, EJ = 26. Significant differences: for $I_{Na,max/A}$ (mA/cm²), E was largest—$p < 0.001$; EB > EJ—$p < 0.001$; for $I_{Na,max/C}$ (mA/μF), EJ was smallest—$p < 0.001$; and for C_m (μF/cm²), E was largest—$p < 0.001$; EB > EJ—$p < 0.05$. Reproduced from reference 10 with permission.

the AChRs, as occurs in clinical and experimental MG, can markedly reduce the number of end plate AChRs.[26–35] The AChRs are closely packed at the end plate so that antibodies can cross-link AChRs (FIGURE 3), which triggers AChR internalization, resulting in a shorter AChR half-life.[30,35–37] In MG, AChRs are lost due to accelerated AChR internalization and loss of end plate membrane.[35,37] Skeletal muscle fibers increase AChR subunit gene expression in response to clinical and experimental MG; however, the increase in AChR production is not able to compensate for the accelerated AChR loss.[35,38]

At the end plate, the AChRs are anchored to the cytoskeleton.[39] The AChRs are connected together in clusters by rapsyn, a 43-kDa protein.[13,40,41] Clusters of AChRs are connected to the cytoskeleton via the dystrophin-glycoprotein complex (DGC).[41] The DGC contains the following: α- and β-dystroglycan; the sarcoglycan complex of α-, β-, γ-, and δ-sarcoglycan; agrin; syntrophin; utrophin (dystrophin-related protein); nitric acid synthetase (NOS); and an 87-kDa protein that is probably the dystrophin-related phosphoprotein, dystrobrevin.[41–47] FIGURE 3 shows a model of the relationships among the AChRs, rapsyn, and the DGC. The DGC connects to the cytoskeleton via F-actin and to the extracellular matrix via connections to laminin and merosin. Rapsyn connects the AChRs to the DGC. β-Spectrin and dystrophin may also participate in anchoring AChRs to the cytoskeleton, but at the end plate dystrophin is predominantly replaced by utrophin.[13,16,17,48,49]

ChE in the extracellular matrix of the basal lamina covers the secondary clefts. Enough ChE is in the secondary synaptic clefts to hydrolyze the nerve terminal–released ACh and prevent repeated binding of ACh to the AChRs. Therefore, AChRs are usually activated only once by ACh released from a nerve terminal.[50]

In addition to AChRs, Na^+ channels are concentrated on the postsynaptic membrane. On mammalian fast-twitch skeletal muscle fibers, Na^+ current (I_{Na}) densities are 5- to 10-fold higher immediately adjacent to the end plate as compared with regions away from the end plate (TABLE 1, FIGURE 2).[11,13,51–54] Fast-twitch fibers have a higher density of Na^+ channels as compared with slow-twitch fibers.[11,53,54] Na^+ channels are concentrated in the depths of the secondary synaptic folds.[13,51,55] Sodium

TABLE 1. Comparison of Maximal I_{Na} Amplitudes of Fast- and Slow-Twitch Rat and Human Skeletal Muscle Fibers on the End Plate (E), End Plate Border (EB), and Extrajunctional Membrane (EJ)[a]

	E $I_{Na,max}$ (mA/μF)	EB $I_{Na,max}$ (mA/μF)	EJ $I_{Na,max}$ (mA/μF)
Rat			
fast-twitch (12 fibers)	26.5 ± 1.7	26.1 ± 1.2	4.33 ± 0.39
slow-twitch (12 fibers)	6.94 ± 0.59	6.75 ± 0.54	2.20 ± 0.31
Human			
fast-twitch (11 fibers)	23.5 ± 2.2	27.3 ± 2.5	4.87 ± 0.62
slow-twitch (10 fibers)	5.51 ± 0.67	6.18 ± 0.51	1.89 ± 0.29
type IIa (10 fibers)	19.6 ± 1.4	23.7 ± 1.5	4.01 ± 0.41
type IIb (11 fibers)	26.9 ± 1.5	30.3 ± 2.7	5.84 ± 0.38

[a]Data based upon reference 57.

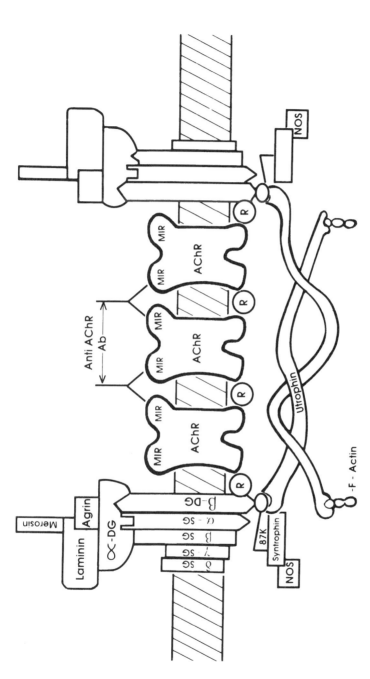

FIGURE 3. Connection of end plate AChRs to the cytoskeleton and extracellular matrix. The AChRs are directly linked via rapsyn (R). AChRs are packed so tightly that IgG and other classes of immunoglobulins can bind to and cross-link AChRs. Clusters of AChRs are linked to the cytoskeleton by connections between rapsyn and a dystrophin-glycoprotein complex (DGC). The DGC contains the sarcoglycans (SG: α-, β-, γ-, and δ-SG, where α-SG was previously called adhalin), agrin, α- and β-dystroglycan, syntrophin, utrophin, an 87-kDa protein that is probably dystrobrevin, and nitric oxide synthase (NOS) bound to syntrophin. The DGC connects to the cytoskeleton via F-actin and to the basal lamina via laminin and merosin.

channels are immobile in the muscle membrane.[56] Ankyrin may attach the Na^+ channels to the cytoskeleton.[13] The increased density of Na^+ channels improves the ability of an end plate potential to trigger an AP.[57] The AP threshold is lower and the rate of rise of the AP is faster at the end plate as compared with extrajunctional membrane (TABLE 2).

MECHANICAL DIFFERENCES BETWEEN END PLATE AND EXTRAJUNCTIONAL SURFACE MEMBRANE

The cytoskeleton at the end plate differs from that on extrajunctional membrane. One of the prominent differences is that, on extrajunctional membrane, dystrophin replaces utrophin (FIGURE 3).[49] As mentioned above, the densities of Na^+ channels and AChRs are many-fold lower on extrajunctional membrane and the membrane folding is more extensive on the end plate as compared with extrajunctional membrane. During changes in muscle fiber length, the fiber dimensions must change to maintain an isovolumic state because the cytosol is a noncompressible fluid.[10] A muscle fiber can be modeled as an isovolumic cylinder to examine how the dimensions of a fiber need to change during length changes. The volume of a model fiber is $\pi R^2 L$, where R is the fiber radius and L is the fiber length. To maintain an isovolumic condition, $R^2 L$ must be constant. Therefore, R varies as $(L)^{-1/2}$.[10] The projected surface area of the model fiber is $2\pi RL$. Therefore, the projected surface area changes during length changes in proportion to $(L)^{1/2}$. The projected surface area increases during lengthening by unfolding of the extrajunctional sarcolemma, while during shortening increased folding of extrajunctional membrane reduces the projected surface area.[10] The folding and unfolding of the extrajunctional membrane can be quantitated by measuring the change in C_m and I_{Na} density as a function of fiber length (FIGURE 4). As fiber length changed, C_m ($\mu F/cm^2$) and I_{Na} density (mA/cm^2) on extrajunctional membrane varied in proportion to $(L)^{-1/2}$. The actual density of Na^+ channels in the sarcolemma did not change as demonstrated by the constancy of I_{Na} normalized to membrane capacitance ($mA/\mu F$). The mechanical properties of the end plate membrane are different from those of the extrajunctional membrane. C_m ($\mu F/cm^2$) and I_{Na} (mA/cm^2) on the end plate and at the end plate border did not vary with changes in fiber length, indicating that the end plate

TABLE 2. Action Potential (AP) Properties[a] on the End Plate Border Compared to Extrajunctional Membrane for 36 Rat Omohyoid Muscle Fibers

	AP Threshold (mV)	AP dV/dt (Vs^{-1})	AP Overshoot (mV)
End plate border	-69.3 ± 1.9	586 ± 22	36.2 ± 2.9
Extrajunctional membrane	-58.7 ± 1.7	352 ± 14	34.5 ± 2.7
	$p < 0.001$	$p < 0.001$	

[a]AP properties: AP threshold is the depolarization from the resting potential required to trigger an AP. AP dV/dt is the maximum rate of rise of the AP. AP overshoot is the most positive membrane potential achieved by the AP. Data based upon reference 57.

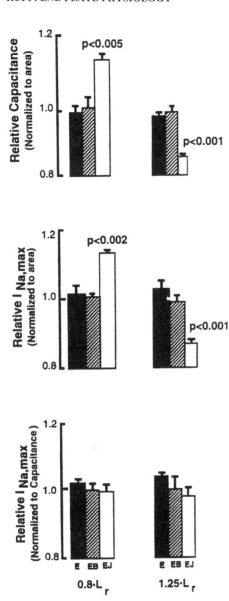

FIGURE 4. The effect of passively changing fiber length on $I_{Na,max/A}$ normalized to projected membrane area (mA/cm^2), $I_{Na,max/C}$ normalized to membrane capacitance (mA/µF), and C_m (µF/cm^2). The regions studied were the end plate (E), the end plate border (EB), and the extrajunctional membrane (EJ) at rest length (L_r), 25% lengthening (1.25·L_r), and 20% shortening (0.8·L_r). Values are shown relative to the values at L_r. Note at the E and the EB that $I_{Na,max}$ and C_m did not change with a change in fiber length. On EJ membrane, $I_{Na,max/A}$ (mA/cm^2) and C_m were larger at 0.8·L_r and smaller at 1.25·L_r, while $I_{Na,max/C}$ (mA/µF) did not change in response to passive changes in fiber length. Twelve omohyoid fibers were studied for each measurement. Reproduced from reference 10 with permission.

membrane does not fold and unfold in response to muscle fiber length changes. Therefore, the end plate membrane is appreciably stiffer than the extrajunctional membrane.[10] The rigidity of the end plate membrane may enable a muscle fiber to maintain a precise relationship with the nerve terminal during muscle stretch and shortening, thereby enabling neuromuscular transmission to be invariant during muscle contraction.

NERVE-MUSCLE SIGNALING

Nerve and muscle have complex influences upon each other. Neuregulins[58] and calcitonin gene–related protein[59] are synthesized by the nerve and can induce muscle AChR subunit gene transcription. Nitric oxide synthase (NOS) is concentrated on the end plate, where it is bound to syntrophin (FIGURE 3).[46,60] Nitric oxide (NO) performs many cell signaling functions and could diffuse from its site of synthesis to affect target proteins in the nerve and muscle.[61] NO activates guanylate cyclase, which could then influence cGMP-dependent systems.[62] In *Xenopus* nerve-muscle cultures, NO donors such as *S*-nitroso-*N*-acetylpenicillamine suppress spontaneous and evoked synaptic currents, and neuronal NOS inhibitors eliminate this effect.[63] If NO functions similarly at the mature mammalian neuromuscular junction, then NO could act as an integrator of neural activity. Cell cytosolic calcium concentration also reflects muscle fiber activity. The AChR is permeable to calcium. Cytosolic calcium concentration rises at the end plate with synaptic depolarization. Therefore, calcium-dependent processes could depend on neuromuscular activity. Calcium activates neuronal NOS, which would increase NO production.

THE SAFETY FACTOR FOR NEUROMUSCULAR TRANSMISSION

The neuromuscular transmission safety factor (SF) can be defined as

$$SF = \frac{EPP}{E_{AP} - E_M},$$

where EPP is the end plate potential amplitude, E_M is the membrane potential, and E_{AP} is the AP threshold.[64] Several factors increase the safety factor of fast-twitch fibers as compared with slow-twitch muscle fibers.[65] The nerve terminals of fast-twitch fibers contain more synaptic vesicles and come in close proximity to the larger end plate area of fast-twitch fibers as compared with nerve terminals innervating slow-twitch fibers.[66] The quantal contents of fast-twitch fibers are larger than slow-twitch fibers.[65,67]

The postsynaptic sensitivities of fast-twitch fibers are greater than slow-twitch fibers. Fast-twitch end plates depolarize more in response to ACh.[68] The increased end plate sensitivity is not because fast-twitch fiber end plates have more AChRs[64] or different types of AChRs.[68] However, AChRs on fast- and slow-twitch fibers have different sensitivities to nicotinic receptor competitive blockers.[69] Consequently, the enhanced sensitivity of fast-twitch end plates to ACh may result from differences in the agonist sensitivities of AChRs in the end plate membranes of fast-twitch compared with slow-twitch fibers.

Fast-twitch end plates on rodents and humans have greater concentrations of Na$^+$ channels compared with slow-twitch end plates (TABLE 1).[11,52–54,57,70–72] The high end plate Na$^+$ channel concentration of fast-twitch fibers increases the safety factor for neuromuscular transmission of the fast-twitch fibers. The AP threshold at the end plate border is about 10 mV lower than on extrajunctional membrane (TABLE 2).[57] The lower end plate border AP threshold increases the safety factor for neuromuscular transmission by about 25% for fast-twitch fibers.[57]

Differences in synaptic transmission for fast- and slow-twitch fibers reflect the different properties of fast- and slow-twitch motor units. Slow-twitch motor units fire tonically at about 10 Hz.[73] Under these conditions, the nerve terminals innervating slow-twitch fibers will not become depleted of ACh. Consequently, slow-twitch fibers do not need a large safety factor.[65,74] The safety factor for rat slow-twitch motor units at a firing rate of 10 Hz is about 1.8.[65] In contrast, fast-twitch motor units are intermittently active at rates $\geq$ 40 Hz.[73] The high firing rates of fast-twitch neuromuscular synapses make them susceptible to neuromuscular transmission failure due to depression of ACh release from depletion of readily releasable synaptic vesicles.[65,74] In addition, at higher rates of stimulation, K^+ can accumulate in the extracellular space around muscle fibers, depolarizing the membrane and resulting in depolarization-induced Na^+ channel inactivation.[57] Muscle fibers in predominantly fast-twitch muscles may be more susceptible to extracellular K^+ accumulation because the capillary networks in these muscles are not well developed.[52,53] The safety factor for fast-twitch rat muscle fibers stimulated at 40 Hz decreases from 3.7 for the first response to 2.0 after 200 stimuli.[65]

SAFETY IS REDUCED IN MG DUE TO LOSS OF ACHRs AND END PLATE Na+ CHANNELS

The major physiological defect in MG is reduced quantal size. The reduced quantal size results from the autoimmune attack directed against AChRs. AChRs are lost from the postsynaptic membrane due to accelerated AChR internalization triggered by antibody cross-linking of AChRs and due to complement-mediated destruction of end plate membrane. The loss of end plate AChRs decreases the postsynaptic sensitivity to ACh.[1,35] Na^+ channels are also lost from the end plate region in MG.[75] End plate Na^+ channels are lost from both fast- and slow-twitch fibers. A reflection of the Na^+ channel loss is that the maximal I_{Na} at the end plate is reduced by 60% for all fiber types in patients with MG[75] and in rats with passively transferred MG[31,76–78] produced by injecting the rats with anti-AChR antibodies. Na^+ channels are probably lost due to complement-mediated destruction of the synaptic folds at the end plate.[75] Due to the loss of end plate Na^+ channels, the AP threshold at the end plate is increased by 8–9 mV in clinical and experimental MG.[79] The increase in the AP threshold at the end plate reduces the safety factor by about 25%. Therefore, the loss of end plate Na^+ channels in MG contributes to the neuromuscular transmission defect in MG by decreasing the safety factor for neuromuscular transmission.

SUMMARY

The safety factor for neuromuscular transmission depends upon the amount of ACh released from the nerve terminal, the number of AChRs, and the concentration of Na^+ channels at the end plate potential. The postsynaptic end plate membrane of the neuromuscular junctions is specialized in three ways: (1) AChRs, Na^+ channels,

ChE, NOS, and other membrane-associated proteins are concentrated at the end plate; (2) the end plate cytoskeleton has a different composition of proteins as compared with extrajunctional membrane; and (3) the end plate membrane is mechanically different as compared with extrajunctional membrane. A blockade of neuromuscular transmission occurs when ACh release is inadequate or the end plate response to ACh is too small to trigger an AP. A safety factor for neuromuscular transmission exists because the EPP is larger than the threshold for generating an AP. The high concentration of Na^+ channels at the end plate increases the safety factor for neuromuscular transmission by reducing the threshold depolarization required to initiate an AP. In MG, the safety factor is reduced due to loss of AChRs and loss of Na^+ channels. The loss of AChRs reduces the EPP and the Na^+ channel loss increases the threshold for triggering an AP.

REFERENCES

1. KAMINSKI, H. J. & R. L. RUFF. 1996. The myasthenic syndromes. *In* Physiology of Membrane Disorders. Volume 1, p. 565–593. Plenum. New York.
2. SALPETER, M. M. 1987. The Vertebrate Neuromuscular Junction. Alan R. Liss. New York.
3. KATZ, B. 1966. Nerve Muscle and Synapse. McGraw–Hill. New York.
4. KATZ, B. & R. MILEDI. 1972. The statistical nature of the acetylcholine potential and its molecular components. J. Physiol. (Lond.) **224:** 665–699.
5. KATZ, B. & R. MILEDI. 1973. The binding of acetylcholine to receptors and its removal from the synaptic cleft. J. Physiol. (Lond.) **231:** 549–574.
6. KATZ, B. & R. MILEDI. 1979. Estimates of quantal content during chemical potentiation of transmitter release. Proc. R. Soc. Lond. **205:** 369–378.
7. MILEDI, R., P. C. MOLENAAR & R. L. POLAK. 1983. Electrophysiological and chemical determination of acetylcholine release at the frog neuromuscular junction. J. Physiol. (Lond.) **334:** 245–254.
8. LAND, B. R., W. V. HARRIS, E. E. SALPETER & M. M. SALPETER. 1984. Diffusion and binding constants for acetylcholine derived from the falling phase of miniature endplate currents. Proc. Natl. Acad. Sci. U.S.A. **81:** 1594–1598.
9. MCMAHAN, U. J., J. R. SANES & L. M. MARSHALL. 1978. Cholinesterase is associated with the basal lamina at the neuromuscular junction. Nature **271:** 172–174.
10. RUFF, R. L. 1996. Effects of length changes on Na^+ current amplitude and excitability near and far from the end-plate. Muscle Nerve **19:** 1084–1092.
11. RUFF, R. L. & D. WHITTLESEY. 1993. Na^+ currents near and away from endplates on human fast and slow twitch muscle fibers. Muscle Nerve **16:** 922–929.
12. KAMINSKI, H. J., J. I. SUAREZ & R. L. RUFF. 1997. Neuromuscular junction physiology in MG: isoforms of the acetylcholine receptor in extraocular muscle and the contribution of sodium channels to the safety factor. Neurology **48(suppl. 5):** S8–S17.
13. FLUCHER, B. E. & M. P. DANIELS. 1989. Distribution of Na^+ channels and ankyrin in neuromuscular junctions is complementary to that of acetylcholine receptors and the 43 kD protein. Neuron **3:** 163–175.
14. LAND, B. R., E. E. SALPETER & M. M. SALPETER. 1981. Kinetic parameters for acetylcholine interaction in intact neuromuscular junction. Proc. Natl. Acad. Sci. U.S.A. **78:** 7200–7204.
15. KUFFLER, S. W. & D. YOSHIKAMI. 1975. The distribution of acetylcholine sensitivity at the post-synaptic membrane of vertebrate skeletal twitch muscles: iontophoretic mapping in the micron range. J. Physiol. (Lond.) **244:** 703–730.

16. MERLIE, J. P. & J. R. SANES. 1985. Concentration of acetylcholine receptor mRNA in synaptic regions of adult muscle fibers. Nature **317:** 66–68.

17. SANES, J. R., Y. R. JOHNSON, P. T. KOTZBAUER, J. MUDD, T. HANLEY, J-C. MARTINOU & J. P. MERLIE. 1991. Selective expression of an acetylcholine receptor–lacZ transgene in synaptic nuclei of adult muscle fibers. Development **113:** 1181–1191.

18. SALPETER, M. M. & R. H. LORING. 1985. Nicotinic acetylcholine receptors in vertebrate muscle: properties, distribution, and neural control. Prog. Neurobiol. **25:** 297–325.

19. KARLIN, A. 1991. Explorations of the nicotinic acetylcholine receptor. Harvey Lect. **85:** 71–107.

20. NUMA, S. 1989. A molecular view of neurotransmitter receptors and ionic channels. Harvey Lect. **83:** 121–165.

21. WITZEMANN, V., B. BARG, Y. NISHIKAWA, B. SAKMANN & S. NUMA. 1987. Differential regulation of muscle acetylcholine receptor γ- and ε-subunit mRNAs. FEBS Lett. **223:** 104–112.

22. WITZEMANN, V., B. BARG, M. CRIADO, E. STEIN & B. SAKMANN. 1989. Developmental regulation of five subunits specific mRNAs encoding acetylcholine receptor subtypes in rat muscle. FEBS Lett. **242:** 419–424.

23. NODA, M., Y. FURUTANI, H. TAKAHASHI, M. TOYOSATO, T. TANABE, S. SHIMIZU, S. KIKYOTANI, T. KAYANO, T. HIROSE, S. INAYAMA & S. NUMA. 1983. Cloning and sequence analysis of calf cDNA and human genomic DNA encoding alpha-subunit precursor of muscle acetylcholine receptor. Nature **305:** 818–823.

24. TAKAI, T., M. NODA, M. MISHINA, S. SHIMIZU, Y. FURUTANI, T. KAYANO, T. IKEDA, K. TAI, H. TAKAHASHI, T. TAKAHASHI, M. KUNO & S. NUMA. 1985. Cloning, sequencing, and expression of cDNA for a novel subunit of acetylcholine receptor from calf muscle. Nature **315:** 761–764.

25. MISHINA, M., T. TAKAI, K. IMOTO, M. NODA, T. TAKAHASHI, S. NUMA, C. METHFESSL & B. SAKMANN. 1986. Molecular distinction between fetal and adult forms of muscle acetylcholine receptor. Nature **321:** 406–411.

26. FAMBROUGH, D. M., D. B. DRACHMAN & S. SATYAMURTI. 1973. Neuromuscular junction in myasthenia gravis: decreased acetylcholine receptors. Science **182:** 293–295.

27. ENGEL, A. 1984. Myasthenia gravis and myasthenic syndrome. Ann. Neurol. **16:** 519–534.

28. LINDSTROM, J. M., M. E. SEYBOLD, V. A. LENNON, S. WHITTINGHAM & D. D. DUANE. 1976. Antibody to acetylcholine receptor in myasthenia gravis: prevalence, clinical correlates, and diagnostic value. Neurology **26:** 1054–1059.

29. DRACHMAN, D. B. 1987. Myasthenia gravis: a model disorder of acetylcholine receptors. Res. Publ. Assoc. Res. Nerv. Ment. Dis. **65:** 65–82.

30. KAO, I. & D. DRACHMAN. 1977. Myasthenic immunoglobulin accelerates acetylcholine receptor degradation. Science **196:** 526.

31. LINDSTROM, J. M., A. G. ENGEL, M. E. SEYBOLD, V. A. LENNON & E. H. LAMBERT. 1976. Pathological mechanisms in experimental autoimmune myasthenia gravis. II. Passive transfer of experimental autoimmune myasthenia gravis in rats with antiacetylcholine receptor antibodies. J. Exp. Med. **144:** 739–753.

32. ENGEL, A. G. 1987. The molecular biology of end-plate diseases. *In* The Vertebrate Neuromuscular Junction. Volume 23, p. 361–424. Alan R. Liss. New York.

33. DRACHMAN, D., C. W. ANGUS, R. N. ADAMS & I. KAO. 1978. Effect of myasthenic patients' immunoglobulin on acetylcholine receptor turnover: selectivity of degradation process. Proc. Natl. Acad. Sci. U.S.A. **75:** 3422–3426.

34. ENGEL, A. G. 1986. Myasthenic syndromes. *In* Myology, p. 1955–1990. McGraw–Hill. New York.

35. DRACHMAN, D. B. 1994. Myasthenia gravis. N. Engl. J. Med. **330:** 1797–1810.

36. MERLIE, J. P., S. HEINEMANN & J. M. LINDSTROM. 1979. Acetylcholine receptor degradation

in adult rat diaphragms in organ culture and the effect of anti-acetylcholine receptor antibodies. J. Biol. Chem. **254:** 6320–6327.

37. ENGEL, A. G. & G. FUMAGALLI. 1982. Mechanisms of acetylcholine receptor loss from the neuromuscular junction. Ciba Found. Symp. **90:** 197–224.

38. ASHER, O., D. NEUMANN, V. WITZEMANN & S. FUCHS. 1990. Acetylcholine receptor gene expression in experimental autoimmune myasthenia gravis. FEBS Lett. **261:** 231–235.

39. RUFF, R. L. 1986. Ionic channels: I. The biophysical basis for ion passage and channel gating. Muscle Nerve **9:** 675–699.

40. FROEHNER, S. C. 1991. The submembrane machinery for nicotinic acetylcholine receptor clustering. J. Cell Biol. **114:** 1–7.

41. APEL, E. D., S. L. ROBERDS, K. P. CAMPBELL & J. P. MERLIE. 1995. Rapsyn may function as a link between the acetylcholine receptor and the agrin-binding dystrophin-associated glycoprotein complex. Neuron **15:** 115–126.

42. SADOULET-PUCCIO, H. M., T. S. KHURANA, J. B. COHEN & L. M. KUNKEL. 1996. Cloning and characterization of the human homologue of a dystrophin-related phosphoprotein found at the *Torpedo* electric organ post-synaptic membrane. Hum. Mol. Genet. **5:** 489–496.

43. OHLENDIECK, K. 1996. Towards an understanding of the dystrophin-glycoprotein complex: linkage between the extracellular matrix and the membrane cytoskeleton in muscle fibers. Eur. J. Cell Biol. **69:** 1–10.

44. CAMPBELL, K. P. & R. H. CROSBIE. 1996. Utrophin to the rescue. Nature **384:** 308–309.

45. KLEIMAN, R. J. & L. F. REICHARDT. 1996. Testing the agrin hypothesis. Cell **85:** 461–464.

46. BRENMAN, J. E., D. S. CHAO, S. H. GEE, A. W. MCGEE, S. E. CRAVEN, D. B. SANTILLANO, Z. WU, F. HUANG, H. XIA, M. F. PETERS, S. C. FROEHNER & D. S. BREDT. 1996. Interaction of nitric oxide synthase with the postsynaptic protein PSD-95 and α1-syntrophin mediated by PDZ domains. Cell **84:** 757–767.

47. CAMPBELL, K. P. 1995. Three muscular dystrophies: loss of cytoskeleton–extracellular matrix linkage. Cell **80:** 675–679.

48. MARTINOU, J-C., D. I. FALLS, G. D. FISCHBACH & J. P. MERLIE. 1991. Acetylcholine receptor–inducing activity stimulates expression of the epsilon-subunit gene of the muscle acetylcholine receptor. Proc. Natl. Acad. Sci. U.S.A. **88:** 7669–7673.

49. DUGGAN, D. J., J. R. GOROSPE, M. FANIN, E. P. HOFFMAN & C. ANGELINI. 1997. Mutations in the sarcoglycan genes in patients with myopathy. N. Engl. J. Med. **336:** 618–624.

50. COLQUHOUN, D. & B. SAKMANN. 1985. Fast events in single-channel currents activated by acetylcholine and its analogues at the frog muscle end-plate. J. Physiol. (Lond.) **369:** 501–557.

51. HAIMOVICH, B., D. L. SCHOTLAND, W. E. FIELES & R. L. BARCHI. 1987. Localization of sodium channel subtypes in rat skeletal muscle using channel-specific monoclonal antibodies. J. Neurosci. **7:** 2957–2966.

52. RUFF, R. L. 1992. Na current density at and away from end plates on rat fast- and slow-twitch skeletal muscle fibers. Am. J. Physiol. **262**(Cell. Physiol. 31): C229–C234.

53. RUFF, R. L. & D. WHITTLESEY. 1992. Na^+ current densities and voltage dependence in human intercostal muscle fibres. J. Physiol. (Lond.) **458:** 85–97.

54. RUFF, R. L. & D. WHITTLESEY. 1993. Comparison of Na^+ currents from type IIa and IIb human intercostal muscle fibers. Am. J. Physiol. **265**(Cell. Physiol. 34): C171–C177.

55. ANGELIDES, K. J. 1986. Fluorescently labeled Na^+ channels are localized and immobilized to synapses of innervated muscle fibres. Nature **321:** 63–66.

56. ALMERS, W., P. R. STANFIELD & W. STÜHMER. 1983. Lateral distribution of sodium and potassium channels in frog skeletal muscle: measurements with a patch-clamp technique. J. Physiol. (Lond.) **336:** 261–284.

57. RUFF, R. L. 1996. Sodium channel slow inactivation and the distribution of sodium channels on skeletal muscle fibres enable the performance properties of different skeletal muscle fibre types. Acta Physiol. Scand. **156:** 159–168.

58. JO, S. A., X. ZHU, M. A. MARCHIONNI & S. J. BURDEN. 1995. Neuregulins are concentrated at nerve-muscle synapses and activate ACh-receptor gene expression. Nature **373:** 158–161.

59. HALL, Z. W. 1992. The nerve terminal. *In* An Introduction to Molecular Neurobiology, p. 148–180. Sinauer Assoc. Sunderland, Massachusetts.

60. KUSHNER, L. L. & H. J. KAMINSKI. 1996. Nitric oxide synthase is concentrated at the skeletal muscle endplate. Brain Res. **730:** 238–242.

61. SCHUMAN, E. M. & D. V. MADISON. 1994. Nitric oxide and synaptic function. Annu. Rev. Neurosci. **17:** 153–183.

62. BREDT, D. S. & S. H. SNYDER. 1992. Nitric oxide, a novel neuronal messenger. Neuron **8:** 3–11.

63. WANG, T., Z. XIE & B. LU. 1995. Nitric oxide mediates activity-dependent synaptic suppression at developing neuromuscular synapses. Nature **374:** 262–266.

64. BANKER, B. Q., S. S. KELLY & N. ROBBINS. 1983. Neuromuscular transmission and correlative morphology in young and old mice. J. Physiol. (Lond.) **339:** 355–375.

65. GERTLER, R. A. & N. ROBBINS. 1978. Differences in neuromuscular transmission in red and white muscles. Brain Res. **142:** 255–284.

66. PADYKULA, H. A. & G. F. GAUTHIER. 1970. The ultrastructure of the neuromuscular junctions of mammalian red, white, and intermediate skeletal muscle fibers. J. Cell Biol. **46:** 27–41.

67. TONGE, D. A. 1974. Chronic effects of botulinum toxin on neuromuscular transmission and sensitivity to acetylcholine in slow and fast skeletal muscle of the mouse. J. Physiol. (Lond.) **241:** 127–139.

68. STERZ, R., M. PAGALA & K. PEPER. 1983. Postjunctional characteristics of the endplates in mammalian fast and slow muscles. Pflügers Arch. **398:** 48–54.

69. STORELLA, R. J., W. F. RIKER & T. BAKER. 1985. *d*-Tubocurarine sensitivities of fast and slow neuromuscular system of the rat. Eur. J. Pharmacol. **118:** 181–184.

70. MILTON, R. L., M. T. LUPA & J. H. CALDWELL. 1992. Fast and slow twitch skeletal muscle fibers differ in their distributions of Na channels near the endplate. Neurosci. Lett. **135:** 41–44.

71. CALDWELL, J. H. & R. L. MILTON. 1988. Sodium channel distribution in normal and denervated rodent and snake skeletal muscle. J. Physiol. (Lond.) **401:** 145–161.

72. CALDWELL, J. H., D. T. CAMPBELL & K. G. BEAM. 1986. Sodium channel distribution in vertebrate skeletal muscle. J. Gen. Physiol. **87:** 907–932.

73. HENNIG, R. & T. LØMO. 1985. Firing patterns of motor units in normal rats. Nature **314:** 164–166.

74. LEV-TOV, A. 1987. Junctional transmission in fast- and slow-twitch mammalian muscle units. J. Neurophysiol. **57:** 660–671.

75. RUFF, R. L. & L. CORSILLO. 1994. Sodium channels near the endplate are lost in myasthenia gravis. Neurology **44:** A189.

76. LINDSTROM, J. M., B. L. EINARSON, V. A. LENNON & M. E. SEYBOLD. 1976. Pathological mechanisms in experimental autoimmune myasthenia gravis. I. Immunogenicity of syngeneic muscle acetylcholine receptor and quantitative extraction of receptor and anti-receptor complexes from muscle of rats with experimental autoimmune myasthenia gravis. J. Exp. Med. **144:** 726–738.

77. LENNON, V. A. & E. H. LAMBERT. 1980. Myasthenia gravis induced by monoclonal antibodies to acetylcholine receptors. Nature **285:** 238–240.

78. LENNON, V. A., M. E. SEYBOLD, J. M. LINDSTROM, C. COCHRANE & R. ULEVITCH. 1978. Role of complement in the pathogenesis of experimental autoimmune myasthenia gravis. J. Exp. Med. **147:** 973–983.

79. RUFF, R. L. 1996. Action potential thresholds are elevated near the end-plate, but not elsewhere in myasthenia gravis and passive transfer experimental myasthenia gravis. Ann. Neurol. **40:** 507–508.

Molecular and Antigenic Structure of Nicotinic Acetylcholine Receptors

JON LINDSTROM,[a] XIAO PENG, ALEXANDER KURYATOV,
EDWARD LEE, RENÉ ANAND,[b] VOLODYMYR GERZANICH, FAN WANG,
GREGG WELLS,[c] AND MARK NELSON[d]

Department of Neuroscience
Medical School of the University of Pennsylvania
Philadelphia, Pennsylvania 19104-6074

INTRODUCTION

The nicotinic acetylcholine receptors (AChRs) in skeletal muscle, which are the target of the autoimmune response that causes myasthenia gravis (MG), are part of a gene family that includes several subtypes of neuronal AChRs.[1,2] In turn, AChRs are part of a gene superfamily that includes ionotropic receptors for the neurotransmitters, glycine, gamma-aminobutyric acid, and serotonin.[3] Subunits of all of these receptors exhibit sequence homologies reflecting their common evolutionary origin.[1] Homologies between the sequences of some subunits of AChRs from muscle and nerves are reflected in the cross-reaction of some mAbs made to muscle AChRs with neuronal AChRs.[4,5] More is known about the structure of subunits of muscle AChRs and their arrangement in the native AChR than is known about any of the other receptors, but all are thought to share a fundamentally similar structure consisting of five homologous rodlike subunits organized like barrel staves to form a central ion channel.[6,7] Aspects of the molecular and antigenic structure of AChRs will be briefly reviewed.

Despite substantial progress in the study of AChR structure, recognition of pathologically important AChR antibody epitopes like the main immunogenic region (MIR),[8,9] and discovery of the mechanisms by which autoantibodies impair neuromuscular transmission in MG,[10] it has not yet been possible to develop a therapy for MG in which only the autoimmune response to AChRs is suppressed. Current therapies for MG consist of four main approaches.[11] One is symptomatic therapy with inhibitors of acetylcholinesterase to compensate for the immune damage to neuromuscular transmission. This is often remarkably useful, but does not treat the basic immunological problem. A second approach is immunosuppressive drug therapy. This can reduce the autoimmune response, but is also nonspecifically immune-suppressive and carries the risk of hormonal or cytotoxic side effects. Thymectomy provides

[a]Research in the laboratory of J. Lindstrom was supported by grants from the National Institutes of Health (NIH) (No. NS11323), the Muscular Dystrophy Association, and the Smokeless Tobacco Research Council, Incorporated.
[b]Supported by NIH Grant No. NS33625.
[c]Supported by NIH Grant No. K08 NSO1903.
[d]Supported by an NRSA fellowship.

a third type of therapy that may result in a reduced autoimmune response, but it is serious surgery, and the effects may be delayed and difficult to evaluate as compared to changes reflecting the natural history of the disease. Plasmapheresis rapidly reduces serum autoantibody levels, but is not antigen-specific and only transiently effective. An ideal therapy for MG might try to take advantage of progress in the study of AChR structure to devise a method for specifically suppressing only the autoimmune response to AChRs. Radically new therapies would need to be first tested in the animal model of MG, experimental autoimmune MG (EAMG),[10] which is typically induced by immunization with *Torpedo* electric organ AChRs in adjuvant. Some success has been reported in inducing tolerance to induction of EAMG by pretreatment of rats orally or nasally with *Torpedo* electric organ AChR.[12–19] The pathological mechanisms of EAMG will be very briefly reviewed. Next, the putative mechanisms of oral tolerance and published experience with it in EAMG will be briefly reviewed. Finally, we will briefly describe our preliminary results with using oral and nasal treatment with bacterially expressed human AChR subunits to try to prevent or treat EAMG in rats induced by active immunization with *Torpedo* AChR.

MOLECULAR STRUCTURE OF AChRs

cDNA sequences for 16 kinds of AChR subunits have been determined.[1,2,7] All are homologous in sequence and are consequently presumed to be basically similar in many aspects of their shapes. These consist of 9 α subunits numbered $\alpha 1$–$\alpha 9$, 4 β subunits numbered $\beta 1$–$\beta 4$, plus a γ, δ, and ε subunit.

AChRs from *Torpedo* electric organ are the best structurally characterized AChRs because they are available in the largest amounts. They have the subunit composition $(\alpha 1)_2 \beta 1 \gamma \delta$.[7] The subunits are thought to be oriented around the central cation channel in the order $\alpha 1$, γ, $\alpha 1$, δ, $\beta 1$.[7] Two ACh binding sites are thought to be formed at the corresponding $\alpha 1/\gamma$ and $\alpha 1/\delta$ interfaces.[7] A similar pattern of 5 subunits with ACh binding sites at particular subunit interfaces is thought to be followed by all AChR subtypes. Fetal muscle AChRs have the subunit composition $(\alpha 1)_2 \beta 1 \gamma \delta$, whereas adult muscle AChRs have the subunit composition $(\alpha 1)_2 \beta 1 \varepsilon \delta$.[7] Electron diffraction analysis of two-dimensional crystalline arrays of AChRs from *Torpedo* electric organ has determined the structure of these proteins to a resolution of 9Å.[6,20,21] This is sufficient to reveal their basic shape, but not sufficient to clearly resolve secondary structures like α helices, much less the atomic resolution of ACh binding sites, epitopes, or the ion channel. The basic shape discovered for electric organ AChRs is thought to apply to all kinds of AChRs and other receptors in this superfamily. Viewed from the top, the *Torpedo* electric organ AChR is roughly pentagonal, about 80 Å in diameter with 25-Å-thick walls, surrounding the 30-Å-diameter extracellular lumen of the central channel.[6,20,21] Viewed from the side, the AChR is roughly cylindrical, about 120 Å long with about 65 Å extending on the extracellular surface of the postsynaptic membrane and about 15 Å extending on the cytoplasmic surface. In cross section, the relatively large extracellular vestibule of the channel narrows to 5–6 Å in diameter as it crosses the membrane before flaring open again on the cytoplasmic surface. Acute binding of ACh to both of its binding sites is thought to produce a transient opening of the channel, whereas prolonged exposure to agonists can cause a desensitized conformation characterized by a closed channel and high-affinity binding of agonists.[22]

Neuronal AChRs, which like muscle AChRs can bind the snake venom toxin α-bungarotoxin (αBgt) at their ACh binding sites, are formed from α7, α8, and α9 subunits.[1,2] These AChRs can function as homomers of α7, α8, or α9 subunits when expressed from cDNAs and may naturally occur as homomers. α7 AChRs are the predominant form of αBgt-binding neuronal AChR in mammals,[23] although small amounts of α9 are found in limited areas.[24] α7 AChRs are found in peripheral ganglia neurons along with a mixture of subtypes containing α3 subunits.[25] The α3 AChRs in ciliary ganglia are located postsynaptically, whereas the α7 AChRs are located perisynaptically and are present in larger amounts.[26] Either subtype is sufficient to ensure transmission in ciliary ganglia.[27] Some α7 AChRs in the hippocampus are located presynaptically where they can modulate the release of glutamate.[28] In general, the functional roles of neuronal AChRs in the central nervous system (CNS) are not well characterized, but it is suspected that many of them may be located presynaptically.[29] α7 AChRs have been found to be expressed in small amounts in muscle[30] and tendon fibroblasts[31] at early developmental times. The functional significance of this is unknown, but it may have to do with regulating Ca^{++}-dependent events during development. All cloned neuronal AChR subtypes that have been studied exhibit greater Ca^{++} permeability than is typical of muscle AChRs.[1,2] However, α7 AChRs are unique in their high Ca^{++} permeability, reportedly exceeding even that of the NMDA subtype of glutamate receptors.[32] However, the other distinguishing feature of α7, α8, and α9 AChRs limits their net Ca^{++} influx. These AChRs are all characterized by very rapid desensitization.[1,2,32] It was primarily for this reason that for many years no functional activity was detected for α7 AChRs. It is suspected that Ca^{++} entering through neuronal AChRs acts as a critical second messenger to activate transmitter release[28] or activate Ca^{++}-sensitive channels (e.g., even K^+ channels that result in a net inhibitory effect[24,33] or trigger signaling cascades that modulate neurite extension or gene regulation).[34,35]

Neuronal AChRs that cannot bind αBgt can be formed by combinations of as few as 2 kinds of subunits or by as many as 4 kinds of subunits. Expression of pairs of cDNAs of α2, α3, α4, or α6 subunits with β2 or β4 subunits will produce functional AChRs.[1,2,36,37] The sequences of α5 and β3 subunits are closely related, and both have been found to form functional AChRs only as a third subunit type in combination with pairs such as α3 and β2 or α3 and β4 subunits.[4,5,38] It is suspected that α5 and β3 subunits may occupy a position around the ion channel comparable to β1 subunits of muscle AChRs, so they do not interface with the part of an α2, α3, α4, or α6 subunit that can form an ACh binding site.[5] AChRs formed from α4 and β2 subunits account for most of the high-affinity nicotine binding sites in brain.[39] When expressed from cloned subunits, they exhibit the subunit stoichiometry of $(α4)_2(β2)_3$,[40] suggesting that, like muscle AChRs, they have two ACh binding sites formed at specific interfaces between α4 and β2 subunits. α3 subunit–containing postsynaptic AChRs are found at many peripheral ganglia, often in combination with α7 AChRs.[1,2,5,25,26] Expression of α3, β4, and α5 subunits has been detected in thymus[41] and α3 AChRs have been reported to be present in keratinocytes.[42] In chick ciliary ganglia, 80% of the α3 AChRs also contain β4 and α5 subunits, and 20% contain α3, β4, α5, and β2 subunits.[43] In the human neuroblastoma line SH-SY5Y, 56% of the α3 AChRs contain β2 subunits.[5] Thus, in many of the neurons that have been charac-terized, complex combinations of AChR subtypes are present, ranging from α7 ho-momers to subtypes of α3 AChRs with as many kinds of subunits as are found in muscle AChRs.

In the mammalian CNS, glutamate is the main excitatory transmitter, in contrast with the peripheral nervous system where ACh predominates. However, AChRs are widespread in the CNS.[23,44] The current lack of evidence for postsynaptic roles for many of these AChRs and evidence for presynaptic roles for some suggest that many are acting presynaptically rather than in the familiar postsynaptic roles of muscle AChRs.[1,2,22,29] In the CNS, there are roughly equal amounts of α4β2 AChRs and α7 AChRs, as well as smaller amounts of other AChR subtypes. Some AChR subtypes containing, for example, α3 or α6 subunits may be found predominantly in limited areas.[45] The detailed localization of CNS AChRs and their functional roles are just beginning to be worked out.

Neuronal AChRs are affected in several diseases. The number of high-affinity nicotine binding sites (presumably α4β2 AChRs) is decreased in both Alzheimer's disease and Parkinson's disease.[46] A rare congenital form of epilepsy has been shown to result from a mutation in α4 subunits.[47] Primarily through the efforts of Engel and coworkers,[48] many congenital myasthenic syndromes have been elegantly character-ized as mutations in subunits of muscle AChRs. It may well be that a similar variety of neuronal AChR mutations remain to be found.

The primary pathological role of neuronal AChRs is mediating addiction to nico-tine. This promotes the use of tobacco, accounting for more than 400,000 premature deaths each year in the United States,[49] a medical impact that dwarfs that of MG, of which there are perhaps a total of 20,000 sufferers in the United States.[11] Nicotine has relatively low affinity for muscle AChRs (EC_{50} for activation is 2×10^{-4} M);[50] thus, its effects on neuromuscular transmission are small at the 2×10^{-7} M average serum concentration typical of smokers or the 1×10^{-6} M concentrations that they might experience transiently.[51] α4β2 AChRs exhibit an EC_{50} for activation by nico-tine of 3×10^{-7} M and, when desensitized, exhibit a K_D for binding of 4×10^{-9} M.[52] Acute exposure to nicotine activates AChRs, but chronic exposure can reversibly de-sensitize or permanently inactivate these AChRs.[52] We have found that chronic expo-sure to 2×10^{-7} M nicotine substantially inactivates human α4β2 AChRs and α7 AChRs, while leaving α3 AChRs able to respond to ACh.[72] Nicotine also causes an increase in the amount of α4β2 AChRs,[52] α7 AChRs, and α3 AChRs.[53] Nicotine in-creases the amount of α4β2 AChRs by causing a decrease in the rate of α4β2 AChR turnover.[52] This is an interesting contrast with MG where antibodies to muscle AChRs cause a decrease in AChRs by increasing the rate of turnover.[10]

All AChR subunits exhibit a characteristic pattern of features in their primary se-quences.[1,7] The N-terminal approximately 200 amino acids are thought to form a large extracellular domain that contains a disulfide-linked loop homologous to that between cysteines 128 and 142 of α1 subunits as well as one or more N-glycosyla-tion sites. All α subunits have a cysteine pair homologous to α1 cysteines 192 and 193. In all α subunits, but α5, this part of the sequence as well as several more N-ter-minal extracellular domain amino acids are thought to contribute to the ACh binding site.[5] Starting at about amino acids 210–220, the subunits begin a series of three hydrophobic sequences of about 30 amino acids each, which are thought to form three largely α helical transmembrane domains.[7] The second of these, termed M2, is thought to contribute much of the lining of the cation channel. It is thought to be oriented as an amphipathic α helix with the hydrophilic amino acids lining the channel.[7] Following M3 is a large cytoplasmic domain consisting of 100–300 amino acids. This region often contains consensus sequences for phosphorylation. It is the most variable in sequence both between subunits and between species. Antibodies to the large cytoplasmic domain often recognize both native and denatured AChRs, suggesting that, in native AChRs, parts of the large cytoplasmic domain are not highly conformationally constrained.[1,54,55] After the large cytoplasmic domain, the M4 transmembrane domain leads to a short C-terminal extracellular domain of 10–20 amino acids.

ANTIGENIC STRUCTURE OF AChRs

At both the B and T cell level, the immune response to muscle AChRs is greater to α1 subunits than to the others, perhaps in part reflecting the antigen doses and orientation resulting from the $(\alpha 1)_2 \beta 1 \gamma \delta$ stoichiometry of the subunits.[10] Immunization with denatured muscle AChR subunits results in an immune response directed primarily at epitopes on the cytoplasmic surface, perhaps by default as a result of the loss of highly immunogenic conformation-dependent epitopes on the extracellular surface.[54,55] Correspondingly, it is very difficult to induce EAMG by immunizing with denatured subunits,[56] and it has been reported that preimmunization with denatured subunits can even protect against induction of EAMG.[57] The most potent epitopes on muscle AChRs are conformation-dependent and are on the extracellular surface. The main immunogenic region (MIR) is on the extracellular surface of α1 subunits.[8,9] The MIR was identified as a consequence of the ability of a single mAb to prevent the binding of many others.[8,9] Half or more of the antibodies in an antiserum to muscle AChR or in MG patient sera are directed at the MIR.[8] mAbs of this specificity can bind to AChRs on the cell surface, cross-link these AChRs to induce antigenic modulation, and fix complement to induce focal lysis and antibody-dependent cell-mediated cytotoxicity.[1,9] Thus, mAbs to the MIR are potent at passively transferring EAMG.[1,9] mAbs to the MIR do not block the ACh binding site or cation channel.[1,9] The functional role, if any, of the MIR is unknown. mAbs to the MIR bind near the extracellular tip of α1 subunits.[21] The MIR is oriented outwards from the axis of the AChR.[21] Thus, mAbs to the MIR do not cross-link the two α1 subunits within an AChR, but are efficient at cross-linking adjacent AChRs.[1,9] The α1 subunit sequence 66–76 may form a hairpinlike structure corresponding to the MIR.[58] Amino acids 68 and 71 in α1 subunits are important to the structure of the MIR in *Torpedo* AChRs.[59] Sequences very similar to the muscle α1 subunit MIR sequence are found in neuronal AChR α3, α5, and β3 subunits.[1] mAbs to muscle α1 MIR react with human α3 and α5 subunits.[5] They also react with β3 subunits, as we discovered only recently (Gerzanich and Lindstrom, unpublished), because until very recently β3 subunits had not been shown to be able to function as part of AChRs.[38] MG patient sera have not been found to react with high-affinity nicotine binding AChRs from human brain (presumably $\alpha4\beta2$ AChRs) or with αBgt binding sites from these brains (presumably $\alpha7$ AChRs).[60] However, these studies would not have detected $\alpha3$ AChRs because they have lower affinity for nicotine and are present in smaller amounts. Neither have we detected immune precipitation of ^{3}H-epibatidine-labeled human $\alpha3\alpha5$ AChRs from neuroblastoma extracts with MG patient sera (Wang and Lindstrom, unpublished experiments). This could be a technical problem reflecting the very low $\alpha3$ AChR concentrations in these extracts ($<10^{-10}$ M) and the low concentrations of MG patient autoantibodies. Alternatively, it could mean that rat mAbs and MG patient autoantibodies recognize different amino acids in the MIR. If there is a cross-reaction that has not yet been detected, its pathological significance might be greatest at peripheral $\alpha3\alpha5$ AChRs not protected by the blood-brain barrier, such as those in the adrenal medulla or the thymus. Such $\alpha3\alpha5$ AChRs might be disrupted by cross-reaction with autoantibodies to muscle AChR or even serve as a source of autoimmunogen in MG.

EXPERIMENTAL AUTOIMMUNE MYASTHENIA GRAVIS

EAMG can be induced in most animals by immunizing with purified electric organ AChRs in adjuvant.[10] As in MG, EAMG results from a T cell–dependent autoantibody response.[10] In rats, there may be a transient acute phase of EAMG between 6 and 10 days after immunization, if appropriate adjuvants are used.[10] The muscular weakness at this time is due to disruption of neuromuscular junctions by an antibody and complement–mediated phagocytic invasion.[10] During the acute phase, antibody titers are low and only a small fraction of the AChRs have antibodies bound.[10] Passive transfer of EAMG by antisera or mAbs to AChRs proceeds by a phagocytic mechanism like that seen during the acute phase of EAMG.[10] Such a phagocytic invasion is not seen in chromic EAMG or MG, nor is an acute phase of EAMG required in order to observe a later chronic phase of EAMG.[10] In rats, the chronic phase of EAMG muscular weakness begins at about day 30.[10] This is characterized by high titers of antibodies to AChR, loss of half or more of the AChRs in muscle, antibodies bound to many of those AChRs that remain, and simplified morphology of the postsynaptic membrane.[10] AChR loss is thought to be mediated by both antibody- and complement-mediated focal lysis of the postsynaptic membrane and an increase in the rate of AChR turnover resulting from antibody cross-linking of AChRs, which facilitates endocytosis and lysosomal destruction of the AChRs.[10] If the dose of AChR is small enough that neither the acute nor chronic phase of EAMG is sufficiently severe to be lethal, then the rats will ultimately recover. The initial autoimmune response to the immunogen does not initiate a continuing response stimulated by muscle AChRs consumed at the end plates.

The great experimental advantage of chronic EAMG is that it provides a model that accurately reflects the pathological mechanisms that impair neuromuscular transmission in MG. It also provides a way to test novel therapies for EAMG.

The great experimental disadvantage of EAMG as a model of MG is that it does not share whatever unknown mechanisms initiate and sustain for years the autoimmune response to AChRs in humans with MG. Thus, when using EAMG to test novel therapies, artificial conditions are encountered. Pretreatment before induction of EAMG may provide a relatively clean and sensitive screen for detecting specific tolerance induction, but it does not model problems encountered in therapy of the ongoing autoimmune response of an MG patient. Posttreatment after induction of EAMG more closely models therapy of MG. However, if the therapy acts on T cells and is started after the T cells have already collaborated with B cells to produce an overwhelming antibody response, then no effect on muscle weakness may be evident over a period of 30 to 50 days, even if the T cell response is diminished, and no response at a longer time would be relevant since the autoimmune response to AChR in EAMG is not self-sustaining as it is in MG. Thus, attempts to model treatment of MG using EAMG may be tricky.

ORAL TOLERANCE

It has long been known that feeding large amounts of antigen can result in suppression of the immune response to this antigen.[61] The resulting tolerance is specific for the antigen given orally.[61] This phenomenon is thought to reflect a natural process whose role is to prevent nonproductive immune responses to the huge array of food antigens to which the gut is exposed. Recently, there has been substantial interest in trying to use oral tolerance to treat autoimmune diseases.[62,63] There has been substantial success in preventing or treating a number of model autoimmune diseases by oral or nasal tolerance.[12–19,61,64–69] What has been published on EAMG[12–19] will be briefly reviewed below. Clinical trials are in progress for multiple sclerosis, diabetes, uveitis, and rheumatoid arthritis, resulting in some early reports of modestly encouraging results.[61–63]

The mechanisms by which oral tolerance is thought to work act at the level of T cells.[61–64] Low doses of orally administered antigen are thought to promote active suppression of the immune response mediated by bystander immunosuppression of T lymphocytes by cytokines like TGF-β that are released by orally induced immunosuppressive T cells at sites where they are stimulated by antigen. Higher doses of antigen are thought to cause clonal anergy. The putative mechanism of active suppression resulting in cytokine-mediated suppression of autoimmune T cells is appealing for several reasons. In theory, it would not require epitope-by-epitope suppression of the immune response to the autoantigen, so a closely related, but not identical, antigen that was available in large amounts might be used to induce tolerance because it shared enough epitopes to induce a sufficient number of suppressor cells. Also, in theory, since T cell receptors only interact with denatured peptide fragments of an antigen, it might be possible to induce tolerance using denatured rather than native antigen. This is the premise behind our preliminary experiments, which will be described subsequently, in which we have undertaken to induce oral tolerance to EAMG with bacterially expressed human AChR subunits.

Tolerance can also be induced by treating animals nasally with antigens.[16,67–69] It has been found that much smaller amounts of antigen are required by this route than are required when the antigen is fed. This makes the nasal route of administration especially attractive for use with antigens available only in small amounts or antigens that might easily be degraded in the gut.

ORAL TOLERANCE STUDIES OF EAMG BY OTHERS

Link and coworkers[12] first reported that oral administration of *Torpedo* AChR to rats prior to immunization with *Torpedo* AChR reduced the incidence and severity of chronic EAMG. Five of 6 rats given 5–20 mg of AChR in a total of four feedings over 8 days exhibited no signs of EAMG weakness, in contrast with all 4 untreated rats or 2 rats fed smaller amounts of AChR. In these experiments, soybean trypsin inhibitor was given in 16-fold weight excess over AChR to inhibit proteolysis in the gut. Subsequently, more detailed experiments by this group confirmed and elaborated these basic observations.[13,14] B cell responses and antibody titers to AChR were reduced by oral pretreatment, as was, to a small degree in some areas, the development of AChR-reactive IFN-γ-secreting T cells.[15] Half of the 27 control rats in these experiments developed acute EAMG and all of them developed chronic EAMG, whereas none of 12 rats developed acute or chronic EAMG after oral pretreatment with four doses of 1.25 mg each over 8 days, ending 3 days before immunization with 50 μg of AChR in complete Freund's adjuvant. Oral treatment reduced the number of AChR-reactive lymphocytes expressing IFN-γ or IL-4, while increasing the number expressing TGF-β.[14] Pretreatment also reduced the number of B cells secreting antibodies to AChR.[15] Link and coworkers found that nasal pretreatment with only 12-μg amounts of *Torpedo* AChR daily for 10 days before induction of EAMG resulted in only 1 of 6 rats developing acute EAMG and only 2 developing chronic EAMG, as compared to 6 out of 7 EAMG controls at the acute phase and all 7 at the chronic phase.[16] Serum antibody titers to AChR were reduced by half as a result of nasal pretreatment.

Drachman and coworkers[18] confirmed that oral pretreatment of rats with purified *Torpedo* AChR suppressed subsequent induction of EAMG. AChR was administered in five oral doses of either 0.25 or 1 mg at 3-day intervals to anesthetized rats without the accompanying trypsin inhibitor that had been used by Link and coworkers.[12–15] Rats were immunized with 50 μg of *Torpedo* AChR in complete Freund's adjuvant at 3 days after the last feeding. Six of 7 untreated rats developed chronic EAMG, whereas none of 6 rats treated with 0.25 mg AChR/dose nor any of 8 rats treated with 1 mg AChR/dose developed chronic EAMG. The weight loss characteristic of EAMG was reduced by the low-dose treatment and prevented by the high-dose treatment. As a specificity control, some rats were pretreated with ovalbumin. These rats were not protected from EAMG, but their antibody responses to ovalbumin were greatly reduced. Pretreatment orally with AChR reduced serum antibody titers to *Torpedo* AChR by 39% at low doses and by 43% at high doses. The antibody titer to rat AChRs was reduced up to 81% by 8 weeks after immunization. Oral pretreatment with AChR was also shown to reduce the AChR-induced T cell proliferation responses in these rats. In a subsequent study,[19] Drachman and coworkers investigated the efficacy of oral treatments with AChR, starting a series of five 1-mg doses every 3 days at 14 days after immunization with AChR. In one set of experiments, the weakness of EAMG was suppressed. However, a second series that food-deprived the rats for 18 hours before each treatment was not successful. It was suggested that food deprivation before treatment may have resulted in more extensive degradation of the antigen in the gut. In both cases, feeding AChR substantially increased the amount of antibodies to AChR in serum. It was suggested that a less immunogenic form might be more effective than native AChR in trying to treat ongoing EAMG through inducing oral tolerance.

OUR PRELIMINARY RESULTS WITH ORAL TOLERANCE OF EAMG

The success of oral pretreatment with AChR purified from *Torpedo* electric organ in suppressing induction of chronic EAMG suggested that induction of oral tolerance might provide an approach to specific immunotherapy of MG. The rationale for our experiments with mucosal induction of tolerance begins with the idea that bacterial expression of cloned human AChR subunits is the only known way to express sufficient amounts of human AChR protein for this purpose. This will result in denatured protein lacking the most potent conformation-dependent B cell epitopes such as the MIR. This would be acceptable if the target of the antigen used for suppression were T cells that only recognized degraded peptide fragments of an antigen, and it might even be a virtue if the absence of the MIR prevented priming or boosting of B cells to produce pathogenic antibodies. An unknown factor would be whether the denatured state of the protein made it more susceptible to degradation than native AChR before it reached antigen-presenting cells or less susceptible to being taken up or properly processed by these cells. The use of human AChR might make for a more potent tolerogen in a human than would the distantly related *Torpedo* AChR. However, in a rat with EAMG induced by native *Torpedo* AChR, sequence differences between the tolerogen, immunogen, and endogenous AChR might also create problems.

The initial problem was to produce large amounts of human AChR subunits in bacteria. Production of large segments, for example, equivalent to the extracellular domain of $\alpha 1$ subunits was quite efficient and provided a useful antigen for stimulating MG patient T lymphocyte cultures.[70] However, the bacteria produced much lower levels of intact $\alpha 1$ subunits. It was suspected that the bacteria did not tolerate the hydrophobic domains of these subunits well. Studies with synthetic peptides had shown that few MG patient T cell epitopes occurred in transmembrane domains.[71] Thus, we simply spliced these transmembrane sequences out and cloned these constructs in pET plasmids. These were transformed into the expression host BL21 (DE3) cells. These bacteria were grown in kanamycin-containing media to ensure retention of the plasmids (which confer kanamycin resistance). Subunit synthesis was induced with 1 mM IPTG at 3 hours before harvesting. The pelleted bacteria were resuspended and then lysed using 1.2% Triton and 0.1 mg/mL lysozyme for 1 hour at room temperature. Centrifuging 5-mL aliquots of lysate through a 20-mL cushion of 40% sucrose for 1 hour at 50,000 rpm at 4 °C produced pellets of washed inclusion bodies containing the subunits. These were solubilized in 3% SDS plus 100 mM dithiothreitol for 5 minutes at 100 °C. Subunits were then purified to homogeneity on an AcA-34 Ultrogel sizing column. Yields of 40–50 mg of purified water-soluble subunit protein per liter of culture have been obtained for human $\alpha 1$, $\beta 1$, γ, δ, and ε subunits. Subunits were concentrated by precipitation with 1.5 M NaC1 at 0 °C and then solubilized in phosphate-buffered saline. Dialysis at room temperature was used to reduce the SDS to a mole ratio of about 13 SDS molecules per subunit.

EAMG was induced using a single dose of 20 μg of *Torpedo* AChR in TiterMax adjuvant given in four sites at the base of the tail. This routinely produced an acute phase as well as a chronic phase of EAMG in a high proportion of young female Lewis rats.

Immunization with the denatured subunits did not produce EAMG, as shown in TABLE 1. Three 100-μg doses at 2-week intervals of α1, β1, γ, δ, or ε produced no acute or chronic EAMG in a total of 30 rats. However, serum antibody titers to muscle AChR in the 100-nM range were produced. This relatively high titer of autoantibodies in the absence of muscle weakness suggests that most of these autoantibodies were not pathologically significant. This would be the case if they were directed primarily at cytoplasmic determinants, as has previously been observed for antibodies to denatured *Torpedo* AChR subunits.[54,55]

Oral treatment with five doses of 5 mg of α1, β1, γ, δ, and ε in the weight ratio of 2:1:1:1:1 at 3-day intervals did not cause signs of EAMG weakness or weight loss in any of 6 rats. It did result in a low level (1.6 ± 1 nM) of serum antibodies to rat muscle AChRs.

Pretreatment with five oral doses of 5 mg of α1 subunits at 3-day intervals until 3 days before immunization with *Torpedo* AChR reduced the incidence of acute EAMG weakness to 4/15 rats as compared to 13/17 untreated. There was no obvious effect on chronic EAMG. This is summarized in TABLE 2. In all cases, oral administration of AChR in 1 mL with a ball-tipped feeding needle was performed under anesthesia after 18 hours with water, but without food. It is unknown whether the 18-hour food deprivation increased the concentration of AChR at Peyer's patches and thus improved uptake, as was intended, or whether this left the AChR protein even more susceptible to proteolysis due to the absence of other food to distract proteases. It may well be that denatured protein is more likely to be proteolyzed than the compact structure of a native protein. Another factor that might explain why oral treatment with just α1 was less effective than had been reported with native AChR is that only a small fraction of the T cell epitopes were represented when using only α1 as tolerogen.

Oral pretreatment with five doses of 5 mg of α1, β1, γ, δ, and ε in a 2:1:1:1:1 weight ratio at 3-day intervals protected all 6 rats tested from an acute phase of EAMG, as compared to 5/5 controls, and reduced the incidence of chronic EAMG to 2/6 as compared to 5/5 controls. This is summarized in TABLE 3. The pretreated rats gained an average of 20 g after immunization, whereas the untreated rats gained an

TABLE 1. Effect of Immunization with Three 100-μg Doses of Bacterially Expressed Human AChR Subunits

Subunit	EAMG Incidence	Anti-AChR Titers (nM)	
		Rat Muscle α1β1εδ AChRs	Human TE671 Cell α1β1γδ AChRs
α1	0/6	152 ± 4.3	119 ± 26
β1	0/6	110 ± 12	84 ± 40
γ	0/6	0	55 ± 39
δ	0/6	4 ± 1.4	117 ± 25
ε	0/6	58 ± 1.7	0

TABLE 2. Effect of Oral Treatment with Five (5-mg) Doses of α1

| | EAMG Incidence | | Anti-AChR Titers | |
	Acute	Chronic	*Torpedo* (μM)	Rat (nM)
EAMG control	13/17	9/17	1.6 ± 1.2	12 ± 20
pretreatment	4/15	7/15	1.2 ± 1.2	21 ± 18

average of only 4 g. There was little effect of pretreatment on AChR loss at the end of the experiment (51 ± 8% loss in treated versus 57 ± 13% in untreated). Antibody titers were virtually identical for both groups.

Oral posttreatment starting on day 14 after immunization with *Torpedo* AChR with the same five-dose regime used for pretreatment resulted in a 3/5 incidence of chronic weakness, an average weight gain of only 6 g, and antibody titers to *Torpedo* AChR of 2.4 ± 2 μM and to rat AChR of 10 ± 3 nM. Thus, the benefit of oral post-treatment on chronic muscle weakness was very modest. On the other hand, neither was there a substantial booster effect of the oral doses on the immune response to AChR. This is summarized in TABLE 3. Oral posttreatment was repeated in two other groups of rats given the same doses as above. In one case, the doses were given on the same 3-day schedule, resulting in a similarly reduced incidence of chronic EAMG of 2/6 as compared to 6/6 in an untreated control group. In the other case, the five doses were given at 6-day intervals, resulting in the same reduced 2/6 incidence of chronic EAMG, but with slightly more weight gain, suggesting the possibility of greater therapeutic effect than with a shorter duration of treatment. Thus, to summarize our experience with posttreatment with five doses of 5 mg of α1, β1, γ, δ, and ε in the weight ratio of 2:1:1:1:1 starting at day 14, only 6/18 treated rats developed chronic EAMG weakness, whereas 11/11 untreated rats did.

In order to investigate whether targeting our treatments to another mucosal com-

TABLE 3. Effect of Oral Treatment with Five (5-mg) Doses of α1, β1, γ, δ, ε

| | EAMG Incidence | | Weight Gain | Anti-AChR Titers | |
	Acute	Chronic	(g)	*Torpedo* (μM)	Rat (nM)
Experiment 1					
adjuvant control	0	0	50 ± 8	0	0
EAMG control	5/5	5/5	4 ± 18	2.2 ± 0.1	6.3 ± 4
pretreatment	0/6	2/6	20 ± 20	2.2 ± 0.1	6.4 ± 4
posttreatment	5/6	3/5	6 ± 25	2.4 ± 0.2	10 ± 3
Experiment 2					
adjuvant control	0	0	15 ± 10	0	0
EAMG control	5/6	6/6	−14 ± 18	1.7 ± 1.6	14 ± 10
posttreatment	4/6	2/6	8.1 ± 18	1.7 ± 1.6	4.9 ± 2.8
posttreatment					
(6-day interval)	6/6	2/6	11 ± 9	1.6 ± 1.0	8.2 ± 6.8

TABLE 4. Effect of Nasal Treatment with Ten (9-μg) Doses of α1, β1, γ, δ, ε

	EAMG Incidence		Weight Gain	Anti-AChR Titers	
	Acute	Chronic	(g)	*Torpedo* (μM)	Rat (nM)
adjuvant control	0	0	15 ± 10	0	0
EAMG control	5/6	6/6	−14 ± 18	1.7 ± 1.6	14 ± 10
pretreatment	1/6	3/6	9.3 ± 26	1.3 ± 1.4	3.9 ± 2.9
posttreatment	6/6	4/4	−14 ± 8.5	1.6 ± 1.8	6.6 ± 4.5

partment might reduce the antigen degradation expected in the gut and thereby increase potency, we investigated nasal treatment. Results are summarized in TABLE 4. Rats were treated with doses of only 9 μg of α1, β1, γ, δ, and ε at a 2:1:1:1:1 ratio divided over 30 μL of saline pipetted into each nostril of the anesthetized animals. Doses were given daily for 10 days preceding immunization with *Torpedo* AChR or starting 14 days afterwards. Nasal pretreatment reduced the incidence of acute EAMG to 1/6 as compared to 5/6 in the untreated group, and reduced the incidence of chronic EAMG to 3/6 as compared to 6/6 in the untreated group. Posttreatment resulted in an incidence of 4/4 chronic EAMG. The encouraging aspect of these experiments is that some nasal pretreatment benefit was seen on both acute and chronic EAMG at a total dose of 90 μg, which is 0.3% of the 25-mg total doses given orally. Thus, we might hope that further studies with larger, but still quite small, nasal doses may prove promising.

In summary, our preliminary experiments with preventing the induction of EAMG and treating ongoing EAMG by mucosal treatment with bacterially expressed human AChR subunits to induce specific tolerance have produced some modestly encouraging results. Many parameters remain to be investigated in hopes of optimizing this approach to developing specific immunosuppressive therapy for MG. Among these are ensuring stability and optimizing the physical state of the tolerogen, targeting it to the most important cells in the most effective compartment, optimizing dose schedules for efficacy and relevance to therapy of MG, and characterizing the immunological mechanisms involved.

REFERENCES

1. LINDSTROM, J. 1996. Neuronal nicotinic acetylcholine receptors. *In* Ion Channels. Volume 4, p. 377–450. Plenum. New York.
2. MCGEHEE, D. & L. ROLE. 1995. Physiological diversity of nicotinic acetylcholine receptors expressed by vertebrate neurons. Annu. Rev. Physiol. **57:** 521–546.
3. BARNARD, E. 1992. Receptor classes and the transmitter-gated ion channels. Trends Biochem. Sci. **17:** 368–374.
4. CONROY, W., A. VERNALLIS & D. BERG. 1992. The α5 gene product assembles with multiple acetylcholine receptor subunits to form distinctive receptor subtypes in brain. Neuron **9:** 1–20.
5. WANG, F., V. GERZANICH, G. WELLS, R. ANAND, X. PENG, K. KEYSER & J. LINDSTROM. 1996.

Assembly of human neuronal nicotinic receptor α5 subunits with α3, β2, and β4 subunits. J. Biol. Chem. **271:** 17656–17665.

6. UNWIN, N. 1995. Acetylcholine receptor channel imaged in the open state. Nature **373:** 37–43.

7. KARLIN, A. & M. AKABAS. 1995. Toward a structural basis for the function of nicotinic acetylcholine receptors and their cousins. Neuron **15:** 1231–1244.

8. TZARTOS, S., M. SEYBOLD & J. LINDSTROM. 1982. Specificity of antibodies to acetylcholine receptors in sera from myasthenia gravis patients measured by monoclonal antibodies. Proc. Natl. Acad. Sci. U.S.A. **79:** 188–192.

9. TZARTOS, S., M. CUNG, P. DEMANGE, H. LOUTRARI, A. MAMALAKI, M. MARRAUD, I. PAPADOULI, C. SAKARELLOS & V. TSIKARIS. 1991. The main immunogenic region (MIR) of the nicotinic acetylcholine receptor and the anti-MIR antibodies. Mol. Neurobiol. **5:** 1–29.

10. LINDSTROM, J., D. SHELTON & Y. FUJI. 1988. Myasthenia gravis. Adv. Immunol. **42:** 233–284.

11. DRACHMAN, D. 1994. Myasthenia gravis. N. Eng. J. Med. **330:** 1797–1810.

12. WANG, Z., J. QIAO & H. LINK. 1993. Suppression of experimental autoimmune myasthenia gravis by oral administration of acetylcholine receptor. J. Neuroimmunol. **44:** 209–214.

13. WANG, Z., J. QIAO, A. MELMS & H. LINK. 1993. T cell reactivity to acetylcholine receptor in rats orally tolerized against experimental autoimmune myasthenia gravis. Cell. Immunol. **152:** 394–404.

14. WANG, Z., H. LINK, A. LJUNGDAHL, B. HOJEBERG, J. LINK, B. HE, J. QIAO, A. MELMS & T. OLSSON. 1994. Induction of interferon-γ, interleukin-4, and transforming growth factor-β in rats orally tolerized against experimental autoimmune myasthenia gravis. Cell. Immunol. **157:** 353–368.

15. WANG, Z., J. HUANG, T. OLSSON, B. HE & H. LINK. 1995. B cell responses to acetylcholine receptor in rats orally tolerized against experimental autoimmune myasthenia gravis. J. Neurol. Sci. **128:** 167–175.

16. MA, C., G. ZHANG, B. XIAO, J. LINK, T. OLSSON & H. LINK. 1995. Suppression of experimental autoimmune myasthenia gravis by nasal administration of acetylcholine receptor. J. Neuroimmunol. **58:** 51–60.

17. MA, C., G. ZHANG, B. XIAO, Z. WANG, J. LINK, T. OLSSON & H. LINK. 1996. Mucosal tolerance to experimental autoimmune myasthenia gravis is associated with down-regulation of AChR-specific IFN-γ-expressing Th1-like cells and up-regulation of TGF-β mRNA in mononuclear cells. Ann. N.Y. Acad. Sci. **778:** 273–287.

18. OKUMURA, S., K. MCINTOSH & D. DRACHMAN. 1994. Oral administration of acetylcholine receptor: effects on experimental myasthenia gravis. Ann. Neurol. **36:** 704–713.

19. DRACHMAN, D., S. OKUMURA, R. ADAMS & K. MCINTOSH. 1996. Oral tolerance in myasthenia gravis. Ann. N.Y. Acad. Sci. **778:** 258–272.

20. UNWIN, N. 1993. Nicotinic acetylcholine receptor at 9 Å resolution. J. Mol. Biol. **229:** 1101–1124.

21. BEROUKHIM, R. & N. UNWIN. 1995. Three-dimensional location of the main immunogenic region of the acetylcholine receptor. Neuron **15:** 323–331.

22. DANI, J. & S. HEINEMANN. 1996. Molecular and cellular aspects of nicotine abuse. Neuron **16:** 905–908.

23. DEL TORO, E., J. JUIZ, X. PENG, J. LINDSTROM & M. CRIADO. 1994. Immunocytochemical localization of the α7 subunit of the nicotinic acetylcholine receptor in the rat central nervous system. J. Comp. Neurol. **349:** 325–342.

24. ELGOYHEN, A., D. JOHNSON, J. BOULTER, D. VETTER & S. HEINEMANN. 1994. α9: an acetylcholine receptor with novel pharmacological properties expressed in rat cochlear hair cells. Cell **79:** 705–715.

25. CONROY, W. & D. BERG. 1995. Neurons can maintain multiple classes of nicotinic acetyl-choline receptors distinguished by different subunit compositions. J. Biol. Chem. **270:** 4424–4431.
26. HORCH, H. & P. SARGENT. 1995. Perisynaptic surface distribution of multiple classes of nicotinic acetylcholine receptors on neurons in the chicken ciliary ganglion. J. Neurosci. **15:** 7778–7795.
27. ZHANG, Z., J. COGGAN & D. BERG. 1996. Synaptic currents generated by neuronal acetyl-choline receptors sensitive to α-bungarotoxin. Neuron **17:** 1231–1240.
28. GRAY, R., A. RAJAN, K. RADCLIFFE, M. YAKEHIRO & J. DANI. 1996. Hippocampal synaptic transmission enhanced by low concentration of nicotine. Nature **383:** 713–716.
29. WONNACOTT, S. 1997. Presynaptic nicotinic ACh receptors. Trends Neurosci. **20:** 92–98.
30. ROMANO, S., P. PUGH, K. McINTOSH & D. BERG. 1997. Neuronal-type acetylcholine recep-tors and regulation of α7 gene expression in vertebrate skeletal muscle. J. Neurobiol. **32:** 69–80.
31. ROMANO, S., R. CORRIVEAU, R. SCHWARZ & D. BERG. 1997. Expression of the nicotinic re-ceptor α7 gene in tendon and periosteum during early development. J. Neurochem. **68:** 640–648.
32. SEGUELA, P., J. WADICHE, K. DINELLY-MILLER, J. DANI & J. PATRICK. 1993. Molecular cloning, functional properties, and distribution of rat brain α7: a nicotinic cation channel highly permeable to calcium. J. Neurosci. **13:** 596–604.
33. FUCHS, P. & B. MURROW. 1992. A novel cholinergic receptor mediates inhibition of chick cochlea hair cells. Proc. R. Soc. Lond. B **248:** 35–40.
34. LIPTON, S. & S. KATER. 1989. Neurotransmitter regulation of neuronal outgrowth, plastici-ty, and survival. TINS **12:** 265–270.
35. PUGH, P. & D. BERG. 1994. Neuronal acetylcholine receptors that bind α-bungarotoxin me-diate neurite retraction in a calcium-dependent manner. J. Neurosci. **14:** 889–896.
36. PAPKE, R. 1993. The kinetic properties of neuronal nicotinic receptor: genetic basis of functional diversity. Prog. Neurobiol. **41:** 509–531.
37. GERZANICH, V., A. KURYATOV, R. ANAND & J. LINDSTROM. 1997. "Orphan" α6 nicotinic AChR subunit can form a functional heteromeric acetylcholine receptor. Mol. Pharma-col. **51:** 320–327.
38. FORSAYETH, J. & E. KOBRIN. 1997. Formation of oligomers containing the β3 and β4 sub-units of the rat nicotinic receptor. J. Neurosci. **17:** 1531–1538.
39. WHITING, P. & J. LINDSTROM. 1988. Characterization of bovine and human neuronal nico-tinic acetylcholine receptors using monoclonal antibodies. J. Neurosci. **8:** 3395–3404.
40. ANAND, R., W. CONROY, R. SCHOEPFER, P. WHITING & J. LINDSTROM. 1991. Chicken neu-ronal nicotinic acetylcholine receptors expressed in *Xenopus* oocytes have a pentameric quaternary structure. J. Biol. Chem. **266:** 11192–11198.
41. MIHOVILOVIC, M. & A. ROSES. 1993. Expression of α3, α5, and β4 neuronal acetylcholine receptor subunit transcripts in normal and myasthenia gravis thymus. J. Immunol. **151:** 6517–6524.
42. GRANDO, S., R. HORTON, E. PEREIRA, B. DIETHELMOKITA, P. GEORGE, E. ALBUQUERQUE & B. CONTI-FINE. 1995. A nicotinic acetylcholine receptor regulating cell adhesion and motil-ity is expressed in human keratinocytes. J. Invest. Dermatol. **105:** 774–781.
43. VERNALLIS, A., W. CONROY & D. BERG. 1993. Neurons assemble acetylcholine receptors with as many as three kinds of subunits while maintaining subunit segregation among re-ceptor subtypes. Neuron **10:** 451–464.
44. SWANSON, L., D. SIMMONS, P. WHITING & J. LINDSTROM. 1987. Immunohistochemical local-ization of neuronal nicotinic receptors in the rodent central nervous system. J. Neurosci. **7:** 3334–3342.
45. LENOVERE, N., M. ZOLI & J. CHANGEUX. 1996. Neuronal nicotinic receptor α6 subunit

mRNA is selectively concentrated in catecholaminergic nuclei of the rat brain. Eur. J. Neurosci. **8:** 2428–2439.

46. WHITEHOUSE, P., A. MARTINO, K. MARCUS, R. ZWEIG, H. SINGER, D. PRICE & K. KELLAR. 1988. Reductions in acetylcholine and nicotine binding in several degenerative diseases. Arch. Neurol. **45:** 722–724.

47. STEINLEIN, O., J. MULLEY, P. PROPPING, R. WALLACE, H. PHILLIPS, G. SUTHERLAND, I. SCHEFFER & S. BERKOVIC. 1995. A missense mutation in the neuronal nicotinic acetylcholine receptor α4 subunit is associated with autosomal dominant nocturnal frontal lobe epilepsy. Nat. Genet. **11:** 201–203.

48. OHNO, K., H. WANG, M. MILONE, N. BREN, J. BRENGMAN, S. NAKANO, P. OUIRAM, J. PRUITT, S. SINE & A. ENGEL. 1996. Congenital myasthenic syndrome caused by decreased agonist binding affinity due to a mutation in the acetylcholine receptor ε subunit. Neuron **17:** 157–170.

49. PETO, R., A. LOPEZ, J. BOREHAM, M. THUN & C. HEATH. 1992. Mortality from tobacco in developed countries: indirect estimation from national vital statistics. Lancet **339:** 1268–1278.

50. LUKAS, R. 1989. Pharmacological distinctions between functional nicotinic acetylcholine receptors in the PC12 rat pheochromocytoma and the TE671 human medulloblastoma. J. Pharmacol. Exp. Ther. **253:** 51–57.

51. BENOWITZ, N., H. PROCHET & P. JACOB. 1990. Pharmacokinetics, metabolism, and pharmacodynamics of nicotine. *In* Nicotine Psychopharmacology, p. 112–157. Oxford Sci. Pub. London/New York.

52. PENG, X., R. ANAND, P. WHITING & J. LINDSTROM. 1994. Nicotine-induced upregulation of neuronal nicotinic receptors results from a decrease in the rate of turnover. Mol. Pharmacol. **46:** 523–530.

53. PENG, X., V. GERZANICH, R. ANAND, F. WANG & J. LINDSTROM. 1997. Chronic nicotine treatment upregulates α3 AChRs and α7 AChRs expressed by the human neuroblastoma cell line SH-SY5Y. Mol. Pharmacol. **51:** 776–784.

54. FROEHNER, S. 1981. Identification of exposed and buried determinants of the membrane-bound acetylcholine receptor from *Torpedo californica*. Biochemistry **20:** 4905–4915.

55. DAS, M. & J. LINDSTROM. 1991. Epitope mapping of antibodies to acetylcholine receptors. Biochemistry **30:** 2470–2477.

56. LINDSTROM, J., B. EINARSON & J. MERLIE. 1978. Immunization of rats with polypeptide chains from *Torpedo* acetylcholine receptor causes an autoimmune response to receptors in rat muscle. Proc. Natl. Acad. Sci. U.S.A. **75:** 769–773.

57. KROLICK, K., T. YEH & S. EDLUND. 1996. Lewis rats given antibodies against denatured acetylcholine receptor become resistant to induction of experimental autoimmune myasthenia gravis. Cell. Immunol. **172:** 10–20.

58. ORLEWSKI, P., M. MARRAUD, M. CUNG, V. TSIKARIS, M. SAKARELLOS DAITSIOTIS, C. SAKARELLOS, E. VATZAKI & S. TZARTOS. 1996. Compared structures of the free nicotinic receptor main immunogenic region (MIR) decapeptide and the antibody bound [A(76)] MIR analogue: a molecular simulation from two-dimensional NMR data. Biopolymers **40:** 419–432.

59. SAEDI, M., R. ANAND, W. CONROY & J. LINDSTROM. 1990. Determination of amino acids critical to the main immunogenic region of intact acetylcholine receptors by *in vitro* mutagenesis. FEBS Lett. **267:** 55–59.

60. WHITING, P., J. COOPER & J. LINDSTROM. 1987. Antibodies in sera from patients with myasthenia gravis do not bind to acetylcholine receptors from human brain. J. Neuroimmunol. **16:** 205–213.

61. WEINER, H. 1997. Oral tolerance for the treatment of autoimmune diseases. Annu. Rev. Med. **48:** 341–351.

62. HOHOL, M., S. KHOURY, S. COOK, E. ORAV, D. HAFLER & H. WEINER. 1996. Three-year open protocol continuation study of oral tolerization with myelin antigens in multiple sclerosis and design of a phase III pivotal trial. Ann. N.Y. Acad. Sci. **778:** 243–250.

63. TRENTHAM, D. 1996. Evidence that type II collagen feeding can induce a durable therapeutic response in some patients with rheumatoid arthritis. Ann. N.Y. Acad. Sci. **778:** 306–314.

64. WHITACRE, C., J. GIENAPP, A. MEYER, K. COX & N. JAVED. 1996. Treatment of autoimmune disease by oral tolerance to autoantigens. Clin. Immunol. Immunother. **80:** 531–539.

65. GREGERSON, D., W. OBRITSCH & L. DONOSO. 1993. Oral tolerance in experimental autoimmune uveoretinitis. J. Immunol. **151:** 5751–5761.

66. SUB, J., C. RASK, T. OLSSON, J. HOLMGREN & C. CZERKINSKY. 1996. Treatment of experimental autoimmune encephalomyelitis by feeding myelin basic protein conjugated to cholera toxin B subunit. Proc. Natl. Acad. Sci. U.S.A. **93:** 7196–7201.

67. DICK, A., Y. CHENG, A. McKINNON, J. LIVERSIDGE & J. FORRESTER. 1993. Nasal administration of retinal antigens suppresses the inflammatory response in experimental allergic uveoretinitis. Br. J. Ophthalmol. **77:** 171–175.

68. HARRISON, L., M. DEMPSEY COLLIER, D. KRAMER & K. TAKAHASHI. 1996. Aerosol insulin induces regulatory CD8 gamma delta T cells that prevent murine insulin-dependent diabetes. J. Exp. Med. **184:** 2167–2174.

69. METZLER, B. & D. WRAITH. 1993. Inhibition of experimental autoimmune encephalomyelitis by inhalation, but not oral administration of the encephalitogenic peptide: influence of MHC binding affinity. Int. Immunol. **5:** 1159–1165.

70. MELMS, A., G. MALCHERIK, U. GERN, H. WIETHOLTER, R. SCHOEPFER & J. LINDSTROM. 1992. T cells from normal and myasthenic individuals recognize the human acetylcholine receptor: heterogeneity of antigenic sites on the α subunit. Ann. Neurol. **31:** 311–318.

71. PROTTI, M., A. MANFREDI, R. HORTON, M. BELLONE & B. CONTI-TRONCONI. 1993. Myasthenia gravis: recognition of a human autoantigen at the molecular level. Immunol. Today **14:** 363–368.

72. OLALE, F., V. GERZANICH, A. KURYATOV, F. WANG & J. LINDSTROM. 1997. Chronic nicotine exposure differentially affects the function of human α3, α4, and α7 neuronal nicotinic receptor subtypes. J. Pharmacol. Exp. Ther. In press.

A Role for α(187–199) in the Conversion of Agonist Binding Energy to the Opening of the Acetylcholine Receptor Ion Channel[a]

ROBERT H. FAIRCLOUGH,[b] ESWARI GUDIPATI,[b] MIKE Y. LIN,[b]
GEORGE M. TWADDLE,[b] DAVID P. RICHMAN,[b] DAVID A. BURKWALL,[c]
AND ROBERT JOSEPHS[c]

[b]Department of Neurology
University of California, Davis
Davis, California 95616

[c]Department of Molecular Genetics and Cell Biology
University of Chicago
Chicago, Illinois 60637

MONOCLONAL ANTIBODY 383C RECOGNIZES α(187–199) OF THE *TORPEDO* AChR

Antiacetylcholine receptor (anti-AChR) monoclonal antibody (mAb) 383C binds selectively to a 13-amino-acid peptide corresponding to α(187–199) of the *Torpedo* AChR.[1] This peptide includes Y190, C192, C193, and Y198, all of which have been affinity-labeled by various agonist/antagonist analogues.[2–5] These amino acids are thought to contribute to the agonist/antagonist binding environment. The structure of this peptide in the context of the AChR was predicted by Fairclough *et al.*[6] to be an antiparallel β-stranded hairpin with a turn at C192–C193. Two-dimensional NMR studies conducted by Basus *et al.*[7] have confirmed that residues α(185–190) are organized as a β strand in complex with α-bungarotoxin (α-Btx). The current picture of the peptide α(187–199) in the AChR resembles the hairpin displayed in FIGURE 1.

CONTRIBUTION OF PEPTIDE CONTACTS TO THE TOTAL 383C EPITOPE

The anti-AChR mAb 383C binds to the SDS-denatured α-subunit of the AChR as well as to the 13-amino-acid peptide synthesized on a plastic pin.[1] Binding to these

[a]This work was supported by grants from the National Institutes of Health: No. NS15462 to D. P. Richman; No. NS24304 to D. P. Richman, R. H. Fairclough, and R. Josephs; and No. HL22654 to R. Josephs. G. M. Twaddle was supported in part by a neuroimmunology training grant to the University of Chicago: No. T32 NS 07113. E. Gudipati was supported in part by an Osserman fellowship from the Myasthenia Gravis Foundation and by a grant from the Chicago chapter of the Myasthenia Foundation. M. Y. Lin was the recipient of a Henry R. Viets fellowship from the Myasthenia Gravis Foundation.

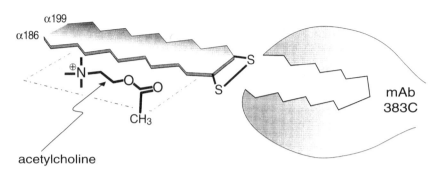

FIGURE 1. Schematic diagram of $\alpha(187-199)$ and a likely agonist orientation in interacting with this peptide. This peptide is also the major component of the epitope for monoclonal antibody 383C.

fragments of the receptor suggests that, independent of the status of the $\alpha(187-199)$ region, if exposed, 383C binds to this peptide. To determine the contribution of the contacts between this peptide and 383C to the entire epitope/383C interaction, we measured the 383C binding affinity to this peptide and compared it to the affinity of 383C to the AChR. The results of this study indicate that the contacts made with the peptide account for all but 3.8 kcal/mole of the 15.2 kcal/mole of stabilization of the 383C/AChR complex.[8]

LOCATION OF 383C EPITOPE ON THE AChR MODEL

Given the central role of the residues of this peptide in binding the neurotransmitter as well as 383C, we have mapped the combining site of 383C onto the 3-D model of the AChR via small-angle X-ray diffraction of AChR-enriched membrane vesicles decorated with 383C along with image processing of electron micrographs of tubular crystalline arrays of AChR decorated with 383C.[1] The image analysis reveals a single decorated α-subunit on the AChR;[1] this is confirmed by measuring the 383C binding stoichiometry to AChR-enriched membrane vesicles, which is one 383C/two toxin sites.[8] The particular α-subunit decorated by 383C is the α_2-subunit[1] located between β and γ in the scheme of Kubalek *et al.*[9] and is illustrated in FIGURE 2a. This subunit is associated structurally and functionally with the high-affinity *d*-tubocurarine (dTc) binding site. The 383C label is located 35 Å above the level of the synaptic side-phosphate groups and on the periphery of the rosette 6° clockwise from the α_2 vertex.[1]

With the peripheral location of this peptide on the AChR, all other residues implicated in the binding of acetylcholine are most likely interior in the rosette from the $\alpha_2(187-199)$ location. Those residues fall into three additional regions as illustrated in FIGURE 2b: the αY93 region, the αW149 region, and the γ/δD,E(174-189) region.

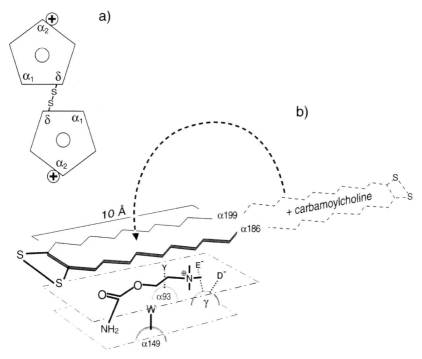

FIGURE 2. (a) Location of the additional stain exclusion ⊕ in the AChR dimeric rosette unit cell with the δ-δ disulfide located between the two pentagons. The location of the two α-subunits is also indicated. (b) Schematic diagram of the proposed structural change that occurs locally in the region of the α_2(187–199) peptide upon binding of carbamoylcholine at the low-affinity agonist binding site.

AChR FUNCTIONAL STATE
AND STOICHIOMETRY OF 383C BINDING

Since in the closed resting state only one α-subunit has residues (187–199) accessible to 383C binding, we explored the 383C binding stoichiometry with the AChR in other functional states. When AChR-enriched membrane vesicles are treated with 10^{-4} M carbamoylcholine, they no longer titrate with 383C, and AChR extracted with Triton X-100 binds twice as much 383C as the AChR in the membranes before extraction.[8]

INFERENCES FROM 383C BINDING STOICHIOMETRY

The 383C binding stoichiometry to AChR-enriched membrane vesicles in the closed resting state of one 383C per two MIR sites reflects a major difference in surface accessibility of the $\alpha(187-199)$ peptide in the two α-subunits. In the α-subunit associated with the high-affinity dTc site, the peptide is readily accessible on the rosette periphery, whereas in the other subunit the peptide is not accessible. Treating the receptor with carbamoylcholine renders the peptide inaccessible in both subunits, while extracting the AChR with Triton X-100 renders the peptide accessible in both subunits.

INTEGRATION OF $\alpha(187-199)$ STRUCTURAL AND FUNCTIONAL DATA WITH AChR AGONIST BINDING DATA

Armed with this structural information, it is interesting to consider the dissociation constants of carbamoylcholine with the receptor in the closed and open states as determined by Meyer Jackson[10] and presented in TABLE 1.[11] In both the closed and open states of the receptor ion channel, there is a low- and high-affinity site for carbamoylcholine (TABLE 1). In the closed resting state, $\alpha_1(187-199)$ is closer to $\alpha_1 Y93$ and $\alpha_1 W149$ than $\alpha_2(187-199)$ is to $\alpha_2 Y93$ and $\alpha_2 W149$ because the α_2 peptide is more peripherally located compared to $\alpha_1(187-199)$. Thus, α_1 very likely corresponds to the high-affinity agonist binding site. α_2, with residues 187–199 protruding like an open door on the periphery of the receptor, anchors the low-affinity agonist site. In the channel-closed state, $\alpha_2 Y93$ and $\alpha_2 W149$, as well as D and E (174–189) from γ, weakly bind agonist > 3.5 mM. The large increase in the affinity for carbamoylcholine at this site results from the additional contacts contributed by $\alpha_2(187-199)$. Following the initial weak association of carbamoylcholine at this site, $\alpha_2(187-199)$ retracts from the surface and wraps itself around carbamoylcholine, and the binding affinity of carbamoylcholine goes up. We propose that this action mechanically pulls the α-subunit residues 10–20 amino acids down the chain in the M1 region of α in or near the extracellular mouth of the ion channel.[12] Binding of agonist reduces the exposure of $\alpha211$, $\alpha215$, $\alpha216$, and $\alpha217$ in a cation-selective region of the receptor.[12] Given the location of $\alpha_2(187-199)$ on the periphery of the receptor and the proposed channel lining/cation-selective location of $\alpha(211-218)$,[12] the α-chain residues 200–211 must go from the outside to the inside of the ACh receptor well by some 25 Å toward the central axis as well as down 35 Å toward the ion channel. We propose that the peptide hairpin, $\alpha_2(187-199)$, acts like a switch to activate channel opening as it hugs the agonist at the low-affinity site, and thereby pulls the α-chain M1 residues 211–217 from the cation-specific well lining, initiating channel activation (see FIGURE 3).

In summary, we propose that the mAb 383C epitope, $\alpha_2(187-199)$, is not only more accessible than the $\alpha_1(187-199)$ counterpart, but this structural difference is at

TABLE 1. AChR/Carbamoylcholine K_d Values

Channel State	High-Affinity	Low-Affinity
closed	5 μM	>3.5 mM
open	0.025 μM	0.110 μM

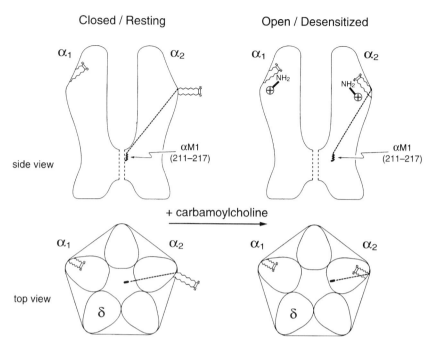

FIGURE 3. Schematic diagram of the proposed structural changes that occur globally upon binding of carbamoylcholine. The retraction of the α_2(187–199) peptide from the AChR surface is accompanied by removal of α_2(211–217) from the cation-specific region at the mouth of the ion channel.

the heart of the differences in agonist affinity at the two sites. We further propose that, as this hairpin retracts about the agonist at the low-affinity site, it pulls residues α_2(211–217), exposed in the mouth of the ion channel, away from this exposure in a process monitored by Akabas and Karlin[12] and likely an integral structural change associated with channel activation/desensitization.

ACKNOWLEDGMENT

We thank Claudia Graham of Illustration Services at UC Davis for graphical insight to the molecular mechanics presented here.

REFERENCES

1. FAIRCLOUGH, R. H., G. M. TWADDLE, E. GUDIPATI, D. P. RICHMAN, D. A. BURKWALL & R. JOSEPHS. 1997. Mapping the mAb 383C epitope to α_2(187–199) of the *Torpedo* acetylcholine receptor on the three-dimensional model. J. Mol. Biol. Submitted.
2. DENNIS, M., J. GIRADAT, F. KOTZYBA-HIBERT, M. GOELDNER, C. HIRTH, J. Y. CHANG, C.

LAZURE, M. CHRÉTIEN & J-P. CHANGEUX. 1988. Amino acids of the *Torpedo marmorata* acetylcholine receptor α subunit labeled by a photoaffinity ligand for the acetylcholine binding site. Biochemistry **27:** 2346–2357.

3. ABRAMSON, S. N., Y. LI, P. CULVER & P. TAYLOR. 1989. An analogue of lophotoxin reacts covalently with Tyr[190] in the α-subunit of the nicotinic acetylcholine receptor. J. Biol. Chem. **264:** 12666–12672.

4. KAO, P. N., A. J. DWORK, R-R. J. KALDANY, M. L. SILVER, J. WIDEMAN, S. STEIN & A. KARLIN. 1984. Identification of the α subunit half-cystine specifically labeled by an affinity reagent for the acetylcholine receptor binding site. J. Biol. Chem. **259:** 11662–11665.

5. MIDDLETON, R. E. & J. B. COHEN. 1991. Mapping of the acetylcholine binding site of the nicotinic acetylcholine receptor: [³H]nicotine as an agonist photoaffinity label. Biochemistry **30:** 6987–6997.

6. FAIRCLOUGH, R. H., J. FINER-MOORE, R. A. LOVE, D. KRISTOFFERSON, P. J. DESMEULES & R. M. STROUD. 1983. Subunit organization and structure of an acetylcholine receptor. Cold Spring Harbor Symp. Quant. Biol. **48:** 9–20.

7. BASUS, V. J., G. SONG & E. HAWROT. 1993. NMR solution structure of an alpha-bungarotoxin/nicotinic receptor peptide complex. Biochemistry **32:** 12290–12298.

8. FAIRCLOUGH, R. H., G. M. TWADDLE, E. GUDIPATI, M. Y. LIN & D. P. RICHMAN. 1997. Differential surface accessibility of α(187–199) in the *Torpedo* ACh receptor α-subunits. J. Mol. Biol. Submitted.

9. KUBALEK, E., S. RALSTON, J. LINDSTROM & N. UNWIN. 1987. Location of subunits within the acetylcholine receptor by electron image analysis of tubular crystals from *Torpedo marmorata*. J. Cell Biol. **105:** 9–18.

10. JACKSON, M. B. 1988. Dependence of acetylcholine receptor channel kinetics on agonist concentration in cultured mouse muscle fibres. J. Physiol. **397:** 555–583.

11. JACKSON, M. B. 1989. Perfection of a synaptic receptor: kinetics and energetics of the acetylcholine receptor. Proc. Natl. Acad. Sci. U.S.A. **86:** 2199–2203.

12. AKABAS, M. H. & A. KARLIN. 1995. Identification of acetylcholine receptor channel-lining residues in the M1 segment of the α-subunit. Biochemistry **34:** 12496–12500.

The Mongoose Neuronal Acetylcholine Receptor (α7) Binds α-Bungarotoxin

SHANY ARIEL,[a] ORNA ASHER,[a] DORA BARCHAN,[a]
MICHAEL OVADIA,[b] AND SARA FUCHS[a]

[a]Department of Immunology
Weizmann Institute of Science
Rehovot 76100, Israel

[b]Department of Zoology
Tel Aviv University
Ramat Aviv 69978, Israel

The acetylcholine receptor (AChR) from animal species that are resistant to α-bungarotoxin (α-BTX) provides an ideal experimental system for elucidating the structural parameters that determine toxin sensitivity. The snake and the mongoose are resistant to α-BTX, and their *muscle* AChRs are unique in their pharmacological properties: they bind cholinergic ligands, but unlike other muscle AChR they do not bind α-BTX.[1–3]

Previous studies in our laboratory have demonstrated that muscle AChR α-subunits (α1) of the toxin-resistant snake,[1] mongoose,[2] and hedgehog[3] differ in unique key positions at the ligand binding site from the α-subunits of toxin-sensitive animals. Such unique substitutions of amino-acid residues were shown to be important in determining the resistance to α-BTX. The contribution of each of these substitutions to α-BTX resistance was determined by site-directed mutagenesis.[4]

It was of interest to find out whether the *neuronal* (α7) AChR of animals that are resistant to α-BTX binds or does not bind α-BTX, and whether there are unique changes in the binding site domain of this neuronal (α7) AChR similar to those observed in the muscle AChR. In the present study, we investigated the neuronal AChR α7-subunit of the mongoose in order to find out whether it is similar to or different from the α7-subunits of α-BTX-sensitive animals.

In order to analyze the characteristics of the nicotinic neuronal AChR of the mongoose, we first tested whether it binds α-BTX. Membrane fractions were prepared from brains of mongoose and rats (for control) and an α-BTX binding assay was performed. Unlike the muscle AChR, the *brain* AChR of mongoose does bind α-BTX specifically, although to a lesser extent than that of the rat (FIGURE 1).

To further analyze the mongoose neuronal AChR, we cloned and sequenced the mongoose AChR α7-subunit. The nucleotide sequence of the coding region (nucleotides 1–1441) of the mongoose α7-subunit is 88.2% homologous to the corresponding subunit of the rat. Most differences observed are at the third position of the codons, thus not affecting the deduced amino acids. The amino-acid sequence of the mongoose α7-subunit is highly homologous to the corresponding subunit of

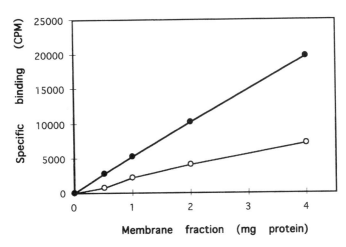

FIGURE 1. α-BTX binding to mongoose and rat brain membrane fractions. Increasing amounts of brain membrane fractions from mongoose (○) and rat (●) were incubated with ^{125}I-α-BTX (specific activity of 200 Ci/mmol, final concentration of 2 nM) for one hour. Non-specific binding values were obtained by incubation of a parallel set of tubes in the presence of 1000-fold (2 mM) unlabeled α-BTX and were subtracted from each value.

human (97.3%), rat (94.8%), mouse (95%), and chick (91.9%). No significant differences were found at the binding site area (amino-acid residues 180–200).

In order to further analyze the binding characteristics of the neuronal AChR α7-subunit of the mongoose, expression in bacteria, Western blot experiments, and overlay with ^{125}I-α-BTX were performed. The amino-terminal extracellular portions of the AChR α7-subunit of the mongoose and rat (for control) were cloned by PCR. The amplified extracellular fragments of the mongoose and rat α7-subunits (amino-acid residues 1–207) were cloned into the pGEX2T expression vector, expressed as fusion proteins with the 29-kDa glutathione S-transferase (GST) protein, purified, and resolved on SDS-PAGE. In addition, a recombinant fragment of the human muscle AChR α1-subunit (residues 1–122), which does not contain the binding site area, and the GST protein were resolved as controls, on the same gels. The proteins were transferred onto nitrocellulose membrane filters and overlaid with ^{125}I-α-BTX. As can be seen in FIGURE 2, α-BTX binding to the mongoose and the rat α7-fragments were similar, in agreement with the high similarity in amino-acid sequence between the species. As expected, the toxin did not bind to the human muscle α1-fragment that does not contain the ligand binding site for α-BTX, nor to the GST protein.

The specificity of the binding of ^{125}I-α-BTX to the recombinant fragments of the neuronal AChR α7-subunit was demonstrated by competition assays. Unlabeled α-BTX (25 μM) and *d*-tubocurarine chloride (12.5 μM) completely abolished the binding of ^{125}I-α-BTX to mongoose and rat AChR α7-subunit extracellular domains. In addition, several 13-mer synthetic peptides derived from the binding site domains of muscle (α1) or neuronal (α7) AChR, or selected from a phage-epitope library with α-

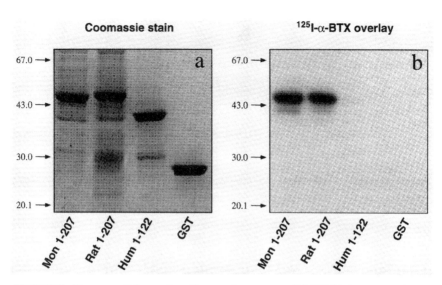

FIGURE 2. The extracellular portion of neuronal mongoose α7 AChR binds α-BTX. The expressed protein fragments were resolved by 10% SDS-PAGE. Mon 1–207 and rat 1–207 represent the extracellular fragments of the mongoose and rat neuronal AChR α7-subunit, respectively. Hum 1–122 represents a human muscle AChR α1-subunit fragment corresponding to residues 1–122. GST represents the glutathione S-transferase protein. The gels were stained for proteins by Coomassie Brilliant Blue (a) or blotted onto nitrocellulose filters and overlaid with 0.6 nM ^{125}I-α-BTX (b).

BTX,[5] were also shown to completely inhibit the binding of α-BTX to the extracellular domains of the mongoose and rat AChR α7-subunit.

Thus, unlike the muscle AChR, the nucleotide and amino-acid sequence of the mongoose neuronal α-BTX-binding AChR is homologous to the sequence of toxin-sensitive species and it binds α-BTX similarly and specifically. It appears that there was no evolutionary pressure on the neuronal AChR to be altered, as is the case with the muscle AChR, since α-BTX most probably does not cross the blood-brain barrier.

REFERENCES

1. NEUMANN, D., D. BARCHAN, M. HOROWITZ, E. KOCHVA & S. FUCHS. 1989. Snake acetylcholine receptor: cloning of the domain containing the four extracellular cysteines of the α-subunit. Proc. Natl. Acad. Sci. U.S.A. **86:** 7255–7259.
2. BARCHAN, D., S. KACHALSKY, D. NEUMANN, Z. VOGEL, M. OVADIA, E. KOCHVA & S. FUCHS. 1992. How the mongoose can fight the snake: the binding site of the mongoose acetylcholine receptor. Proc. Natl. Acad. Sci. U.S.A. **89:** 7717–7721.
3. BARCHAN, D., M. OVADIA, E. KOCHVA & S. FUCHS. 1995. The binding site of the nicotinic acetylcholine receptor in animal species resistant to α-bungarotoxin. Biochemistry **34:** 9172–9176.

4. KACHALSKY, S. G., B. S. JENSEN, D. BARCHAN & S. FUCHS. 1995. Two subsites in the binding domain of the acetylcholine receptor: an aromatic subsite and a proline subsite. Proc. Natl. Acad. Sci. U.S.A. **92:** 10801–10805.
5. BALASS, M., E. KATCHALSKI-KATZIR & S. FUCHS. 1997. The α-bungarotoxin binding site on the nicotinic acetylcholine receptor: analysis using a phage-epitope library. Proc. Natl. Acad. Sci. U.S.A. **94:** 6054–6058.

How Does the Mongoose Cope with α-Bungarotoxin?

Analysis of the Mongoose Muscle AChR α-Subunit

ORNA ASHER,[a] MONICA LUPU-MEIRI,[b] BO S. JENSEN,[a]
TAMAR PAPERNA,[a] YORAM ORON,[b] AND SARA FUCHS[a]

[a]Department of Immunology
Weizmann Institute of Science
Rehovot 76100, Israel

[b]Department of Physiology and Pharmacology
Sackler Faculty of Medicine
Tel Aviv University
Ramat Aviv 69978, Israel

The muscle acetylcholine receptor (AChR) α-subunit has been cloned from the mongoose. This subunit is highly homologous to the mouse and rat AChR α-subunits, with only six differences in amino-acid residues at positions that are conserved in animal species that bind α-bungarotoxin (α-BTX). Four of these six substitutions cluster in the ligand binding site and, of these four, Asn-187 forms a putative N-glycosylation site. The mongoose α-subunit cRNA was injected together with the rat β-, γ-, and δ-subunit cRNAs into *Xenopus* oocytes. Oocytes expressing this mongoose/rat AChR hybrid bind α-BTX with 200 times lower affinity than oocytes expressing the rat receptor and, on the other hand, exhibit a higher apparent affinity to ACh (EC_{50} of 1.3 ± 0.3 μM) than that of the rat AChR (EC_{50} of 23.3 ± 2.1 μM). Thus, it appears that both the decreased affinity of the mongoose AChR to α-BTX and the increased affinity to ACh contribute to the toxin resistance of the mongoose.

RESULTS AND DISCUSSION

For the analysis of the binding site of muscle AChR, and in particular for elucidating the structural requirements for α-BTX binding, our lab has been studying AChRs from animal species that are resistant to α-BTX, such as the snake,[1] mongoose,[2] and hedgehog.[3] We have previously cloned, sequenced, and expressed a 250-bp fragment corresponding to amino-acid residues 122–205 of the AChR α-subunit from these three species as well as from the mouse. We have now cloned and sequenced the entire mongoose AChR α-subunit gene and have analyzed its glycosylation potential and the ligand binding properties of the corresponding translated protein.

The mongoose AChR α-subunit cDNA has been amplified by PCR on mongoose muscle cDNA, cloned into pBluescript, and sequenced. This AChR α-subunit clone has an open reading frame of 1374 bp, which translates to form a protein of 437 residues. Alignment of the amino-acid sequence of the mongoose α-subunit with those of the mouse and rat α-subunits shows 93% and 92% homology with these two species, respectively. There are only six differences in amino-acid residues in the mongoose α-subunit, at positions that are conserved in animal species that are sensitive to α-BTX. These six differences include four residues within the binding site domain at positions 187 (Trp to Asn), 189 (Phe to Thr), 194 (Pro to Leu), and 197 (Pro to His), and two others at positions 112 (Tyr to His) and 153 (Gly to Ser). Five of these six substitutions (153, 187, 189, 194, and 197) are within the previously cloned 250-bp fragment (corresponding to residues 122–205 of the mongoose α-subunit; see reference 2), and only one additional difference at a conserved position (112) has been identified, following the cloning of the entire α-subunit. Asn-187 in the mongoose α-subunit is a putative N-glycosylation site, in addition to the single N-glycosylation site (Asn-141), which is present in all muscle AChR α-subunits.

To follow the glycosylation pattern of the mongoose α-subunit, *in vitro* translation was carried out in the presence of canine microsomal membranes that allow glycosylation to take place. Indeed, when *in vitro* translation was carried out in the presence of microsomes, the glycosylated mongoose α-subunit displayed a higher apparent molecular mass of 46 kDa and an additional band at 44 kDa, whereas the glycosylated form of the rat α-subunit yielded only a band of a molecular mass of 44 kDa. The higher molecular mass of the glycosylated mongoose α-subunit (46 kDa) is most likely due to an additional glycosylation at position 187. *In vitro* translation products of the mongoose and rat α-subunit have been applied onto α-BTX-Sepharose columns. The mongoose α-subunit protein did not adsorb to the α-BTX column, whereas the rat α-subunit did adsorb to such a column. These results indicate that the *in vitro* translated α-subunit of the mongoose AChR, even in its nonglycosylated form, does not bind to α-BTX and that glycosylation within the binding site by itself may not be essential for determining the resistance to α-BTX. Nevertheless, it is possible that, in the intact animal, this glycosylation is an important factor in defining the level of resistance to α-BTX and provides an additional protection against the toxin.

Mongoose/rat AChR hybrid has been expressed in *Xenopus* oocytes following injection of cRNAs encoding the mongoose α-subunit together with rat β-, γ-, and δ-subunits. For comparison, wild-type rat AChR was expressed following injection of cRNAs encoding the rat α-, β-, γ-, and δ-subunits. ACh-induced currents were measured at different ACh concentrations (FIGURE 1). At all ACh concentrations, the amplitudes of the currents for the mongoose/rat AChR were higher than those observed in oocytes expressing the rat AChR. The dose-response curves revealed that the mongoose/rat hybrid has a higher apparent affinity to ACh than that of the rat AChR. The EC_{50} values of ACh for the rat AChR and for the mongoose/rat AChR are 23.3 ± 2.1 μM and 1.3 ± 0.3 μM, respectively (TABLE 1).

To analyze the interaction of α-BTX with the mongoose/rat AChR hybrid, we measured the effect of α-BTX on the ACh-induced currents. Oocytes expressing the mongoose/rat hybrid or the rat AChR were incubated for 20 minutes in various α-BTX concentrations, the ACh-induced currents were recorded, and the inhibition by α-BTX was calculated (FIGURE 2). The ACh concentrations employed were 1 μM

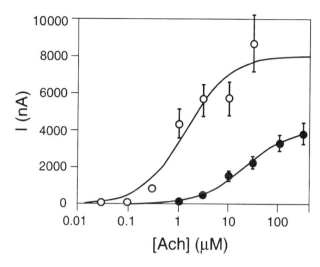

FIGURE 1. ACh dose-response curves for mongoose/rat hybrid AChR and for rat AChR. Oocytes were injected with mongoose α-subunit together with rat β-, γ-, and δ-subunit cRNAs (mongoose/rat hybrid), or with rat α-, β-, γ-, and δ-subunit cRNAs, and assayed after 3 days. ACh at the indicated concentrations was added and the peak current, at a holding potential of –60 to –40 mV, was recorded. The points represent the mean ± SEM ($n \geq 10$) current amplitudes for the mongoose/rat hybrid (○) and rat (●) AChR, respectively.

and 10 μM for the mongoose/rat hybrid and the rat AChR, respectively, and they approximately correspond to the EC_{50} for each of the receptors, calculated from the dose-response curve (FIGURE 1 and TABLE 1). The affinity of the mongoose/rat AChR to α-BTX is about 200 times lower than the affinity of the rat AChR (IC_{50} of 80.4 ± 15.7 and 0.4 ± 0.1 nM for the mongoose/rat and rat AChR, respectively). Thus, the affinity for α-BTX is markedly decreased, while the affinity for ACh is increased in the mongoose. This may give a much better chance for ACh to compete with α-BTX for the receptor under equilibrium binding conditions. This advantage is even greater under nonequilibrium conditions, the conditions usually observed in the nicotinic synapse.

TABLE 1. Response of Oocytes Expressing AChRs to ACh and α-BTX[a]

cRNAs Injected	EC_{50} (μM)	I_{max} (μA)	IC_{50} (nM)
$\alpha_M\beta\gamma\delta_R$	1.3 ± 0.3	6.6 ± 0.7	80.4 ± 15.7
$\alpha\beta\gamma\delta_R$	23.3 ± 2.1	4.0 ± 0.1	0.4 ± 0.1

[a]The calculated values of EC_{50} and I_{max} for ACh and of IC_{50} for α-BTX were obtained from experiments described in FIGURES 1 and 2.

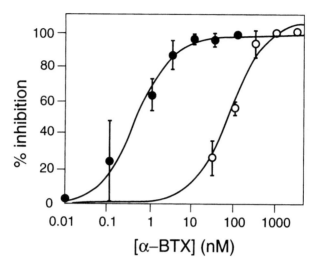

FIGURE 2. Inhibition of AChR currents by α-BTX in oocytes. Oocytes expressing mongoose/rat AChR hybrid or wild-type rat AChR were exposed for 20 min to the indicated concentrations of α-BTX. Responses to 10 μM and 1 μM ACh (for the rat and the mongoose/rat hybrid AChR, respectively) were measured. The results are presented as the mean ± SEM ($n \geq$ 5) percent inhibition when compared to controls without α-BTX. Symbols: (○) mongoose/rat hybrid AChR; (●) rat AChR.

REFERENCES

1. NEUMANN, D., D. BARCHAN, M. HOROWITZ, E. KOCHVA & S. FUCHS. 1989. Snake acetylcholine receptor: cloning of the domain containing the four extracellular cysteines of the α-subunit. Proc. Natl. Acad. Sci. U.S.A. **86:** 7255–7259.
2. BARCHAN, D., S. KACHALSKY, D. NEUMANN, Z. VOGEL, M. OVADIA, E. KOCHVA & S. FUCHS. 1992. How the mongoose can fight the snake: the binding site of the mongoose acetylcholine receptor. Proc. Natl. Acad. Sci. U.S.A. **89:** 7717–7721.
3. BARCHAN, D., M. OVADIA, E. KOCHVA & S. FUCHS. 1995. The binding site of the nicotinic acetylcholine receptor in animal species resistant to α-bungarotoxin. Biochemistry **34:** 9172–9176.

MAb 383C Binds to the α-Subunit of the Acetylcholine Receptor Associated with the High-Affinity Tubocurarine Site

MIKE Y. LIN,[a] GEORGE M. TWADDLE, ESWARI GUDIPATI,[b]
DAVID P. RICHMAN, AND ROBERT H. FAIRCLOUGH

Department of Neurology
University of California, Davis
Davis, California 95616

INTRODUCTION

The antiacetylcholine monoclonal antibody 383C (383C) binds to the membrane-bound acetylcholine receptor (AChR) and blocks all α-bungarotoxin (α-Btx) and 50% of carbamoylcholine binding.[1] However, binding of α-Btx or carbamoylcholine to the AChR completely inhibits the binding of 383C to the AChR.[1,2] 383C binds to the α-subunit(s) of the AChR in Western blots, and the binding stoichiometry of both 383C and its Fab fragments to the membrane-embedded AChR is one IgG/Fab per two toxin sites and one IgG/Fab per two anti-MIR MAb 132A sites. Here, we investigate which α-subunit of membrane-embedded AChR the 383C binds to: the α-subunit associated with the high-affinity *d*-tubocurarine (dTc) site or the α-subunit associated with the low-affinity dTc site.

METHODS

dTc Titration of AChR-embedded Membranes

Nonalkali-stripped AChR-enriched membranes were prepared from *Torpedo californica* using a modification of the procedure previously described.[2] The resulting membrane preparation was characterized using a modified Lowry protein assay and a centrifugation toxin site assay using rhodamine-labeled α-Btx (R-Btx). The membrane preparation was further characterized by dTc titration, monitored by the inhibition of R-Btx binding: AChR/dTc complexes formed by preincubating 18 pmol of toxin sites with increasing concentrations of dTc were incubated with 10-fold excess of R-Btx. After separating the membrane complexes from unbound ligands via airfuge ultracentrifugation, the pellets were resuspended in SDS/borate and the rhodamine-fluorescent emissions were quantitated.

[a]Supported by the Myasthenia Gravis Foundation through a Henry R. Viets Summer Fellowship.
[b]Supported by the Myasthenia Gravis Foundation through a Kermit G. Osserman Postdoctoral Fellowship for the academic year 1994–1995.

Titration of the AChR α-Subunit Associated with the High-Affinity dTc Site with 383C

Via an ELISA, one can characterize 383C binding to the AChR-enriched membranes with and without α-Btx bound to the low-affinity dTc site. To selectively bind fluorescein-labeled α-Btx (F-Btx) to the AChR α-subunit associated with the low-affinity dTc site, membrane-bound AChR was adsorbed onto a 96-well microtiter plate and preincubated with 5×10^{-6} M dTc and incubated with 1×10^{-7} M F-Btx in 5×10^{-6} M dTc, followed by washing with PBS. ELISA titrations were subsequently performed using 383C, antifluorescein MAb 147, and anti-MIR MAb 132A. The titrations were then analyzed with the Softmax® ELISA curve-fitting program.

RESULTS AND DISCUSSION

The dTc titration of AChR using R-BTX was biphasic, indicating two dTc affinities to the AChR (FIGURE 1). ELISA titration of the toxin/membrane complex with

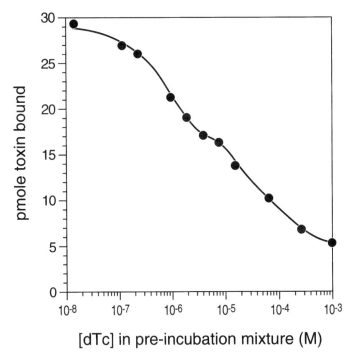

[dTc] in pre-incubation mixture (M)

FIGURE 1. dTc titration of membrane-bound AChR monitored by the inhibition of R-Btx binding: AChR/dTc complexes formed by preincubating membrane-bound AChR with increasing concentrations of dTc were incubated with 10-fold excess of R-Btx. After separation of the membrane complexes from unbound ligands, the rhodamine emission was quantitated.

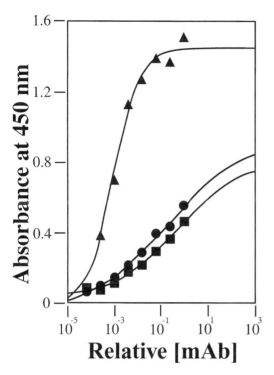

FIGURE 2. ELISA titrations of membrane-bound AChR adsorbed onto a 96-well microtiter plate: (■) F-Btx/AChR complex titrated with MAb 383C; (●) nontreated AChR titrated with MAb 383C; (▲) F-Btx/AChR complex titrated with anti-MIR MAb 132A.

antifluorescein MAb 147 in the presence of 5×10^{-6} M dTc revealed a plateau value slightly greater than one-half the value obtained for F-Btx binding in the absence of dTc.[2] This indicates successful covering of the low-affinity dTc site by F-Btx. The same toxin/membrane complex, when titrated with 383C, reveals a plateau value that is virtually the same with or without F-Btx covering the low-affinity dTc site (FIGURE 2). In addition, the 383C titration curve in the presence of F-Btx is shifted to higher 383C concentrations by 0.35 log units. This suggests that the 383C/AChR/α-Btx complexes are characterized by a K_d value that is approximately 3.5 times the K_d value for 383C/AChR complexes. Hence, the AChR/383C complex is weakened slightly by α-Btx binding to the low-affinity dTc site, but binding of 383C still occurs at the α-subunit associated with the high-affinity dTc site.

REFERENCES

1. MIHOVILOVIC, M. & D. P. RICHMAN. 1987. Monoclonal antibodies as probes of the α-bungarotoxin and cholinergic binding regions of the acetylcholine receptor. J. Biol. Chem. **262:** 4978–4986.
2. FAIRCLOUGH, R. H., G. M. TWADDLE, E. GUDIPATI, M. Y. LIN & D. P. RICHMAN. 1997. Differential surface accessibility of $\alpha(187–199)$ in the *Torpedo* acetylcholine receptor α-subunit. J. Mol. Biol. Submitted.

Distance between α-Cys 192 of the Acetylcholine Receptor and Rhodamine-labeled α-Bungarotoxin Complexed to the Receptor

ESWARI GUDIPATI,[a,b] LAURA SILVIAN,[c] VISWANATHAM KATTA,[d] AND ROBERT H. FAIRCLOUGH[b]

[b]Department of Neurology
University of California, Davis
Davis, California 95616

[c]Department of Molecular Biophysics and Biochemistry
Yale University
New Haven, Connecticut 06520

[d]Division of Protein Structure
Amgen Incorporated
Thousand Oaks, California 91320

INTRODUCTION

The nicotinic acetylcholine receptor (AChR) from *Torpedo californica* is an integral-membrane five-subunit protein that contains two copies of the α-subunit. Each α-subunit, when separated from the other subunits, can bind α-bungarotoxin (α-Btx).[1] Residues 185–190 of the α-subunit interact directly with α-Btx as demonstrated by NMR spectroscopy.[2] However, the toxin contacts other residues as well in complexes with the receptor.[3]

Each α-subunit contains a unique disulfide between residues Cys 192 and Cys 193,[4] which upon mild reduction with DTT can react with bromoacetylcholine.[5] This reaction occurs far more readily at the α-subunit associated with the high-affinity tubocurarine site than that associated with the low-affinity site.[6,7] We have observed similar selective alkylation of one of the two AChR α-subunits with iodoacetamidofluorescein (IAF), whose site of reactivity has been mapped to α-Cys 192/Cys 193.[8]

In addition, we have labeled Lys 51 and Lys 70 of α-Btx with the hydroxysuccinimide ester of 5-(and 6-)carboxytetramethylrhodamine (R-Btx).[8] The isomer mixture in R-Btx contained 50% unlabeled, 35% singly labeled, and 15% doubly labeled α-Btx as determined by mass spectrometry.

To measure the distance between receptor-bound α-Btx and α-Cys 192–193 of the AChR α-subunit, we used resonance energy transfer between the fluorescein on IAF-labeled AChR (F-AChR) and the rhodamines on AChR-bound R-Btx.

[a]Supported by the Myasthenia Gravis Foundation through a Kermit G. Osserman Postdoctoral Fellowship for the academic year 1994–1995.

RESULTS

The emission spectrum of F-AChR in *Torpedo* Ringer's buffer was recorded (FIG-
URE 1) followed by the addition of a threefold excess of the isomer mix of R-Btx, and
the fluorescein spectrum was recorded a second time after a one-hour incubation.
The control experiment recorded the fluorescein emission after a one-hour incubation of unlabeled α-Btx. The energy transfer result observed was an average transfer
efficiency of $E = 0.069$. This small transfer efficiency with the particular mixture of
rhodamine-labeled α-Btx isomers translates into a measured distance of 77 ± 17 Å
between the fluorescein and rhodamine dyes. The ± 17 Å results primarily from the
Dale-Eisinger[9] limits imposed on the R_0 of 55 Å by the measured limiting anisotropy
of the fluorescein and rhodamine emissions in the AChR/Btx complex.

DISCUSSION

The observed transfer efficiency of 0.069 between the fluorescein on α-Cys
192/193 and the rhodamines attached to Lys 51 and/or Lys 70 of α-Btx is quite small.
The incorporation of fluorescein into the receptor of 3.7 pmol/μg was comparable to
the toxin binding specific activity of 3 pmol/μg. Furthermore, the dye labeling of the
receptor did not alter the toxin binding specific activity to any measurable extent.

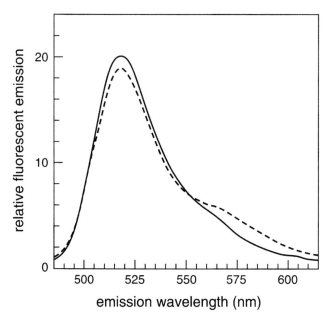

FIGURE 1. Fluorescence emission spectra of IAF-labeled, alkali-stripped, AChR-enriched
membranes in the presence of α-Btx (——) and R-Btx (– – –). Fluorescence was excited at 480
nm.

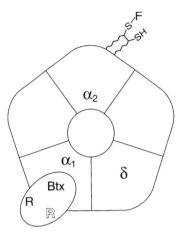

FIGURE 2. The distance measured between the fluorescein and rhodamine dyes of 77 ± 17 Å is the same as the entire distance across the AChR rosette. The fluorescein is covalently attached at Cys 192/Cys 193 to the peptide loop 187–199 and α-Btx is modified at Lys 51 and Lys 70 with rhodamine. The distance is consistent with the fluorescein being attached to the α-subunit that is across the rosette from the one that is binding R-Btx.

The measured distance of 77 ± 17 Å with the 40-Å-long dimension of the toxin suggested that R-Btx is not binding to the α-subunit labeled with fluorescein. If it were binding, one would expect with the 55-Å R_0 to observe substantial transfer efficiency at least on the order of 0.25–0.3 with the labeling statistics of the R-Btx sample used in this experiment. The distance measured in this experiment, 77 ± 17 Å, between the fluorescein and the sites on the α-Btx labeled with rhodamine, Lys 51 and Lys 70, means that both these residues are at the far reaches of the receptor/toxin complex from the fluorescein label on α-Cys 192/193 as indicated in FIGURE 2.

REFERENCES

1. GERSHONI, J. M., E. HAWROT & T. L. LENTZ. 1983. Binding of α-bungarotoxin to isolated α-subunits of the acetylcholine receptor of *Torpedo californica*: quantitative analysis with protein blots. Proc. Natl. Acad. Sci. U.S.A. **80:** 4973–4977.
2. BASUS, V. J., G. SONG & E. HAWROT. 1993. NMR solution structure of an alpha-bungarotoxin/nicotinic receptor peptide complex. Biochemistry **32:** 12290–12298.
3. HAMILTON, S. L., D. R. PRATT & D. C. EATON. 1985. Arrangement of the subunits of the nicotinic acetylcholine receptor of *Torpedo californica* as determined by α-neurotoxin cross-linking. Biochemistry **24:** 2210–2219.
4. KAO, P. N. & A. KARLIN. 1986. Acetylcholine receptor binding site contains a disulfide crosslink between adjacent half-cystinyl residues. J. Biol. Chem. **261:** 8085–8088.
5. MOORE, H-P. H. & M. A. RAFTERY. 1979. Studies of reversible and irreversible interactions of an alkylating agonist with *Torpedo californica* acetylcholine receptor in membrane-bound and purified states. Biochemistry **18:** 1862–1867.
6. RATNAM, M., W. GULLICK, J. SPIESS, K. WAN, M. CRIADO & J. LINDSTROM. 1986. Structural heterogeneity of the α subunits of the nicotinic acetylcholine receptor in relation to agonist affinity alkylation and antagonist binding. Biochemistry **25:** 4268–4275.
7. PEDERSEN, S. E., E. B. DREYER & J. B. COHEN. 1986. Location of ligand-binding sites on the nicotinic acetylcholine receptor α-subunit. J. Biol. Chem. **261:** 13735–13743.

8. GUDIPATI, E., L. SILVIAN, V. KATTA & R. H. FAIRCLOUGH. 1998. The distance between fluorescein labeled α-Cys 192 of the acetylcholine receptor and isomers of rhodamine labeled α-bungarotoxin complexed to the receptor. In preparation.
9. DALE, R. E. & J. EISINGER. 1975. Polarized excitation energy transfer. *In* Biochemical Fluorescence: Concepts. Volume I, chapter 4, p. 115–284. Dekker. New York.

Measurement of the Dissociation Rate Constants of α-Bungarotoxin from the Acetylcholine Receptor Low- and High-Affinity Tubocurarine Sites

MIKE Y. LIN,[a] GEORGE M. TWADDLE, ESWARI GUDIPATI,[b]
AND ROBERT H. FAIRCLOUGH

Department of Neurology
University of California, Davis
Davis, California 95616

INTRODUCTION

α-Bungarotoxin (α-Btx) binds to acetylcholine receptor (AChR)–enriched membranes as well as to detergent-solubilized AChR. Affinity-purified AChR binds α-Btx with a specific activity of 7.2–7.4 pmol of toxin/μg of protein, which translates to two toxin sites per AChR. One site binds the toxin with an association rate constant of 10^6 M^{-1} s^{-1}, whereas the other site binds the toxin with a rate constant of 10^5 M^{-1} s^{-1}. Triton X-100–solubilized AChR appears to bind the toxin irreversibly, whereas membrane-bound AChR is reported to bind the toxin in two modes: reversibly and irreversibly.[1] To further characterize the toxin binding sites on membrane-bound AChR, we have loaded rhodamine-labeled α-Btx (R-Btx) at the toxin site correlated with the low-affinity *d*-tubocurarine (dTc) binding site and fluorescein-labeled α-Btx (F-Btx) at the correlate of the high-affinity dTc site. We then isolated the doubly labeled complexes and monitored the release of each of the fluorescent toxins in the presence of excess unlabeled toxin as a function of time.

METHODS

F-Btx and R-Btx were prepared using the hydroxysuccinimide ester of 5- and 6-carboxyl derivatives of fluorescein and tetramethylrhodamine. The dye:α-Btx ratios were close to 1:1 for both derivatives. Four hundred eighty-five pmol of toxin sites of a 4-month-old nonalkali-stripped membrane preparation[2] was preincubated with dTc for 30 minutes followed by the addition of R-Btx. The concentrations of toxin sites, dTc, and R-Btx after the addition of R-Btx were 9×10^{-8} M, 9×10^{-6} M, and 2.4×10^{-7} M, respectively. The resulting membrane complex was separated from unbound ligands by ultracentrifugation using a Beckman SW55Ti rotor at 28,600 rpm. The pellet was

[a]Supported by the Myasthenia Gravis Foundation through a Henry R. Viets Summer Fellowship.
[b]Supported by the Myasthenia Gravis Foundation through a Kermit G. Osserman Postdoctoral Fellowship for the academic year 1994–1995.

then resuspended in a solution containing 3×10^{-7} M F-Btx. As indicated in FIGURE 1, this selectively puts R-Btx on the AChR α-subunit associated with the low-affinity dTc site and F-Btx on the AChR α-subunit associated with the high-affinity dTc site. The R-Btx/F-Btx/AChR complex was again separated from the unbound ligands by ultracentrifugation, and the pellet was resuspended in a solution containing 10-fold excess of unlabeled α-Btx. At various times over the next 3 days, the amount of each fluorescent derivative left in the complex was assayed by removing a 200-μL aliquot from the incubating mixture and immediately pelleting the membrane/toxin complex using airfuge ultracentrifugation. The resulting pellet was resuspended in 2.0 mL SDS/borate, followed by recording the fluorescent emission intensity of the two dyes. Fluorescein was excited using 494-nm light and its emission at 516 nm was recorded; rhodamine was excited using 550-nm light and its emission at 575 nm was recorded. The kinetic data were plotted as log emission versus time and the curve fitted using Delta Graph®. The slopes of the linear plots were obtained from a least-squares fit of the data to $f(t) = C \cdot e^{(-k \cdot t)}$, and τ was calculated by taking the inverse of the rate constant, k.

RESULTS AND DISCUSSION

The kinetic data illustrated in FIGURE 2 show that α-Btx dissociates very slowly from both sites on the membrane-bound AChR, but that two dissociation rates are distinguishable. Single exponential decay analysis of the rhodamine component gives a first-order rate constant of 3.76×10^{-2} days^{-1}, which corresponds to a complex lifetime of 26.6 days. Similarly, single exponential decay analysis of the fluorescein component gives a first-order rate constant of 8.54×10^{-2} days^{-1}, which corresponds to a complex lifetime of 11.7 days.

These values indicate that toxin binding to the receptor in our hands is irreversible at both sites. This is in accord with the findings of Conti-Tronconi *et al.*[1] demonstrating that a membrane preparation loses the reversible toxin binding site subsequent to

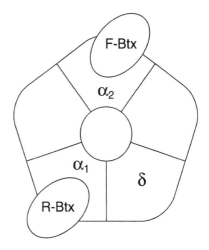

FIGURE 1. A representation of the acetylcholine receptor molecule viewed from the synaptic side with borders arbitrarily drawn between subunits. The loadings of F-Btx and R-Btx on the α-subunit associated with the respective high- and low-affinity dTc sites are shown.

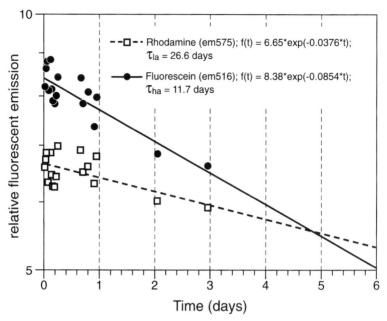

FIGURE 2. Semilog kinetic plot of rhodamine and fluorescein emission remaining in complex at time t. The dissociation of Btx from the two sites is slow, but distinguishable.

incubation at 4 °C. The double labeling of the receptor/toxin complex using two fluorescent bungarotoxin derivatives has enabled us to differentiate the two seemingly irreversible toxin sites. Each fluorescent derivative appears to be displaced slowly by unlabeled α-Btx. However, the F-Btx at the correlate of the high-affinity dTc site dissociates more rapidly than the R-Btx at the correlate of the low-affinity dTc site. This is just the reverse of what one would expect if the toxin/receptor complexes followed the same stability paradigm as the two dTc complexes on the AChR.

Previously, we investigated the ability of both R-Btx and F-Btx to compete with unlabeled α-Btx for binding to the AChR. Both derivatives compete equally well with unlabeled α-Btx. We are currently investigating the dissociation kinetics of the complexes produced by switching the two labeled α-Btx derivatives with respect to the two dTc sites.

REFERENCES

1. CONTI-TRONCONI, B. M., F. TANG, S. WALGRAVE & W. GALLAGHER. 1990. Nonequivalence of α-bungarotoxin binding sites in the native nicotinic receptor molecule. Biochemistry **29:** 1046–1054.
2. FAIRCLOUGH, R. H., G. M. TWADDLE, E. GUDIPATI, M. Y. LIN & D. P. RICHMAN. 1997. Differential surface accessibility of α(187–199) in the *Torpedo* AChR α-subunit. J. Mol. Biol. Submitted.

Control of Gene Expression of Human Muscle Acetylcholine Receptor[a]

P. P. NICHOLS AND D. M. W. BEESON

Neurosciences Group
Institute of Molecular Medicine
John Radcliffe Hospital
University of Oxford
Oxford OX3 9DS, United Kingdom

INTRODUCTION

The development of the mature mammalian nicotinic acetylcholine receptor (AChR) at the neuromuscular junction (NMJ) involves the coordinated transcriptional expression of the five AChR subunits (α, β, γ, δ, and ϵ). Any hypothesis to explain this process must address the transcriptional changes occurring at three stages (see below).

First, myoblast fusion to myotubes and fetal AChR expression: Prior to myotube formation, AChR subunit mRNAs are only expressed at low levels in undifferentiated myoblasts. Following myoblast fusion, fetal AChR is expressed along the entire length of the myotube. The evidence suggests that this change involves the binding of myogenic regulatory factors (MRF) of the MyoD family (MyoD, myf5, myogenin, and MRF4) to specific nucleotide target sequences, called E boxes (-CANNTG-), in the promoter regions of the AChR subunits. The MyoD proteins are helix-loop-helix (HLH) DNA-binding proteins involved in the activation of many muscle-specific genes and they play a key role in skeletal myogenesis.

Transfection experiments in animals using constructs containing the five AChR subunit promoter regions cloned into expression vectors have shown that each contains control sequences defining muscle-specific expression and that, in the α, β, γ, and δ promoters, this function is E box–dependent. In the species that have been studied (rat/mouse) the ϵ promoters also contain E boxes that bind myogenic factors, but are not involved in the control of the level of expression in muscle. Mutation of the ϵ promoter E boxes in the rat leads to expression in nonmuscle tissue, suggesting that E boxes can act as sites of both negative and positive regulation.

Second, the effect of electrical activity on AChR transcription: If adult skeletal muscle is denervated, fetal AChRs reappear in the extrasynaptic membrane. If then stimulated by reinnervation or artificial chronic electrical stimulation, they are lost again. Hybridization and nuclear run-on experiments have shown an increase in AChR subunit mRNA transcription following muscle denervation and have confirmed earlier work showing that electrical activity affects transcriptional control.

[a]This work was supported by the Medical Research Council and the Myasthenia Gravis Association of Great Britain.

111

Studies using promoter expression constructs (α chick, δ mouse) in transfected muscle cell cultures and transgenic mice demonstrated that electrical activity–dependent gene expression is also E box–dependent. The mechanism of control is thought to involve the MyoD family, in particular myogenin, whose levels change in parallel with that of AChR subunit mRNA; that is, during postnatal mouse and rat development, the level of myogenin mRNA decreases rapidly in parallel with the α subunit mRNA and rises again in parallel on denervation.[1]

Third, increased synthesis of adult AChR at the NMJ: Maturation from fetal ($\alpha_2\beta\gamma\delta$) to adult AChR ($\alpha_2\beta\epsilon\delta$) involves localized upregulation of mRNA transcription and a switch from γ to ϵ subunit expression. Experiments using AChR promoter expression constructs in transgenic mice and muscle cultures have shown that the upregulation in subunit transcription is tightly restricted to subsynaptic nuclei and is independent of E boxes in the subunits studied (mouse δ and ϵ).[2,3] Another promoter nucleotide target sequence called an N box (-TTCCGG-) has been proposed as the site for regulation of synapse-specific expression of the AChR subunits. Preliminary evidence using mouse δ and ϵ promoter expression constructs suggests that mutation of N box regions leads to disruption of normal subunit expression at the synapse.[4,5] This is unlikely to be the whole story since a recent study showed that ARIA (heregulin β1) induces mouse ϵ expression via a promoter sequence called an ARE element (ARIA responsive element),[6] which is close to, but distinct from, the N box. The transcription factors acting at the level of the N box or ARE element have not yet been identified. Further complicating the picture is evidence to suggest that an agrin-mediated pathway may also increase ϵ subunit expression.[7]

THE HUMAN NICOTINIC AChR PROMOTER REGIONS

Prior to this study, all the investigations into AChR transcriptional control were based on animal models. To investigate the transcriptional control of the human nicotinic AChR, the promoter regions of human α, β, γ, δ, and ϵ subunit genes were subcloned and a minimum of 735 nucleotides upstream of the translation initiation site were sequenced (EMBL database accession numbers: β, δ, γ Z79610–12; α Z82984; and ϵ Z84811). Transcriptional control target sequences were then compared with those identified in other species. In animal studies, it has been noted that not all E boxes in any given promoter region are required for full activation of transcription. The E boxes closest to the transcription start site are, in general, the most important. This probably reflects the fact that it is not only the presence of the -CANNTG- nucleotide sequence, but also the surrounding nucleotides that are required for MyoD factor binding and transcriptional activation. With this in mind, the E boxes and contiguous areas of the human promoter sequences have been compared with those regions known to be important in muscle-specific transcriptional regulation in animals (FIGURE 1). E boxes and contiguous areas present in the α, β, γ, and δ subunit promoters show over 75% sequence identity between human and rat/mouse/chick. The relative positions of the "control" E boxes are highly conserved across the species studied, consistent with their role in muscle-specific transcriptional regulation. One E box in the ϵ promoter is highly conserved between species, human/rat/mouse, con-

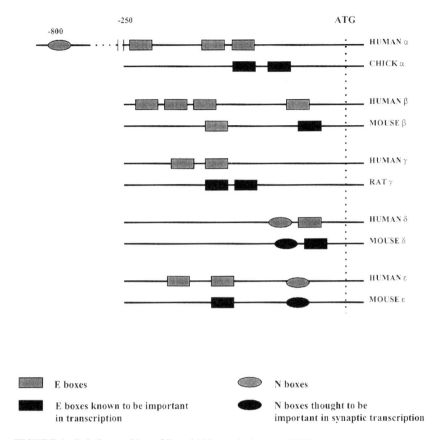

FIGURE 1. Relative position of E and N boxes in human AChR promoter sequences compared with reported animal sequences.

sistent with a suggested role in restricting expression to muscle. N box regions are present in the α, δ, and ε promoters, but not in the γ. This further implicates the N box in the regulation of synaptic expression and the switch from fetal to adult AChR. Comparing the region overlapping the N box and ARE element in the mouse ε promoter with the human sequence, there is a striking degree of conservation, emphasizing the importance of this region in interactions leading to transcription initiation (FIGURE 2).

This initial study suggests that transcriptional regulation of the human AChR will closely mimic that seen in other species and will involve a differential mechanism of extrasynaptic expression based around E box regulation and synaptic expression probably based on a number of different interacting transcription factors binding to regions including the N box, the ARE element, and several areas and regulatory pathways as yet undefined.

```
                  ·                 ·        E box    ·                ·                  ·
gggcaggaaacacaggatggggcagctgcctctggaagcagccaaaatgt
 |  |  |         | | | | | | | | | | | | | | | | | | | |                          |
ggg . . . . . . acacaggatggggcagctgcc . . . . . . . . . . . . . . . accc
   ,      E box   ·                  ·                ·                ·                ·
cccagctgcagcaggggtgagcagaggattaggtgacagtcccctaac.
 | |  |   |    | | | | | | | | | |        | | | | | | | | | |·| | | | | | | | | | | | |   | | |
ccacccccacagcaggggt . . . cagaggattaggtgacagtccccaaacc
                     ARE     ·                    ·                ·                ·
.agcccggaactaacaccctcctcccctcacacaggcaccctggcatgc
 | | | | | | | | | | | | | | | | | | | | | | | | | | | | | | | | | |  | | | | | | | | | | | | | |  |  | |   | |
tagcccggaactaacaccctcctccccttcacacaggcacctttgcctgt
              N box          ▲      Transcription start site                      ·                ·
cccctccaagcctgccagagctcagaataaccctgagaaccacgcagcag
 | | | |   | | | | |   | |    | |   | | | | | | | | | | | |   | | | | | | | | | |     | |   | | |
tccct.caagcttgtcaaagctcagaataa.cctgagaaccagacatcag


gATG   Human ε
 | | | |
gatg   Mouse ε
```

FIGURE 2. Comparison of human and mouse ε promoter regions.

REFERENCES

1. DUCLERT, A. & J-P. CHANGEUX. 1995. Acetylcholine receptor gene expression at the developing neuromuscular junction. Physiol. Rev. **75:** 339–368.
2. TANG, J., S. A. JO & S. J. BURDEN. 1994. Separate pathways for synapse-specific and electrical activity–dependent gene expression in skeletal muscle. Development **120:** 1799–1804.
3. DUCLERT, A., N. SAVATIER & J-P. CHANGEUX. 1993. An 83-nucleotide promoter of the acetylcholine receptor ε-subunit gene confers preferential synaptic expression in mouse muscle. Proc. Natl. Acad. Sci. U.S.A. **90:** 3043–3047.
4. KOIKE, S., L. SCHAEFFER & J-P. CHANGEUX. 1995. Identification of a DNA element determining synaptic expression of the mouse acetylcholine receptor δ-subunit gene. Proc. Natl. Acad. Sci. U.S.A. **92:** 10624–10628.
5. DUCLERT, A., N. SAVATIER, L. SCHAEFFER et al. 1996. Identification of an element crucial for the sub-synaptic expression of the acetylcholine receptor ε-subunit gene. J. Biol. Chem. **271:** 17433–17438.
6. SI, J., D. S. MILLER & L. MEI. 1997. Identification of an element required for acetylcholine receptor–inducing activity (ARIA)–induced expression of the acetylcholine receptor ε subunit gene. J. Biol. Chem. **272:** 10367–10371.
7. JONES, G., A. HERCZEG, M. A. RUEGG et al. 1996. Substrate-bound agrin induces expression of acetylcholine receptor ε-subunit gene in cultured mammalian muscle cells. Proc. Natl. Acad. Sci. U.S.A. **93:** 5985–5990.

Isolation of Ca^{2+} Channel α_{1A}, α_2, and β Subunit Segments from Human Spinal Cord RNA[a]

RAVINDRA K. HAJELA AND WILLIAM D. ATCHISON[b]

Neuroscience Program
and
Department of Pharmacology and Toxicology
Michigan State University
East Lansing, Michigan 48824-1317

Voltage-gated Ca^{2+} channels play critical roles in neurotransmitter secretion from nerve terminals, providing a rapid influx of Ca^{2+} in response to an arriving action potential. The impairment of this stimulus secretion coupling at motor nerve terminals is thought to underlie the neuromuscular disorder, Lambert-Eaton myasthenic syndrome (LEMS).[1] Autoantibodies directed against Ca^{2+} channels are believed to disrupt release of acetylcholine (ACh) and cause the subsequent muscle weakness in LEMS.[1] We are interested in identifying and characterizing the types of Ca^{2+} channels of the human neuromuscular junction. Because it is not currently possible to isolate mammalian motor nerve terminals for biochemical characterization, we chose to isolate molecular clones of Ca^{2+} channels from human motor neurons for study via heterologous expression. These clones would include those for channels expressed at the nerve terminals.

Consensus sequences were culled from published nucleotide sequences of cDNA copies of various subunits of different subtypes of Ca^{2+} channels from mammalian neuronal tissue to synthesize polymerase chain reaction (PCR) primer pairs with 5′ extensions containing uracil residues to allow uracil DNA glycosylase–mediated cloning of amplified DNA[2] in pAMP1 (GIBCO-BRL Life Technologies). Reverse transcription followed by PCR (RTPCR) was performed on human fetal (18–20-week) spinal cord[c] RNA using these primers. Spinal cord was used as a source of template RNA because motor neuron soma and nuclei reside here and messenger RNA isolated from this tissue would include messages for proteins expressed at the nerve terminals.

The primers for the α_1 subunit were selected to amplify a segment of the α_{1A} that is thought to be expressed phenotypically in the P/Q-subtypes of Ca^{2+} channels. These subtypes have been shown to be responsible for ACh release at the mammalian neuromuscular junction.[3,4] These primers represented the 5′ and 3′ ends of the 343-nucleotide sequence isolated from a small cell lung carcinoma (SCLC) cell line.[5] An-

[a]This work was supported by NIH Grant No. NS 33006 and a travel grant to R. K. Hajela from the Detroit Chapter of the Myasthenia Gravis Association.

[b]To whom all correspondence should be addressed.

[c]Fetal spinal cord tissue was obtained from the Brain and Tissue Bank for Developmental Disorders, University of Maryland, Baltimore, Maryland.

tipeptide antibodies against the translated sequence blocked a current in SCLC cells that was also blocked by ω-agatoxin IVA, suggesting it to be a segment of a P/Q-type Ca^{2+} channel α_{1A} subunit.[5] The $\alpha_2\delta$ and β subunit primers were from conserved consensus regions designed to amplify unique regions in between.

We successfully amplified cDNA segments from human fetal spinal cord RNA using primers from α_{1A}, $\alpha_2\delta$, and β_3 subunits of voltage-gated Ca^{2+} channels (FIGURE 1). Similar RTPCR amplifications using these primers have also been performed on various tissues (brain, heart, lung, liver, and muscle) from human fetuses, as well as from rats, and similarly sized DNA fragments have been recovered. No DNA was amplified in controls in which reverse transcriptase was omitted from the cDNA synthesis reaction, assuring that the PCR product resulted from cDNA made from RNA in the reverse transcription step and not from any contaminating DNA. The RTPCR products were cloned in pAMP1; several recombinants were analyzed by restriction digestion and agarose gel electrophoresis as well as DNA sequencing from both ends. Almost all the clones were found to be identical to the others in each of the three groups corresponding to RTPCR performed using the α_1, $\alpha_2\delta$, or β subunit primers. BLASTN (basic local alignment search tool for nucleotides)[6] homology search was performed with nucleotide sequences in the databases available via NCBI (National Center for Biotechnology Information). The three segments showed a high degree of homology with sequences of the corresponding subunits of Ca^{2+} channels only. These results indicated that we have RTPCR-amplified and cloned pieces of cDNA corresponding to the α_1, $\alpha_2\delta$, and β subunits of Ca^{2+} subunits from human spinal cord RNA.

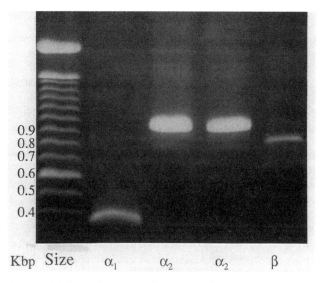

FIGURE 1. Agarose gel electropherogram of RTPCR products of a typical reaction using human fetal spinal cord RNA as template and primer pairs for the α_{1A} (lane 2), $\alpha_2\delta$ (lanes 3 and 4), or β subunit (lane 5). Lane 1 shows size markers in kbp.

```
α₁
pHA1-8     -----------  -----------  ...........  ...........  ...........  ...........  ..........        20
S76537     -----------  -----------  ...........  ...G.......  ...........  ...........  ..........        21
X99897     -----------  -----------  ...........  ...C.......  ...........  ...........  ..........      5100
Consensus  GGTTACACCA  TCCGCATTCT  TCTCTGGACC  TTTGTGCAGT  CCTTCAAGGC  CCTGSCTTAT  GTCTGTCTGC  TGATC      5100

pHA1-8     '          ...........  ...........  ...........  ...........  ...........  ..........        95
S76537     ...........  ...........  ...........  ...........  ...........  ...........  ..........        96
X99897     ...........  ...........  ...........  ...........  ...........  ...........  ..........      5175
Consensus  GCCATGCTCT  TCTTCATCTA  TGCCATCATT  GGGATGCAGG  TGTTTGGTAA  CATTGGCATC  GACGTGGAGG  ACGAG      5175

α₂
M21948     ...........  ........C..  ...TA.A..C  ...........  G.........  ...........  ..........      2154
M76559     ...........  ........A..  ..CG.G..T   ...........  T.........  ...........  ..........      2109
pHA2-1     ...........  ........A..  ..CG.G..T   ...........  T.........  ...........  ..........       311
Consensus  ACTCCAAACA  ACCCATCMTG  TAAYRCRGAY  TTGATTAATA  GAGTCTTGCT  KGATGCAGGC  TTTACAAATG  AACTT      2175

M21948     ..T.......  ...........  ......G...  ...........  ..G.......  ...........  ..........      2228
M76559     ..C.......  .....-.....  ......A...  ...........  ..A.......  ...........  ..:.......      2183
pHA2-1     ..C.......  ...........  ......-...  ...........  ..A.......  ...........  ---------       336
Consensus  GTYCAAAATT  ACTGGGAGTA  AGCAGAARAA  TATCAAGGGA  GTGAAAGCAC  GRTTTGTTGT  GACTGATGGT  GGGAT      2250

β
pHA3-1     -----------  -----------  ...........  ...C......  ...........  ..........        23
U07139     -----------  -----------  ...........  ...A......  ...........  ..........       525
Consensus  GAACCCTTCC  AGCCTGAGTG  ACATTGGCAA  CCGACGCTCC  CTCTMGCCAA  GCGAGAAGCAA  AGCA      525

pHA3-1     ...........  ...........  ...........  ...........  ...........  ..........        98
U07139     ...........  ...........  ...........  ...........  ...........  ..........       600
Consensus  GGCGGAACAT  GTTCCCCCAT  ATGACGTGGT  GCCCTCCATG  CGGCCTGTGG  TGCTGGTGGG  ACCCTCTCTG  AAAGG      600
```

FIGURE 2. Nucleotide sequence comparison of relevant regions of α_{1A} (pHA1-8), $\alpha_2\delta$ (pHA2-1), and β (pHA3-1) subunit segments cloned from human fetal spinal cord RNA with some corresponding rabbit and human sequences previously published. The only differences shown between pHA1-8 (a human SCLC cell line sequence) and X99897 (a human cerebellar sequence) result in inconsequential amino-acid changes. The pHA2-1 and M76559 (a human neuronal sequence) are identical; all the differences are with the rabbit skeletal muscle sequence M21948. The pHA3-1 and U07139 (a human fetal brain sequence) are essentially identical. The sequence differences in our pHA1-8 and pHA3-1 may also be PCR and/or cloning artifacts.

We next sequenced in from both ends to get an additional nucleotide sequence of cloned inserts and did alignments of the respective clones with α_1, $\alpha_2\delta$, or β subunit sequences from the NCBI databases. The 341-nucleotide α_1 segment clone pHA1-8 is essentially identical to a human SCLC clone[5] S776537 and the corresponding part of a human cerebellar clone[7] X99897, reported to be cDNAs encoding the P/Q-type α_1 subunit. We therefore conclude that we have isolated part of the cDNA of the α_{1A} type. The approximately 980-nucleotide $\alpha_2\delta$ segment clone pHA2-1 shows total identity with the corresponding part of M76559,[8] a human neuronal, and near identity with M21948,[9] a rabbit skeletal muscle cDNA sequence of the $\alpha_2\delta$ subunit, suggesting that we have isolated a part of the cDNA of this subunit. The approximately 890-nucleotide pHA3-1 also shows a very high degree of homology with U07139,[10] a human fetal brain novel β subunit cDNA (FIGURE 2).

Based on the above observations, we conclude that we have isolated fragments of an α_{1A}, an $\alpha_2\delta$, and a β subunit of a voltage-gated Ca^{2+} channel from human spinal cord using RTPCR. These clones are being used as homologous probes to isolate full-length copies of the cDNAs for these subunits that will be used for expression studies.

REFERENCES

1. SMITH, D. O., M. W. CONKLIN, P. J. JENSEN et al. 1995. Decreased calcium currents in motor nerve terminals of mice with Lambert-Eaton myasthenic syndrome. J. Physiol. (Lond.) **487:** 115–132.

2. NISSON, P. E., A. RASHTCHIAN & P. C. WATKINS. 1991. Rapid and efficient cloning of Alu-PCR products using uracil DNA glycosylase. PCR Methods Appl. **1:** 120–123.

3. UCHITEL, O. D., D. A. PROTTI, V. SANCHEZ et al. 1992. P-type voltage-dependent calcium channel mediates presynaptic calcium influx and transmitter release in mammalian synapses. Proc. Natl. Acad. Sci. U.S.A. **89:** 3330–3333.

4. XU, Y-F. & W. D. ATCHISON. 1996. Effects of ω-agatoxin-IVA and ω-conotoxin-MVIIC on perineurial Ca^{2+} and Ca^{2+}-activated K^+ currents on mouse motor nerve terminals. J. Pharmacol. Exp. Ther. **279:** 1229–1236.

5. BARRY, E. L. R., M. P. VIGLIONE, Y. I. KIM et al. 1995. Expression and antibody inhibition of P-type calcium channels in human small cell lung carcinoma cells. J. Neurosci. **15:** 274–283.

6. ALTSCHUL, S. F., W. GISCH, W. MILLER et al. 1990. Basic alignment search tool. J. Mol. Biol. **219:** 403–410.

7. OPHOFF, R. A., G. M. TERWINDT, M. N. VERGOUWE et al. 1996. Familial hemiplegic migraine and episodic ataxia type-2 are caused by mutations in the Ca^{2+} channel gene CACNL1A4. Cell **87:** 543–552.

8. WILLIAMS, M. E., D. H. FELDMAN, A. F. McCUE et al. 1992. Structure and functional expression of α_1, α_2, and β subunits of a novel human neuronal calcium channel subtype. Neuron **8:** 71–84.

9. ELLIS, S. B., M. E. WILLIAMS, N. R. WAYS et al. 1988. Sequence and expression of mRNAs encoding the α_1 and α_2 subunits of a DHP-sensitive calcium channel. Science **241:** 1661–1664.

10. FURNEAUX, H. M. 1994. Accession no. U07139. Direct submission.

Transient Translocation of N-type Calcium Channels from Secretory Granules to the Cell Surface[a]

MARIA PASSAFARO,[b] ELENA TAVERNA,[c] ELENA MORLACCHI,[c]
PATRIZIA ROSA,[c] FRANCESCO CLEMENTI,[c] AND EMANUELE SHER[c,d]

[b]CNR Institute of Biotechnology Applied to Pharmacology
88021 Roccelletta di Borgia (CZ), Italy

[c]CNR Cellular and Molecular Pharmacology Center
20129 Milan, Italy

INTRODUCTION

Multiple voltage-operated calcium channel (VOCC) subtypes, with different biophysical and pharmacological properties, have been characterized in vertebrate secretory cells.[1] Among these, the N-type is selectively blocked by the marine snail toxin, ω-conotoxin GVIA (ωCtx), and is expressed in many neurons and endocrine cells.[2] The N-type VOCC plays a crucial role in the control of neurotransmitter release[3] and represents a major autoantigen in Lambert-Eaton myasthenic syndrome.[4] Given their importance, it is not surprising that N-type VOCCs represent the target of various forms of modulation of both their gating properties and their actual expression. G protein–mediated modulation of the gating of N-type VOCCs by hormones and neurotransmitters has been characterized extensively in several cell types.[5] In contrast, few data are available on the biosynthesis and intracellular trafficking of N-type VOCCs in neuronal and endocrine cells. We have recently described the presence of an intracellular pool of N-type VOCCs in rat pheochromocytoma PC12 and human neuroblastoma IMR32 cells.[6] Here, we have investigated the presence, localization, and regulated translocation to the plasma membrane of the intracellular pool of N-type VOCCs in IMR32, PC12, RINm5F, and primary cultures of bovine adrenal chromaffin cells. We have found that intracellular N-type VOCCs (revealed as [^{125}I]-ωCtx binding sites) are accumulated in subcellular fractions enriched in secretory granules and translocate to the plasma membrane after exposure to secretagogue agents (high KC1, TPA, and high Ba^{2+}).

METHODS

Subcellular fractionation by velocity and equilibrium gradient centrifugation was performed as described.[7] Western blotting and [^{125}I]-ωCtx binding to intact adherent cells were performed as described.[6]

[a]This work was supported by Telethon-Italy (Grant No. 858 to E. Sher).
[d]To whom all correspondence should be addressed. Present address: Lilly Research Centre, Erl Wood Manor, Windlesham, Surrey GU20 6PH, United Kingdom.

RESULTS AND DISCUSSION

In order to identify the intracellular compartment(s) where the N-type VOCCs are accumulated, we subjected PC12 cells to subcellular fractionation on sucrose gradients and detected, in parallel, the distribution of different organelle markers and the presence of [125I]-ωCtx binding sites. Following published procedures for secretory granule purification from PC12 cells,[7] we performed two subsequent sucrose gradients: (i) a velocity and (ii) an equilibrium gradient. Aliquots of each collected fraction were processed for either Western blots or [125I]-ωCtx binding assays. At equilibrium, both the plasma membrane marker Na^+/K^+ ATPase and the small synaptic-like microvesicle and endosome marker synaptophysin were highly concentrated in the first fractions containing the less-dense organelles. On the other hand, chromogranin B (CgB), a marker of the more-dense secretory granules, had a bell-shaped distribution with a peak in fractions 5–6. We found that fractions 7, 8, and 9 from the second gradient were almost pure in secretory granules, containing CgB and no contamination by the plasma membrane or small vesicles.

In parallel, we found that the [125I]-ωCtx binding distribution was very similar to the distribution of CgB, in both the first and second gradient. The distribution was bell-shaped and broad, with a peak in fractions 5–6 and 5 in the first and second gradient, respectively. [125I]-ωCtx binding sites are normally expressed on the cell surface. However, the distribution of [125I]-ωCtx in our gradients did not superimpose with the distribution of the plasma membrane marker, suggesting that a significant amount of the intracellular [125I]-ωCtx binding sites in PC12 cells are accumulated in the secretory granules. To further demonstrate that the membrane component of binding sites did not compromise our data, we performed fractionation experiments and sucrose gradients on cells in which surface binding sites were saturated by a preincubation with unlabeled ωCtx. Since ωCtx binds irreversibly to the channels, after fractionation of the cells only intracellular binding sites should be revealed. Although the total recoverable [125I]-ωCtx binding was reduced by around one-fourth, the relative distribution of [125I]-ωCtx binding in presaturated cells was not significantly different from the control (data not shown). The fact that we did not see a significant difference in [125I]-ωCtx binding distribution, regardless of whether the surface component was present or not, is in line with an even distribution of the plasma membrane throughout the velocity gradients and a small amount of plasma membrane loaded on the equilibrium gradients.

The presence of [125I]-ωCtx binding sites in subcellular fractions of PC12 cells enriched in secretory granules implies that these binding sites should be translocated to the plasma membrane when the cells are stimulated to undergo exocytosis. We found that cell depolarization with 55 mM KCl or treatment with 100 nM TPA or 10 mM barium stimulated an increase in the number of surface [125I]-ωCtx binding sites in PC12, IMR32, and RINm5F and in primary cultures of chromaffin cells (TABLE 1). This recruitment of [125I]-ωCtx binding sites to the cell surface shares several similarities with the KCl-stimulated release of chromogranin B and [3H]-serotonin from PC12 and RINm5F, respectively (data not shown). Our results suggest that N-type VOCCs are present in the membrane of secretory granules and that they can be translocated to the plasma membrane via a process that has all of the characteristics of a regulated secretion.

TABLE 1. Recruitment of Surface [^{125}I]-ωCtx Binding Sites after Different Treatments[a]

| | [^{125}I]-ωCtx GVIA Surface Binding (% of Control) | | |
Cell Type	55 mM K$^+$ (2 mM Ca^{2+})	10 mM Ba^{2+}	100 nM TPA
IMR32 human neuroblastoma	212 ± 9.8 (7)	ND	218 ± 27.6 (7)
PC12 rat pheochromocytoma	204 ± 3.6 (7)	ND	199 ± 9.5 (6)
RINm5F rat insulinoma	190 ± 2.5 (5)	175 ± 2 (5)	ND
Bovine adrenal chromaffin cells	173 ± 1.4 (4)	199 ± 2.4 (4)	ND

[a][^{125}I]-ωCtx binding to intact adherent cells was performed as described.[6] ND = not determined. Numbers in parentheses indicate the number of experiments.

REFERENCES

1. BEAN, B. P. 1989. Classes of calcium channels in vertebrate cells. Annu. Rev. Physiol. **51:** 367–384.
2. SHER, E. & F. CLEMENTI. 1991. ω-Conotoxin-sensitive voltage-operated calcium channels in vertebrate cells. Neuroscience **42:** 301–307.
3. MILLER, R. J. 1992. Voltage-sensitive Ca^{2+} channels. J. Biol. Chem. **267:** 1403–1406.
4. SHER, E., C. GOTTI, N. CANAL, C. SCOPPETTA, G. PICCOLO, A. EVOLI & F. CLEMENTI. 1989. Specificity of calcium channel autoantibodies in Lambert-Eaton myasthenic syndrome. Lancet **II:** 640–643.
5. CARBONE, E. & D. SWANDULLA. 1989. Neuronal calcium channels: kinetics, blockade, and modulation. Prog. Biophys. Mol. Biol. **54:** 31–58.
6. PASSAFARO, M., P. ROSA, C. SALA, F. CLEMENTI & E. SHER. 1996. N-type Ca^{2+} channels are present in secretory granules and are transiently translocated to the plasma membrane during regulated exocytosis. J. Biol. Chem. **271:** 30096–30104.
7. STINCHCOMBE, J. C. & W. B. HUTTNER. 1994. Purification of secretory granules from PC12 cells. *In* Cell Biology: A Laboratory Handbook, p. 557–566. Academic Press. New York.

Pathogenesis of Human Botulism

RICARDO A. MASELLI

Department of Neurology
University of California, Davis
Davis, California 95616

INTRODUCTION

Historical Perspective

Although botulism has been known since ancient times, it was not until two centuries ago when accurate descriptions of this disease started to emerge in the German literature.[1] Because of the frequent association of botulism with the consumption of sausages, it was initially called sausage disease. However, this name was later changed to botulism, from the Latin word *botulus*, which means sausage. A turning point in the history of botulism occurred about 100 years ago when Van Ermengem published the results of an extensive study that he conducted on an outbreak of botulism that took place in the small Belgian village of Ellezelles.[2] The intoxication occurred among a group of amateur musicians who ate raw ham at a funeral gathering. From the ham and from the spleen of one of the patients who died of the intoxication, Van Ermengem isolated a spore-forming obligately anaerobic bacterium. He called this organism *Clostridium botulinum*. He also showed that extracts of the ham were toxic to laboratory animals. Another astute observation that he made was that not all species of animals were equally susceptible to the toxin. For instance, some species like mice, monkeys, and rabbits were extremely susceptible, while cats and pigeons were less susceptible and dogs and chickens were relatively resistant.

Neurotoxin Serotypes

In subsequent years, it was found that often antitoxins prepared against the culture fluid from one strain did not cross-neutralize those from different strains. That led to the recognition of several different toxin serotypes designated A to G. TABLE 1 presents a list of the seven serotypes that have been so far described along with a summary of the species and the most common regions of occurrence of the outbreaks. Type A is distributed worldwide, but especially in the western part of the United States, Russia, Asia, and South America. Type B is also distributed worldwide, but is most common in the eastern part of the United States, Europe, and Russia. Types C and D are responsible for outbreaks in animals only. Type E has been associated with outbreaks in Northern Europe, Scandinavia, Canada, Alaska, Japan, and Russia, usually in association with the consumption of fish.[3] Only two outbreaks have been detected for type F: one in Denmark and the other in the United States.[4,5] Type G was found to be produced by a strain recovered from cornfield soil in the western province of Mendoza in Argentina, but no outbreaks have been so far recognized.[6,7]

TABLE 1. Types of *C. botulinum*, Susceptible Species, and Sites of Outbreaks

Type	Species	Sites of Outbreaks
A	human	United States, Russia, China, South America
B	human, horse	United States, Northern Europe, Russia
C alpha	birds, turtles	worldwide
C beta	cattle, sheep, horse	worldwide
D	cattle, sheep	Australia, South Africa
E	human, birds	Northern Europe, Canada, United States, Japan, Russia
F	human	Denmark, United States
G		no outbreaks have been recognized

The Organism

Three factors make *Clostridium botulinum* an extremely powerful pathogenic organism: (i) its ability to proliferate in anaerobic environments; (ii) its power to generate spores, which guarantees survival even in extreme weather conditions; and (iii) the capability to fabricate the most powerful neurotoxin on earth. The spores of *Clostridium botulinum* are among the most resistant bacterial spores. They are surrounded by thick inner and outer coats formed by a keratin-like structure rich in disulfide bonds, making them extremely resistant to environmental factors.[8] They can survive more than 30 years in a fluid medium and probably even longer in the dry state.[9] They can also survive well in conditions reproducing the weather environment of Mars for a total test period of 10 months.[10] This raises a safety concern of contamination for future interplanetary expeditions.

Clinical Forms

There are several forms of botulism, but three are the most common—**(1) Foodborne botulism:** This is the classical form of the disease. It results from the ingestion of food contaminated with spores that have been maintained in anaerobic conditions, allowing germination and toxin production. Botulinum neurotoxins have a high molecular weight; therefore, they are rapidly inactivated by heat, but not by the acid and proteolytic activity of stomach fluids.[11] This is due to the fact that botulinum toxins are released from the bacteria and form complexes with other proteins that protect them from proteolysis.[12] This property is not shared by the tetanus toxin, thus explaining why tetanus is not a foodborne disease.[13] In the alkaline environment of the intestine, the toxin is dissociated from these accessory proteins, absorbed, and directly transported by the circulation to nerve terminals of the neuromuscular junction and the peripheral autonomic nervous system. Confirmation of the diagnosis is accomplished most quickly by performing a toxin determination in the patient's blood. Additional tests can be performed in ingested food, stomach fluids, and feces, looking for both the toxin and the clostridium itself. Foodborne botulism is still a disease of concern: more than 12,000 cases of foodborne botulism have been recorded worldwide since 1951. The case/fatality ratio worldwide is 20%.[14] More than 90% of foodborne botulism is caused by home-prepared or home-preserved foods: 34% type A, 52% type B, and 12% type E.[15]

(2) Wound botulism: For about 50 years, we have known that there is another form of human botulism, the so-called wound botulism.[16] This form of botulism, like tetanus, results from the contamination of wounds with bacterial spores that proliferate and produce the toxin locally. The toxin is in turn transported via the circulation to peripheral synapses. The diagnosis is confirmed by identifying the toxin in serum or the clostridium in the wound or serum. Except for isolated cases reported from a few other countries, most of the cases have been reported in the United States, with an overwhelming majority of cases in the state of California.[17] In recent years, most of the cases of wound botulism have been reported in drug addicts, especially in association with subcutaneous tissue injections using a technique termed "popping". This technique produces a slow release of the drug as the subcutaneous tissue acts as a depot.[18,19] This form of botulism is markedly underdiagnosed and underreported because usually wounds do not appear seriously infected; moreover, even if the diagnosis is entertained, the detection of toxin in the serum is less than 33%.

(3) Infant botulism: The third and most important form of botulism in the United States is infant botulism.[20] This variant of botulism was first recognized in 1976.[21,22] In this situation, botulism results from the ingestion of viable spores that germinate and colonize the intestinal tract of infants between 3 weeks to 8 months of age. The toxin is produced locally, absorbed through the intestinal tract, and transported via the circulation to the peripheral nerve terminals. The toxin and the organism can be identified in the stools, but rarely in the serum. More than 90% of the cases of infant botulism have been reported in the United States, where it is the most commonly accounted form of botulism. Half of the United States cases have been identified in the state of California. In the rest of the world, except for Argentina, Japan, and Australia, there have been only sporadic reports.[23]

Pathogenic Mechanism

At synapses of the peripheral nervous system, the toxin that is formed by disulfide-linked heavy and light chains (FIGURE 1) binds via the carboxy-terminal of the heavy chain to an as yet unidentified receptor.[24] Recently, neurotoxin B was shown to bind to synaptotagmin II complexed with gangliosides.[25] The toxin is introduced inside the nerve terminal through a receptor-mediated endocytosis process.[26] Once inside the nerve terminal, the toxin crosses the hydrophobic barrier of the vesicle membrane through a mechanism that is poorly understood. Apparently, acidification of the vesicle lumen is required for this step. The proteolytic activity is exerted by the light chain (FIGURE 1).

Molecular Targets

Another turning point in the history of botulism, ironically close to 100 years after Van Ermengem's observation, was the discovery by Schiavo, Blasi, and associates that botulinal toxins cleave three key proteins involved in the process of neurotrans-

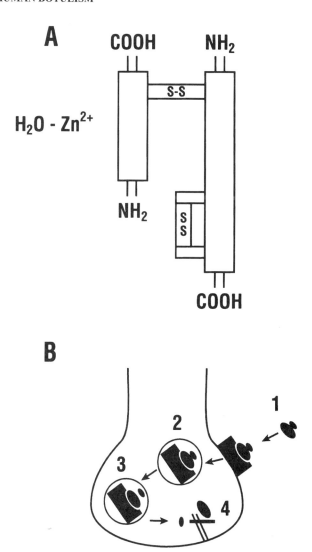

FIGURE 1. Structure of *C. botulinum* neurotoxins and cell intoxication mechanisms: (A) The neurotoxin consists of a heavy (H, 100 kDa) and a light (L, 50 kDa) chain bridged by a single interchain disulfide bond. (B) The cell intoxication mechanism consists of four different steps: (1) cell binding, (2) endocytotic internalization, (3) vesicular membrane translocation, and (4) enzymatic cleavage of target proteins. The carboxy-terminal of the H chain is responsible for cell binding, whereas the amino-terminal of the H chain is responsible for membrane translocation.

mitter release: VAMP or synaptobrevin of the synaptic vesicle and SNAP-25 and Syntaxin in the presynaptic membrane.[27,28] Botulinal toxin A and E hydrolyze SNAP-25, whereas B, D, F, and G cleave VAMP. Botulinal toxin C cleaves both SNAP-25 and Syntaxin (FIGURE 2). A number of arguments such as the immediate death of neurons in culture indicate that this is the main action mechanism of the toxins; however, additional effects may be responsible for the intoxication in humans.[29] The sites of cleavage are specific and a difference of even a single amino acid of the cleavage site of the synaptic protein of a given species may be responsible for the resistance of that particular species to the toxin.[30] This provides an explanation for the early observation of Van Ermengem in terms of the variability of species susceptibility. Another interesting point recently shown by Dolly's group was that even a single mutation of the light chain of botulinum neurotoxin A abolishes its ability to cleave SNAP-25 and to produce neurotoxicity.[31]

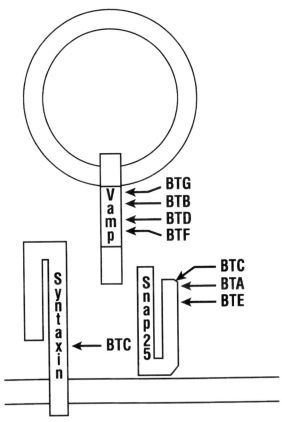

FIGURE 2. Molecular targets: *C. botulinum* neurotoxin B, D, F, and G cleave the conserved central portion of the vesicular protein VAMP/synaptobrevin. *C. botulinum* neurotoxin A, C, and E cleave the presynaptic membrane protein SNAP-25. *C. botulinum* neurotoxin C cleaves the cytosolic protein Syntaxin.

METHODS

Patient Population

Six drug users seen at the University of California Davis Medical Center (UCDMC) with symptoms compatible with botulism were studied with conventional electromyogram, muscle biopsy, and mouse bioassay for botulinum toxins. A six-week-old female seen at the University of Chicago with symptoms consistent with infant botulism was studied in similar fashion.

Electrodiagnostic Studies

These studies included nerve conduction velocity measurements, repetitive stimulation of multiple nerves using frequencies of 1–30 Hz, and conventional needle EMG. Stimulated single-fiber EMG (SSFEMG) was performed in two patients using microstimulation of distal nerve branches. Recording and analysis of SSFEMG data was done as previously described.

Muscle Biopsy; In Vitro Microelectrode

All patients underwent anconeus muscle biopsy. This technique is suitable for exploring the physiology of neuromuscular transmission *in vitro*.[32] Structural and *in vitro* microelectrode studies were performed following previously described techniques.[33]

RESULTS AND DISCUSSION

Clinical Presentation

All of our patients were chronic drug addicts with a mean age of 43 years (TABLE 2). All presented with symptoms of blurred vision, dysphagia, and dysarthria. This

TABLE 2. Clinical Findings[a]

Patient	Age	Sex	Subcutaneous Abscesses	Pupil Function	Deep Tendon Reflexes	Serum Botulism
1	44	M	absent	loss of accommodation	absent	A
2	41	F	present	normal	decrement	A
3	42	M	absent	sluggish	decrement	negative
4	31	F	absent	normal	decrement	negative
5	56	M	present	normal	normal	A
6	44	M	present	sluggish	absent	A

[a]All exhibited blurred vision, dysphagia, and dysarthria.

was followed by descending generalized weakness and acute respiratory failure, which required intubation and mechanical ventilation in five of them. It should be noted that symptoms of autonomic dysfunction such as blurred vision due to loss of accommodation, dry mouth, orthostatic hypotension, and constipation are common in botulism. This is due to the fact that the synapses of the autonomic nervous system are also involved.[34] Constipation was present in our infant patient. Constipation is another common symptom in infant botulism. Gastrointestinal symptoms are less common, except with type E toxin, which is usually associated with nausea and vomiting.[35] Pupillary abnormalities and subcutaneous abscesses were present in only half of our patients. The last finding is consistent with the notion that, in wound botulism, the wounds are often undetectable. In fact, this is one of the reasons for underdiagnosis of wound botulism.[36] Deep tendon reflexes were decreased or absent in the majority of the patients. Using the mouse bioassay, we were able to confirm the presence of type A toxin in the serum of four of our patients.

Electrodiagnostic Studies

Neurophysiologic testings were performed usually within hours of admission. Typically, the working diagnosis was not botulism, but rather a different one. Most common speculations were a myasthenic crisis or the Miller-Fisher ophthalmoplegic variance of Guillain-Barré syndrome. However, nerve conduction velocities and F-wave latencies were normal in all the patients (TABLE 3). Compound muscle action potential amplitudes (CMAPs) were reduced in our patients. This is characteristic of the three forms of botulism when the intoxication is severe and when the appropriate muscles, especially proximal muscles, are tested. However, testing of only distal muscles as is done with routine studies would have shown abnormalities only in half of our patients. Repetitive stimulation, the classical test for neuromuscular transmission disorders, provided mixed results. Decremental responses at slow rates were present only in half of the patients. Incremental responses stimulating at 30 Hz were more common, but not invariably present either. In one patient, there was decrement in the response to both slow and fast rates of stimulation. These findings led to the erroneous diagnosis of myasthenia gravis and to the incorrect treatment with plasmapheresis for several weeks without results. In botulism, the needle examination paradoxically showed a myopathic pattern consisting of short-duration, small-amplitude

TABLE 3. Electrodiagnostic Findings[a]

Patient	CMAP Amplitude	Repetitive Stimulation (2 Hz)	Repetitive Stimulation (30 Hz)
1	decrease	decrement	normal
2	decrease	normal	increment
3	decrease	decrement	decrement
4	normal	normal	increment
5	normal	decrement	normal
6	normal	normal	increment

[a]All exhibited normal nerve conduction velocities; EMG: decreased-amplitude, short-duration motor unit potentials.

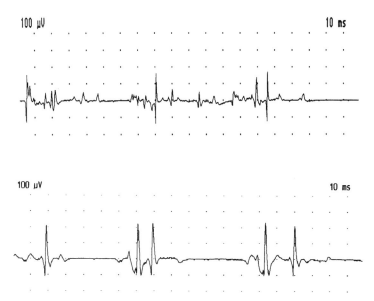

FIGURE 3. Electromyogram in botulism: (Top) Myopathic-like motor unit potentials (decreased amplitude, short duration) in an adult patient with botulism. (Bottom) Recording from the same muscle of an age-matched control.

motor unit potentials (FIGURE 3). This was present in all the patients and it was not associated with denervation activity except in one. The explanation of this apparently incongruent finding is as follows: due to the blocking of neuromuscular transmission, a large percentage of muscle fibers of a motor unit fail to generate action potentials and the resultant field potential generated by the motor unit is diminished in amplitude and duration in a similar way as occurs in acute myopathic processes. Of course, in an acute myopathic process, there is muscle necrosis and denervation activity, which were not present in our patients. In our case of infant botulism, there was a clear incremental response stimulating at 30 Hz[37] (FIGURE 4). In general, incre-

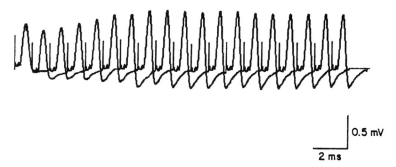

0.5 mV

2 ms

FIGURE 4. Repetitive stimulation in infant botulism: Incremental response to 30-Hz stimulation recorded from an infant intoxicated with *C. botulinum* toxin B.

TABLE 4. *In Vitro* Microelectrode Studies

Patient	MEPP Frequency	MEPP Amplitude	EPP (1 Hz) Quantal Content
1	0.6 ± 0.57	0.3 ± 0.01	11.4
2	1	0.81 ± 0.47	3.24
3[a]	11.83 ± 5.42[b]	0.59 ± 0.07	4.36 ± 2.59
4	1.03 ± 1.04	0.44 ± 0.1	8.24 ± 6.54
5	1.24 ± 0.98	0.62 ± 0.2	7.17 ± 4.93
6	2	0.34 ± 0.1	4.82 ± 3.84
average	1.17 ± 0.51	0.53 ± 0.17	6.53 ± 3.0
control	4.0 ± 5.1[c]	0.81 ± 0.08[d]	22.2 ± 2.8[d]

[a]Performed 8 weeks after the onset of symptoms.
[b]Not considered for the average.
[c]$P = 0.01$.
[d]$P = 0.001$.

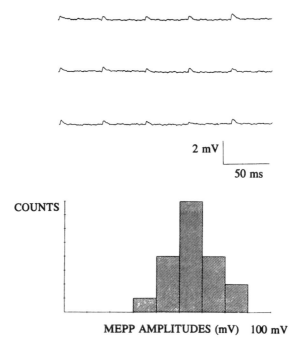

FIGURE 5. Miniature end plate potentials (MEPPs) in wound botulism: Examples of small-amplitude MEPPs recorded from the muscle biopsy of a patient with wound botulism (type A). There is a homogeneous distribution of MEPP amplitudes. Notice the absence of large-amplitude MEPPs.

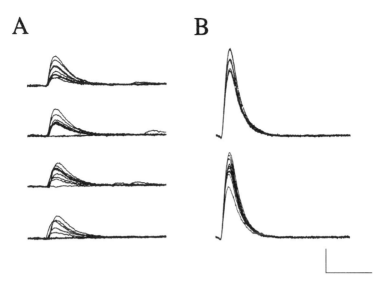

FIGURE 6. End plate potentials (EPPs) in wound botulism: (A) Examples of small-amplitude EPPs recorded from a patient intoxicated with *C. botulinum* toxin A. Ten EPPs recorded from an unblocked preparation are superimposed. Notice also the reduction of MEPP amplitudes and the stepwise variation of EPP amplitudes consisting of very low quantal content. (B) Examples of EPPs recorded from a control patient. Calibration bars are 3 mV and 10 ms.

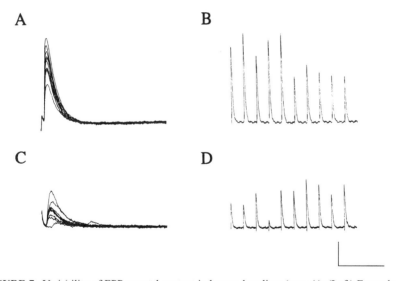

FIGURE 7. Variability of EPP quantal content in human botulism (type A): (Left) Examples of superimposed EPPs recorded from a neuromuscular junction with high (A) and low (C) quantal content. (Right) Stimulation at fast rates elicited a decremental response at the neuromuscular junction with high quantal content (B) and an incremental response at the neuromuscular junction with low quantal content (D). Calibration bars are 10 mV and 15 ms in A and C and 10 mV and 150 ms in B and D.

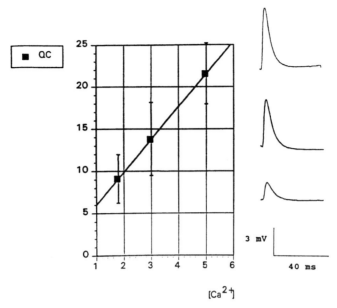

FIGURE 8. Effect of increasing concentrations of extracellular calcium on EPP quantal content in human botulism (type A): A linear increase of the EPP quantal content is shown on the left. On the right, there are examples of averaged EPPs recorded at calcium concentrations of 1.8 mM (bottom), 3 mM (middle), and 5 mM (top). QC = quantal content.

mental responses appear to be more constant in infant botulism as reported by Cornblath,[38] who conducted a large electrodiagnostic study of infant botulism. Fakadej and Gutmann reported that stimulation at fast rates for several seconds was needed to elicit an incremental response in an infant intoxicated with type B toxin.[39] Long runs of stimulation were tested in some of our patients intoxicated with type A toxin, but this failed to elicit further incremental responses.

Microelectrode Study

Frequencies of MEPPs were reduced in all the patients in whom the study was conducted during the acute phase of the illness (TABLE 4). As shown in FIGURE 5, which displays MEPPs recorded from a single end plate, the amplitudes of MEPPs were also reduced. The distribution of MEPP amplitudes was either normal or skew-deviated to the left due to the presence of small-amplitude MEPPs. We looked very carefully for the presence of very large amplitude, slow-raising-phase MEPPs, often referred to as giant MEPPs, which have been reported to occur in experimental models of botulinal intoxication and in other situations such as prolonged immobilization.[40,41] However, we did not find them in any of the patients.

The most constant finding during the acute period and even several weeks after

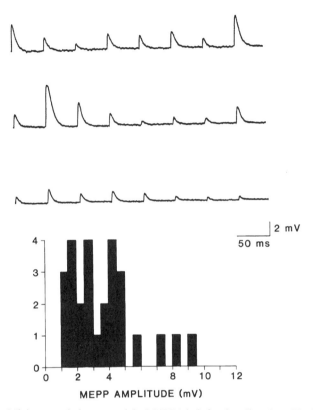

FIGURE 9. Miniature end plate potentials (MEPPs) in infant botulism (type B): (Top) Examples of MEPPs recorded from a single end plate. Notice the marked variability of MEPP amplitudes. (Bottom) Wide dispersion of the MEPP amplitude distribution.

the onset of the illness was the severe reduction of the EPP quantal content (FIGURE 6). Not only were the amplitudes of the EPPs severely reduced, but the EPPs tended to vary in quantal steps following Poisson's prediction, implying a severe reduction of the quantal content or number of vesicles being released with each nerve stimulation. The synchronization of the onsets of the EPPs was relatively intact. In addition, the amplitudes of the MEPPs were often lower than the amplitudes of the quantal component of the EPP. This has been described in several publications on animal models and in one abstract about a human case of foodborne botulism type A studied by Lambert, Engel, and Cherington.[42] As in Lambert's case, we also found that there was a wide range of involvement of different end plates. For instance, FIGURE 7 shows the recording from one end plate stimulating the nerve at 1 Hz and 20 Hz. The quantal content of this particular junction is high and a train of fast rate stimulation elicited, as in normal junctions, a decremental response. In contrast, on the bottom there is another recording from a different end plate of the same patient with low quantal content. In this example, EPPs vary following Poisson's distribution and fast rate stimulation elicited an incremental response. The percentage of high- versus low-quantal-content end plates likely determines whether an incremental response to fast rate stimulation would be present or not. This explains the great variability of the results of the repetitive stimulation studies.

Another interesting finding was that an increase in the calcium concentration in the bath solution could revert the presynaptic process and normalize completely the quantal content (FIGURE 8). This has also been found in animal models of botulism type A.[43]

Contrasting these findings were those that we obtained in the patient with infant botulism.[37] The ultrastructure of the neuromuscular junction was normal in this infant. MEPP amplitudes were also normal; however, there was a marked variability of amplitudes with very large amplitudes reminiscent of giant MEPPs, but with normal rise time. This resulted in very distorted amplitude distribution histograms (FIGURE 9). In contrast with type A, the MEPP frequencies in this patient intoxicated with type B toxin were normal. EPPs obtained by stimulating nerve terminals at 1 Hz were very small in amplitude, with most of the stimulations resulting in failures. Most of the stimuli failed to result in any release of neurotransmitter and even those that did resulted in the release of one or only a few quanta. In addition and in contrast with type A, there was impressive desynchronization of the onsets of EPPs (FIGURE 10). This has also been seen in animal models of type B toxicity.[44] At several end plates, we found that the loss of synchronization of the EPP often involved a single quantal element.

These observations led us to hypothesize that, in human type B intoxication, the site of involvement was downstream from the peak entry of calcium elicited by the stimulus-evoked depolarization of the nerve terminal because the loss of synchronization appeared to involve individual vesicles or quanta and not all the EPP quantal components (FIGURE 11A). Furthermore, the site of involvement was upstream from

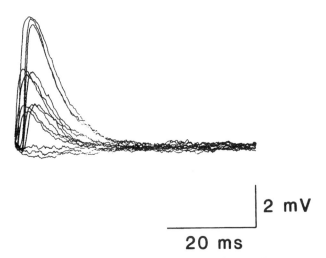

2 mV

20 ms

FIGURE 10. Dispersion of EPP onsets or "EPP jitter" in infant botulism type B: Example of superimposed EPPs recorded from a patient with infant botulism type B. Note the marked variability of EPP onsets.

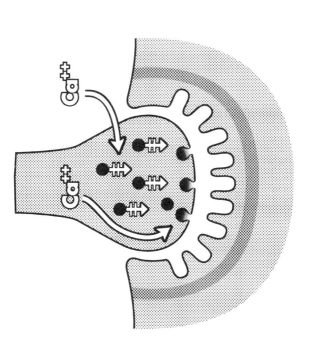

FIGURE 11. Proposed mechanism of action of *botulinum* neurotoxin A and B: (Left) The proposed site of involvement for *botulinum* type B neurotoxin is downstream from the peak entry of calcium to the nerve terminal, but upstream from the actual docking of vesicles to the nerve terminal. (Right) The postulated site of action of *botulinum* type A neurotoxin is downstream from that of type B. This is suggested by the fact that there is equal impairment in the release of vesicles activated by the action potential–linked entry of calcium to the nerve terminal and in the spontaneous release of vesicles mobilized by endogenous calcium.

the actual fusion of the vesicle to the synaptic membrane because quantal elements activated by endogenous calcium exhibited no difficulties to form normal quantal sizes and to be spontaneously released in full as suggested by the normal MEPP amplitudes and MEPP frequencies. This hypothesis tides up well with the molecular finding that type B toxin cleaves the synaptic protein VAMP/synaptobrevin.[45,46] Synaptotagmin, another synaptic protein, has been thought to act as a calcium sensor and to respond to the calcium trigger by removing a temporary clamp that inhibits the fusion of vesicles to the presynaptic membranes.[47,48] Physiologically, type B toxin also appears to interfere with this process. In contrast, type A seems to act downstream from type B because both vesicles activated by the peak entry of calcium with an action potential and those mobilized by endogenous calcium encounter equal difficulties to be released (FIGURE 11B). In support of this are the findings of diminished EPP quantal content as well as low frequencies and amplitudes of MEPPs in type A intoxication. This view also fits well with the known cleavage effect of toxin A over the presynaptic protein SNAP-25.[28,49] The fact that several physiologic maneuvers aiming to increase calcium in the nerve terminal (i.e., tetanic nerve stimulation or increased external calcium) can restore normal neurotransmitter release supports the hypothesis recently put forward by Montecucco and Schiavo that perhaps SNAP-25 is also a calcium-binding protein and that the toxin simply lowers its calcium-binding affinity.[50]

CONCLUSIONS

(1) Botulism continues to be a threat to public health around the world.

(2) In the United States, there has been a change in the pattern of reported cases of botulism. The most frequently reported form is infant botulism. More than half of the cases of infant botulism have been reported in the state of California. In recent years, wound botulism has been largely affecting needle-injecting drug addicts.

(3) There are still several aspects of the pathogenesis of botulism that are poorly understood, especially the receptor protein in the nerve terminal and the process of translocation of the toxin from inside endocytotic vesicles to the cytosol of the nerve terminal. Answers to these basic questions may explain the curious patchy distribution of nerve terminal involvement in this disease.

(4) Clinically, a descending paralysis in a self-injecting drug addict is very likely to result from wound botulism.

(5) The most constant and often disregarded finding of the electrodiagnostic assessment of botulism is the presence of small-amplitude, short-duration motor unit potentials (i.e., myopathic type). Myopathic-like units and a recruitment pattern without denervation activity in a patient with an acute episode of weakness are highly suggestive of botulism.

(6) Physiologically, type B induces a loss of synchronization of individual quantal elements. Our findings suggest that the most likely site of type B blockade is downstream from the action potential–linked depolarization of the nerve terminal, but upstream from vesicle fusion because the spontaneous quantal release is unaffected.

(7) Type A seems to act downstream from type B because both vesicles activated

by peak calcium entry and those mobilized by endogenous calcium encounter equal difficulties to be released.

REFERENCES

1. KERNER, C. A. J. 1820. Neue Beobachtungen uber die in Wurttemberg so haufig vorfallen-den todtlichen Vergiftungen durch in den Genuss geraucherter Wurste, Tübingen. (Cited in Dickson, 1918.)

2. VAN ERMENGEM, E. 1897. Ueber einen neuen anaeroben Bacillus und seine Beziehungen zum Botulismus. Z. Hyg. Infekt. **26:** 1–56.

3. SAKAGUCHI, G., S. SAKAGUCHI & T. KARASHIMADA. 1970. Characterization of *Clostridium botulinum* type E toxin in "izuchi." *In* Toxic Microorganisms. U.S. Dept. of Interior. Washington, District of Columbia.

4. MOLLER, V. & I. SCHEIBEL. 1960. Preliminary report on the isolation of an apparently new type of *Cl. botulinum*. Acta Pathol. Microbiol. Scand. **48:** 80.

5. SMITH, L. D. S. & H. SUGIYAMA. 1988. Botulism: The Organism, Its Toxins, The Disease. Second edition. Thomas. Springfield, Illinois.

6. GIMENEZ, D. F. & A. S. CICCARELLI. 1970. Studies on strain 84 of *Clostridium botulinum*. Zbl. Bakt. I Abt. Orig. **215:** 212–220.

7. GIMENEZ, D. F. & A. S. CICCARELLI. 1970. Another type of *Clostridium botulinum*. Zbl. Bakt. I Abt. Orig. **215:** 212–220.

8. DURBAN, E. E., M. DURBAN & N. GRECZ. 1974. Production of spore spheroplasts of *Clostridium botulinum* and DNA extraction for density gradient centrifugation. Can. J. Microbiol. **20:** 353–358.

9. HOFER, J. W. & J. DAVIS. 1972. Survival and dormancy. Tex. Med. **68:** 80–81.

10. HAWRYLEWICZ, E., B. GOWDY & R. EHRLICH. 1962. Microorganisms under simulated Martian environment. Nature **193:** 497.

11. MONTECUCCO, C., G. SCHIAVO, V. TUGNOLI & D. DE GRANDIS. 1996. Botulinum neurotoxins: mechanism of action and therapeutic applications. Mol. Med. Today **October:** 418–424.

12. OGOMA, K. *et al.* 1996. Structure and function of progenitor toxins produced by *Clostridium botulinum* types A, C, D, and E. *In* Biomedical Aspects of Clostridial Neurotoxins. Oxford University Press. London/New York.

13. SINGH, B. R., B. LI & D. READ. 1995. Botulinum versus tetanus neurotoxins: why is botulinum neurotoxin but not tetanus neurotoxin a food poison? Toxicon **33:** 1541–1547.

14. HATHEWAY, C. L. 1995. Botulism: the present state of the disease. Curr. Top. Microbiol. Immunol. **195:** 55–75.

15. HAUSCHILD, A. H. W. 1992. Epidemiology of human foodborne botulism. *In Clostridium botulinum*: Ecology and Control in Foods. Dekker. New York.

16. DAVIS, J. B., L. H. MATTMAN & M. WILEY. 1951. *Clostridium botulinum* in a fatal wound infection. JAMA **146:** 646–648.

17. WEBER, J. T., H. C. GOODPASTURE, H. ALEXANDER, S. B. WERNER, C. L. HATHEWAY & R. V. TAUXE. 1993. Wound botulism in a patient with a tooth abscess: case report and review. Clin. Infect. Dis. **16:** 635–639.

18. DAVIS, L. E. 1993. Botulinum toxin—from poison to medicine. West. J. Med. **158:** 25–29.

19. WOUND BOTULISM—CALIFORNIA. 1995. MMWR CDC Surveill. Summ. **44:** 889–892.

20. ARNON, S. S. 1992. Infant botulism. *In* Textbook of Pediatric Infectious Diseases. Third edition. Saunders. Philadelphia.

21. PICKETT, J., B. BERG, E. CHAPLIN & M. A. BRUNSTETTER. 1976. Syndrome of botulism in infancy: clinical and electrophysiologic study. N. Engl. J. Med. **295:** 770–772.

22. MIDURA, T. F. & S. S. ARNON. 1976. Infant botulism: identification of *Clostridium botulinum* and its toxin in faeces. Lancet **ii:** 934–936.
23. DODDS, K. L. 1992. Worldwide incidence and ecology of infant botulism. *In Clostridium botulinum*: Ecology and Control in Foods. Dekker. New York.
24. MONTECUCCO, C. & G. SCHIAVO. 1995. Structure and function of tetanus and botulinum neurotoxins. Q. Rev. Biophys. **28:** 423–472.
25. NISHIKI, T., Y. KAMATA, Y. NEMOTO, A. OMORI, T. ITO, M. TAKAHASHI & S. KOZAKI. 1994. Identification of protein receptor for *Clostridium botulinum* type B neurotoxin in rat brain synaptosomes. J. Biol. Chem. **269:** 10498–10503.
26. BLACK, J. D. & J. O. DOLLY. 1986. Interaction of ^{125}I-labeled neurotoxins with nerve terminals. II. Autoradiographic evidence for its uptake into motor nerves by acceptor-mediated endocytosis. J. Cell Biol. **103:** 535–544.
27. SCHIAVO, G., F. BENEFENATI, B. POULAIN, O. ROSSETTO, P. POLVERINO DE LAURETO, B. R. DASGUPTA & C. MONTECUCCO. 1992. Tetanus and botulinum-B neurotoxins block neurotransmitter release by a proteolytic cleavage of synaptobrevin. Nature **359:** 832–835.
28. BLASI, J., E. R. CHAPMAN, E. LINK, T. BINZ, S. YAMASAKI, P. DECAMILLI, T. C. SUDHOF, H. NIEMANN & R. JAHN. 1993. Botulinum neurotoxin A selectively cleaves the synaptic protein SNAP-25. Nature **365:** 160–163.
29. MACDONALD, K. L., M. L. COHEN & P. A. BLAKE. 1986. The changing epidemiology of adult botulism in the United States. Am. J. Epidemiol. **124:** 794–799.
30. PATARNELLO, T., L. BARGELLONI, O. ROSSETTO, G. SCHIAVO & C. MONTECUCCO. 1993. Neurotransmission and secretion. Nature **364:** 581–582.
31. ZHOU, L., A. DE PAIVA, D. LIU, R. AOKI & J. O. DOLLY. 1995. Expression and purification of the light chain of botulinum neurotoxin A: a single mutation abolishes its cleavage of SNAP-25 and neurotoxicity after reconstitution with the heavy chain. Biochemistry **34:** 15175–15181.
32. MASELLI, R. A., D. P. MASS, B. J. DISTAD & D. P. RICHMAN. 1991. Anconeus muscle: a human muscle preparation suitable for *in-vitro* microelectrode studies. Muscle Nerve **14:** 1189–1192.
33. MASELLI, R. A., R. L. WOLLMANN, D. LEUNG, B. DISTAD, S. PALOMBI, D. P. RICHMAN, E. F. SALAZAR-GRUESO & R. P. ROOS. 1993. Neuromuscular transmission in amyotrophic lateral sclerosis. Muscle Nerve **16:** 1193–1203.
34. HUGHES, J. M., J. R. BLUMENTHAL, M. H. MERSON, G. L. LOMBARD, V. R. DOWELL, JR. & E. J. GANGAROSA. 1981. Clinical features of type A and B food-borne botulism. Ann. Intern. Med. **95:** 442–445.
35. EISENBERG, M. S. & T. R. BENDER. 1976. Plastic bags and botulism: a new twist to an old hazard of the North. Alaska Med. **18:** 47–49.
36. DAVIS, L. E. 1993. Botulinum toxin—from poison to medicine. West. J. Med. **158:** 25–29.
37. MASELLI, R. A., M. E. BURNETT & J. H. TONSGARD. 1992. *In vitro* microelectrode study of neuromuscular transmission in a case of botulism. Muscle Nerve **15:** 273–278.
38. CORNBLATH, D. R., J. T. SHADKY & A. J. SUMMER. 1983. Clinical electrophysiology of infantile botulism. Muscle Nerve **6:** 448–452.
39. FAKADEJ, A. V. & L. GUTMANN. 1982. Prolongation of post-tetanic facilitation in infant botulism. Muscle Nerve **5:** 727–729.
40. SELLIN, L. C., S. THESLEFF & B. R. DASGUPTA. 1983. Different effects of types A and B botulinum toxin on transmitter release at the neuromuscular junction. Acta Physiol. Scand. **119:** 127–133.
41. THESLEFF, S., J. MOLGO & H. LUNDH. 1983. Botulinum toxin and 4-aminoquinoline induce a similar abnormal type of spontaneous quantal transmitter release at the rat neuromuscular junction. Brain Res. **264:** 89–97.
42. LAMBERT, E. H., A. G. ENGEL & M. CHERINGTON. 1974. End-plate potentials in human botulism [abstract]. Excerpta Med. (Amsterdam) **334:** 65.

43. MOLGO, J., J. X. COMELLA, D. ANGAUT-PETIT, M. PEQCOT-DECHAVASSINE, N. TABTI, L. FAILLE, A. MALLART & S. THESLEFF. 1990. Presynaptic actions of botulinal neurotoxins at vertebrate neuromuscular junctions. J. Physiol. (Paris) **84:** 152–166.

44. GANSEL, M., R. PENNER & F. DREYER. 1987. Distinct sites of action of clostridial neurotoxins revealed by double-poisoning of mouse motor nerve terminals. Pflügers Arch. **409:** 533–539.

45. TONELLO, F., S. MORANTE, O. ROSSETTO, G. SCHIAVO & C. MONTECUCCO. 1996. Tetanus and botulism neurotoxins: a novel group of zinc-endopeptidases. Adv. Exp. Med. Biol. **389:** 251–260.

46. RHEE, S. D., H. H. JUNG, G. H. YANG, Y. S. MOON & K. H. YANG. 1997. Cleavage of the synaptobrevin/vesicle-associated membrane protein (VAMP) of the mouse brain by the recombinant light chain of *Clostridium botulinum* type B toxin. FEMS Microbiol. Lett. **150:** 203–208.

47. LITTLETON, J. T., M. STERN, M. PERIN & H. J. BELLEN. 1994. Calcium dependence of neurotransmitter release and rate of spontaneous vesicle fusions are altered in *Drosophila* synaptotagmin mutants. Proc. Natl. Acad. Sci. U.S.A. **91:** 10888–10892.

48. WISER, O., D. TOBI, M. TRUS & D. ATLAS. 1997. Synaptotagmin restores kinetic properties of a Syntaxin-associated N-type voltage sensitive calcium channel. FEBS Lett. **404:** 203–207.

49. SCHIAVO, G., O. ROSSETTO, S. CATSICAS, P. POLVERINO DE LAURETO, B. R. DASGUPTA, F. BENEFENATI & C. MONTECUCCO. 1993. Identification of the nerve-terminal targets of botulinum neurotoxin serotypes A, D, and E. J. Biol. Chem. **268:** 23784–23787.

50. SCHIAVO, G., O. ROSSETTO, F. TONELLO & C. MONTECUCCO. 1995. The metalloproteinase activity of tetanus and botulinum neurotoxins. Curr. Top. Microbiol. Immunol. **195:** 257–274.

Congenital Myasthenic Syndromes

New Insights from Molecular Genetic and Patch-Clamp Studies[a]

ANDREW G. ENGEL,[b] KINJI OHNO,[b] MARGHERITA MILONE,[b]
AND STEVEN M. SINE[c]

[b]Muscle Research Laboratory
and
Department of Neurology
[c]Department of Physiology and Biophysics
and
Receptor Biology Laboratory
Mayo Clinic and Mayo Foundation
Rochester, Minnesota 55905

INTRODUCTION

Congenital myasthenic syndromes (CMS) are heterogeneous disorders arising from presynaptic, synaptic, or postsynaptic defects. In each CMS, the specific defect compromises the safety margin of neuromuscular transmission by one or more mechanisms.[1] With few exceptions, the clinical features of diverse CMS are similar and the precise diagnosis requires the correlation of clinical, *in vitro* electrophysiological, morphological, and (whenever possible) molecular genetic studies.[1,2] In three CMS, namely, the slow-channel CMS (SCCMS),[3] end plate (EP) acetylcholinesterase (AChE) deficiency,[4,5] and the disorder attributed to a defect in acetylcholine (ACh) resynthesis or packaging,[6,7] clinical and electromyography clues alone can suggest the correct diagnosis. These clues, however, are not consistently reliable and do not distinguish between different subtypes of the three syndromes. TABLE 1 lists the studies that we use to investigate CMS, and TABLE 2 shows a classification of CMS based on 71 index patients investigated by these studies to date.

MUTATIONS IN AChR SUBUNITS CAUSE POSTSYNAPTIC CMS

Prior to 1990, our studies of CMS patients were based on clinical, morphologic, conventional microelectrode, and noise analysis studies. In the early 1990s, we succeeded in patch-clamping EPs in excised intercostal muscles of humans and could evaluate the kinetic properties of AChR at the single channel level.[8] Coincident with this, we hypothesized that a kinetic abnormality of AChR predicts one or more muta-

[a]This work was supported by National Institutes of Health grants to A. G. Engel (No. NS6277) and S. M. Sine (No. NS31744), an MDA Research Grant to A. G. Engel, an MDA postdoctoral fellowship to K. Ohno, and an Italian Telethon Award to M. Milone.

TABLE 1. Investigation of Congenital Myasthenic Syndromes[a]

Clinical
History, examination, response to AChE inhibitor
EMG: conventional, stimulation studies, SFEMG
Serologic tests (AChR antibodies, tests for botulism)
Morphologic studies
Routine histochemical studies
Cytochemical and immunocytochemical localizations of AChE, AChR, AChR subunits, agrin, β_2-laminin, utrophin, rapsyn, IgG, C3, C5b-9 at the EP
Estimate of the size, shape, and two-dimensional profile of AChE-reactive EP regions on teased muscle fibers
Quantitative electron microscopy and electron cytochemistry
^{125}I-α-Bungarotoxin binding sites/EP
In vitro electrophysiology studies
Conventional microelectrode studies: MEPP, MEPC, evoked quantal release (m, n, p)
Noise analysis: channel kinetics
Single-channel patch-clamp recordings
Molecular genetic studies
Mutation analysis (if candidate gene or protein identified)
Expression studies (if mutation identified)
Linkage analysis (if no candidate gene or protein recognized)

[a]AChE, acetylcholinesterase; AChR, acetylcholine receptor; EMG, electromyography; SFEMG, single-fiber EMG; EP, end plate; MEPP, miniature EP potential; MEPC, miniature EP current; m, no. of transmitter quanta released by nerve impulse; n, no. of readily releasable transmitter quanta; p, probability of quantal release.

tions of an AChR subunit.[1,2] This hypothesis was subsequently confirmed by the discovery of mutations in different subunits of AChR that either increase[9–13] or decrease[13,14] the response to ACh. Subsequently, we postulated, and then demonstrated, that severe EP AChR deficiency can be due to mutations in an AChR subunit gene.[13,15–20] Although EP AChR deficiency could also arise from defects in molecules that regulate the synthesis,[21–23] aggregation,[24–26] or cytoskeletal attachment[27–30] of AChR, mutations in genes encoding these molecules have not been detected in humans to date.

Since 1994, we have identified 40 AChR subunit gene mutations in 38 CMS kinships. TABLE 3 classifies the identified mutations according to their functional consequences and subunit locations. Functional consequences range from augmented response to ACh (slow channel) to decreased response (fast channel and reduced or null expression). A surprising number of mutations fall into the category of decreased response to ACh, which necessarily arises from recessive inheritance. Further, nearly three-quarters of the mutations are found in the ε subunit, highlighting the importance of this subunit in receptor activation and susceptibility of the gene to mutation. FIGURE 1 illustrates locations of the mutations reported by us to date ac-

TABLE 2. Classification of CMS and Index Patients Studied at Mayo[a]

	Index Patients (No.)
Presynaptic defects	
Defect in ACh resynthesis or packaging[6]	4
Paucity of synaptic vesicles and reduced quantal release[50]	1
Synaptic defects	
End plate acetylcholinesterase deficiency[4,5,51]	9
Postsynaptic defects	
Primary kinetic abnormality of AChR with secondary AChR deficiency[3,9–12,32,33]	15
Primary kinetic abnormality of AChR without AChR deficiency[14,38,52]	5
Severe deficiency of AChR with or without kinetic abnormality[15–20]	35
No identified defect	2
Total	71

[a]Fifty-nine index patients had intercostal biopsies at Mayo; the remaining 12, mostly from other countries, had genetic studies that identified pathogenic mutation in DNA isolated from blood.

cording to functional domain. Gain-of-function mutations are found in portions of the extracellular domain contributing to the ACh binding site, in the M1 and M2 domains contributing to the ion channel, and in the short extracellular loop between transmembrane domains M2 and M3. Sites of null mutations are concentrated either in the long cytoplasmic loop or in the extracellular domain that harbors residues governing subunit folding, assembly, and glycosylation.

TABLE 3. Forty AChR Subunit Gene Mutations in 38 Kinships[a]

Mutation	α	β	δ	ε	Total
Point mutations					
slow-channel mutation	5	1		3	9
fast-channel mutation	1			1	2
null mutation				2	2
reduced expression	2		1	4	7
In-frame rearrangement		1		2	3
Premature chain termination (null mutations)					
frameshifting rearrangement				11	11
splice-site mutation				4	4
nonsense mutation				2	2
Total	8	2	1	29	40

[a]Italicized numbers indicate mutations that severely decrease AChR expression.

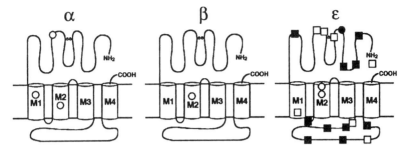

O   Slow channel mutations
●   Fast channel mutation
❑   Missense mutations, reduced expression
■   Premature chain termination, null mutations

Subunits	Mutations	Domains	References
α subunit	O αG153S	Near ACh binding site	(10)
	O αN217K	M1 domain	(11)
	O αV249F	M2 domain	(12)
β subunit	O βV266M	M2 domain	(11)
ε subunit	❑ εG-8R	Signal peptide	(14)
	■ εR64X	Extracellular domain	(13)
	■ ε70insG	Extracellular domain	(20)
	■ ε127ins5	Extracellular domain	(13)
	● εP121L	Near ACh binding site	(14)
	❑ εC128S	Disulfide loop	(19)
	❑ εS143L	N-glycosylation site	(14)
	❑ εR147L	Extracellular domain	(13)
	■ ε553del7	Extracellular domain	(13, 15, 16)
	❑ εP245L	M1 domain	(13)
	■ εIVS7+2T→C	Link between M1 and M2	(20)
	O εT264P	M2 domain	(9)
	O εL269F	M2 domain	(11)
	❑ εR311W	Long cytoplasmic loop	(13)
	■ εIVS9-1G→C	Long cytoplasmic loop	(15)
	■ ε1012del20	Long cytoplasmic loop	(17)
	■ ε1101insT	Long cytoplasmic loop	(18)
	■ ε1206ins19	Long cytoplasmic loop	(20)
	❑ ε1254ins18	Long cytoplasmic loop	(19)
	■ ε1293insG	Long cytoplasmic loop	(18)

FIGURE 1. Twenty-four mutations in the α, β, and ε subunits of AChR reported from our laboratories to date.

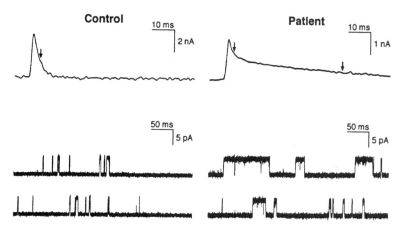

FIGURE 2. Miniature EP currents (MEPC) (top traces) and channel events (bottom traces) from normal human EPs (left) and from EPs of an SCCMS patient harboring αV249F. Note markedly prolonged and biexponentially decaying MEPC and some highly prolonged channel events in the SCCMS. Vertical arrows indicate the decay time constants. MEPCs filtered at 500 Hz and channel currents at 5.8 kHz; –80 mV; temperature, 22 °C. (Reproduced from reference 12 by permission.)

INCREASED RESPONSE TO ACh: SLOW-CHANNEL MUTATIONS

The clues for the diagnosis of an SCCMS consist of selectively severe weakness of the forearm extensor muscles, a repetitive compound muscle action potential response to single nerve stimuli that is accentuated by edrophonium, a prolonged and biexponentially decaying miniature EP current (MEPC) (FIGURE 2, upper panels), and an EP myopathy. The EP myopathy, which stems from calcium overloading of the postsynaptic region,[3] is evidenced by degeneration of junctional folds with loss of AChR and widening of the synaptic space (FIGURE 3A), junctional folds honey-combed by membranous networks (FIGURE 3B), degenerating organelles (FIGURE 3C) and apoptotic nuclei (FIGURE 3D) in the junctional sarcoplasm, and focal myofibrillar degeneration and sometimes vacuolar change near the EPs.[3,9–12,31] The safety margin of neuromuscular transmission is compromised by loss of AChR, by altered synaptic geometry, by a depolarization block caused by temporal summation of prolonged EP potentials during activity, and in some cases by desensitization of a fraction of the AChR even in the resting state.[11,12]

Patch-clamp analysis of EP AChR reveals activities of both wild-type and mutant AChRs, and the channel opening events generated by the mutant AChRs are markedly prolonged (FIGURE 2, lower panels). A third and minor population of channel events, with the 46-pS conductance and prolonged open duration typical of AChR containing the fetal γ instead of the adult ε subunit (γ-AChR), is detected in some cases.[9–12]

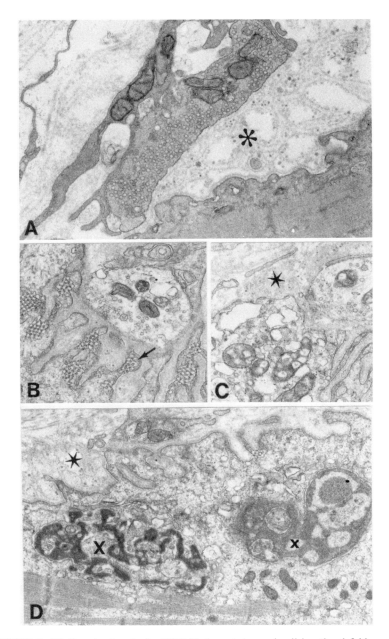

FIGURE 3. EP fine structure in the SCCMS. In part **A,** nearly all junctional folds are destroyed. The widened synaptic space (asterisk) contains globular residues of the degenerated folds and loops of basal lamina that had invested the preexisting folds. In part **B,** many junctional folds are honeycombed by membranous networks. In part **C,** the junctional sarcoplasm (left) is filled with degenerating organelles. The star indicates remnants of degenerated junctional folds. In part **D,** the junctional sarcoplasm harbors nuclei in early (x) and advanced (X) stages of apoptosis. The star indicates remnants of degenerated junctional folds. EP in part **A** is from a patient harboring βV266M; EPs in parts **B–D** are from a patient harboring αV249F. **A,** ×25,900; **B,** ×18,100; **C,** ×17,500; **D,** ×14,800. [Figure reduced to 87%.] (Parts **B–D** are reproduced from reference 12 by permission.)

Genetic Heterogeneity

Ten SCCMS mutations have been reported to date. Six were described by us (ϵT264P,[9] αG153S,[10] ϵL269F,[11,32] βV266M,[11] αN217K,[11,33] and αV249F[12]), one by Gomez et al.[34] (βL262M), and three by Croxen et al.[35] (αV156M, αT254I, and αS269I). One mutation (ϵL269F), first reported by us,[32] was also reported by Gomez,[36] and another mutation described by us, αG153S, was subsequently also detected by Croxen et al.[35] The different mutations occur in different AChR subunits and in different functional domains of the subunits (FIGURES 1 and 4). Each is dominant, causing a pathologic gain of function.

Physiologic Heterogeneity

AChRs harboring different SCCMS mutations display a number of physiologic differences:

(1) Each SCCMS mutation is associated with a prolonged and biexponential decay of EP currents and potentials, but the greatest prolongations are caused by M2 mutations that introduce a phenylalanine residue into the M2 domain (i.e., ϵL269F and αV249F). With these mutations the longer component of the MEPC decay time constant is 40 to 50 ms, whereas with the other SCCMS mutations it is 17 to 26 ms (normal = 2.8–3.6 ms). The markedly prolonged MEPCs predict staircase summation

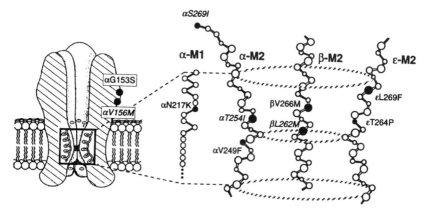

FIGURE 4. AChR subunit mutations causing SCCMS reported to date. Six of the mutated residues (ϵT264P, ϵL269F, αV249F, βV266M, αT254I, and βL262M) are in M2 transmembrane domains lining the channel pore. αN217K is in a segment of M1 that likely lines the channel lumen and may face the lumen in the absence of ACh. These mutations slow the rate of channel closure and have a variable effect on apparent agonist binding affinity. αG153S, which is in the extracellular domain near residues that contribute to agonist binding, enhances agonist binding affinity, allowing an increased number of reopenings during ACh occupancy; by contrast, it only modestly affects channel-gating rate constants. αV156M,[35] which is close to αG153S, may have similar effects. Mutations first reported from other laboratories are shown in italics.

of the EP potentials (which are even more prolonged than the MEPCs) and a depolarization block of transmission at physiologic rates of stimulation, similar to that demonstrated in organophosphate poisoning.[37]

(2) The M2 SCCMS mutations are associated with spontaneous openings of the AChR channel.[9,11,12] The leaky channel should have at least two adverse effects: (i) partial depolarization of the postsynaptic region at rest, which would partially inactivate the perijunctional Na^+ channels and further reduce the safety margin of neuromuscular transmission; (ii) enhanced cationic overloading of the postsynaptic region, which would exacerbate the EP myopathy.

(3) Expression studies in HEK cells indicate that each mutation enhances the apparent affinity of ACh binding at equilibrium. Equilibrium ACh affinity can be enhanced through several mechanisms, including increased probability of channel opening, increased extent of desensitization, and increased affinity for ACh for a particular functional state: resting, open channel, or desensitized. For example, αV249F enhances the apparent affinity for ACh more than the other mutations, but it does this through channel desensitization, enhanced probability of channel opening, and enhanced intrinsic affinity of ACh for the resting state of the receptor.[12] Other M2 mutations, εL269F and βV266M, enhance the apparent ACh affinity to a much lesser extent, owing to lesser enhancement of desensitization.[11] αG153S and αN217K have little effect on the probability of channel opening, but enhance apparent affinity by enhancing both desensitization and intrinsic affinity of ACh for the resting state.[10,11,33]

(4) All M2 mutations prolong the duration of channel open intervals and bursts by slowing the rate of channel closing.[9,11,12] By contrast, αG153S, which is located in the extracellular domain, prolongs burst durations by a distinctly different mechanism. It decreases the rate of ACh dissociation from the binding site without affecting the rate of channel closing, allowing repeated reopening of the channel during each ACh occupancy.[10] Effects of M1 mutations are intermediate to the M2 and the extracellular domain mutations. M1 mutations also slow the rate of channel closing, although to a lesser extent than the M2 mutations, and the major effect of one of these (αN217K) is to slow the rate of ACh dissociation from the binding site.[33]

Clinical Heterogeneity

From the patients observed thus far, it appears that mutations in the M2 domain are more disabling than those in the M1 domain and that αG153S in the extracellular domain has the least severe consequences. For example, our patient with the εT264P mutation in M2 has been wheelchair-dependent since her teens; our patient with the αN217K mutation in M1 is less severely affected and can walk about 100 yards before having to rest; and some members of the family with the αG153S mutation can still ski and play tennis into their sixties.

DECREASED RESPONSE TO ACh: THE LOW-AFFINITY FAST-CHANNEL MUTATION

We observed the first patient with this CMS in 1991.[38] She was a young woman with moderately severe myasthenic symptoms since birth, normal EP ultrastructure, normal evoked quantal release, and normal number of AChR per EP, but very small miniature EP potentials. The power spectrum of ACh-induced current noise was best fitted by a double Lorentzian, suggesting a kinetic abnormality of AChR or two populations of AChRs at the EPs. We attributed the disorder to an abnormal interaction of ACh with AChR.[38] In 1995, we observed a second patient, a 4-year-old boy (FIGURE 5), with similar electrophysiologic and morphologic (FIGURE 6) findings.

Patch-clamp studies in the second patient demonstrated infrequent AChR channel events; diminished channel reopenings during ACh occupancy, resulting in abnormally brief bursts of openings (FIGURE 7); and an increased resistance to desensitization by ACh.[14]

Mutation analysis revealed that each patient had two heteroallelic AChR ε subunit gene mutations: a common εP121L mutation in both patients as well as a signal peptide mutation (εG-8R) in patient 1 and a glycosylation consensus site mutation (εS143L) in patient 2 (FIGURE 1). All three mutations are recessive, loss-of-function mutations.[14]

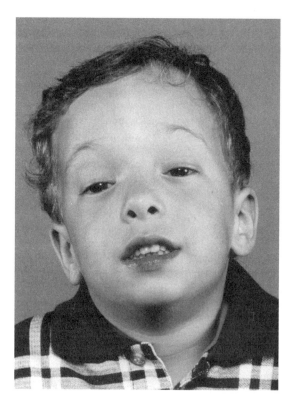

FIGURE 5. A 4-year-old boy harboring the εP121L low-affinity fast-channel mutation and the εS143L null mutation. Note ptosis, ophthalmoparesis, and hyperactive frontalis muscle.

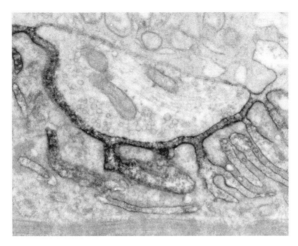

FIGURE 6. Ultrastructural localization of EP AChR with peroxidase-labeled α-bungarotoxin in the low-affinity fast-channel syndrome. The density and distribution of AChR on the junctional folds is normal; ×21,500. (Reproduced from reference 14 by permission.)

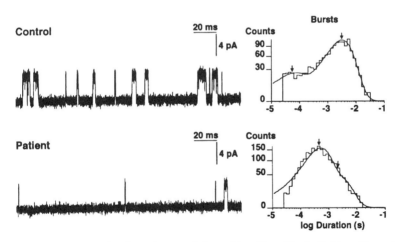

FIGURE 7. Representative channel events *(left panels)* and logarithmically binned burst duration histograms *(right panels)* fitted by the sum of exponentials from a control EP *(upper panels)* and from a low-affinity fast-channel syndrome EP in which the AChR harbors the εP121L mutation *(lower panels)*. Channel events are less frequent in the patient than in the control. In the control, the mean duration of the dominant burst component is 2.1 ms; in the patient, the corresponding value is only 0.46 ms. $T = 22 \pm 0.5$ °C; ACh concentration = 1 μM; bandwidth = 12 kHz. (Reproduced from reference 14 by permission.)

The amount of AChR expressed in HEK fibroblasts was normal with εP121L, but was severely reduced with the other two mutations, indicating that the clinical phenotype is defined by the εP121L mutation. Studies of genetically engineered εP121L AChR expressed in HEK cells revealed a markedly decreased rate of channel opening; AChR affinity for ACh was little changed in the resting state, but was greatly reduced in the open-channel and desensitized states. The reduced affinity for ACh in these functional states accounts for the resistance to both channel opening and desensitization.[14]

It is interesting to note that the εP121L mutation and the SCCMS mutations have opposite effects: the SCCMS mutations increase the burst open duration, enhance ACh binding affinity, increase desensitization by ACh, and cause an EP myopathy; by contrast, εP121L decreases the burst open duration, reduces ACh binding affinity, decreases desensitization by ACh, and leaves no anatomic footprint.

AChR DEFICIENCY CAUSED BY RECESSIVE MUTATIONS IN AChR SUBUNITS

Genetic Heterogeneity

Severe EP AChR deficiency can result from different types of recessive mutations in AChR subunit genes. The mutations are either homozygous or, more frequently, heterozygous. Morphologic studies show an increased number of EP regions distributed over an increased span of the muscle fiber (FIGURES 8A and 8B). The integrity of the junctional folds is preserved, but some EP regions are simplified and smaller than normal (FIGURE 8C). The distribution of AChR on the junctional folds is patchy and the density of the reaction for AChR is attenuated (FIGURES 8C and 8D). Conventional microelectrode studies reveal a decreased amplitude of the miniature EP potentials and currents, as well as high or higher than normal quantal release by nerve impulses. Single channel recordings at the EP[13,16,19] or immunocytochemical studies[18] often reveal the presence of γ-AChR at the EPs (also see below).

Different types of recessive mutations causing severe EP AChR deficiency have now been identified (FIGURE 1 and TABLE 3):

(1) Mutations causing premature termination of the translational chain. These mutations are frameshifting,[13,17,18,20] occur at a splice site,[15,20] or produce a stop codon directly.[13]

(2) Missense mutation in a signal peptide region (εG-8R).[14]

(3) Missense mutations in residues essential for assembly of the pentameric receptor. Mutations of this type were observed in an N-glycosylation site (εS143L);[14] in cysteine 128 (εC128S), a residue that is an essential part of the C128–C142 disulfide loop in the extracellular domain;[19] and in arginine 147 (εR147L) in the extracellular domain, which lies between isoleucine 145 and threonine 150, residues that contribute to subunit assembly.[13]

(4) Missense mutations affecting both AChR expression and kinetics. For example, εR311W[13] and ε1254ins18[19] in the long cytoplasmic loop between M3 and M4 decrease, whereas εP245L in the M1 domain[13] increases the open

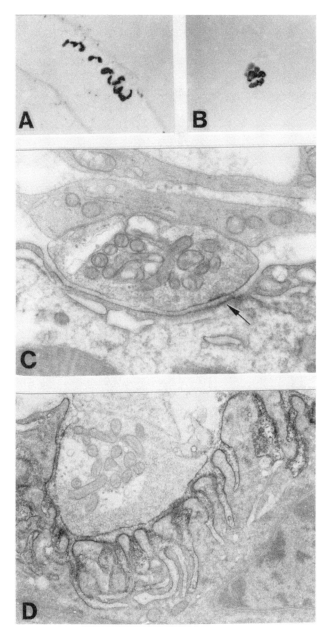

FIGURE 8. (A & B) Cholinesterase-reactive EP regions from a patient harboring a frameshifting null mutation (ε127ins5) and a missense mutation that reduces AChR expression (εP245L) **(A)** and from a control subject **(B)**. Note the dispersion of EP regions over an extended length of the muscle fiber in the patient. **(C & D)** Ultrastructural localization of AChR with peroxidase-labeled α-bungarotoxin at an EP of the same patient **(C)** and at a control EP **(D)**. The control EP shows heavy reaction for AChR on the terminal expansions of the junctional folds. At the patient's EP, the junctional folds are simplified and the reaction for AChR is patchy and attenuated (arrow). **A & B**, ×310; **C**, ×21,900; **D**, ×6,500. (Parts **B** and **D** are reproduced from reference 13 by permission.)

duration of channel events. In these instances, the kinetic consequences are modest and are likely overshadowed by the reduced expression of the mutant gene.

Recessive Mutations Causing Severe AChR Deficiency Are Concentrated in the ε Subunit

Thus far, we have observed 29 recessive mutations in CMS patients that markedly decrease the surface expression of pentameric AChR. Interestingly, 25 of these mutations reside in the ε subunit gene (TABLE 3 and FIGURE 1). A possible reason for this is that substitution of the γ for the ε subunit may rescue the phenotype from a fatal null mutation in ε, whereas patients harboring null mutations in subunits other than ε might not survive for lack of a substituting subunit. AChR at adult EPs is a pentamer of homologous subunits with the composition of $\alpha_2\beta\delta\varepsilon$. Fetal AChR, which contains the chromosome 2–encoded γ instead of the chromosome 17–encoded ε subunit (γ-AChR), is normally expressed at human EPs until the 31st week of gestation.[39] We have now obtained both patch-clamp and immunocytochemical evidence demonstrating that γ-AChR reappears at the CMS EP when there are null mutations in the ε subunit gene.[13,16,18] This finding is consistent with the observation that homozygous deletion of the ε subunit in mice results in persistent, but reduced γ-subunit gene expression in the adult mutants.[40] Although γ-AChR has prolonged channel openings, the postsynaptic region is protected from cationic overloading because the synaptic current is restricted by the severe AChR deficiency, the γ-AChR channel opens to a reduced conductance, and γ-AChR passes threefold less calcium than the mature ε-AChR.[41]

Compensatory Mechanisms

In addition to persistent expression of the fetal γ-AChR at the EPs, three other mechanisms may help improve neuromuscular transmission in CMS patients with mutations that severely reduce AChR expression.

First, the nerve sprouts, associated with the increased number of EP regions on individual muscle fibers, have an imprinting influence on the underlying nuclei to induce transcription of AChR subunit genes,[42–44] augmenting the total amount of EP AChR.

Second, the postsynaptic AChR deficiency causes an increase in the number of ACh quanta released by nerve impulse.[13,18,45,46] This may be due to a trophic influence of muscle on nerve; alternatively, the increased quantal release stems from an increased number of active zones per EP due to the increased number of EP regions.

Third, in the presence of null mutations of the ε subunit, the ε-omitted species of $\alpha_2\beta\delta_2$-AChR could be expressed at the EPs.[13,16,18] However, even if $\alpha_2\beta\delta_2$-AChR were expressed at the EPs, it would not function well because it has a reduced affinity for ACh[14] and is prone to become desensitized even at low concentrations of ACh.[47]

CLINICAL AND BASIC SCIENCE IMPLICATIONS

The CMS are not uncommon, but are commonly misdiagnosed or treated incorrectly. Combined clinical, morphological, electrophysiological, as well as molecular genetic investigations can provide a correct diagnosis and a rational basis for therapy. For example, patients harboring slow-channel syndrome mutations are significantly improved by quinidine, a long-lived AChR channel blocker.[48,49] Patients with frameshifting mutations in AChR subunit genes benefit from AChE inhibitors, which prolong the lifetime of ACh in the synaptic space, as well as from 3,4-diaminopyridine (3,4-DAP), an agent that increases the quantal release of acetylcholine (ACh). Patients with mutations that reduce the affinity of AChR for ACh are strikingly improved by 3,4-DAP.[14]

A kinetic abnormality or a severe deficiency of EP AChR is presumptive evidence for one or more mutations in an AChR subunit gene. Identification of these mutations is relevant to genetic counseling and prevention.

Spontaneous mutations in human AChR subunits that cause CMS are experiments of nature that highlight functionally significant residues or domains in the subunits. Correlation of a change in the sequence of an AChR subunit with a specific alteration of AChR function yields exquisitely precise structure-function correlations.[9–14]

REFERENCES

1. ENGEL, A. G. 1994. Myasthenic syndromes. *In* Myology: Basic and Clinical, p. 1798–1835. McGraw–Hill. New York.
2. ENGEL, A. G. 1993. The investigation of congenital myasthenic syndromes. Ann. N.Y. Acad. Sci. **681:** 425–434.
3. ENGEL, A. G., E. H. LAMBERT, D. M. MULDER, C. F. TORRES, K. SAHASHI, T. E. BERTORINI & J. N. WHITAKER. 1982. A newly recognized congenital myasthenic syndrome attributed to a prolonged open time of the acetylcholine-induced ion channel. Ann. Neurol. **11:** 553–569.
4. ENGEL, A. G., E. H. LAMBERT & M. R. GOMEZ. 1977. A new myasthenic syndrome with end-plate acetylcholinesterase deficiency, small nerve terminals, and reduced acetylcholine release. Ann. Neurol. **1:** 315–330.
5. HUTCHINSON, D. O., T. J. WALLS, S. NAKANO, S. CAMP, P. TAYLOR, C. M. HARPER, R. V. GROOVER, H. A. PETERSON, D. G. JAMIESON & A. G. ENGEL. 1993. Congenital endplate acetylcholinesterase deficiency. Brain **116:** 633–653.
6. MORA, M., E. H. LAMBERT & A. G. ENGEL. 1987. Synaptic vesicle abnormality in familial infantile myasthenia. Neurology **37:** 206–214.
7. ENGEL, A. G. & E. H. LAMBERT. 1987. Congenital myasthenic syndromes. Electroencephalogr. Clin. Neurophysiol. Suppl. **39:** 91–102.
8. MILONE, M., D. O. HUTCHINSON & A. G. ENGEL. 1994. Patch-clamp analysis of the properties of acetylcholine receptor channels at the normal human endplate. Muscle Nerve **17:** 1364–1369.
9. OHNO, K., D. O. HUTCHINSON, M. MILONE, J. M. BRENGMAN, C. BOUZAT, S. M. SINE & A. G. ENGEL. 1995. Congenital myasthenic syndrome caused by prolonged acetylcholine receptor channel openings due to a mutation in the M2 domain of the ε subunit. Proc. Natl. Acad. Sci. U.S.A. **92:** 758–762.

10. SINE, S. M., K. OHNO, C. BOUZAT, A. AUERBACH, M. MILONE, J. N. PRUITT & A. G. ENGEL. 1995. Mutation of the acetylcholine receptor α subunit causes a slow-channel myasthenic syndrome by enhancing agonist binding affinity. Neuron **15:** 229–239.

11. ENGEL, A. G., K. OHNO, M. MILONE, H-L. WANG, S. NAKANO, C. BOUZAT, J. N. PRUITT, D. O. HUTCHINSON, J. M. BRENGMAN, N. BREN *et al.* 1996. New mutations in acetylcholine receptor subunit genes reveal heterogeneity in the slow-channel congenital myasthenic syndrome. Hum. Mol. Genet. **5:** 1217–1227.

12. MILONE, M., H-L. WANG, K. OHNO, T. FUKUDOME, J. N. PRUITT, N. BREN, S. M. SINE & A. G. ENGEL. 1997. Slow-channel syndrome caused by enhanced activation, desensitization, and agonist binding affinity due to mutation in the M2 domain of the acetylcholine receptor alpha subunit. J. Neurosci. **17:** 5651–5665.

13. OHNO, K., P. QUIRAM, M. MILONE, H-L. WANG, C. M. HARPER, J. N. PRUITT, J. M. BRENGMAN, L. PAO, K. H. FISCHBECK, T. O. CRAWFORD, S. M. SINE & A. G. ENGEL. 1997. Congenital myasthenic syndromes due to heteroallelic nonsense/missense mutations in the acetylcholine receptor ε subunit gene: identification and functional characterization of six new mutations. Hum. Mol. Genet. **6:** 753–766.

14. OHNO, K., H-L. WANG, M. MILONE, N. BREN, J. M. BRENGMAN, S. NAKANO, P. QUIRAM, J. N. PRUITT, S. M. SINE & A. G. ENGEL. 1996. Congenital myasthenic syndrome caused by decreased agonist binding affinity due to a mutation in the acetylcholine receptor ε subunit. Neuron **17:** 157–170.

15. OHNO, K., A. G. ENGEL, M. MILONE, J. M. BRENGMAN, J. P. SIEB & IANNACCONE. 1995. A congenital myasthenic syndrome with severe acetylcholine receptor deficiency caused by heteroallelic frameshifting mutations in the epsilon subunit. Neurology **45(suppl. 4):** A283.

16. MILONE, M., K. OHNO, J. N. PRUITT, J. M. BRENGMAN, S. M. SINE & A. G. ENGEL. 1996. Congenital myasthenic syndrome due to frameshifting acetylcholine receptor epsilon subunit mutation. Soc. Neurosci. Abstr. **22:** 1942.

17. OHNO, K., T. FUKUDOME, S. NAKANO, M. MILONE, T. E. FEASBY, G. M. TYCE & A. G. ENGEL. 1996. Mutational analysis in a congenital myasthenic syndrome reveals a novel acetylcholine receptor epsilon subunit mutation. Soc. Neurosci. Abstr. **22:** 234.

18. ENGEL, A. G., K. OHNO, C. BOUZAT, S. M. SINE & R. G. GRIGGS. 1996. End-plate acetylcholine receptor deficiency due to nonsense mutations in the ε subunit. Ann. Neurol. **40:** 810–817.

19. MILONE, M., K. OHNO, T. FUKUDOME, X-M. SHEN, J. BRENGMAN, R. C. GRIGGS & A. G. ENGEL. 1998. Congenital myasthenic syndrome caused by novel loss of function mutations in the human AChR ε subunit gene. This volume.

20. OHNO, K., B. ANLAR, E. ÖZDIRION, J. M. BRENGMAN & A. G. ENGEL. 1998. Frameshifting and splice-site mutations in acetylcholine receptor ε subunit gene in three Turkish kinships with congenital myasthenic syndromes. This volume.

21. SANDROCK, A. W., S. E. DRYER, K. M. ROSEN, S. M. GOZANI, R. KRAMER, L. E. THEILL & G. D. FISCHBACH. 1997. Maintenance of acetylcholine receptor number by neuregulins at the neuromuscular junction *in vivo*. Science **276:** 599–603.

22. TANSEY, M. G., G. C. CHU & J. P. MERLIE. 1996. ARIA/HRG regulates AChR epsilon subunit gene expression at the neuromuscular synapse via activation of phosphatidylinositol 3-kinase and RAS/MAPK pathway. J. Cell Biol. **134:** 465–476.

23. SI, J., Z. LUO & L. MEI. 1996. Induction of acetylcholine receptor gene expression by ARIA requires activation of mitogen-activated protein kinase. J. Biol. Chem. **271:** 19752–19759.

24. GAUTAM, M., P. G. NOAKES, L. MOSCOSO, F. RUPP, R. H. SCHELLER, J. P. MERLIE & J. R. SANES. 1996. Defective neuromuscular synaptogenesis in agrin-deficient mutant mice. Cell **85:** 525–535.

25. DeChiara, T. M., D. C. Bowen, D. M. Valenzuela, M. V. Simmons, W. T. Poueymirou, S. Thomas, E. Kinetz, D. L. Compton, E. Rojas, J. S. Park *et al.* 1996. The receptor tyrosine kinase MuSK is required for neuromuscular junction formation *in vivo*. Cell **85:** 501–512.

26. Glass, D. J., D. C. Bowen, T. N. Stitt, C. Radziejewski, J. Bruno, T. E. Ryan, D. R. Gies, H. Shah, K. Mattson, S. J. Burden *et al.* 1996. Agrin acts via MuSK receptor complex. Cell **85:** 513–523.

27. Gautam, M., P. G. Noakes, J. Mudd, M. Nichol, G. C. Chu, J. R. Sanes & J. P. Merlie. 1995. Failure of postsynaptic specialization to develop at neuromuscular junctions of rapsyn-deficient mice. Nature **377:** 232–236.

28. Phillips, W. D. 1995. Acetylcholine receptors and the cytoskeletal connection. Clin. Exp. Pharmacol. Physiol. **22:** 961–965.

29. Deconinck, A. E., A. C. Potter, J. M. Tinsley, S. J. Wood, R. Vater, C. Young, L. Metzinger, A. Vincent, C. R. Slater & K. E. Davies. 1997. Postsynaptic abnormalities at the neuromuscular junction of utrophin-deficient mice. J. Cell Biol. **136:** 883–894.

30. Grady, R. M., J. P. Merlie & J. R. Sanes. 1997. Subtle neuromuscular defects in utrophin-deficient mice. J. Cell Biol. **136:** 871–882.

31. Engel, A. G., K. Ohno, M. Milone & S. M. Sine. 1997. Congenital myasthenic syndromes caused by mutations in acetylcholine receptor genes. Neurology **48(suppl. 5)**: S28–S35.

32. Ohno, K., D. O. Hutchinson, M. Milone, S. Nakano, J. P. Sieb, J. M. Brengman & A. G. Engel. 1995. Molecular genetic basis of a slow-channel syndrome. Muscle Nerve **18:** 463 (abstract).

33. Wang, H-L., A. Auerbach, N. Bren, K. Ohno, A. G. Engel & S. M. Sine. 1997. Mutation in the M1 domain of the acetylcholine receptor alpha subunit decreases the rate of agonist dissociation. J. Gen. Physiol. **109:** 757–766.

34. Gomez, C. M., R. Maselli, J. Gammack, J. Lasalde, S. Tamamizu, D. R. Cornblath, M. Lehar, M. McNamee & R. Kuncl. 1996. A beta-subunit mutation in the acetylcholine receptor gate causes severe slow-channel syndrome. Ann. Neurol. **39:** 712–723.

35. Croxen, R., C. Newland, D. Beeson, H. Oosterhuis, G. Chauplanaz, A. Vincent & J. Newsom-Davis. 1997. Mutations in different functional domains of the human muscle acetylcholine receptor α subunit in patients with the slow-channel congenital myasthenic syndrome. Hum. Mol. Genet. **6:** 767–773.

36. Gomez, C. M. & J. T. Gammack. 1995. A leucine-to-phenylalanine substitution in the acetylcholine receptor ion channel in a family with the slow-channel syndrome. Neurology **45:** 982–985.

37. Maselli, R. A. & C. Leung. 1993. Analysis of anticholinesterase-induced neuromuscular transmission failure. Muscle Nerve **16:** 548–553.

38. Uchitel, O., A. G. Engel, T. J. Walls, A. Nagel, Z. M. Atassi & V. Bril. 1993. Congenital myasthenic syndromes. II. A syndrome attributed to abnormal interaction of acetylcholine with its receptor. Muscle Nerve **16:** 1293–1301.

39. Hesselmans, L. F. G. M., F. G. I. Jennekens, C. J. M. Van Den Oord, H. Veldman & A. Vincent. 1993. Development of innervation of skeletal muscle fibers in man: relation to acetylcholine receptors. Anat. Rec. **236:** 553–562.

40. Witzemann, V., H. Schwartz, M. Koenen, C. Berberich, A. Villarroel, A. Wernig, H. R. Brenner & B. Sakmann. 1996. Acetylcholine receptor epsilon subunit deletion causes muscle weakness and atrophy in juvenile and adult mice. Proc. Natl. Acad. Sci. U.S.A. **93:** 13286–13291.

41. Villarroel, A. & B. Sakmann. 1996. Calcium permeability increase of endplate channels in rat muscle during postnatal development. J. Physiol. (Lond.) **496:** 331–338.

42. Sakmann, B., V. Witzemann & H. Brenner. 1992. Developmental changes in acetyl-

choline receptor channel structure and function as a model for synaptic plasticity. Fidia Res. Found. Neurosci. Award Lect. **6:** 51–103.

43. HALL, Z. W. & J. R. SANES. 1993. Synaptic structure and development: the neuromuscular junction. Cell **72(suppl.):** 99–121.

44. MOSCOSO, L. M., G. C. CHU, M. GAUTAM, P. G. NOAKES, J. P. MERLIE & J. R. SANES. 1995. Synapse-associated expression of an acetylcholine receptor–inducing protein, ARIA/Heregulin, and its putative receptors, Erb2 and Erb3, in developing mammalian muscle. Dev. Biol. **172:** 158–169.

45. PLOMP, J. J., G. T. H. VAN KEMPEN & P. C. MOLENAAR. 1992. Adaptation of quantal content to decreased postsynaptic sensitivity at single endplates in α-bungarotoxin treated rats. J. Physiol. (Lond.) **458:** 487–499.

46. PLOMP, J. J., G. T. H. VAN KEMPEN, M. B. DE BAETS, Y. M. F. GRAUS, J. B. M. KUKS & P. C. MOLENAAR. 1995. Acetylcholine release in myasthenia gravis: regulation at single endplate level. Ann. Neurol. **37:** 627–636.

47. LIU, Y. & P. BREHM. 1993. Expression of subunit-omitted mouse nicotinic acetylcholine receptors in *Xenopus laevis* oocytes. J. Physiol. (Lond.) **470:** 349–363.

48. FUKUDOME, T., K. OHNO, J. M. BRENGMAN & A. G. ENGEL. 1997. Quinidine sulfate normalizes the open duration of slow channel congenital myasthenic syndrome acetylcholine receptor channels expressed in human embryonic kidney cells. Neurology **48:** A72 (abstract).

49. HARPER, C. M. & A. G. ENGEL. 1997. Quinidine sulfate in the treatment of the slow channel congenital myasthenic syndrome. Neurology **48:** A72 (abstract).

50. WALLS, T. J., A. G. ENGEL, A. S. NAGEL, C. M. HARPER & V. F. TRASTEK. 1993. Congenital myasthenic syndrome associated with paucity of synaptic vesicles and reduced quantal release. Ann. N.Y. Acad. Sci. **681:** 461–468.

51. CAMP, S., S. BON, Y. LI, D. K. GETMAN, A. G. ENGEL, J. MASSOULIÉ & P. TAYLOR. 1995. Patients with congenital myasthenia associated with end-plate acetylcholinesterase deficiency show normal sequence, mRNA splicing, and assembly of catalytic subunits. J. Clin. Invest. **95:** 333–340.

52. ENGEL, A. G., O. UCHITEL, T. J. WALLS, A. NAGEL, C. M. HARPER & J. BODENSTEINER. 1993. Newly recognized congenital myasthenic syndrome associated with high conductance and fast closure of the acetylcholine receptor channel. Ann. Neurol. **34:** 38–47.

Congenital Myasthenic Syndrome (CMS) Type Ia

Clinical and Genetic Diversity[a]

LEFKOS T. MIDDLETON,[b] KYPROULA CHRISTODOULOU,[b]
FEZA DEYMEER,[c] PIRAYE SERDAROGLU,[c] COSKUN OZDEMIR,[c]
ABDEL KARIM AL-QUDAH,[d] AHMAD AL-SHEHAB,[d]
IOANNIS MAVROMATIS,[e] IOANNIS MYLONAS,[e] AMELIA EVOLI,[f]
MARIOS TSINGIS,[b] ELENI ZAMBA,[b] AND KYRIAKOS KYRIALLIS[b]

[b]The Cyprus Institute of Neurology and Genetics
1683 Nicosia, Cyprus

[c]Istanbul University
Istanbul, Turkey

[d]University of Jordan
Amman, Jordan

[e]Aristotelion University
Thessaloniki, Greece

[f]Universita Cattolica del Sarco Cuore
Rome, Italy

INTRODUCTION

Congenital myasthenic syndromes (CMS) form a group of inherited congenital disorders, affecting the neuromuscular junction. They contrast with the autoimmune disorders, myasthenia gravis and the Eaton-Lambert syndrome, in which, respectively, antibodies to acetylcholine receptors (AChRs) and voltage-gated calcium channels are present in the majority of cases. CMS are uncommon, with an estimated prevalence of less than 1:500,000.[1]

Morphologic and *in situ* neurophysiological observations have allowed for a better understanding of the pathological changes of the neuromuscular junction and the kinetic abnormalities of neuromuscular transmission, in selected patients with CMS. Based on this information, they were classified with regard to presynaptic, synaptic, and postsynaptic defects.[2] In each of these groups, syndromes were further classified according to recognized physiopathogenic mechanisms. Familial infantile myasthenia (FIM) was listed as a presynaptic defect due to a "defect in ACh resynthesis or packaging".

[a]This work was supported by a grant from the Muscular Dystrophy Association (U.S.A.) to L. T. Middleton.

TABLE 1. ENMC Classification of Congenital Myasthenic Syndromes (Modified)

Type I: autosomal recessive	
Ia	familial infantile myasthenia
Ib	limb girdle myasthenia
Ic	acetylcholinesterase deficiency
Id	acetylcholine receptor deficiency
Ie	benign CMS with facial dysmorphism
Type II: autosomal dominant	
IIa	slow-channel syndrome
Type III	
sporadic cases with no family history, excluding myasthenia gravis	

A classification of CMS has recently been proposed by the 34th International ENMC Workshop,[3] based on clinical features and the mode of inheritance (TABLE 1). Type I includes autosomal recessive (AR) disorders, that is, Ia, encompassing familial infantile myasthenia; Ib, limb girdle myasthenia; Ic, corresponding to acetylcholinesterase (AChE) deficiency; and Id, including cases of acetylcholine receptor (AChR) deficiency. Type II is autosomal dominant (AD) and includes one entity, namely the "classic slow-channel syndrome". Type III groups sporadic cases with no family history, excluding myasthenia gravis. For each of the above CMS types, diagnostic criteria have been defined. CMSIa is mainly characterized by its temporal profile with onset at birth to early childhood of fluctuating ptosis, poor cry and suck, feeding difficulties, and possible respiratory distress. In early childhood, there is variable ophthalmoparesis and ptosis as well as mild to moderate fatigable weakness. Episodic exacerbations may occur, resulting in respiratory distress and apnea. Later in life, patients present with ophthalmoparesis, associated with fluctuating ptosis and mild to moderate fatigable weakness of bulbar and limb muscles. Symptoms partially improve with anticholinesterase medication. Otherwise, the neurological examination shows no objective findings. CMSIb has a later age of onset and a characteristic distribution of fatigable weakness, mainly of limb girdle muscles. CMSIc has distinct clinical and neurophysiological features, including selective involvement of axial muscles leading to fixed scoliosis in all the patients, slow pupillary responses to light, and reduced tendon reflexes. Symptoms are refractory or worsened by anticholinesterase medication. Cases of congenital benign, nonprogressive myasthenia mainly involving oculomotricity, with onset at birth and early infancy persisting into adult life without significant exacerbations, were grouped as CMSId. Another benign form of CMS with facial malformations was reported in Oriental Jews,[4] which was not linked to known CMS loci.[5] This form may be assigned as subtype Ie.

We have recently studied the largest reported series of patients with autosomal recessive CMS, conforming to the ENMC diagnostic criteria of CMS Type Ia, in an attempt to map the gene(s) responsible for this disorder.[6]

CLINICAL ASPECTS

Thirteen pedigrees were included in the study; 7 families originated from Turkey, 3 from Greece, 2 from Jordan, and 1 from Italy. The 3 Greek families and 1 of the Turkish families are of Gypsy origin. Consanguinity was noted in 6 of the 7 Turkish families and in the Jordanian and the Italian families. The 38 patients were 22 males and 16 females aged 5 to 56 years of age (mean, 22.75). Clinical history was obtained and neurological examination was performed in 105 individuals from the 13 families. Twenty affected individuals had nerve conduction studies (NCS), needle electromyography (EMG), and repetitive stimulation studies (RSS) before and after exercise. In 6 patients, stimulated single-fiber EMG (SFEMG) was performed. Antiacetylcholine receptor antibodies were measured in at least 1 affected individual from each family (Institute of Molecular Medicine, J. Radcliffe Hospital, Oxford, United Kingdom).

The early history of the disease in infancy and childhood could be obtained in 33 patients. The remaining 5 patients were aged between 31 and 56 years. Onset at birth was reported in 20 individuals and was characterized by variable ptosis and poor suck and cry. Three of the above also had generalized hypotonia. The onset was within the first month in 2 patients, within 12 months in 4 patients, and within 1–2 years in the remaining patients. Initial symptoms mainly included ptosis, feeding, and respiratory difficulties. Definite history of episodic myasthenic exacerbations in infancy and childhood was obtained in 15 patients from 10 families. Two children were reported to have died from respiratory distress at the age of 6 and 8 months. In childhood and adult life, there was fluctuating ptosis and prominent ophthalmoparesis/ophthalmoplegia without diplopia. There was mild to moderate fatigable weakness of limb muscles, with mild bulbar involvement in the majority of patients. A significant degree of intrafamilial variability in myasthenic symptoms was noted. The Greek family 3210 includes a male patient of 36 years of age who had a severe presentation from birth with persistence of significant proximal limb weakness. A second male patient of this family had, at the age of 46, mild symptoms of ptosis and ophthalmoparesis; he continued working as a farmer without significant functional difficulties and with no need for treatment. Anticholinesterase medication improved symptoms in all patients; 19 patients required chronic treatment.

The neurological examination showed no abnormalities of tendon reflexes, and cutaneoplantar reflexes were normal; sensory examination was also normal and there were no signs of muscle atrophy of a generalized or focal distribution. There were no significant signs of facial dysmorphism or foot deformities. Two Turkish patients had mild scoliosis at the age of 8 and 13 years of age, but both had episodic exacerbations during infancy.

Twenty patients underwent neurophysiological investigations. RSS showed significant decremental response at 2–3 Hz in affected segments in all patients studied. Nerve conduction studies and needle EMG were within normal limits in all patients. Double CMAP responses to single nerve stimuli were not observed; 6 patients underwent single-fiber EMG studies, which were normal in all patients. Antiacetylcholine receptor antibody assays showed negative titers in all patients.

MOLECULAR GENETICS–LINKAGE STUDIES

We recently reported mapping of the CMS Ia gene to the telomeric region of 17p.[6] One hundred five individuals from 13 families with CMS Ia, including 38 patients, were analyzed for linkage search through the genome. More than 70% of the genome was excluded after screening with microsatellite polymorphic marker loci in an average of 30-cM distances. Homozygosity mapping, using DNA pooled from the affected individuals of each family, was then employed to screen the nonexcluded regions of the genome at 10-cM distances. Five candidate regions were detected, of which one was subsequently confirmed by linkage analysis as the CMS Ia region. A lod score of 6.48 at $\Theta = 0.054$ was obtained between the disease and marker locus D17S1298. Linkage to the region was confirmed with additional marker loci, and a maximum two-point lod score of 9.28 at $\Theta = 0.034$ was obtained between the disease and marker locus D17S1537. Representative two-point linkage analysis results are shown in TABLE 2. Genetic heterogeneity in this set of families could not be a priori excluded; thus, in linkage analysis and homozygosity mapping on DNA pools, families were studied both as a group and individually. All families were found positive for at least one of the marker loci from this region, suggesting genetic homogeneity within our group of families.

The linkage map of marker loci from the region was established using 7 CEPH-type families from our DNA bank. Haplotypes were constructed in our FIM families following the order in which the above marker loci were mapped on chromosome 17p, and a number of recombination events were identified. Homozygosity by descent in 2 consanguineous families (FIGURE 1) enabled restriction of the candidate region within the interval between marker loci D17S1298 and D17S1537, estimated to be approximately 4.0 cM. Multipoint linkage analysis confirmed the confinement of the CMS Ia region within the above interval, with a maximum multipoint lod score of 12.07 (FIGURE 2).

The CMS Ia locus was mapped at the telomeric region of chromosome 17p, within an interval of 4.0 cM, with finding indicative of genetic homogeneity within this group of families.

TABLE 2. Two-Point lod Scores Obtained between the Disease and Six Microsatellite Polymorphic Marker Loci from the Telomeric Region of Chromosome 17p[a]

				Θ Values					
Locus	0.00	0.01	0.05	0.1	0.2	0.3	0.4	Z_{max}	Θ_{max}
D17S926	$-\infty$	1.78	4.48	4.83	3.87	2.40	1.01	4.84	0.091
D17S849	$-\infty$	−5.16	0.85	2.53	2.77	1.87	0.81	2.91	0.156
D17S1298	$-\infty$	5.25	6.47	6.12	4.46	2.64	1.11	6.84	0.054
D17S1537	$-\infty$	8.67	9.18	8.23	5.61	3.05	1.07	9.28	0.034
D17S578	$-\infty$	6.79	7.97	7.30	4.92	2.55	0.82	7.98	0.046
D17S938	$-\infty$	6.36	7.63	7.05	4.90	2.68	0.94	7.63	0.048

[a]The sum of the lod scores of the 12 FIM families is presented.

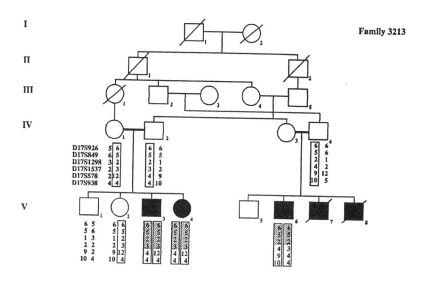

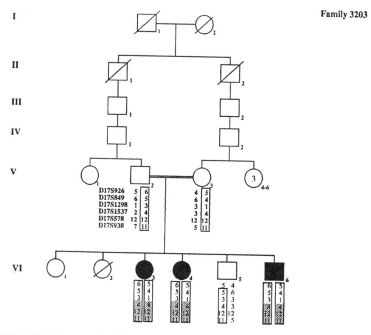

FIGURE 1. Haplotype analysis in families 3213 and 3203. Affected individuals are designated by black symbols. The disease-bearing chromosomes are shown in boxes. The homozygous regions are shown as shaded areas.

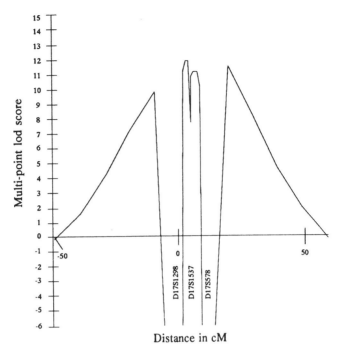

FIGURE 2. Multipoint linkage analysis results. The multipoint lod score of the disease locus is plotted against the fixed map of loci D17S1298, D17S1537, and D17S578.

DISCUSSION AND SUMMARY

The present clinical data of Mediterranean families represent the largest reported series of patients with congenital myasthenic syndromes. Our patients conformed with the recently reported diagnostic criteria of CMS Ia.[3]

Early reports on the clinical aspects of congenital myasthenias were scarce and were based on a limited number of patients. Infants with myasthenic symptoms at birth or early infancy born to nonmyasthenic mothers were first reported in 1949.[7,8] The term of "congenital myasthenia gravis" was employed to differentiate the above from "neonatal myasthenia gravis", a transient disease of infants born to mothers with myasthenia gravis. The two siblings described by Levin,[8] a boy and a girl, suggested a Mendelian autosomal recessive inheritance and had significant variation in their symptomatology. Greer and Schotland[9] studied an infant of 12 weeks of age, with a neonatal history of episodes of respiratory distress, associated with generalized hypotonia, ptosis, and facial weakness, who was responsive to anticholinesterase medication; the apneic episodes regressed within a week and no further myasthenic manifestations were reported, until last seen at the age of 12 weeks. His sister had a similar neonatal history and died of apnea at the age of 3½ months. The authors found their patient unusual, compared to 10 previously reported cases of congenital myasthenia, in the mode of onset, frequency, and severity of the episodes of respiratory distress and in the paucity of intercurrent myasthenic symptoms and signs. They cautiously admitted that recurrence of myasthenia later in life could not be ruled out, as previously noted in a case of neonatal myasthenia.[10]

Namba *et al.*[11] described "familial myasthenia gravis" as a disease occurring among siblings with onset at birth or early infancy, characterized by impairment of extraocular movements, ptosis, long survival, little demand for medication, and a nonfluctuating course. For Conomy *et al.*,[12] "familial infantile myasthenia" (FIM) may have a more severe presentation, characterized by episodes of early respiratory distress requiring chronic anticholinesterase treatment, as noted in their own family. They commented on the significant degree of intrafamilial and interfamilial variability in FIM and emphasized the need for follow-up. They suggested possible genetic associations with an unusual facial appearance and "triple furrowing of the tongue", not reported by others. Robertson *et al.*[13] reported a patient with significant abnormal fatigability at the age of 14 years; RSS showed a decremental response after 60 seconds of exercise, and anti-AChR antibodies were negative. His sibling, who also had apneic episodes during infancy, had no significant symptoms after the age of 2 years. Intrafamilial and interfamilial variability was also evident in 7 patients of Seybold and Lindstrom[14] with family histories of similar illness and negative anti-AChR antibody titers. In 1 of their patients aged 18, an intercostal muscle biopsy was performed, with findings consistent with a presynaptic defect of acetylcholine resynthesis or mobilization.[15] The 3 cases reported by Gieron and Korthals[16] were remarkable in that they were last seen in early adult life. Following a history suggestive of FIM during infancy and childhood, they persisted in having respiratory exacerbations as well as ophthalmoparesis, ptosis, and proximal muscle weakness in early adult life. The validity of the distinction of FIM as a separate entity has been disputed by others.[17]

Following the development of sophisticated morphologic and electrophysiologic techniques for the study of the neuromuscular junction by Engel and coworkers, subsequent studies on congenital myasthenic syndromes were focused on these features. CMS were assigned descriptive morphologic and/or neurophysiologic terms rather than clinical terms, based on remarkably accurate and elegant studies of selected patients. The first report of AChE deficiency was published in 1977 as "a new myasthenic syndrome with end plate acetylcholinesterase deficiency, small nerve terminals, and reduced acetylcholine release".[18] The autosomal dominant form "attributed to a prolonged open-time of the acetylcholine-induced ion channel"[19] was later termed "slow-channel congenital myasthenic syndrome" (SCCMS). The above conditions have distinctive clinical and neurophysiological features.

Three patients with a phenotype similar to the patient of Greer and Schotland underwent *in vitro* neurophysiological and morphological studies.[20] The miniature end plate potential (MEPP) amplitudes were normal at rest, but were reduced after prolonged stimulation at 10 Hz. A similar phenomenon was observed in normal muscle treated with hemicholinium, an inhibitor of choline uptake by the nerve terminal.[21] Therefore, a defect in ACh reuptake and synthesis or packaging has been suggested. No histological or ultrastructural abnormalities of the neuromuscular junction or of the AChR folds were noted. The number of synaptic vesicles in the resting nerve terminals was normal, but their size was smaller, compared to control muscles. The synaptic vesicle size increased or did not change after 10-Hz stimulation, whereas in controls the synaptic vesicles decreased or remained unchanged. Following these observations, a presynaptic syndrome of "defect in ACh resynthesis or packaging" was defined.

A number of observations of postsynaptic defects with and without AChR deficiency and with and without kinetic deficiencies have been reported over the last five years. Clinically, patients are characterized by an onset at birth or early infancy with poor cry and suck and episodes of respiratory distress in some patients and a subsequent course of fluctuating weakness involving ocular, facial, bulbar, and limb muscles. No deaths in infancy were reported. An autosomal recessive inheritance could be documented in a case "associated with high conductance and fast closure of the acetylcholine receptor channel",[22] whose younger sister had similar features. The "syndrome of deficiency and short open-time of the acetylcholine receptor"[23] and the "syndrome attributed to abnormal interaction of acetylcholine with its receptor"[24,25] were studied in children devoid of relevant family history. "AChR deficiency" could be demonstrated in a series of 22 patients with autosomal recessive CMS.[26] The majority of patients had an onset at birth or early infancy. They all had generalized weakness and 16/22 had ocular symptoms. In favor of AChR deficiency were findings of small miniature end plate potentials (MEPPs) and end plate potentials (EPPs) and reduced numbers of AChR, often distributed abnormally along the muscle fibers. Engel et al.[27] reported 2 unrelated patients with negative family history. They had moderate ptosis and ophthalmoparesis, as well as fatigable weakness of facial, neck flexor, and limb muscles, in adult age. Evidence of a mutation affecting the ε subunit of AChR, resulting in end plate AChR deficiency "with prolonged open-time and reduced conductions of the AChR channel", was obtained in these cases. These mutations have recently been characterized as nonsense mutations in the ε subunit with evidence of the γ isoform replacing the ε subunit (γ-AChR) at the EPs, as a protective mechanism from the potentially fatal nonsense mutations in the ε subunit gene.[28]

Two putative candidate genes already mapped to the telomeric region of chromosome 17p encode presynaptic and postsynaptic proteins. Synaptobrevin-2 (syb-2), an 18-kDa intrinsic membrane protein of synaptic vesicles,[29] is encoded by a gene mapped to this region.[30] The syb-2 participates in exocytosis at a step between docking and fusion,[31] forming a stable complex with syntaxin and synaptotagmin[32,33] and also forming a distinct complex with synaptophysin.[34] Tetanus and botulinum neurotoxin types B, D, F, and G block exocytosis by cleaving syb-2 at specific peptide bonds.[35] The role of syb-2 in synaptogenesis still remains unknown.[36] The ε subunit of AChR (ε-AChR) is also encoded by a gene located in the telomeric region of chromosome 17p. A physical map of the region of interest in the telomeric part of chromosome 17p is now being constructed, using YAC clones. We also are in the process of screening our CMS Ia patients for mutations in the syb-2 genes and are initiating screening for mutations in the ε subunit of the AChR gene.

Detailed studies of phenotypic/genotypic correlations will be necessary steps in the elucidation of the nosological and clinical boundaries between the autosomal recessive familial myasthenic syndromes.

REFERENCES

1. VINCENT, A. *et al.* 1997. Genes at the junction—candidates for congenital myasthenic syndromes. Trends Neurosci. **20:** 15–22.
2. ENGEL, A. G. 1994. Congenital myasthenic syndromes. *In* Myology. Volume 1, p. 1806–1835. McGraw–Hill. New York.
3. MIDDLETON, L. T. 1996. Report of the 34th ENMC International Workshop—congenital myasthenic syndromes. Neuromusc. Disord. **6:** 133–136.
4. GOLDHAMMER, Y. *et al.* 1990. Congenital myasthenia associated with facial malformations in Iraqi and Iranian Jews. Brain **113:** 1291–1306.
5. MENOLD, M. M. *et al.* 1996. Genetic analysis of congenital myasthenic syndrome [abstract]. Am. J. Hum. Genet. **59**(4)**:** A386.
6. CHRISTODOULOU, K. *et al.* 1997. Mapping of the familial infantile myasthenia (congenital myasthenic syndrome type Ia) gene to chromosome 17p with evidence of genetic homogeneity. Hum. Mol. Genet. In press.
7. BOWMAN, J. R. 1948. Myasthenia gravis in young children. Pediatrics **1:** 472.
8. LEVIN, P. M. 1949. Congenital myasthenia in siblings. Arch. Neurol. Psychiatry **62:** 745.
9. GREER, M. & M. SCHOTLAND. 1960. Myasthenia gravis in the newborn. Pediatrics **26:** 101–108.
10. TENG, P. & K. E. OSSERMAN. 1956. Studies in myasthenia gravis: neonatal and juvenile types—a report of 21 and a review of 188 cases. J. Mt. Sinai Hosp. **23:** 711–727.
11. NAMBA, T. *et al.* 1971. Familial myasthenia gravis. Arch. Neurol. **25:** 49.
12. CONOMY, J. P., M. LEVINSOHN & A. FANAROFF. 1975. Familial infantile myasthenia gravis: a cause of sudden death in young children. J. Pediatr. **87:** 428–429.
13. ROBERTSON, W. C., R. W. M. CHUN & S. E. KORNGUTH. 1980. Familial infantile myasthenia. Arch. Neurol. **37:** 117–119.
14. SEYBOLD, M. E. & J. M. LINDSTROM. 1981. Myasthenia gravis in infancy. Neurology **31:** 476–480.
15. HART, Z. H. *et al.* 1979. A congenital familial myasthenic syndrome caused by a presynaptic defect of transmitter resynthesis or mobilization [abstract]. Neurology **29:** 559.
16. GIERON, M. A. & J. K. KORTHALS. 1985. Familial infantile myasthenia gravis: report of three cases with follow-up into adult life. Arch. Neurol. **42:** 143–144.
17. SCOPPETTA, C., C. CASALI & M. PIANTALLI. 1983. Congenital myasthenia gravis. Muscle Nerve **5:** 493.
18. ENGEL, A. G., E. H. LAMBERT & M. R. GOMEZ. 1977. A new myasthenic syndrome with end-plate acetylcholinesterase deficiency, small nerve terminals, and reduced acetylcholine release. Ann. Neurol. **1:** 315–330.
19. ENGEL, A. G. *et al.* 1982. A newly recognized congenital myasthenic syndrome attributed to a prolonged open time of the acetylcholine-induced ion channel. Ann. Neurol. **11:** 553–569.
20. MORA, M., E. H. LAMBERT & A. G. ENGEL. 1987. Synaptic vesicle abnormality in familial infantile myasthenia. Neurology **37:** 206–214.
21. ELMQVIST, D. & D. M. J. QUASTEL. 1965. Presynaptic action of hemicholinium at the neuromuscular junction. J. Physiol. (Lond.) **177:** 463–482.
22. ENGEL, A. G. *et al.* 1993. Newly recognized congenital myasthenic syndrome associated with high conductance and fast closure of the acetylcholine receptor channel. Ann. Neurol. **34:** 38–47.
23. ENGEL, A. G. *et al.* 1993. Congenital myasthenic syndromes. I. Deficiency and short open-time of the acetylcholine receptor. Muscle Nerve **16:** 1284–1292.
24. UCHITEL, O. *et al.* 1993. Congenital myasthenic syndromes. II. A syndrome attributed to abnormal interaction of acetylcholine with its receptor. Muscle Nerve **16:** 1293–1301.

25. OHNO, K. *et al.* 1996. Congenital myasthenic syndrome caused by decreased agonist binding affinity due to a mutation in the acetylcholine receptor ε subunit. Neuron **17:** 157–170.
26. VINCENT, A. *et al.* 1993. Clinical and experimental observations in patients with congenital myasthenic syndromes. Ann. N.Y. Acad. Sci. **681:** 451–460.
27. ENGEL, A. G. *et al.* 1993. Myasthenic syndromes attributed to mutations affecting the epsilon subunit of the acetylcholine receptor. Ann. N.Y. Acad. Sci. **681:** 496–508.
28. ENGEL, A. G. *et al.* 1996. End-plate acetylcholine receptor deficiency due to nonsense mutations in the subunit. Ann. Neurol. **40:** 810–817.
29. BAUMERT, M. *et al.* 1989. Synaptobrevin: an integral membrane protein of 18,000 daltons present in small synaptic vesicles of rat brain. EMBO J. **8:** 379–384.
30. ARCHER, B. T. *et al.* 1990. Structures and chromosomal localizations of two human genes encoding synaptobrevins 1 and 2. J. Biol. Chem. **265:** 17267–17273.
31. HUNT, J. M. *et al.* 1994. A post-docking role for synaptobrevin in synaptic vesicle fusion. Neuron **12:** 1269–1279.
32. HAYASHI, T. *et al.* 1994. Synaptic vesicle membrane fusion complex: action of clostridial neurotoxins on assembly. EMBO J. **13:** 5051–5061.
33. EL FAR, O. *et al.* 1995. Interaction of a synaptobrevin (VAMP)–syntaxin complex with presynaptic calcium channels. FEBS Lett. **361:** 101–105.
34. WASHBOURNE, P., G. SCHIAVO & C. MONTECUCCO. 1995. Vesicle-associated membrane protein-2 (synaptobrevin-2) forms a complex with synaptophysin. Biochem. J. **305:** 721–724.
35. SCHIAVO, G. *et al.* 1992. Tetanus and botulinum-B neurotoxins block neurotransmitter release by proteolytic cleavage of synaptobrevin. Nature **359:** 832–835.
36. ANHERT-HILGER, G. *et al.* 1996. Synaptobrevin is essential for secretion, but not for the development of synaptic processes. Eur. J. Cell Biol. **70:** 1–11.

Genetic Manipulation of AChR Responses Suggests Multiple Causes of Weakness in Slow-Channel Syndrome[a]

CHRISTOPHER M. GOMEZ,[b,c] RICARDO MASELLI,[d]
JOAN M. WILLIAMS,[b] BULA B. BHATTACHARYYA,[e]
ROBERT L. WOLLMANN,[f] AND JOHN W. DAY[b]

[b]Department of Neurology
[c]Institute of Human Genetics
University of Minnesota
Minneapolis, Minnesota 55455

[d]Department of Neurology and Center for Neuroscience
University of California, Davis
Davis, California 95616

[e]Department of Ophthalmology
Northwestern University Medical School
Chicago, Illinois 60611

[f]Section of Neuropathology
University of Chicago School of Medicine
Chicago, Illinois 60637

INTRODUCTION

The slow-channel congenital myasthenic syndrome (SCCMS) is a dominantly in-herited disorder of neuromuscular transmission that is characterized by progressive muscle weakness, fatigability, and a constellation of electrophysiological and patho-logical findings attributed to inherited abnormalities of acetylcholine receptor (AChR) ion channel function.[1–3] Recently, several distinct point mutations either in the sequences encoding the ion channel domain (M1 and M2)[4–10a] or in the region encoding the acetylcholine-binding domain[8,10a,10b] have been identified within AChR subunit genes of patients with SCCMS. Point mutations believed responsible for SC-CMS have been found in the α, β, and ε subunits. In this laboratory, we have shown that the point mutation, εL269F, is present in the three affected members of one of the kindreds in the original clinical report on SCCMS.[1,5] When expressed in oocytes, the εL269F mutation causes 6- to 8-fold increases in single-channel open time, with-out affecting channel conductance.[8,11,12]

Although these studies firmly establish the connection between AChR mutations and abnormal AChR channel kinetics, they do not clarify the basis for the weakness

[a]This work was supported by grants from the National Institutes of Health (Nos. NS01540 and NS32201) and the Muscular Dystrophy Association.

and fatigability. The clinical features of the SCCMS are most likely due to a reduced safety factor of neuromuscular transmission. In theory, missense mutations that affect AChR ion channel function could reduce the miniature end plate current (MEPC) amplitude through several possible mechanisms, including effects on single-channel conductance, AChR desensitization, depolarization blockade, and degeneration of the postsynaptic region secondary to excessive Ca^{2+} entry through mutant AChRs. Some spontaneous AChR mutations in SCCMS are known to cause increased AChR desensitization,[9] while many cause prolonged open time.

Ultrastructural study of motor end plates in SCCMS has demonstrated the presence of a localized degenerative process, termed end plate myopathy.[1,2,6] In this condition, the synaptic cleft is widened and contains electron-dense, granular debris; the junctional basal lamina is highly reduplicated in some areas; the postsynaptic folds are simplified or are frankly degenerating; and the junctional sarcoplasm contains increased pinocytotic vesicles, autophagic vacuoles, myeloid structures, areas of myofibrillar disruption, and varying numbers of degenerating organelles, such as mitochondria and junctional myonuclei. These ultrastructural abnormalities are believed to arise from the effects of Ca^{2+} overload of the junctional sarcoplasm through slowly closing AChRs and may lead to reduced function of the neuromuscular junction.

The basic molecular defect produced by a given mutation may be assessed well by studying the function of the mutant AChRs *in vitro*. However, the relative contribution of each mechanism underlying reduced neuromuscular transmission in SCCMS cannot be well defined from *in vitro* studies alone. For a full understanding of the pathological consequences of the mutant AChRs, a more native setting is essential, with the mutant AChRs packed in dense arrays at the tips of end plate postsynaptic folds and exposed transiently to high concentrations of acetylcholine. For this reason, we have developed transgenic mouse models of the SCCMS. The desire for a detailed understanding of the pathogenesis of this disease is not merely academic. The SCCMS and AChR mutations serve as prototypes for the growing number of other channelopathies that affect synapses or excitable membranes that are far less understood than the neuromuscular junction. Our ability to study the molecular, ultrastructural, and electrophysiological aspects of neuromuscular junctions expressing mutant AChRs may aid in understanding disorders ranging from periodic paralysis and myotonia to migraine, ataxia, and epilepsy.

MATERIALS AND METHODS

Establishment of Transgenic Lines

The design for the transgene constructs that were used to express mutant AChRs have been described previously.[13] Briefly, the cDNAs encoding the δS262T or εL269F mutant AChR subunits were joined to the 3' end of a 3.3-kb portion of the mouse creatine kinase promoter.[14] The 3' untranslated ends of the AChR were removed and replaced with the 3' untranslated region of the bacterial neomycin resistance gene (NEO) and the SV40 small-t intron to allow distinction of transgene mRNA.

Transgenic mice were generated by microinjection of purified transgene into single-cell mouse embryos.[15] Mice bearing the transgenes were identified by analysis of tail DNA by the polymerase chain reaction,[16] using primers corresponding to sequences in the transgene subunit[17] and the NEO gene.[18]

Clinical Evaluation of Muscle Strength

Muscle strength was assessed using two tests.[12] In the first test, mice were observed for 60 seconds after they had been placed on top of a 6-mm wooden dowel that was suspended at a height of 35 cm. In the second test, mice were placed with front claws gripping a suspended wire and observed for 60 seconds. The possible outcomes of each test consisted of not falling for the entire observation period (score of 100%) or falling before 1 minute was reached (scored as a percentage of a minute). For each test, five sets of three repetitions were conducted. The mean and standard error for 15 tests were calculated. Mice were tested blindly using littermate controls.

Electromyography

Compound muscle action potentials (CMAPs) were studied as described.[13] For hindlimb recordings, animals were anesthetized with pentobarbital or Avertin[15] and the sciatic nerve was exposed. Wounds were closed with stainless-steel wound clips. Subdermal stainless-steel pin electrodes were used to measure the CMAP amplitude and waveform produced by supramaximal stimulation of the sciatic nerve. During repetitive stimulation of the sciatic nerve at rates of greater than 5 Hz, the initial CMAP amplitude ($CMAP_1$) was greatest, and decrement was maximal by the eighth CMAP ($CMAP_8$). Fractional decrement was calculated as follows: ($CMAP_1 - CMAP_8$)/$CMAP_1$. The baseline responses to stimulation rates of 5, 10, and 20 Hz were recorded in mice that were then injected with curare (0.3 mg/kg, subcutaneous). Fifteen minutes after the injection, the responses to repetitive stimulation at 5 and 10 Hz were recorded at 5-min intervals until the peak decrement in CMAP was reached ($\sim$30 min).

Voltage-Clamp

Previously reported methods were employed.[13] In brief, the phrenic nerve and diaphragm muscles were removed and perfused at room temperature (22–25 °C) with Tyrode's solution [composition (mM): NaCl, 137; KCl, 2.8; $CaCl_2$, 1.8; $MgCl_2$, 1.1; $NaHCO_3$, 11.9; NaH_2PO_4, 0.33; dextrose, 11.2; pH 7.4] when bubbled with a mixture of 95% O_2 and 5% CO_2 (V/V). A cut muscle preparation was used for end plate current (EPC) recording using a two-microelectrode voltage-clamp system.[19–21] Intracellular potentials were measured with a 3 M KCl microelectrode of 8–15 MΩ resistance using an Axoclamp-2A amplifier system. Currents were obtained at a holding potential of –50 mV, digitized at 50 μs per point, and stored in computer memory

(IBM PC/AT) by using SCAN software (J. Dempster, Glasgow). EPCs were elicited by stimulating the phrenic nerve with rectangular pulses of 0.05-ms duration. During single-shock stimulation, the nerve was stimulated at 0.2 Hz, while tetanic stimulation was performed at either 20 or 40 Hz for 0.5 to 2 s. For some experiments, MEPCs were recorded just before and immediately after (2–5 s) tetanic stimulation.

The time constants of decay of MEPCs and EPCs were determined using biexponential decay analyses according to the Marquardt-Levenberg algorithm.[22] The "rundown" of a train of EPCs was defined as the fractional decrease in EPC amplitude from the peak response to the plateau (usually by 50 responses). The plateau was estimated as the mean of the last 10 responses. Quantal content was calculated using the following equation: Q direct = Avg(PkEPC)/Avg(PkMEPC), where Avg(PkMEPC) is the average MEPC amplitude and Avg(PkEPC) is the average EPC amplitude evoked at 0.2 Hz stimulation.

Measurement of α-Bungarotoxin Binding Sites

The number of α-bungarotoxin (αBT) binding sites in muscle was quantitated either by immunoprecipitation[20] or by surface binding in freshly excised limb muscle using ^{125}I-αBT exactly as described,[23] except that diaphragm and brachioradialis muscle were used.

Pathological Studies

Muscle was fixed in phosphate buffer with 2% glutaraldehyde by either immersion or perfusion following cardiac puncture. For immersion fixation, the right forelimb flexor muscles were teased apart to bundles of ~100 fibers and immersed in phosphate buffer with 2% glutaraldehyde. Following perfusion fixation, forelimb flexor muscles were removed and fixed overnight in fresh glutaraldehyde. The muscle bellies were rinsed in 0.1 M phosphate buffer, teased into 1-mm bundles, osmicated, and embedded in epon.

RESULTS

δS262T-Transgenic Mice: Reduced MEPCs and AChR Desensitization

δS262T-Transgenic Mice Have Impaired Neuromuscular Transmission

We established three transgenic lines, each of which expresses the mutant δ subunit (δS262T) mRNA in skeletal muscle, although the steady state level of mutant mRNA differs between lines over a 50-fold range.[13] Transgenic mice from all three lines had electrophysiological evidence of a kinetic disturbance of AChR function, including repetitive CMAPs evoked by a single sciatic nerve stimulus and prolonged decay phases of the MEPCs.[13] The amplitudes of the MEPCs were reduced to 33% of normal.[13] δS262T-transgenic mice did not develop clinically evident weakness, but

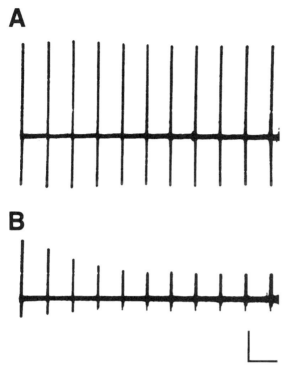

FIGURE 1. δS262T-transgenic mice show increased sensitivity to curare. The effect of a low dose of curare (0.3 mg/kg) on the amplitude of the CMAP during repetitive stimulation at 5 Hz is shown for a control (A) and a transgenic mouse (B). In A, the decrement is only 1.3%. In B, the initial CMAP amplitude is reduced and there is a decrement of 58% by the eighth response. Calibration: 0.2 s, 20 mV.

did show abnormal sensitivity to low doses of curare. FIGURE 1 displays the effect of low-dose curare on CMAPs recorded over the gastrocnemius during 5 Hz sciatic nerve stimulation in control (A) and transgenic (B) mice. In A, there is 1.3% decrement in amplitude. In B, the amplitude of the initial response is reduced compared with predrug amplitude and there is 58% decrement. At this dose, δS262T-transgenic mice manifested 21.3 ± 6.5% decrement (mean ± SE), while control mice had less than 0.26 ± 0.77% decrement ($p < 0.005$).[13] Thus, the reduced MEPC amplitudes cause a significant impairment of neuromuscular transmission.

No Structural Basis for Reduced MEPCs in δS262T-Transgenic Mice

We investigated the basis for the reduction in MEPC amplitude in δS262T-transgenic mice and showed that diminished MEPC amplitudes were not due to a decrease in ion channel conductance. Patch-clamp recordings of single channels recorded from acutely dissociated muscle fibers of the flexor digitorum brevis demonstrated that AChRs of δS262T-transgenic mice have a channel conductance of 61.8 pS,[21] which was identical to that of control end plate AChRs.

Reduced MEPC amplitudes in δS262T-transgenic mice are not due to degeneration or changes in the end plate architecture. End plates of δS262T-transgenic mice are ultrastructurally normal. FIGURE 2 is an electron micrograph of a neuromuscular junction from a forelimb muscle of a 6-month-old δS262T-transgenic mouse, showing normal synaptic cleft, postsynaptic folds, and junctional sarcoplasm.[21]

Finally, as determined by immunoprecipitation of α-bungarotoxin (αBT) binding sites from solubilized muscle, there is no reduction in skeletal muscle AChR content in δS262T-transgenic mice to account for the reduced MEPC amplitudes. The number of αBT binding sites in transgenic muscle was normal or slightly increased relative to control (0.32 ± 0.04 pmol/g, $n = 30$ versus 0.22 ± 0.03 pmol/g, $n = 11$, $p > 0.1$).[21]

δS262T-Transgenic Mice Have Reduced MEPC Amplitude Associated with Rundown

To test the hypothesis that MEPC amplitude in δS262T-transgenic mice falls during repetitive nerve-evoked activity, we used a preparation similar to one used to demonstrate *in situ* AChR desensitization during esterase inhibition.[24] EPCs were recorded from the cut diaphragm preparation[20] while stimulating the phrenic nerve at physiologic rates. The amplitude of EPCs diminished in both transgenic and control mice during 20 and 40 Hz stimuli, but the reduction was significantly greater in the transgenic mice (FIGURE 3). FIGURE 3A is a representative recording of the EPC rundown for transgenic and control mice during 20 and 40 Hz stimulation. At –50 mV holding potential, EPC amplitudes of δS262T-transgenic mice diminished to 69.4 ±

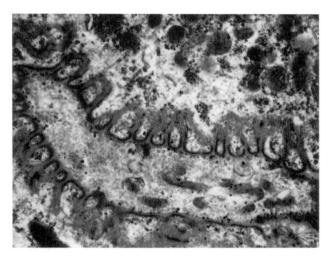

FIGURE 2. δS262T-transgenic mice have ultrastructurally normal end plates. Motor end plate from a diaphragm of a 6-month-old δS262T-transgenic mouse. No pathological changes or ultrastructural abnormalities are present.

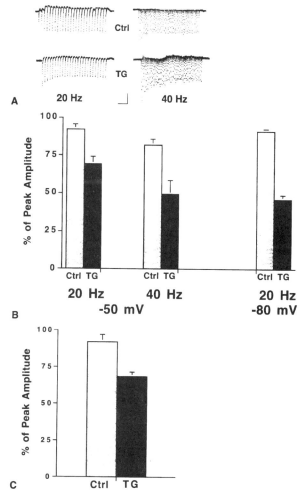

FIGURE 3. EPCs and MEPCs in δS262T-transgenic mice desensitize with nerve stimulation. (A) Trains of EPCs evoked in transgenic and control diaphragm by stimulation at 20 and 40 Hz. In these recordings, the EPC amplitude in the transgenic mouse reduces by 36% and 45.4% at 20 and 40 Hz, while the control reduces by only 7.6% and 26% at the same stimulus frequencies. Calibration: 50 nA, 500 ms. (B) Percent reduction of EPC amplitude from the initial peak response in transgenic mice (dark bars) compared with control mice (light bars) at 20 and 40 Hz, at –50 mV and –80 mV holding potentials. EPC amplitudes of δS262T-transgenic mice (TG, dark bars) diminish to 69 ± 4.7% (30.6% reduction, $n = 9$) and to 49.6 ± 9.2% (50.4% reduction, $n = 5$) of the peak amplitude, during 20 and 40 Hz stimulation, compared with reductions in control diaphragm (Ctrl, light bars) to 92 ± 3.2% (8% reduction, $n = 6$) and to 82 ± 4.1% (18.3% reduction, $n = 6$) of peak response, respectively ($p < 0.01$). At –80 mV, the difference in rundown was even greater at 20 Hz, with transgenic EPCs diminishing to 44 ± 2.8% (56% reduction, $n = 4$) and control EPCs diminishing to 69.4 ± 4.7% (30.6% reduction, $p < 0.01$, $n = 9$). (C) After a 20 Hz stimulus, MEPCs in transgenic mice (dark bars) reduce to 68.7 ± 3% (31.3% reduction, $n = 14$), while those of control mice (light bars) reduce only to 91.9 ± 5% (8.1% reduction, $n = 10$) ($p < 0.01$). Values for B and C are means ± SEM.

4.7% of peak amplitude ($n = 9$) with 20 Hz stimulation and to $49.6 \pm 9.2\%$ of peak amplitude ($n = 5$) with 40 Hz stimulation, while control EPC amplitudes fell only to $92 \pm 3.2\%$ ($n = 6$) and $81.7 \pm 4.1\%$ ($n = 6$) during 20 and 40 Hz stimulation, respectively ($p < 0.01$) (FIGURE 3B). Furthermore, the reduction in EPC amplitude in δS262T-transgenic mice during 20 Hz stimulation was voltage-dependent, falling to $69.4 \pm 4.7\%$ of peak amplitude ($n = 9$) at –50 mV and to $44 \pm 2.8\%$ of peak amplitude ($n = 4$, $p < 0.01$) at –80 mV. In comparison, control mouse EPCs declined to $92 \pm 3.2\%$ of peak response at –50 mV ($n = 6$) and to $90.9 \pm 0.71\%$ of peak response at –80 mV ($n = 3$).

To test whether repetitive activity had a similar effect on MEPCs, we recorded MEPCs immediately before and after (2–5 s) trains of stimuli at physiological rates. The MEPC amplitudes in δS262T-transgenic diaphragms ($n = 14$) were only $68.7 \pm 3\%$ of the prestimulus amplitude following 20 Hz phrenic nerve stimulation, while MEPC amplitudes in control mouse diaphragm ($n = 10$) minimally decreased to $91.9 \pm 5\%$ of the prestimulus amplitude ($p < 0.01$) (FIGURE 3C). This change in MEPC amplitude can account for the magnitude of the EPC rundown. Thus, in comparison to studies showing normal end plate morphology, AChR content, and AChR ion channel conductance for δS262T-transgenic mice, both nerve-evoked and spontaneously occurring postsynaptic responses in the diaphragm were significantly reduced by previous nerve activity. These findings suggest that the reduced MEPC and EPC amplitudes in δS262T-transgenic mice are due to an increased rate of desensitization manifested by the mutant AChRs. While desensitization of wild-type AChRs probably plays no significant role in shaping synaptic responses under normal conditions, these findings in δS262T-transgenic mice indicate that certain mutations alter AChR channel kinetics and increase the rate of desensitization, thus reducing the safety factor of neuromuscular transmission.

εL269F-Transgenic Mice: Weakness from Multiple Factors

εL269F-Transgenic Mice Have Reduced AChR Numbers Soon after Birth

We established three lines that express the mutant mouse ε subunit, εL269F, a mutation found in two families with SCCMS.[5,8] Levels of expression range 8-fold.[12] Mice from all three lines developed progressive weakness, fatigability, and end plate myopathy. Degeneration and simplification of the postsynaptic membrane, as seen in myasthenia gravis and SCCMS, are usually associated with AChR loss. To better understand the time course of the changes, we followed clinical and morphological features as well as AChR number in mice from 3 weeks to 15 months of age. At 3 weeks, εL269F-transgenic mice could be distinguished from their littermate controls by the presence of a more rapid respiratory rate. Ultrastructurally, the singular abnormality at this age was the presence of myriads of vacuolar structures in the junctional sarcoplasm (FIGURE 4A). The vacuoles ranged in size from 0.5 to 10 nm and did not contain any electron-dense material. The synaptic cleft, postsynaptic folds, junctional nuclei, and mitochondria all appeared normal at this age. Thus, the first ultrastructural change of the synapse was the accumulation of vacuoles.

We next determined the number of end plate AChRs in both 3- and 6-week-old

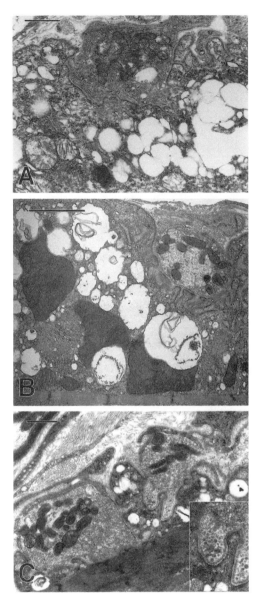

FIGURE 4. Progressive end plate myopathy in εL269F-transgenic mice. The typical ultra-structural findings in forelimb neuromuscular junctions of εL269F-transgenic mice aged 3 weeks (A), 4 months (B), and 15 months (C) are displayed. (A) At 3 weeks, the synaptic cleft, basement membrane, and postsynaptic folds are normal. The junctional sarcoplasm is filled with empty-appearing vacuoles that presumably derive from dilated sarcoplasmic reticulum. (B) At 4 months, the postsynaptic folds are blunted, numerous mitochondria in the junctional sarcoplasm are massively enlarged and have densely packed cristae, and the vacuoles are filled with membranous and granular debris. In other views, the subjunctional nuclei are degenerating. (C) At 15 months, the postsynaptic folds still appear blunted in some places and the synaptic cleft is widened and contains granular debris (inset). The basement membrane is obviously thickened (inset). Scale bars: 1 μM.

mice. In both age groups, AChRs were 80–84% of control AChRs. Thus, in spite of the lack of degenerative changes in 3-week-old εL269F-transgenic mice, the number of AChRs at the end plate was less than control (FIGURE 5). The reduction in AChR number in transgenic motor end plates that have been functional for 1–2 weeks and have no evidence of degeneration suggests the role of developmental factors in determining the AChR number.

Adult εL269F-Transgenic Mice Have Progressive Weakness and End Plate Degeneration

At 3–4 months of age, εL269F-transgenic mice were obviously weak. Transgenic mice at this age had less spontaneous locomotor activity, and performance on standardized strength tests was clearly abnormal (FIGURE 6). Transgenic mice remained on the dowel perch for an average of 25 seconds, while control mice endured an average of 55 seconds ($p < 0.001$).

Ultrastructurally, end plates of 3–4-month-old mice showed marked degenerative changes (FIGURE 4B) The principal features of the synaptic degeneration at this age were the presence of lysosomes filled with membranous debris, abnormal or degenerating subsarcolemmal nuclei and mitochondria, and short, blunt postsynaptic folds with shallow secondary synaptic clefts. In mice aged 4–5 months, MEPC amplitudes were diminished from a control mean of 2.9 ± 0.26 pA ($n = 33$) to 2.0 ± 0.18 pA ($n = 105$), a reduction of approximately 31%.[12] In mice of the same age range, 4–6

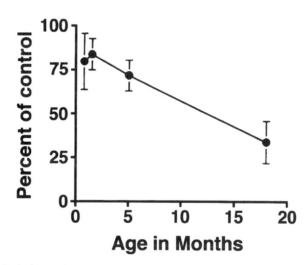

FIGURE 5. End plate AChRs diminish throughout the life of εL269F-transgenic mice. The AChR numbers expressed as the fraction (percent) of normal are plotted for each age group. Mice aged 4–6 months were pooled for the 5-month group, and mice aged 15–21 months were pooled for the 18-month group. Numbers of mice for each group were as follows—controls: 3 wk, $n = 2$; 6 wk, $n = 3$; 4–6 mos, $n = 6$; 15–21 mos, $n = 4$; transgenic: 3 wk, $n = 3$; 6 wk, $n = 3$; 4–6 mos, $n = 6$; 16–20 mos, $n = 4$.

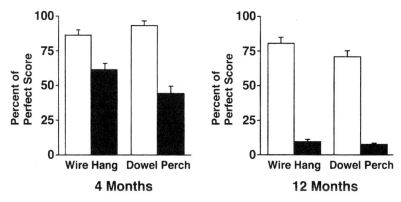

FIGURE 6. εL269F-transgenic mice have progressive skeletal muscle weakness. At 4–5 months of age, transgenic mice (dark bars) performed significantly more poorly than control mice (light bars) both on the wire hang test (61.5% compared with 86.7% for control) and on the dowel perch test (44.1% compared with 93.4% for control, $n = 15$, $p \ll 0.001$). By 8–15 months of age, strength had deteriorated further. Transgenic mice performed poorly both on the wire hang test (9.5% compared with 74.4% for control) and on the dowel test (7.6% compared with 63.6% for control, $n = 10$ transgenic mice, $n = 33$ control, $p \ll 0.001$). Perfect score (100%) = 1 min hang or escape.

months, AChR numbers were reduced significantly to 72% of normal (a reduction of 28%) (FIGURE 5). The reduction in MEPC amplitudes corresponds well with the reduction in AChR number. However, this modest reduction in MEPC amplitude and AChR number is not alone sufficient to explain the weakness. Other factors, such as depolarization block or desensitization, must be responsible.

Progressive End Plate Degeneration in εL269F-Transgenic Mice Influences the Efficiency of Neuromuscular Transmission through Mechanical Effects

In εL269F-transgenic mice of advanced age, the picture was even more complicated. Mice aged 12 to 18 months showed no more weakness than younger mice when observed during normal cage activity. However, on formal strength testing, weakness was significantly increased (FIGURE 3). Many mice could no longer grasp the wire at all. Average time on the dowel was 4.4 seconds for transgenic mice as compared with 38 seconds for control ($p < 0.001$). MEPC amplitudes have not yet been measured in these older mice. As assessed by αBT binding, AChR number in mice aged 15–21 months was diminished to 34% of control. In addition, ultrastructurally, end plates in older mice had significant degenerative and reactive change: postsynaptic folds were flattened in some areas, the synaptic cleft was widened, and the basement membrane was thickened (FIGURE 4C and inset). The widened synaptic cleft and thickened basement membrane most likely exacerbate the effect of the reduced AChR number and contribute to the reduction in safety factor and muscle weakness.

DISCUSSION

Spontaneous AChR mutations associated with different forms of congenital myasthenic syndrome give rise to several types of changes in AChR function, including null mutations or mutant AChRs with increased spontaneous channel openings in the unbound state, prolonged channel openings, increased agonist affinity, slowed rate of agonist dissociation, increased rate of desensitization, slowed rate of channel opening or decreased rate of channel opening, and desensitization with increased rate of agonist dissociation.[4,6,8–10,25,26] In some cases, the manner by which the subsequent defect in neuromuscular transmission arises from these mutations seems straightforward. In others, multiple factors may play a role. These *in vivo* studies provide evidence for the possible participation of several mechanisms in the reduction in the neuromuscular safety factor.

For δS262T-transgenic mice, we found that direct stimulation of the phrenic nerve *in vitro* had two important consequences not seen in control mice. First, during stimulation at low rates, the amplitude of the EPCs fell by 30.6%. Under identical conditions, control EPC amplitudes diminished by only 8%. At –80 mV, transgenic EPCs were even more sensitive to 20 Hz stimulation, falling by 56% compared to only 9.1% in control mice. Second, MEPC amplitudes recorded after stimulation decreased by 31% in δS262T-transgenic mice versus only 8% for controls. These findings suggest that, like wild-type AChRs exposed to esterase inhibitors,[24] the δS262T-AChRs in these mice desensitize *in vivo* in response to physiological amounts of ACh.

For εL269F-transgenic mice, detailed evaluation over the lifetime of the mice demonstrated the presence of several factors likely to contribute to impaired neuromuscular transmission. First, we observed that, in end plates of 1–2-week-old εL269F-transgenic mice, there were dilated vacuoles in the junctional sarcoplasm, but no other evidence of end plate myopathy. In spite of this, the AChR number was only 84% of control. This suggests that the first effect of mutant AChRs with prolonged open time may be to reduce AChR expression and AChR number. This is a reasonable hypothesis given that gene expression at the neuromuscular junction is regulated in part by Ca^{2+} (see reference 27) and εL269F-AChRs cause increased entry of Ca^{2+} into the junctional sarcoplasm.[12]

Second, while the modest reduction in MEPC amplitude in adult εL269F-transgenic mice correlates roughly with the decrease in AChR number, the weakness of the mice seems more severe than expected. Since reductions in MEPC amplitudes of up to 70% in rats do not cause overt weakness,[28] the severe weakness in adult mice implies the presence of an additional effect of the mutation on neuromuscular transmission. Possibilities include the occurrence of desensitization and depolarization block or a direct effect of the end plate myopathy on muscle contractility. The effect of the localized contracture seen at many neuromuscular junctions has not yet been evaluated.

Third, while increased weakness in older εL269F-transgenic mice correlates with further reduction in AChR number, ultrastructural changes probably play an additional role. The widened synaptic cleft and the increase in basement membrane thickness may alter the total number and synchrony of the quanta that reach the postsynaptic membrane. Also, the greater thickness of the basement membrane could mean a larger concentration of AChE in the synaptic cleft. These reactive changes could affect both the amplitude and the rise time of the EPCs, further lowering the safety factor.

These studies demonstrate the potential importance of a wide variety of factors that may impair neuromuscular transmission following a single point mutation in one of the AChR subunit genes. Certain factors may gain in importance during the progression of the disease. Different mutations may have entirely distinct consequences. These findings will affect the approach to potential therapies and the understanding of the pathogenesis of these and other so-called channelopathies.

REFERENCES

1. ENGEL, A. G., E. H. LAMBERT, D. M. MULDER *et al.* 1982. A newly recognized congenital myasthenic syndrome attributed to a prolonged open time of the acetylcholine-induced ion channel. Ann. Neurol. **11**(6): 553–569.
2. OOSTERHUIS, H. J., J. NEWSOM-DAVIS, J. H. WOKKE *et al.* 1987. The slow channel syndrome: two new cases. Brain **110**: 1061–1079.
3. ENGEL, A. G. 1994. Myasthenic syndromes. *In* Myology. Second edition. Vol. 2, p. 1798–1835. McGraw–Hill. New York.
4. OHNO, K., D. HUTCHINSON, M. MILONE *et al.* 1995. Congenital myasthenic syndrome caused by prolonged acetylcholine receptor channel openings due to a mutation in the M2 domain of the ε subunit. Proc. Natl. Acad. Sci. U.S.A. **92**: 758–762.
5. GOMEZ, C. M. & J. T. GAMMACK. 1995. A leucine-to-phenylalanine substitution in the acetylcholine receptor ion channel in a family with the slow-channel syndrome. Neurology **45**(5): 982–985.
6. GOMEZ, C. M., R. MASELLI, J. LASALDE *et al.* 1996. A β subunit mutation in the acetylcholine receptor channel gate causes severe slow-channel syndrome. Ann. Neurol. **39**(6): 717–723.
7. OHNO, K., M. MILONE, H-L. WANG *et al.* 1996. Identification of neuromuscular junction acetylcholine receptor mutations in the slow-channel congenital myasthenic syndrome. Neurology **46**: A214.
8. ENGEL, A. G., K. OHNO, M. MILONE *et al.* 1996. New mutations in acetylcholine receptor subunit genes reveal heterogeneity in the slow-channel congenital myasthenic syndrome. Hum. Mol. Genet. **5**(9): 1217–1227.
9. MILONE, M., H-L. WANG, K. OHNO *et al.* 1997. Slow-channel myasthenic syndrome caused by enhanced activation, desensitization, and agonist binding affinity attributable to mutation in the m2 domain of the acetylcholine receptor alpha subunit. J. Neurosci. **17**(15): 5651–5665.
10. (a) CROXEN, R., C. NEWLAND, D. BEESON *et al.* 1997. Mutations in different functional domains of the human muscle acetylcholine receptor α subunit in patients with the slow-channel congenital myasthenic syndrome. Hum. Mol. Genet. **6**(5): 767–774; (b) SINE, S. M., K. OHNO, C. BOUZAT *et al.* 1995. Mutation of the acetylcholine receptor α subunit causes a slow-channel myasthenic syndrome by enhancing agonist binding affinity. Neuron **15**: 229–239.
11. GOMEZ, C. M., S. TAMAMIZU, J. LASALDE *et al.* 1996. *In vitro* and *in vivo* properties of an acetylcholine receptor (AChR) mutation in a family with the slow-channel syndrome (SCS). Neurology **46**(2): A310.
12. GOMEZ, C. M., R. MASELLI, J. E. GUNDECK *et al.* 1997. Slow-channel transgenic mice: a model of postsynaptic organellar degeneration at the neuromuscular junction. J. Neurosci. **17**(11): 4170–4179.

13. GOMEZ, C. M., B. B. BHATTACHARYYA, P. CHARNET et al. 1996. A transgenic mouse model of the slow-channel syndrome. Muscle Nerve **19:** 79–87.

14. JOHNSON, J. E., B. J. WOLD & S. D. HAUSCHKA. 1989. Muscle creatine kinase sequence elements regulating skeletal and cardiac muscle expression in transgenic mice. Mol. Cell. Biol. **9**(8): 3393–3399.

15. HOGAN, R., F. COSTANTINI & E. LACEY. 1986. Manipulating the Mouse Embryo: A Laboratory Manual. Cold Spring Harbor Laboratory. Cold Spring Harbor, New York.

16. SAIKI, R. K., D. H. GELFAND, S. STOFFEL et al. 1988. Primer-directed enzymatic amplification of DNA with a thermostable DNA polymerase. Science **239**(4839): 487–491.

17. GARDNER, P. D. 1990. Nucleotide sequence of the mouse muscle nicotinic acetylcholine receptor. Nucleic Acids Res. **18**(22): 100.

18. GORMAN, C. M., L. F. MOFFAT & B. H. HOWARD. 1982. Recombinant genomes which express chloramphenicol acetyltransferase in mammalian cells. Mol. Cell. Biol. **2:** 1044–1051.

19. DIONNE, V. E. & C. F. STEVENS. 1975. Voltage dependence of agonist effectiveness at the frog neuromuscular junction: resolution of a paradox. J. Physiol. **251:** 245–270.

20. GLAMINOVIC, M. I. 1979. Voltage clamping of unparalysed cut diaphragm for the study of transmitter release. J. Physiol. **290:** 467–480.

21. BHATTACHARYYA, B. B., J. DAY, J. E. GUNDECK, S. LEONARD, R. WOLLMANN & C. GOMEZ. 1997. Desensitization of mutant acetylcholine receptors in transgenic mice reduces the amplitude of synaptic currents. Synapse **27**(4): 367–377.

22. DEMPSTER, J. 1993. Computer Analysis of Electrophysiological Signals. Harcourt Brace Jovanovich/Academic Press. New York.

23. PESTRONK, A., D. B. DRACHMAN & S. G. SELF. 1985. Measurement of junctional acetylcholine receptors in myasthenia gravis: clinical correlates. Muscle Nerve **8**(3): 245–251.

24. MAGLEBY, K. L. & B. S. PALLOTTA. 1981. A study of desensitization of acetylcholine receptors using nerve-released transmitter in the frog. J. Physiol. **316:** 225–250.

25. OHNO, K., P. A. QUIRAM, M. MILONE et al. 1997. Congenital myasthenic syndromes due to heteroallelic nonsense/missense mutations in the acetylcholine receptor epsilon subunit gene—identification and functional characterization of six new mutations. Hum. Mol. Genet. **6**(5): 753–766.

26. WANG, H-L., A. AUERBACH, N. BREN, K. OHNO, A. G. ENGEL & S. M. SINE. 1997. Mutation in the m1 domain of the acetylcholine receptor alpha subunit decreases the rate of agonist dissociation. J. Gen. Physiol. **109**(6): 757–766.

27. WALKE, W., J. STAPLE, L. ADAMS, M. GNEGY, K. CHAHINE & D. GOLDMAN. 1994. Calcium-dependent regulation of rat and chick muscle nicotinic acetylcholine receptor (nAChR) gene expression. J. Biol. Chem. **269**(30): 19447–19456.

28. LAMBERT, E. H., J. M. LINDSTROM & V. A. LENNON. 1976. End-plate potentials in experimental autoimmune myasthenia gravis in rats. Ann. N.Y. Acad. Sci. **274:** 300–318.

Congenital Myasthenic Syndromes

Studies of the AChR and Other Candidate Genes[a]

D. BEESON,[b] C. NEWLAND,[b] R. CROXEN,[b] A. BUCKEL,[b] F-Y. LI,[c]
C. LARSSON,[c] M. TARIQ,[d] A. VINCENT,[b] AND J. NEWSOM-DAVIS[b]

[b]Neurosciences Group
Institute of Molecular Medicine
John Radcliffe Hospital
Headington, Oxford OX3 9DS, United Kingdom

[c]Karolinska Institute
Stockholm, Sweden

[d]Pakistan Institute of Medical Sciences
Islamabad, Pakistan

INTRODUCTION

Congenital myasthenic syndromes (CMS) are a rare heterogeneous group of disorders affecting neuromuscular transmission. They may involve abnormalities of presynaptic, synaptic, or postsynaptic proteins. We are employing a variety of techniques to identify mutations responsible for these syndromes. At present, the most clearly defined CMS involve mutations in the AChR that have been shown to underlie the altered kinetic properties of the AChR typically evident in the slow-channel syndrome, and the reduced numbers of functional AChR found in some patients with AChR deficiency.

MUTATIONS WITHIN THE AChR GENES

In patients with slow-channel syndrome, we have used SSCP analysis to screen for mutations within the AChR genes. Four abnormal conformers were located; two in exon 5 and two in exon 7 of the AChR α-subunit gene. DNA sequence analysis of the respective exons showed that each patient had a heterozygous single-nucleotide change that alters an amino acid. These were nucleotide (n)457 G→A, G153S; (n)466 G→A, V156M; (n)761 T→C, T254I; and (n)806 G→T, S269I.[1] Three of these mutations are novel and a fourth (G153S) has previously been shown to underlie two independent cases of the slow-channel syndrome.[2] αV156M and αG153S are located in the vicinity of αW149, which contributes to the ACh-binding pocket;[3] αT254I is located in the pore-lining region, like five out of six previously reported slow-channel mutations; and αS269I is within the short extracellular loop between M2 and M3.

[a]This work was supported by MGA/MDG of Great Britain and Action Research.

To ascertain if the three novel mutations, αV156M, αT254I, and αS269I, affect channel function, we constructed expression vectors containing the respective mutations in the human α-subunit cDNA. Wild-type and mutant α-subunit cRNAs were injected separately into *Xenopus* oocytes in combination with cRNAs encoding the human AChR β-, δ-, and ϵ-subunits,[4] and single-channel recordings were analyzed. Each of the novel mutations prolongs channel activation episodes. Thus, mutations in different functional domains of the α-subunit may cause a similar pathogenic gain of function of the AChR.

A reduction in AChR number is the most common form of CMS in the United Kingdom. In four pedigrees, we have shown that AChR deficiency associates with the recessive inheritance of a single G nucleotide deletion at position 1267 within the AChR ϵ-subunit gene. An additional case, where the patient was adopted, was also homozygous for this deletion. The mutation results in a frameshift in translation of the AChR ϵ-subunit at position 423 and generates an ϵ-subunit polypeptide of 485 amino acids containing 63 missense C-terminal amino acids. A more-detailed account of these cases is described by Croxen *et al.* in this volume.

OTHER CANDIDATE GENES

In AChR deficiency, there may be changes in the structure of the neuromuscular junction (NMJ) as well as in the number and density of the AChR. Some cases of

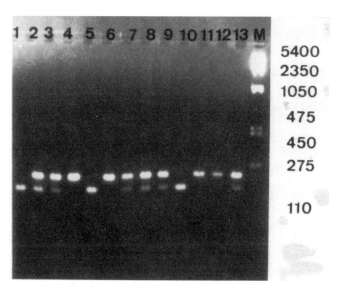

FIGURE 1. Detection of the R58C polymorphism at nucleotide position 172 within the human rapsyn gene. PCR amplifications of exon 1 were digested with *Hae* III, run on a 1.2% agarose gel, stained with ethidium bromide, and visualized under UV. Amplified products cut by *Hae* III indicate a C nucleotide at position 172.

AChR deficiency may arise from mutations in proteins involved in maintaining NMJ structure or in the control of AChR synthesis. Rapsyn has been shown to play a key role in the organization of the NMJ. We have isolated cDNA and genomic clones encoding human rapsyn,[5] characterized sequences flanking the intron/exon boundaries, and used this information in screening for mutations within the rapsyn gene.

In 20 patients with AChR deficiency, screening by SSCP analysis of 6 of the 8 exons that encode rapsyn failed to reveal mutations that might underlie the disease, although two coding polymorphisms, at (n)172 C→T within exon 1 (FIGURE 1) and at (n)1038 G→A within exon 7, were identified. The former results in a substitution of cysteine for arginine at amino-acid position 58, R58C, and the latter substitutes glutamate for arginine at position 346, R346Q.

Although screening for mutations within the rapsyn gene has not yet revealed any mutations, linkage analysis performed on two extended congenital myasthenic pedigrees has excluded the genes encoding muscle AChR located on chromosomes 2 and 17, providing further evidence that mutations in proteins other than the AChR are likely to be responsible for some of the heterogeneity of congenital myasthenic syndromes.

REFERENCES

1. CROXEN, R., C. NEWLAND, D. BEESON, H. OOSTERHUIS, G. CHAUPLANNAZ, A. VINCENT & J. NEWSOM-DAVIS. 1997. Mutations in different functional domains of the human muscle acetylcholine receptor α subunit in patients with the slow-channel congenital myasthenic syndrome. Hum. Mol. Genet. **6:** 767–774.
2. SINE, S., K. OHNO, C. BOUZAT, A. AUERBACH, M. MILONE, J. PRUITT & A. G. ENGEL. 1995. Mutations of the acetylcholine receptor α subunit cause a slow-channel myasthenic syndrome by enhancing agonist binding affinity. Neuron **15:** 229–239.
3. DENNIS, M., J. GIRAUDAT, F. KOTZYBA-HIBERT, M. GOELDNER, C. HIRTH, J-Y. CHANG, C. LAZURE, M. CRETIEN & J-P. CHANGEUX. 1988. Amino acids of the *Torpedo marmorata* acetylcholine receptor α subunit labeled by photoaffinity ligand for the acetylcholine binding site. Biochemistry **27:** 2346–2357.
4. BEESON, D., M. BRYDSON, M. BETTY, S. JEREMIAH, S. POVEY, A. VINCENT & J. NEWSOM-DAVIS. 1993. Primary structure of the human muscle acetylcholine receptor: cDNA cloning of the γ and ε subunits. Eur. J. Biochem. **215:** 229–238.
5. BUCKEL, A., D. BEESON, M. JAMES & A. VINCENT. 1996. Cloning of cDNA encoding human rapsyn and mapping of the RAPSN gene locus to chromosome 11p11.2–p11.1. Genomics **35:** 613–616.

Congenital Myasthenic Syndrome Caused by Novel Loss-of-Function Mutations in the Human AChR ε Subunit Gene[a]

MARGHERITA MILONE,[b] KINJI OHNO,[b] TAKAYASU FUKUDOME,[b]
XIN-MING SHEN,[b] JOAN BRENGMAN,[b] ROBERT C. GRIGGS,[c]
AND ANDREW G. ENGEL[b,d]

[b]Muscle Research Laboratory
and
Department of Neurology
Mayo Clinic
Rochester, Minnesota 55905

[c]Department of Neurology
University of Rochester School of Medicine
Rochester, New York 14642

INTRODUCTION

Congenital myasthenic syndromes (CMS) are heterogeneous disorders in which the safety margin of neuromuscular transmission is compromised by one or more presynaptic, synaptic, or postsynaptic mechanisms.[1] In our experience, the majority of CMS are postsynaptic in origin, and most postsynaptic CMS are caused by one or more mutations in an acetylcholine receptor (AChR) subunit gene (see paper by Engel *et al.* elsewhere in this volume). Most mutations causing a marked decrease in expression, or loss of function, or both, of endplate (EP) AChR are observed in the ε subunit, presumably because the fetal AChR γ subunit can substitute for the adult ε subunit and thus can serve as means of phenotypic rescue.[2–4] We here describe our electrophysiological, morphological, and molecular genetic studies in a 39-year-old woman who had myasthenic symptoms involving the ocular, bulbar, and limb muscles since early childhood. She had difficulty climbing steps, could not keep up with her peers in sports, and fatigued easily. At age 36, exposure to a curariform muscle relaxant during surgery caused paralysis lasting several hours. She had negative tests for anti-AChR antibodies, a decremental EMG response on stimulation of motor nerves, and a favorable (but incomplete) response to cholinesterase inhibitors. The propositus' brother, age 36, and sister, age 38, are similarly affected; her 7-month-old son and 2-year-old daughter have no myasthenic symptoms.

[a]This work was supported by a National Institutes of Health grant to A. G. Engel (No. NS6277), an MDA research grant to A. G. Engel, an MDA postdoctoral fellowship to K. Ohno, and an Italian Telethon award to M. Milone.
[d]To whom all correspondence should be addressed.

RESULTS

Morphology

Routine histologic studies revealed only type-2 muscle fiber atrophy. The configuration of the EPs, evaluated from the cytochemical reaction for acetylcholinesterase on longitudinally oriented teased single muscle fibers, was abnormal, with an increased number of small EP regions distributed over a 2- to 5-fold increased span of the muscle fiber surface. The reaction for AChR, detected in cryostat sections with rhodamine-labeled α-bungarotoxin (α-bgt), was markedly attenuated. Electron microscopy revealed that the structural integrity of the junctional folds was preserved, but a number of EPs had a simplified postsynaptic architecture. The reaction for AChR, detected with peroxidase-labeled α-bgt, was patchy and attenuated. The AChR index [defined as the ratio of the length of the postsynaptic membrane reacting for AChR to the length of the primary synaptic cleft[5]] was only 17% of the control mean. The number of ^{125}I-α-bgt sites per EP was also markedly decreased (TABLE 1).

In Vitro *Electrophysiologic Studies*

The number of ACh quanta released by nerve impulse was 1.9-fold higher than the control mean, perhaps as an adaptive response to decreased postsynaptic sensitiv-

TABLE 1. EP Studies[a]

	Patient	Controls
^{125}I-α-bgt binding sites/EP	1.03 E6	12.82 ± 0.79 E6 (13)
AChR index	0.56 ± 0.07 (36)	3.3 ± 0.08 (155)
EPP quantal content (1 Hz)[b]	59 ± 6 (18)	31 ± 1 (190)
MEPP amplitude (mV)[c]	0.31 ± 0.02 (29)	1.00 ± 0.025 (164)
MEPC amplitude (nA)[d]	1.13 ± 0.07 (45)	3.95 ± 0.10 (79)
τ_{noise} (ms)[d]	(i) 1.58 ± 0.25 (6)	2.3 ± 0.043 (52)
	(ii) 11.18 ± 1.41 (6)	
Patch-clamp $\tau_{open\ interval}$ (ms)[e]	0.88 ± 0.05 (8)	1.13 ± 0.10 (7)
Patch-clamp τ_{burst} (ms)[e]	1.61 ± 0.09 (8)	2.99 ± 0.26 (7)

[a]Values represent the mean ± SE; numbers in parentheses indicate the number of EPs, except for ^{125}I-α-bgt binding sites/EP where they indicate the number of controls. $T = 29 ± 0.5$ °C for EPP and MEPP recordings and $22 ± 0.5$ °C for noise analysis, MEPC, and patch-clamp studies.

[b]Quantal content of EPP at 1-Hz stimulation corrected for resting membrane potential of −80 mV, nonlinear summation, and non-Poisson release.

[c]Corrected for resting membrane potential of −80 mV and normalized for a fiber diameter of 50 μm.

[d] −80 mV.

[e]Patch-clamp data for 60-pS channels indicate the predominant open interval and burst durations assigned to openings of AChR liganded by two ACh molecules; −80 mV; ACh = 0.1 to 5.0 μM. Open interval and burst durations were not significantly affected by the indicated range of ACh concentrations. Data for 46-pS channels are not shown in the table.

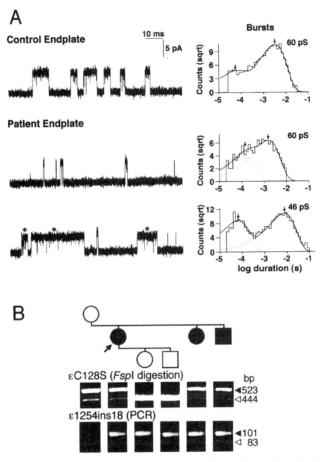

FIGURE 1. (A) Representative channel events (left panels) and logarithmically binned burst duration histograms (right panels) from a control EP and from a patient EP. Both 60-pS and 46-pS (asterisks) channels appear at the patient EP. The predominant burst open duration of the 60-pS channels at the patient EP is shorter than at the control EP (1.59 versus 3.24 ms). The predominant burst open duration of the 46-pS channels at the patient EP is 7.8 ms. (B) Restriction analysis with *Fsp*I to detect εC128S and gel size-fractionation to detect ε1254ins18 in PCR-amplified fragments of genomic DNA obtained from patient's muscle and relatives' blood. For εC128S (upper panel), the wild-type allele gives rise to 444-bp (open arrowhead) and 79-bp fragments, whereas the mutant allele remains 523 bp (closed arrowhead). The 79-bp fragment is not shown. For ε1254ins18 (lower panel), the sizes of the respective wild-type and mutant fragments are 83 bp (open arrowhead) and 101 bp (closed arrowhead). The patient's mother is heterozygous for εC128S, her unaffected children are heterozygous for ε1254ins18, and the patient and her affected siblings have both mutations. The arrow indicates the patient. Closed symbols show affected individuals.

ity to ACh.[6,7] The amplitude of the MEPPs and MEPCs was reduced to about 30% of normal, consistent with the degree of postsynaptic AChR deficiency.[8] Spectral analysis of the ACh-induced current noise revealed two channel-open times, with one τ_{noise} briefer than normal and one severalfold prolonged (TABLE 1).

To examine the kinetic properties of AChR, we recorded single-channel currents from the patient's EPs. Forty percent of the AChR channel events had a conductance of 60 pS and briefer-than-normal open durations (TABLE 1), whereas 60% of the channel events had a conductance of 46 pS and prolonged open durations, typical of AChR containing the γ instead of the ε subunit (γ-AChR) (FIGURE 1A).

Molecular Genetic Studies

Expression of γ-AChR and the AChR deficiency at the patient's EPs strongly suggested one or more mutations in the ε subunit gene.[2–4] Indeed, direct sequencing of all exons and flanking intronic regions of the patient's ε subunit gene revealed two heterozygous mutations. The first mutation was a T-to-A transversion in ε exon 5 at nucleotide 382 (ε382T→A) that converts a cysteine to a serine codon at position 128 (εC128S). The mutated cysteine at codon 128 forms a disulfide bond with the cysteine at codon 142. Both cysteines are conserved in all AChR subunits and all species, as well as across all subunits of the AChR superfamily of ion channels.[9] The second mutation was a duplication of 18 nucleotides at 1237 to 1254 in ε exon 11 (ε1254ins18) that predicted a duplication of Ser-Thr-Arg-Asp-Gln-Glu codons at positions 413 to 418 in the long cytoplasmic loop between the M3 and M4 domains. Two affected siblings harbored the same mutations as the patient, and her unaffected mother and two children were respectively heterozygous for εC128S and ε1254ins18. Neither mutation was detected in 72 other CMS patients. Expression studies in human embryonic kidney (HEK) cells revealed the following: (1) εC128S is a null mutation; (2) ε1254ins18 reduces expression of surface AChRs and the mutated AChR has shorter-than-normal opening episodes, like the 60-pS channels detected at the patient's EPs. Further studies revealed other unusual kinetic properties of this mutation and these will be reported separately.

REFERENCES

1. ENGEL, A. G. 1994. Myasthenic syndromes. *In* Myology: Basic and Clinical, p. 1798–1835. McGraw–Hill. New York.
2. ENGEL, A. G., K. OHNO, C. BOUZAT, S. M. SINE & R. G. GRIGGS. 1996. End-plate acetylcholine receptor deficiency due to nonsense mutations in the ε subunit. Ann. Neurol. **40:** 810–817.
3. OHNO, K., P. QUIRAM, M. MILONE, H-L. WANG, C. M. HARPER, J. N. PRUITT, J. M. BRENGMAN, L. PAO, K. H. FISCHBECK, T. O. CRAWFORD *et al.* 1997. Congenital myasthenic syndromes due to heteroallelic nonsense/missense mutations in the acetylcholine receptor ε subunit gene: identification and functional characterization of six new mutations. Hum. Mol. Genet. **6:** 753–766.
4. WITZEMANN, V., H. SCHWARTZ, M. KOENEN, C. BERBERICH, A. VILLARROEL, A. WERNIG, H. R. BRENNER & B. SAKMANN. 1996. Acetylcholine receptor epsilon subunit deletion caus-

es muscle weakness and atrophy in juvenile and adult mice. Proc. Natl. Acad. Sci. U.S.A. **93:** 13286–13291.

5. ENGEL, A. G. 1994. Quantitative morphological studies of muscle. *In* Myology: Basic and Clinical, p. 1018–1045. McGraw–Hill. New York.

6. PLOMP, J. J., G. T. H. VAN KEMPEN & P. C. MOLENAAR. 1992. Adaptation of quantal content to decreased postsynaptic sensitivity at single endplates in α-bungarotoxin treated rats. J. Physiol. (Lond.) **458:** 487–499.

7. PLOMP, J. J., G. T. H. VAN KEMPEN, M. B. DE BAETS, Y. M. F. GRAUS, J. B. M. KUKS & P. C. MOLENAAR. 1995. Acetylcholine release in myasthenia gravis: regulation at single endplate level. Ann. Neurol. **37:** 627–636.

8. PENNEFATHER, P. & D. M. J. QUASTEL. 1981. Relation between subsynaptic receptor blockade and response to quantal transmitter at the mouse neuromuscular junction. J. Gen. Physiol. **78:** 313–344.

9. KARLIN, A. & M. H. AKABAS. 1994. Toward a structural basis for the function of nicotinic acetylcholine receptors and their cousins. Neuron **15:** 1231–1244.

Frameshifting and Splice-Site Mutations in the Acetylcholine Receptor ε Subunit Gene in Three Turkish Kinships with Congenital Myasthenic Syndromes[a]

KINJI OHNO,[b] BANU ANLAR,[c] EMIRE ÖZDIRIM,[c]
JOAN M. BRENGMAN,[b] AND ANDREW G. ENGEL[b,d]

[b]Muscle Research Laboratory
and
Department of Neurology
Mayo Clinic
Rochester, Minnesota 55905

[c]Department of Pediatric Neurology
Hacettepe University
Ankara 06100, Turkey

INTRODUCTION

Recent genetic studies have elucidated molecular bases of congenital myasthenic syndromes (CMS) associated with severe endplate (EP) acetylcholine receptor (AChR) deficiency and/or kinetic abnormalities of AChR (see main paper by Engel *et al.* earlier in this volume). CMS due to a kinetic abnormality of AChR stem from missense mutations in the α, β, or ε subunit genes of AChR. Except for a recessive missense mutation in the ε subunit that reduces the affinity of AChR for ACh, the kinetic abnormalities in AChR are caused by dominant gain-of-function mutations that prolong the opening episodes of the AChR channel. By contrast, mutations that cause severe EP AChR deficiency are recessive mutations and are concentrated in the ε subunit of AChR. Prompted by these observations, we searched for mutations in the ε subunit gene in three recessively inherited CMS observed in Turkish kinships. We here report three new mutations in the ε subunit gene and prove their pathogenicity by expression studies in human embryonic kidney (293 HEK) fibroblasts.

[a]This work was supported by a National Institutes of Health grant to A. G. Engel (No. NS6277), by an MDA research grant to A. G. Engel, and by an MDA postdoctoral fellowship to K. Ohno.
[d]To whom all correspondence should be addressed.

RESULTS

Patients

A woman (patient 1), a girl (patient 2), and a girl (patient 3), 29, 16, and 12 years of age, respectively, had myasthenic symptoms since birth or early childhood and no anti-AChR antibodies. Each patient had an affected sibling. All three patients have negative tests for anti-AChR antibodies, have abnormal single-fiber electromyograms or a decremental electromyographic response on stimulation of motor nerves, and respond favorably (but only partially) to anticholinesterase medication. The parents of patient 2 are first cousins. None of the parents is affected and the three kinships are not known to be related.

Mutation Analysis

We sequenced all exons and flanking intronic regions of genomic DNA of the AChR ε subunit gene in each patient. Patient 1 has a homozygous 19-bp duplication in exon 11 at nucleotides 1188–1206 (ε1206ins19) in the long cytoplasmic loop, predicting 38 missense codons followed by a stop codon (FIGURES 1D and 1E). An affected brother is homozygous, and the parents and a brother are heterozygous for ε1206ins19 (FIGURE 1A). Patient 2 has a homozygous "G" insertion in exon 2 after nucleotide 70 (ε70insG) in the extracellular domain that predicts conversion of the wild-type Glu-Pro-Glu codons at 24–26 to Gly-Ala-Stop codons (FIGURES 1D and 1E). An affected sister is homozygous and the consanguineous parents are heterozygous for ε70insG (FIGURE 1B). Patient 3 has heteroallelic ε70insG (same as patient 2) and a T-to-C transition at the second nucleotide of intron 7 (εIVS7+2T→C) (FIGURE 1D). The splice-site mutation predicts retention of intron 7 or skipping of exon 7.[1] Retention of intron 7 (82 bp) is a frameshift and skipping of exon 7 (201 bp) is an in-frame deletion (FIGURE 1E). An affected brother has both mutations and each parent has one of the mutations (FIGURE 1C), indicating that the patient is a compound heterozygote. No polymorphisms of the ε subunit gene were detected in any patient. None of the above mutations was observed in 51 non-Turkish CMS kinships.

Expression Studies of Mutant ε Subunits

To examine the effects of the identified mutations, we engineered ε1206ins19, ε70insG, and two predicted aberrant transcripts due to εIVS7+2T→C (skipped exon 7 or retained intron 7) into the human ε subunit cDNAs and coexpressed these with complementary wild-type α, β, and δ subunit cDNAs in 293 HEK cells.

Measurements of $[^{125}I]\alpha$-bungarotoxin (bgt) binding to cell surface receptors revealed reduced expression of AChRs in the absence of the ε subunit or in the presence of ε70insG, εIVS7+2T→C (– exon 7), εIVS7+2T→C (+ intron 7), and ε1206ins19 (FIGURE 2A). To distinguish between lack of incorporation and reduced expression of the mutant subunits, we measured ACh binding by competition against the initial rate of $[^{125}I]\alpha$-bgt binding.[2] Omitting the ε subunit leads to ex-

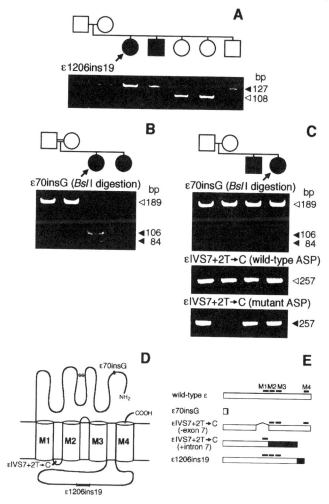

FIGURE 1. (**A**) Size fractionation of PCR products amplified from genomic DNA of the blood of patient 1 and her relatives. PCR products from the wild-type and mutant alleles contain 108 bp and 127 bp, respectively. Both parents and an asymptomatic brother are heterozygous for ε1206ins19, patient 1 and an affected brother are homozygous for ε1206ins19, and two sisters have no mutation. The arrow indicates patient 1. Closed symbols show affected individuals. (**B**) Restriction analysis using genomic DNA from the blood of patient 2 and her relatives. The ε70insG mutation results in the gain of a *Bsl*I site. The wild-type allele gives rise to 189- and 27-bp fragments, whereas the mutant allele yields 106-, 84-, and 27-bp fragments. The 27-bp fragment is not shown. The consanguineous parents are heterozygous, and patient 2 and an affected sister are homozygous for ε70insG. The arrow indicates patient 2. Closed symbols show affected individuals. (**C**) Restriction analysis and allele-specific PCR using genomic DNA from the blood of patient 3 and her relatives. For the ε70insG analysis, the wild-type and mutant fragments are the same as in part B. The mother, an affected brother, and patient 3 are heterozygous for ε70insG. Allele-specific PCR (ASP) shows that the father, an affected brother, and patient 3 are heterozygous for εIVS7+2T→C. (**D**) Schematic representation of the identified AChR ε subunit gene mutations. (**E**) Schematic diagram of predicted ε subunits for each mutant transcript. Open and closed bars indicate wild-type and missense amino acids, respectively; skipped exon 7 is shown as a gap. Positions of transmembrane domains M1–M4 are also indicated.

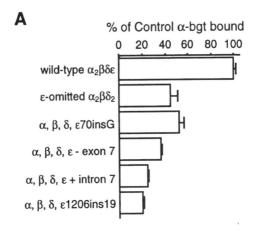

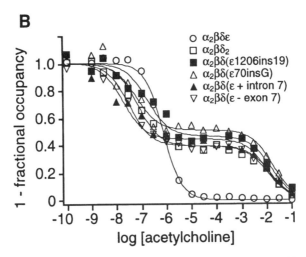

FIGURE 2. (A) Specific α-bgt binding to intact 293 HEK cells transfected with the indicated AChR subunit cDNAs. The results are normalized for α-bgt binding to wild-type $\alpha_2\beta\delta\varepsilon$ pentamers and represent the mean ± SD of 2–3 experiments. **(B)** Acetylcholine binding to intact 293 HEK cells transfected with the indicated AChR subunit cDNAs as determined by competition against the initial rate of $[^{125}I]\alpha$-bgt binding. For $\alpha_2\beta\delta\varepsilon$, the smooth curve is a fit to the monophasic Hill equation: $1 - Y = 1/\{1 + ([ACh]/K_{OV})^n\}$, with $K_{OV} = 7.51 \times 10^{-7}$ and $n = 1.20$, where Y is the fractional occupancy by ACh, n is the Hill coefficient, and K_{OV} is an overall dissociation constant for a monophasic binding profile. For the other AChRs, the curves are fitted by the sum of two distinct binding sites: $1 - Y = \text{fract}_A\{1/(1 + [ACh]/K_A)\} + (1 - \text{fract}_A)\{1/(1 + [ACh]/K_B)\}$, where K_A and K_B are intrinsic dissociation constants for the two binding sites, and fract_A is the fraction of sites with dissociation constant K_A. For $\alpha_2\beta\delta_2$, $K_A = 7.29 \times 10^{-8}$, $K_B = 1.12 \times 10^{-2}$, and $\text{fract}_A = 0.61$.

pression of $\alpha_2\beta\delta_2$ pentamers, which bind ACh in a biphasic manner, with a plateau at 50% occupancy extending over three decades of ACh concentration; this contrasts with a monophasic binding profile of wild-type $\alpha_2\beta\delta\varepsilon$ pentamers (FIGURE 2B). When each ε mutant is cotransfected with the complementary α, β, and δ subunit cDNAs, ACh binding closely mimics that observed with ε-omitted $\alpha_2\beta\delta_2$ pentamers, indicating that none of the ε mutants is incorporated into cell surface pentamers (FIGURE 2B).

DISCUSSION

Implications of the AChR ε Subunit Gene Mutations in Turkish Kinships

Recently, Christodoulou *et al.*[3] investigated 12 Mediterranean CMS kinships, of which 7 were Turkish. In all families, the CMS locus was mapped between marker loci D17S1537 and D17S1298. They considered synaptobrevin, a presynaptic protein, as a likely candidate gene in their CMS kinships. The same chromosomal region, however, overlaps with the locus for the AChR ε subunit gene (human STS SHGC-11989, accession number G19458) that lies between D17S1828 and D17S1810.[4] This suggests that some or all kinships investigated by Christodoulou *et al.* have ε subunit gene mutations.

Mutations Causing Severe AChR Deficiency Are Concentrated in the ε Subunit Gene

The findings in the CMS kinships investigated in this study support the notion that recessive mutations affecting the expression of EP AChR are concentrated in the ε subunit gene. There are two possible reasons for this: (1) The fetal-type γ-AChRs appear at the EP to compensate for deficiency of ε-AChR (see Engel *et al.* earlier in this volume), whereas patients harboring null mutations in subunits other than ε might not survive for lack of a substituting subunit. (2) The GC content of the ε coding region (61.2%) exceeds that of the other AChR subunit genes, and DNA rearrangements are clustered in the GC-rich regions.[5] The GC contents in a 40-bp window of genomic DNA around seven DNA rearrangements observed by us in this and previous studies (ε70insG, ε127ins5, ε553del7, ε1012del20, ε1101insT, ε1206ins19, and ε1293insG) range from 55.0% to 92.5% (mean $\pm$ SD, 68.2 $\pm$ 13.2%).

REFERENCES

1. MAQUAT, L. E. 1996. Defects in RNA splicing and the consequence of shortened translational reading frames. Am. J. Hum. Genet. **59:** 279–286.
2. SINE, S. & P. TAYLOR. 1979. Functional consequences of agonist-mediated state transitions in the cholinergic receptor: studies in cultured muscle cells. J. Biol. Chem. **254:** 3315–3325.

3. CHRISTODOULOU, K., M. TSINGIS, F. DEYMEER, P. SERDAROGLU, C. OZDEMIR, A. ALSHEHAB, C. BAIRACTARIS, I. MAVROMATIS, I. MYLONAS, A. EVOLI, K. KYRIALLIS & L. T. MIDDLETON. 1997. Mapping of the familial infantile myasthenia (congenital myasthenic syndrome type Ia) gene to chromosome 17p with evidence of genetic homogeneity. Hum. Mol. Genet. **6:** 635–640.

4. COLLINS, A., J. FREZAL, J. TEAGUE & N. E. MORTON. 1996. A metric map of humans: 23,500 loci in 850 bands. Proc. Natl. Acad. Sci. U.S.A. **93:** 14771–14775.

5. KRAWCZAK, M. & D. N. COOPER. 1991. Gene deletions causing human genetic disease: mechanisms of mutagenesis and the role of the local DNA sequence environment. Hum. Genet. **86:** 425–441.

A Single Nucleotide Deletion in the ε Subunit of the Acetylcholine Receptor (AChR) in Five Congenital Myasthenic Syndrome Patients with AChR Deficiency[a]

REBECCA CROXEN, DAVID BEESON, CLAIRE NEWLAND, MARIA BETTY, ANGELA VINCENT, AND JOHN NEWSOM-DAVIS

Neurosciences Group
Institute of Molecular Medicine
John Radcliffe Hospital
University of Oxford
Oxford OX3 9DS, United Kingdom

INTRODUCTION

The congenital myasthenic syndromes (CMS) are a group of rare, genetically determined disorders in which neuromuscular transmission is impaired. These disorders are clinically and genetically heterogeneous. Syndromes identified to date include end plate acetylcholinesterase (AChE) deficiency, presynaptic abnormalities that affect the release or size of transmitter quanta, postsynaptic abnormalities associated with marked acetylcholine receptor (AChR) deficiency, and kinetic abnormalities of the AChR (see Engel *et al.* in this volume).[1] Several mutations underlying AChR kinetic abnormalities have now been characterized[2,3] and, recently, mutations that underlie AChR deficiency have been detected.[4,5] Here, we identify a novel homozygous deletion (ε1267delG) in exon 12 of the ε subunit gene that is present in five unrelated cases of AChR deficiency.

PATIENT DETAILS

The patients first showed symptoms at birth or during infancy. Symptoms include limb weakness, bilateral ptosis, and facial weakness. Muscle biopsies from two of the patients showed reduced numbers of AChRs at the end plate (as determined by [^{125}I]α-bungarotoxin binding), elongated end plates, and significantly reduced miniature end plate potentials. Four of the patients are from consanguineous pedigrees; the fifth is adopted and parentage is unknown. All patients are negative for anti-AChR antibodies and respond favorably to anticholinesterase treatment.

[a]This work was supported by the Myasthenia Gravis Association/Muscular Dystrophy Group of Great Britain.

195

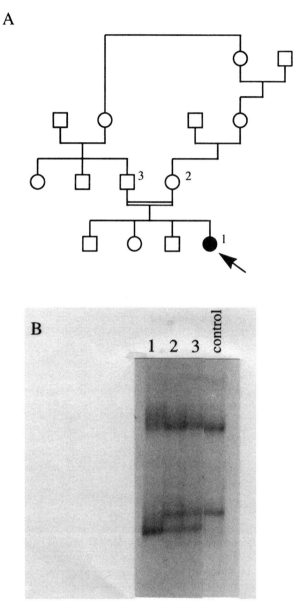

FIGURE 1. Single-strand conformation polymorphism (SSCP) analysis of exon 12 of the ε subunit gene from an AChR deficiency pedigree. (**A**) Family pedigree. The arrow indicates the index patient. (**B**) SSCP analysis using the primer set $\varepsilon_1 11F$-$\varepsilon 12R$ (see text). The lanes correspond to the numbered family members in part A. The control sample is from an unrelated healthy individual.

METHODS AND RESULTS

Microsatellite repeat markers corresponding to repeats in, or closely linked to, the AChR α, β, δ, and ε subunit genes respectively were used to analyze homozygosity by descent in the consanguineous pedigree of patient 1. This enabled the β and δ subunit genes to be excluded and, although uninformative for the α subunit gene, analysis implicated the AChR ε subunit gene as the candidate for the underlying mutation.

Single-strand conformation polymorphism (SSCP) analysis was used to screen regions of the ε subunit gene. An abnormal conformer was identified for patient 1 using a primer set corresponding to a sequence at the 3′ of intron 11 ($\varepsilon_1$11F) and a sequence downstream of the stop codon in exon 12 (ε12R). Subsequently, it was also identified in four independent AChR deficiency cases. This abnormal conformer was not seen in 60 controls of similar ethnic background or 60 other CMS cases. The unaffected parents of the patients, for whom DNA was available, had both the normal and abnormal conformers, indicating heterozygosity (example in FIGURE 1).

Genomic DNA from patient 1, the parents of patient 1, and a control were PCR-amplified using the primer set $\varepsilon_1$11F-ε12R. Direct cycle sequencing of the amplified products showed that the abnormal SSCP conformer was caused by a single G nucleotide deletion; the patient was homozygous for the deletion and the parents were heterozygous and clinically asymptomatic. Sequencing of AChR ε subunit cDNA derived from patient 1 confirmed the presence of the single nucleotide deletion within the mRNA at position 1267, the first nucleotide of exon 12 (FIGURE 2). The same homozygous mutation was identified in the four additional AChR deficiency cases.

DISCUSSION

The loss of a single nucleotide at position 1267 would lead to a frameshift in the translation of the ε subunit from amino acid 423 in the long cytoplasmic loop that

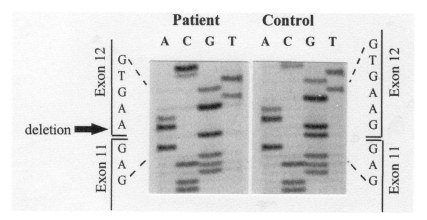

FIGURE 2. cDNA sequence analysis of patient 1 showing the single nucleotide deletion ε1267delG. The sequence of the sense strand is shown.

precedes the M4 transmembrane region. This would result in 63 missense amino acids that terminate at a new TAG stop site at nucleotide position 1457–1459. It would generate a longer ε subunit polypeptide of 485 amino acids. Expression studies to examine the effects of the mutant ε subunit clones *in vitro* are in progress.

REFERENCES

1. VINCENT, A., C. NEWLAND, R. CROXEN & D. BEESON. 1997. Genes at the junction—candidates for congenital myasthenic syndromes. Trends Neurosci. **20:** 15–22.
2. ENGEL, A. G., K. OHNO, M. MILONE, H-L. WANG, S. NAKANO, C. BOUZAT, J. N. PRUITT II, D. O. HUTCHINSON, J. M. BRENGMAN, N. BREN, J. P. SIEB & S. M. SINE. 1996. New mutations in acetylcholine receptor subunit genes reveal heterogeneity in the slow-channel congenital myasthenic syndrome. Hum. Mol. Genet. **5:** 1217–1227.
3. CROXEN, R., C. NEWLAND, D. BEESON, H. OOSTERHUIS, G. CHAUPLANNAZ, A. VINCENT & J. NEWSOM-DAVIS. 1997. Mutations in different functional domains of the human muscle acetylcholine receptor α subunit in patients with the slow-channel myasthenic syndrome. Hum. Mol. Genet. **6:** 767–774.
4. ENGEL, A. G., K. OHNO, C. BOUZAT, S. M. SINE & R. C. GRIGGS. 1996. End-plate acetylcholine receptor deficiency due to nonsense mutations in the ε subunit. Ann. Neurol. **40:** 810–817.
5. OHNO, K., P. A. QUIRAM, M. MILONE, H-L. WANG, M. C. HARPER, J. N. PRUITT II, J. M. BRENGMAN, L. PAO, K. H. FISCHBECK, T. O. CRAWFORD, S. M. SINE & A. G. ENGEL. 1997. Congenital myasthenic syndromes due to heteroallelic nonsense/missense mutations in the acetylcholine receptor ε subunit gene: identification and functional characterization of six new mutations. Hum. Mol. Genet. **6:** 753–766.

AChR Channel Blockade by Quinidine Sulfate Reduces Channel Open Duration in the Slow-Channel Congenital Myasthenic Syndrome[a]

TAKAYASU FUKUDOME, KINJI OHNO, JOAN M. BRENGMAN, AND ANDREW G. ENGEL[b]

Muscle Research Laboratory
and
Department of Neurology
Mayo Clinic
Rochester, Minnesota 55905

INTRODUCTION

The slow-channel congenital myasthenic syndrome (SCCMS) is characterized by prolonged opening episodes of the acetylcholine receptor (AChR) channel due to mutations in AChR subunit genes.[1–6] The prolonged channel opening events cause cationic overloading of the postsynaptic region, resulting in an endplate myopathy with destruction of the junctional folds, loss of AChR, and alteration of the endplate geometry.[7] In addition, physiologic stimulation causes staircase summation of the markedly prolonged endplate potentials, thus inducing a depolarization block.[1–3]

We have previously shown that quinidine sulfate (QS) is a long-lived open-channel blocker of the AChR channel.[8] We also demonstrated that 5 μM of QS reduces the open duration of wild-type AChR, but has no significant effect on the amplitude of the miniature endplate potential or on quantal release by nerve impulse.[8] Because this concentration of QS can be achieved in clinical practice, we tested the hypothesis that clinically attainable levels of QS can significantly reduce the open duration of channel events in the SCCMS.

METHODS

We genetically engineered five AChR subunit cDNAs harboring five well-characterized SCCMS mutations: εT264P,[1] εL269F,[3] αG153S,[2] αN217K,[3] and βV266M.[3] We transfected each mutant cDNA together with complementary wild-type AChR subunit cDNAs and with plasmid-encoding green fluorescent protein into 293 human embryonic kidney (HEK) cells.[6,9] Single-channel recordings were obtained in the cell-attached mode at 22 °C, at 10–12-kHz bandwidth, with 5–250 nM acetylcholine

[a]This work was supported by a National Institutes of Health grant to A. G. Engel (No. NS6277) and by an MDA postdoctoral fellowship to K. Ohno.
[b]To whom all correspondence should be addressed.

(ACh) and a range of QS concentrations in the patch pipette. Dwell-time histograms were plotted on a logarithmic abscissa and fitted to the sum of exponentials by maximum likelihood.[10]

RESULTS

Increasing concentrations of QS progressively decreased the predominant burst open duration (τ_b) of both wild-type and mutant AChRs in a concentration-dependent manner (FIGURE 1, A and B). In the absence of QS, the respective mean τ_b values for

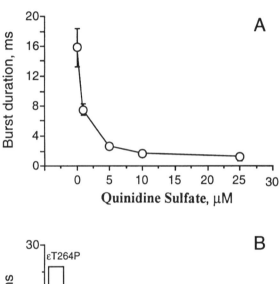

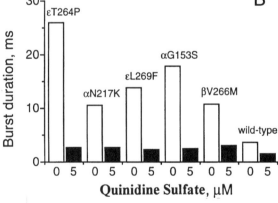

FIGURE 1. (A) The effect of increasing concentration of quinidine sulfate on the predominant burst duration of the five genetically engineered slow-channel mutants expressed in 293 HEK cells. Vertical lines indicate the SE. Note that even 1 μM of the drug significantly reduces the burst duration of the mutant channels. **(B)** The effect of 5 μM quinidine sulfate on the predominant burst duration of mutant and wild-type AChR channels. Note the proportionately greater effect on the mutant than on the wild-type channels.

wild-type and mutant channels were 3.6 and 15.8 ms. In the presence of 5 μM QS, the respective mean τ_b values were 1.7 and 2.6 ms. From these values and FIGURE 1B, it is clear that the effect of QS is proportionately greater on the τ_b's of the mutant than those of the wild-type AChRs. Moreover, even 1 μM QS significantly reduces the τ_b's of the mutant AChRs.

FIGURE 2 illustrates the ACh-elicited channel activity of wild-type AChR and εT264P slow-channel AChR in the absence and presence of 5 μM QS. In the pres-

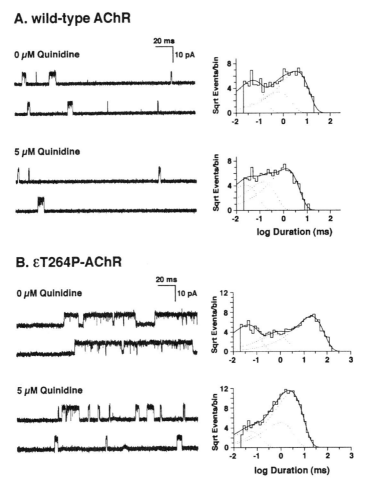

FIGURE 2. The effect of 5 μM quinidine sulfate on channel events of wild-type AChR (**A, left**) and εT264P-AChR (**B, left**). The very long bursts characteristic of the slow-channel mutation become much shorter in the presence of 5 μM of the drug, approaching the duration of wild-type bursts. The burst duration histograms (**A and B, right**) indicate that the drug shifts the predominant burst duration to the left and that the shift is greater for mutant (**B, right**) than for wild-type (**A, right**) AChR.

ence of QS, the opening bursts of the εT264P-AChR (FIGURE 2B, bottom) resemble those of wild-type AChR in the absence of QS (FIGURE 2A, top).

DISCUSSION

One to 5 μM of QS significantly shortens or normalizes the opening episodes of the slow-channel AChRs expressed in HEK cells. These drug levels are readily attainable in clinical practice and do not reduce the amplitude of the miniature endplate potential or the quantal release by nerve impulse. Therefore, our findings predict a therapeutic effect for QS in the SCCMS. This prediction has now been validated (see presentation by C. M. Harper and A. G. Engel in this volume).

REFERENCES

1. OHNO, K., D. O. HUTCHINSON, M. MILONE, J. M. BRENGMAN, C. BOUZAT, S. M. SINE & A. G. ENGEL. 1995. Congenital myasthenic syndrome caused by prolonged acetylcholine receptor channel openings due to a mutation in the M2 domain of the ε subunit. Proc. Natl. Acad. Sci. U.S.A. **92:** 758–762.
2. SINE, S. M., K. OHNO, C. BOUZAT, A. AUERBACH, M. MILONE, J. N. PRUITT & A. G. ENGEL. 1995. Mutation of the acetylcholine receptor α subunit causes a slow-channel myasthenic syndrome by enhancing agonist binding affinity. Neuron **15:** 229–239.
3. ENGEL, A. G., K. OHNO, M. MILONE, H-L. WANG, S. NAKANO, C. BOUZAT, J. N. PRUITT, D. O. HUTCHINSON, J. M. BRENGMAN, N. BREN et al. 1996. New mutations in acetylcholine receptor subunit genes reveal heterogeneity in the slow-channel congenital myasthenic syndrome. Hum. Mol. Genet. **5:** 1217–1227.
4. GOMEZ, C. M., R. MASELLI, J. GAMMACK, J. LASALDE, S. TAMAMIZU, D. R. CORNBLATH, M. LEHAR, M. MCNAMEE & R. KUNCL. 1996. A beta-subunit mutation in the acetylcholine receptor gate causes severe slow-channel syndrome. Ann. Neurol. **39:** 712–723.
5. CROXEN, R., C. NEWLAND, D. BEESON, H. OOSTERHUIS, G. CHAUPLANAZ, A. VINCENT & J. NEWSOM-DAVIS. 1997. Mutations in different functional domains of the human muscle acetylcholine receptor alpha subunit in patients with the slow-channel congenital myasthenic syndrome. Hum. Mol. Genet. **6:** 767–774.
6. MILONE, M., H-L. WANG, K. OHNO, T. FUKUDOME, J. N. PRUITT, N. BREN, S. M. SINE & A. G. ENGEL. 1997. Slow-channel syndrome caused by enhanced activation, desensitization, and agonist binding affinity due to mutation in the M2 domain of the acetylcholine receptor alpha subunit. J. Neurosci. **17:** 5651–5665.
7. ENGEL, A. G., E. H. LAMBERT, D. M. MULDER, C. F. TORRES, K. SAHASHI, T. E. BERTORINI & J. N. WHITAKER. 1982. A newly recognized congenital myasthenic syndrome attributed to a prolonged open time of the acetylcholine-induced ion channel. Ann. Neurol. **11:** 553–569.
8. SIEB, J. P., M. MILONE & A. G. ENGEL. 1996. Effects of the quinoline derivatives quinine, quinidine, and chloroquine on neuromuscular transmission. Brain Res. **712:** 179–189.
9. BOUZAT, C., N. BREN & S. M. SINE. 1994. Structural basis of different gating kinetics of fetal and adult acetylcholine receptors. Neuron **13:** 1395–1402.
10. SIGWORTH, F. J. & S. M. SINE. 1987. Data transformation for improved display and fitting of single-channel dwell time histograms. Biophys. J. **52:** 1047–1054.

Safety and Efficacy of Quinidine Sulfate in Slow-Channel Congenital Myasthenic Syndrome[a]

C. MICHEL HARPER AND ANDREW G. ENGEL

Department of Neurology
Mayo Clinic and Foundation
Rochester, Minnesota 55905

INTRODUCTION

Slow-channel congenital myasthenic syndrome (SCCMS) is an autosomal dominant disorder characterized by prolonged single-channel openings of the AChR and a prolonged decay constant of the end plate potential.[1] The weakness in SCCMS is unresponsive to cholinesterase inhibitors and results from depolarization block of the AChR as well as an end plate myopathy caused by cationic overload of the postsynaptic region.[1–3] Nerve conduction studies show repetitive compound muscle action potentials (R-CMAP) with single stimuli and a rate-dependent decrement of the main CMAP (M-CMAP) with repetitive stimulation.

We recently demonstrated that quinidine sulfate shortens the open time of the AChR without reducing the MEPP amplitude or quantal content at concentrations < 5 μM, while at concentrations > 10 μM progressive neuromuscular blockade is observed.[4] We report improvement in clinical strength and electrophysiologic measures of neuromuscular transmission in a series of six patients treated with quinidine sulfate.

METHODS

Six patients with SCCMS (ages 12–65 years) were enrolled in an open label prospective IRB-approved trial of quinidine sulfate. Patients were hospitalized in the Mayo General Clinical Research Center for the first 2–7 days with continuous ECG and pulse oximetry monitoring as well as daily measurements of respiratory muscle strength and manual muscle testing. Quinidine sulfate was administered at a dose of 200 mg three times daily. After the first week, the dose was gradually increased to maintain a serum level of 1.0–2.5 μg/mL.

The efficacy of quinidine sulfate therapy was assessed by measuring the following: (1) forward arm elevation time, (2) number of deep knee bends performed in 1 minute, (3) muscle subset of the neuropathy impairment score (NIS), (4) presence

[a]This study was supported by Human Health Services Grant No. M01-RR00585, General Clinical Research Centers, Division of Research Resources, and by the Mayo Clinic Foundation.

and size of the R-CMAP following single electrical stimulus, and (5) decrement of the M-CMAP with low (2 Hz) and high (10–50 Hz) rates of repetitive stimulation. In the NIS, manual muscle strength is graded bilaterally against normal for age, sex, and muscle as assessed by the examiner: normal strength = 0, mild weakness (25% weaker than normal) = 1, moderate weakness (50% weaker than normal) = 2, severe weakness (75% weaker than normal) = 3, and unable to generate any force = 4. The scores for each muscle are summated to give a total numerical score between 0 and 176. This scale has been validated in patients with peripheral neuropathy[5] and has been used to assess the effects of 3,4-diaminopyridine in Lambert-Eaton syndrome.[6] All outcome measures were assessed at 30-minute intervals for a total of 2 hours following oral administration of 200 mg quinidine sulfate on the first and second day, and then 60 minutes after the morning dose of quinidine sulfate on day 7 and day 30 of continuous therapy. The Wilcoxon ranked-sign test was used to determine the statistical significance ($p < 0.05$) of results at days 1, 2, 7, and 30 compared to baseline.

RESULTS

Four patients tolerated the drug well and have taken quinidine continuously in daily doses ranging from 600 to 900 mg with a length of follow-up from 6 to 14 months. Despite improvement, quinidine was discontinued in one patient (patient 6 in TABLE 1) on day 7 of therapy due to an allergic reaction (fever and elevated liver enzymes) that resolved rapidly after the drug was discontinued. In another patient (patient 4 in

TABLE 1. Patient Response to Quinidine[a]

	Patient 1	Patient 2	Patient 3	Patient 4	Patient 5	Patient 6
			Patient Characteristics			
Age (years)/sex	19/F	30/F	64/M	12/M	16/M	22/F
Mutation	βV266M	αN217K	αG153S	αV249F	εL269F	εT264P
Onset	childhood	childhood	childhood	neonate	neonate	neonate
Distribution of weakness	neck, UE, F > EOM, LE	neck, UE, F > EOM, LE	neck, UE, F > EOM, LE	neck, UE, F = EOM, LE	neck, UE, F = EOM, LE	neck, UE, F = EOM, LE
			Response to 200 mg Quinidine po tid: Baseline/30 Days of Rx			
NIS	54/20[b]	58/20[b]	26/10[b]	106/41[b]	89/74[b]	78/67[c]
No. R-CMAP	1/1	1/1	1/0	3/2	3/1	0/0[c]
Dec. 2 Hz (%)	12/14	18/13	5/4	47/27	48/28	58/54[c]
Dec. 10–50 Hz (%)	60/53[b]	52/30[b]	45/15[b]	56/32[b]	77/34[b]	72/59[c]

[a]Terms: UE, upper extremity; F, face; EOM, extraocular muscles; LE, lower extremity; NIS, neuropathy impairment score; R-CMAP, repetitive compound muscle action potential; Dec., decrement of CMAP area.
[b]$p < 0.05$.
[c]Day 7 compared to baseline in patient 6.

TABLE 1), the quinidine was temporarily discontinued when the patient developed nocturnal hypoventilation after 3 months of quinidine therapy (900 mg/day, serum level of 2.0 μg/mL). This occurred at a time when significant improvement in limb strength and overall endurance was demonstrated. The quinidine was discontinued, but this resulted in an increase in extremity weakness and further decline in respiratory reserve, despite treatment with nocturnal oxygen under positive pressure. Placement of a tracheostomy was considered, but became unnecessary after the patient improved significantly on a combination of quinidine sulfate (800 mg/day) and nocturnal oxygen under positive pressure.

All six patients exhibited objective improvement in measures of muscle strength, endurance, and neuromuscular transmission after quinidine therapy (TABLE 1 and FIGURE 1). Acutely, the peak effect was observed 60–90 minutes after a single oral dose of quinidine (FIGURE 1). Additional improvement was noted at 7 and 30 days of continuous therapy (TABLE 1). Arm elevation time improved in two of five patients and statistically significant improvement was observed in the NIS and in the number of deep knee bends performed in 1 minute after 30 days of therapy in all patients. All patients have reported subjective improvement in strength and endurance. Two of the patients who were wheelchair-dependent have drastically reduced the need for wheelchair assistance.

DISCUSSION

This study shows that quinidine sulfate improves clinical measures of strength and neurophysiological measures of neuromuscular transmission in SCCMS when

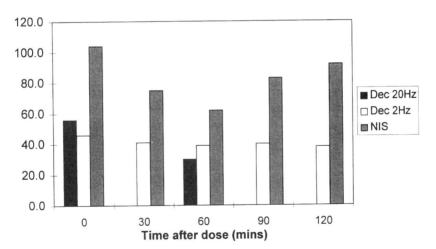

FIGURE 1. Response of patient 4 (see TABLE 1) to a single 200-mg oral dose of quinidine sulfate. Neuropathy impairment score (NIS) and decrement with 2-Hz and 20-Hz repetitive nerve stimulation assessed at 30-minute intervals for 120 minutes after a single dose of quinidine.

administered in doses sufficient to produce serum concentrations of 1–2.5 μg/mL. Acutely, the peak effect occurred 60–90 minutes after oral administration of the drug and was associated with a reduction in the M-CMAP decrement at high rates of repetitive stimulation as well as with a reduction in the number, amplitude, and duration of the R-CMAP observed after single stimuli. The acute effect is likely caused by a direct shortening of the AChR opening episodes, which would reduce the depolarization block at the neuromuscular junction. Chronic quinidine therapy may improve the end plate myopathy associated with SCCMS by reducing the influx of cations into the end plate region. This hypothesis is supported by our observations of continued clinical improvement in all five of the patients who have continued to take the medication for 8–14 months.

Quinidine sulfate should be used with caution in patients with SCCMS because of the potential for adverse effects such as drug allergy, exacerbation of weakness at concentrations higher than 2.5 μg/mL, and the possible development of respiratory failure in patients with borderline baseline respiratory function. The mechanism of the temporary decline in respiratory function in one of our patients in the setting of improved extremity strength is unknown. We suspect that the increased metabolic demands of stronger limb muscles lead to increased respiratory muscle fatigue and to eventual decompensation of borderline respiratory function.

REFERENCES

1. ENGEL, A. G., E. H. LAMBERT, D. M. MULDER, C. F. TORRES, K. SAHASHI, T. E. BERTORINI & J. N. WHITAKER. 1982. A newly recognized congenital myasthenic syndrome attributed to a prolonged open time of the acetylcholine-induced ion channel. Ann. Neurol. **11:** 553–569.
2. SINE, S. M., K. OHNO, C. BOUZAT, A. AUERBACH, M. MILONE, J. N. PRUITT & A. G. ENGEL. 1995. Mutation of the acetylcholine receptor alpha subunit causes a slow-channel myasthenic syndrome by enhancing agonist binding affinity. Neuron **15:** 229–239.
3. ENGEL, A. G., K. OHNO, M. MILONE, H-L. WANG, S. NAKANO, C. BOUZAT, J. N. PRUITT, D. O. HUTCHINSON, J. M. BRENGMAN, N. BREN et al. 1996. New mutations in acetylcholine receptor subunit genes reveal heterogeneity in the slow-channel congenital myasthenic syndrome. Hum. Mol. Genet. **5:** 1217–1227.
4. SIEB, J. P., M. MILONE & A. G. ENGEL. 1996. Effects of the quinoline derivatives quinine, quinidine, and chloroquine on neuromuscular transmission. Brain Res. **712:** 179–189.
5. DYCK, P. J., W. J. LITCHY, K. A. LEHMAN, J. L. HOKANSON, P. A. LOW & P. C. O'BRIEN. 1995. Variables influencing neuropathic endpoints: The Rochester Diabetic Neuropathy Study of Healthy Subjects. Neurology **45:** 1115–1121.
6. MCEVOY, K. M., A. J. WINDEBANK, J. R. DAUBE & P. A. LOW. 1989. 3,4-Diaminopyridine in the treatment of Lambert-Eaton myasthenic syndrome. N. Engl. J. Med. **321:** 1567–1571.

Rhodamine-labeled Alpha-Bungarotoxin Allows Visualization of End Plates in Congenital End Plate Acetylcholinesterase Deficiency (CEAD)

MARK A. AGIUS, RICARDO A. MASELLI, SHAN ZHU,
ROBERT H. FAIRCLOUGH, MIKE Y. LIN, AND WILLIAM ELLIS

Department of Neurology
University of California at Davis
Davis, California 95616

INTRODUCTION

The severe deficiency of cholinesterase at the neuromuscular junction is associated with a syndrome of congenital myasthenia gravis (MG). We describe two recently diagnosed patients with a diagnosis of congenital MG secondary to cholinesterase deficiency. We have developed a method of measuring the number of acetylcholine receptors (AChRs) per end plate in the neuromuscular junction of these patients that allows for the visualization and counting of end plates.

CASE REPORTS

Patient 1 (CG) is a 42-year-old female with weakness since early childhood. An older and a younger brother are also involved. She had repetitive motor response to a single shock with median nerve stimulation. *In vivo* electrophysiology, staining for acetylcholinesterase, as well as electron microscopy were consistent with the diagnosis of congenital end plate acetylcholinesterase deficiency (CEAD). Electron microscopy revealed focal degeneration of the postsynaptic membrane, small nerve terminals, and encasement of the nerve terminal with Schwann cells.

Patient 2 (SA) is a 41-year-old female with weakness since 8 months of age. She had delayed motor milestones. Weakness has been slowly progressive over several years. She has had severe ptosis since early childhood and, over the past several years, has had progressive difficulty with extremity strength. An older brother has a similar illness. Both parents and two half-siblings are normal. Repetitive stimulation produced marked decrement. There was no repetitive responses to a single stimulus. However, *in vitro* studies performed in anconeus muscle showed no change in the decay of end plate potentials during perfusion of neostigmine at concentrations of 1 μM, 2 μM, 0.1 mM, and 2 mM. Staining for acetylcholinesterase was markedly reduced.

MATERIALS AND METHODS

AChR Density

Measurements were performed on serially consecutive muscle fiber bundles of freshly dissected human anconeus of equivalent size and weight. Intact muscle fibers were obtained from origin to insertion. Analysis of specific α-bungarotoxin (α-bgtx) binding sites was done on two of the consecutive serial sections. Total gamma counts were determined by incubating one bundle with ^{125}I-labeled α-bgtx, whereas nonspecific counts were determined by incubating a second bundle with radiolabeled α-bgtx after first incubating with unlabeled α-bgtx. The number of end plates per muscle fiber bundle was determined under fluorescence microscopy by incubating a consecutive serial muscle fiber bundle with rhodamine-labeled α-bgtx. Nonspecific rhodamine-labeled α-bgtx binding was assessed by preincubating a fourth muscle fiber bundle with unlabeled α-bgtx. Microscopic analysis was performed without the need for embedding or fixing.

Confocal Microscopy

The end plates of muscle fibers, incubated with rhodamine-labeled α-bgtx, were visualized by dual-laser, confocal microscopy. This allowed the generation of three-dimensional images of the postsynaptic membrane at the end plates. Furthermore, this technology has the potential of allowing the determination of AChR density per end plate by integration and quantification of the intensity of fluorescence.

RESULTS

AChR density was 4.7×10^7 α-bgtx binding sites per end plate (CG) and $5.4 \pm 0.5 \times 10^7$ α-bgtx binding sites per end plate (SA) (see TABLE 1). AChR density from a control individual without neuromuscular disease was $1.8 \pm 1.8 \times 10^7$ α-bgtx binding

TABLE 1. AChR Density[a]

Patient Tested	α-bgtx (Moles)	α-bgtx Binding Sites (Molecules)	End Plate Number	AChR/End Plate $\times 10^7$
(1) CG	7.3×10^{-15}	4.49×10^9	188	4.70
(2) SA	8.53×10^{-15}	5.14×10^9	102	5.04
	3.5×10^{-15}	2.10×10^9	36	5.80
				5.42 ± 0.54[b]
(3) Control	1.56×10^{-14}	9.39×10^9	360	2.60
	5.27×10^{-15}	3.17×10^9	340	0.93
				1.77 ± 1.77[b]

[a]Measured in terms of α-bgtx binding sites/end plate.
[b]Mean ± standard deviation determined from duplicate experiments.

sites per end plate. Acetylcholinesterase staining revealed markedly diminished staining for acetylcholinesterase at the neuromuscular junctions. In contrast, rhodamine-labeled α-bgtx allowed the visualization of end plates by confocal microscopy.

DISCUSSION

The conventional assay for measuring AChR density involves the enumeration of end plates visualized after staining for acetylcholinesterase.[1] In CEAD, this determination is difficult. We have developed a modification of the standard assay involving the labeling of consecutive serial sections of muscle fibers with rhodamine-labeled α-bgtx and radioiodinated α-bgtx. This procedure allows the counting of both AChRs and end plate numbers in CEAD. Furthermore, labeling with rhodamine-labeled bgtx allows the utilization of confocal microscopy to measure the number of end plates, evaluate the morphology of the postsynaptic membrane, and provide a measurement of AChR density in individual end plates.

REFERENCE

1. ENGEL, A. G., A. NAGEL, T. J. WALLS, C. M. HARPER & H. A. WAISBURG. 1993. Congenital myasthenic syndromes: I. Deficiency and short open-time of the acetylcholine receptor. Muscle Nerve **16:** 1284–1292.

Immune Regulation and Myasthenia Gravis

SAMIA RAGHEB AND ROBERT P. LISAK

Department of Neurology
Division of Neuroimmunology
Wayne State University School of Medicine
and
The Detroit Medical Center
Detroit, Michigan 48201

INTRODUCTION

The hallmarks of an adaptive immune response are its specificity and its memory. Both of these properties are attributable to the lymphocyte. Two major subsets of lymphocytes exist: T cells and B cells. In order for the immune response to operate in an appropriate manner, both T and B cell function must be tightly regulated. This regulation is first achieved centrally during lymphocyte development. Peripherally, lymphocyte function may also be regulated through intrinsic regulatory pathways or through extrinsic intervention.

CENTRAL REGULATION OF THE IMMUNE RESPONSE

The specificity of the immune response is due to the presence of antigen-specific receptors on T and B cells. Both the T cell receptor (TCR) and the B cell receptor (BCR) arise from somatic recombination of separate multiple gene segments.[1] This allows lymphocytes to be able to recognize and respond to an infinite number of antigenic determinants. However, somatic recombination may also produce TCRs and BCRs that recognize self antigens. The immune system has evolved so that exposure to an antigen during lymphocyte development would result in clonal deletion or anergy (nonresponsiveness) to maintain a state of tolerance to that antigen.[2–4] Therefore, lymphocytes that would encounter an abundant circulating self antigen during development would become tolerized to that antigen. However, tissue-restricted antigens may not be accessible to a developing lymphocyte; it is not clearly understood how tolerance to these antigens is achieved. Lack of tolerance or loss of tolerance to a self antigen would result in autoimmunity.

During lymphocyte development, T cell tolerance occurs in the thymus and B cells are tolerized in the bone marrow. Some lymphocytes that express self-reactive antigen receptors fail to be tolerized during development and escape into the periphery. There is evidence that the mechanisms of clonal deletion and clonal anergy also operate in the periphery to induce tolerance. There are additional mechanisms to maintain peripheral tolerance. Circulating lymphocytes that have not been anergized and are therefore capable of responding to a self antigen may not encounter the antigen if it is in a sequestered site; this is termed clonal ignorance. Recent evidence also suggests that self-reactive B cells compete with other B cells for entry into lymphoid follicles;[5] the self-reactive B cells are excluded from the follicles and therefore they subsequently die. This has been termed follicular exclusion. Even though tolerance to self antigens is maintained under normal circumstances, genetic, hormonal, and/or environmental factors may bypass or breakdown tolerance, leading to an autoimmune response.

INITIATION OF THE IMMUNE RESPONSE

In an adaptive immune response, T cells play a central role in initiating, coordinating, and regulating the response to an antigen. The initiation of an immune response ultimately relies on the capacity of the T cell to recognize the antigen through its TCR. Professional antigen-presenting cells (APC) are specialized at breaking down or "processing" complex antigens and at "presenting" small antigenic determinants on their cell surface in the context of major histocompatibility complex (MHC) molecules.[6] The TCR recognizes this antigen/MHC complex, thereby activating the T cell to respond.[7] Since the MHC is polygenic and polymorphic,[8] MHC molecules differ in their capacity to bind and present antigenic peptides. Therefore, MHC molecules control and determine what will be presented to the TCR. The initial interaction between the APC and the T cell is weak and involves cellular adhesion molecules (CAMs): lymphocyte function–associated antigen-1 (LFA-1) on the T cell surface and intercellular adhesion molecule-1 (ICAM-1) on the APC surface. The binding of the antigen/MHC complex by the TCR is strengthened by the binding of the CD4 molecule on the T cell with MHC class II molecules on the APC.

The critical event in T cell activation is the recognition of antigen/MHC by the TCR. However, other molecular interactions provide important costimulatory signals for T cells. B7-1 and B7-2 are structurally related glycoproteins that are expressed on the APC surface. The interaction of B7 molecules with CD28 on the T cell surface provides a costimulatory signal[9,10] that allows T cells that have recognized antigen to produce and secrete interleukin-2 (IL-2), a cytokine important for T cell growth. T cells that have recognized antigen, but have not received a costimulatory signal, fail to produce an appreciable amount of IL-2 and become anergic.[11,12] However, they may be stimulated when exogenous IL-2 is provided. Therefore, T cell activation requires two signals:[13] the first is recognition of antigen and the second is costimulation. There is experimental evidence to suggest that B7-1 costimulation promotes TH1 responses, whereas B7-2 costimulation promotes TH2 responses[9] (see discussion below).

ACTIVATION OF B CELLS

The initial step in B cell activation also requires the recognition of antigen by the BCR. However, unlike the TCR, the antigenic determinants recognized by the BCR are not processed. B cells recognize three-dimensional conformational determinants. Cross-linking of the BCR by antigen provides the first signal required for B cell activation. However, the B cell response to most antigens also requires a second signal.

This is provided by the T cell in the form of "help".[14] CD4+ T cells provide help in two ways: first, cognate interactions that involve cell-surface molecules on the T cell and B cell surfaces; second, soluble cytokine signals.

Of the cognate interactions, the best described is the interaction of CD40 on the B cell surface with the CD40 ligand (CD40L) on the T cell surface.[15,16] CD40 is constitutively expressed on B cells; however, CD40L expression is induced upon T cell activation. The molecular interaction between CD40 and its ligand delivers a stimulatory signal that allows the B cell to respond to soluble cytokines that are produced and secreted by the T cell. These activated B cells then proliferate and some differentiate into antibody-secreting plasma cells, while some remain as antigen-specific memory B cells. The interaction of CD40 and CD40L also drives isotype switching in B cells so that they may produce antibody isotypes other than IgM. Without T cell help, antigen-stimulated B cells can only produce IgM antibodies; this is the case in X-linked hyper-IgM syndrome.[17]

Soluble cytokine signals that are secreted by antigen-activated T cells are important for B cell growth and differentiation.[14] These include IL-4, IL-5, IL-6, IL-10, and IL-13. IL-4 is a B cell growth factor and it also promotes isotype switching from IgM to IgG1 and IgE production. IL-5 promotes IgA production and also promotes B cell differentiation into antibody-secreting cells. Both IL-6 and IL-10 are potent growth and differentiation factors for activated B cells and promote immunoglobulin secretion. IL-13 is very similar to IL-4 in its activity.

It is important to note that the interaction of B cells with T cells is not a one-way interaction, but a two-way interaction. Because B cells express both MHC class II and B7 molecules on the cell surface, they can present antigen and provide costimulatory signals for antigen-specific T cells.[18] Furthermore, since the BCR is antigen-specific and can bind antigen, B cells are especially efficient at presenting the antigen to which they have specificity. Therefore, an antigen-specific B cell may bind antigen to its BCR, thereby receiving its first activating signal. The B cell may then present that antigen to an antigen-specific T cell in the context of MHC class II and also may provide a costimulatory signal to the T cell. The activated T cell in turn will express CD40L and secrete soluble cytokines that provide the second signal for B cell stimulation.

TWO SUBSETS OF CD4+ T CELLS: TH1 VERSUS TH2

Studies of T cell clones have shown that CD4+ T cells are segregated into two subsets based on the types of cytokines that they produce.[19] TH1 cells tend to produce interferon-γ (IFN-γ), IL-2, and tumor necrosis factor (TNF). TH2 cells tend to produce IL-4, IL-5, IL-6, IL-10, and IL-13. These cells, therefore, have very different functions during an immune response. TH1 cells produce cytokines that enhance cell-mediated immunity, whereas TH2 cells produce cytokines that enhance humoral immunity.

Both TH1 and TH2 cells arise from naive T cells that produce and secrete IL-2.[20] After antigen priming, these naive cells may differentiate into TH1 or TH2 cells. The priming conditions greatly influence this differentiation step. In the response to a protein antigen, the nature and amount of antigen can have an effect on the differentiation of naive T cells into TH1 versus TH2 cells. The use of adjuvants may also have an effect. Furthermore, costimulation via B7-1 versus B7-2 may favor differentiation of TH1 versus TH2 cells, respectively.[9] The presence of cytokines during T cell priming will also influence TH1 versus TH2 cell differentiation.[21,22] IL-12 promotes priming for IFN-γ production (TH1 profile), whereas IL-4 promotes priming for IL-4 production (TH2 profile). Moreover, these cytokines cross-regulate each other's function. Therefore, IL-4 inhibits the IL-12-driven priming of TH1 cells and, vice versa, IFN-γ inhibits the IL-4-driven priming of TH2 cells. However, primed T cells that have already differentiated into TH1 or TH2 cells tend to retain their cytokine production profile.

TH2 cells produce and secrete IL-10, which not only is a B cell growth and differentiation factor, but also has potent anti-inflammatory properties.[23] IL-10 inhibits cytokine synthesis by TH1 cells, particularly IFN-γ production. This indirectly results in inhibition of MHC class II expression on APCs and in inhibition of macrophage function. Therefore, CD4+ T cells, through the cytokines that they produce, are able to cross-regulate each other's priming, growth, differentiation, and effector function.[21,22] Moreover, the balance of TH1 versus TH2 cells will shift the immune response to a particular antigen towards a T cell–mediated or a B cell–mediated response.

PERIPHERAL REGULATION OF THE IMMUNE RESPONSE

If an ongoing immune response remains unchecked, immune cells and their secreted products are likely to cause damage or destruction of surrounding cells and tissues. Various intrinsic pathways may regulate the immune response: (a) feedback inhibition, (b) cytokine shifts, (c) suppressor T cells, and (d) idiotypic networks.

Feedback Inhibition

One of the simplest, most-effective ways of abating an immune response is to eliminate the stimulus, that is, the antigen. Activated T and B cells will then become resting cells. In the case of autoimmune disease, however, there is a continuous supply of self antigen. There is a feedback inhibition pathway for stimulated T cells. Once activated, T cells express CTLA-4 on the cell surface.[9,24] This molecule closely resembles CD28 and also binds to B7 molecules. However, while the binding of CD28 to B7 delivers a costimulatory signal, the binding of CTLA-4 to B7 delivers an inhibitory signal to the T cell.

Cytokine Shifts

As discussed above, CD4+ T cells can be divided into two subsets, TH1 and TH2 cells, that enhance cellular immunity or humoral immunity through the production and secretion of soluble cytokines. Therefore, an autoimmune disease whose pathology is mediated primarily by a TH1 response may be ameliorated by a shift to a TH2 response. This has been demonstrated in experimental autoimmune encephalomyelitis (EAE).[25] It is not certain that a B cell–mediated disease such as myasthenia gravis (MG) would be ameliorated by a shift to a TH1 response. IL-2 enhances B cell growth and IFN-γ enhances B cell differentiation.[26]

Suppressor T Cells

Antigen-specific suppressor cells have been described that may downregulate an immune response. These T cells exert their inhibitory activities through the production and secretion of soluble suppressor factors. Both CD4+ and CD8+ T cells have been shown to secrete transforming growth factor-β (TGF-β), an immunoregulatory cytokine that is inhibitory for both T cell and B cell function.[27]

Idiotypic Networks

Each T cell and B cell clone expresses a unique antigen-specific receptor on the cell surface, which is termed the idiotype (id). The idiotypic network theory[28] states that, for every id, there is a clone that expresses an anti-id. Therefore, id/anti-id interactions serve to check the growth of a clone undergoing expansion. Id/anti-id interactions have been shown to operate at the antibody level and they presumably operate at the cellular level *in vivo*.

BREAKDOWN OF IMMUNE TOLERANCE

It is important to maintain tolerance to a self antigen to avoid pathologic autoimmune responses. Various mechanisms have been proposed to account for the breakdown of immune tolerance. The *disruption of a cellular or tissue barrier* may expose a sequestered self antigen to circulating lymphocytes; if these lymphocytes have not been tolerized to that antigen, they may become activated and initiate an autoimmune response.

Historically, there has been an association between a *recent infection* and the onset of autoimmune disease, in a genetically susceptible host. Antigenic determinants that are expressed by infectious agents may closely resemble determinants on self antigens. Therefore, mounting an immune response against the infectious agent(s) would result in the activation of B cells and T cells that are cross-reactive to self antigens. This is termed *molecular mimicry.* Furthermore, there is a possibility that *determinants from infectious agents may bind to a self antigen.* This would create new antigenic determinants that were not present during lymphocyte development and to which tolerance has not been established. Both bacteria and viruses also produce *superantigens*[29] that can activate many clones of lymphocytes in an antigen-independent manner. Tolerance to self antigens that is maintained through anergy may be overridden via superantigen activation. Superantigens that serve as polyclonal activators of T and B cells have been described. Finally, *infection of APCs* upregulates the expression of costimulatory molecules, which may result in the activation of anergic T cells. These mechanisms offer possible explanations for the frequent onset of autoimmune disease following infectious disease. However, under these circumstances, autoimmune disease will not develop without the genetic background that predisposes an individual to mount a self-directed immune response. This "background" includes genes for the MHC, TCR, and BCR.

Hormonal factors may also contribute to the breakdown of immune tolerance. It is well established that the frequency of autoimmune disease in females is greater than the frequency in males. The mechanisms by which hormonal factors influence the development of autoimmunity are not understood. During lymphocyte development, it is possible that the hormonal environment may affect the central induction of tolerance. Peripherally, hormonal factors may be involved in the breakdown of lymphocyte anergy. *Age* is also a contributing factor in the breakdown of immune tolerance as the incidence of autoimmune disease increases with age. This may reflect a failure of both central and peripheral immunoregulatory pathways. Many of the factors that contribute to the breakdown of immune tolerance are not "antigen-specific," which may explain why an individual may develop more than one autoimmune disease.

IMMUNOPATHOGENESIS OF MYASTHENIA GRAVIS

Autoimmune myasthenia gravis (MG) is a B cell–mediated disease in which the target autoantigen is the acetylcholine receptor (AChR) at the neuromuscular junction.[30] Antibody-mediated pathology at the postsynaptic muscle membrane[31] leads to deficits in neuromuscular transmission and progressive weakness. T cells do not appear to contribute to the pathology of the myasthenic neuromuscular junction. However, the *in vitro* production of AChR-specific antibodies by B cells is T cell–dependent; that is, T cell "help" is necessary (reviewed in reference 30). Furthermore, the induction of experimental autoimmune myasthenia gravis (EAMG), the animal model of MG, is also T cell–dependent. This experimental evidence demonstrates that T cells are required and do participate in the induction and development of autoimmune MG. Removal of the thymus, the organ of T cell development, leads to clinical improvement in patients with MG.

While both AChR-specific B cells and T cells are required for the development of autoimmune MG, the antigenic determinants that are recognized by the BCR and TCR have not been easy to identify. The AChR is a multichain molecular complex composed of two alpha (α), one beta (β), one delta (δ), and either a gamma (γ) or an epsilon (ε) subunit.[32] Numerous antigenic determinants are found on each subunit, some of which are immunodominant, while others are cryptic. The majority of determinants that are recognized by B cells and T cells appear to be on the α subunit.[30] Studies in MG patients have shown that different antigenic determinants appear to be immunodominant in different patients and that individual patients respond to multiple determinants. This reflects the heterogeneity and polymorphism of the MHC molecules in the patients. Both the B cell and T cell responses to AChR determinants are heterogeneous and polyclonal in MG.[30]

IMMUNOREGULATION IN MYASTHENIA GRAVIS

Idiotypic Networks

Approximately 60% of AChR-specific antibodies bind to an extracellular segment of the α subunit that has been named the main immunogenic region (MIR).[30] It is possible that these antibodies share idiotypes, and the existence of anti-id antibodies has been demonstrated in MG patients. Anti-id antibodies have been used to treat animals with EAMG; however, in some cases, because the anti-id antibodies may mimic or resemble the antigen, treatment of EAMG with anti-id antibodies may result in exacerbation of the disease rather than improvement.

Suppressor T Cells (Ts)

AChR-specific Ts cell cultures[30] have been established from animals with EAMG and these cells produce and secrete soluble "suppressor factors." The Ts cells inhibited the capacity of TH cells to provide "help" to AChR-specific B cells.

Role of CD8+ T Cells

CD8+ T cells comprise two major subsets: cytotoxic T cells and suppressor T cells. It has been suggested that MG patients have a deficient Ts cell population. Studies of lymphocyte populations in the blood do show a higher CD4+:CD8+ T cell ratio in patients when compared to healthy controls.[30] Peripheral blood mononuclear cells from patients with MG produce anti-AChR antibodies in culture. The depletion of CD8+ cells from these *in vitro* cultures results in an increased production of AChR-specific antibodies and in increased production of total IgG. Cell cultures from healthy controls do not produce detectable levels of anti-AChR antibodies. The depletion of CD8+ cells from these cultures results in an increased production of total IgG, but the cultures still do not produce detectable levels of AChR-specific antibodies. These experiments demonstrate that, while CD8+ T cells may regulate immunoglobulin production, the inability of cells from healthy subjects to produce AChR-specific antibodies is not simply due to CD8+ T cell regulation. Stated differently, the production of AChR-specific antibodies by cell cultures from MG patients is not simply due to a functionally defective CD8+ T cell population.[30]

In EAMG, the role of CD8+ T cells in induction of disease remains unclear. EAMG was induced in mice in which the β$_2$-microglobulin gene was disrupted.[33] These animals had a deficiency in MHC class I molecules and hence a deficiency in CD8+ cells. The incidence of EAMG in homozygous mice was higher than in heterozygous mice. These data demonstrate a regulatory role of CD8+ T cells in induction of EAMG. In Lewis rats, animals in which CD8+ cells were depleted developed EAMG. However, there was a decrease in AChR-specific antibody production. These data demonstrate that CD8+ T cells may play a role in the development of EAMG.[34]

IS THERE CLONAL DELETION OF AChR-SPECIFIC CELLS?

During lymphocyte development, exposure to an antigen should result in deletion or anergy of clones that are specific to that antigen. For T cells, this occurs in the thymus; for B cells, this occurs in the bone marrow.

T Cells

Tolerance to a self antigen occurs as T cells develop in the thymus if the self antigen is present during development. Epithelial and myoid cells within the thymus have been shown to express the AChR or a molecule that is very similar to the AChR.[30] However, AChR in the thymus contains the γ subunit instead of the ε subunit, which is present in adult skeletal muscle AChR. Despite the presence of AChR within the thymus, AChR-responsive T cells are not deleted and they emerge into the periphery. There is some recent evidence that apoptosis mechanisms[35] may not be operating normally in the MG thymus; a decreased expression of Fas has been reported.[36] Other experimental evidence also demonstrates that clonal deletion is not the mechanism by which tolerance to the AChR is maintained. *In vitro* studies have shown that peripheral blood mononuclear cells from patients with MG and from healthy controls are responsive to the AChR, to the α subunit of the AChR, and to synthetic peptide sequences of the AChR. Furthermore, AChR-specific T cell lines have been established.[30] These data demonstrate that AChR-specific T cells are present in the peripheral circulation, even in nonmyasthenic healthy individuals who do not exhibit any symptoms of MG and who do not have detectable anti-AChR antibodies in the serum. What then are the mechanisms that maintain peripheral tolerance in nonmyasthenics? There are several mechanisms that may be operating separately or in concert: (1) *in vivo*, AChR-specific T cells are anergic and incapable of responding; unlike clonal deletion, anergy is reversible, allowing the cells to respond and leading to development of MG; (2) AChR-specific T cells are present in a frequency that is too low to lead to the immunopathologic manifestations of MG; (3) the TH1 versus TH2 balance of AChR-specific T cells may be such that there are insufficient cognate and soluble cytokine signals for the activation of B cells; (4) regardless of what the T cells are doing, AChR-specific B cells are not present in nonmyasthenics; for reasons that are discussed later, this is highly unlikely since it is easier to maintain tolerance in T cells than in B cells.

B Cells

MG patients clearly have AChR-specific B cells circulating in the periphery. Patients with generalized MG have AChR-specific antibodies in the serum and cell cultures from these patients produce anti-AChR antibodies *in vitro*. Healthy nonmyasthenic controls do not have detectable levels of AChR-specific antibodies in the serum and cell cultures from nonmyasthenics do not produce the antibody *in vitro*.[30] These experimental results imply that AChR-specific B cells either are absent (clonally deleted) or are anergic in nonmyasthenics. It is unlikely that there are no AChR-specific B cells in nonmyasthenic controls due to the nature of the BCR. Unlike the TCR, the BCR undergoes somatic hypermutation.[37] This allows affinity maturation of antibodies. Therefore, even when self-reactive B cell clones are deleted during development, other B cell clones that express closely related BCRs may become self-reactive via somatic hypermutation of the BCR. It is more likely that AChR-specific B cells are present in nonmyasthenics and are either anergic or nonpathogenic due to regulation by T cells. There is experimental evidence that AChR-specific B cells are present in nonmyasthenic controls at a low frequency.[38] Given T cell "help," AChR-reactive B cell clones could be activated, leading to the production of self-reactive antibodies.

EXTRINSIC INTERVENTION FOR TREATMENT OF MYASTHENIA GRAVIS

Tremendous progress has been made in understanding the pathogenesis of MG; yet, there is no cure for MG or for any other autoimmune disease. Therapy for MG consists of cholinesterase inhibitors, plasmapheresis, thymectomy, cytotoxic/immunosuppressive drugs, and (more recently) intravenous IgG. Recent efforts have concentrated on manipulating the immune response in EAMG and MG.

Lymphocyte Toxicity

This approach to therapy aims at targeting and eliminating antigen-specific or activated lymphocytes: (a) In EAMG, AChR-specific T cell or TCR vaccination has been used in an attempt to induce an anticlonotypic response. This has not been very successful in EAMG.[39] (b) AChR-specific T cells from C57BL6 mice that are susceptible to the induction of EAMG preferentially utilize a TCR with Vβ6.[40] A Vβ-specific toxin that consists of an anti-Vβ6 monoclonal antibody coupled to ricin A has been used to target and selectively kill Vβ6-expressing T cells,[41] which are the AChR-reactive T cells. (c) Both activated T and B cells express cell-surface IL-2 receptors. Recently, an IL-2 toxin that would target cells expressing IL-2 receptors has been used to kill B cell cultures from patients with MG.[42]

Induction of Tolerance/Anergy

The immune response to a protein antigen is influenced by several factors, including the form of the antigen, the dose of the antigen, and the route of administration: (a) It is well documented that mucosal administration of an antigen will usually result in antigen-specific tolerance. In EAMG, both nasal and oral administration of AChR have been used successfully to tolerize rats.[43–45] Tolerance induction was accompanied by an increase in the frequency of cells that produce transforming growth factor-β (TGF-β), which is an immunoregulatory cytokine for T and B cells.[46] However, oral administration of antigen may lead to B cell priming.[44,47] (b) As discussed earlier, the presentation of an antigen to a T cell in the absence of costimulation will induce T cell anergy. Soluble MHC class II/AChR peptide complexes have been used *in vitro* to induce anergy of peptide-specific T cell lines and clones.[48,49]

Interference with T Cell Activation

CD4+ T cells recognize antigen in the context of MHC class II molecules and they require costimulation to be activated. Various experimental approaches are designed to interfere with T cell activation: (a) C57BL6 mice are normally susceptible to induction of EAMG. The disruption of MHC class II genes in these mice results in a decrease in the percentage of CD4+ T cells and prevents EAMG induction.[50] The *in vivo* administration of anti-MHC class II antibodies also inhibits EAMG.[51] (b) Interference with costimulation will inhibit T cell activation. CTLA-4-Ig is a soluble molecule that competes with CD28 for binding to B7 molecules on the APC surface. The *in vitro* use of CTLA-4-Ig on cell cultures from rats with EAMG results in decreased IL-2 production, decreased lymphocyte proliferation, and decreased antibody production.[52] (c) Antigen-unrelated competitor peptides may be used in excess to saturate MHC class II molecules and compete with or prevent the antigen from binding. In the EAMG model, rats were coimmunized with AChR and ovalbumin as competitor; this approach inhibited EAMG.[53] (d) Antigen antagonists consist of peptides that would normally bind to MHC class II molecules and activate T cells; however, these peptides have been altered through one or several amino-acid substitutions that allow the peptides to bind MHC class II molecules, but fail to activate the T cells.[54,55] Altered peptide ligands have been shown to inhibit the *in vitro* T cell response in MG and EAMG.[56–58]

Altering the Cytokine Balance

Many cytokines have pleiotropic functions; therefore, altering the cytokine balance will influence APC and lymphocyte function, thereby altering the immune response. *In vivo* therapy of EAMG with IFN-α has been successful.[59,60]

Other Approaches to Therapy

These include the following: (a) Daily intraperitoneal injections of a soluble complement receptor have inhibited EAMG.[61] This experimental treatment would prevent the antibody plus complement–mediated damage to the AChR, but would have no effect on antibodies that block the ACh binding site or those that increase AChR turnover. (b) Intravenous injections of IgG (IvIg) have been used in the treatment of MG patients in crisis. Mechanisms by which IvIg may be beneficial have been reviewed.[62] (c) In EAMG, the α subunit sequence of 61–76 has been defined as a main immunogenic region (MIR) for antibody production. The complementary peptide to AChR 61–76 has been synthesized and named RhCA 67–16. Complementary peptide therapy has been beneficial in EAMG. Mechanistically, it has been shown that the complementary peptide induces the production of antibodies that react with MIR-specific antibodies.[63,64] Therefore, complementary peptide therapy induces anti-id antibody production.

FUTURE IMMUNOREGULATORY THERAPEUTIC APPROACHES IN MYASTHENIA GRAVIS

The ideal therapy for MG should be targeted at AChR-specific lymphocytes. This is a daunting task since there are multiple epitopes, some of which are immunodominant and some are cryptic.[65,66] Restoring tolerance to these epitopes is the goal. This may be more feasible for T cells rather than B cells. Clonal deletion is one approach to restoring tolerance, but is difficult to achieve where there is a polyclonal T cell response.[30] Experiments in the EAMG model have demonstrated that, even when the T cell response is predominated by Vβ6+ cells, the elimination of Vβ6+ T cells results in the generation of new clones to replace them.[67] Some of the experimental approaches that induce anergy and/or interfere with AChR-specific T cell activation show promise. These approaches rely on identifying T cell "ligands" that consist of peptide plus MHC. If proven to be successful in patients, they would provide antigen-specific treatment alternatives, but not a cure.

REFERENCES

1. SEIDMAN, J. G. & P. LEDER. 1978. The arrangement and rearrangement of antibody genes. Nature **276:** 790–795.
2. MILLER, J. F. A. P. & G. MORAHAN. 1992. Peripheral T cell tolerance. Annu. Rev. Immunol. **10:** 51–69.
3. MACLENNAN, I. C. M. 1995. Deletion of autoreactive B cells. Curr. Biol. **5:** 103–106.
4. SPRENT, J. & S. R. WEBB. 1995. Intrathymic and extrathymic clonal deletion of T cells. Curr. Opin. Immunol. **7:** 196–205.
5. CYSTER, J. G., S. B. HARTLEY & C. C. GOODNOW. 1994. Competition for follicular niches excludes self-reactive cells from the recirculating B-cell repertoire. Nature **371:** 389–395.
6. BARBER, L. D. & P. PARHAM. 1993. Peptide binding to major histocompatibility complex molecules. Annu. Rev. Cell Biol. **9:** 163–206.
7. JORGENSEN, J. L., P. A. REAY, E. W. EHRICH & M. M. DAVIS. 1992. Molecular components of T-cell recognition. Annu. Rev. Immunol. **10:** 835–873.
8. KLEIN, J., Y. SATTA & C. O'HUIGIN. 1993. The molecular descent of the major histocompatibility complex. Annu. Rev. Immunol. **11:** 269–295.
9. BLUESTONE, J. A. 1995. New perspectives of CD28-B7-mediated T cell costimulation. Immunity **2:** 555–559.
10. LENSCHOW, D. J., T. L. WALUNAS & J. A. BLUESTONE. 1996. CD28/B7 system of T cell costimulation. Annu. Rev. Immunol. **14:** 233–258.
11. HARDING, F. A., J. G. MCARTHUR, J. A. GROSS, D. H. RAULET & J. P. ALLISON. 1992. CD28-mediated signalling co-stimulates murine T cells and prevents induction of anergy in T-cell clones. Nature **356:** 607–609.
12. GIMMI, C. D., G. J. FREEMAN, J. G. GRIBBEN, G. GRAY & L. M. NADLER. 1993. Human T-

cell clonal anergy is induced by antigen presentation in the absence of B7 costimulation. Proc. Natl. Acad. Sci. U.S.A. **90:** 6586–6590.

13. JANEWAY, C. A., JR. & K. BOTTOMLY. 1994. Signals and signs for lymphocyte responses. Cell **76:** 275–285.

14. PARKER, D. C. 1993. T cell–dependent B cell activation. Annu. Rev. Immunol. **11:** 331–360.

15. BANCHEREAU, J., F. BAZAN, D. BLANCHARD, F. BRIÈRE, J. P. GALIZZI, C. VAN KOOTEN, Y. J. LIU, F. ROUSSET & S. SAELAND. 1994. The CD40 antigen and its ligand. Annu. Rev. Immunol. **12:** 881–922.

16. FOY, T. M., A. ARUFFO, J. BAJORATH, J. E. BUHLMANN & R. J. NOELLE. 1996. Immune regulation by CD40 and its ligand GP39. Annu. Rev. Immunol. **14:** 591–617.

17. ALLEN, R. C., R. J. ARMINTAGE, M. E. CONLEY, H. ROSENBLATT, N. A. JENKINS, N. G. COPELAND, M. A. BEDELL, S. EDELHOFF, C. M. DISTECHE, D. K. SIMONEAUX, W. C. FANSLOW, J. BELMONT & M. K. SPRIGGS. 1993. CD40-ligand gene defects responsible for X-linked hyper IgM syndrome. Science **259:** 990–993.

18. LANZAVECCHIA, A. 1990. Receptor-mediated antigen uptake and its effect on antigen presentation to class II–restricted T lymphocytes. Annu. Rev. Immunol. **8:** 773–793.

19. STREET, N. E. & T. R. MOSMANN. 1991. Functional diversity of T lymphocytes due to secretion of different cytokine patterns. FASEB J. **5:** 171–177.

20. SAD, S. & T. R. MOSMANN. 1994. Single IL-2-secreting precursor CD4 T cell can develop into either Th1 or Th2 cytokine secretion phenotype. J. Immunol. **153:** 3514–3522.

21. FITCH, F. W., M. D. MCKISIC, D. W. LANCKI & T. F. GAJEWSKI. 1993. Differential regulation of murine T lymphocyte subsets. Annu. Rev. Immunol. **11:** 29–48.

22. PAUL, W. E. & R. A. SEDER. 1994. Lymphocyte responses and cytokines. Cell **76:** 241–251.

23. MOORE, K. W., A. O'GARRA, R. DE WAAL MALEFYT, P. VIEIRA & T. R. MOSMANN. 1993. Interleukin-10. Annu. Rev. Immunol. **11:** 165–190.

24. TIVOL, E. A., F. BORRIELLO, A. N. SCHWEITZER, W. P. LYNCH, J. A. BLUESTONE & A. H. SHARPE. 1995. Loss of CTLA-4 leads to massive lymphoproliferation and fatal multiorgan tissue destruction, revealing a critical negative regulatory role of CTLA-4. Immunity **3:** 541–547.

25. KENNEDY, M. K., D. S. TORRANCE, K. S. PICHA & K. M. MOHLER. 1992. Analysis of cytokine mRNA expression in the central nervous system of mice with experimental autoimmune encephalomyelitis reveals that IL-10 mRNA expression correlates with recovery. J. Immunol. **149:** 2496–2505.

26. ARAI, K., F. LEE, A. MIYAJIMA, S. MIYATAKE, N. ARAI & T. YOKOTA. 1990. Cytokines: coordinators of immune and inflammatory responses. Annu. Rev. Biochem. **59:** 783–836.

27. SPORN, M. B. & A. B. ROBERTS. 1990. TGF-β: problems and prospects. Cell Regul. **1:** 875–882.

28. JERNE, N. K. 1974. Towards a network theory of the immune system. Ann. Inst. Pasteur **125C:** 373–389.

29. SCHERER, M. T., L. IGNATOWICZ, G. M. WINSLOW, J. W. KAPPLER & P. MARRACK. 1993. Superantigens: bacterial and viral proteins that manipulate the immune system. Annu. Rev. Cell Biol. **9:** 101–128.

30. RAGHEB, S. & R. P. LISAK. 1994. The immunopathogenesis of acquired (autoimmune) myasthenia gravis. *In* Handbook of Myasthenia Gravis and Myasthenic Syndromes, p. 239–276. Dekker. New York.

31. LOPATE, G. & A. PESTRONK. 1994. The myasthenic neuromuscular junction. *In* Handbook of Myasthenia Gravis and Myasthenic Syndromes, p. 225–237. Dekker. New York.

32. SCHUETZE, S. M. & L. W. ROLE. 1987. Developmental regulation of nicotinic acetylcholine receptors. Annu. Rev. Neurosci. **10:** 403–457.

33. SHENOY, M., R. KAUL, E. GOLUSZKO, C. DAVID & P. CHRISTADOSS. 1994. Effect of MHC

    class I and CD8 cell deficiency on experimental autoimmune myasthenia gravis patho-
genesis. J. Immunol. **152:** 5330–5335.

34. ZHANG, G. X., C. G. MA, B. G. XIAO, M. BAKHIET, H. LINK & T. OLSSON. 1995. Depletion
of CD8+ T cells suppresses the development of experimental autoimmune myasthenia
gravis in Lewis rats. Eur. J. Immunol. **25:** 1191–1198.

35. NAGATA, S. & P. GOLSTEIN. 1995. The Fas death factor. Science **267:** 1449–1456.

36. MASUNAGA, A., T. AIAI, T. YOSHITAKE, S. ITOYAMA & I. SUGAWARA. 1994. Reduced expression of apoptosis-related antigens in thymuses from patients with myasthenia gravis. Immunol. Lett. **39:** 169–172.

37. WAGNER, S. D. & M. S. NEUBERGER. 1996. Somatic hypermutation of immunoglobulin
genes. Annu. Rev. Immunol. **14:** 441–457.

38. YI, Q., R. PIRSKANEN & A. K. LEFVERT. 1993. Human muscle acetylcholine receptor reactive T and B lymphocytes in the peripheral blood of patients with myasthenia gravis. J.
Neuroimmunol. **42:** 215–222.

39. KAHN, C. R., K. R. MCINTOSH & D. B. DRACHMAN. 1990. T-cell vaccination in experimental myasthenia gravis: a double-edged sword. J. Autoimmun. **3:** 659–669.

40. INFANTE, A. J., H. LEVCOVITZ, V. GORDON, K. A. WALL, P. A. THOMPSON & K. A. KROLICK.
1992. Preferential use of a T cell receptor Vβ gene by acetylcholine receptor–reactive T
cells from myasthenia gravis susceptible mice. J. Immunol. **148:** 3385–3390.

41. THOMPSON, P. A., R. MCATEE, A. J. INFANTE, P. CURRIER, W. BENINATI & K. A. KROLICK.
1994. Vβ-specific immunotoxin selectively kills acetylcholine receptor–reactive T lymphocytes from mice with experimental autoimmune myasthenia gravis. Int. Immunol. **6:**
1807–1815.

42. STEINBERGER, I., T. BRENNER & H. LORBERBOUM-GALSKI. 1995. Interleukin-2
Pseudomonas exotoxin chimeric protein is cytotoxic to B cell cultures derived from
myasthenia gravis patients. J. Neurol. Sci. **133:** 183–191.

43. WANG, Z. Y., J. QIAO & H. LINK. 1993. Suppression of experimental autoimmune myasthenia gravis by oral administration of acetylcholine receptor. J. Neuroimmunol. **44:**
209–214.

44. OKUMURA, S., K. MCINTOSH & D. B. DRACHMAN. 1994. Oral administration of acetylcholine receptor: effects on experimental myasthenia gravis. Ann. Neurol. **36:** 704–713.

45. MA, C. G., G. X. ZHANG, B. G. XIAO, J. LINK, T. OLSSON & H. LINK. 1995. Suppression of
experimental autoimmune myasthenia gravis by nasal administration of acetylcholine receptor. J. Neuroimmunol. **58:** 51–60.

46. WANG, Z. Y., H. LINK, Å. LJUNGDAHL, B. HÖJEBERG, J. LINK, B. HE, J. QIAO, A. MELMS & T.
OLSSON. 1994. Induction of interferon-γ, interleukin-4, and transforming growth factor-
β in rats orally tolerized against experimental autoimmune myasthenia gravis. Cell. Immunol. **157:** 353–368.

47. HUSBY, S., J. MESTECKY, Z. MOLDOVEANU, S. HOLLAND & C. O. ELSON. 1994. Oral tolerance in humans: T cell, but not B cell tolerance after antigen feeding. J. Immunol. **152:**
4663–4670.

48. NICOLLE, M. W., B. NAG, S. D. SHARMA, N. WILLCOX, A. VINCENT, D. J. P. FERGUSON & J.
NEWSOM-DAVIS. 1994. Specific tolerance to an acetylcholine receptor epitope induced *in
vitro* in myasthenia gravis CD4+ lymphocytes by soluble major histocompatibility complex class II–peptide complexes. J. Clin. Invest. **93:** 1361–1369.

49. SPACK, E. G., M. MCCUTCHEON, N. CORBELLETTA, B. NAG, D. PASSMORE & S. D. SHARMA.
1995. Induction of tolerance in experimental autoimmune myasthenia gravis with solubilized MHC class II: acetylcholine receptor peptide complexes. J. Autoimmun. **8:**
787–807.

50. KAUL, R., M. SHENOY, E. GOLUSZKO & P. CHRISTADOSS. 1994. Major histocompatibility

complex class II gene disruption prevents experimental autoimmune myasthenia gravis. J. Immunol. **152:** 3152–3157.

51. WALDOR, M. K., S. SUBRAMANIAM, H. O. McDEVITT & L. STEINMAN. 1983. *In vivo* therapy with monoclonal anti-I-A antibody suppresses immune responses to acetylcholine receptors. Proc. Natl. Acad. Sci. U.S.A. **80:** 2713–2717.

52. McINTOSH, K. R., P. S. LINSLEY & D. B. DRACHMAN. 1995. Immunosuppression and induction of anergy by CTLA4Ig *in vitro*: effects on cellular and antibody responses by lymphocytes from rats with experimental autoimmune myasthenia gravis. Cell. Immunol. **165:** 103–112.

53. WAUBEN, M. H. M., A. C. W. E. HOEDEMAEKERS, Y. M. F. GRAUS, J. P. A. WAGENAAR, W. VAN EDEN & M. H. DEBAETS. 1996. Inhibition of experimental autoimmune myasthenia gravis by major histocompatibility complex class II competitor peptides results not only in a suppressed, but also in an altered immune response. Eur. J. Immunol. **26:** 2866–2875.

54. SETTE, A., J. ALEXANDER, J. RUPPERT, K. SNOKE, A. FRANCO, G. ISHIOKA & H. M. GREY. 1994. Antigen analogs/MHC complexes as specific T cell receptor antagonists. Annu. Rev. Immunol. **12:** 413–431.

55. JAMESON, S. C. & M. J. BEVAN. 1995. T cell receptor antagonists and partial agonists. Immunity **2:** 1–11.

56. WALL, K. A., J. Y. HU, P. CURRIER, S. SOUTHWOOD, A. SETTE & A. J. INFANTE. 1994. Residues involved in I-A^b binding, self-nonself discrimination, and TCR antagonism. J. Immunol. **152:** 4526–4536.

57. KIRSHNER, S. L., E. ZISMAN, M. FRIDKIN, M. SELA & E. MOZES. 1996. Altered peptide ligands of a myasthenogenic epitope as modulators of specific T-cell responses. Scand. J. Immunol. **44:** 512–521.

58. ZISMAN, E., Y. KATZ-LEVY, M. DAYAN, S. L. KIRSHNER, M. PAAS-ROZNER, A. KARNI, O. ABRAMSKY, C. BRAUTBAR, M. FRIDKIN, M. SELA & E. MOZES. 1996. Peptide analogs to pathogenic epitopes of the human acetylcholine receptor alpha subunit as potential modulators of myasthenia gravis. Proc. Natl. Acad. Sci. U.S.A. **93:** 4492–4497.

59. SHENOY, M., S. BARON, B. WU, E. GOLUSZKO & P. CHRISTADOSS. 1995. IFN-α treatment suppresses the development of experimental autoimmune myasthenia gravis. J. Immunol. **154:** 6203–6208.

60. DENG, C., E. GOLUSZKO, S. BARON, B. WU & P. CHRISTADOSS. 1996. IFN-α therapy is effective in suppressing the clinical experimental myasthenia gravis. J. Immunol. **157:** 5675–5682.

61. PIDDLESDEN, S. J., S. JIANG, J. L. LEVIN, A. VINCENT & B. P. MORGAN. 1996. Soluble complement receptor 1 (sCR1) protects against experimental autoimmune myasthenia gravis. J. Neuroimmunol. **71:** 173–177.

62. DURELLI, L. 1994. High-dose intravenous immunoglobulin G treatment of myasthenia gravis. *In* Handbook of Myasthenia Gravis and Myasthenic Syndromes, p. 375–388. Dekker. New York.

63. ARAGA, S., R. D. LEBOEUF & J. E. BLALOCK. 1993. Prevention of experimental autoimmune myasthenia gravis by manipulation of the immune network with a complementary peptide for the acetylcholine receptor. Proc. Natl. Acad. Sci. U.S.A. **90:** 8747–8751.

64. ARAGA, S., F. SHAWN GALIN, M. KISHIMOTO, A. ADACHI & J. E. BLALOCK. 1996. Prevention of experimental autoimmune myasthenia gravis by a monoclonal antibody to a complementary peptide for the main immunogenic region of the acetylcholine receptor. J. Immunol. **157:** 386–392.

65. GAMMON, G., E. E. SERCARZ & G. B. BENICHOU. 1991. The dominant self and the cryptic self: shaping the autoreactive T-cell repertoire. Immunol. Today **12:** 193–195.

66. SERCARZ, E. E., P. V. LEHMANN, A. AMETANI, G. BENICHOU, A. MILLER & K. MOUDGIL. 1993. Dominance and crypticity of T cell antigenic determinants. Annu. Rev. Immunol. **11:** 729–766.

67. WU, B., M. SHENOY, E. GOLUSZKO, R. KAUL & P. CHRISTADOSS. 1995. TCR gene usage in experimental autoimmune myasthenia gravis pathogenesis: usage of multiple TCRBV genes in the H-2^b strains. J. Immunol. **154:** 3603–3610.

Mechanisms and Genetics of Autoimmunity[a]

ARGYRIOS N. THEOFILOPOULOS AND DWIGHT H. KONO

Department of Immunology
The Scripps Research Institute
La Jolla, California 92037

Much progress has been made in recent years in delineating the editing processes by which self-reactive cells are eliminated or inactivated to achieve self-tolerance. Despite this progress, however, our understanding of the etiologic and genetic bases of autoimmune diseases remains far from resolved. In the following, we will review some of the dominant mechanisms of autoimmunity, and then, as an example, we will outline efforts to identify the number and nature of predisposing loci in lupus, the prototypic autoimmune disease.

MECHANISTIC THEORIES

Several nonmutually exclusive mechanistic theories have been proposed,[1] the most prominent of which will be discussed. A well-established form of autoimmune disease resulting from the absence of self-tolerance is that against peripheral tissue antigens normally sequestered behind anatomic barriers. Such antigens are unavailable to the developing immune system inside the thymus and, therefore, tolerance for them does not exist. Any release of such antigens into the circulation, however, caused by trauma or inflammation, can provide the opportunity for an autoimmune response.

Sequestration of peripheral tissue antigens behind anatomic barriers has been clearly documented in recent experiments with mice transgenic for the hepatitis B surface antigen (HBsAg).[2] Thus, intravenous injection of $CD8^+$ cytotoxic T cell lines and clones specific for this antigen into transgenic animals with widespread tissue expression of HBsAg failed to cause disease or infiltration of any organ but the liver. This indicates that the vascular endothelium and basement membranes constitute an extremely effective barrier that normally precludes access of T cells to most peripheral tissue antigens.

Additional findings have clearly established that experimentally induced thymic availability of peripheral tissue-associated antigens leads to tolerance and loss of susceptibility to autoimmune disease. For example, streptozotocin-induced diabetes in mice is inhibited by prior elimination of mature T cells with anti-CD3 mAb and tolerization of the newly emerging T cells by intrathymic injection of streptozotocin-treated islet cells.[3] Similarly, intrathymic injection of islet cells prevents autoimmune disease in the diabetes-prone BB rat and the NOD mouse.[4,5] Diabetes in NOD mice

[a]This is Publication No. 11338IMM from the Department of Immunology, The Scripps Research Institute. The work reported herein was supported in part by NIH Grant Nos. AR39555, AR31203, and AR42242.

has also been reported to be inhibited by the intrathymic or intravenous administration of glutamic acid decarboxylase, apparently a major autoantigen in this disease.[6,7] Prevention of experimental encephalomyelitis by intrathymic injection of myelin basic protein or its major encephalitogenic epitope has also been reported,[8] and we recently showed inhibition of antichromatin autoantibody induction in lupus mice by intrathymic injection of polynucleosomes.[9]

The available evidence indicates that anatomically sequestered antigens that are not presented in the thymus may not induce tolerance, and that availability of such antigens in the periphery can lead to autoimmune disease. If this is an important mechanism, as supported by the mentioned findings, then certain autoimmune diseases can be viewed as representing a conventional immunologic response against normally sequestered peripheral tissue self-antigens for which there is no need to become tolerant. Tissue-tropic pathogens, such as viruses, of course, will be important in inducing the initial organ damage and antigen availability as well as the production of costimulatory factors necessary for the immune response.

A corollary hypothesis that addresses molecular rather than anatomic sequestration is that of "cryptic" self-determinants.[10] Overall, the theory posits that (a) each self-protein presents a small minority of dominant determinants; (b) these well-displayed self-determinants, constituting the dominant self, are involved in thymic negative selection and the organism is tolerant to them; (c) the poorly displayed majority of subdominant or cryptic determinants, constituting the cryptic self, do not induce tolerance and, therefore, a large cohort of potentially self-reactive T cells exists. Thus, notwithstanding anatomically sequestered antigens, the theory proposes that the available T cell repertoire is directed against cryptic self-determinants and, therefore, pathogenic autoimmune responses must be directed against such determinants. Several interesting experimental examples of this mechanism have been presented[11,12] and several mechanisms by which such cryptic antigens may become available to the immune system have been proposed,[13] but their relevance to the pathogenesis of spontaneous autoimmune diseases is unclear.

Another model is that of invoking self-ignorance by T cells. This model refutes the concept that delivery of one instead of the required two signals for T cell activation (one by cognate interaction and one by a costimulatory molecule) leads to T cell anergy and instead suggests that mature resting T cells specific for extrathymic antigens presented by nonprofessional antigen-presenting cells (APCs) simply ignore such antigens and remain quiescent. If adequate antigen presentation and costimulation occur through professional APCs, then it follows that these quiescent self-ignoring cells may be activated and cause tissue damage. The validity of this theory is supported by the results of studies with lymphocytic choriomeningitis virus (LCMV) glycoprotein (GP)–transgenic animals in the induction of diabetes.[14,15] Using LCMV-GP-specific T cell antigen receptor and pancreas-expressed GP double-transgenic mice, it was shown that the GP-specific T cells were not deleted, modulated, or anergized, as documented by their presence in sufficient numbers using appropriate anticlonotypic TCR antibodies and by their efficient GP-specific proliferative and cytotoxic responses *in vitro*. Under normal conditions, these cells did not attack the GP-expressing pancreatic cells. However, upon infection with the appropriate GP-expressing LCMV, T cell attraction to the pancreas and damage ensued, leading to hyperglycemia.

The interpretation of these findings was that extrathymic tissue-reactive helper and cytotoxic T cells were not activated, deleted, or rendered anergic because the "self" antigen-expressing β cells did not display MHC class II–GP peptide complexes or costimulatory molecules. However, when infection occurs with the virus that bears an epitope mimicking the tissue-expressed "self" epitope, effective presentation and costimulation by infected APCs occur, leading to activation of the previously quiescent helper, and then cytotoxic, T cells. Obviously, some tissue damage must also occur in order for the activated T cells to gain access to the tissue.

The theories of cryptic or ignored self are compatible with the antigen mimicry hypothesis of autoimmunity,[16] particularly as it pertains to infectious agents. Because of the constraints imposed upon construction of coding sequences, closely related or identical polypeptides are often found in unrelated proteins, and many peptide fragments of infectious agents are homologous with host proteins, including MHC molecules. Autoreactive B cells may be activated through stimulation by a foreign antigen that contains a foreign T cell epitope and a B cell epitope that mimics the self.[17,18] Alternatively, autoreactive T cells may be activated directly by a foreign T cell peptide that mimics the self–T cell peptide.[19–23] Disease expression may then be dependent on spreading of the response to additional self-determinants,[24–26] which may be localized within a subcellular particle.[27]

It should be noted that mimicry has been primarily addressed on the basis of autoantibody cross-reactivities, but most likely is applicable to T cells, since T cells recognize linear peptides, whereas antibodies recognize conformational epitopes created by discontinuous sequences. However, even with T cells, mimicry does not necessarily require complete concordance in sequence between a foreign mimic and a self-molecule because of degeneracy in TCR-MHC interactions and the dependence of such interactions on peptide conformation rather than linear sequence characteristics. This has been illustrated in recent experiments by Wucherpfennig and Strominger.[19] Thus, the immunodominant epitope for MBP has been defined as being located at residues 85–99. When residues necessary for TCR or MHC contact were substituted with various aliphatic and aromatic amino acids in a manner that maintained their overall capacity to bind MHC and TCR, and when searches for corresponding common viral/bacterial peptides were made on available protein databases, several (EBV, β cells; papillomavirus, epithelial cells; herpes simplex, neurons) were found that were capable of being presented by the susceptible DR2 MHC and that stimulated MBP-specific T cell clones established from the blood of two patients with MS.[19] The importance of peptide conformational characteristics in defining T cell epitope molecular mimicry has also been documented by others.[28] These findings are important because (a) they indicate that mimeotopes and aggretopes cannot be predicted on simple alignments; (b) T cells actually recognize not only a single peptide, but a limited repertoire of structurally related peptides derived from different antigens; and (c) if applicable *in vivo*, they suggest that it is unlikely that a single pathogen is responsible for the initiation of a given autoimmune disease, and they explain why it has been so difficult to link autoimmune diseases with a particular pathogen.

Finally, an additional mechanism implicated in the pathogenesis of systemic and organ-specific autoimmune diseases is that related to apoptosis, either decreased or increased apoptosis. Thus, Nagata and associates found that the lupuslike syndrome associated with lymphoaccumulation in *lpr*, *lpr*[cg], and *gld* mutant mice is characterized by defective expression of these molecules.[29] The *lpr* mutation, mapped on chromosome 19, was shown to be associated with an intronic insertion of an early retroviral transposon in the Fas gene, leading to abnormal transcription. The related *lpr*[cg] mutation was associated with a single point mutation at the intracellular "death" domain of this gene, leading to a lack of functionality, and the *gld* mutation, mapped on chromosome 1, was associated with a single point mutation in the carboxyl terminus of the type II membrane protein, FasL, which negatively impacts on its ability to bind to Fas. Recently, rare human counterparts of Fas mutations, some manifesting systemic autoimmunity, have been identified.[30–32]

In addition, expression of Fas and FasL in tissues has been shown to promote organ-specific autoimmunity, as recently shown in Hashimoto's thyroiditis[33] and in the NOD diabetes model.[34] Although many cell types can express Fas, FasL initially seemed to be expressed only on activated T cells. However, it was subsequently shown that FasL is expressed in a small number of other cell types, such as cells in the eye chamber, parts of the nervous system, and the testis.[29] It was then demonstrated that these cells use FasL to protect themselves from immune attack by promoting apoptosis of Fas-expressing attacking T cells (immune privilege).[35–37] Now, however, Giordano and colleagues have shown that thyroid cells (both normal and from Hashimoto's thyroiditis patients) express FasL and that, upon induction of Fas in such cells following incubation with IL-1, there is a fratricidal killing by apoptosis.[33] Similarly, Chervonsky *et al.*[34] showed that NOD diabetic mice rendered transgenic for FasL expression in the pancreas developed severe rapid disease upon passive transfer of a diabetogenic T cell clone, which promoted Fas expression by the β cells. Moreover, NOD mice bred for homozygosity in the *lpr* (Fas-defective) mutation did not develop spontaneous diabetes, nor were they susceptible to early disease induction by transfer of the diabetogenic CD8[+] clones.

GENETIC STUDIES

Regardless of the actual mechanisms, propensity to autoimmunity is highly dependent on genetic factors. However, attempts to define the precise genetic defects of these multigenic diseases in humans are hindered by several problems,[38–40] including the following: (a) possible heterogeneity of causation (genetic heterogeneity), such that a different constellation of mutated genes may lead to the same disease phenotype; (b) high incidence of disease-prone alleles in the population, wherein an identified allele may not be contributing to the disease process in all individuals with that allele; (c) small contributions by any given gene to the disease process, so large numbers of samples may be required and any biases in patient selection may obscure the contribution by that gene; (d) diagnoses are based on observations far removed from the basic physiologic process, causing both false-positive and false-negative classifications of individuals; (e) the suspect genomic region may be too large to permit careful analysis of the role of all the embedded genes within this region; (f) a suspected gene may not be the actual culprit, but may be in linkage disequilibrium with another important gene located in close proximity; and (g) for statistical and other factors such as race and environmental effects, replication of results may be difficult and erratic.

Because of these difficulties and despite the possibility that animal models may not fully reflect the human disorders, we and others have attempted first to identify the number and nature of genes predisposing to autoimmune diseases in appropriate spontaneous or experimental models of rodents. These models offer the advantage that large numbers of animals can be studied under well-defined conditions, and congenic, transgenic, and gene knockout mice can be created to establish the role of a suspected gene.

Three approaches are commonly used to define the genetic basis of diseases—candidate or functional cloning, positional cloning, and positional candidate cloning. The candidate cloning approach screens genes with structural and biochemical properties that fit the disease phenotype. Positional cloning relies first on mapping the phenotype to a small segment of a chromosome, and then systematically cloning and screening all genes within that region. Although very laborious, this approach has the advantage of not requiring prior knowledge of gene identity and function, and having closure. Finally, the positional candidate cloning approach is, as the same implies, a combination of the two strategies and involves screening known genes in the delineated chromosomal segment, thereby significantly reducing the required effort. Thus far, the candidate gene approach, with very few exceptions (Fas/FasL mutations in *lpr/gld* mice,[29] PTP1C mutations in motheaten mice[41,42]), has been unsuccessful in identifying the exact autoimmunity-predisposing genes despite extensive analyses of appropriate candidates, such as Ig, TCR, and cytokine genes.

Recent significant advances in methods to identify genes based on genome-wide searches have, however, provided the hope that the task of identifying these genes will be feasible.

Genome-wide searches to identify predisposing genes are based on the use of dense chromosomal maps that are, in turn, based on microsatellite polymorphisms. Microsatellites or single-sequence length polymorphisms (SSLP) are repeats of usually dinucleotides that exhibit a high degree of polymorphism in the number of repeats at a given chromosomal site and from one individual to another.[43] SSLP are abundant (>100,000) and randomly dispersed throughout the mammalian genome, thereby providing an enormous pool from which to derive markers. Thus far, more than 6000 microsatellite markers have been identified within the 1600-cM mouse genome. Specific SSLP loci can easily be defined by the polymerase chain reaction using oligonucleotide primers to the conserved sequences flanking the repeats, and length polymorphisms among individuals are identified by electrophoresis of the amplified products on agarose or polyacrylamide gels. As an example of the application of this approach to unraveling the genetics of autoimmune diseases, we summarize below our recent efforts with mice that spontaneously develop lupuslike syndromes,[44,45] but similar approaches have been utilized to define the genetics of other autoimmune syndromes, including insulin-dependent diabetes,[46] experimental encephalomyelitis,[47–49] multiple sclerosis,[50–52] autoimmune ovarian dysgenesis,[53] autoimmune orchitis,[54] and others.

To establish an exclusion linkage map for NZB and NZW mice, 315 microsatellites were screened and 91 markers were selected for maximum coverage and discernible separation in agarose gels. Based on distances between markers and loci not exceeding 20 cM, coverage for 97% of the genome was achieved. With these markers at hand, we then analyzed 150 female (NZB×NZW) F_2 mice for segregation with early mortality, glomerulonephritis (GN), and antichromatin autoantibodies. We identified eight loci, designated *Lbw-1* to *-8* (*Lbw*, lupus B×W) on chromosomes 17, 4, 5, 6, 7, 18, 1, and 11, respectively, that contributed to the B×W lupus susceptibility.[44] Four of these loci were NZB dominant, two were NZB recessive, two were NZW recessive, and one was NZW dominant. Three loci, *Lbw-1* (corresponding to the MHC locus), *-7*, and *-8* on chromosomes 17, 1, and 11, respectively, were linked to increased antichromatin response. GN was linked to three loci, *Lbw-1*, *-2*, and *-6* on chromosomes 17, 4, and 18, respectively, all of which also had linkage to mortality consistent with GN being the major cause of death. The two non-MHC GN-predisposing loci had no linkage to autoantibody production, suggesting that their contribution to GN involves a stage beyond the initial autoantibody formation. Six loci, *Lbw-1* to *-6* on chromosomes 17, 4, 5, 6, 7, and 18, respectively, were linked to early mortality, three of which were also associated with GN. The loci that are unlinked to GN may play a role in other pathologic conditions such as vascular disease, neoplasias, and others that might contribute to the overall mortality susceptibility. Similar studies with New Zealand lupus mice have been performed by others[55–58] with considerable concordance of overall results. Using congenic lines of mice, Wakeland and associates have also begun to dissect the means by which each of the predisposing loci affects the NZ mouse lupuslike disease, with one locus shown to be associated with loss of tolerance to chromatin, another with hyperresponsiveness of B cells to stimuli, and a third with end-stage organ damage.[59,60]

We have also recently conducted a genome-wide search for loci predisposing to lymphoaccumulation and immunopathologic manifestations in 274 F_2 intercrosses between the MRL-*lpr* (severe disease) and C57BL/6-*lpr* (mild disease) strains.[45] Among the various strains of *lpr* mice, the MRL-*lpr* develops the most severe manifestations, with early onset of autoantibodies, GN, systemic vasculitis, arthritis, and 50% mortality at 5.5 months, while the C57BL/6-*lpr* has a much milder disease course with late-onset autoantibody production and little or no histopathologic manifestations. These findings indicate that genes other than the Fas are important contributors to disease expression in *lpr* mice. Using markers covering 98% of the genome, four loci were identified with significant linkage to lymphadenopathy and/or splenomegaly on chromosomes 4, 5, 7, and 10 (named *Lmb1–4*, respectively). *Lmb1*, *2*, and *3* were also linked to the production of anti-dsDNA antibodies, but not to GN, whereas *Lmb4* was linked to GN. Disease-predisposing *Lmb2*, *3*, and *4* alleles were inherited from the MRL background, whereas the lupus susceptibility *Lmb1* allele was derived from the B6. Regardless of the strain of origin, each of the loci appeared to contribute to disease susceptibility in an additive manner, although certain combinations had a greater effect. A single locus on chromosome 1 was linked to inflammatory arthritis.

Lmb2 and *Lmb4* have no overlap with known mouse lupus susceptibility loci and define new susceptibility genes. *Lmb1* overlaps with other lupus susceptibility loci on chromosome 4, for which the disease-predisposing alleles are derived from the NZW[55] and NZB[44,56–58] strains. Although *Lmb1* cannot be the same as the locus derived from the NZW strain (this locus was identified using an NZ cross with the B6 strain), there is a possibility that it may be the same as the NZB locus. *Lmb3* is probably the same as the *Lrdm1* locus previously described in a cross between the MRL-

lpr and *Mus castaneous* strains[61] and maps to the same region as an NZW locus associated with lupus.[44,55] The identification of these loci with highly significant linkages will facilitate the cloning of genetic defects contributing to autoimmunity. Interestingly, the *Lmb1* locus on chromosome 4 also overlaps *Idd9*, a locus associated with insulin-dependent diabetes mellitus.[46] This suggests that different autoimmune diseases may share common genetic defects and may explain the higher incidence of different autoimmune diseases among relatives of affected individuals. Their potential applicability to a broad range of autoimmune diseases may make such susceptibility genes particularly useful as targets for intervention. Future studies will be directed toward generating and characterizing congenic mice, more precise chromosomal localization of loci, and the identification of susceptibility alleles. Definition of the nature of genetic susceptibility should help delineate the mechanistic theories most applicable to spontaneous disease. Finally, the relevance of these mouse models for human genetic studies was recently shown in a study by Tsao *et al.*[62] wherein screening based on synteny to a mouse lupus susceptibility locus[44,55] resulted in the identification of a human candidate chromosome 1 region linked to SLE. Studies similar to those outlined in several models of autoimmunity can also be performed in the animal models of myasthenia gravis, to which MHC and other genes appear to contribute.[63,64]

REFERENCES

1. THEOFILOPOULOS, A. N. 1995. The basis of autoimmunity: Part I. Mechanisms of aberrant self-recognition. Immunol. Today **16:** 90–98.
2. ANDO, K., L. G. GUIDOTTI, A. CERNY, T. ISHIKAWA & F. V. CHISARI. 1994. CTL access to tissue antigen is restricted *in vivo*. J. Immunol. **153:** 482–488.
3. HEROLD, K. C., A. G. MONTAG & F. BUCKINGHAM. 1992. Induction of tolerance to autoimmune diabetes with islet antigens. J. Exp. Med. **176:** 1107–1114.
4. POSSELT, A. M., C. F. BARKER, A. L. FRIEDMAN & A. NAJI. 1992. Prevention of autoimmune diabetes in the BB rat by intrathymic islet transplantation at birth. Science **256:** 1321–1324.
5. GERLING, I. C., D. V. SERREZE, S. W. CHRISTIANSON & E. H. LEITER. 1992. Intrathymic islet cell transplantation reduces beta-cell autoimmunity and prevents diabetes in NOD/Lt mice. Diabetes **41:** 1672–1676.
6. KAUFMAN, D. L., M. CLARE-SALZLER, J. TIAN, T. FORSTHUBER, G. S. TING, P. ROBINSON, M. A. ATKINSON, E. E. SERCARZ, A. J. TOBIN & P. V. LEHMANN. 1993. Spontaneous loss of T-cell tolerance to glutamic acid decarboxylase in murine insulin-dependent diabetes. Nature **366:** 69–72.
7. TISCH, R., X. D. YANG, S. M. SINGER, R. S. LIBLAU, L. FUGGER & H. O. MCDEVITT. 1993. Immune response to glutamic acid decarboxylase correlates with insulitis in non-obese diabetic mice. Nature **366:** 72–75.
8. KHOURY, S. J., M. H. SAYEGH, W. W. HANCOCKM, L. GALLON, C. B. CARPENTER & H. L. WEINER. 1993. Acquired tolerance to experimental autoimmune encephalomyelitis by intrathymic injection of myelin basic protein or its major encephalitogenic peptide. J. Exp. Med. **178:** 559–566.
9. DUNCAN, S. R., R. L. RUBIN, R. W. BURLINGAME, S. B. SINCLAIR, K. W. PEKNY & A. N. THEOFILOPOULOS. 1996. Intrathymic injection of polynucleosomes delays autoantibody production in BXSB mice. Clin. Immunol. Immunopathol. **79:** 171–181.

10. SERCARZ, E. E., P. V. LEHMANN, A. AMETANI, G. BENICHOU, A. MILLER & K. MOUDGIL. 1993. Dominance and crypticity of T cell antigenic determinants. Annu. Rev. Immunol. **11:** 729–766.

11. MOUDGIL, K. D. & E. E. SERCARZ. 1994. The T cell repertoire against cryptic self determinants and its involvement in autoimmunity and cancer. Clin. Immunol. Immunopathol. **73:** 283–289.

12. MILICH, D. R., F. SCHODEL, D. L. PETERSON, J. E. JONES & J. L. HUGHES. 1995. Characterization of self-reactive T cells that evade tolerance in hepatitis B antigen transgenic mice. Eur. J. Immunol. **25:** 1663–1672.

13. LANZAVECCHIA, A. 1997. Understanding the mechanisms of sustained signaling and T cell activation. J. Exp. Med. **185:** 1717–1719.

14. OHASHI, P. S., S. OEHEN, K. BUERKI, H. PIRCHER, C. T. OHASHI, C. ODERMATT, B. MALISSEN, R. M. ZINKERNAGEL & H. HENGARTNER. 1991. Ablation of "tolerance" and induction of diabetes by virus infection in viral antigen transgenic mice. Cell **65:** 305–317.

15. OLDSTONE, M. B., M. NERENBERG, P. SOUTHERN, J. PRICE & H. LEWICKI. 1991. Virus infection triggers insulin-dependent diabetes mellitus in a transgenic model: role of anti-self (virus) immune response. Cell **65:** 319–331.

16. OLDSTONE, M. B. 1996. Principles of viral pathogenesis. Cell **87:** 799–801.

17. LIN, R. H., M. J. MAMULA, J. A. HARDIN & C. A. JANEWAY, JR. 1991. Induction of autoreactive B cells allows priming of autoreactive T cells. J. Exp. Med. **173:** 1433–1439.

18. MAMULA, M. J., R. H. LIN, C. A. JANEWAY, JR. & J. A. HARDIN. 1992. Breaking T cell tolerance with foreign and self co-immunogens: a study of autoimmune B and T cell epitopes of cytochrome c. J. Immunol. **149:** 789–795.

19. WUCHERPFENNIG, K. W. & J. L. STROMINGER. 1995. Molecular mimicry in T cell–mediated autoimmunity: viral peptides activate human T cell clones specific for myelin basic protein. Cell **80:** 695–705.

20. GAUTAM, A. M., C. I. PEARSON, D. E. SMILEK, L. STEINMAN & H. O. MCDEVITT. 1992. A polyalanine peptide with only five native myelin basic protein residues induces autoimmune encephalomyelitis. J. Exp. Med. **176:** 605–609.

21. EVAVOLD, B. D., J. SLOAN-LANCASTER, K. J. WILSON, J. B. ROTHBARD & P. M. ALLEN. 1995. Specific T cell recognition of minimally homologous peptides: evidence for multiple endogenous ligands. Immunity **2:** 655–663.

22. BHARDWAJ, V., V. KUMAR, H. M. GEYSEN & E. E. SERCARZ. 1993. Degenerate recognition of a dissimilar antigenic peptide by myelin basic protein–reactive T cells: implications for thymic education and autoimmunity. J. Immunol. **151:** 5000–5010.

23. HEMMER, B., B. T. FLECKENSTEIN, M. VERGELLI, G. JUNG, H. MCFARLAND, R. MARTIN & K. H. WIESMULLER. 1997. Identification of high potency microbial and self ligands for a human autoreactive class II–restricted T cell clone. J. Exp. Med. **185:** 1651–1659.

24. LEHMANN, P. V., E. E. SERCARZ, T. FORSTHUBER, C. M. DAYAN & G. GAMMON. 1993. Determinant spreading and the dynamics of the autoimmune T-cell repertoire. Immunol. Today **14:** 203–408.

25. TOPFER, F., T. GORDON & J. MCCLUSKEY. 1995. Intra- and intermolecular spreading of autoimmunity involving the nuclear self-antigens La (SS-B) and Ro (SS-A). Proc. Natl. Acad. Sci. U.S.A. **92:** 875–879.

26. GARZA, K. M., N. D. GRIGGS & K. S. TUNG. 1997. Neonatal injection of an ovarian peptide induces autoimmune ovarian disease in female mice: requirement of endogenous neonatal ovaries. Immunity **6:** 89–96.

27. CASIANO, C. A. & E. M. TAN. 1996. Recent developments in the understanding of antinuclear autoantibodies. Int. Arch. Allergy Immunol. **111:** 308–313.

28. QUARATINO, S., C. J. THORPE, P. J. TRAVERS & M. LONDEI. 1995. Similar antigenic surfaces, rather than sequence homology, dictate T-cell epitope molecular mimicry. Proc. Natl. Acad. Sci. U.S.A. **92:** 10398–10402.

29. NAGATA, S. 1997. Apoptosis by death factor. Cell **88:** 355–365.
30. BETTINARDI, A., D. BRUGNONI, E. QUIROS-ROLDAN, A. MALAGOLI, S. LAGRUTTA, A. COR-RERA & L. D. NOTARANGELO. 1997. Missense mutations in the Fas gene resulting in autoimmune lymphoproliferative syndrome: a molecular and immunological analysis. Blood **89:** 902–909.
31. FISHER, G. H., F. J. ROSENBERG, S. E. STRAUS, J. K. DALE, L. MIDDLETON, A. Y. LIN, W. STROBER, M. J. LENARDO & J. M. PUCK. 1995. Dominant interfering Fas gene mutations impair apoptosis in a human autoimmune lymphoproliferative syndrome. Cell **81:** 935–946.
32. RIEUX-LAUCAT, F., F. LE DEIST, C. HIVROZ, I. A. G. ROBERTS, K. M. DEBATIN, A. FISCHER & J. P. DE VILLARTAY. 1995. Mutations in Fas associated with human lymphoproliferative syndrome and autoimmunity. Science **268:** 1347–1349.
33. GIORDANO, C., G. STASSI, R. DE MARIA, M. TODARO, P. RICHIUSA, G. PAPOFF, G. RUBERTI, M. BAGNASCO, R. TESTI & A. GALLUZZO. 1997. Potential involvement of Fas and its ligand in the pathogenesis of Hashimoto's thyroiditis. Science **275:** 960–963.
34. CHERVONSKY, A. V., Y. WANG, F. S. WONG, I. VISINTIN, R. A. FLAVELL, C. A. JANEWAY, JR. & L. A. MATIS. 1997. The role of Fas in autoimmune diabetes. Cell **89:** 17–24.
35. GRIFFIN, T. S., T. BRUNNER, S. M. FLETCHER, D. R. GREEN & T. A. FERGUSON. 1995. Fas ligand-induced apoptosis as a mechanism of immune privilege. Science **270:** 1189–1192.
36. BELLGRAU, D., D. GOLD, H. SELAWRY, J. MOORE, Z. FRANZUSOFF & R. C. DUKE. 1995. A role for CD95 ligand in preventing graft rejection. Nature **377:** 630–632.
37. STREILEIN, J. W. 1995. Unraveling immune privilege. Science **270:** 1158–1159.
38. WEISSMAN, S. M. 1995. Genetic bases for common polygenic diseases. Proc. Natl. Acad. Sci. U.S.A. **92:** 8543–8544.
39. RISCH, N. & K. MERIKANGAS. 1996. The future of genetic studies of complex human diseases. Science **273:** 1516–1517.
40. LANDER, E. S. & L. KRUGLYAK. 1995. Genetic dissection of complex traits: guidelines for interpreting and reporting linkage results. Nat. Genet. **11:** 241–247.
41. SHULTZ, L. D., P. A. SCHWEITZER, T. V. RAJAN, T. YI, J. N. IHLE, R. J. MATTHEWS, M. L. THOMAS & D. R. BEIER. 1993. Mutations at the murine motheaten locus are within the hematopoietic cell protein–tyrosine phosphatase (*Hcph*) gene. Cell **73:** 1445–1454.
42. TSUI, H. W., K. A. SIMINOVITCH, L. DESOUZA & F. W. L. TSUI. 1995. Motheaten and viable motheaten mice have mutations in the hematopoietic cell phosphatase gene. Nat. Genet. **4:** 124–129.
43. STALLINGS, R. L., D. C. TORNEY, C. E. HILDERBRAND, J. L. LONGMIRE, L. L. DEAVEN, J. H. JETT, N. A. DOGGETT & R. K. MOYZIS. 1990. Physical mapping of human chromosomes by repetitive sequence fingerprinting. Proc. Natl. Acad. Sci. U.S.A. **87:** 6218–6222.
44. KONO, D. H., R. W. BURLINGAME, D. G. OWENS, A. KURAMOCHI, R. S. BALDERAS, D. BALOMENOS & A. N. THEOFILOPOULOS. 1994. Lupus susceptibility loci in New Zealand mice. Proc. Natl. Acad. Sci. U.S.A. **91:** 10168–10172.
45. VIDAL, S., D. H. KONO & A. N. THEOFILOPOULOS. 1997. Loci predisposing to autoimmunity in MRL-*Fas*^lpr and C57BL/6-*Fas*^lpr mice. J. Clin. Invest. In press.
46. VYSE, T. J. & J. A. TODD. 1996. Genetic analysis of autoimmune disease. Cell **85:** 311–318.
47. ENCINAS, J. A., M. B. LEES, R. A. SOBEL, C. SYMONOWICZ, J. M. GREER, C. L. SHOVLIN, H. L. WEINER, C. E. SEIDMAN, J. G. SEIDMAN & V. K. KUCHROO. 1996. Genetic analysis of susceptibility to experimental autoimmune encephalomyelitis in a cross between SJL/J and B10.S mice. J. Immunol. **157:** 2186–2192.
48. BAKER, D., O. A. ROSENWASSER, J. K. O'NEILL & J. L. TURK. 1995. Genetic analysis of experimental allergic encephalomyelitis in mice. J. Immunol. **155:** 4046–4051.
49. SUNDVALL, M., J. JIRHOLT, H. T. YANG, L. JANSSON, A. ENGSTROM, U. PETTERSSON & R. HOLMDAHL. 1995. Identification of murine loci associated with susceptibility to chronic experimental autoimmune encephalomyelitis. Nat. Genet. **10:** 313–317.

50. KUOKKANEN, S., M. SUNDVALL, J. D. TERWILLIGER, P. J. TIERNARI, J. WIKSTROM, R. HOLM-DAHL, U. PETTERSSON & L. PELTONEN. 1996. A putative vulnerability locus to multiple sclerosis maps to 5p14-p12 in a region syntenic to the murine locus Eae2. Nat. Genet. **13:** 477–480.

51. EBERS, G. C., K. KUKAY, D. E. BULMAN, A. D. SADOVNICK, G. RICE, C. ANDERSON, H. ARM-STRONG, K. COUSIN, R. B. BELL, W. HADER, D. W. PATY, S. HASHIMOTO, J. OGER, P. DUQI-ETTE, S. WARREN, T. GRAY, P. O'CONNOR, A. NATH, A. AUTY, L. METZ, G. FRANCIS, J. E. PAULSETH, T. J. MURRAY, W. PRYSE-PHILLIPS, N. RISCH et al. 1996. A full genome search in multiple sclerosis. Nat. Genet. **13:** 472–476.

52. HAINES, J. L., M. TER-MINASSIAN, A. BAZYK, J. F. GUSELLA, D. J. KIM, H. TERWEDOW, M. A. PERICAK-VANCE, J. B. RIMMLER, C. S. HAYNES, A. D. ROSES, A. LEE, B. SHANER, M. MENOLD, E. SEBOUN, R. P. FITOUSSI, C. GARTIOUX, C. REYES, F. RIBIERRE, G. GYAPAY, J. WEISSENBACH, S. L. HAUSER, D. E. GOODKIN, R. LINCOLN, K. USIJU, J. R. OKSENBERG et al. 1996. A complete genomic screen for multiple sclerosis underscores a role for the major histocompatibility complex: The Multiple Sclerosis Genetics Group. Nat. Genet. **13:** 469–471.

53. WARDELL, B. B., S. D. MICHAEL, K. S. TUNG, J. A. TODD, E. P. BLANKENHORN, K. MCENTEE, J. D. SUDWEEKS, W. K. HANSEN, N. D. MEEKER, J. S. GRIFFITH et al. 1995. Aod1, the im-munoregulatory locus controlling abrogation of tolerance in neonatal thymectomy-in-duced autoimmune ovarian dysgenesis, maps to mouse chromosome 16. Proc. Natl. Acad. Sci. U.S.A. **92:** 4758–4762.

54. MEEKER, N. D., W. F. HICKEY, R. KORNGOLD, W. K. HANSEN, J. D. SUDWEEKS, B. B. WARDELL, J. S. GRIFFITH & C. TEUSCHER. 1995. Multiple loci govern the bone marrow–derived immunoregulatory mechanism controlling dominant resistance to au-toimmune orchitis. Proc. Natl. Acad. Sci. U.S.A. **92:** 5684–5688.

55. MOREL, L., U. H. RUDOFSKY, J. A. LONGMATE, J. SCHIFFENBAUER & E. K. WAKELAND. 1994. Polygenic control of susceptibility to murine systemic lupus erythematosus. Immunity **1:** 219–229.

56. DRAKE, C. G., S. K. BABCOCK, E. PALMER & B. L. KOTZIN. 1994. Genetic analysis of the NZB contribution to lupus-like autoimmune disease in (NZB × NZW)F1 mice. Proc. Natl. Acad. Sci. U.S.A. **91:** 4062–4066.

57. VYSE, T. J., S. J. ROZZO, C. G. DRAKE, S. IZUI & B. L. KOTZIN. 1997. Control of multiple autoantibodies linked with a lupus nephritis susceptibility locus in New Zealand black mice. J. Immunol. **158:** 5566–5574.

58. JIANG, Y., S. HIROSE, Y. HAMANO, S. KODERA, H. TSURUI, M. ABE, K. TERASHIMA, S. ISHIKAWA & T. SHIRAI. 1997. Mapping of a gene for the increased susceptibility of B1 cells to Mott cell formation in murine autoimmune disease. J. Immunol. **158:** 992–997.

59. MOREL, L., C. MOHAN, Y. YU, B. P. CROKER, N. TIAN, A. DENG & E. K. WAKELAND. 1997. Functional dissection of systemic lupus erythematosus using congenic mouse strains. J. Immunol. **158:** 6019–6028.

60. MOHAN, C., L. MOREL, P. YANG & E. K. WAKELAND. 1997. Genetic dissection of systemic lupus erythematosus pathogenesis: Sle2 on murine chromosome 4 leads to B cell hyper-activity. J. Immunol. **159:** 454–465.

61. WATSON, M. L., J. K. RAO, G. S. GILKESON, P. RUIZ, E. M. EICHER, D. S. PISETSKY, A. MAT-SUZAWA, J. M. ROCHELLE & M. F. SELDIN. 1992. Genetic analysis of MRL-lpr mice: rela-tionship of the Fas apoptosis gene to disease manifestations and renal disease–modifying loci. J. Exp. Med. **176:** 1645–1656.

62. TSAO, B. P., R. M. CANTOR, K. C. KALUNIAN, C. J. CHEN, H. BADSHA, R. SINGH, D. J. WAL-LACE, R. C. KITRIDOU, S. L. CHEN, Y. W. SONG, D. A. ISENBERG, C. L. YU, B. H. HAHN & J. I. ROTTER. 1997. Evidence for linkage of a candidate chromosome 1 region to human systemic lupus erythematosus. J. Clin. Invest. **99:** 725–731.

63. DJABIRI, F., S. CAILLAT-ZUCMAN, P. GAJDOS, J. P. JAIS, L. GOMEZ, I. KHALIL, D. CHARRON, J. F. BACH & H. J. GARCHON. 1997. Association of the AChRalpha-subunit gene (CHRNA), DQA1*0101, and the DR3 haplotype in myasthenia gravis: evidence for a three-gene disease model in a subgroup of patients. J. Autoimmun. **10:** 407–413.

64. CHRISTODOULOU, K., M. TSINGIS, F. DEYMEER, P. SERDAROGLU, C. OZDEMIR, A. AL-SHEHAB, C. BAIRACTARIS, I. MAVROMATIS, I. MYLONAS, A. EVOLI, K. KYRIALLIS & L. T. MIDDLE-TON. 1997. Mapping of the familial myasthenia (congenital myasthenic syndrome type Ia) gene to chromosome 17p with evidence of genetic homogeneity. Hum. Mol. Genet. **6:** 635–640.

T Cell Tolerance and the Thymus[a]

JONATHAN SPRENT AND HIDEHIRO KISHIMOTO[b]

Department of Immunology
The Scripps Research Institute
La Jolla, California 92037

INTRODUCTION

Production of mature T cells expressing $\alpha\beta$ T cell receptors (TCR) occurs in the thymus and involves a complex process of positive and negative selection directed to self peptides bound to major histocompatibility complex (MHC) molecules.[1-3] Positive selection generates a diverse repertoire of T cells with specificity for foreign antigens, whereas negative selection (central tolerance) deletes T cells with overt reactivity to self antigens. This article provides a brief overview of the mechanisms involved in thymic selection and central tolerance induction.

POSITIVE SELECTION

Positive selection occurs at an intermediate stage of thymocyte differentiation when CD4$^-$ 8$^-$ precursors have differentiated into the major population of TCR^{lo} CD4$^+$ 8$^+$ cells situated in the cortex.[1-5] Differentiation of "double-positive" (DP) CD4$^+$ 8$^+$ thymocytes into the mature "single-positive" (SP) CD4$^+$ 8$^-$ and CD4$^-$ 8$^+$ TCR^{hi} cells found in the medulla and extrathymic environment requires contact with MHC molecules. Thus, mice lacking both MHC class I (MHC I) and class II (MHC II) molecules generate almost no functional mature SP cells, but contain normal numbers of DP cells in the cortex.[6]

MHC I and II molecules drive DP cells to form SP cells by a process of positive selection.[5] This process is not directed to MHC molecules per se, but to various self peptides bound to MHC molecules.[7-10] TCR recognition of peptide/MHC complexes is aided by corecognition of nonpolymorphic epitopes on MHC I and II molecules by CD8 and CD4 molecules, respectively. Combined TCR and CD4/CD8 recognition of MHC peptide complexes occurs during the interaction of DP cells with cortical epithelial cells. Of the large numbers of DP cells generated in the cortex, a small proportion of these cells have low, but significant binding avidity for the peptide/MHC complexes expressed on cortical epithelium. If recognition of these complexes is directed to MHC II/peptide complexes, involvement of the CD4 coreceptor induces the reactive DP cells to retain CD4 expression, but to downregulate CD8, thus causing

[a]This work was supported by Grant Nos. CA38355, CA25803, AI21487, AI32068, and AG01743 from the United States Public Health Service. It is Publication No. 10858-IMM from the Scripps Research Institute.

[b]H. Kishimoto is the recipient of a fellowship from the Cancer Research Institute.

the cells to differentiate into mature CD4$^+$ 8$^-$ cells. These cells move to the medulla where the cells are screened for overt autoreactivity before being exported to the periphery. Similarly, recognition of MHC I/peptide complexes on cortical epithelium induces differentiation of DP cells into mature CD4$^-$ 8$^+$ cells.

Positive selection to MHC/peptide complexes in the cortex affects only a very small proportion of the total DP thymocytes, that is, about 1–2%.[2,11] The vast majority of DP cells lack binding specificity for the MHC/peptide complexes on cortical epithelial cells and these "neglected" DP cells die within 3–4 days via apoptosis.[12] Positive selection appears to rescue DP cells from death by delivering a low-level survival signal that induces the cells to differentiate and mature. Such signaling is manifested by upregulation of CD69 molecules on the cell surface.[13]

The raison d'être of positive selection requires comment.[2] Thus, why does the immune system generate enormous numbers of DP cells, but allow only a tiny fraction of these cells to mature into functional T cells? The prevailing view here is that the specificity of mature T cells is self MHC–restricted, that is, T cell specificity is skewed towards recognition of foreign peptides binding to self MHC molecules (the MHC molecules seen during positive selection). Because most of the peptides inducing positive selection are probably derived from ubiquitous self proteins,[14] the peptides eliciting positive selection will continue to be recognized in the extrathymic environment. However, recognition of these peptides by mature T cells seems to be covert (nonimmunogenic), implying some degree of desensitization after positive selection.[15,16] Nevertheless, covert recognition of self peptides on APC might serve to amplify recognition of foreign peptides on the same APC. Positive selection could thus be a device for generating a repertoire of T cells that is operationally self tolerant, but highly sensitive to slight perturbations of "self," that is, to the altered self determinants created by MHC binding of foreign peptides.

Most of the DP cells in the thymus lack fine specificity for self MHC molecules plus bound peptides and these cells are discarded. Because MHC molecules are highly polymorphic, in any given thymus the particular subset of DP cells undergoing positive selection is small and is determined by the particular "self" MHC molecules expressed in the thymus. The total repertoire of DP precursor cells can thus be viewed as collectively embracing specificity for all of the different MHC alleles expressed in the species as a whole. In the individual thymus, only a small fraction of these cells are useful and the rest of the cells are destroyed.

In recent years, particular attention has been focused on which particular self peptides are responsible for positive selection.[3,5,7–10,15] Based on the results of several different experimental models, the current view is that positive selection is directed largely to "weak" (antagonist) peptides, that is, to peptides that bind well to MHC molecules, but relatively poorly to TCR molecules. Whether stronger (agonist or partial agonist) peptides contribute to positive selection is still debatable.

NEGATIVE SELECTION AND SELF TOLERANCE INDUCTION

As discussed above, positive selection produces a repertoire of cells with significant, but covert reactivity for self peptide/MHC complexes. Some DP thymocytes have overt reactivity for these complexes, and such potentially autoaggressive T cells have to be destroyed to prevent autoimmunity. For the most part, the elimination of autoreactive T cells occurs within the thymus.[17–20] This process of negative selection or central tolerance is restricted to self components that are synthesized within the thymus or reach the thymus from the bloodstream.

Of the multiplicity of different self peptides displayed throughout the body, most of these peptides are probably derived from ubiquitous proteins and are thus expressed on all cells.[14] It is highly likely therefore that negative selection to the bulk of self peptides occurs within the thymus. However, it is well recognized that some self peptides are tissue-specific, for example, myelin basic protein (MBP).[21,22] Since the concentration of tissue-specific antigens reaching the thymus is presumably quite low, "tolerance" to these antigens cannot be explained solely by central tolerance. Yet, it is well recognized that injecting tissue-specific antigens in a high dose together with some form of adjuvant can lead to autoimmune disease, for example, of the brain after injection of MBP.[22]

Since organ-specific autoimmune disease is relatively rare, mature T cells display operational tolerance to tissue-specific antigens while retaining the potential to respond to these antigens under experimental conditions. The simplest explanation for tolerance to tissue-specific antigens is that, for the most part, these antigens are sequestered, whereas T cells remain within the confines of the lymphoid tissues, blood, and lymph.[20,23] Such segregation prevents T cells from contacting tissue-specific antigens, thus leading to a state of "ignorance". As the result of trauma or infection, however, nontolerant T cells will inevitably come into contact with tissue-specific antigens. Yet, despite transient antibody production, such contact rarely leads to the production of overt T-mediated autoimmune disease. The prevailing explanation for this paradox is that breaking self tolerance to tissue-specific antigens usually leads to an abortive response where the reactive T cells rapidly become anergic, are destroyed, or are subject to some form of immune deviation.[18–20,23] The main problem with this scenario is that it is difficult to explain why a blanket of immunoregulation selectively inhibits responses to self antigens, but generally does not inhibit responses to foreign antigens (which are usually unrestrained until the waning stages of the primary response). However, with the appreciation that certain tissue-specific antigens can be found in the thymus,[24,25] an alternative explanation is that the repertoire of T cells reactive to tissue-specific antigens consists largely of low-affinity cells (high-affinity cells having been removed in the thymus via central tolerance). This idea could explain why inducing experimental autoimmune disease in animal models is often quite difficult except in defined strains.

NEGATIVE SELECTION IN THE CORTEX

Since cortical DP cells are highly sensitive to death following TCR ligation,[26,27] the cortex has long been considered an important site for negative selection. Data from several models are consistent with this idea. Thus, in the case of the HY (male antigen)–specific TCR transgenic line, crossing these mice to a male (HY$^+$) background produces a small thymus with marked atrophy of the cortex.[1] Likewise, prominent atrophy of the cortex occurs when lymphocytic choriomeningitis virus

(LCMV)–specific TCR transgenic mice are injected with live virus[28] or when TCR transgenic mice specific for protein antigens are injected with specific peptide.[29] In the latter situation, injection of peptide causes striking collapse of the cortex and prominent induction of apoptosis.

There are two potential problems with these data. First, the fact that TCR expression in TCR transgenic mice tends to be higher than normal and occurs very early in ontogeny makes it difficult to extrapolate to negative selection occurring in the normal thymus. Second, finding that the injection of specific antigen into TCR transgenic mice causes destruction of DP cells does not necessarily indicate that the antigen destroys these cells as the result of direct TCR ligation. Thus, there is the concern that the injected antigen could stimulate mature extrathymic T cells to produce toxic cytokines and release corticosteroids that then destroy cortical DP cells nonspecifically.[30] In support of this idea, we have recently found that injection of anti-TCR mAb causes massive destruction of DP thymocytes in adult mice, but not in neonates, perhaps reflecting the lower numbers of mature T cells in neonatal mice and reduced steroid levels in these mice (unpublished data of the authors and C. D. Surh).

These data certainly do not rule out the possibility that negative selection can occur in the cortex. Nevertheless, definitive evidence that negative selection does occur in the cortex under normal physiological conditions is very limited. Moreover, it is striking that no negative selection was observed in a recent transgenic model in which MHC molecules were expressed solely by cortical epithelium.[31]

THE MEDULLA AS A SITE FOR NEGATIVE SELECTION

In the case of endogenous superantigens (Sags), it has long been recognized that negative selection to these antigens is inconspicuous for most DP cells, but prominent for SP cells.[17] Since SP cells are found largely in the medulla, this region is a likely site for negative selection to endogenous Sags. In fact, direct support for this idea has come from the finding that negative selection of Vβ5[+] TCR transgenic T cells for certain endogenous Sags is associated with the appearance of large numbers of apoptotic cells in the medulla.[12]

The medulla is a logical site for negative selection because, unlike the cortex, the medulla is relatively open to the circulation and is packed with bone-marrow-derived cells with antigen-presenting cell (APC) function.[20] Therefore, the medulla is well equipped to present circulating self antigens to maturing T cells. A problem with this idea, however, is that the medulla is generally viewed as a site for mature thymocytes, that is, for cells that are beyond the stage of being tolerance-susceptible. Nevertheless, it is well established that medullary SP cells show considerable heterogeneity in terms of their surface markers.[32–35] Thus, some medullary T cells have the typical HSA[lo] Qa-2[hi] phenotype of fully mature T cells, whereas others (60–70%) retain the HSA[hi] Qa-2[lo] phenotype of DP cells and are therefore partly immature. These semimature SP cells are presumed to be the direct descendants of DP cells undergoing positive selection in the cortex. We have recently tested the tolerance susceptibility of semimature HSA[hi] CD4[+] 8[−] SP cells by studying the effects of injecting mice with anti-TCR mAb and then FACS-analyzing thymocyte subsets.[16] The data are summarized below.

When normal adult mice are injected intravenously with anti-TCR mAb, the total cellularity of the thymus decreases by 20-fold within two days and most of the residual cells are SP cells. In contrast to normal SP cells, however, nearly all of the SP cells surviving after anti-TCR mAb injection are fully mature HSA^{lo} cells. For SP cells, anti-TCR mAb thus causes selective destruction of semimature HSA^{hi} cells. In contrast to DP cells, the disappearance of HSA^{hi} SP cells does not seem to be a nonspecific consequence of stress because injection of corticosteroids reduces the cellularity of the thymus by 10-fold, but does not alter the ratio of HSA^{hi} to HSA^{lo} SP cells.

Direct evidence that anti-TCR mAb selectively destroys HSA^{hi} SP cells has been obtained by culturing whole thymocytes with a combination of anti-TCR and anti-CD28 mAb in culture.[16] When cross-linked on plastic, this combination of mAbs is highly effective in inducing apoptosis of thymocytes, presumably because anti-CD28 mAb provides costimulation for TCR-mediated death (see below).[26] The key finding is that, in addition to destroying DP cells, combined TCR/CD28 ligation *in vitro* causes extensive elimination of HSA^{hi} CD4$^+$ 8$^-$ cells, but does not affect HSA^{lo} CD4$^+$ 8$^-$ cells.

The finding that HSA^{hi} CD4$^+$ 8$^-$ thymocytes retain tolerance susceptibility, both *in vitro* and *in vivo*, indicates that negative selection can be delayed until a relatively late stage of thymocyte differentiation, that is, after the transition of DP cells to SP cells, but before SP cells have become fully mature. This late-onset form of negative selection presumably occurs in the medulla and corticomedullary junction at a time when early SP cells first enter the medulla from the cortex.

To examine the susceptibility of individual thymocyte subsets to TCR-mediated apoptosis, purified populations of CD4$^+$ 8$^+$ cells, HSA^{hi} CD4$^+$ 8$^-$ cells, and HSA^{lo} CD4$^+$ 8$^-$ cells were subjected to combined TCR/CD28 ligation or to TCR ligation alone *in vitro*;[16] HSA^{lo} CD4$^+$ 8$^-$ lymph node (LN) cells were used as a control. Confirming the results of other workers,[26] purified DP cells die rapidly (within 24 hours) via apoptosis when exposed to combined TCR/CD28 ligation, but are unaffected by TCR ligation alone. Diametrically opposite findings apply with fully mature HSA^{lo} CD4$^+$ 8$^-$ thymus or LN cells; that is, induction of apoptosis occurs with TCR ligation alone, but not with combined TCR/CD28 ligation. Interestingly, apoptosis of HSA^{lo} SP cells fails to occur with T cells from Fas-defective *lpr/lpr* mice, indicating that apoptosis is Fas-mediated. Our working hypothesis for this finding is that, with normal mature HSA^{lo} cells, TCR ligation induces rapid upregulation of Fas-L, which then induces apoptosis through interaction with surface Fas.[36] With combined TCR/CD28 ligation, however, signaling via CD28 induces upregulation of the anti-apoptotic molecule Bcl-X$_L$, which counteracts death mediated via Fas/Fas-L interaction.[37] It should be emphasized that rapid induction of TCR-mediated apoptosis of mature T cells *in vitro* is prevented when even very small numbers of APC are present, presumably because these cells express B7, the counterreceptor for CD28.[38] Hence, Fas-mediated death of mature T cells following TCR ligation alone may never occur under normal *in vivo* conditions (where bystander APC are plentiful).

In the case of HSA^{hi} CD4$^+$ 8$^-$ cells, these cells display properties that are intermediate between immature DP cells and fully mature HSA^{lo} cells.[16] Thus, under *in vitro* conditions, HSA^{hi} CD4$^+$ 8$^-$ cells resemble mature HSA^{lo} CD4$^+$ cells in being susceptible to Fas-mediated apoptosis following TCR ligation alone. However, like DP cells, HSA^{hi} CD4$^+$ 8$^-$ cells are susceptible to apoptosis induced by combined TCR/CD28 ligation. A key issue is whether apoptosis of HSA^{hi} CD4$^+$ 8$^-$ cells following TCR/CD28 ligation is Fas-dependent. This question is discussed below.

ROLE OF Fas IN NEGATIVE SELECTION OF HSA^{hi} CD4$^+$ 8$^-$ CELLS

Many groups have searched for a role for Fas in negative selection, but without success.[39,40] Thus, the susceptibility of *lpr/lpr* mice to negative selection is reported to be the same as for normal mice (although one recent study found that *lpr/lpr* mice showed a deficit in negative selection of cortical thymocyte when examined early after antigen injection[41]). In view of these findings, we expected that Fas would play no role in inducing apoptosis of HSA^{hi} CD4$^+$ 8$^-$ cells by combined TCR/CD28 ligation. This turned out to be true, but only in part. Thus, when HSA^{hi} CD4$^+$ 8$^-$ cells are exposed to a low-to-moderate concentration of anti-TCR mAb plus a fixed high concentration of anti-CD28 mAb, apoptosis of cells from normal and *lpr/lpr* mice is identical.[16] However, with a high concentration of anti-TCR mAb (plus anti-CD28 mAb), apoptosis is prominent with normal cells, but undetectable with *lpr/lpr* cells. Thus, apoptosis is Fas-independent at a low concentration of anti-TCR mAb, but Fas-dependent at a high concentration.

Culturing purified subsets of thymocytes with cross-linked anti-TCR and anti-CD28 mAbs *in vitro* is clearly a highly artificial situation. Nevertheless, essentially similar findings have been obtained *in vivo*. Thus, more recent studies have shown that injecting a low concentration of anti-TCR mAb into normal and *lpr/lpr* mice causes equivalent selective elimination of HSA^{hi} CD4$^+$ 8$^-$ cells in the thymus (unpublished data of the authors). By contrast, a high dose of mAb causes marked elimination of HSA^{hi} CD4$^+$ 8$^-$ cells in normal mice, but no elimination of these cells in *lpr/lpr* mice. Similar findings apply when mice are injected with *Staphylococcus* enterotoxin B (SEB). In this situation, negative selection is restricted to Vβ8$^+$ cells.

Collectively, the above data indicate that Fas does play an important role in negative selection, but only when the dose of antigen concerned is expressed at a high concentration. At low-to-moderate concentrations of antigen—which may apply to most self antigens expressed in the thymus—Fas-independent pathways operate effectively and cause normal negative selection in both normal and *lpr/lpr* mice. The problem arises when the antigen is expressed at a high level. In normal animals, a Fas-dependent mechanism comes into play and negative selection continues to operate efficiently. In *lpr/lpr* mice, by contrast, we can envisage that exposure to a high dose of self antigen, for example, to nucleoprotein peptides, allows T cells reactive to this antigen to escape and be released into the extrathymic environment. These nontolerant T cells would then be able to respond to the antigen in the periphery. The key issue here is whether the peculiar syndrome of lymphadenopathy seen in *lpr/lpr* mice[40] does indeed reflect a chronic response to self antigens by nontolerant T cells. This notion remains to be proved.

CELL-SURFACE MOLECULES CONTROLLING
NEGATIVE SELECTION

Although it is generally agreed that negative selection requires some form of co-stimulation,[42,43] which particular costimulatory molecules are involved is still unclear. CD28 expression does not seem to be essential because CD28 "knockout" mice show no obvious defect in negative selection.[43–46] Likewise, deletion of a number of other molecules with potential costimulatory function has failed to prevent negative selection;[6] impairing CD40/CD40L interaction does reduce negative selection, but this finding is thought to reflect that T cell CD40L interaction with CD40 on APCs maintains upregulation of various costimulatory molecules.[46]

In future studies, it is conceivable that deleting an as yet unknown costimulatory molecule will result in a clear defect for negative selection. A more-likely possibility in our view is that negative selection is controlled by multiple costimulatory molecules. According to this view, elimination of individual molecules, for example, CD28, would not impair negative selection because other molecules would fill in functionally.

The notion that negative selection involves the combined action of several different costimulatory molecules raises the question of which particular molecules on thymocytes can provide costimulation for death. For CD4$^+$ 8$^+$ cells, we have so far found only one molecule with this property, namely, CD28. For HSA^{hi} medullary T cells, however, two additional molecules, CD5 and CD43, have this property (unpublished data of the authors).

INHIBITION OF NEGATIVE SELECTION BY CYTOKINES

The finding that three different molecules, CD28, CD5, and CD43, can provide costimulation for TCR-mediated death of HSA^{hi} CD4$^+$ 8$^-$ cells raises the question of whether these molecules induce apoptosis via similar or different pathways. Although direct information on this point is not yet available, recent studies have shown that coculturing HSA^{hi} CD4$^+$ 8$^-$ cells with either IL-4 or IL-7 *in vitro* prevents TCR-mediated death of HSA^{hi} CD4$^+$ 8$^-$ cells, irrespective of whether the cells are subjected to coligation via CD28, CD5, or CD43 (unpublished data of the authors). The implication therefore is that injecting mice with antigen, for example, SEB, together with IL-4 or IL-7, might block negative selection *in vivo*. This is indeed the case. Thus, preliminary work has shown that the elimination of Vβ8$^+$ HSA^{hi} CD4$^+$ 8$^-$ cells induced by injection of a low-to-moderate dose of SEB can be prevented by coinjecting IL-4.

CONCLUDING COMMENTS

The finding that certain cytokines, namely, IL-4 and IL-7, can block negative selection could possibly be relevant to the defective self tolerance induction observed in myasthenia gravis. As discussed elsewhere in this volume, CD4$^+$ cells from patients with myasthenia gravis appear to be sensitized to peptides derived from the acetylcholine receptor (AChR). This observation might seem surprising because, at least at the level of mRNA, low levels of AChR are apparent in the normal thymus and also in the thymus of myasthenia gravis patients (A. Levinson *et al.*, this volume).

In view of this finding, exposure of immature T cells to low levels of AChR peptides in the thymus presumably eliminates high-affinity T cells, but may allow low-affinity cells to escape to the periphery. Sensitization of these low-affinity T cells in myasthenia gravis is likely to hinge on these cells encountering high concentrations of AChR in the periphery, for example, in muscle (perhaps as the end result of a viral infection). If so, we can envisage that some of these cells switch to an IL-4-producing Th-2 phenotype and then migrate into the thymic medulla (which is permeable to activated T cells).[47] In line with the suggestion of Levinson *et al.* (this volume), these or other cells might induce upregulation of AChR expression in the myasthenia thymus through local release of IFN-γ. Enhanced AChR expression in the thymus would then stimulate IL-4 production by immigrant AChR-reactive Th-2 cells, which in turn would impair clonal elimination of newly formed AChR-reactive thymocytes. Local IL-4 production in the thymus would thus allow *de novo* production and release of a new cohort of AChR-reactive T cells, including high-affinity cells, thus amplifying the peripheral response to AChR. This "vicious circle" concept is clearly highly hypothetical, but it could be tested by measuring the TCR affinity of AChR-reactive T cells in normal people versus patients with early or advanced myasthenia gravis.

ACKNOWLEDGMENTS

We thank Barbara Marchand for typing the original manuscript.

REFERENCES

1. VON BOEHMER, H. 1990. Developmental biology of T cells in T cell receptor transgenic mice. Annu. Rev. Immunol. **8:** 531–556.
2. SPRENT, J. 1993. T lymphocytes and the thymus. *In* Fundamental Immunology. Volume 3, p. 75–110. Raven Press. New York.
3. JAMESON, S. C., K. A. HOGQUIST & M. J. BEVAN. 1995. Positive selection of thymocytes. Annu. Rev. Immunol. **13:** 93–126.
4. SPRENT, J., D. LO, E. K. GAO & Y. RON. 1988. T cell selection in the thymus. Immunol. Rev. **101:** 173–190.
5. FINK, P. J. & M. J. BEVAN. 1995. Positive selection of thymocytes. Adv. Immunol. **59:** 99–133.
6. PFEFFER, K. & T. W. MAK. 1994. Lymphocyte ontogeny and activation in gene-targeted mice. Annu. Rev. Immunol. **12:** 367–411.
7. HOGQUIST, K. A., S. C. JAMESON, W. R. HEATH, J. L. HOWARD, M. J. BEVAN & F. R. CARBONE. 1994. T cell receptor antagonist peptides induce positive selection. Cell **76:** 17–27.
8. SEBZDA, E., V. A. WALLACE, J. MAYER, R. S. YEUNG, T. W. MAK & P. S. OHASHI. 1994. Positive and negative thymocyte selection induced by different concentrations of a single peptide. Science **263:** 1615–1618.
9. ASHTON-RICKARDT, P. G. & S. TONEGAWA. 1994. A differential-avidity model for T-cell selection. Immunol. Today **15:** 362–366.

10. JANEWAY, C. A., JR. 1994. Thymic selection: two pathways to life and two to death. Immunity **1:** 3–6.
11. SHORTMAN, K., M. EGERTON, G. J. SPANGRUDE & R. SCOLLAY. 1990. The generation and fate of thymocytes. Semin. Immunol. **2:** 3–12.
12. SURH, C. D. & J. SPRENT. 1994. T-cell apoptosis detected *in situ* during positive and negative selection in the thymus. Nature **372:** 100–103.
13. SWAT, W., M. DESSING, H. VON BOEHMER & P. KISIELOW. 1993. CD69 expression during selection and maturation of CD4$^+$ 8$^+$ thymocytes. Eur. J. Immunol. **23:** 739–746.
14. MARRACK, P., L. IGNATOWICZ, J. W. KAPPLER, J. BOYMEL & J. H. FREED. 1994. Comparison of peptides bound to spleen and thymus class II. J. Exp. Med. **178:** 2173.
15. SEBZDA, E., T. M. KUNDIG, C. T. THOMSON, K. AOKI, S-Y. MAK, J. P. MAYER, T. ZAMBORELLI, S. G. NATHENSON & P. S. OHASHI. 1996. Mature T cell reactivity altered by peptide agonist that induces positive selection. J. Exp. Med. **183:** 1093–1104.
16. KISHIMOTO, H. & J. SPRENT. 1997. Negative selection in the thymus includes semi-mature T cells. J. Exp. Med. **185:** 263–272.
17. KAPPLER, J. W., N. ROEHM & P. MARRACK. 1987. T cell tolerance by clonal elimination in the thymus. Cell **49:** 273–280.
18. NOSSAL, G. J. V. 1994. Negative selection of lymphocytes. Cell **76:** 229–239.
19. SPRENT, J. & S. R. WEBB. 1995. Intrathymic and extrathymic clonal deletion of T cells. Curr. Opin. Immunol. **7:** 196–205.
20. SPRENT, J. 1995. Central tolerance of T cells. Int. Rev. Immunol. **13:** 95–105.
21. WEIGLE, W. O. 1973. Immunological unresponsiveness. Adv. Immunol. **16:** 61–122.
22. SINHA, A. A., M. T. LOPEZ & H. O. MCDEVITT. 1990. Autoimmune diseases: the failure of self tolerance. Science **248:** 1380–1388.
23. MILLER, J. F. A. P. & W. R. HEATH. 1993. Self-ignorance in the peripheral T-cell pool. Immunol. Rev. **133:** 131–150.
24. JOLICOEUR, C., D. HANAHAN & K. M. SMITH. 1994. T-cell tolerance toward a transgenic beta-cell antigen and transcription of endogenous pancreatic genes in thymus. Proc. Natl. Acad. Sci. U.S.A. **91:** 6707–6711.
25. ANTONIA, S. J., T. GEIGER, J. MILLER & R. A. FLAVELL. 1995. Mechanisms of immune tolerance induction through the thymic expression of a peripheral tissue-specific protein. Int. Immunol. **7:** 715–725.
26. PUNT, J. A., B. A. OSBORNE, Y. TAKAHAMA, S. O. SHARROW & A. SINGER. 1994. Negative selection of CD4$^+$ CD8$^+$ thymocytes by T cell receptor–induced apoptosis requires a costimulatory signal that can be provided by CD28. J. Exp. Med. **179:** 709–713.
27. VASQUEZ, N. J., L. P. KANE & S. M. HEDRICK. 1994. Intracellular signals that mediate negative selection. Immunity **1:** 45–56.
28. PIRCHER, H., K. BURKI, R. LANG, H. HENGARTNER & R. M. ZINKERNAGEL. 1989. Tolerance induction in double specific T cell receptor transgenic mice varies with antigen. Nature **342:** 559–561.
29. MURPHY, K. M., A. B. HEIMBERGER & D. H. LOH. 1990. Induction by antigen of intrathymic apoptosis of CD4$^+$ CD8$^+$ TCR^{lo} thymocytes *in vivo*. Science **250:** 1720–1723.
30. JONDAL, M., S. OKRET & D. MCCONKEY. 1993. Killing of immature CD4$^+$ CD8$^+$ thymocytes *in vivo* by anti-CD3 or 5′(N-ethyl)-carboxamide-adenosine is blocked by glucocorticoid receptor antagonist RU-486. Eur. J. Immunol. **23:** 1246–1250.
31. LAUFER, T. M., J. DEKONING, J. S. MARKOWITZ, D. LO & L. H. GLIMCHER. 1996. Unopposed positive selection and autoreactivity in mice expressing class II MHC only on thymic cortex. Nature **383:** 81–85.
32. CRISPE, I. N. & M. J. BEVAN. 1987. Expression and functional significance of the J11d marker on mouse thymocytes. J. Immunol. **138:** 2013–2018.
33. VERNACHIO, J., M. LI, A. D. DONNENBERG & M. J. SOLOSKI. 1989. Qa-2 expression in the

adult murine thymus: a unique marker for a mature thymic subset. J. Immunol. **142:** 48–56.

34. NIKOLIC-ZUGIC, J. & M. J. BEVAN. 1990. Functional and phenotypic delineation of two subsets of CD4 single positive cells in the thymus. Int. Immunol. **2:** 135–141.

35. RAMSDELL, F., M. JENKINS, Q. DINH & B. J. FOWLKES. 1991. The majority of CD4$^+$ 8$^-$ thymocytes are functionally immature. J. Immunol. **147:** 1779–1785.

36. NAGATA, S. & P. GOLSTEIN. 1995. The Fas death factor. Science **267:** 1449–1456.

37. BOISE, L. H., A. J. MINN, P. J. NOEL, C. H. JUNE, M. A. ACCAVITTI, T. LINDSTEN & C. B. THOMPSON. 1995. CD28 costimulation can promote T cell survival by enhancing the expression of Bcl-x$_L$. Immunity **3:** 87–98.

38. LINSLEY, P. S. & J. A. LEDBETTER. 1993. The role of the CD28 receptor during T cell responses to antigen. Annu. Rev. Immunol. **11:** 191–212.

39. SINGER, G. G. & A. K. ABBAS. 1994. The Fas antigen is involved in peripheral, but not thymic deletion of T lymphocytes in T cell receptor transgenic mice. Immunity **1:** 365–371.

40. THEOFILOPOULOS, A. N. 1995. The basis of autoimmunity: Part I. Mechanisms of aberrant self-recognition. Immunol. Today **16:** 90–98.

41. CASTRO, J. E., J. A. LISTMAN, B. A. JACOBSON, Y. WANG, P. A. LOPEZ, S. JU, P. W. FINN & D. L. PERKINS. 1996. Fas modulation of apoptosis during negative selection of thymocytes. Immunity **5:** 617–627.

42. PAGE, D. M., L. P. KANE, J. P. ALLISON & S. M. HEDRICK. 1993. Two signals are required for negative selection of CD4$^+$ CD8$^+$ thymocytes. J. Immunol. **151:** 1868–1880.

43. AIBA, Y., O. MAZDA, M. M. DAVIS, S. MURAMATSU & Y. KATSURA. 1994. Requirement of a second signal from antigen presenting cells in the clonal deletion of immature T cells. Int. Immunol. **6:** 1475–1483.

44. SHAHINIAN, A., K. PFEFFER, K. P. LEE, T. M. KUNDIG, K. KISHIHARA, A. WAKEHAM, K. KAWAI, P. S. OHASHI, C. B. THOMPSON & T. W. MAK. 1993. Differential T cell costimulatory requirements in CD28-deficient mice. Science **261:** 609–612.

45. WALUNAS, T. L., A. I. SPERLING, R. KHATTRI, C. B. THOMPSON & J. A. BLUESTONE. 1996. CD28 expression is not essential for positive and negative selection of thymocytes or peripheral T cell tolerance. J. Immunol. **156:** 1006–1013.

46. FOY, T. M., D. M. PAGE, T. J. WALDSCHMIDT, A. SCHONEVELD, J. D. LAMAN, S. R. MASTERS, L. TYGRETT, J. A. LEDBETTER, A. ARUFFO, E. CLAASSEN, J. C. XU, R. A. FLAVELL, S. OEHEN, S. M. HEDRICK & R. J. NOELLE. 1995. An essential role for gp39, the ligand for CD40, in thymic selection. J. Exp. Med. **182:** 1377–1388.

47. AGUS, D. B., C. D. SURH & J. SPRENT. 1991. Reentry of T cells to the adult thymus is restricted to activated T cells. J. Exp. Med. **173:** 1039–1046.

Principles of Paraneoplastic Syndromes

EDWARD J. DROPCHO[a]

Department of Neurology
Indiana University Medical Center
and
Neuro-Oncology Program
Indiana University Cancer Center
and
Neurology Service
The Richard Roudebush Veterans Affairs Medical Center
Indianapolis, Indiana

THE AUTOIMMUNE HYPOTHESIS

Several neurologic paraneoplastic disorders are believed to be autoimmune diseases. The central theory of autoimmunity for paraneoplastic disorders postulates that tumor cells express "onconeural" antigen(s) identical or antigenically related to molecules normally expressed by neurons and that, in rare instances, an autoimmune response initially arising against the tumor "spills over" to attack neurons expressing the same or related antigen(s). If true, this theory should be supported by several lines of evidence: (1) patients should have specific antibody and/or cellular immune autoreactivity; (2) the neuropathology should be consistent with an immune or inflammatory process; (3) tumor cells in affected patients should express the onconeural antigen(s); (4) there should be a demonstrable antitumor immune response; (5) immunosuppressive treatment should produce a beneficial clinical effect; and (6) the clinical and neuropathologic features should be reproduced in an experimental model. Of the various syndromes, these lines of evidence are most solidly fulfilled for the Lambert-Eaton myasthenic syndrome. The purpose of this chapter is to examine the present evidence for autoimmunity in the paraneoplastic disorders affecting the central nervous system (CNS).

CLINICAL SYNDROMES AND AUTOANTIBODIES

The bulk of recent research on autoimmunity in neurologic paraneoplastic syndromes has focused on the specific presence of circulating antineuronal antibodies in some affected patients. A number of protein autoantigens have been identified and cloned by using sera from these patients to screen human cDNA expression libraries (TABLE 1).[1] There are good, but not perfect correlations among paraneoplastic syndromes, antineuronal antibody specificities, and the associated tumor types. The antineuronal antibodies have become a very useful clinical tool, both for diagnosing a

[a]Address for correspondence: Department of Neurology, Clinical Building 365, Indiana University Medical Center, Indianapolis, Indiana 46202.

TABLE 1. Antineuronal Antibodies and Antigens in CNS Paraneoplastic Syndromes

Antibody	Clinical Syndrome	Associated Tumor(s)	Immunocytochemical Pattern	Protein Autoantigen	Molecular Weight	Cellular Function
APCA (anti-Yo)	cerebellar degeneration	breast, ovarian	Purkinje cell cytoplasm	CDR34	34 kDa	unknown
				PCD-17	52 kDa	leucine zipper
				CDR62	62 kDa	leucine zipper
				CDR3	?	leucine zipper
				CZF	58 kDa	zinc finger
anti-Hu (ANNA-1)	encephalomyelitis, sensory neuronopathy	small cell lung	pan-neuronal nuclear > cytoplasmic	HuD	35–40 kDa	RNA binding
				ple21	35–40 kDa	RNA binding
				Hel-N1	35–40 kDa	RNA binding
				Hel-N2	35–40 kDa	RNA binding
anti-Ri (ANNA-2)	opsoclonus-myoclonus	breast, ovarian	CNS neurons nuclear > cytoplasmic	Nova-1	54 kDa	RNA binding
antiamphiphysin	stiff-person, encephalomyelitis	breast, small cell lung	CNS neuropil	amphiphysin	128 kDa	synaptic vesicle–associated
anti-CAR	retinal degeneration	small cell lung	photoreceptors and nuclear layer	recoverin	23 kDa	calcium binding

patient's condition as paraneoplastic and for guiding a search for the underlying tumor. These antineuronal antibody assays, however, do have important practical clinical limitations: (1) a small percentage of patients have high-titer antineuronal autoantibodies and yet never develop a demonstrable tumor; (2) several of the autoantibodies are present at low titers in tumor patients without any accompanying clinical manifestations; (3) a considerable proportion of patients with the paraneoplastic syndromes described below either do not have demonstrable antineuronal antibodies or have atypical antibodies that may not be detected in commercially available assays.

For paraneoplastic syndromes affecting the CNS, there is presently little direct evidence regarding the actual role of autoantibodies in producing clinical disease. It is not known whether the antibodies can by themselves cause neuronal injury, or act in concert with cellular immunity or other immune effectors, or whether they are an epiphenomenon or "footprint" for autoimmunity, but not directly involved in pathogenesis of clinical disease. The high degree of specificity of an autoantibody for a particular syndrome does not in itself prove that the antibodies are pathogenic.

Encephalomyelitis and Anti-Hu Antibodies

A large proportion of patients with paraneoplastic disorders can be grouped into the clinicopathologic entity known as paraneoplastic encephalomyelitis (PEM).[1] Small cell lung carcinoma is by far the tumor most commonly associated with PEM, with a scattering of patients with a variety of other neoplasms. Nearly all patients display signs and symptoms of multifocal involvement of the CNS and dorsal root ganglia. The most-common clinical manifestation of PEM is a disabling subacute sensory neuronopathy (SSN).[2,3] SSN Is not clinically evident or is a minor component in approximately 20–30% of patients with PEM. These patients have predominant involvement of other parts of the CNS, leading to a clinical diagnosis of subacute cerebellar degeneration, limbic encephalitis, brain stem encephalitis, paraneoplastic motor neuron disease, or autonomic system failure. By far, the most-common clinical course of PEM/SSN is for patients to deteriorate over a period of weeks to months and then to stabilize at a level of severe neurologic disability.

A high percentage of patients with PEM/SSN have polyclonal IgG anti-Hu antibodies (also called type 1 antineuronal nuclear antibodies or ANNA-1).[1,3,4] Anti-Hu antibodies produce diffuse staining of the nuclei and to a lesser degree the cytoplasm of all neurons in human brain, spinal cord, dorsal root ganglia, and autonomic ganglia. In immunoblots of human neuronal extracts, anti-Hu antibodies react with a group of closely spaced proteins with apparent molecular weight of 35–40 kDa. Intrathecal synthesis of anti-Hu antibodies out of proportion to the serum titer is common and is probably more prevalent among patients with clinically overt PEM plus SSN than among patients with relatively "pure" SSN.[5] High-titer anti-Hu antibodies have been reported in a few patients with sensory neuronopathy and encephalomyelitis in whom no tumor was detected, even at autopsy.[3] Depending on the methodology used, low serum titers of anti-Hu antibodies can be detected in 20–50% of patients with small cell lung carcinoma, but without clinically overt PEM/SSN.[6,7]

Anti-Hu antibodies react with a group of very closely related RNA-binding proteins that are believed to play an essential role in posttranscriptional processing of genes that participate in the development, maturation, and maintenance of neurons (TABLE 1).[8–10] The HuD and Hel-N1 proteins can bind to the 3'-untranslated regulatory region of mRNA encoding several oncoproteins and cytokines, including c-fos and c-myc.[9,11] Alternative splicing of mRNA transcripts produces multiple isoforms of the Hu autoantigen proteins, which probably differ in their neuronal distribution and antigenicity.[11,12] It is not yet known whether some of the polyclonal anti-Hu antibody response is targeted specifically to one neuronal autoantigen or whether individual PEM/SSN patients' anti-Hu antibodies react preferentially with one Hu autoantigen over another.[7] Differences in the fine specificity of the anti-Hu autoimmune response among different individuals may in part explain the clinical heterogeneity of patients with PEM/SSN.

Cerebellar Degeneration and Anti–Purkinje Cell Antibodies

Ninety percent of patients with paraneoplastic cerebellar degeneration (PCD) have small cell lung carcinoma, Hodgkin's lymphoma, or carcinomas of the breast, ovary, or female genital tract.[1,13,14] Patients typically have a subacute onset and progression of pancerebellar dysfunction. In addition to the cerebellar deficits, many patients show symptoms or signs of a multifocal PEM, including lethargy, cognitive deterioration, bulbar palsy, and limb weakness. The neurologic deficits in PCD generally worsen over a period of several weeks to months and then stabilize at a level of severe disability. Significant neurologic improvement, either spontaneously or after successful treatment of the associated tumor, is distinctly unusual.

The most-prevalent autoantibodies in patients with PCD are high-titer, polyclonal IgG anti–Purkinje cell antibodies (APCA) (also called "anti-Yo" antibodies).[1,4,14] In most patients, the APCA titers are disproportionately higher in the CSF than in serum, indicating intrathecal synthesis or selective concentration of the antibodies within the CNS. APCA characteristically stain the cytoplasm and proximal dendrites of Purkinje cells in a coarsely clumped pattern. Except for faint staining of neurons in the molecular and granular layers of the cerebellar cortex, these antibodies do not stain other neurons in the CNS or any extraneural tissues. In immunoblots of isolated human Purkinje cells, the APCA react specifically with a 58–62-kDa protein and (less strongly and consistently) with a 34–38-kDa protein.

To date, APCA with these immunocytochemical and immunoblotting characteristics are entirely restricted to women with PCD and carcinomas of the breast, ovary, or genital tract, and to a few women or men with adenocarcinoma of unknown origin. The only reported false-positives for APCA are a few patients in whom no tumor can be found after extended follow-up and a few patients with APCA and ovarian carcinoma, but no neurologic symptoms. APCA have not been found in patients with a wide variety of cerebellar disorders unrelated to a neoplasm.

Several distinct proteins reacting with APCA have been identified and cloned.[1] The 34-kDa CDR34 protein autoantigen features a distinctive pattern of inexact tandem repeats of a hexapeptide unit, extending over 90% of its primary sequence. The normal cellular function of the CDR34 protein is still unknown. The PCD-17, CDR62, and CDR3 autoantigens share a very high degree of sequence homology with one another and feature a 22-amino-acid "leucine zipper" region that probably contains the immunodominant epitope(s).[15–17] Several leucine zipper proteins, including the oncoproteins jun and fos, bind to DNA and regulate transcription, but localization of the PCD-17 protein to membrane-bound and free ribosomes suggests that it functions to regulate protein synthesis rather than DNA transcription.[18]

Opsoclonus-Myoclonus and Anti-Ri Antibodies

Small cell lung cancer and breast carcinoma together account for approximately 70% of adults with paraneoplastic opsoclonus.[1] Opsoclonus may occur in the setting of pure or relatively pure pancerebellar dysfunction; some of these patients have typical APCA. In other patients, some of whom have anti-Hu antibodies, the opsoclonus is part of a multifocal PEM, with or without truncal or limb ataxia, myoclonus, or altered mental status. A separate group of patients with breast cancer and ataxia (mainly truncal), most of whom also have opsoclonus, have anti-Ri antibodies (also called type 2 antineuronal nuclear antibodies or ANNA-2) in the serum and CSF.[1,4,19] By immunocytochemistry, anti-Ri antibodies stain nuclei of all neurons in the CNS in a pattern identical to that of anti-Hu antibodies. Anti-Ri antibodies are distinguished, however, by their lack of reactivity with neurons in the dorsal root ganglia, sympathetic ganglia, and myenteric plexus. In neuronal immunoblots, anti-Ri antibodies react with two groups of 53–61-kDa and 79–84-kDa proteins. There are individual reports of high-titer anti-Ri antibodies in women presenting with opsoclonus with ataxia, encephalomyelitis with rigidity, or sensory neuronopathy, in whom no tumor is detected even after extended follow-up.

As with anti-Hu antibodies in PEM, the multiplicity of protein bands that react with anti-Ri antibodies on neuronal immunoblots suggests that the Ri autoantigens are related, but distinct members of a family of proteins. To date, a single 54-kDa autoantigen termed the Nova-1 protein has been cloned by screening a human cerebellum cDNA library with anti-Ri serum.[20,21] The Nova-1 protein shares sequence homology with a group of nuclear RNA-binding proteins that are distinct from the RNA-binding proteins that react with anti-Hu antibodies. Alternative splicing of Nova-1 gives rise to different RNA transcripts. Expression of the Nova-2 gene in the mouse is largely restricted to the diencephalon, brain stem, and cerebellum.

Stiff-Person Syndrome and Antiamphiphysin Antibodies

A syndrome of muscle rigidity and spasms that clinically resembles the "stiff-person syndrome" has been reported in several patients with small cell lung carcinoma, thymoma, Hodgkin's disease, or carcinomas of the breast or colon.[1,22] In at least some of these patients, the rigidity is believed to be caused by multifocal PEM affecting spinal cord interneurons. Several patients with paraneoplastic rigidity or stiff-person syndrome have serum and CSF IgG antibodies directed against the synaptic vesicle–associated protein, amphiphysin.[23–26] Antiamphiphysin antibodies diffusely stain the CNS neuropil and to a lesser degree stain the cytoplasm of large neurons in the cerebral and cerebellar cortex. Antiamphiphysin antibodies have also been detected in the serum and CSF of a few patients with small cell lung cancer and PEM mainly manifesting as SSN, without rigidity.[26]

Retinal Degeneration and Antirecoverin Antibodies

The diagnosis "paraneoplastic retinal degeneration" encompasses patients with heterogeneous tumor associations and clinical features, and probably represents more than one pathophysiologic mechanism. More than 90% of reported patients with carcinoma-associated retinopathy (CAR) have small cell lung carcinoma, with individual case reports of patients with non–small cell lung carcinoma, breast carcinoma, and a variety of gynecologic tumors. Patients develop bilateral, but often asymmetric dimming or blurring of vision with loss of visual acuity and impaired color vision. Many patients develop night blindness and/or "positive symptoms" described as visual glare, distortions, sparkles, shimmering, or bizarre images. The symptoms generally deteriorate over several weeks to months in a gradual or stepwise course to a level of severe visual impairment.

The most-prevalent antiretinal antibodies in patients with carcinoma-associated retinopathy are polyclonal IgG antirecoverin (also called anti-CAR) antibodies.[27,28] Nearly all patients with antirecoverin antibodies have small cell lung carcinoma. Antirecoverin antibodies stain the inner and outer segment layers and the outer nuclear layer of the retina, and to a lesser degree the inner nuclear layer. In immunoblots of retinal extracts, the antibodies react with the 23-kDa calcium-binding protein, recoverin, which functions in the phototransduction cascade initiated by rhodopsin.

Other Syndromes and Antibodies

There are numerous reports of patients with the clinical syndromes who have "atypical" autoantibodies that do not fit the specificities described above. These include antibodies in patients with SSN or PEM and small cell lung carcinoma or other tumors, or antibodies in patients with paraneoplastic opsoclonus and small cell lung carcinoma.[29] The clinical features in these patients do not differ from the spectrum of signs and symptoms in patients with typical anti-Hu or anti-Ri antibodies.

Patients who develop PCD in association with Hodgkin's disease, non–small cell lung cancer, gastrointestinal carcinomas, or a number of other neoplasms either have no demonstrable antineuronal antibodies or have "atypical" antineuronal antibodies whose immunocytochemical and immunoblotting staining patterns differ from those of typical APCA.[13,30] There are no major clinical differences among PCD patients with typical APCA, those with other antineuronal antibodies, and those who are antibody-negative, including abruptness of neurologic onset, tempo of progression, additional CNS involvement, or ultimate neurologic outcome.[30] One exception to this is that patients with PCD and Hodgkin's disease are slightly more likely to show neurologic improvement, either spontaneously or after antitumor treatment, than patients with carcinoma and APCA.[13]

Approximately two-thirds of reported patients with paraneoplastic limbic encephalitis have small cell lung carcinoma. In most of these patients, the limbic encephalitis is part of an anti-Hu antibody-positive multifocal PEM. Some patients with small cell lung cancer and most patients with other tumors have clinically "pure" limbic system involvement. Other associated neoplasms include thymoma, Hodgkin's disease, non–small cell lung cancer, germ cell tumors, and carcinomas of the colon, breast, and bladder. There are individual case reports of "atypical" antineuronal autoantibodies in patients with colon carcinoma,[31] germ cell tumors,[32] and thymoma.[33,34]

One of the best-known paraneoplastic syndromes is the opsoclonus-myoclonus syndrome occurring in approximately 2–3% of children with neuroblastoma.[1] In nearly all of these patients, it is the neurologic syndrome that leads to discovery of an otherwise occult neoplasm. The syndrome typically has an abrupt onset and most children develop irritability, vomiting, and ataxia of the trunk and limbs, in addition to opsoclonus and myoclonus. The concept of an autoimmune response against onconeural antigens makes intuitive sense for this neuroectodermal tumor and is supported by indirect evidence (see below). With the exception of a few reported children with anti-Hu antibodies or atypical antibodies, however, there is to date no direct evidence for a consistent and specific humoral or cellular antineuronal immune response in children with opsoclonus-myoclonus and neuroblastoma.

A minority of patients with carcinoma-associated retinopathy do not have antirecoverin antibodies, but rather have antibodies against enolase[35] or antibodies with atypical specificities.[36] Second to small cell lung carcinoma, melanoma is the tumor most commonly associated with paraneoplastic retinal degeneration.[37–39] The clinical features of patients with retinal degeneration and melanoma differ somewhat from patients with CAR. Nearly all reported patients developed visual symptoms after the diagnosis of melanoma, after intervals of up to ten years. Subacute night blindness is a universal feature, and patients often additionally report floaters or shimmering lights. Visual acuity, visual fields, color vision, and funduscopic exam are usually normal. Sera from some patients with melanoma-associated retinal degeneration stain a subset of retinal bipolar cells and to a lesser degree the outer rod segments.[37–39] To date, the retinal autoantigen target of these antibodies has not been identified.

Recent studies indicate that some patients with paraneoplastic disorders develop more than one autoantibody response. Moderate titers of serum antibodies against N-type and/or P/Q-type voltage-gated calcium channels have been reported in up to 50% of patients with PEM or PCD, most of whom had APCA, anti-Hu, or anti-Ri antibodies as well.[40] Whether these antibodies differ in fine specificity from the antibodies against calcium channels in the Lambert-Eaton syndrome is not known. Antibodies against one or more glutamate receptor subunit proteins have been detected in patients with APCA or anti-Hu antibodies in some studies, but not in others.[41]

NEUROPATHOLOGY

PEM is characterized by patchy, multifocal neuronal loss in any or all areas of the cerebral hemispheres, limbic system, cerebellum, brain stem, spinal cord, dorsal root ganglia, and autonomic ganglia. The neuronal loss is accompanied by a variable degree of perivascular and leptomeningeal infiltration of mononuclear cells, including

T lymphocytes (both CD4+ and CD8+ cells), B lymphocytes, and plasma cells.[42,43] There is only a rough correlation between individual patients' clinical manifestations and the degree of neuronal loss and inflammatory changes in different sites seen at autopsy.

Direct immunoperoxidase studies of brains from several patients with PEM/SSN and small cell lung cancer show intraneuronal deposition of IgG in a pattern similar to that seen when patient anti-Hu serum is used to stain sections of normal brain.[42,43] The pattern of distribution of intraneuronal anti-Hu antibodies varies among different brain regions and among different PEM patients, without a tight correlation between the amount of IgG present in a given region, histologic abnormalities, and clinical manifestations.

The most striking and consistent neuropathologic finding in PCD is a severe, diffuse loss of Purkinje cells.[1,14] There may also be some neuronal loss in the granular cell layer and deep cerebellar nuclei. Perivascular cuffing and mononuclear cell infiltrates may be present in the cerebellum and overlying leptomeninges, but are often scanty or absent despite severe Purkinje cell loss. Patchy neuronal loss and inflammatory infiltrates are scattered through the cerebral hemispheres, brain stem, and spinal cord in up to one-half of autopsied PCD cases.

There are no distinctive or uniformly present neuropathologic abnormalities in patients with paraneoplastic opsoclonus.[1] Diffuse dropout of Purkinje cells, ranging from mild to nearly complete, is present in approximately one-half of reported autopsies. Neuronal loss in the inferior olivary nuclei and perivascular mononuclear cell infiltrates in the cerebellum, brain stem, and/or leptomeninges may be present, with or without Purkinje cell loss. In a significant proportion of autopsied children and adults with paraneoplastic opsoclonus, there are no identifiable histopathologic abnormalities in either the cerebellum or brain stem. These findings suggest that there are multiple sites in the cerebellum or brain stem that can result in opsoclonus when disrupted structurally or functionally.

In a single autopsied patient with opsoclonus, ataxia, and anti-Ri antibodies, there was severe Purkinje cell loss and pervascular and interstitial infiltrates of B lymphocytes and CD4+ T lymphocytes in the brain stem. Direct immunocytochemistry showed intraneuronal deposits of IgG predominantly in the basis pontis and dorsal midbrain.[44]

The histopathology of carcinoma-associated retinopathy includes severe, sometimes total, loss of inner and outer segments of rods and cones and widespread degeneration of the outer nuclear layer.[36] Some cases show patchy, mild infiltration of mononuclear cells around retinal arterioles. Ganglion and bipolar cells are usually preserved.

EXPRESSION OF AUTOANTIGENS BY TUMOR CELLS

Expression of one or more Hu autoantigens is very common, if not universal, among small cell lung carcinomas, including tumors from patients with PEM/SSN and anti-Hu antibodies as well as tumors from neurologically unaffected patients.[45] There is marked heterogeneity in the level of expression of mRNA for individual Hu proteins among individual tumors.[46,47] To date, no definite genetic mutations or antigenic differences have been identified between Hu autoantigen(s) expressed by tumors from PEM/SSN patients and the proteins from neurologically unaffected small cell carcinoma patients.[12] Small cell lung carcinomas from patients with PEM/SSN and anti-Hu antibodies are more likely to express cell surface class I and class II major histocompatibility complex antigens than are tumors from patients without PEM.[45] It is possible that this facilitates presentation of Hu onconeural antigens to the immune system and development of an anti-Hu immune response.

Expression of one or more autoantigens for APCA is fairly common, but not universal, among breast and ovarian carcinomas.[1] A higher proportion of tumors is positive for mRNA expression than for expression of the corresponding protein as detected by immunoreactivity with patients' APCA sera. Some studies suggest differences in protein expression or protein antigenicity in carcinomas from patients with PCD versus tumors from neurologically unaffected patients,[48] but this needs to be better clarified.

Less is known about tumor expression of onconeural antigens associated with other paraneoplastic syndromes. Amphiphysin is expressed by the majority of small cell lung cancers and by a lesser percentage of breast carcinomas from patients without antiamphiphysin antibodies or neurologic symptoms.[26] To date, recoverin has been detected in cell lines derived from the small cell lung carcinomas of a few patients with CAR, but has not been found in a small number of cell lines derived from "control" tumors.[28]

ANTITUMOR IMMUNE RESPONSE

There are several pieces of circumstantial evidence indicating an effective antitumor immune response in patients with paraneoplastic disorders. For all of the syndromes under discussion, it is not at all unusual for the underlying neoplasm to remain undetectable for one year or more after onset of neurologic symptoms despite repeated searching, supporting the theory of an autoimmune response against onconeural antigen(s) that simultaneously suppresses the tumor and attacks neurons.

Anti-HuD-specific lymphocytes have been identified as infiltrating the small cell lung carcinoma of a patient with PEM.[8] In a disproportionately high percentage of patients with PEM/SSN and anti-Hu antibodies, the underlying small cell lung carcinoma is limited to the lung and mediastinum, compared with neurologically unaffected small cell cancer patients.[6] This indirectly supports the presence of an effective antitumor immune response, but the alternative explanation is that the occurrence of neurologic symptoms leads to early tumor diagnosis. There are a few reports of spontaneous regression of small cell lung carcinoma accompanying or shortly preceding the onset of anti-Hu antibody-positive PEM/SSN;[49] the role of the anti-Hu immune response in this process is intriguing, but speculative.

In several patients with PCD and APCA, the associated breast or ovarian carcinoma contained an unusually prominent intratumoral mononuclear cell infiltrate.[14] Patients with PCD, APCA, and ovarian or fallopian tube carcinoma have a smaller metastatic tumor volume and a lower incidence of peritoneal tumor implants than neurologically unaffected "control" patients.[50]

The tumors of an unusually high percentage of children with paraneoplastic opsoclonus-myoclonus and neuroblastoma show intratumoral mononuclear cell infiltrates, evidence for maturation to ganglioneuromas, or both.[51,52] It has been known for 20 years that the occurrence of opsoclonus-myoclonus in children with neuroblastoma generally carries a good prognosis for survival independent of patient age, tumor site, or tumor stage, although a good oncologic outcome is not universal. As noted above, the antigen target(s) of the postulated onconeural immune response remains unknown.

RESPONSE TO IMMUNOSUPPRESSIVE TREATMENT

PEM/SSN very rarely remits despite successful tumor treatment and/or a variety of immunosuppressive therapies, including prednisone, cyclophosphamide, intravenous immunoglobulin (IVIg), or plasmapheresis.[2,3,53,54] Many patients attain a remission or apparent cure of the underlying tumor, but are permanently neurologically disabled. In patients with concomitant PEM/SSN and Lambert-Eaton myasthenic syndrome, the central nervous system manifestations rarely improve despite a good response of the neuromuscular symptoms to chemotherapy and immunosuppression.[55] Exceptional patients with PEM/SSN and anti-Hu antibodies (probably fewer than 10%) do in fact have significant neurological improvement with prednisone and/or IVIg; there is nothing distinctive about the clinical presentation of these responders.

Similarly, fewer than 10% of patients with PCD and APCA show significant neurologic improvement after plasmapheresis, IVIg, corticosteroids, or cyclophosphamide, despite reductions in serum autoantibody titers.[1,14,54] There are reports of neurologic improvement in individual patients treated with IVIg or cyclophosphamide.[56] There are no apparent differences in the clinical features of the few responders versus the large majority of PCD patients who do not improve following antitumor or immunosuppressive therapy.

The disappointing response of most patients with PEM/SSN or PCD to immunosuppressive therapies is open to several possible interpretations and does not necessarily refute an autoimmune etiology. It is possible that plasmapheresis or systemic immunosuppressive drugs do not adequately treat an autoimmune response that started in the periphery, but then became established and "sequestered" within the CNS. This is supported by the finding that plasmapheresis in patients with PEM/SSN or PCD reduces serum anti-Hu or APCA titers, but often fails to affect the level of autoantibodies in the CSF.[57] Unfortunately, an alternative explanation is that, at the time of diagnosis, many patients with PEM/SSN or PCD have already suffered irreversible neuronal damage or loss. This is supported by the typical monophasic clinical course in which patients deteriorate subacutely and then "level off" at a level of severe disability. Patients who receive "early" tumor treatment and immunosuppressive therapy do not seem to fare significantly better than patients with a longer lag between onset of neurologic symptoms and initiation of therapy.

Patients with other paraneoplastic syndromes have a somewhat better outlook. At least two-thirds of children with neuroblastoma and opsoclonus-myoclonus show rapid and dramatic neurologic improvement with ACTH or corticosteroids, independent of the status of the tumor. There are anecdotal reports of improvement with

IVIg. A sizable proportion of children become dependent on ACTH or steroids, however, or suffer exacerbations of neurologic symptoms during febrile illnesses.[51,52,58] Most children are left with residual motor deficits, speech delay, cognitive impairment, or behavior problems despite an initial good response to ACTH or complete tumor resection.

As a group, adults with paraneoplastic opsoclonus have a better neurologic outcome than patients with PCD or PEM. Spontaneous improvement of the opsoclonus and other neurologic features occasionally occurs, and there are reports of neurologic improvement following tumor treatment or corticosteroids.[1] A few patients with small cell lung cancer or breast carcinoma, opsoclonus-myoclonus, and atypical autoantibodies improved following immunoadsorption therapy with a protein A column;[29] the mechanism of this response is unknown. Of the small number of reported patients with paraneoplastic opsoclonus and anti-Ri antibodies (most of whom had breast carcinoma), approximately half showed significant improvement following antitumor chemotherapy and/or prednisone.[1,19] There are reports of individual patients with anti-Ri antibodies who improved after IVIg or low-dose oral cyclophosphamide.

Approximately one-half of the small number of reported patients with paraneoplastic rigidity and antiamphiphysin antibodies had neurologic improvement following tumor treatment and prednisone.[23,26] Other patients, including some with rigidity and others with prominent sensory neuronopathy, failed to improve despite successful tumor treatment and reductions in the antiamphiphysin titers.

Most patients with carcinoma-associated retinopathy show mild to moderate improvement in visual acuity and visual fields within days to weeks of beginning prednisone treatment, often prior to discovery of the underlying neoplasm.[27,36] There does not seem to be a difference in the likelihood of response to prednisone between patients with antirecoverin antibodies and patients with other antiretinal antibodies or no antibodies. Of the handful of reported patients with melanoma-associated retinal degeneration who were treated with prednisone, approximately one-half showed partial improvement in vision.[37]

Some patients with small cell lung cancer and clinically "pure" limbic encephalitis improve after tumor treatment and corticosteroids, or show spontaneous neurologic improvement independent of their tumor status. Several reported patients with limbic encephalitis and thymoma or Hodgkin's disease had significant neurologic improvement following successful tumor treatment, with or without concomitant immunosuppressive treatment.[33] Among patients with anti-Hu antibodies and prominent limbic encephalitis as part of multifocal PEM, the "limbic" features may improve following tumor treatment, prednisone, and/or plasmapheresis, while other signs and symptoms of PEM/SSN do not.[3]

EXPERIMENTAL MODELS

Thus far, it has been difficult to prove that the antineuronal autoantibodies described above are directly involved in causing neuronal injury and clinical disease. One major argument against a direct pathogenetic role for the antibodies outlined above is that the known autoantigens are primarily intracytoplasmic or intranuclear.

Autoantibodies against intracellular antigens are generally not thought to be pathogenetic unless the antigen is released from the cell and binds to the surface, or the antigen is "aberrantly" expressed on the cell surface, or if the relevant antigenic target is actually a cross-reacting cell surface molecule.[59]

To date, there is not a fully successful experimental model for PEM/SSN. Passive transfer of human anti-Hu antibodies into mice fails to produce any histopathologic changes in the cerebellum, spinal cord, or dorsal root ganglia. There are conflicting reports of the effects of anti-Hu antibodies *in vitro*. In one laboratory, incubation of rat cerebellar neuronal cultures with patients' anti-Hu sera (but not with anti-Ri sera) produced cytotoxicity,[60] but other laboratories have not reproduced these results. A monoclonal antibody against the HuD protein has been reported to cause apoptosis in human neuroblastoma cells. Conversely, in another study, patients' anti-Hu IgG was specifically taken up into the nucleus and cytoplasm of NCI-H69 human small cell lung carcinoma cells, but did not inhibit cell proliferation nor cause complement-dependent lysis or antibody-dependent cell-mediated cytotoxicity.[61] The mechanism by which anti-Hu antibodies are internalized into cells is unknown.[62] Hu autoantigens have been shown to be expressed on the surface of human Colo-688 small cell lung carcinoma cells;[63] whether neurons also express these proteins on their surface is not known. In studies reported to date, animals actively immunized with recombinant Hu antigens produce anti-Hu antibodies, but do not develop the clinical or pathologic features of PEM/SSN.[64]

Attempts at reproducing PCD in an experimental model have been unsuccessful. APCA IgG injected into the lateral ventricles or peritoneal cavity of rats or guinea pigs is taken up into the cytoplasm of Purkinje cells and other cerebellar neurons, but the animals show no clinical effects or neuropathologic changes.[65–67] The actual intracellular fate of immunoglobulin molecules taken up by Purkinje cells is unknown. *In vitro* incubation of human breast carcinoma cell lines with APCA sera from PCD patients does not cause significant cytotoxicity. Mice immunized with recombinant PCD-17 protein mount a good APCA response, but show no clinical or pathologic signs of disease, and have only minimal uptake of antibodies into Purkinje cells.[66]

In contrast to the studies of PEM and PCD, there has been success in establishing an animal model for CAR. Rats immunized with a segment of recoverin develop antirecoverin antibodies, uveoretinitis with cellular infiltrates, and degeneration of photoreceptors.[28] The same histopathological changes can be reproduced by passive transfer of stimulated lymphocytes from rats immunized with recoverin into naive animals, indicating that a combination of antibody-mediated injury and cellular immune effector cells is at work.

REFERENCES

1. DROPCHO, E. J. 1995. Autoimmune CNS paraneoplastic disorders: mechanisms, diagnosis, and therapeutic options. Ann. Neurol. **37(suppl. 1):** S102–S113.

2. CHALK, C. H., A. J. WINDEBANK, D. W. KIMMEL & P. G. McMANIS. 1992. The distinctive clinical features of paraneoplastic sensory neuronopathy. Can. J. Neurol. Sci. **19:** 346–351.

3. DALMAU, J., F. GRAUS, M. K. ROSENBLUM & J. B. POSNER. 1992. Anti-Hu-associated para-

neoplastic encephalomyelitis/sensory neuronopathy: a clinical study of 71 patients. Medicine **71:** 59–72.

4. MOLL, J. W., J. C. ANTOINE, H. R. BRASHEAR *et al.* 1995. Guidelines on the detection of paraneoplastic anti-neuronal-specific antibodies. Neurology **45:** 1937–1941.

5. VEGA, F., F. GRAUS, Q. M. CHEN *et al.* 1994. Intrathecal synthesis of the anti-Hu antibody in patients with paraneoplastic encephalomyelitis or sensory neuronopathy: clinical-immunologic correlations. Neurology **44:** 2145–2147.

6. DALMAU, J., H. M. FURNEAUX, R. J. GRALLA *et al.* 1990. Detection of the anti-Hu antibody in the serum of patients with small cell lung cancer: a quantitative Western blot analysis. Ann. Neurol. **27:** 544–552.

7. DROPCHO, E. J. & P. H. KING. 1994. Autoantibodies against the Hel-N1 RNA-binding protein among patients with lung carcinoma: an association with type I anti-neuronal nuclear antibodies. Ann. Neurol. **36:** 200–205.

8. SZABO, A., J. DALMAU, G. MANLEY *et al.* 1991. HuD, a paraneoplastic encephalomyelitis antigen, contains RNA-binding domains and is homologous to Elav and sex-lethal. Cell **67:** 325–333.

9. KING, P. H., T. D. LEVINE, R. T. FREMEAU & J. D. KEENE. 1994. Mammalian homologs of *Drosophila* ELAV localized to a neuronal subset can bind *in vitro* to the 3'-UTR of mRNA encoding the Id transcriptional repressor. J. Neurosci. **14:** 1943–1952.

10. SAKAI, K., M. GOFUKU, Y. KITAGAWA *et al.* 1994. A hippocampal protein associated with paraneoplastic neurologic syndrome and small cell lung carcinoma. Biochem. Biophys. Res. Commun. **199:** 1200–1208.

11. LIU, J., J. DALMAU, A. SZABO *et al.* 1995. Paraneoplastic encephalomyelitis antigens bind to the AU-rich elements of mRNA. Neurology **45:** 544–550.

12. SEKIDO, Y., S. A. BADER, D. P. CARBONE *et al.* 1994. Molecular analysis of the HuD gene encoding a paraneoplastic encephalomyelitis antigen in human lung cancer cell lines. Cancer Res. **54:** 4988–4992.

13. HAMMACK, J. E., H. KOTANIDES, M. K. ROSENBLUN & J. B. POSNER. 1992. Paraneoplastic cerebellar degeneration: clinical and immunologic findings in 21 patients with Hodgkin's disease. Neurology **42:** 1938–1943.

14. PETERSON, K., M. K. ROSENBLUM, H. KOTANIDES & J. B. POSNER. 1992. Paraneoplastic cerebellar degeneration: a clinical analysis of 55 anti-Yo antibody-positive patients. Neurology **42:** 1931–1937.

15. SAKAI, K., D. J. MITCHELL, T. TSUKAMOTO & L. STEINMAN. 1990. Isolation of a cDNA clone encoding an autoantigen recognized by an anti-neuronal cell antibody from a patient with paraneoplastic cerebellar degeneration. Ann. Neurol. **28:** 692–698.

16. FATHALLAH-SHAYKH, H., S. WOLF, E. WONG *et al.* 1991. Clining of a leucine-zipper protein recognized by the sera of patients with antibody-associated paraneoplastic cerebellar degeneration. Proc. Natl. Acad. Sci. U.S.A. **88:** 3451–3454.

17. SAKAI, K., T. OGASAWARA, G. HIROSE *et al.* 1993. Analysis of autoantibody binding to 52-kd paraneoplastic cerebellar degeneration–associated antigen expressed in recombinant proteins. Ann. Neurol. **33:** 373–380.

18. HIDA, C., T. TSUKAMOTO, H. AWANO & T. YAMAMOTO. 1994. Ultrastructural localization of anti–Purkinje cell antibody-binding sites in paraneoplastic cerebellar degeneration. Arch. Neurol. **51:** 555–558.

19. LUQUE, A., H. M. FURNEAUX, R. FERZIGER *et al.* 1991. Anti-Ri: an antibody associated with paraneoplastic opsoclonus and breast cancer. Ann. Neurol. **29:** 241–251.

20. BUCKANOVICH, R. J., J. B. POSNER & R. B. DARNELL. 1993. Nova, the paraneoplastic Ri antigen, is homologous to an RNA-binding protein and is specifically expressed in the developing motor system. Neuron **11:** 657–672.

21. BUCKANOVICH, R. J., Y. Y. YANG & R. B. DARNELL. 1996. The onconeural antigen Nova-1 is

a neuron-specific RNA-binding protein, the activity of which is inhibited by paraneo-plastic antibodies. J. Neurosci. **16:** 1114–1122.

22. GRIMALDI, L. M., G. MARTINO, S. BRAGHI *et al.* 1993. Heterogeneity of autoantibodies in stiff-man syndrome. Ann. Neurol. **34:** 57–64.

23. FOLLI, F., M. SOLIMENA, R. COFIELL *et al.* 1993. Autoantibodies to a 128-kd synaptic pro-tein in three women with the stiff-man syndrome and breast cancer. N. Engl. J. Med. **328:** 546–551.

24. DE CAMILLI, P., A. THOMAS, R. COFIELL *et al.* 1993. The synaptic vesicle–associated pro-tein amphiphysin is the 128-kD autoantigen of stiff-man syndrome with breast cancer. J. Exp. Med. **178:** 2219–2223.

25. DAVID, C., M. SOLIMENA & P. DE CAMILLI. 1994. Autoimmunity in stiff-man syndrome with breast cancer is targeted to the C-terminal region of human amphiphysin, a protein similar to the yeast proteins, Rvs167 and Rvs161. FEBS Lett. **351:** 73–79.

26. DROPCHO, E. J. 1996. Antiamphiphysin antibodies with small cell lung carcinoma and paraneoplastic encephalomyelitis. Ann. Neurol. **39:** 659–667.

27. THIRKILL, C. E., J. L. KELTNER, N. K. TYLER & A. M. ROTH. 1993. Antibody reactions with retina and cancer-associated antigens in 10 patients with cancer-associated retinopathy. Arch. Ophthalmol. **111:** 931–937.

28. POLANS, A. S., D. WITKOWSKA, T. L. HALEY *et al.* 1995. Recoverin, a photoreceptor-specif-ic calcium-binding protein, is expressed by the tumor of a patient with cancer-associated retinopathy. Proc. Natl. Acad. Sci. U.S.A. **92:** 9176–9180.

29. CHER, L. M., F. H. HOCHBERG, J. TERUYA *et al.* 1995. Therapy for paraneoplastic neurolog-ic syndromes in six patients with protein A column immunoadsorption. Cancer **75:** 1678–1683.

30. HAMMACK, J. E., D. W. KIMMEL, B. P. O'NEILL & V. A. LENNON. 1990. Paraneoplastic cere-bellar degeneration: a clinical comparison of patients with and without Purkinje cell cy-toplasmic antibodies. Mayo Clin. Proc. **65:** 1423–1431.

31. TSUKAMOTO, T., R. MOCHIZUKI, H. MOCHIZUKI *et al.* 1993. Paraneoplastic cerebellar degen-eration and limbic encephalitis in a patient with adenocarcinoma of the colon. J. Neurol. Neurosurg. Psychiatry **56:** 713–716.

32. AHERN, G. L., M. O'CONNOR, J. DALMAU *et al.* 1994. Paraneoplastic temporal lobe epilep-sy with testicular neoplasm and atypical amnesia. Neurology **44:** 1270–1274.

33. ANTOINE, J. C., J. HONNORAT, C. T. ANTERION *et al.* 1995. Limbic encephalitis and immuno-logical perturbations in two patients with thymoma. J. Neurol. Neurosurg. Psychiatry **58:** 706–710.

34. HONNORAT, J., J. C. ANTOINE, E. DERRINGTON *et al.* 1996. Antibodies to a subpopulation of glial cells and a 66-kDa developmental protein in patients with paraneoplastic neurologi-cal syndromes. J. Neurol. Neurosurg. Psychiatry **61:** 270–278.

35. ADAMUS, G., N. APTSIAURI, J. GUY *et al.* 1996. The occurrence of serum autoantibodies against enolase in cancer-associated retinopathy. Clin. Immunol. Immunopathol. **78:** 120–129.

36. RIZZO, J. F. & J. W. GITTINGER. 1992. Selective immunohistochemical staining in the para-neoplastic retinopathy syndrome. Ophthalmology **99:** 1286–1295.

37. MILAM, A. H., J. C. SAARI, S. G. JACOBSON *et al.* 1993. Autoantibodies against retinal bipo-lar cells in cutaneous melanoma-associated retinopathy. Invest. Ophthalmol. Visual Sci. **34:** 91–100.

38. KIM, R. Y., S. RETSAS, F. W. FITZKE *et al.* 1994. Cutaneous melanoma-associated retinopa-thy. Ophthalmology **101:** 1837–1843.

39. WEINSTEIN, J. M., S. E. KELMAN, G. H. BRESNICK & S. E. KORNGUTH. 1994. Paraneoplastic retinopathy associated with antiretinal bipolar cell antibodies in cutaneous malignant melanoma. Ophthalmology **101:** 1236–1243.

40. LENNON, V. A., T. J. KRYZER, G. E. GRIESMANN *et al.* 1995. Calcium-channel antibodies in the Lambert-Eaton syndrome and other paraneoplastic syndromes. N. Engl. J. Med. **332:** 1467–1474.

41. GAHRING, L. C., R. E. TWYMAN, J. E. GREENLEE & S. W. ROGERS. 1995. Autoantibodies to neuronal glutamate receptors in patients with paraneoplastic neurodegenerative syndrome enhance receptor activation. Mol. Med. **1:** 245–253.

42. DALMAU, J., H. M. FURNEAUX, M. K. ROSENBLUM *et al.* 1991. Detection of the anti-Hu antibody in specific regions of the nervous system and tumor from patients with paraneoplastic encephalomyelitis/sensory neuronopathy. Neurology **41:** 1757–1764.

43. JEAN, W. C., J. DALMAU, A. HO & J. B. POSNER. 1994. Analysis of the IgG subclass distribution and inflammatory infiltrates in patients with anti-Hu-associated paraneoplastic encephalomyelitis. Neurology **44:** 140–147.

44. HORMIGO, A., J. DALMAU, M. K. ROSENBLUM *et al.* 1994. Immunological and pathological study of anti-Ri-associated encephalopathy. Ann. Neurol. **36:** 896–902.

45. DALMAU, J., F. GRAUS, N. K. CHEUNG *et al.* 1995. Major histocompatibility proteins, anti-Hu antibodies, and paraneoplastic encephalomyelitis in neuroblastoma and small cell lung cancer. Cancer **75:** 99–109.

46. MANLEY, G. T., P. S. SMITT, J. DALMAU & J. B. POSNER. 1995. Hu antigens: reactivity with Hu antibodies, tumor expression, and major immunogenic sites. Ann. Neurol. **38:** 102–110.

47. KING, P. H. & E. J. DROPCHO. 1996. Expression of Hel-N1 and Hel-N2 in small cell lung carcinoma. Ann. Neurol. **39:** 679–681.

48. FURNEAUX, H. M., M. K. ROSENBLUM, J. DALMAU *et al.* 1990. Selective expression of Purkinje cell antigens in tumor tissue from patients with paraneoplastic cerebellar degeneration. N. Engl. J. Med. **322:** 1844–1851.

49. DARNELL, R. B. & L. M. DEANGELIS. 1993. Regression of small-cell lung carcinoma in patients with paraneoplastic neuronal antibodies. Lancet **341:** 21–22.

50. HETZEL, D. J., R. STANHOPE, B. P. O'NEILL & V. A. LENNON. 1990. Gynecologic cancer in patients with subacute cerebellar degeneration predicted by anti–Purkinje cell antibodies and limited in metastatic volume. Mayo Clin. Proc. **65:** 1558–1563.

51. TELANDER, R. L., W. A. SMITHSON & R. V. GROOVER. 1989. Clinical outcome in children with acute cerebellar encephalopathy and neuroblastoma. J. Pediatr. Surg. **24:** 11–14.

52. MITCHELL, W. G. & S. R. SNODGRASS. 1990. Opsoclonus-ataxia due to childhood neural crest tumors: a chronic neurologic syndrome. J. Child Neurol. **5:** 153–158.

53. GRAUS, F., F. VEGA, J. Y. DELATTRE *et al.* 1992. Plasmapheresis and antineoplastic treatment in CNS paraneoplastic syndromes with antineuronal autoantibodies. Neurology **42:** 536–540.

54. UCHUYA, M., F. GRAUS, F. VEGA *et al.* 1996. Intravenous immunoglobulin treatment in paraneoplastic neurological syndromes with antineuronal antibodies. J. Neurol. Neurosurg. Psychiatry **60:** 388–392.

55. GOLDSTEIN, J. M., S. G. WAXMAN, T. L. VOLLMER *et al.* 1994. Subacute cerebellar degeneration and Lambert-Eaton myasthenic syndrome associated with antibodies to voltage-gated calcium channels: differential effect of immunosuppressive therapy on central and peripheral defects. J. Neurol. Neurosurg. Psychiatry **57:** 1138–1139.

56. STARK, E., U. WURSTER, U. PATZOLD *et al.* 1995. Immunological and clinical response to immunosuppressive treatment in paraneoplastic cerebellar degeneration. Arch. Neurol. **52:** 814–818.

57. GRAUS, F., J. ABOS, J. ROQUER *et al.* 1990. Effect of plasmapheresis on serum and CSF autoantibody levels in neurologic paraneoplastic syndromes. Neurology **40:** 1621–1623.

58. KOH, P. S., J. G. RAFFENSPERGER, S. BERRY *et al.* 1994. Long-term outcome in children with opsoclonus-myoclonus and ataxia and coincident neuroblastoma. J. Pediatr. **125:** 712–716.

59. NAPARSTEK, Y. & P. H. PLOTZ. 1993. The role of autoantibodies in autoimmune disease. Annu. Rev. Immunol. **11:** 79–104.

60. GREENLEE, J. E., T. N. PARKS & K. A. JAECKLE. 1993. Type IIa ("anti-Hu") antineuronal antibodies produce destruction of rat cerebellar granule neurons *in vitro*. Neurology **43:** 2049–2054.

61. HORMIGO, A. & F. LIEBERMAN. 1994. Nuclear localization of anti-Hu antibody is not associated with *in vitro* cytotoxicity. J. Neuroimmunol. **55:** 205–212.

62. HORMIGO, A., C. BALL & F. S. LIEBERMAN. 1996. Internalization of anti-Hu IgG is not FcR mediated. Neurology **46:** 607–609.

63. TORA, M., F. GRAUS, C. DE BOLOS & F. X. REAL. 1997. Cell surface expression of paraneoplastic encephalomyelitis/sensory neuronopathy–associated Hu antigens in small-cell lung cancers and neuroblastomas. Neurology **48:** 735–741.

64. SILLEVIS SMITT, P. A., G. T. MANLEY & J. B. POSNER. 1995. Immunization with the paraneoplastic encephalomyelitis antigen HuD does not cause neurologic disease in mice. Neurology **45:** 1873–1878.

65. GRAUS, F., I. ILLA, M. AGUSTI et al. 1991. Effect of intraventricular injection of an anti–Purkinje cell antibody (anti-Yo) in a guinea pig model. J. Neurol. Sci. **106:** 82–87.

66. TANAKA, K., M. TANAKA, O. ONODERA et al. 1994. Passive transfer and active immunization with the recombinant leucine-zipper (Yo) protein as an attempt to establish an animal model of paraneoplastic cerebellar degeneration. J. Neurol. Sci. **127:** 153–158.

67. GREENLEE, J. E., J. B. BURNS, J. W. ROSE et al. 1995. Uptake of systemically administered human anticerebellar antibody by rat Purkinje cells following blood-brain barrier disruption. Acta Neuropathol. **89:** 341–345.

Factors That Determine the Severity of Experimental Myasthenia Gravis[a]

DANIEL B. DRACHMAN, KEVIN R. McINTOSH,[b] AND BINGZHI YANG

Neuromuscular Unit
Department of Neurology
The Johns Hopkins University School of Medicine
Baltimore, Maryland 21287-7519

INTRODUCTION

Although the mechanisms of immune pathogenesis of myasthenia gravis (MG) have been studied extensively, the factors that influence the *susceptibility* to MG and the *severity* of clinical disease manifestations are still poorly understood. This study was undertaken to learn more about the molecular, cellular, and humoral interactions that determine susceptibility to experimental myasthenia (EAMG) and its clinical severity. To this end, we have taken advantage of a congenic pair of mouse strains, one of which—B6 (C57BL/6)—is highly susceptible to the development of severe EAMG when immunized with *Torpedo* acetylcholine receptor (AChR), while a mutant variant—bm12 (B6.C-H-2^{bm12})—is relatively resistant.[1–4] The mutation in the bm12 mouse is isolated to its MHC Class II and consists of a change of three amino acids due to a gene conversion event.[5] The difference in susceptibility to EAMG has been the subject of much valuable previous research[2–8] and has been attributed to the genetically determined change in the MHC Class II. This change is associated with an altered repertoire of AChR-specific T cells in immunized bm12 mice.[6,8–10] It is likely that the altered T cell repertoire, in turn, plays a pivotal role in the reduced susceptibility to EAMG in the bm12 strain. However, any explanation of differential susceptibility to MG must take into account the fact that the pathogenetic mechanisms that lead to loss of AChRs in MG and EAMG are *antibody-mediated*.[11–14] How differences in Class II expression can lead to differences in antibody-mediated loss of AChRs, and hence differences in clinical expression of weakness, is not yet clear and is the subject of this report.

In order to address this multifaceted question, we carried out a comprehensive analysis of the sequence of immunological events, from antigen presentation to clinical EAMG, in B6 and bm12 mice, focusing particularly on the pivotal role of T cells in these responses. The new data, combined with previous information about this model, allow us to propose a plausible scheme to explain how a relatively subtle difference in MHC Class II can translate into differential severity of an antibody-mediated autoimmune disease. As described below, we conclude that the differences in

[a]This work was supported in part by a grant from the NIH (No. 5T32NS07368), grants from the Muscular Dystrophy Association, and gifts from the Ann and Donald Brown Family Foundation and the Eleanor Denmead Ingram Foundation.
[b]Present affiliation: Osiris Therapeutics, Incorporated, Baltimore, Maryland 21231.

susceptibility and severity are determined by the efficiency of a series of cognate interactions, first between antigen-presenting cells (APCs) and T cells and then between T cells and the antibody-producing B cells. At the molecular level, the trimolecular complex—that is, MHC Class II, peptide, and T cell receptor (TCR)—are critically involved. The end result—clinical weakness of EAMG—depends on how well the three components of the system fit together. This has important implications for understanding some of the factors that influence the severity of MG as well as other autoimmune diseases, and also provides insights into possible strategies for specific immunotherapy of MG.

EXPERIMENTAL DESIGN

Our working hypothesis is that (a) genetic differences between the *MHC Class II* of B6 and bm12 mice can lead to (b) differences in *AChR-specific T cell repertoires*, which in turn play a key role in (c) *the AChR antibody response*, which determines (d) the *susceptibility* to development of EAMG and its *severity* in these animals. In order to evaluate each of these steps, we undertook a series of studies outlined in TABLE 1.

T Cell Hybridomas

To compare the T cell responses of B6 and bm12 mice in detail, we used an experimental strategy involving the preparation of relatively large numbers of AChR-specific T cell hybridomas of each strain. The hybridoma strategy[15] avoids certain problems inherent in the study of T cells derived either from primed lymph node populations,[3,16] which give an averaged composite view of T cell responses, or from antigen-stimulated T cell clones or lines,[4,8] which include a potentially biased and limited population.[17] Hybridomas have the advantages of being randomly selected from the AChR-specific T cell pool and having replicative properties that are inde-

TABLE 1. Outline of Experimental Protocol

- Production of representative populations of *AChR-specific T cell hybridomas* from B6 and bm12 mice:
    - Determination of the *specific AChR epitope* recognized by each hybridoma
    - Evaluation of *cross-presentation* of the appropriate epitopes by antigen-presenting cells of the opposite strain
    - Analysis of the *T cell receptor* (TCR) α and β chains and their epitope contact domains (CDR3 loops) for each hybridoma

- Measurement of AChR antibodies in groups of B6 and bm12 mice:
    - *Torpedo* AChR
    - Mouse AChR
    - Isotype distribution of AChR antibodies

- Clinical incidence and severity of EAMG in B6 and bm12 mice

pendent of antigen stimulation. Therefore, they can provide representative populations of AChR-specific T cells from each strain, which allow examination of their relevant molecular structures and functional properties.

Production of T Cell Hybridomas

In order to obtain hybridomas that were as representative of the overall T cell populations as possible, we carried out seven separate sets of fusions (four for the B6 strain and three for bm12) and used multiple mice for each fusion experiment. Groups of four mice each were immunized with 50 μg of purified *Torpedo* AChR. Ten days later, the regional lymph nodes from groups of four mice were pooled, processed into single-cell suspensions (LNC), and cultured in serum-free medium (HL-1, Hycor Company, Portland, Maine). LNC were stimulated with AChR (5 μg/mL AChR) for 48 hours in bulk cultures (4×10^6 LNC/mL) and then expanded in medium containing recombinant IL2 (20 IU/mL, Genzyme, Cambridge, Massachusetts) for 16 hours. The activated T cells were mixed at a ratio of 1:1 with the thymoma fusion partner BW5147 (a kind gift of W. Born, University of Colorado Health Sciences Center, Denver, Colorado). These thymoma cells do not express their own T cell receptor α or β chains, but can only express the antigen receptors of the T cells with which they are fused.[18,19] Hybridomas were produced by fusion in the presence of polyethylene glycol (PEG 1500) and were selected by culture in HAT medium.[20]

Hybridomas were tested for antigen specificity by assay of their production of IL2 in response to stimulation *in vitro* with AChR. AChR-specific hybridomas were cloned, and then subcloned by limiting dilution at 0.3 cells per well, and tested for antigen specificity at each step. Only one AChR-specific subclone descended from each original well was used in order to avoid selection bias. Forty subcloned hybridomas (20 each from B6 and bm12 mice) were cryopreserved and 31 that continued to respond briskly to antigen stimulation after thawing were used for further immunological and molecular analyses (described below).

Responses of Hybridomas to AChR Peptides

We tested the responses of each hybridoma to purified *Torpedo* AChR, the extracellular domain of the α subunit of AChR (amino acids 1–210) prepared in our lab by recombinant methods, and four peptides from the α subunit that were previously reported[3,4,21] to stimulate T cell responses from B6 or bm12 mice (amino acids α111–126; α146–162; α181–200; and α360–378) (see FIGURE 1). Stimulation of hybridomas was carried out using 5×10^4 hybridoma cells cultured with 5×10^5 mononuclear spleen cells as APCs. The cells were cultured in DMEM complete medium containing high glucose, 25 mM Hepes (pH 7.2), 2 mM L-glutamine, 10% fetal bovine serum (FBS), 1× nonessential amino acids, 100 units/mL penicillin, and 100 μg/mL streptomycin at 37 °C in a humidified incubator with 5% CO_2. Each hybridoma was stimulated in triplicate with three different concentrations of each antigen, as follows: control culture medium only (complete DMEM with 10% FBS); purified *Torpedo* AChR at 0.5 μg/mL, 2.5 μg/mL, and 12.5 μg/mL; recombinant extra-

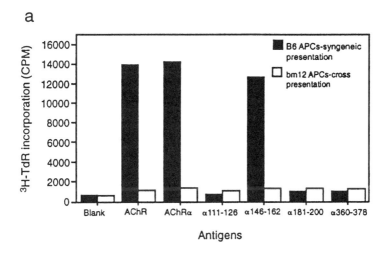

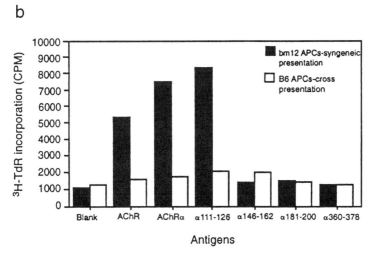

FIGURE 1. Responses of a typical B6 hybridoma (a) and a typical bm12 hybridoma (b). Conditions of stimulation are described in the text. APCs were either syngeneic (black bars) or opposite strain (white bars). Each T cell hybridoma was stimulated with several concentrations of whole purified AChR, recombinant extracellular α subunit domain (AChRα), each of the four peptides indicated, or medium only (blank). Culture supernatant medium was assayed for IL2 by CTLL bioassay. Results are given for the optimal responses, as ^{3}H-TdR incorporated by CTLL cells (CPM). Note that the B6 hybridoma responded to whole AChR, α1–210, and α146–162 peptides, presented by B6 APCs only. In contrast, bm12 hybridomas responded to whole AChR, α1–210, and α111–126 peptides, presented by bm12 APCs only.

cellular domain of the AChR α subunit (aa 1–210) at 0.2 μg/mL, 1 μg/mL, and 5 μg/mL; and the α subunit peptides α111–126, α146–162, α181–200, and α360–378 at 0.2 μM, 2 μM, and 20 μM. The supernatant medium was assayed for production of IL2 using the CTLL cell assay described below. We evaluated the ability of each of the AChR peptides, α111–126, α146–162, α181–200, and α360–378, and the AChR α subunit 1–210 to stimulate each of the hybridomas as follows: The IL2 production of each hybridoma in response to the optimal concentration of each individual peptide was compared statistically with the IL2 production of the same hybridoma to two peptides to which it did not respond.

Cross-Presentation of AChR Antigens to Hybridomas

These experiments were performed simultaneously with the stimulation experiments described above. The experimental design was exactly the same, except that APCs from the strain opposite that of the hybridoma were used: that is, bm12 spleen cells were used as APCs for presentation of antigens to B6 hybridomas, and B6 spleen cells were used as APCs for antigen presentation to bm12 hybridomas.

Interleukin-2 Assay

The amount of IL2 in cell culture supernatants was determined by bioassay using the IL2-dependent murine T cell line CTLL (ATCC, Rockville, Maryland). In brief, 100 μL of supernatant was harvested from hybridoma culture wells at 72 h after stimulation with antigen. The supernatant from each well was added to an equal volume of RPMI medium containing 10% horse serum (JRH Biosciences, Lenexa, Kansas). CTLL cells (7.5×10^3) were added to each well. The cultures were pulsed with ^{3}H-thymidine for the final 18 hours of a 2-day culture period and harvested, and the incorporated radioactivity was counted. Results are expressed as ^{3}H-TdR incorporated by CTLL cells (CPM).

Analysis of TCR α and β Chains of T Cell Hybridomas

We determined the molecular structure of the TCR of each hybridoma by (1) preparing cDNA for the rearranged α and β chains by RT-PCR, (2) amplifying the cDNAs, (3) sequencing the cDNAs, and (4) comparing the resulting sequences with known sequences of mouse TCR α and β chains in Genbank, as follows:

(1) *cDNA synthesis*: Total RNA was purified from hybridoma cells using 6 M guanidine thiocyanate.[22] RNA was incubated with reverse transcriptase (BRL Company, Gaithersburg, Maryland), using oligo-dT 12–18 as the primer, under the conditions described by the manufacturer (Pharmacia, Piscataway, New Jersey), at 42 °C for 1 hour. The reaction was stopped by boiling for 8 minutes.

(2) *PCR amplification*: PCR was carried out using the high-fidelity PFU DNA polymerase, as described.[23] For amplification of all α chains, we used three

degenerate Vα primers (VαA, VαB, and VαC) and a single primer for the α chain constant region (Cα) as described by Osman *et al.*[15] For amplification of the β chains, we used a complete set of primers for Vβ 1–17 (kindly provided by A. B. Peck and J-M. Wu, University of Florida, Gainesville, Florida) and a β chain constant region (Cβ) primer. Initial studies using a "universal" primer described for the β chains[15] resulted in omissions and artifacts (Yang and Drachman, in preparation).

(3) *DNA sequencing*: In about half the cases, PCR resulted in a single clear-cut band of the correct length, and the cDNA was directly sequenced using the Sequenase® PCR Product Sequencing kit (U.S. Biochemicals, Cleveland, Ohio). When necessary for preparation of sufficient amounts of DNA, the PCR products were cloned into a double-stranded plasmid vector (pT7 blue— Novagen, Madison, Wisconsin) and each strand was sequenced, either by the Sequenase® Quick-Denature Plasmid Sequencing kit or in The Johns Hopkins Genetic Core Facility. All sequencing methods used were based on the principles of dideoxy-chain termination.[24]

(4) *Sequence analysis*: The TCR Vα, Jα, Vβ, and Jβ chain sequences obtained were identified by comparison with sequences available through Genbank (see TABLES 2–5). Designation of the CDR3 loop sequences was based on cri-

TABLE 2. Amino-Acid Sequences of the TCR Vα and Jα Regions of AChR-specific B6 T Cell Hybridomas Deduced from the Rearranged Gene Sequences[a]

B6 Hybrids	Vα Gene	Peptide Specificity	Vα Sequence	CDR3 Loop	Jα Sequence	Jα Gene
5	8.4	146–162	AQLSDSALYYCAL	SSHNSGAKL	TFGGGT	39
6	8.4	146–162	AQLSDSALYYCAL	SDYNAGAKL	TFGGGT	39
8	8.5	146–162	AQLSDSALYYCAL	SGSNMGYKL	TSGQEQ	9
11	8.5	146–162	AQLSDSALYYCAL	SAHNAGAKL	TFGGGT	39
12	8.4	146–162	AQQSDSALYYCAL	SDNNAGAKL	TFGGGT	39
13	8.4	146–162	AQ SDSALYYCAL	S NNAGAKL	TFGGGT	39
14	8.5	146–162	AQLSDSALYYCAL	SGSNMGYKL	TSGQEQ	9
15	8.3	146–162	VQLSDSALYFCAL	SGSNMGYKL	TSGQEQ	9
19	8.3	146–162	VQLSDSALYFCAL	RRGSNLGRL	HFGAGT	18
7	1.3	181–200	SQPSDSALYFCAV	TYSNF	LRGGPL	34
9	10	360–378	AQLEDSDTYFCAT	EAGCRCPA	HIRRGT	39
1	3	–	VHWSDSTVYICAL	ASSGNCQL	IFGSGT	22
3	8.5	–	AQ SDSALYYCAL	SKGNTG KL	IFGLGT	37
4	1.1	–	PQPSDSALYLCAV	SNRGSALGRL	HFGAGT	18
10	1.3	–	SQPSDSALYLCAV	STGTNAYKV	IFGKGT	30
16	8.5	–	AQLSDSALYYCAL	SESNNRI	FFGDGT	31
18	8.3	–	VQLSDSALYFCAL	GSPNYAQGL	TFGLGT	26
20	nd	–	TLATDTAVYFCAT	ERGNTGKL	IFGLGT	37

[a]The Vα gene designation was according to Wang *et al.*[50] and the Jα gene designation was according to Koop *et al.*[51] The underlined amino acids constituted a sequence motif—SXXNX-GA(Y)KL—that was conserved among B6 hybridomas specific for peptide α146–162 of AChR.

TABLE 3. Amino-Acid Sequences of the TCR Vβ and Jβ Regions of AChR-specific B6 T Cell Hybridomas Deduced from the Rearranged Gene Sequences[a]

B6 Hybrids	Vβ Gene	Peptide Specificity	Vβ Sequence	CDR3 Loop	Jβ Sequence	Jβ Gene
5	6	146–162	SQKNEMAGFLCSI	TRDRGNSPL	YFSAGTR	1.6
6	6	146–162	SQKNEMAGFLCAS	STGEDTQ	YFGPGTR	2.1
8	6	146–162	SQKNEMAVFLCAS	SMGENTGQL	YFGEGSK	2.2
11	6	146–162	PQKNEMAVFLCAS	TRDRGNSPL	YFAAGTR	1.6
12	6	146–162	SQKNEMAGFLCAS	SPYRGREQ	YFGPGTR	2.1
13	6	146–162	SQKDEMAGFLCAS	SPYRGREQ	YFGPGTR	2.1
14	6	146–162	SQEDEMPVGLCAS	SMGENTGQL	YFGEGSK	2.2
15	6	146–162	SQKNEMAGFLCAS	STGEDTQ	YFGPGTR	2.1
19	6	146–162	SQKNEMAVFLCAS	SIEENSDY	TFGSGTR	1.2
7	1	181–200	VDPEDSAVYLCTI	NRSKRKDSK	LLDSRSR	nd
9	16	360–378	TALEDSAVDFCAS	SLNTEI	FFGKGTR	1.1
1	2	–	SQGRTLVRRS	ADAGDTEV	FFGKGTR	1.1
3	14	–	LLLNHSGFYLCAS	SLIGTGEETP	LFGEGTR	1.5
4	4	–	LKPDDSATYFCAI	NQPGQNYAEQ	FFGPGTR	2.1
10	8.1	–	ASLSQTAVYFCAS	SEGTLDTQ	YFGPGTR	2.1
16	nd	–	LSLNQSAPVPQLI	RESTYAEV	FFGKGTR	1.1
18	6	–	SQKNEMAVFLCAS	SITGDQDTQ	YFGPGTR	2.1
20	12	–	TETKDSAVYLCAS	SSGTGGDTQ	YFGPGTR	2.1

[a]The Vβ gene designation was according to Wilson et al.[52] and the Jβ gene designation was according to Pannetier et al.[53] Within the CDR3 loop, the conserved glutamic acid (E) or aspartic acid (D) is underlined.

TABLE 4. Amino-Acid Sequences of TCR Vα and Jα Regions of AChR-specific bm12 T Cell Hybridomas Deduced from the Rearranged Gene Sequences[a]

bm12 Hybrids	Vα Gene	Peptide Specificity	Vα Sequence	CDR3 Loop	Jα Sequence	Jα Gene
1	4.2	111–126	ESDSAVYYCAL	TNTGYQNF	YFGKGT	49
9	8.1	111–126	LSDSALYYCAL	SENTNTGKL	TFGDGT	27
13	nd	111–126	GVKTPLCTSVL	LHQGRKQCKA	NFGKGT	42
5	3	111–126 146–162	WSDSAKYFCAL	EGRAGGSNA	KLTSGT	42
11	4.2	146–162	ESDSAVYYCAL	SENTGYQNF	YFGKGT	49
2	4.2	–	ESDSAVYYCAL	GNTGYQNF	YFGKGT	49
3	4.2	–	ESDSAVYYCAL	GNTGYQNF	YFGKGT	49
7	nd	–	PVTPLSTSVQL	VTNTGANTGKL	TFGHGT	52
8	8.4	–	LSDSALYYCAL	KTNNTNAYKV	IFGKGT	30
10	3	–	WSDSAKYFCAL	LTGNTGKL	IFGLGT	37
17	4.0	–	ESDSTVFNCAL	GHPGYQNF	YFGQRY	7
18	4.3	–	ESDSAVYYCAL	SDRGSNNRI	FFGDGT	31
19	1.2	–	PSDSALYFCAE	DSNYQL	IWGSGT	33

[a]Gene designations were determined as described for TABLE 2. The conserved CDR3 loop sequence motif—GYQNF—is underlined.

TABLE 5. Amino-Acid Sequences of TCR Vβ and Jβ Regions of AChR-specific bm12 T Cell Hybridomas Deduced from the Rearranged Gene Sequences[a]

bm12 Hybrids	Vβ Gene	Peptide Specificity	Vβ Sequence	CDR3 Loop	Jβ Sequence	Jβ Gene
1	14	111–126	LLLNHSGFYLCAW	SLLGAGTEV	FFGKGTR	1.1
9	16	111–126	TALEDSTVYFCAS	SSTGVNYSEQ	FFGPGTR	2.1
13	14	111–126	LLLNHSGFYLCAW	SGTGSYEQ	YFGPGTR	2.1
5	8.2	111–126	ATPSQTSVYFCAS	GDAGQIYEQ	YFGPGTR	2.1
		146–162				
11	6	146–162	SQKNEMAGFLCAS	TKGLSYKSPL	YFSAGTR	1.6
2	16	–	TTLEDSTVYFCAS	SLTLRGDTQ	YFGPGTR	2.1
3	7	–	AKTNQTSVYFCAI	SLSPGNTL	YFGAGTR	2.4
7	8.2	–	ATPSQTSVYFCAS	GDLGQQNSDY	TFGSGTR	1.2
8	8.1	–	ASLSQTAVYFCAS	GQQNTL	YFGAGRL	2.4
10	16	–	TALEDSTVYFCAS	SLSLRGDTQ	YFGPGTR	2.1
17	7	–	AKTNQTSVYFCAS	SLSPGNTL	YFGAGTR	2.4
18	8.2	–	ATPSQTSVYFCAS			na
19	3.2	–	SEEDDSTLYLCAS	QSSTGTQKS	CFGKGTR	1.1

[a]Gene designations were determined as described for TABLE 3. Where present in the CDR3 loop, the glutamic acid (E) or aspartic acid (D) is underlined.

teria outlined by Rock *et al.*[25] The CDR3 loop is defined as beginning 2 amino acids downstream from the conserved cysteine in the V region and ending 2 amino acids upstream of the conserved GXG motif in the J region.

Clinical Evaluation of EAMG in Mice

At frequent intervals after immunization, mice were observed for signs of EAMG according to the following scale: 0 = no weakness; 1+ = weak grip or cry, with fatigability; 2+ = hunched posture, with lowered head and uncoordinated movements; 3+ = severe weakness, tremulous, moribund.

Antibody Assays

Two types of antibody assays were used in this study. A kinetic enzyme-linked immunosorbent assay (ELISA) was used to determine antibody titers to *Torpedo* AChR, as previously described.[26] In brief, this method uses a computer-driven 96-channel kinetic microplate reader (Molecular Devices Corporation, Menlo Park, California) to measure the maximum rate of increase of optical density in an enzyme-linked assay. Antibody titers are determined from the linear portion of the dilution curve. They are expressed as units per milliliter, relative to a standard of pooled high-titer sera from mice immunized with AChR. The standard, which was used throughout this study, is arbitrarily assigned a value of 1×10^6 U/mL.

Measurement of IgG Isotypes of AChR Antibodies by ELISA

Procedures for measurement of IgG subclasses by ELISA are similar to those previously described for measurement of total IgG antibodies to AChR.[26] Briefly, 96-well plates were coated with AChR and washed with PBS Tween. Mouse sera were diluted serially from 1:20 to 1:2560 and incubated in the wells overnight at 4 °C. After washing five times, affinity-purified rat IgG antibodies specific for mouse isotypes IgG1, IgG2a, or IgG2b were added to the plates (1:2000, Bio-source Company, Camarillo, California) overnight at 4 °C. Affinity-purified goat anti-rat IgG conjugated with HRP (Jackson Labs) was added to the plates and incubated in the dark at room temperature for 4 h. TMB substrate was added, and kinetic ELISA results were determined as above.

Measurement of Autoantibodies to Mouse AChR

An immunoprecipitation radioimmunoassay (RIA) was used to determine autoantibody levels, using AChR from denervated mouse limb muscles as the antigen, as described previously.[27] Individual sera from each mouse, diluted serially, were assayed separately. Pooled normal mouse serum was serially diluted and assayed simultaneously as a "background". The background counts, which were negligible, were subtracted from the values for the experimental sera before calculation of the antibody levels. Antibody levels, determined from the linear portion of the dilution curves, are expressed as moles $\times 10^{-9}$ of α-BuTx sites precipitated per liter of serum.

Statistical Analysis

Student's two-tailed t test or the Mann-Whitney U test was used for comparisons of group data (Abstat® statistical program). For comparison of the time course of development of AChR antibodies in B6 and bm12 mice, a paired t test was used.

RESULTS AND DISCUSSION

Clinical EAMG in B6 and bm12 Mice

During the course of two sets of immunizations in this study, 17 B6 and 19 bm12 mice were monitored daily for signs of muscle weakness characteristic of EAMG of grade 1 or more. Clinical weakness developed at 1 to 2 weeks after the first boost, paralleling the increased levels of AChR antibodies at that time (see below). In the B6 mice, 88% developed EAMG (15/17), compared to only 21% of the bm12 mice (4/19). These findings are consistent with previous reports of the greater susceptibility of B6 mice to the development of EAMG.[2–4,7]

Epitope Recognition by B6 and bm12 Hybridomas

Our results (see FIGURE 1 and TABLES 2–5) demonstrate striking differences in the AChR-specific T cells of the two strains, which confirms and extends previous reports.[3,4,8,9,16] Half of our B6 hybridomas recognized the AChR α146–162 epitope, which has been reported to be immunodominant and to play an important role in determining the "myasthenogenicity" of the immune response. Although the T cell hybridoma responses showed considerable restriction to this important epitope, the restriction was not absolute since 50% of the B6 hybridomas recognized other AChR epitopes (TABLES 2 and 3). By contrast, only two of the bm12 hybridomas responded to α146–162, and one of these was promiscuous, recognizing another epitope as well. Four of the bm12 hybridomas recognized α111–126. Epitope recognition by bm12 hybridomas was not only different, but also more heterogeneous than that of B6 hybridomas (TABLES 4 and 5).

Cross-Presentation of Antigens to B6 and bm12 Hybridomas

We examined the ability of APCs of each strain to present the appropriate antigens to hybridomas of the opposite strain (see FIGURE 1 for example). None of the B6 hybridomas responded to *Torpedo* AChR presented by bm12 APCs. Only three of the hybridomas responded to the recombinant fragment α1–210, and one responded to α360–378 presented by the bm12 APCs. None of the bm12 hybridomas responded to native AChR, α1–210, or any of the peptides when presented by B6 APCs. The virtually complete inability of opposite strain APCs to present appropriate peptides to T cell hybridomas suggests (1) that the APC did not bind the antigen adequately or (2) that the TCR did not recognize the peptide when complexed with the opposite strain MHC Class II. Indeed, both of these mechanisms may prevent effective cross-presentation, as discussed further below.

Structure of TCR α and β Chains Deduced from Gene Sequences

The TCR gene usage was also strikingly different in hybridomas from the two strains (TABLES 2–5). More than half of the B6 hybridomas (10/18) used the Vβ6 gene, in confirmation of previous reports.[8–10,28–30] However, the Vα gene usage, which has not previously been studied in mice with EAMG, was even more strikingly restricted in the B6 hybridomas since two-thirds of these hybridomas used Vα8 family members. Most significant was the fact that all B6 hybridomas that recognized the α146–162 epitope used exclusively the TCR heterodimer consisting of Vα8 and Vβ6. By contrast, there was no consistent TCR gene usage pattern in the bm12 strain, although half of the hybridomas used Vα4 and one-third used Vβ8 family members. Neither the relationship to epitope recognition nor the heterodimer pairing followed any consistent pattern. Perhaps most relevant were the CDR3 sequence patterns in the two strains. The CDR3 loops are the domains of TCR α and β chains that make direct physical contact with the particular peptide recognized by the T cell, in the context of the MHC

Class II.[31,32] In the B6 hybridomas, we found that the α chain CDR3s were relatively restricted in length and had a highly conserved amino-acid motif (TABLE 2), which was present in all but one of the hybridomas that recognized α146–162. The CDR3 of the β chain showed greater variation in length and sequence pattern, but invariably had either glutamic acid or the structurally similar aspartic acid residue in every hybridoma that recognized α146–162 (see references 28 and 29; TABLE 3). Both glutamic acid and aspartic acid are strongly negatively charged, which is a key element in binding to the strongly positively charged lysine at position 155 within the 146–162 epitope (see below). The glutamic and aspartic acid residues in the β chain CDR3 were coded for by both alternative codons. This suggests that the selection of AChR-specific T cell receptors in B6 mice is antigen-driven and is preferentially selected by interaction with the dominant epitope, α146–162 in association with its MHC Class II (I-A[b]). It is highly unlikely that the marked degree of TCR restriction observed in the hybridomas that recognize α146–162 could be accounted for by extremely narrow limitation of the pre-existing T cell repertoire. By contrast, the CDR3 domains of bm12 hybridomas varied in length and sequence, and only 50% had a glutamic or aspartic acid, as compared to 100% of the B6 hybridomas.

The foregoing observations allow us to draw two inferences regarding the T cells: (1) The epitope α146–162 plays an important role in the AChR-specific T cell repertoire of B6 mice, but not in the repertoire of bm12 mice, in agreement with previous reports.[3,4,8,16,28–30] (2) The T cell receptor selection in B6 mice results from an antigen-driven process rather than from a preexisting hole in the T cell repertoire of bm12 mice due to negative selection. The possibility of deletion of the relevant T cells by a dominant negative gene is excluded by observations that preexisting T cell repertoires of bm12 and B6 × bm12 F1 hybrid mice include T cells that are potentially capable of responding to the α146–162 epitope[8] and express the same proportion of Vβ6 T cells as are present in the B6 strain,[9] and the F1 mice develop clinical manifestations of EAMG as frequently as mice of the parent B6 strain.[8,9]

These conclusions raise the key question of how the process of specific TCR selection is influenced by the MHC Class II of B6 mice. The principle that T cell stimulation is dependent on interactions of the trimolecular complex—MHC Class II, peptide epitope, and TCR— is illustrated diagrammatically in FIGURE 2. Previous work has shown that the MHC Class II molecule that is present in B6 mice (I-A[b]) binds the epitope α146–162 with high affinity.[33,34] Changes in either the sequence of the I-A[b] molecule[34] or the amino-acid sequence of the peptide 146–162[33] have been shown to reduce the binding affinity. As noted above, the dominant peptide α146–162 has a strongly positively charged lysine at position 155. One of the alterations in the MHC Class II of the bm12 mouse is the substitution of lysine for threonine at position 71. This change results in markedly reduced binding of α146–162[34] due to mutual repulsion of the strongly positively charged lysines in both the peptide and the altered MHC. This would predict that APCs from bm12 mice should not be able to present α146–162 to T cells from B6 mice. Our studies of cross-strain presentation support this prediction, in contrast to previous reports.[3,4] APCs from bm12 mice completely failed to present α146–162 to any of the B6 hybridomas, even at high peptide concentrations (see FIGURE 1a). This suggests that the antigen-driven selection of T cells specific for α146–162 in B6 mice is attributable to the propensity of APCs of B6 (but not of bm12) mice to present this epitope (FIGURE 2). The MHC II/α146–162 complex must fit the

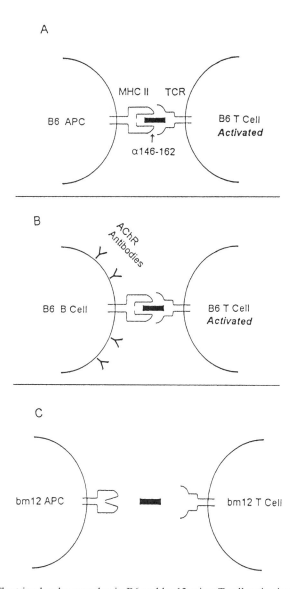

FIGURE 2. The trimolecular complex in B6 and bm12 mice: T cell activation and antibody production. The "better fit" of MHC Class II, peptide, and TCR in B6 mice enhances cognate interactions of APCs with T cells, and T cells with B cells, resulting in a more abundant and pathogenic AChR antibody response and thus more severe EAMG than in bm12 mice. (A) APCs of B6 mice have MHC Class II that fits peptide α146–162 very well and presents it. B6 mice have T cells with receptors (TCRs) that fit the MHC II/peptide complex very well. These T cells are strongly activated and proliferate more than other T cells. (B) B cells of B6 mice also present α146–162 very well. They interact strongly with the activated B6 T cells and are induced to produce AChR antibodies abundantly. (C) APCs of bm12 mice do not fit α146–162 well. Although potentially appropriate T cells are present (note the similar TCRs), they are not stimulated. However, bm12 APCs can present other peptides to other bm12 T cells. The reciprocal activation of T cells and B cells is not as effective, resulting in less abundant and less pathogenic AChR antibody production.

appropriate TCR extremely well, resulting in stimulation and expansion of these T cells. We also asked whether T cells from bm12 mice can ever respond to α146–162. Although two of our bm12 hybridomas responded to α146–162, their TCR sequences were completely different from those of the B6 cells that recognized the same peptide. Undoubtedly, the configuration of this same peptide in the context of the bm12 MHC Class II differed from its configuration in the B6 MHC II context. Although the involvement of α146–162-specific T cells has a strong influence in determining the severity of EAMG in these mice, it is by no means absolutely required. As we have seen, even bm12 mice, whose T cells respond only minimally (and differently) to this epitope, can be induced to develop clinical EAMG, although in a lower fraction of immunized animals (see references 2–4 and 7, and present results). Similarly, mice that have been treated either immunologically or genetically[30,35,36] to eliminate TCR Vβ6, or mice that have been neonatally tolerized to α146–162,[16] can develop clinical weakness of EAMG, although with variably reduced incidence and severity.

We next considered several possible ways by which the T cell epitope specificity might influence the incidence and severity of the antibody-mediated autoimmune disease process in EAMG: (1) the overall T cell response of B6 mice to AChR, as measured by proliferation, might be greater than that of bm12 mice; (2) the overall AChR antibody responses of B6 mice may be quantitatively greater than those of bm12 mice; (3) the AChR antibody responses in B6 and bm12 mice may differ in certain specific characteristics, involving the production of autoantibodies (i.e., anti-mouse AChR), IgG isotype representation, or epitope specificity.

Overall T Cell Response

Previous reports presented conflicting data concerning AChR-specific proliferation of T cells from AChR-primed B6 and bm12 mice. While some investigators reported relatively reduced responses in bm12 mice,[2,17] others found no difference in the overall proliferative responses to AChR.[3,4] Review of the published reports suggested that weak immunization (up to 20 μg AChR per mouse) might enhance differences in T cell responses of the two strains,[2,7,35] while such differences might be masked by strong immunization. We therefore compared AChR-specific proliferative responses of T cells from B6 and bm12 mice that had been primed with either low-dose (20 μg) or high-dose (50 μg) AChR. Our results, repeated several times, showed no significant difference between the responses of T cells from B6 and bm12 mice, although priming with the higher dose resulted in more vigorous responses in both strains (data not shown; see reference 37). Thus, differential proliferation of the overall populations of T cells cannot be implicated in the different susceptibility of B6 and bm12 mice to develop EAMG. However, it is well known that proliferation may not correlate either with the ability of T cells to provide help or with their effector function.

Overall Antibody Responses to AChR

Previous publications have reported conflicting data regarding differences in AChR antibody responses in B6 and bm12 mice after immunization with *Torpedo*

AChR.[2–4,7,8] In order to reexamine this important question, we compared the antibody responses in B6 and bm12 mice to *Torpedo* AChR and to mouse (self) AChR following primary immunization and subsequent antigen challenge boosts. Our findings showed that B6 mice had consistently and significantly higher mean titers of antibodies to both *Torpedo* AChR and mouse AChR throughout the time course observed (FIGURES 3–5). Autoantibodies to mouse (self) AChR play a more important role in the pathogenesis of EAMG than antibodies to *Torpedo* (foreign) AChR. In human MG, AChR antibody levels in different patients do not correspond with the severity of myasthenic weakness,[13] but a change in the level in a given individual patient generally correlates well with a change in clinical severity.[38] Since these inbred mice are congenic, the higher levels of AChR autoantibodies in B6 mice (see below) can account, at least in part, for the differences in incidence and severity of EAMG in the two strains.

Antibody Isotypes

Since certain antibody isotypes are more pathogenic than others, we compared the IgG isotype distribution of AChR antibodies in sera of B6 and bm12 mice. Our results showed that the levels of IgG2b antibodies to AChR were significantly higher in B6 mice than in bm12 mice (FIGURE 4). Recent evidence indicates that the particular isotype produced may be influenced by the characteristics of the helper T cell (T_H)

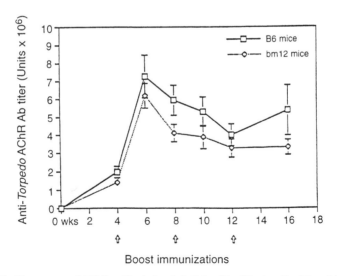

FIGURE 3. Time course of AChR antibody levels in B6 and bm12 mice. Ten B6 and 11 bm12 mice were immunized with AChR in CFA (50 μg/mouse) and boosted at 4-week intervals (20 μg in IFA [arrows]). Serum antibodies to AChR were measured by kinetic ELISA, and mean values ± SEM at each time point are expressed as units (see text for details). The levels for immunized B6 mice were significantly higher than those for bm12 mice ($p < 0.01$, paired t test).

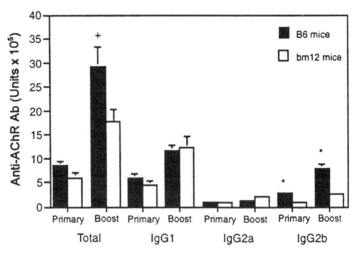

FIGURE 4. Isotypes of AChR antibodies in B6 and bm12 mice. Isotypes of AChR antibodies were determined by kinetic ELISA, as described in the text. Measurement of antibody levels was carried out separately in sera from 7 B6 mice and 8 bm12 mice at 4 weeks after the primary immunization and 2 weeks after the boost. Black bars indicate the mean results ± SEM for B6 mice, and white bars indicate the mean results ± SEM for bm12 mice. Total IgG anti-AChR was significantly higher in B6 mice than in bm12 mice after the boost ($p < 0.05$), and IgG2b was highly significantly greater after the priming immunization and after the boost in B6 mice ($p < 0.01$).

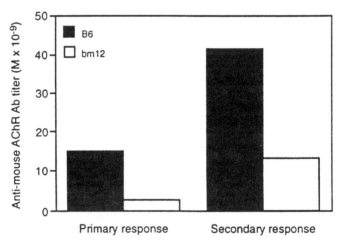

FIGURE 5. Autoantibodies to mouse AChR in B6 and bm12 mice. B6 and bm12 mice were immunized with AChR in CFA and boosted as in FIGURE 4. Measurement of antibodies was performed by immunoprecipitation RIA (see text) and is expressed as moles × 10^{-9} of ^{125}I-α-bungarotoxin precipitated per liter of serum. Black bars represent the mean values for B6 mice, and white bars for bm12 mice. Differences at both time points were significant ($p < 0.05$, Mann-Whitney).

(reviewed in reference 39). T_{H1} cells produce IFNγ and IL2, and provide help for production of IgG2 isotypes by B cells, while T_{H2} cells produce IL4, IL6, and IL10, and provide help for production of IgG1 isotype antibodies by B cells.[39] It has been shown that the specific peptide presented to the T cell may play a key role in determining its T_H type.[40–42] Our findings indicate a bias in B6 mice towards the production of IgG2b, which suggests a predominance of T_{H1}-type help. It is tempting to speculate that the selective response of T cells from B6 mice to the peptide α146–162 may induce T_{H1}-type responses and thus favor IgG2b production. Although we wanted to test this hypothesis directly, it was not feasible using the hybridoma system since the cytokine profile of hybridomas is determined by the parent thymoma cell (not the incorporated TCR). Further studies are needed to elucidate the roles of the helper T cell type and the IgG isotype in determining the severity of EAMG.

Anti-Mouse AChR Autoantibody Levels in B6 and bm12 Mice

Sera collected 4 weeks after the primary immunization and 2 weeks after the boost were assayed for autoantibodies to mouse AChR by radioimmunoassay (RIA). At both time points, the anti-mouse AChR autoantibody levels were significantly higher than those of bm12 mice ($p < 0.05$, FIGURE 5). Following the boost, antibody levels of both B6 and bm12 mice increased markedly.

Epitope Specificity

It has been suggested that production of antibodies of particular epitope specificities may result from "preferential pairing", or the preferred interaction of specific T cells with B cells that produce certain specific antibodies.[43,44] The factors thought to influence such pairing include "protection" of epitopes that are bound to the B cell's specific surface immunoglobulin receptor or an advantage afforded by the particular distance between potential T cell and B cell epitopes within the antigen molecule.[43,44] The possibility that fine specificity of antibodies, resulting from "T-B pairing", may play a role in determining the severity of EAMG in these mice remains to be tested.

SUMMARY AND CONCLUSIONS

Based on our current information, the robust differences in responses of B6 and bm12 mice after immunization with AChR are as follows: (1) The AChR-specific T cell repertoires are strikingly different. The epitope specificities, as well as the rearranged TCR α and β chains and their CDR3 domains, are virtually nonoverlapping in the two strains of mice. (2) The AChR antibody responses are quantitatively different, both to *Torpedo* AChR and to the autoantigen—mouse AChR. (3) The isotype distribution of AChR antibodies favors IgG2b in B6 mice, but not in bm12 mice. (4) The clinical manifestations of EAMG are qualitatively and quantitatively different in the two strains.

These considerations have led to the following scheme, illustrated diagrammatically in FIGURE 2, to explain the differences in EAMG in B6 and bm12 mice:

(1) The MHC Class II of B6 mice binds the α146–162 peptide of *Torpedo* AChR with high affinity, while the genetically altered MHC Class II of bm12 mice does not, as previously suggested[33,34] (see FIGURE 2).

(2) The α146–162/MHC Class II complex occurs only in B6 mice and interacts with T cells having appropriate TCRs, resulting in their stimulation and expansion. Although T cells of appropriate specificity are also available in the bm12 strain,[8,9] the relevant peptide/MHC Class II complex is not present. Therefore, very few T cells with specificity for α146–162 are stimulated, and those that are stimulated have different TCRs. T cells with specificity for other AChR peptides are also present and expanded in both strains of mice, but they have less influence on the outcome of the immune response.

(3) The α146–162-specific T cells of B6 mice, in turn, interact strongly with AChR-specific B cells of B6 mice. These B cells present the same epitope/MHC Class II complex as the APCs and therefore interact well with the α146–162-specific T cells (FIGURE 2). Thus, T cells of this specificity appear to provide more efficient help for AChR antibody production than T cells with specificity for other *Torpedo* AChR epitopes.[36] This results in production of greater amounts of AChR antibodies, including a critical subset that cross-reacts with autologous mouse AChR. The higher autoantibody levels contribute to the greater susceptibility to EAMG and to the greater severity of manifestations in the B6 strain compared with the bm12 strain.

(4) There is a bias in B6 mice toward the production of AChR antibodies of IgG2b isotype. We suggest that T cells specific for α146–162 may contribute to this isotype bias. The IgG2b antibodies appear to have particularly potent "myasthenogenic" effects in rats and mice.[37,45,46]

(5) Finally, it should be emphasized that these differences in immunological and clinical aspects of EAMG in B6 and bm12 mice are relative rather than absolute. T cells that respond to AChR epitopes other than α146–162 can also provide help for AChR antibody production, albeit less potent.

In a sense, this model represents a special case of molecular mimicry.[47] In this case, the source of the foreign antigenic molecule is injection rather than the more usual route of infection. The antigen (*Torpedo* AChR) is one that these mice would never naturally encounter, and the critical amino acid (lysine 155) of the key epitope (α146–162) is present only in the AChR of electric organs of electric fish and not in the AChR of mice, chickens, cows, or humans. The important point is that a detail of the structure of the foreign antigen—that is, a particular peptide of *Torpedo* AChR—can determine the severity of an antibody-mediated autoimmune disease, depending on how it interacts with a detail of the structure of the MHC Class II molecule and, in turn, on how the peptide/MHC Class II complex interacts with the available T cell repertoire.

What principles derived from this model may be applicable to MG and other autoimmune diseases? The fact that the interaction of a single peptide, MHC Class II, and TCR strongly influences the clinical manifestations in this experimental autoimmune disease might provide some hope that similar unique interactions could be involved in MG (or other autoimmune diseases) in human patients and could therefore be manipulated therapeutically. However, even in this highly simplified inbred mouse model, with a fully defined antigenic trigger molecule and a single defined MHC Class II, the factors that contribute to disease severity are extremely complex. Furthermore, even though the most influential peptide (α146–162), the MHC Class II to which it binds (I-A^b), and the details of the relevant TCR (Vα8/Vβ6) have been defined in this model, it is important to recognize that they are not essential to the development of EAMG, but only affect its incidence and severity. In other strains of mice and rats, *Torpedo* AChR may not induce clinical EAMG at all,[1,48] or peptides other than 146–162 may be the clinically important ones.[49] In spontaneous autoimmune diseases in humans, such as MG, the triggering antigens are not known, and the vast polymorphism and multiplicity of MHC Class II molecules in different individuals make the prospect of identifying the relevant interactions staggering. Indeed, the example of EAMG in B6 and bm12 mice underlines the principle of heterogeneity: that is, that the immune system can utilize multiple pathways to produce, modulate, and regulate the level of response. The concept that a single antigenic peptide, or a single MHC Class II molecule, may represent the "key" to pathogenesis and the route to therapy of human autoimmune diseases is at best simplistic. The complexities of the autoimmune response dictate that specific treatment will require co-opting the immune system itself to modify or eliminate the pathogenic reaction.

ACKNOWLEDGMENTS

We are grateful to Sheila Moran and Robert N. Adams for skilled technical help and to Noel Rose and Gary Ketner for helpful discussions throughout these investigations. Toni Claudio, Bianca Conti-Fine, Michael Lenardo, and Jian-Ming Wu generously provided materials and advice, as noted in the text. TABLES 2–5 and FIGURES 1 and 3–5 are reprinted from reference 37 with permission by Academic Press. FIGURE 2 is modified from reference 54 with permission by Saunders.

REFERENCES

1. FUCHS, S., D. NEVA, R. TARRAB-HAZDAI & F. YAAR. 1976. Strain differences in the autoimmune response of mice to acetylcholine receptors. Nature **263:** 329–330.
2. CHRISTADOSS, P., J. M. LINDSTROM, R. W. MELVOLD & N. TALAL. 1985. Mutation at I-A beta chain prevents experimental autoimmune myasthenia gravis. Immunogenetics **21:** 33–38.
3. BELLONE, M., N. OSTLIE, S. LEI, X-D. WU & B. M. CONTI-TRONCONI. 1991. The I-A^{bm12} mutation, which confers resistance to experimental myasthenia gravis, drastically affects the epitope repertoire of murine CD4$^+$ cells sensitized to nicotinic acetylcholine receptor. J. Immunol. **147:** 1484–1491.
4. INFANTE, A. J., P. A. THOMPSON, K. A. KROLICK & K. A. WALL. 1991. Determinant selection in murine experimental autoimmune myasthenia gravis: effect of the bm12 mutation on T cell recognition of acetylcholine receptor epitopes. J. Immunol. **146:** 2977–2982.
5. MCINTYRE, K. & J. SEIDMAN. 1984. Nucleotide sequence of mutant I-A β bm12 gene is ev-

idence for genetic exchange between mouse immune response genes. Nature **308**: 551–553.

6. BELLONE, M., N. OSTLIE, S. LEI & B. M. CONTI-TRONCONI. 1991. Experimental myasthenia gravis in congenic mice: sequence mapping and H-2 restriction of T helper epitopes on the α subunits of *Torpedo californica* and murine acetylcholine receptors. Eur. J. Immunol. **21**: 2303–2310.

7. CHRISTADOSS, P., V. A. LENNON, C. J. KRCO, E. H. LAMBERT & C. S. DAVID. 1981. Genetic control of autoimmunity to acetylcholine receptors: role of Ia molecules. Ann. N.Y. Acad. Sci. **377**: 258–277.

8. KARACHUNSKI, P. I., N. OSTLIE, M. BELLONE, A. J. INFANTE & B. M. CONTI-TRONCONI. 1995. Mechanisms by which the I-A^{bm12} mutation influences susceptibility to experimental myasthenia gravis: a study in homozygous and heterozygous mice. Scand. J. Immunol. **42**: 215–225.

9. INFANTE, A. J., H. LEVCOVITZ, V. GORDON, K. A. WALL, P. A. THOMPSON & K. A. KROLICK. 1992. Preferential use of a T cell receptor Vβ gene by acetylcholine receptor reactive T cells from myasthenia gravis–susceptible mice. J. Immunol. **148**: 3385–3390.

10. INFANTE, A. J., J. FALER, S. CHANG, P. CURRIER, P. THOMPSON, K. KROLICK, K. ZBOROWSKI & E. KRAIG. 1993. T-cell receptor expression in murine myasthenia gravis. Ann. N.Y. Acad. Sci. **681**: 292–294.

11. DRACHMAN, D. B. 1994. Myasthenia gravis. N. Engl. J. Med. **330**: 1797–1810.

12. DRACHMAN, D. B., R. N. ADAMS, E. F. STANLEY & A. PESTRONK. 1980. Mechanisms of acetylcholine receptor loss in myasthenia gravis. J. Neurol. Neurosurg. Psychiatry **43**: 601–610.

13. DRACHMAN, D. B., R. N. ADAMS, L. F. JOSIFEK & S. G. SELF. 1982. Functional activities of autoantibodies to acetylcholine receptors and the clinical severity of myasthenia gravis. N. Engl. J. Med. **307**: 769–775.

14. ENGEL, A. G. & K. ARAHATA. 1987. The membrane attack complex of complement at the endplate in myasthenia gravis. Ann. N.Y. Acad. Sci. **505**: 326–332.

15. OSMAN, G. E., M. TODA, O. KANAGAWA & L. E. HOOD. 1993. Characterization of the T cell receptor repertoire causing collagen arthritis in mice. J. Exp. Med. **177**: 387–395.

16. SHENOY, M., M. OSHIMA, M. Z. ATASSI & P. CHRISTADOSS. 1993. Suppression of experimental autoimmune myasthenia gravis by epitope-specific neonatal tolerance to synthetic region α146–162 of acetylcholine receptor. Clin. Immunol. Immunopathol. **66**: 230–238.

17. LODGE, P. A., M. ALLEGRETTA, L. STEINMAN & S. SRIRAM. 1994. Myelin basic protein peptide specificity and T cell receptor gene usage of HPRT mutant T cell clones in patients with multiple sclerosis. Ann. Neurol. **36**: 734–740.

18. KAPPLER, J. W., B. SKIDMORE, J. WHITE & P. MARRACK. 1981. Antigen-inducible, H-2-restricted, interleukin-2-producing T cell hybridomas: lack of independent antigen and H-2 recognition. J. Exp. Med. **153**: 1198–1214.

19. BORN, W., J. WHITE, R. O'BRIEN & R. KUBO. 1988. Development of T cell receptor expression: studies using T cell hybridomas. Immunol. Res. **7**: 279–291.

20. KRUISBEEK, A. M. 1994. Production of mouse T cell hybridomas. *In* Current Protocols in Immunology. Chapter 3.14, p. 3.14.1–3.14.11. Wiley. New York.

21. YOKOI, T., B. MULAC-JERICEVIC, J. KURISAKI & M. Z. ATASSI. 1987. T lymphocyte recognition of acetylcholine receptor: localization of the full T cell recognition profile on the extracellular part of the α chain of *Torpedo californica* acetylcholine receptor. Eur. J. Immunol. **17**: 1697–1702.

22. CHOMCZYNSKI, P. & N. SACCHI. 1987. Single step method of RNA isolation by acid guanidinium-thiocyanate-phenol-chloroform extraction. Anal. Biochem. **162**: 156–159.

23. YANG, B., R. YOLKEN & R. VISCIDI. 1993. Quantitative polymerase chain reaction by monitoring enzymatic activity of DNA polymerase. Anal. Biochem. **208**: 110–116.

24. SANGER, F., S. NICKLEN & A. R. COULSON. 1977. DNA sequencing with chain terminating inhibitors. Proc. Natl. Acad. Sci. U.S.A. **74:** 5463–5466.

25. ROCK, E. P., P. R. SIBBALD, M. M. DAVIS & Y. CHIEN. 1994. CDR3 length in antigen-specific immune receptors. J. Exp. Med. **179:** 323–328.

26. MCINTOSH, K. R. & D. B. DRACHMAN. 1992. Tolerance to acetylcholine receptor induced by AChR-coupled syngeneic cells. J. Neuroimmunol. **38:** 75.

27. OKUMURA, S., K. MCINTOSH & D. B. DRACHMAN. 1994. Oral administration of acetylcholine receptor: effects on experimental myasthenia gravis. Ann. Neurol. **36:** 704–713.

28. PIERCE, J. L., K. A. ZBOROWSKI, E. KRAIG & A. J. INFANTE. 1994. Highly conserved TCR β chain CDR3 sequences among immunodominant acetylcholine receptor–reactive T cells in murine myasthenia gravis. Int. Immunol. **6:** 775–783.

29. KRAIG, E., J. L. PIERCE, K. Z. CLARKIN, N. E. STANDIFER, P. CURRIER, K. A. WALL & A. J. INFANTE. 1996. Restricted T cell receptor repertoire for acetylcholine receptor in murine myasthenia gravis. J. Neuroimmunol. **71:** 87–95.

30. WU, B., M. SHENOY, E. GOLUSZKO, R. KAUL & P. CHRISTADOSS. 1995. TCR gene usage in experimental autoimmune myasthenia gravis pathogenesis usage of multiple TCRBV. J. Immunol. **154:** 3603–3610.

31. JORGENSEN, J. L., U. ESSER, S. FAZEKAS, B. GROTH, P. A. REAY & M. M. DAVIS. 1992. Mapping T-cell receptor–peptide contacts by variant peptide immunization of single-chain transgenics. Nature **355:** 224–230.

32. CHIEN, Y. & M. M. DAVIS. 1993. How α/β T cell receptors "see" peptide/MHC complexes. Immunol. Today **14:** 597–602.

33. WALL, K. A., J. HU, P. CURRIER, S. SOUTHWOOD, A. SETTE & A. J. INFANTE. 1994. A disease-related epitope of *Torpedo* acetylcholine receptor: residues involved in I-A^b binding, self discrimination, and TCR antagonism. J. Immunol. **152:** 4526–4536.

34. OSHIMA, M. & M. Z. ATASSI. 1995. Effects of amino acid substitutions within the region 62–76 of I-A$^b_\beta$ on binding with and antigen presentation of *Torpedo* acetylcholine receptor α-chain peptide 146–162. J. Immunol. **154:** 5245.

35. KRCO, C. J., C. S. DAVIS & V. A. LENNON. 1992. Mouse T lymphocyte response to acetylcholine receptor determined by T cell receptor for antigen Vβ gene products recognizing Mls-a. J. Immunol. **147:** 3303–3305.

36. THOMPSON, P. A., R. MCATEE, A. J. INFANTE, P. CURRIER, W. BENINATI & K. A. KROLICK. 1994. Vβ-specific immunotoxin selectively kills acetylcholine receptor–reactive lymphocytes from mice with experimental autoimmune myasthenia gravis. Int. Immunol. **6:** 1807–1815.

37. YANG, B., K. R. MCINTOSH & D. B. DRACHMAN. 1998. How subtle differences in MHC class II affect the severity of experimental myasthenia gravis. Clin. Immunol. Immunopathol. **86:** 45–58.

38. DAU, P. C., J. M. LINDSTROM, C. K. CASSEL & E. C. CLARK. 1979. Plasmapheresis in myasthenia gravis and polymyositis. *In* Plasmapheresis and the Immunobiology of Myasthenia Gravis, p. 229–247.

39. MOSMANN, T. R. & R. L. COFFMAN. 1989. Th1 and Th2 cells: different patterns of lymphokine secretion lead to different functional properties. Annu. Rev. Immunol. **7:** 145–173.

40. NICHOLSON, L. B., J. M. GREER, R. A. SOBEL, M. B. LEES & V. K. KUCHROO. 1995. An altered peptide ligand mediates immune deviation and prevents autoimmune encephalomyelitis. Immunity **3:** 397–405.

41. WINDHAGEN, A., C. SCHOLZ, P. HOLLSBERG, H. FUKAURA, A. SETTE & D. A. HAFLER. 1995. Modulation of cytokine patterns of human autoreactive T cell clones by a single amino acid substitution of their peptide ligand. Immunity **2:** 373–380.

42. CHATURVEDI, P., Q. YU, S. SOUTHWOOD, A. SETTE & B. SINGH. 1996. Peptide analogs with

different affinities for MHC alter the cytokine profile of T helper cells. Int. Immunol. **8:** 745–755.

43. PALMER, M. & E. SERCARZ. 1989. Determinant preferences in the relationship between T and B cells specific for lysozyme. *In* The Immune Response to Structurally Defined Proteins: The Lysozyme Model, p. 285. Adenine Press. Boston.

44. BELLONE, M., P. I. KARACHUNSKI, N. OSTLIE, S. LEI & B. M. CONTI-TRONCONI. 1994. Preferential pairing of T and B cells for production of antibodies without covalent association of T and B epitopes. Eur. J. Immunol. **24:** 799–804.

45. WAUBEN, M. H. M., A. C. W. E. HOEDEMAEKERS, Y. M. F. GRAUS, J. P. A. WAGENAAR, W. VAN EDEN & M. H. DE BAETS. 1996. Inhibition of experimental autoimmune myasthenia gravis by major histocompatibility complex class II competitor peptides results not only in a suppressed, but also in an altered immune response. Eur. J. Immunol. **26:** 2866–2875.

46. MCINTOSH, K. R., P. S. LINSLEY, P. A. BACHA & D. B. DRACHMAN. 1997. Immunotherapy of experimental autoimmune myasthenia gravis: selective effects of CTLA4Ig and synergistic combination with an IL2–diphtheria toxin fusion protein. Submitted.

47. VON HERRATH, M. G. & M. B. OLDSTONE. 1996. Virus-induced autoimmune disease. Curr. Opin. Immunol. **8:** 878–885.

48. BERMAN, P. W., J. PATRICK, S. HEINEMANN, F. G. KLIER & J. H. STEINBACH. 1981. Factors affecting the susceptibility of different strains of mice to experimental myasthenia gravis. Ann. N.Y. Acad. Sci. **377:** 237–257.

49. YEH, T-M. & K. A. KROLICK. 1990. T cells reactive with a small synthetic peptide of the acetylcholine receptor can provide help for a clonotypically heterogeneous antibody response and subsequently impaired muscle function. J. Immunol. **144:** 1654–1660.

50. WANG, K., J. L. KLOTZ, G. KISER, G. BRISTOL, E. HAYS, E. LAI, E. GESE, M. KRONENBERG & L. HOOD. 1994. Organization of the V gene segments in mouse T cell antigen receptor α/δ locus. Genomics **20:** 419–428.

51. KOOP, B. F., L. ROWEN, K. WANG, C. L. KUO, D. SETO, J. A. LENSTRA, S. HOWARD, W. SHAN, P. DESHPANDE & L. HOOD. 1994. The human T-cell receptor TCRAC/TCRDC (Cα/Cδ) region: organization, sequence, and evolution of 97.6 kb of DNA. Genomics **19:** 478–493.

52. WILSON, R. K., E. LAI, P. CONCANNON, R. K. BARTH & L. E. HOOD. 1988. Structure, organization, and polymorphism of murine and human T-cell receptor α and β chain gene families. Immunol. Rev. **101:** 149–172.

53. PANNETIER, C., M. COCHET, S. DARCHE, A. CASROUGE, M. ZOLLER & P. KOURILSKY. 1993. The sizes of the CDR3 hypervariable regions of the murine T cell receptor β chains vary as a function of the recombined germ-line segments. Proc. Natl. Acad. Sci. U.S.A. **90:** 4319–4323.

54. ABBAS, A. K., A. H. LICHTMAN & J. S. POBER. 1994. Cellular and Molecular Immunology. Second edition. Saunders. Philadelphia.

T Cell Recognition of the Acetylcholine Receptor in Myasthenia Gravis[a]

BIANCA M. CONTI-FINE,[b,c] DURAISWAMY NAVANEETHAM,[c]
PETER I. KARACHUNSKI,[c] RAGHAVANPILLAI RAJU,[c,d]
BRENDA DIETHELM-OKITA,[c] DAVID OKITA,[c]
JAMES HOWARD, JR.,[e] AND ZENG-YU WANG[c,f]

[c]Department of Biochemistry
College of Biological Sciences
University of Minnesota
St. Paul, Minnesota 55108
and
Department of Pharmacology
School of Medicine
University of Minnesota
Minneapolis, Minnesota 55455

[e]Department of Neurology
University of North Carolina at Chapel Hill
Chapel Hill, North Carolina 27599

INTRODUCTION

Although the symptoms of myasthenia gravis (MG) and its experimental model, experimental autoimmune myasthenia gravis (EAMG), induced by immunization with nicotinic acetylcholine receptor (AChR), are due to the binding of autoantibodies to muscle AChR,[1–5] the anti-AChR CD4+ T cells have been the subject of intense investigations because they may be the prime movers in MG pathogenesis, and specific immunosuppressive treatments of autoimmune CD4+ cells were successful in experimental animals.[6,7]

MG patients have anti-AChR CD4+ cells in the blood and thymus, and anti-AChR CD4+ cell lines that have T helper function can be propagated *in vitro* from these tissues.[1,2,5] In EAMG, the necessity of CD4+ cells for synthesis of anti-AChR antibod-

[a]This work was supported by NINCDS Grant No. NS 23919 and a research grant from the Muscular Dystrophy Association (to B. M. Conti-Fine).
[b]Previously known as Bianca M. Conti-Tronconi.
[d]Present address: Department of Immunology, Mayo Clinic, Rochester, Minnesota 55905.
[f]Z-Y. Wang was a recipient of a postdoctoral fellowship from the Muscular Dystrophy Association.

ies and development of myasthenic symptoms has been demonstrated by different approaches. EAMG can be prevented or ameliorated by interfering with formation of the molecular complexes involved in activation of CD4+ T cells, such as by administration of antibodies against the MHC class II molecules, thus affecting presentation of the AChR epitopes, or of antibodies against the CD4+ marker, thus affecting the interaction between the CD4+ protein and the MHC class II molecules.[8,9] The crucial role of CD4+ cells in EAMG was demonstrated by the finding that disruption of the MHC class II locus in B6 mice, thus eliminating the expression of class II molecules, drastically reduced the T cell and antibody responses against the AChR and prevented EAMG.[10]

Circumstantial evidence suggests that CD4+ T helper cells must have an important role in the pathogenesis of human MG. First, anti-AChR antibodies in MG patients, including those bound to the neuromuscular junction, are primarily high-affinity IgG:[11,12] the presence of high-affinity anti-AChR IgG antibodies implies that T helper factors led to a switch to synthesis of antibodies of the IgG isotype by the anti-AChR B cells and to "maturation" of their affinity. Second, anti-AChR reactive CD4+ T cells are present in the blood and thymus of MG patients, can be propagated in vitro from these tissues, and have T helper function.[1–5] Third, the only obvious and early effect on the anti-AChR immune response of thymectomy—a staple in the treatment of MG—is an immediate and pronounced decrease in the anti-AChR reactivity of circulating T cells.[13] Fourth, treatment of MG patients with anti-CD4+ antibodies abolishes the T cell response in vitro to the AChR and causes clinical and electrophysiological improvement.[14]

We will summarize here studies that we have carried out from 1992 onwards on the AChR recognition by CD4+ T cells in MG patients and on the pathogenic role of CD4+ cells in MG; studies prior to that time are reviewed in the previous volume on MG of this series.[15] Those studies had the following goals: (i) to obtain direct evidence on a pathogenic role of CD4+ T cells in human MG; (ii) to identify the AChR subunits and the individual epitopes recognized by anti-AChR CD4+ T cells; (iii) to investigate whether ocular MG (oMG) and generalized MG (gMG) have distinct characteristics of the CD4+ recognition of the AChR that are related to the pathogenic mechanisms of these different forms of MG; (iv) to investigate how the CD4+ repertoire evolves with time; (v) to determine whether Th1 CD4+ cells, which secrete proinflammatory cytokines and have a role in other autoimmune diseases, are involved in the anti-AChR response; (vi) to identify the characteristics of the T cell receptor (TCR) genes used by the anti-AChR CD4+ cells.

In the course of those studies, we found that a few sequence segments of the AChR form "universal" CD4+ epitopes recognized by most or all MG patients. Thus, we investigated whether the CD4+ cells recognizing those regions can drive the synthesis of pathogenic anti-AChR antibodies and how the ability of the different sequence regions of the AChR to interact with different HLA DR molecules correlates with the presence of universal CD4+ epitopes.

Finally, we carried out similar studies on the normal CD4+ response in humans to two exogenous antigens to which we are commonly exposed, tetanus toxoid (TTD) and diphtheria toxoid (DTD), to compare and contrast the characteristics of a human autoimmune CD4+ response with those of normal responses to exogenous antigens.

CD4+ T CELLS ARE NECESSARY FOR DEVELOPMENT OF ANTI-AChR ANTIBODIES AND MG SYMPTOMS

The severe combined immunodeficiency (SCID) mice have a deletion of the J region,[16] lack mature B and T cells, and tolerate xenografts:[17,18] they are a useful tool to investigate the pathogenic mechanisms of autoimmune diseases because they can be transplanted with human tissues and/or lymphocytes. They can be used to investigate in a simplified experimental setting *in vivo* the mechanisms by which the anti-AChR response in MG patients leads to impairment of the neuromuscular transmission.

Human peripheral blood mononuclear cells (PBMC) can be transplanted successfully in the peritoneal cavity of SCID mice. They survive for at least 12 weeks and produce human antibodies[17–19] because they include all the cellular components necessary for an immune response: CD4+ and CD8+ T cells, B cells, and professional antigen-presenting cells. SCID mice engrafted with PBMC from MG patients developed serum anti-AChR IgG, had human antibody bound to the mouse muscle, and had ultrastructural damage at the end plate, although those studies did not detect clinical signs of EAMG.[20]

We have used SCID mice to investigate the role of CD4+ cells in the pathogenesis of MG. We engrafted SCID mice with PBMC from 17 gMG patients and 5 healthy controls and investigated the appearance of myasthenic weakness, of human IgG and IgM in the blood and at the neuromuscular junctions, and of human anti-AChR antibodies in the blood. We studied the mice for approximately 12 weeks following the engraftment of PBMC in the peritoneal cavity.

Mice engrafted with PBMC of healthy humans developed serum human IgG and IgM, but never had anti-AChR antibodies in the serum or at the neuromuscular junction, nor myasthenic symptoms. Mice engrafted with PBMC from gMG patients developed serum concentrations of human IgG and IgM significantly higher than those observed following engraftment of PBMC from normal subjects, indicating the presence of abnormally active B cells in the PBMC from gMG patients. The higher blood levels of human IgM in mice engrafted with PBMC from gMG patients than from controls suggest that activation of naive B cells by the AChR occurs in gMG patients, prior to the B cell interaction with the T helper cells, and shifts to production of IgG.

Approximately 53% of the mice engrafted with PBMC from gMG patients developed anti-AChR antibody in the blood and 65% had muscle AChR complexed by human antibody. Approximately 66% of the mice developed myasthenic symptoms: several were tested for the presence of human antibodies at the neuromuscular junctions and they were all positive (FIGURE 1).

We investigated the role of CD4+ cells in this form of passively transferred MG by engrafting SCID mice with either PBMC or PBMC depleted of CD4+ cells from 4 gMG patients. Mice engrafted with CD4+-depleted PBMC never developed myasthenic symptoms or anti-AChR antibodies, while mice treated with PBMC from the same patients developed anti-AChR antibodies and MG symptoms with the frequency described above.

Those results directly prove a crucial role of CD4+ cells for the production of pathogenic anti-AChR antibodies and development of MG symptoms.

Patient #1

Patient #2

Patient #3

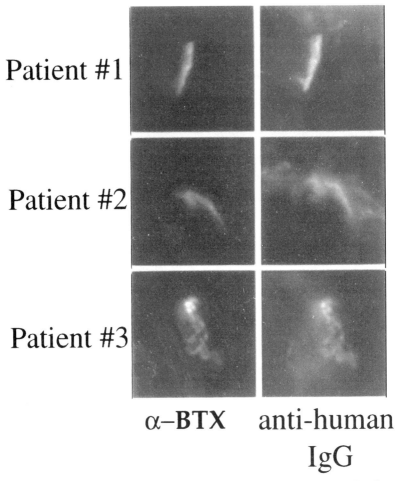

α–BTX   anti-human IgG

FIGURE 1. SCID mice engrafted with PBMC from gMG patients have human IgG at the neuromuscular junctions. The figure shows biopsies of hind limb muscles from three mice, each engrafted from PBMC from a different patient, as indicated on the left. The neuromuscular junctions are identified from the binding of rhodamine-labeled α-bungarotoxin (α-BTX); the presence of human IgG is identified from the binding of a specific phycoerythrin-labeled antibody.

ALL AChR SUBUNITS ARE RECOGNIZED BY ANTI-AChR CD4+ CELLS

Muscle AChR is formed by four homologous subunits and it exists in two developmentally regulated isoforms.[5] Embryonic muscle AChR contains α, β, γ, and δ subunits.[5] Upon innervation, the γ subunit is replaced by a homologous ε subunit.[21] Adult extra ocular muscles (EOM) still express the γ subunit and the embryonic form of the AChR.[22,23]

The α subunit has an important role in MG and EAMG because it forms a domain recognized by most anti-AChR antibodies (main immunogenic region, MIR) and several epitopes recognized by CD4[+] cells.[1-5] In rodent EAMG, the anti-AChR response involves also subunits other than the α: immunization of rats with individual purified AChR α, β, γ, or δ subunits causes EAMG[24] and antibodies and CD4[+] cells of rodents immunized with AChR recognize the α subunit preferentially, but they recognize also other AChR subunits.[25-27]

Little is known about the role of non-α subunits in the anti-AChR response in MG. CD4[+] T cell lines specific for the β, γ, and δ subunits have been propagated from MG patients:[4,5] this suggests a role of those subunits in the anti-AChR CD4[+] response, but does not prove it because the high antigen concentration used for propagation of the lines might cause T cell activation *in vitro* and might yield lines that are not representative of the clonal anti-AChR CD4[+] population *in vivo*.[28] Nothing is known about a role of the ε subunit in MG pathogenesis. The thymus, where the anti-AChR sensitization might start,[29] expresses an AChR-like protein (or proteins) similar or identical to embryonic muscle AChR, containing the γ and not the ε subunit:[30,31] thus, the anti-AChR CD4[+] cells in MG might not recognize the ε subunit at all.

We studied whether anti-AChR CD4[+] cells in MG patients recognize subunits other than the α and whether T cells in gMG and oMG recognize the AChR subunits differently by investigating the human muscle AChR subunits recognized by the blood CD4[+] cells in 25 gMG and 4 oMG patients. We used CD4[+] T cells directly obtained from the blood to avoid misrepresentations of the CD4[+] repertoire resulting from biased clonal propagation *in vitro*. As representative antigens of the human AChR subunits, we used pools of synthetic peptides spanning the sequences of each of the human AChR subunits. We tested the response of CD4[+] cells to those AChR subunit peptide pools in proliferation assays *in vitro*.

The synthetic peptides that we used were approximately 20 residues long, a length that compares with that of naturally processed class II–restricted epitopes, which are 9–14 residues.[32] Extra residues at either end of the epitope sequence do not affect the attachment of the peptide to the binding cleft of the presenting HLA class II molecule, which is open at both its ends. The peptides overlapped by 5–10 residues to reduce the risk of missing epitopes "broken" between peptides. Peptides thus designed are a reasonable compromise between the conflicting needs of reducing the risk of missing epitopes and using peptide panels of manageable size.

Most gMG patients without thymoma recognized all AChR subunits (FIGURE 2). The intensity of the T cell response to the AChR peptide pools was comparable to that of the normal response to TTD. Only 6 out of 22 gMG patients did not recognize all AChR subunits and they were patients whose disease had started recently: as discussed below, the recent onset of their disease is likely related to the recognition of a limited T epitope repertoire on the AChR. One of the 22 gMG patients without thymoma did not recognize the γ subunit and another did not recognize the α subunit. In gMG patients without thymoma, the δ subunit was recognized slightly, yet significantly less than the α and γ subunits: we do not have an explanation for this finding, which might be related to the mechanisms by which the anti-AChR response is triggered and evolves.

The CD4[+] cells of oMG patients recognized consistently only the γ subunit and

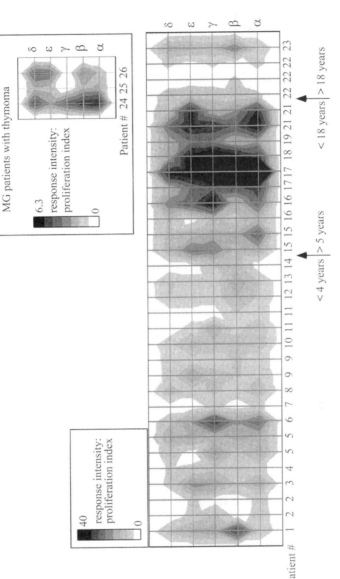

FIGURE 2. Spreading of the T cell response to all AChR subunits during the course of gMG. The results of a proliferation assay using PBMC and CD4+-enriched PBMC from gMG patients are compared with the years elapsed between the first appearance of the symptoms and the time of the assay. We report only the proliferative indices (PI) that were significant, as compared to the spontaneous cell proliferation: they are represented as a contour map. Each vertical line represents the PI obtained with the different AChR subunit peptide pools for one subject in one experiment, as indicated at the bottom of the plot. The subjects, and the different experiments carried out with the same subjects, are arranged in the order determined by the length of time during which they had MG symptoms, starting at the left with the patients whose symptoms had the most recent onset, as indicated at the bottom of the plot. Each horizontal line represents the recognition by the different subjects of one AChR subunit, as indicated at the right of the plot. The intensity of the responses to the peptide pools is represented by the gradations. The main plot reports the results obtained for gMG patients without thymoma; the insert reports those for three thymoma patients.

they never recognized the ε subunit significantly. They occasionally recognized the α, β, and δ subunits. The proliferative responses to the different AChR subunits of the CD4+ cells from oMG patients were much lower than those observed for gMG patients. A low CD4+ T cell response agrees with the low serum concentrations of anti-AChR antibodies in oMG patients.[33]

Thus, oMG and gMG patients differ in the recognition of the γ and the ε subunits. While in gMG the T cell sensitization to these two subunits is comparable, in oMG the γ subunit is recognized predominantly as compared to the other AChR subunits, and the ε subunit is not recognized detectably. The differential recognition of the γ and the ε subunits in oMG and gMG might be related to the distribution of the muscle weakness in these two forms of MG: all the *en grappe* synapses of multiterminal toxic fibers and many *en plaque* synapses of singly innervated fibers in the EOM express an embryonic-like AChR;[23] they are the only synapses of adult muscle that express the fetal AChR isoform, in addition to the adult isoform,[23] and for that reason they might be preferential targets of an anti-AChR response that involves the γ subunit. The finding that some oMG patients have antibodies that uniquely recognize EOM synapses[33] supports the possibility that in oMG the anti-AChR response might focus on the γ subunit.

The thymus expresses an AChR similar to that of embryonic muscle.[30,31,34] Although the thymus may express RNA transcripts for the ε subunit,[35] the lack of reactivity of thymus AChR with antibodies specific for the ε subunit[30] makes it unlikely that the ε subunit protein is expressed significantly in that tissue. If oMG is a form of MG "frozen" in its initial stage, without spreading of the CD4+ response to the adult muscle AChR isotype and of the symptoms to muscle groups other than the EOM, those findings support the possibility that the anti-AChR response is triggered by an embryonic-like AChR within the thymus. Also, the widespread recognition of γ subunit epitopes in both gMG and oMG indicates that a true sensitization of CD4+ cells to the embryonic form of the AChR takes place in MG, and is consistent with the possibility that such sensitization may occur in the thymus. The finding that the adult ε subunit is recognized consistently and vigorously in gMG is well explained by spreading of the T cell response to all parts of the AChR expressed by adult skeletal muscle.

We studied 3 gMG patients with thymoma. One of them recognized all AChR subunits strongly, while the other 2 did not recognize the γ subunit (FIGURE 2). Although the number of thymoma patients that we tested is too small to allow conclusions, those results suggest that gMG patients with thymoma, at difference with all the other MG patients, might recognize the γ subunit to a lesser extent than the other AChR subunits: this might be related to the unique antigenic properties of the AChR-like protein or proteins expressed in thymoma tissue.[5,29]

SPREADING OF THE ANTI-ACHR CD4+ RESPONSE IN MG

In B6 mice, hyperimmunization with AChR focuses the CD4+ response onto one epitope of the AChR α subunit,[25] recognized by highly pathogenic CD4+ cells.[36] Also in Lewis rat EAMG, the pathogenic T cells recognize primarily one epitope on the AChR α subunit.[26,37] On the other hand, in rat experimental autoimmune encephalomyelitis (EAE), the CD4$^+$ response to myelin components may be initiated by sensitization to one epitope and it spreads later to other epitopes within the same or other myelin antigens.[38]

We investigated whether or not anti-AChR CD4$^+$ cells in gMG recognize increasingly larger parts of the AChR molecule as the disease progresses. The population of gMG patients without thymoma that we used for the studies described in the previous section comprised patients in which the onset of the symptoms had occurred from 1 month to 30 years prior to the testing: we compared the ability to recognize the different AChR subunit peptide pools with the duration of the disease (FIGURE 2). The patients that did not recognize some AChR subunits were clustered among those who developed MG less than 4 years prior to the test. Among the patients that had the disease for 5–18 years, all but one recognized all AChR subunits and they had significantly ($p < 0.05$) stronger responses to all AChRs than the patients that had the disease for less than 4 years. One patient did not recognize the ε pool. The patients whose disease had started more than 18 years prior to the test had relatively low responses, which for all but the β subunit were significantly lower than those obtained for the 5–18 year group; the response to the α pool of the patients who had the disease for more than 18 years was also significantly lower than that of the patients that had symptoms for less than 4 years.

Thus, the autoimmune CD4$^+$ response in MG involves the whole AChR molecule, and this results from spreading of the CD4$^+$ sensitization to increasing larger parts of the AChR molecule as the disease progresses and sensitization to an increasing number of AChR subunits. The finding that the responses to the AChR subunit pools were higher in the patients whose disease had lasted for 5 years or longer than in those whose disease had lasted for less than 4 years suggests that also the number of T cells that respond to each AChR subunit increases with time. Longitudinal studies of the same patients[39,40] also indicated that the number of AChR epitopes recognized by CD4$^+$ cells and the number of AChR-specific CD4$^+$ cells change as the disease progresses, consistent with the possibility that T epitope spreading occurs in MG.

The different characteristics of evolution and epitope repertoire of the anti-AChR CD4$^+$ response in MG as compared to rodent EAMG underscore the different immunobiology of spontaneous human autoimmune diseases as compared to their experimental models, induced by immunization with purified autoantigens and adjuvants.

CD4$^+$ T REPERTOIRE ON THE AChR:
IMMUNODOMINANT SEQUENCE REGIONS RECOGNIZED
BY MOST OR ALL MYASTHENIC PATIENTS

We have studied the epitope repertoire of AChR-specific CD4$^+$ cells in MG patients by testing the response to individual overlapping synthetic AChR peptides spanning the sequence of each AChR subunit, of unselected blood CD4$^+$ T cells, and of CD4$^+$ T cell lines enriched with AChR-specific cells by culture *in vitro* with AChR antigens. The use of those two cell populations has different advantages and limitations. AChR-specific CD4$^+$ lines have strong, consistent responses to individual peptides that allow a clear-cut assessment of their epitope repertoire. However, they may have an epitope repertoire different from that of the original CD4$^+$ population due to biased clonal propagation *in vitro*. Also, denatured forms of the antigen such as synthetic and biosynthetic peptides, which are commonly used for propagation of CD4$^+$ cells specific for rare antigens, may be processed into peptide epitopes different from those obtained from processing of the native antigen *in vivo* and may expand CD4$^+$ clones irrelevant for the immune process *in vivo*. The use of unselected T cells or CD4$^+$ T cells from the blood of MG patients avoids the risk of detecting a biased repertoire due to the selective clonal loss or enrichment, but, because of the low frequency of antigen-specific CD4$^+$ cells, reliable testing of nonselected blood CD4$^+$ T cells is not always successful, especially when assessing the response to individual epitopes.

Due to the "orthogonal" advantages and shortcomings of unselected blood CD4$^+$ cells and of AChR-specific CD4$^+$ lines, it was from the combined results of those two approaches that many AChR sequence regions forming CD4$^+$ epitopes could be confidently identified. We tested the response to the individual AChR peptides of the anti-AChR cell lines by proliferation assay, and that of unselected blood CD4$^+$ cells by both proliferation and enzyme-linked immunospot (ELISPOT) assays. The latter assay detects the antigen-induced secretion of interferon-γ (IFN-γ) by individual CD4$^+$ Th1 cells, demonstrating their role in the anti-AChR CD4$^+$ response. These different approaches have given consistent and complementary results.

We have studied the CD4$^+$ epitope repertoire on the AChR α subunit by all three approaches listed above: testing of unselected blood CD4$^+$ cells by proliferation assay and by IFN-γ immunospot assay, and propagation of α subunit–specific CD4$^+$ cell lines and determination of their epitope repertoire. We investigated the CD4$^+$ epitope repertoire on the other AChR subunits using only one or two of those approaches: although less extensive than for the α subunit, those studies yielded repertoires with similar overall characteristics for all of the AChR subunits—a number of sequence regions on each AChR subunit form CD4$^+$ epitopes (TABLE 1); each patient had an individual repertoire, yet a few sequences on each AChR subunit are recognized by all or most patients, irrespective of the MHC haplotype.[39–46] The results of studies on the response of blood CD4$^+$ cells[39,40] or of the CD4$^+$ Th1 subset, discussed below, indicated that those "universal" epitope sequences are recognized by high numbers of T cells. Thus, they should be considered both universal and immunodominant epitope sequences (indicated by bold characters in TABLE 1). Their immunodominance may be related to easy cleavage and processing, and to the ability of human DR molecules to interact with many unrelated peptides, as discussed later.

Thus, while the anti-AChR antibody response in MG is focused on the MIR,[5,6] the anti-AChR CD4$^+$ cells in MG patients recognize a very complex epitope repertoire that involves a large part of the AChR molecule. This reduces the hope for easy development of specific immunosuppressive procedures targeted on epitopes recognized by autoimmune T cells because even the immunodominant epitopes recognized by most MG patients are quite a few.

An interesting question is the transmembrane topology of the sequence regions forming epitopes recognized most frequently by CD4$^+$ cells, and whether those se-

TABLE 1. Sequence Segments of the α, β, γ, δ, and ε Subunits of Human Muscle AChR Forming Epitopes Frequently Recognized by CD4[+] Cells in MG Patients

α Subunit[a]

Region α1–80	Region α101–168	Region α191–207	Region α293–337	Region α387–437
α1–14	**α101–120**	α191–207	α293–308	α387–405
α19–34	**α118–137**		α304–322	**α403–421**
α32–51	α135–154		α320–337	**α419–437**
α48–67	α151–168			
α63–80				

β Subunit[b]

Region β16–50	Region β181–200	Region β271–290	Region β316–350	Region β361–425
β16–35	**β181–200**	**β271–290**	**β316–335**	β361–380
β31–50			**β331–350**	β376–395
				β391–410
				β406–425

γ Subunit[c]

Region γ30–49	Region γ60–124	Region γ135–154	Region γ248–288	Region γ297–355	Region γ366–400	Region γ411–430	Region γ470–495
γ30–49	γ60–79	γ135–154	γ248–267	γ297–312	γ366–385	γ411–430	γ470–489
	γ75–94		γ263–273	γ306–325	γ381–400		γ476–495
	γ90–109		γ269–288	**γ321–340**			
	γ105–124			γ336–355			

δ Subunit[d]

Region δ1–20	Region δ61–80	Region δ91–185	Region δ196–290	Region δ346–392	Region δ461–496
δ1–20	δ61–80	δ91–110	δ196–215	δ346–362	δ461–480
		δ106–125	δ213–230	δ363–386	δ476–496
		δ121–140	δ226–245	δ373–392	
		δ136–155	δ241–260		
		δ151–170	δ256–275		
		δ166–185	δ271–290		

ε Subunit[e]

Region ε51–70	Region ε91–110	Region ε121–170	Region ε231–320	Region ε351–370	Region ε431–473
ε51–70	**ε91–110**	ε121–140	ε231–250	ε351–370	ε431–450
		ε141–160	ε241–260		ε451–470
		ε151–170	ε261–280		ε461–473
			ε281–300		
			ε291–310		
			ε301–320		

[a]From references 39, 42, and 46.
[b]From reference 43.
[c]From references 40 and 45.
[d]From references 40 and 44.
[e]From an unpublished study by Z-Y. Wang *et al.*

quences are likely exposed on the AChR surface. We will discuss here those possible structural features for the CD4[+] epitopes that we have identified on the α subunit: given the similar overall characteristics of the CD4[+] epitope repertoire on all AChR subunits, similar considerations apply to the subunits other than the α. Four AChR α subunit sequences—α48–67, α101–137, α304–322, and the carboxyl-terminal sequence α403–437—are recognized by the majority of the patients, irrespective of their HLA class II type, and by a high number of cells. We will refer to them as universal epitope sequences (UES). The strong response to them is the tip of a response to sequence regions that may include peptide sequences on either side of the UES (see figure 1 of Wang *et al.*[47] elsewhere in this volume). The peptide sequences recognized by 50% or more of the MG patients are clustered in five sequence regions. One corresponds to residues 1–14; the second corresponds to residues α48–80 and comprises peptides α48–67 and α63–80; the third corresponds to residues α101–154 and includes peptides α101–120, α118–137, and α135–154; the fourth corresponds to residues α304–337 and includes peptides α304–322 and α320–337; and the fifth corresponds to residues α403–437 and includes peptides α403–421 and α419–437. Most of the α subunit sequences recognized by the CD4[+] cells correlate with the sequence regions that form nontransmembrane domains, which are believed to be at least partially exposed on the AChR surface. Three UES should be extracellular or should include extracellular parts. The UES region α48–80 neighbors with, and includes, residues α67–76, which are involved in formation of the MIR.[5] The sequence region α101–154 includes a putative extracellular sequence region between two cysteine residues at positions 128 and 142, which must be at least partially exposed on the AChR surface because it is glycosylated.[5] Sequence regions homologous to the UES α304–322 are exposed on the cytoplasmic surface in other AChRs.[48] The amino-terminus of all AChR subunits is extracellular, although it is not clear whether it is exposed on the AChR surface because it is accessible to the binding of Ab only after mild denaturation of the AChR.[48] The fifth UES, α403–437, includes both the carboxyl-terminal end of the α subunit (residues α428–437), which is hydrophilic and likely exposed on the extracellular surface, and the hydrophobic segment α409–427, which is believed to form a transmembrane α helix, called M4.[5,48] Three other transmembrane segments are believed to exist in α and in the other AChR subunits, called M1 (residues α211–236), M2 (residues α242–261), and M3 (residues α277–298).[5,48] These putative transmembrane regions largely correspond to three peptides that were recognized by the CD4[+] cells of MG patients: α214–234, α246–264, and α280–297 (see figure 1 of Wang *et al.*[47] elsewhere in this volume). Hydrophobic sequences in the core of a protein may form epitopes and even UES for human CD4[+] T cells, provided that they are flanked by sequence loops exposed on the surface of the molecule and accessible to the processing enzymes.[49]

The UES identified by the use of CD4[+] T cell lines propagated from MG patients by stimulation with a pool of synthetic peptides spanning the α subunit sequence[42] and those identified by the use of unselected blood CD4[+] cells[39,46] corresponded very well. This verifies that, as shown in many other human and experimental systems,[28] synthetic peptides can be used for propagation of antigen-specific CD4[+] cell lines. The use of nonselected CD4[+] blood cells identified a broader repertoire than that detectable with α subunit–specific CD4[+] cell lines, indicating that the use of peptide sequences as stimulators results in preferential propagation of the CD4$^+$ cells specific for the most immunogenic parts of the antigen.

TH1 CELLS ARE INVOLVED IN THE ANTI-AChR RESPONSE IN MG

CD4$^+$ cells comprise different subpopulations (Th0, Th1, and Th2), which differ in the cytokines that they produce and in their effector functions. Th1 cells secrete interleukin-2 and interferon-γ (IFN-γ), provide helper function only for particular immunoglobulin classes and subclasses, and have cytolytic activity against antigen-presenting cells. Th2 cells secrete interleukin-4 and interleukin-5, provide help for most immunoglobulin classes, and do not have cytolytic potential. Th0 cells have features of both the Th1 and the Th2 cells and they may be precursors of either of those subsets.[50]

Th1 cells secrete cytokines that stimulate inflammatory responses, while Th2 cells secrete anti-inflammatory cytokines.[50] In multiple sclerosis and EAE, the pathogenic CD4$^+$ cells are Th1: the acute phases of those diseases are associated with high activity of the Th1 subset and with release of proinflammatory cytokines, while remission of the symptoms correlates with high activity of the Th2 subset and with release of anti-inflammatory factors.[51–53]

Two studies investigated the cytokines expressed by the PBMC of MG patients after exposure to AChR:[54,55] a variety of cytokines was expressed and it was not possible to identify which CD4$^+$ subset(s) responded to the AChR. The antigen-specific T cells in the PBMC are but a very small fraction and their response was likely obfuscated by that of nonspecific T cells.

We investigated the role of Th1 cells in MG using two approaches. In the first studies, we propagated from MG patients anti-AChR CD4$^+$ T cell lines specific for different AChR subunits or for individual AChR epitopes and tested the lines for interleukin-2 or interleukin-4 production after challenge with the relevant AChR sequences.[43–46] Most lines uniquely secreted interleukin-2, indicating that they comprised Th1 cells only. Recently, we investigated the presence and frequency in the blood of MG patients of Th1 cell precursors specific for individual epitopes of the AChR α subunit.[46] We used overlapping synthetic peptides to screen the α subunit sequence and an ELISPOT assay that detects antigen-induced IFN-γ secretion of individual Th1 cells. This approach is sensitive, allows direct detection of the Th1 response, and gives a qualitative assessment of the relative frequency of the epitope-specific clones. Thus, it allows conclusions on the relative importance of different AChR epitope sequences for sensitization of the autoimmune anti-AChR CD4$^+$ cells. All patients recognized a pool of all the α subunit peptides. All but one patient recognized numerous peptides. Each patient had an individual pattern of peptide recognition, but most or all patients recognized four sequences (residues 48–67, 101–137, 304–322, and 403–437) that stimulated relatively large numbers of Th1 cells. They included the previously identified UES recognized by CD4$^+$ T cell lines and blood CD4$^+$ T cells from MG patients discussed in the previous section. Peptide 1–14 was also recognized frequently. The healthy controls recognized with a low precursor frequency the pool of α peptides and a few individual peptide sequences that frequently included the immunodominant sequences described above.

Those results demonstrated that Th1 cells are involved in the anti-AChR response in MG and that their epitope repertoire is very complex. The finding that all of the sequence regions of the α subunit previously identified as forming epitopes recognized by T cells or CD4[+] T cells in MG[4,5] are included in the repertoire recognized by the Th1 cells[46] suggests that the results obtained by studying the response of the total T cell or the total CD4[+] population might have reflected the response of the Th1 subset. Other observations implicate IFN-γ, secreted by the Th1 cell, in the development of MG and EAMG. Both MG patients and Lewis rats with EAMG have high levels of AChR-reactive lymphocytes that secrete IFN-γ and express IFN-γ mRNA.[55,57,58] Transgenic mice that produce IFN-γ at the neuromuscular junction develop functional disruption of the junction and clinical weakness reminiscent of MG.[59]

All of the healthy subjects that we tested had low numbers of CD4[+] Th1 cells that responded to the AChR α subunit. Several studies demonstrated that normal subjects frequently have T cells that respond *in vitro* to different autoantigens, including the AChR.[5] T cells that recognize self epitopes with low affinity may escape clonal deletion[60] and they may never be activated due to the low affinity of their TCR. Also, priming of naive CD4[+] cells requires costimulatory signals[61] that can be delivered only by professional antigen-presenting cells: in their absence, engagement of the TCR, as might occur in healthy people, leads to T cell tolerization rather than to activation.

AChR RESIDUES FORMING UNIVERSAL CD4[+] EPITOPES

The finding that a few sequence regions of the AChR, 20 residues long, are the most-frequent target of autoimmune CD4[+] T cells in all or most MG patients has potential implications for development of epitope-specific immunosuppressive procedures.[6,7] Also, it raises questions related to the immunobiology of MG, such as whether the T cells that recognize these immunodominant regions are oligoclonal or polyclonal, and whether they recognize one epitope or different overlapping epitopes within those regions.

Short-term polyclonal lines specific for the immunodominant AChR sequence regions can be easily propagated *in vitro* by cycles of stimulation with synthetic AChR peptides.[5] Given the short time of propagation and the limited potential for biased clonal selection, they should be representative of the clonal repertoire of the CD4[+] cells recognizing epitopes within each immunodominant sequence region.[28] We challenged those lines with single residue–substituted analogues of the relevant immunodominant sequence regions to define the residues involved in formation of "universal" epitopes, to obtain clues about the clonality of the lines, and (if they are polyclonal) to understand whether they recognize one epitope or different overlapping epitopes:[56] the response to the peptide analogues of polyclonal lines recognizing overlapping epitopes would be abolished by substitutions of "core" residues, common to all epitopes, and only partially affected by substitutions of residues included in some, but not all epitopes.

We investigated four UES—α48–67, α304–322, γ75–94, and γ321–340.[56] That study indicated that CD4$^+$ T cells from different MG patients, of the same or different DR haplotypes, recognize the same 10–12-residue sequence segments (FIGURE 3). In the same patient, the CD4$^+$ T cells recognizing a given UES were polyclonal and recognized overlapping epitopes: their response was abolished by some substitutions, identifying residues common to all epitopes within a given region, while other substitutions reduced (but did not obliterate) the response, indicating residues included in some, but not all epitopes recognized by the line. Comparison of the residues involved in epitope formation for different lines supported the conclusion that, within the 20-residue UES that we investigated, the same sequence segment is involved in formation of universal epitope(s) in DR-discordant patients. Within region α48–67, the segment 55–63 contained most or all of the residues involved in T cell activation for all lines from two different patients (DR4/w53 and DR7/w53 restricted). Within the region α304–322, residues 311–318 were involved in formation of all or most of the epitopes recognized by four lines from two different patients, both DR4/w53 restricted. Epitope recognition by one line from each patient was susceptible to substitutions outside the segment α311–318. Within region γ75–94, the segment 76–88 contained all residues involved in epitope(s) formation for three different patients, restricted by DR2/w51 and DR1. Within region γ321–340, the segment 324–332 contained residues involved in epitope formation for three lines from two different patients, all restricted by DR2/w51.

Since each DR molecule can bind a broad range of peptides, which largely overlap the peptide repertoire bound by other DR molecules, a universal DR-binding motif has been proposed, composed of an aromatic or hydrophobic residue (W, F, Y, V, I, L) at position 1, a noncharged and relatively small residue (A, V, I, L, P, C, S, T) at position 6, and another relatively hydrophobic residue (A, V, I, L, C, T, S, Y) at position 9.[62] Perusal of the residues crucial for CD4$^+$ activation within the AChR UES that we studied indicates that at least residues 1 and 6 of that proposed motif are present in all of them.[56] Within the sequence α48–67, they could be L_{56} and V_{61}, both necessary for activation of the lines. Within the sequence α304–322, they could be V_{312} and I_{317}. Within the sequence γ75–94, they could be W_{76} and P_{81}, V_{77} and S_{82}, or L_{78} and W_{83}. The sequence region γ321–340 seems to have all three residues of the proposed motif, that is, V_{324} (position 1), L_{329} (position 6), and L_{332} (position 9).

Comparison of the residues crucial for epitope formation within the sequence regions α48–67 and α304–322 (FIGURE 3) revealed a curious common motif: the residues crucial for CD4$^+$ cell activation of all the lines tested included a hydrophobic residue followed by a positively charged residue (L_{56} and K_{57}; V_{312} and R_{313}; we refer to them as position 1 and 2), followed at position 5 by an aromatic residue (W_{60}, F_{316}), at position 6 by a hydrophobic residue (V_{61}, I_{317}), and at position 7 by a negatively charged residue (D_{62}, D_{318}). In most cases, substitutions of any of these residues obliterated or strongly decreased the response of the lines. Because all lines recognizing those consequence regions were restricted by the DR4 or DR7 alleles, which both coexpress the DRw53 molecules, this common sequence motif might be due to presentation of epitope(s) by the common isotype DRw53.

The finding that the same sequence segments within the UES are involved in

Sequence region α 48-67

			I49 V50 T51 T52 N53 V54 R55 L56 K57 Q58 Q59 W60 V61 D62 Y63 N64 L65 K66 W67
DR4,DRw53	Pat. #1	Line 1	- - - + ‡ - - ‡ ‡ - ‡ ‡ ‡ + + - - -
		Line 2	- - - - - - ‡ ‡ + ‡ ‡ + ‡ + ‡ - - - - -
DR7,DRw53	Pat. #2	Line 1	- - - - - - ‡ ‡ ‡ ‡ ‡ ‡ ‡ ‡ ‡ - - - -
		Line 2	- - - - - - - ‡ ‡ ‡ ‡ ‡ ‡ ‡ + - - - -

Sequence region α 304-322

			S304 T305 H306 V307 M308 P309 N310 V311 V312 R313 K314 V315 F316 D317 D318 L319 I320 P321 N322
DR4,DRw53	Pat. #1	Line 1	- - - + + + - ‡ ‡ ‡ ‡ ‡ ‡ ‡ ‡ + - ‡ +
		Line 2	- - - - - - - - + ‡ ‡ ‡ ‡ ‡ ‡ ‡ - - - -
	Pat. #3	Line 1	- - - - - - + ‡ ‡ ‡ ‡ ‡ - ‡ - + ‡ ‡ -
		Line 2	- - - - - - - + ‡ ‡ ‡ ‡ ‡ ‡ ‡ - - - -

Sequence region γ 75-94

			L75 W76 V77 T78 Q79 L80 R81 P82 V83 S84 S85 M86 V87 W88 R89 P90 D91 L92 E93 N94
DR2,DRw51	Pat. #4	Line 1	- ‡ ‡ ‡ ‡ + ‡ - + - - - - - - - - - - -
		Line 2	- - + ‡ + + + - - - - - ‡ + - - - - - -
	Pat. #5	Line 1	- ‡ ‡ ‡ ‡ ‡ ‡ + ‡ + - - ‡ + - - - - - -
		Line 2	- ‡ ‡ ‡ ‡ ‡ ‡ ‡ + ‡ ‡ ‡ - - ‡ ‡ - - - + -
DR1	Pat. #6		- ‡ ‡ + ‡ + - - ‡ + + + + + - - - - ‡ -

Sequence region γ 321-340

			V321 R322 K323 V324 F325 L326 R327 L328 Q329 P330 L331 L332 G333 L334 M335 H336 V337 R338 P339 L340
DR2,DRw51	Pat. #1		- - - ‡ ‡ ‡ ‡ ‡ ‡ ‡ ‡ ‡ ‡ ‡ ‡ ‡ + - + - -
	Pat. #4	Line 1	- - - ‡ ‡ ‡ ‡ - ‡ ‡ + ‡ - - - - - - + - -
		Line 2	- - - ‡ ‡ ‡ ‡ - ‡ ‡ - ‡ - ‡ - - - - - - -

FIGURE 3. Effect of single-residue substitutions of peptide sequences of the AChR α and γ subunits containing UES on the response of the specific CD4+ lines propagated from MG patients. The response of the lines was abolished by some substitutions, identifying residues common to all epitopes within a given region and including those involved in interaction with the DR molecule(s), while other substitutions reduced, but did not obliterate the response, indicating residues included in some, but not all of the epitopes recognized by the line. The plus or minus symbols represent the effect of the individual substitution of the response of the line, as compared to the unmodified peptide, as follows: –, the response of the line to the analogue was 75% or more of that to the unmodified peptide; +, the response to the analogue was 50–75% of that to the unmodified peptide; ++, the response to the analogue was 25–50% of that to the unmodified peptide; +++, the response to the analogue was 25% or less of that to the unmodified peptide. Figure and legend reprinted with permission from reference 56.

CD4$^+$ epitope formations in all MG patients is potentially useful for development of peptide analogues able to inhibit pathogenic T cell response.

CD4$^+$ CELLS THAT RECOGNIZE UNIVERSAL AChR EPITOPES CAN DRIVE THE SYNTHESIS OF PATHOGENIC ANTI-AChR ANTIBODIES

Some AChR epitopes dominate also the sensitization of CD4$^+$ cells in mice, and tolerization of the CD4$^+$ cells recognizing even just one of those dominant epitopes can protect from development of EAMG.[63] On the other hand, other AChR sequences sensitize mouse CD4$^+$ cells of lesser or no pathogenic potential, whose tolerization does not affect EAMG development.[63] To understand whether similar epitope-specific tolerization of pathogenic CD4$^+$ cells could be suitable for the treatment of MG, we investigated whether the immunodominant universal sequences described above are recognized by CD4$^+$ cells able to drive the synthesis of pathogenic antibodies.

We used the SCID mouse model of MG and determined the effects on appearance of human IgG, anti-AChR antibodies, and MG symptoms of engraftment into SCID mice of PBMC, CD4$^+$-depleted PBMC from the same patient, or CD4$^+$-depleted PBMC supplemented with a CD4$^+$ line from the same patient that was specific for a given immunodominant universal epitope of the α subunit. The lines were propagated by cycles of stimulations *in vitro* with individual 20-residue synthetic peptides, corresponding to a given α subunit universal CD4$^+$ epitope. As controls, we used DTD- or TTD-specific CD4$^+$ lines from the same patients.

SCID mice engrafted with PBMC developed anti-AChR antibodies and myasthenic symptoms, while the mice engrafted with CD4$^+$-depleted PBMC or with PBMC supplemented with CD4$^+$ cell lines specific for DTD or TTD did not present myasthenic weakness. Addition to the CD4$^+$-depleted PBMC of any (but one) of the CD4$^+$ cell lines specific for α subunit universal epitopes induced myasthenic weakness in 25–50% of the engrafted mice and appearance of human anti-AChR antibody in the serum and at the neuromuscular junction of most mice.

Those findings clearly demonstrate that most of the anti-AChR CD4$^+$ T cells specific for the UES of the α subunit can drive the synthesis of pathogenic anti-AChR antibodies that cause myasthenic weakness and strongly support an important role of those immunodominant sequence regions in the pathogenesis of MG. Those results underline the usefulness of synthetic epitope sequences for the propagation and study of autoimmune CD4$^+$ cells of pathogenic relevance.

CD4$^+$ CELLS THAT RECOGNIZE UNIVERSAL AChR EPITOPES HAVE A RESTRICTED, BUT INDIVIDUAL USAGE OF THE TCR Vβ GENE FAMILIES

An important question in the biology of both normal and autoimmune T cells is how the structure of the TCR relates to the peptide epitope/MHC molecule complex that is specifically recognized.

We analyzed the TCR Vβ usage of 16 anti-AChR CD4$^+$ polyclonal cell lines specific for immunodominant AChR epitopes, using a semiquantitative polymerase chain reaction assay.[64] The lines had been propagated from MG patients using pools of overlapping peptides corresponding to the sequence of an AChR subunit or individual synthetic peptides containing immunodominant epitopes: in either case, the lines recognized the peptides that we identified previously as forming UES (see previous sections). The lines had been propagated for relatively short periods of time (12 lines for less than two months, 4 lines for less than five months) to reduce the risk of biased clonal propagation. We found that most lines had limited Vβ usage: in most cases, different Vβ regions were used for different epitopes in the same patient and for the same epitope in different patients. A few patients used the same Vβ regions for recognition of different epitopes. The Vβ4 and Vβ6 regions were used most frequently.

Those results agree well with those of a previous study, which also concluded that there is a restricted, but individual heterogeneity among the TCR Vβ and Vα gene transcripts used by anti-AChR T cells from MG patients.[65] Thus, the potentially autoimmune T cells that survive clonal deletion have a limited TCR repertoire. The finding that different Vβ families were used in different patients does not support an important role of a superantigen in maintenance of the anti-AChR CD4$^+$ response, but does exclude the intervention of a superantigen in triggering the anti-AChR response because, in principle, activation of autoimmune CD4$^+$ cells specific for one epitope might start an autoimmune response:[66] the epitope spreading that occurs as autoimmune responses develop[66,67] may obfuscate the epitope specificity and TCR usage of the CD4$^+$ populations originally expanded by a superantigen.

BINDING OF AChR α AND γ SUBUNIT SEQUENCES TO PURIFIED DR MOLECULES

We investigated the relationship between immunodominance of AChR sequences for sensitization of CD4$^+$ T cells and ability to bind to different DR molecules—the most-common restriction elements of AChR epitopes.[4,5]

In one study,[68] we first identified the alleles DR2/w51, DR4/w53, and DR7/w53 as the restriction elements for CD4$^+$ recognition of immunodominant AChR epitopes on the α subunit. Then, we investigated the ability of overlapping synthetic peptides spanning the α subunit sequence to bind to the corresponding purified DR molecules and to the DR1 molecule (DRB1*0101, DRB1*0201, DRB1*0401, and DRB1*0701). The binding assay that we used assessed the ability of the test peptide to competitively block the binding to different purified DR molecules of two radiolabeled test peptides of known DR-binding characteristics. FIGURE 4 shows the percentage of inhibition caused by the different AChR peptides. The AChR peptides that stimulated anti-AChR autoimmune CD4$^+$ cells all bound to the relevant DR molecules. Among them, the α subunit peptides forming immunodominant CD4$^+$ epitopes consistently bound to most or all of the molecules tested. However, some AChR peptides that were never recognized by CD4$^+$ cells of MG patients also bound well to one or more DR molecules. We obtained similar results in another study that investigated

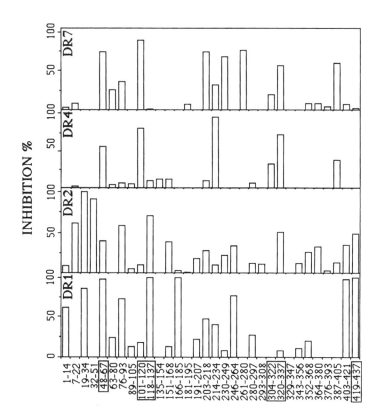

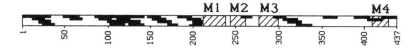

FIGURE 4. Inhibition of the binding of the ^{125}I-radiolabeled test peptides TT830–849 (to DR2/w51, DR4/w53, DR7/w53) and YH 307–324 (to DR1) to purified DR molecules, as indicated in the different panels, by 100 µM of different AChR synthetic sequences, as indicated along the abscissa. The columns represent the percent of inhibition of the binding of the ^{125}I-radiolabeled probe peptides. The peptides comprised within the AChR sequence regions known to contain epitopes important for CD4+ cell sensitization, that is, recognized by CD4+ cells of all or most MG patients, are indicated in open boxes. At the bottom of the figure, we depict a schematic representation of the CD4+ epitopes so far identified in different studies on the human AChR α subunit: the sequence regions identified as forming CD4+ epitopes are indicated as black boxes; those forming the putative transmembrane segments M1–M4 are also indicated. Figure and legend reprinted with permission from reference 68.

the binding to the same purified DR molecules of overlapping synthetic peptides spanning the human γ subunit sequence.[69] All peptides recognized by CD4[+] cells bound[40,45] to the relevant DR molecule, and the UES γ75–94 and γ321–340 bound to most or all of the DR molecules studied. Some γ subunit peptides not recognized by CD4[+] cells of MG patients bound well to one or more DR molecules.

Similar studies on DR binding of exogenous antigen peptides[70] yielded results similar to those that we obtained with the AChR: some sequence regions uniquely bound to one DR molecule; others bound to several DR molecules; others still did not bind any of the DR molecules used.

CD4[+] RESPONSES TO TETANUS AND DIPHTHERIA TOXOIDS: SIMILARITIES AND DIFFERENCES WITH THE ANTI-AChR RESPONSE

Two interesting characteristics of the CD4[+] response to the AChR in MG are the presence on the AChR of immunodominant epitopes, recognized by most or all MG patients, and the restricted TCR Vβ usage of the CD4[+] cells recognizing the UES. To find out whether those features are shared by normal CD4[+] responses to exogenous antigens, we studied the CD4[+] response of healthy subjects to TTD and DTD—two protein antigens to which we are all exposed due to mass vaccination against diphtheria and tetanus. Also, the three-dimensional structure of DTD is known[71] and this allowed us to correlate structural properties of the antigen with presence of UES, and to find out whether intrinsic structural properties of the antigen have a role in determination of the CD4[+] immunodominance of particular sequence regions of the antigen. That possibility was suggested by the consistent findings, summarized above, that promiscuous DR binding is necessary, but not sufficient, for a sequence to form a UES.

In one study[72] we identified the sequence regions of TTD-forming CD4[+] epitopes in eight HLA-disparate subjects. The TTD molecule includes two subunits, the L chain (456 residues) and the H chain (858 residues).[73] We used 87 overlapping synthetic peptides, similar in length and overlap to those used to test the anti-AChR CD4[+] cells, spanning the sequences of both TTD subunits, to test in proliferation assay unselected blood CD4[+] cells and CD4[+] lines propagated by stimulation with TTD of the PBMC of the same subjects. The peptides are indicated with codes that include the letter L or H for the L and H chain, and two numbers referring to the position of the first and the last residue of the peptide of the L and H chain sequences. The CD4[+] lines recognized most of the peptides recognized by the blood CD4[+] cells, plus additional peptides. Their responses were stronger than those of unselected blood CD4[+] cells. Several peptides were recognized by each of the subjects studied (FIGURE 5). Two peptides, corresponding to residues H176–195 and H491–510 of the TTD heavy chain, were recognized by all subjects: they elicited vigorous responses by the CD4[+] lines and were frequently recognized better than most other TTD sequences by the blood CD4[+] cells. The response of the CD4[+] lines to those two peptides alone accounted for 8–40% of the total response of the cell lines to the TTD sequences: thus, they can be considered UES. Peptide H491–510 overlaps a TTD sequence region previously identified[74] as a universal T epitope, and peptide H176–195 overlaps a se-

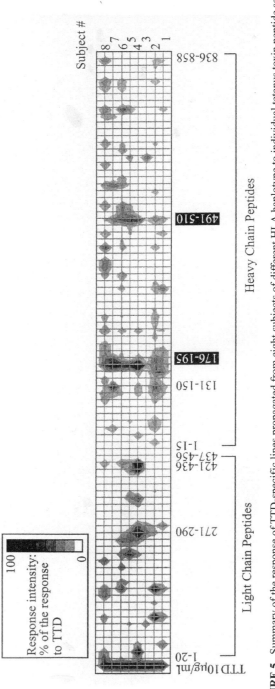

FIGURE 5. Summary of the response of TTD-specific lines propagated from eight subjects of different HLA haplotype to individual tetanus toxin peptide sequences, represented as a contour map. Each horizontal strip represents the results obtained with the CD4+ line of one subject, as indicated at the right of the plot. The response of the lines to TTD is reported at the extreme left of the plot and it is followed by the response to the individual peptides (one peptide for each vertical line), starting with the amino-terminal sequence of the L chain and ending, at the extreme right, with the carboxyl-terminal sequence of the H chain. The responses to the peptide are represented relative to the response to TTD, using the gradations. Figure and legend reprinted with permission from reference 72.

quence region that another study found to be frequently recognized by PBMC of humans.[75] Thirteen other peptides elicited a CD4+ response in six or seven of the eight subjects studied and another ten peptides did so in five of the eight subjects. Similar to what occurs for the CD4+ recognition of AChR sequences, the strong response to the UES in the TTD molecule is the "tip" of a response to sequence regions that include peptide sequences on either side of the UES (FIGURE 5). Other TTD sequence regions strongly recognized by most subjects are those flanking and including peptides L271–290 and H131–150 (FIGURE 5). The sequence region comprising the overlapping peptides L406–425 and L421–436 was recognized by only five subjects, but very strongly (FIGURE 5).

Many TTD epitopes were preferentially or uniquely presented by only one of the DR/DQ alleles of the donor, while the immunodominant peptides H176–195 and H491–510 were always presented by both alleles of the subject.[72] Thus, the UES peptides might be "universally" recognized because of their ability to bind different class II isotypes and different alleles of the same isotype.

In another study,[49] we used the same approach to identify sequence regions of the DTD molecule recognized by CD4+ cells of seven healthy humans of different HLA haplotype. Overlapping synthetic peptides, screening the DTD sequence, were used to test in proliferation assays unselected blood CD4+ cells or DTD-specific CD4+ lines propagated by stimulation with DTD of the PBMC of those same subjects. Blood CD4+ cells and DTD-specific CD4+ lines gave consistent results. Although each subject had an individual pattern of peptide recognition, six peptide sequences (residues 271–290, 321–340, 331–350, 351–370, 411–430, and 431–450) were recognized by all subjects. Recognition of those peptides accounted for a substantial fraction of the total response of the CD4+ lines to DTD sequences (28–57%). Also, the unselected blood CD4+ cells recognized those peptides strongly, at levels comparable to the response induced by the complete DTD molecule, in spite of the overall low responses of the unselected blood CD4+ cells. Those UES peptides were frequently presented by more than one class II isotype.

In the native DTD molecule, all the UES include, or are flanked by at the amino- and carboxyl-terminal ends, sequence regions forming relatively unstructured loops fully exposed to the solvent, which may be easily accessible targets for the proteolytic enzymes involved in antigen processing, even in the absence of any substantial denaturation of the antigen. Like for the AChR, in the DTD some UES are hydrophobic and are contained in the core of the molecule. Those findings directly demonstrate that sequence segments "hidden" in the hydrophobic core of a protein antigen might be important targets of immune recognition by CD4+ T cells and underscore the importance for UES formation of flanking exposed loops, which would make an easy target for processing enzymes, resulting in the fast release of even sequence segments embedded in the hydrophobic core of the antigen molecule.

The UES must have characteristics compatible with binding to a large number of different class II molecules. X-ray diffraction study of the DR1 molecule indicated that several residues involved in formation of the peptide binding site are conserved in most or all class II isotypes, suggesting that all class II molecules bind peptides with similar mechanisms.[32] In agreement with that prediction, the UES of both DTD and TTD were frequently recognized in association with different class II isotypes.[49,72] Peptides bind to DR molecules in an extended conformation, which allows extensive hydrophobic interactions between the peptide backbone and the binding groove of the DR molecules, thus providing a mode of peptide binding independent of the peptide sequence.[32] Specificity and further affinity of the binding between peptides and different DR alleles are due to interactions between pockets on the DR molecules, whose surfaces have shapes and charges characteristic for a given DR allele, and anchor residues of suitable size, hydropathic properties, and charge in the peptide.[32,76] Although as many as seven anchor residues have been identified, at least for a DR4 subtype,[76] only one or very few residues are crucial for binding,[76] and the others, while improving the affinity of the binding, tolerate a broad range of substitutions without obliterating the peptide/DR interaction.[76,77] While anchor residues are frequently uncharged or hydrophobic, both positively and negatively charged anchor residues have been identified for peptide binding to individual DR alleles, fitting in pockets, on the DR molecule, lined by residues of complementary charge.[32,76,77] Because the lining of DR-binding pockets may have charges,[76,78] the presence of the wrong charge on a peptide residue aligned with that pocket likely destabilizes peptide/DR binding.

All the UES that we identified on the DTD sequence overlap four of the five DTD sequence segments which are mostly hydrophobic: four of those segments do not contain any charged residue and one (segment 353–371) contains one charge.[49] However, the uncharged nature of a DTD peptide sequence is not predictive of a UES because some peptides that largely overlapped an uncharged sequence region were not recognized by all the subjects.[49] Also, all the UES included residues outside the hydrophobic regions described above, some of which are charged.[49] Keeping in mind the *caveats* listed above, it is possible that the presence of a stretch of uncharged residues might be related with UES formation because, although charged residues may be present in DR-binding pockets and may function as anchor residues in DR-binding peptides, uncharged sequence segments might be preferred as "universal" DR binders since charged residues carrying a "wrong" charge would strongly and negatively affect peptide binding to some class II molecules.

Recently, we investigated in a population of 21 healthy subjects the ability of blood CD4$^+$ cells to recognize the UES identified previously on the DTD and TTD sequences. CD8$^+$-depleted, CD4$^+$-enriched PBMC of 21 healthy subjects were challenged in proliferation assay with each of the DTD and TTD UES peptides and with the complete DTD and TTD molecules. All subjects recognize the two TTD UES and most of the DTD UES. The responses to those peptides were in general comparable to those induced by the complete DTD and TTD molecules.

Thus, the presence of sequence regions forming universal, immunodominant epitopes appears to be a common occurrence for CD4$^+$ recognition of protein antigens in humans. The structural properties identified for UES on the DTD molecule (presence of exposed residues, easily accessible sequence loop at both ends, and preference for uncharged residues) may be general requirements for immunodominance in CD4$^+$ cell sensitization in humans.

We have studied the TCR Vβ regions used by the CD4$^+$ cells of six donors, which recognized each of the two UES on the TTD. For one donor, we also investigated the TCR Vβ usage of CD4$^+$ cells lines recognizing TTD sequences other than the UES. Most of the latter lines had a completely nonrestricted TCR Vβ usage. In all donors, the CD4$^+$ lines recognizing one or the other UES had a TCR Vβ usage that was very moderately restricted: they generally used six to eight different Vβ regions. Thus, the restricted Vβ usage of autoimmune CD4⁺ cells that recognize UES on the AChR is likely due to the limited number of potential autoreactive cells that survive clonal deletion and not to the ability of the cell to recognize universal epitopes.

REFERENCES

1. LINDSTROM, J. *et al.* 1988. Myasthenia gravis. Adv. Immunol. **42:** 233–284.
2. SCHONBECK, S. *et al.* 1990. Myasthenia gravis: prototype of the antireceptor autoimmune diseases. Int. Rev. Neurobiol. **32:** 175–200.
3. DRACHMAN, D. B. 1994. Myasthenia gravis. N. Engl. J. Med. **330:** 1797–1810.
4. PROTTI, M. P. *et al.* 1993. Myasthenia gravis: recognition of a human autoantigen at the molecular level. Immunol. Today **14:** 363–368.
5. CONTI-TRONCONI, B. M. *et al.* 1994. The nicotinic acetylcholine receptor: structure and autoimmune pathology. Crit. Rev. Biochem. Mol. Biol. **29:** 69–123.
6. VANDENBARK, A. *et al.* 1992. TCR peptide therapy in autoimmune diseases. Int. Rev. Immunol. **2:** 251–277.
7. SETTE, A. *et al.* 1994. Antigen analogs/MHC complexes as specific T cell receptor antagonists. Annu. Rev. Immunol. **12:** 413–431.
8. WALDOR, M. K. *et al.* 1983. *In vivo* therapy with monoclonal anti-I-A antibody suppresses immune response to acetylcholine receptor. Proc. Natl. Acad. Sci. U.S.A. **80:** 2713–2717.
9. CHRISTADOSS, P. *et al.* 1986. Immuno-therapy for myasthenia gravis: a murine model. J. Immunol. **136:** 2437–2440.
10. KAUL, R. *et al.* 1994. Major histocompatibility complex class II gene disruption prevents experimental autoimmune myasthenia gravis. J. Immunol. **152:** 3152–3157.
11. ENGEL, A. G. *et al.* 1977. Immune complexes (IgG and C3) at the motor end-plate in myasthenia gravis: ultrastructural and light microscopic localization and electrophysiological correlation. Mayo Clin. Proc. **55:** 2647–2680.
12. LENNON, V. A. *et al.* 1983. Autoantibodies to acetylcholine receptors in myasthenia gravis. N. Engl. J. Med. **308:** 402–403.
13. MORGUTTI, M. *et al.* 1979. Cellular immune response to acetylcholine receptor in myasthenia gravis: thymectomy and corticosteroids. Neurology **29:** 734–738.
14. ÅHLBERG, R. *et al.* 1994. Treatment of myasthenia gravis with anti-CD4⁺ antibody: improvement correlates to decreased T-cell autoreactivity. Neurology **44:** 1732–1737.
15. PENN, A., D. RICHMAN, R. RUFF & V. LENNON, Eds. 1993. Myasthenia Gravis and Related Disorders: Experimental and Clinical Aspects. Volume 681. Ann. N.Y. Acad. Sci. New York.
16. BOSMA, G. C. *et al.* 1983. A severe combined immunodeficiency mutation in the mouse. Nature **301:** 527–530.
17. MCCUNE, J. M. *et al.* 1988. The SCID-hu mouse: murine model for the analysis of human hematolymphoid differentiation and function. Science **241:** 1632–1639.
18. MOSIER, D. E. *et al.* 1988. Transfer of a functional human immune system to mice with severe combined immunodeficiency. Nature **335:** 256–259.
19. PFEFFER, K. *et al.* 1989. Adoptive transfer of human peripheral blood lymphocytes (PBL) into SCID mice. Curr. Top. Microbiol. Immunol. **152:** 211–217.
20. MARTINO, G. *et al.* 1993. The human SCID myasthenic mouse model: a new approach for the study of myasthenia gravis. Ann. Neurol. **34:** 48–56.
21. GU, Y. *et al.* 1988. Immunological evidence for a change in subunits of the acetylcholine receptor in developing and denervated rat muscle. Neuron **1:** 117–125.

22. HORTON, R. H. *et al.* 1993. The "embryonic" γ subunit of the nicotinic acetylcholine receptor is expressed in adult extrinsic ocular muscles. Neurology **43:** 983–986.
23. KAMINSKI, H. J. *et al.* 1996. Expression of acetylcholine receptor isoforms at extraocular muscle endplates. Invest. Ophthalmol. Visual Sci. **37:** 345–351.
24. LINDSTROM, J. *et al.* 1978. Immunization of rats with polypeptide chains from *Torpedo* acetylcholine receptor causes an autoimmune response to receptors in rat muscle. Proc. Natl. Acad. Sci. U.S.A. **75:** 769–773.
25. BELLONE, M. *et al.* 1993. Cryptic epitopes on nicotinic acetylcholine receptor are recognized by autoreactive CD4+ cells. J. Immunol. **151:** 1025–1038.
26. FUJII, Y. *et al.* 1988. Specificity of the T cell immune response to acetylcholine receptor in experimental autoimmune myasthenia gravis: response to subunits and synthetic peptides. J. Immunol. **140:** 1830–1837.
27. LINDSTROM, J. *et al.* 1991. Monoclonal antibody probes for nicotinic receptors of muscles and nerves. Biochem. Soc. Trans. **19:** 115–120.
28. RAJU, R. *et al.* 1996. Epitopes repertoire of human CD4+ T lines propagated with tetanus toxoid or with synthetic tetanus toxoid sequences. J. Autoimmun. **9:** 79–88.
29. HOHLFELD, R. 1994. The thymus in myasthenia gravis. Neurol. Clin. North Am. **12:** 331–343.
30. NELSON, S. *et al.* 1990. Adult thymus expresses an embryonic muscle acetylcholine receptor–like protein. J. Neuroimmunol. **29:** 81–92.
31. GEUDER, K. I. *et al.* 1992. Pathogenetic significance of fetal-type acetylcholine receptors on thymic myoid cells in myasthenia gravis. Dev. Immunol. **2:** 69–75.
32. STERN, L. J. *et al.* 1994. Crystal structure of the human class II MHC protein HLA-DR1 complexed with an influenza virus peptide. Nature **368:** 215–221.
33. ODA, K. *et al.* 1981. Myasthenia gravis: antibodies to acetylcholine receptor in ocular myasthenia gravis. J. Neurol. **225:** 251–258.
34. HARA, H. *et al.* 1993. Nicotinic acetylcholine receptor mRNAs in myasthenic thymuses: association with intrathymic pathogenesis of myasthenia gravis. Biochem. Biophys. Res. Commun. **194:** 1269–1275.
35. KAMINSKI, H. J. *et al.* 1993. Acetylcholine receptor subunit gene expression in thymic tissue. Muscle Nerve **16:** 1332–1337.
36. SHENOY, M. *et al.* 1994. The pathogenic role of acetylcholine receptor α chain epitope within α146–162 in the development of experimental autoimmune myasthenia gravis in C57BL6 mice. Clin. Immunol. Immunopathol. **73:** 338–343.
37. YEH, T. M. *et al.* 1990. T cells reactive with a small synthetic peptide of the acetylcholine receptor can provide help for a clonotypically heterogeneous antibody response and subsequently impaired muscle function. J. Immunol. **144:** 1654–1660.
38. MILLER, S. D. *et al.* 1995. Evolution of the T cell repertoire during the course of experimental immuno-mediated demyelinating diseases. Immunol. Rev. **144:** 225–244.
39. MANFREDI, A. *et al.* 1992. CD4+ T epitope repertoire on the human acetylcholine receptor α subunit in severe myasthenia gravis: a study with synthetic peptides. Neurology **42:** 1092–1100.
40. MANFREDI, A. *et al.* 1993. T helper cell recognition of muscle acetylcholine receptor in myasthenia gravis: epitopes on the γ and δ subunits. J. Clin. Invest. **92:** 1055–1067.
41. PROTTI, M. P. *et al.* 1990. CD4+ T cell response to human acetylcholine receptor α subunit correlates with myasthenia gravis severity: a study with synthetic peptides. J. Immunol. **144:** 1276–1281.
42. PROTTI, M. P. *et al.* 1990. Immunodominant regions for T helper sensitization on the human nicotinic receptor α subunit in myasthenia gravis. Proc. Natl. Acad. Sci. U.S.A. **87:** 7792–7796.
43. MOIOLA, L. *et al.* 1994. Epitopes on the β subunit of human muscle acetylcholine receptor

recognized by CD4$^+$ cells of myasthenia gravis patients and healthy subjects. J. Clin. Invest. **93:** 1020–1028.

44. PROTTI, M. P. *et al.* 1991. Myasthenia gravis: T epitopes of the δ subunit of human muscle acetylcholine receptor. J. Immunol. **146:** 2253–2261.

45. PROTTI, M. P. *et al.* 1992. Myasthenia gravis: CD4$^+$ T epitopes on the embryonic γ subunit of human muscle acetylcholine receptor. J. Clin. Invest. **90:** 1558–1567.

46. WANG, Z-Y. *et al.* 1997. Th1 epitope repertoire on the α subunit of human muscle acetylcholine receptor in myasthenia gravis. Neurology **48:** 1643–1653.

47. WANG, Z-Y. *et al.* 1998. Th1 cells of myasthenia gravis patients recognize multiple epitopes on the muscle acetylcholine receptor α subunit. This volume.

48. CONTI-FINE, B. M. *et al.* 1996. Antibodies as tools to study the structure of membrane proteins: the case of the nicotinic acetylcholine receptor. Annu. Rev. Biophys. Biomol. Struct. **25:** 197–229.

49. RAJU, R. *et al.* 1995. Epitopes for human CD4$^+$ T cells on diphtheria toxin: structural features of sequence segments forming epitopes recognized by most subjects. Eur. J. Immunol. **25:** 3207–3214.

50. ROMAGNANI, S. 1995. Biology of human Th1 and Th2 cells. J. Clin. Immunol. **15:** 121–129.

51. VOSKUHL, R. R. *et al.* 1993. T helper 1 (TH1) functional phenotype of human myelin basic protein–specific T lymphocytes. Autoimmunity **15:** 137–143.

52. CORREALE, J. *et al.* 1995. Patterns of cytokine secretion by autoreactive proteolipid protein–specific T cell clones during the course of multiple sclerosis. J. Immunol. **154:** 2959–2968.

53. VAN DER VEEN, R. *et al.* 1993. Fine specificity differences in the recognition of an encephalitogenic peptide by T helper 1 and 2 cells. J. Neuroimmunol. **48:** 221–226.

54. YI, Q. *et al.* 1994. Acetylcholine receptor–reactive T cells in myasthenia gravis: evidence for the involvement of different subpopulations of T helper cells. J. Neuroimmunol. **50:** 177–186.

55. LINK, J. *et al.* 1994. Organ-specific autoantigens induce interferon-γ and interleukin-4 mRNA expression in mononuclear cells in multiple sclerosis and myasthenia gravis. Neurology **44:** 728–734.

56. MOIOLA, L. *et al.* 1994. Myasthenia gravis: residues of the α and γ subunits of muscle acetylcholine receptor involved in formation of immunodominant CD4$^+$ epitopes. J. Immunol. **152:** 4686–4698.

57. LINK, H. *et al.* 1991. Acetylcholine receptor–reactive T and B cells in myasthenia gravis and controls. J. Clin. Invest. **87:** 2191–2196.

58. WANG, Z-Y. *et al.* 1994. Induction of interferon-γ, interleukin-4, and transforming growth factor-β in rats orally tolerized against experimental autoimmune myasthenia gravis. Cell. Immunol. **157:** 353–368.

59. GU, D. *et al.* 1995. Myasthenia gravis–like syndrome induced by expression of interferon-γ in the neuromuscular junction. J. Exp. Med. **181:** 547–557.

60. GAMMON, G. 1989. How some T cells escape tolerance induction. Nature **342:** 183–185.

61. MONDINO, A. *et al.* 1994. Surface protein involved in T cell costimulation. J. Leukocyte Biol. **55:** 805–815.

62. O'SULLIVAN, D. T. *et al.* 1991. On the interaction of promiscuous antigenic peptides with different DR alleles. J. Immunol. **147:** 2663.

63. KARACHUNSKI, P. I. *et al.* 1997. Nasal administration of synthetic acetylcholine receptor T epitopes affects the immune response to the acetylcholine receptor and prevents experimental myasthenia gravis. J. Clin. Invest. In press.

64. RAJU, R. *et al.* 1997. Preferential TCR Vβ usage by acetylcholine receptor specific CD4$^+$ T cells in myasthenia gravis. J. Autoimmun. **10:** 203–217.

65. MELMS, A. *et al.* 1993. T-cell receptor gene usage of acetylcholine receptor–specific T-helper cells. Ann. N.Y. Acad. Sci. **681:** 313–314.
66. LANZAVECCHIA, A. *et al.* 1995. How can cryptic epitopes trigger autoimmunity? J. Exp. Med. **181:** 1945–1948.
67. LEHMANN, P. V. *et al.* 1993. Determinant spreading and the dynamics of the autoimmune T-cell repertoire. Immunol. Today **14:** 203–208.
68. MANFREDI, A. *et al.* 1994. Human acetylcholine receptor presentation in myasthenia gravis: DR restriction of autoimmune T epitopes and binding of synthetic receptor sequences to DR molecules. J. Immunol. **152:** 4165–4174.
69. YUEN, M. H. 1996. MHC class II presentation of human acetylcholine receptor in myasthenia gravis: binding of synthetic γ subunit sequences to DR molecule. J. Autoimmun. **9:** 67–77.
70. O'SULLIVAN, P. J. *et al.* 1990. Characterization of the specificity of peptide binding to four DR haplotypes. J. Immunol. **145:** 1799–1808.
71. CHOE, S. *et al.* 1992. The crystal structure of diphtheria toxin. Nature **357:** 216–222.
72. DIETHELM-OKITA, B. M. *et al.* 1996. Epitope repertoire of human CD4$^+$ T cells on tetanus toxin: identification of immunodominant sequence segments. J. Infect. Dis. **175:** 382–391.
73. EISEL, Y. *et al.* 1986. Tetanus toxin: primary structure, expression in *E. coli*, and homology with botulinum toxins. EMBO J. **5:** 2495–2502.
74. PANINA-BORDIGNON, P. *et al.* 1989. Study on the immunogenicity of human class-II-restricted T-cell epitopes: processing constraints degenerate binding, and promiscuous recognition. Cold Spring Harbor Symp. Quant. Biol. **54:** 445–469.
75. REECE, J. C. *et al.* 1993. Mapping the major human T helper epitopes of tetanus toxin. J. Immunol. **151:** 6175–6184.
76. HAMMER, J. *et al.* 1995. Peptide binding specificity of HLA-DR4 molecules: correlation with rheumatoid arthritis association. J. Exp. Med. **181:** 1847–1855.
77. HAMMER, J. *et al.* 1994. High-affinity binding of short peptides to major histocompatibility complex class II molecules by anchor combinations. Proc. Natl. Acad. Sci. U.S.A. **91:** 4456–4460.
78. WUCHERPFENNIG, K. W. *et al.* 1995. Selective binding of self peptides to disease-associated major histocompatibility complex (MHC) molecules: a mechanism for MHC-linked susceptibility to human autoimmune diseases. J. Exp. Med. **181:** 1597–1601.

Acetylcholine Receptor Epitopes in Ocular Myasthenia[a]

HENRY J. KAMINSKI[b]

Department of Neurology
Case Western Reserve University School of Medicine
Department of Veterans Affairs Medical Center in Cleveland
University Hospitals of Cleveland
Cleveland, Ohio

Myasthenia gravis (MG) shows a propensity to involve the ocular muscles. Ocular muscle weakness is the initial sign of MG in the majority of patients and ultimately occurs in at least 90% of myasthenics. About 10–15% of myasthenics have weakness restricted to the ocular muscles.[1] Clinical classifications of MG do not differentiate between the occurrence of diplopia and ptosis in the characterization of ocular muscle involvement. This clearly is an oversimplification. The levator palpebrae (LP), the muscle responsible for eyelid elevation, is anatomically and physiologically distinct from the four recti and two obliques, which generate eye movements. To dissect the pathogenesis of ocular muscle manifestations of MG, future investigations will need to differentiate between the involvement of these muscles.[2]

For the purpose of this review, the term "extraocular muscle" (EOM) will refer only to the muscles of ocular movement, while "ocular muscle" will include these muscles and the LP. This terminology differs from the standard definition of EOM, which includes the LP. The reasons for these distinctions and their importance in understanding the pathogenesis of the ocular manifestations of MG will become clear after a review of ocular muscle anatomy and physiology. This article will discuss how the unique properties of the ocular muscles predispose them to MG and emphasize evidence that adult EOM expresses unique acetylcholine receptor (AChR) epitopes that may target these muscles for immune-mediated damage.

REVIEW OF EXTRAOCULAR MUSCLE AND LEVATOR PALPEBRAE ANATOMY AND PHYSIOLOGY

The muscle fiber classification used in skeletal muscle cannot be applied to EOM. Six distinct EOM fiber types based on anatomic location, histochemical staining, and innervational pattern are identified. EOM is divided anatomically into a global region, adjacent to the globe, and an orbital region, next to the bony orbit. The majority of EOM fibers are singly innervated fibers (SIFs) and share a similar endplate morphology with other skeletal muscle, having a single *en plaque* neuromuscu-

[a]This work was supported by NIH Grant No. EY-00332 and the Office of Research and Development, Medical Research Service of the Department of Veterans Affairs.
[b]Address for correspondence: Department of Neurology, University Hospitals of Cleveland, 11100 Euclid Avenue, Cleveland, Ohio 44106.

lar junction. In response to a single nerve stimulation, SIFs produce a synchronized contraction and a propagated action potential. Certain SIFs have greater contraction speeds and fatigue resistance (with associated higher mitochondrial content) than the twitch fibers of other skeletal muscle. Detailed descriptions of EOM fiber properties can be found in references 3–5.

Approximately 20% of EOM fibers are innervated at multiple points, the multiply innervated fibers (MIFs, FIGURE 1). MIFs have been studied best in nonmammalian species; in humans, other than EOM, MIFs are present only in the pharyngeal, tensor tympani, and stapedius muscles. In amphibians and reptiles, the MIFs are divided into tonic and intermediate fibers. Tonic fibers are distinguished by three physiological characteristics. First, they cannot propagate action potentials. Second, they maintain a graded contraction to depolarization, and the amplitude of the contraction is proportional to the degree of membrane depolarization. Third, tonic fibers contract and relax very slowly compared with twitch fibers. Intermediate fibers share properties of twitch and tonic fibers. In mammalian EOM, two MIFs are present, one in each of the anatomic regions. The orbital MIF has multiple, small *en grappe* endplates at its ends and a single *en plaque* endplate at its center. This fiber's contractile characteristics correlate with its innervation pattern, contracting in a graded fashion in the region of the *en grappe* endplates and in a twitch manner around the *en plaque* endplate.[6] The global MIF has *en grappe* endplates along its length and contracts in a graded or "tonic" fashion.[7]

The LP shares a common embryological origin and innervation with the superior rectus; however, it differs from EOM. Four muscle fiber types are evident in LP, three similar to the three global SIFs of EOM and an additional fiber similar to slow-twitch fibers. No MIFs are present and no anatomic division is evident.[8] LP fibers have

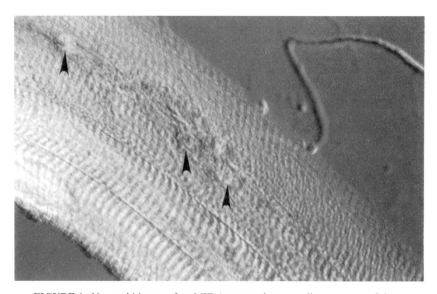

FIGURE 1. Nomarski image of rat MIF. Arrows point to small *en grappe* endplates.

twitch characteristics and, based on their histological appearance, some are highly fatigue-resistant.

FUNCTIONAL AND PHYSIOLOGIC SUSCEPTIBILITY OF OCULAR MUSCLES TO MYASTHENIA GRAVIS

Prior to the discussion of AChR epitopes, nonimmunological factors will be reviewed that may make ocular muscle susceptible to MG.[5,9,10] First, slight EOM weakness will sufficiently misalign the visual axes to produce symptoms. Second, the high firing frequencies of EOM motor units may increase EOM susceptibility to fatigue. Third, physiological properties of EOM fibers may make them more susceptible to the block of muscular excitation produced by MG. Ocular myasthenics have lower concentrations of antibody and have higher frequencies of seronegativity than generalized myasthenics.[11,12] This observation supports the idea that ocular muscles are physiologically more susceptible to low titers of antibody. LP is subject to near-constant neuronal stimulation and has physiological characteristics that may predispose to MG.

Only slight weakness of an EOM is necessary to cause symptoms. The visual axes must be aligned precisely; otherwise, a slight discrepancy in retinal images occurs, and symptoms, such as diplopia or visual confusion, develop.[13] Extraocular motor neuron activity is primarily efferently coded, and the extent of proprioceptive feedback is not clear.[14] During limb movements, continuous correction of motor neuron activity occurs due to feedback of position, velocity, and muscle tension information. A slight reduction in force generation of extremity muscles, as would occur in the early phases of MG, may be compensated for prior to a patient's appreciation of weakness. The ocular motor system may be particularly susceptible to MG because its central control mechanism, utilizing primarily visual feedback, cannot adapt quickly to asymmetric or variable weakness of the EOMs. Dramatic visual manifestations result that lead the patient to seek medical attention.

EOM motor neuron activity would be expected to make EOM fibers susceptible to the neuromuscular transmission failure of MG. EOM twitch motor units operate at very high firing frequencies. Fast EOM motor units fire at frequencies exceeding 600 Hz during saccades, while the maximum firing frequencies of other motor units do not exceed 100 Hz.[3,5] Further, EOM motor units are active even when the eye is positioned outside the direction of action of a given EOM.[15] This repetitive stimulation at high frequencies would be expected to make EOM susceptible to myasthenic fatigue.[16] In normal EOM, the safety factor is sufficient to prevent fatigue during repeated saccades or maintained eccentric gaze.

EOM twitch fibers possess anatomic characteristics that may make them more susceptible to neuromuscular blockade. EOM twitch fibers have less prominent secondary synaptic folds and therefore may have fewer AChRs and sodium channels on their postsynaptic membrane.[4] In addition, the mean quantal content is decreased in EOM twitch fibers compared with extremity muscle.[17] A reduction in AChR, sodium channels, and quantal content would reduce the safety factor for neuromuscular transmission of EOM twitch fibers as compared to other skeletal twitch fibers.[16] Proximal and distal muscles differ in their response to repetitive stimulation, which reflects variations in the safety factor for neuromuscular transmission. Variations in AChR and sodium channel density and in quantal release also could help explain differential involvement of other skeletal muscles by MG.

Assuming EOM MIFs share characteristics of amphibian and reptilian MIFs, they would be predisposed to MG for structural and physiological reasons. Force generation in tonic fibers is directly proportional to the membrane depolarization caused by the synaptic potential. Hence, unlike the twitch fibers, no safety factor exists for neuromuscular transmission in tonic fibers, and any reduction of synaptic depolarization could lead to symptomatic weakness.[5,10] Junctional folds are sparse to nonexistent in the tonic fibers of reptiles, and the AChR receptor density is lower by a factor of 1.3 to 1.5. With a lower density of AChR, force of contraction of a tonic EOM fiber would be compromised by any AChR loss or inhibition produced by MG.

Evidence from ocular motility studies exists demonstrating that MIFs are preferentially involved by MG. The role of the various EOM fibers in generation of the various types of eye movements is not known. MIFs are thought to play a role in maintaining gaze and in performing small eye movements from mid-position, while SIFs are responsible for rapid eye movements.[13,18] Saccades are generally spared in myasthenics,[19,20] and this finding suggests that MIFs are preferentially effected by the disease. This view is further supported by a computer model of eye movements of myasthenics. In this model, the ocular motility disorders of myasthenics could be simulated by a defect in the component of EOM force generation that is responsible for holding the eyes fixed with sparing of the fibers that generate a saccade.[21]

The reasons for the frequency of LP involvement in MG are not well understood. During eye opening, LP fibers are subject to constant neuronal stimulation, making neuromuscular fatigue more likely to occur than in limb muscles. Junctional folds of LP endplates are sparse[8] as in EOM, which could suggest a lower AChR number and a reduction in safety factor. Functional reasons are likely to exist for LP's susceptibility to the neuromuscular transmission defect of MG because LP, as is EOM, is subject to involvement by nonimmune disorders of neuromuscular transmission.[22,23]

ACETYLCHOLINE RECEPTOR EXPRESSION IN EOM

The fetal isoform of the mammalian AChR is a pentameric protein composed of α-, β-, δ-, and γ-subunits. An ϵ-subunit substitutes for the γ-subunit in the adult AChR, and this subunit substitution confers specific electrophysiological and antigenic characteristics to the receptor. Developing myotubes express the fetal AChRs along their length. The fetal AChR supports spontaneous contractile activity in embryonic muscle and appears to be essential for normal muscle development.[24] With innervation, AChRs cluster at the synaptic contact. As the endplate matures, the fetal AChR concentration decreases and the adult form appears.[25] Coincident with these changes, γ-subunit gene expression declines and ϵ-subunit transcripts are localized to subsynaptic nuclei.[26–28] With denervation, the fetal AChR and γ-subunit gene expression reappear. Limb muscles of animals with experimentally induced MG, however, do not express the γ-subunit gene.[29] All these observations are limited to nonocular mammalian skeletal muscle.

We postulated that the MIFs of mammalian EOM would express the fetal AChR, which would offer a unique antigenic target for immune damage of EOM.[5,10] This theory is based on single-channel recordings from snake MIFs that demonstrate the presence of two channels with characteristics similar to the mammalian adult and fetal AChR.[30,31] Using polymerase chain reaction and Northern hybridization, we[32,33] and Horton *et al.*[34] identified γ-subunit mRNA expression in adult rat and bovine EOM (FIGURE 2). Despite LP's and EOM's common embryological origin and certain structural similarities, the LP does not contain γ-subunit gene transcripts.[33] Fetal AChR expression may be limited to muscles that contain MIFs. Missias *et al.* using a different method confirmed γ-subunit gene expression in adult murine EOM.[35] Mice with a transgene containing a promoter element of the γ-subunit linked to a reporter gene show activity of the reporter in adult EOM fibers. AChR protein expression is thought to be primarily transcriptionally regulated and, therefore, detection of γ-subunit gene transcripts suggests expression of the fetal AChR.[36] MacLennan and colleagues using RNase protection assays also found expression of the γ-subunit gene in human EOM.[37] In contrast to previous investigations, this study also found γ-subunit gene expression in gastrocnemius and intercostal muscles. This discrepancy could be explained by species differences in AChR gene expression and by the greater sensitivity of the Rnase protection assay compared to RNA blot hybridization. However, immunocytochemical studies suggest that the γ-subunit gene transcription in non-EOMs identified by MacLennan is not translated into AChR at the endplate. It is

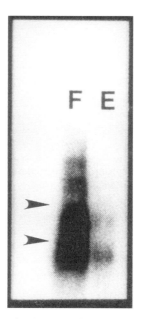

FIGURE 2. γ-subunit gene expression in bovine fetal gluteus (F) and adult EOM (E). Five μg of Poly(A)+ RNA was applied to the gel. The blot was probed with a ^{32}P-labeled fragment from a plasmid containing the bovine γ-subunit gene sequence. Arrows point to migration positions of 28S and 18S rRNA. For a detailed description of methods, see reference 33.

likely that the γ-subunit transcripts identified are synthesized in the extrasynaptic region and do not contribute to AChR protein expression at the endplate.

Consistent with our identification of γ- and ε-subunit gene transcripts, we found γ- and ε-subunit immunoreactivity at rat EOM endplates.[38] γ- and ε-subunit antisera bound all *en grappe* endplates of the MIFs. All SIFs bound ε-subunit antibodies. Surprisingly, the orbital SIFs and certain global SIF endplates expressed the γ-subunit of the fetal AChR. Missias *et al.*[35] performed an extensive evaluation of the developmental time course of ε- and γ-subunit protein expression among various muscles in mice. By postnatal day 17, tibialis anterior, extensor digitorum longus, sternomastoid, and diaphragm endplates showed only ε-subunit expression. γ-subunit expression persisted to postnatal day 21 in soleus, a predominantly slow-twitch muscle, but was absent by day 50. Only EOM endplates contained γ-subunit immunoreactivity at day 50. In contrast to our study, this group found prominent γ-subunit protein expression only at *en grappe* endplates. ε-subunit immunoreactivity was found at all *en plaque* and some *en grappe* endplates. γ-subunit transgene expression was evident at subsynaptic nuclei of some *en plaque* endplates,[35] in keeping with our observation of γ-subunit immunoreactivity at such endplates. (See FIGURE 3.)

The role of the fetal AChR in EOM is unknown, but it may serve to improve contractile function. The fetal AChR has a longer open time than the adult isoform and would prolong the endplate potential at *en grappe* endplates, which would serve to prolong tonic contraction. The function of the fetal AChR at the SIFs is less clear. The expression of the fetal AChR does provide a unique AChR epitope that could lead to preferential damage of EOM by MG. The next section reviews information regarding immunological targeting of EOM and the fetal AChR.

IMMUNOLOGICAL REACTION OF MYASTHENIA GRAVIS TO EXTRAOCULAR MUSCLE AND THE FETAL ACETYLCHOLINE RECEPTOR

The standard radioimmunoassay to detect AChR antibodies among patients uses denervated leg muscle as a source of antigen. Some studies demonstrate that ocular myasthenics' sera react more strongly when human EOM is used as a source of antigen.[39,40] Oda[41,42] found a subgroup of seronegative ocular myasthenics who were positive when tested against EOM-derived antigen. By immunohistochemistry, two sera bound only the *en grappe* synapses, four bound the *en plaque* and *en grappe* synapses, and two bound the *en plaque* synapses of EOM and extremity muscle. The sera that only reacted with *en grappe* endplates presumably were binding the fetal AChR. When bovine EOM and foot muscles are used as a source of antigen, no difference in antibody detection is evident;[43] however, the interspecies differences between the human and bovine AChR likely mask the significance of the type of muscle used for antigen preparation.

Some myasthenic sera react selectively with fetal AChRs and some myasthenic T cells respond to fetal AChR epitopes. Schuetze *et al.* studied the effects of myasthenic serum on AChR in developing rat muscle.[44] A certain myasthenic serum blocked function of the AChR with a long open time, but not the adult AChR with the short open time. Other investigations have identified preferential binding of myas-

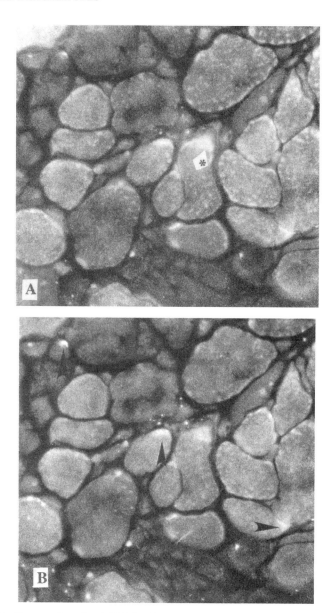

FIGURE 3. Cross section of rat EOM showing two SIF endplates (small arrows) stained with biotin-labeled α-bungarotoxin (A) and anti-γ antibody (B). One en plaque endplate is seen without anti-γ antibody staining (*). An en grappe endplate of an MIF is also seen (large arrow). Binding was detected by fluorescein isothiocyanate streptavidin (A) and anti-rabbit IgG tetramethyl rhodamine isothiocyanate (B).

thenic sera to extrajunctional AChRs,[45–48] which are now appreciated to be primarily fetal AChRs. Tzartos *et al.*[49] found that a small number of myasthenic sera reacted to regions of the γ-subunit, although this did not correlate with ocular symptoms. Myasthenics also have T cells that are activated by epitopes on the γ-subunit, and T cell activation correlates with ocular manifestations (see reference 50 and the paper by Conti-Fine elsewhere in this volume).

MacLennan and coworkers[37] utilized a novel source of antigen for detection of AChR antibodies. They stably transfected TE671 cells with a cDNA encoding the ε-subunit and used the cell line as a rich source of adult AChR in a radioimmunoassay. Thirty-three of 53 ocular myasthenic sera contained detectable AChR antibodies using this assay as compared to only 18 with the conventional assay using denervated muscle. Therefore, these patients had antibodies directed against the adult AChR. The adult AChR is the isoform found in all skeletal muscles and the predominant form found in EOM, and myasthenic antibodies would be expected to be directed towards this isoform.[2] AChR antibodies from ocular myasthenic sera were detected more frequently using the new assay, suggesting ocular manifestations are not correlated with antibodies toward the fetal AChR. The investigators concluded that the expression of the fetal AChRs in EOM could not explain their susceptibility to MG. One difficulty with this conclusion is that ocular myasthenics were not divided clinically into those with and without diplopia. Fetal AChR antibodies may only correlate with diplopia. Perhaps, the fetal AChR is the inciting antigen, but rapid diversification of antibody specificity leads to the adult AChR antibodies being the most readily detectable.

It is possible that non-AChR epitopes are important in directing the immune response towards ocular muscle. Ocular and generalized myasthenic sera contain antibodies directed towards other muscle proteins and the antibody specificities differ between ocular and generalized myasthenics.[51] These non-AChR antibodies may be particularly important in the explanation of LP involvement by MG. LP differs from both EOM and other skeletal muscle and unique antigenic targets could be present.

CONCLUDING REMARKS

The question remains why myasthenics possess antibodies directed only toward the fetal AChR. As mentioned, myasthenic muscle is not denervated and does not express the fetal AChR.[29] The thymus may be the source of fetal AChR; however, data regarding AChR epitope expression in the myasthenic thymus are contradictory. EOM is the only mature, innervated skeletal muscle that expresses the fetal AChR and the only muscle that myasthenic antibodies to the fetal AChR could bind. Further investigations will be needed to clarify these issues.

REFERENCES

1. GROB, D., E. L. ARSURA, N. G. BRUNNER & T. NAMBA. 1987. The course of myasthenia gravis and therapies affecting outcome. Ann. N.Y. Acad. Sci. **505:** 472–499.
2. KAMINSKI, H. J. & R. L. RUFF. 1997. Ocular muscle involvement by myasthenia gravis. Ann. Neurol. **41:** 419–420.

3. PORTER, J. D. & R. BAKER. 1996. Muscles of a different "color": the unusual properties of the extraocular muscles may predispose or protect them in neurogenic and myogenic disease. Neurology **46**: 30–37.

4. SPENCER, R. F. & J. D. PORTER. 1988. Structural organization of the extraocular muscles. *In* Neuroanatomy of the Oculomotor System, p. 33–79. Elsevier. Amsterdam/New York.

5. RUFF, R. L., H. J. KAMINSKI, E. MAAS & P. SPIEGEL. 1989. Ocular muscles: physiology and structure-function correlations. Bull. Soc. Belge Ophtalmol. **237**: 321–352.

6. JACOBY, J., K. KO, C. WEISS & J. RUSHBROOK. 1989. Systematic variation in myosin expression along extraocular muscle fibers of the adult rat. J. Muscle Res. Cell Motil. **11**: 25–40.

7. CHIARANDINI, D. & E. STEFANI. 1979. Electrophysiological identification of two types of fibre in rat extraocular muscles. J. Physiol. (Lond.) **290**: 453–465.

8. PORTER, J. D., L. A. BURNS & P. J. MAY. 1989. Morphological substrate for eyelid movements: innervation and structure of primate levator palpebrae superioris and oblicularis oculi muscles. J. Comp. Neurol. **287**: 64–81.

9. KAMINSKI, H., C. KERNICH & L. KUSNER. 1996. Ocular myasthenia. Adv. Clin. Neurosci. **6**: 37–54.

10. KAMINSKI, H. J., E. MAAS, P. SPIEGEL & R. L. RUFF. 1990. Why are eye muscles frequently involved by myasthenia gravis? Neurology **40**: 1663–1669.

11. HOWARD, F. M., V. LENNON, J. FINLEY, J. MATSUMOTO & L. ELVEBACK. 1987. Clinical correlations of antibodies that bind, block, or modulate human acetylcholine receptors in myasthenia gravis. Ann. N.Y. Acad. Sci. **505**: 526–538.

12. LIMBURG, P. C., T. C. THE, E. HUMMEL-TEPPEL & H. OOSTERHUIS. 1983. Antiacetylcholine receptor antibodies in myasthenia gravis. I. Relation to clinical parameters in 250 patients. J. Neurol. Sci. **58**: 357–370.

13. LEIGH, R. & D. ZEE. 1991. The Neurology of Eye Movements. Davis. Philadelphia.

14. BUISSERET, P. 1995. Influence of extraocular muscle proprioception on vision. Physiol. Rev. **75**: 323–338.

15. ROBINSON, D. 1970. Oculomotor unit behavior in the monkey. J. Neurophysiol. **33**: 393–404.

16. KAMINSKI, H., J. SUAREZ & R. RUFF. 1997. Neuromuscular junction physiology in myasthenia gravis: isoforms of the acetylcholine receptor in extraocular muscle and the contribution of sodium channels to the safety factor. Neurology **48**(suppl.): 8–17.

17. KIM, Y., D. ZAHM, H. LIU & T. JOHNS. 1982. Safety margin of neuromuscular transmission in rat extraocular muscle. Soc. Neurosci. **8**: 616.

18. KELLER, E. & D. ROBINSON. 1972. Abducens unit behavior in the monkey during vergence movements. Vision Res. **12**: 369–382.

19. BARTON, J., A. HUAMAN & J. SHARPE. 1994. Effects of edrophonium on saccadic velocity in normal subjects and nonmyasthenic ocular palsies. Ann. Neurol. **36**: 585–594.

20. YEE, R. D., D. G. COGAN, D. S. ZEE, R. W. BALOH & V. HONRUBIA. 1976. Rapid eye movements in myasthenia gravis. II. Electro-oculographic analysis. Arch. Ophthalmol. **94**: 1465–1472.

21. ABEL, L., L. F. DELL'OSSO, D. SCHMIDT & R. B. DAROFF. 1980. Myasthenia gravis: analog computer model. Exp. Neurol. **68**: 378–389.

22. ENGEL, A. 1994. Myasthenic syndromes. *In* Myology, p. 1798–1835. McGraw–Hill. New York.

23. KAMINSKI, H. J. & R. L. RUFF. 1996. The myasthenic syndromes. *In* Molecular Biology of Membrane Transport Disorders. Plenum. New York.

24. JARAMILLO, F., S. VICINI & S. M. SCHUETZE. 1988. Embryonic acetylcholine receptors guarantee spontaneous contractions in rat developing muscle. Nature **335**: 66–68.

25. GU, Y. & Z. HALL. 1988. Immunological evidence for a change in subunits of the acetylcholine receptor in developing and denervated rat muscle. Neuron **1**: 117–125.

26. Witzemann, V., B. Barg, Y. Nishikawa, B. Sakmann & S. Numa. 1987. Differential regulation of muscle acetylcholine receptor γ- and ε-subunit mRNAs. FEBS Lett. **223:** 104–112.

27. Witzemann, V., B. Barg, M. Criado, E. Stein & B. Sakmann. 1989. Developmental regulation of five subunits specific mRNAs encoding acetylcholine receptor subtypes in rat muscle. FEBS Lett. **242:** 419–424.

28. Mishina, M., T. Takai, K. Imoto, M. Noda, T. Takahashi, S. Numa, C. Methfessl & B. Sakmann. 1986. Molecular distinction between fetal and adult forms of muscle acetylcholine receptor. Nature **321:** 406–411.

29. Asher, O., D. Neumann, V. Witzemann & S. Fuchs. 1990. Acetylcholine receptor gene expression in experimental autoimmune myasthenia gravis. FEBS Lett. **261:** 231–235.

30. Dionne, V. E. 1989. Two types of nicotinic acetylcholine receptor channels at slow fibre end-plates of the garter snake. J. Physiol. (Lond.) **409:** 313–331.

31. Ruff, R. L. & P. Spiegel. 1990. Ca sensitivity and AChR currents of twitch and tonic snake muscle fibers. Am. J. Physiol. **259:** C911–C919.

32. Kaminski, H. J., R. Fenstermaker & R. L. Ruff. 1991. Adult extraocular and intercostal muscles express the gamma-subunit of fetal AChR. Biophys. J. **59:** 444a.

33. Kaminski, H. J., L. L. Kusner, K. V. Nash & R. L. Ruff. 1995. The γ-subunit of the acetylcholine receptor is not expressed in the levator palpebrae superioris. Neurology **45:** 516–518.

34. Horton, R. M., A. A. Manfredi & B. M. Conti-Tronconi. 1993. The "embryonic" gamma subunit of the nicotinic acetylcholine receptor is expressed in adult extraocular muscle. Neurology **43:** 983–986.

35. Missias, A. C., G. C. Chu, B. J. Klocke, J. R. Sanes & J. P. Merlie. 1996. Regulation of the acetylcholine receptor gamma subunit gene in developing skeletal muscle: analysis with subunit-specific antibodies, transgenic mice, and cultured cells. Dev. Biol. **179:** 223.

36. Hall, Z. W. & J. R. Sanes. 1993. Synaptic structure and development: the neuromuscular junction. Cell **72:** 99–121.

37. MacLennan, C., D. Beeson, A-M. Buijs, A. Vincent & J. Newsom-Davis. 1997. Acetylcholine receptor expression in human extraocular muscles and their susceptibility to myasthenia gravis. Ann. Neurol. **41:** 423–431.

38. Kaminski, H. J., L. L. Kusner & C. H. Block. 1996. Expression of acetylcholine receptor isoforms at extraocular muscle endplates. Invest. Ophthalmol. Visual Sci. **37:** 345–351.

39. Compston, D. A. S., A. Vincent, J. Newsom-Davis & J. R. Batchelor. 1980. Clinical, pathological, HLA antigen, and immunological evidence for disease heterogeneity in myasthenia gravis. Brain **103:** 579–601.

40. Vincent, A. & J. Newsom-Davis. 1982. Acetylcholine receptor antibody characteristics in myasthenia gravis. I. Patients with generalized myasthenia or disease restricted to ocular muscles. Clin. Exp. Immunol. **49:** 257–265.

41. Oda, K. & H. Shibasaki. 1988. Antigenic difference of acetylcholine receptor between single and multiple form endplates of human extraocular muscle. Brain Res. **449:** 337–340.

42. Oda, K. 1993. Differences in acetylcholine receptor–antibody interactions between extraocular and extremity muscle fibers. Ann. N.Y. Acad. Sci. **681:** 238–255.

43. Hayashi, M., K. Kida, I. Yamada, H. Matsuda, M. Tsuneishi & O. Tamura. 1989. Differences between ocular and generalized myasthenia gravis: binding characteristics of anti-acetylcholine receptor antibody against bovine muscles. J. Neuroimmunol. **21:** 227–233.

44. Schuetze, S., S. Vicini & Z. Hall. 1985. Myasthenic serum selectively blocks acetylcholine receptors with long channel open times at developing rat endplates. Proc. Natl. Acad. Sci. U.S.A. **82:** 504–508.

45. WEINBERG, C. & Z. HALL. 1979. Antibodies from patients with myasthenia gravis recognize determinants unique to extrajunctional acetylcholine receptors. Proc. Natl. Acad. Sci. U.S.A. **76:** 504–508.

46. LENNON, V. & G. GRIESMANN. 1989. Evidence against acetylcholine receptor antibodies having a main immunogenic region as target for antibodies in myasthenia gravis. Neurology **39:** 1069–1076.

47. DWYER, D. S., R. BRADLEY, R. FURNER & G. KEMP. 1981. Immunochemical properties of junctional and extrajunctional acetylcholine receptor. Brain Res. **217:** 23–40.

48. VINCENT, A. 1987. Disorders affecting the acetylcholine receptor: myasthenia gravis and congenital myasthenia. J. Recept. Res. **7:** 599–616.

49. TZARTOS, S., M. SEYBOLD & J. LINDSTROM. 1982. Specificities of antibodies to acetylcholine receptors in sera from myasthenia gravis patients measured by monoclonal antibodies. Proc. Natl. Acad. Sci. U.S.A. **79:** 188–192.

50. YUEN, M., K. MACKLIN & B. CONTI-FINE. 1996. MHC class II presentation of human acetylcholine receptor in myasthenia gravis: binding of synthetic gamma subunit. J. Autoimmunol. **9:** 67–77.

51. ZIMMERMANN, C. & F. EBLEN. 1993. Repertoires of autoantibodies against homologous eye muscle in ocular and generalized myasthenia gravis differ. Clin. Invest. **71:** 445–451.

Biosynthetic and Synthetic AChR Sequences to Study T Cells in Myasthenia Gravis[a]

B. DIETHELM-OKITA,[b] G. WELLS,[c] A. KURYATOV,[c] D. OKITA,[b]
J. HOWARD,[d] J. LINDSTROM,[c] AND B. M. CONTI-FINE[b,e,f]

[b]Department of Biochemistry
College of Biological Sciences
University of Minnesota
St. Paul, Minnesota 55108
and
Department of Pharmacology
School of Medicine
University of Minnesota
Minneapolis, Minnesota 55455

[c]Department of Neuroscience
University of Pennsylvania Medical Center
Philadelphia, Pennsylvania

[d]Department of Neurology
University of North Carolina at Chapel Hill
Chapel Hill, North Carolina 27599

Antigen (Ag)–specific T cell lines and clones are important tools to understand the molecular interactions occurring in the T cell compartment in both normal and autoimmune responses. Propagation *in vitro* of polyclonal cell lines specific for a given Ag yields populations of T cells enriched in Ag-specific cells and allows studies on the Ag sequence regions forming T epitopes. Such studies would be of dubious success if using unselected blood CD4+ cells, given the low frequency of T cells specific for one individual epitope.[1,2] Also, Ag-specific T cell lines and clones are necessary to investigate the functional properties of the CD4+ cells recognizing a given Ag or epitope, as well as the structural properties of their T cell receptor.

For human autoimmune diseases involving autoantigens (autoAg) of known identity and sequence, given the scarcity of the relevant autoAg, synthetic and biosynthetic autoAg sequences have been used to propagate specific T cell lines. Anti-AChR CD4+ T cells from myasthenia gravis (MG) patients have been studied using synthetic or recombinant AChR sequences, sometimes yielding inconsistent results and raising questions about the suitability of those AChR Ag for the study of T cells.[1,3]

[a]This work was supported by NINCDS Grant No. NS 23919 (to B. M. Conti-Fine), NIH Grant No. NS 11323 (to J. Lindstrom), NIH Grant No. K08 NSO 1903 (to G. Wells), and research grants from the Muscular Dystrophy Association (to B. M. Conti-Fine and J. Lindstrom).
[e]Previously known as B. M. Conti-Tronconi.
[f]To whom all correspondence should be addressed.

In this study, we compared the efficacy for stimulation of CD4[+] T cells from MG patients, of pools of overlapping synthetic peptides spanning the human muscle AChR α_1 subunit sequence[4] (α pool) or its extracellular domain (residues 1–218, α1–218 pool), and of biosynthetic preparations of the α_1 subunit sequence comprising residues 1–209, obtained in *E. coli*.[5] The biosynthetic construct was obtained as inclusion bodies partially purified by differential extraction with sequential washes at pH 8 in 50 mM Tris, 1 M NaCl, and 3 M KSCN ($ib\alpha_1$1–209), or further purified by SDS-polyacrylamide gel electrophoresis[6,7] followed by desalting for removal of free detergent ($pur\alpha_1$1–209). A biosynthetic extracellular domain of the neuronal α_7 subunit ($ib\alpha_7$1–206), isolated from *E. coli* as inclusion bodies following the procedure used for $ib\alpha_1$1–209, served as control for potential bacterial contaminants in $ib\alpha_1$1–209.

Blood CD4[+] cells from six MG patients were tested with increasing concentrations of $ib\alpha_1$1–209, $pur\alpha_1$1–209, and α pool. Peripheral blood lymphocytes (PBL) were depleted in CD8[+] cells using mouse anti-CD8 antibody and paramagnetic beads coated with goat antibody against mouse immunoglobulin.[8] The resulting CD4[+]-enriched population was tested in five-day proliferation assays using triplicate cultures and 1–20 µg/mL of construct proteins or α pool.[8] Both biosynthetic preparations elicited consistent, strong responses that were frequently higher for $ib\alpha_1$1–209 than $pur\alpha_1$1–209. The α pool elicited low and inconsistent responses.

The α pool, $ib\alpha_1$1–209, $pur\alpha_1$1–209, and the α1–218 pool were used as Ag to propagate CD4[+] lines from the PBL of two MG patients whose CD4[+] epitope repertoire on the α subunit sequence had been characterized previously, using CD4[+] lines propagated with a pool of synthetic peptides identical to the α pool.[4] The lines were propagated with cycles of stimulation with the Ag followed by interleukin-2 expansion[4] and tested for recognition of antigens in three-day proliferation assays.[4] We obtained similar results for both patients: FIGURE 1 reports the results obtained with the lines propagated from one of them. The lines obtained using $pur\alpha_1$1–209, the α pool, or the α1–218 pool cross-reacted well with both the peptide pools and the biosynthetic α_1 sequences and did not cross-react with $ib\alpha_7$1–206. The lines recognized the peptide sequences previously identified as forming CD4[+] epitopes in these patients.[4] The lines propagated with $ib\alpha_1$1–209 cross-reacted poorly with the other synthetic and biosynthetic α_1 sequences and recognized strongly and to a similar extent $ib\alpha_1$1–209 and $ib\alpha_7$1–206. Thus, the use of $ib\alpha_1$1–209 may preferentially propagate CD4[+] cells sensitized to *E. coli* contaminants. This also explains the higher stimulation of unselected blood CD4[+] cells with $ib\alpha_1$1–209 versus $pur\alpha_1$1–209.

In conclusion, biosynthetic sequences of human autoAg used as an alternative to the native molecule for the study of autoimmune CD4[+] responses have the important caveat that great attention needs to be paid to eliminating any contamination from bacterial Ag. Contaminants from bacterial or yeast cells are likely recognized by human CD4[+] cells, and their presence may cause misleading results. Synthetic peptide sequences are also suitable Ag for propagation *in vitro* of autoimmune CD4[+] lines. As previously demonstrated for a variety of exogenous antigens, such as tetanus and diphtheria toxin,[2,9] the use of short synthetic AChR sequences resulted in propagation of cells that recognize the cognate Ag, as shown here by the cross-reactivity with the biosynthetic α_1 constructs of the lines propagated with the α subunit peptide

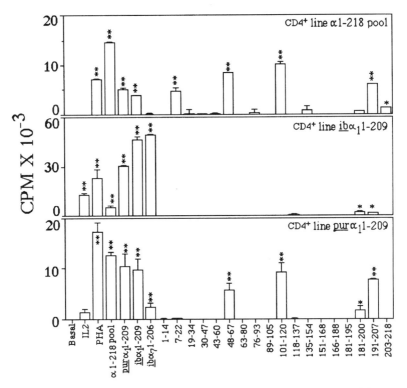

FIGURE 1. Response of a CD4[+] line propagated by an MG patient by the use of the α1–218 pool or the biosynthetic constructs, $ib\alpha_1$1–209 or $pur\alpha_1$1–209, tested in three-day proliferation assays, with the stimulants indicated along the abscissa. The columns represent the average incorporation ± standard deviation of ^{3}H-thymidine of triplicate cultures. The asterisks indicate the significance of the response, compared to the basal rate of ^{3}H-thymidine incorporation in the absence of any stimulus, determined using a two-tailed Student's t test (*$p < 0.05$, **$p < 0.01$).

pools. These results agree with those of previous studies, namely, that CD4[+] lines propagated from MG patients by stimulation with synthetic AChR sequences cross-reacted with purified muscle AChR.[1] The use of a short synthetic autoAg sequence will be especially useful to propagate the autoimmune CD4[+] cells that recognize one individual epitope sequence.

REFERENCES

1. Protti, M. P. *et al.* 1993. Myasthenia gravis: recognition of an autoantigen at the molecular level. Immunol. Today **14:** 363–368.
2. Raju, R. *et al.* 1996. Epitope repertoire of human CD4[+] lines propagated with tetanus toxoid or with synthetic tetanus toxin sequences. J. Autoimmun. **9:** 79–88.

3. HAWKE, S. *et al.* 1996. Autoimmune T cell in myasthenia gravis: heterogeneity and potential for specific immunotargeting. Immunol. Today **17:** 307–311.

4. PROTTI, M. P. *et al.* 1990. Immunodominant regions for T-helper sensitization of the human nicotinic receptor α subunit in myasthenia gravis. Proc. Natl. Acad. Sci. U.S.A. **87:** 7792–7796.

5. MELMS, A. *et al.* 1992. T cells from normal and myasthenic individuals recognize the human acetylcholine receptor: heterogeneity of antigenic sites on the α-subunit. Ann. Neurol. **31:** 311–318.

6. FERNANDEZ, A. *et al.* 1992. Reverse staining of sodium dodecyl sulfate polyacrylamide gels by imidazole-zinc salts: sensitive detection of unmodified proteins. Biotechniques **12:** 564–573.

7. CONTI-TRONCONI, B. M. *et al.* 1982. Subunit structure of the acetylcholine receptor from *Electrophorus electricus*. Proc. Natl. Acad. Sci. U.S.A. **79:** 6489–6493.

8. MANFREDI, A. A. *et al.* 1992. CD4$^+$ epitope repertoire on the human acetylcholine receptor α subunit in severe myasthenia gravis: a study with synthetic peptides. Neurology **42:** 1092–1100.

9. RAJU, R. *et al.* 1995. Epitopes for human CD4$^+$ T cells on diphtheria toxin: structural features of sequence segments forming epitopes recognized by most subjects. Eur. J. Immunol. **25:** 3207–3214.

Acetylcholine Receptor–specific CD4⁺ T Cells in Myasthenia Gravis Patients Have Individual, but Restricted TCR Vβ Usage[a]

RAGHAVANPILLAI RAJU,[b,c] DURAISWAMY NAVANEETHAM,[b]
MARIA PIA PROTTI,[b,d,e] ROBERT M. HORTON,[b,f,g] BOBBI L. HOPPE,[b]
JAMES HOWARD, JR.,[h] AND BIANCA M. CONTI-FINE[b,i,j]

[b]Department of Biochemistry
College of Biological Sciences
University of Minnesota
St. Paul, Minnesota 55108
and
Department of Pharmacology
School of Medicine
University of Minnesota
Minneapolis, Minnesota 55455

[h]Department of Neurology
University of North Carolina
Chapel Hill, North Carolina 27599

INTRODUCTION

Myasthenia gravis (MG) is an ideal system to study the T cell receptor (TCR) gene usage and its relationship with the CD4⁺ epitope repertoire in human autoimmunity because the target autoantigen (autoAg)—the muscle acetylcholine receptor (AChR)—is known and well characterized.[1] Previous studies on the TCR usage of T cells isolated from tissues and blood of autoimmune patients yielded conflicting results.[2] This was likely due to the use of unselected T cells that, even if eluted from the affected tissues, may have included "bystander" T cells, in addition to autoimmune T cells specific for the autoAg. Investigations on these matters should strive to use pop-

[a]This work was supported by NINCDS Grant No. NS 23919 and a research grant from the Muscular Dystrophy Association (to B. M. Conti-Fine).
[c]Present address: Department of Immunology, Mayo Clinic, Rochester, Minnesota 55905.
[d]Present address: Laboratorio di Immunologia, Medicina II Department, H. San Raffaele Scientific Institute, University of Milano, Milano 20132, Italy.
[e]M. P. Protti was a recipient of a Sidney Blackmer Fellowship from the Muscular Dystrophy Association.
[f]Present address: Attotron Biosensor Corporation, Carson City, Nevada 89701.
[g]R. M. Horton was a recipient of a Robert G. Sampson Neuromuscular Disease Research Fellowship from the Muscular Dystrophy Association.
[i]Previously known as B. M. Conti-Tronconi.
[j]To whom all correspondence should be addressed.

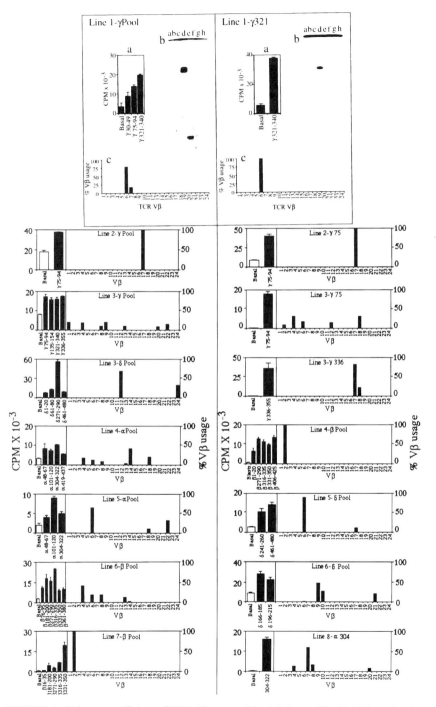

FIGURE 1. Epitope specificity and TCR Vβ usage of the AChR-specific CD4[+] lines. Results of one of at least two consistent RT-PCR assay experiments for each of the CD4[+] lines, as indicated in each panel. The lines are grouped according to the patient from which the lines were

ulations of T cells enriched as much as possible in Ag-specific autoimmune T cells. The goal of this study was to determine whether anti-AChR autoimmune CD4$^+$ cells in MG have a preferred use of TCR Vβ genes, using CD4$^+$ T cell lines propagated *in vitro* from MG patients and specific for muscle AChR epitopes. The Vβ usage was determined by a semiquantitative reverse transcriptase PCR (RT-PCR) assay.

MATERIALS AND METHODS

Antigens and T Cell Lines

CD4$^+$ lines were propagated using pools of synthetic peptides, ~20 residues long, spanning the sequences of the human AChR α, β, γ, and δ subunits, or individual peptides corresponding to immunodominant sequence regions of the α and γ subunits (α48–67, α118–137, α304–322, γ75–94, γ321–340, and γ336–355) of human AChR.[3–8] Propagation and characterization of the lines were described previously.[4–8] The lines are indicated with a code that includes a number referring to the patient from which they were derived [from 1 to 8] and the Ag used for propagation of the line (α, β, γ, or δ pool, or individual peptide sequence: for the latter lines, the code includes only the number of the sequence position of the first peptide residue). All lines tested for reactivity to purified muscle AChR responded strongly to that Ag, indicating that they recognize epitopes derived from AChR processing.[3–7]

RT-PCR

Total RNA was isolated from the CD4$^+$ lines (1×10^6 cells) or from PBL (5×10^6 cells) and cDNA was reverse-transcribed.[8] The TCR Vβ usage was determined by RT-PCR as described previously.[8] Family-specific 5′ primers were used with a constant region 3′ primer to amplify each of the 24 human Vβ families. The specific primers were mixed into eight pools of three primers, yielding products of different sizes, plus the constant region primer. The constant region primer was end-labeled with γ-^{32}P-ATP and T4 polynucleotide kinase. The RT-PCR products were resolved on a denaturing high-resolution acrylamide gel and autoradiographed. Their identity was confirmed by eluting and reamplifying the bands using an internal constant region primer.[9]

---

obtained. For each line, we report the result of a proliferation assay, carried out to verify the peptide specificity of the line. We report only the responses of the lines to peptides that were recognized significantly. The basal rate of cell proliferation of each line is also reported. For the lines of patient 1 (top panels), we report the radiogram (b), whose densitometric scan[8,9] yielded the data used to calculate the percent usage of the different Vβ gene families, reported in graph c. The signal-to-noise ratio obtained in this experiment is representative of that obtained in all RT-PCR experiments carried out with the CD4$^+$ lines. For all the other lines, we report a plot of the relative Vβ usage, determined from densitometric scans of autoradiograms of RT-PCR experiments.[8,9] Reprinted with permission from RAJU, R. *et al.* 1997. J. Autoimmun. **10:** 203–217.

RESULTS AND DISCUSSION

We assayed the Vβ usage of PBL from several healthy controls and from MG patients along with that of the CD4+ lines. PCR products of expected size were obtained for each family-specific primer. The relative Vβ usage of PBL from MG patients and healthy controls was comparable. Some Vβ families appeared to be used more than others, but even the most used Vβ families (e.g., Vβ2, Vβ4, Vβ5, Vβ13) were always less than 19% of the overall usage.

The result of RT-PCR analysis of the anti-AChR CD4+ lines is illustrated in FIGURE 1. Most lines had a limited Vβ usage. For several lines, the number of Vβ gene families used correlated with the number of epitopes recognized. For example, we studied two lines from patient 1, one propagated with the γ pool and recognizing three γ subunit epitopes, and the other propagated with and specific for peptide γ321–340 (top panels of FIGURE 1): the line 1-γPool used primarily Vβ6 and Vβ7, and the Vβ6 primers yielded two bands of similar intensity, indicating the presence of at least two clonal populations that rearranged Vβ6 genes differently, to yield V regions of different size; the line 1-γ321 used only Vβ6, whose RT-PCR product was a single band of the same MW as that of the top band observed for the Vβ6 products of the line 1-γPool. Both lines propagated from patient 2 (lines 2-γPool and 2-γ75) recognized only peptide γ75–94 and both used only Vβ17. The two lines from patient 5 (lines 5-αPool and 5-δPool) also had a good correspondence between the number of epitopes recognized and the number of Vβ families used.

For other lines, this correlation did not hold. Two lines (lines 4-βPool and 7-βPool) recognized several β subunit sequences, yet both used only Vβ2 genes. Other lines had opposite behavior: for example, lines 3-γ336 and 8-α304 recognized only one epitope, and they used two or more Vβ families, although one Vβ family was predominantly used. The Vβ4 and Vβ6 regions were used most frequently (in five of the lines studied: 3-γPool, 8-α304, 1-γPool, 5-αPool, and 5-δPool, respectively).

Thus, in spite of the limited Vβ usage of the individual lines, in most cases different Vβ regions were used for different epitopes in the same patient and for the same epitope in different patients. These findings suggest that the potentially autoimmune T cells that survive clonal deletion have a limited TCR repertoire. Although the present data do allow conclusions on the role of a superantigen in triggering the anti-AChR autoimmune response, the finding that different Vβ regions were used in different patients does not support an important role of a superantigen in the maintenance of the CD4+ response in MG.

REFERENCES

1. CONTI-FINE, B. M. *et al.* 1994. The nicotinic acetylcholine receptor: structure and autoimmune pathology. Crit. Rev. Biochem. Mol. Biol. **29:** 69–123.
2. NAVARRETE, C. & G. F. BOTTAZZO. 1993. In search of TCR restriction in autoreactive T cell in human autoimmunity: why is it so elusive? Clin. Exp. Immunol. **91:** 189–192.
3. PROTTI, M. P. *et al.* 1990. Immunodominant regions for T helper sensitization on the human nicotinic acetylcholine receptor α subunit in myasthenia gravis. Proc. Natl. Acad. Sci. U.S.A. **87:** 7792–7796.

4. PROTTI, M. P. *et al.* 1991. Myasthenia gravis: T epitopes of the δ subunit of human muscle acetylcholine receptor. J. Immunol. **146:** 2253–2261.
5. PROTTI, M. P. *et al.* 1992. Myasthenia gravis: CD4+ epitopes on the embryonic γ subunit of human muscle acetylcholine receptor. J. Clin. Invest. **90:** 1558–1567.
6. MOIOLA, L. *et al.* 1994. Epitopes on the β subunit of human muscle acetylcholine receptor recognized by CD4+ cells of myasthenia gravis patients and healthy subjects. J. Clin. Invest. **93:** 1020–1028.
7. MOIOLA, L. *et al.* 1994. Myasthenia gravis: residues of the α and γ subunits of muscle acetylcholine receptor involved in formation of immunodominant CD4+ epitopes. J. Immunol. **152:** 4686–4698.
8. HORTON, R. M. *et al.* 1996. Designing PCR primers to amplify specific members or subgroups of multigene families. *In* Methods in Molecular Biology. Humana Press. Clifton, New Jersey. In press.
9. RAJU, R. *et al.* 1995. Rapid method for the elution and analysis of PCR products separated on high resolution acrylamide gels. Biotechniques **18:** 33–35.

Th1 Cells of Myasthenia Gravis Patients Recognize Multiple Epitopes on the Muscle Acetylcholine Receptor α Subunit[a]

ZENG-YU WANG,[b,c] DAVID K. OKITA,[b] JAMES F. HOWARD, JR.,[d]
AND BIANCA M. CONTI-FINE[b,e]

[b]Department of Biochemistry
College of Biological Sciences
and
Department of Pharmacology
School of Medicine
University of Minnesota
Twin Cities Campus, Minnesota 55108

[d]Department of Neurology
University of North Carolina at Chapel Hill
Chapel Hill, North Carolina 27599

INTRODUCTION

In myasthenia gravis (MG), the muscle acetylcholine receptor (AChR) is the target of an autoimmune response, with production of anti-AChR antibodies (Ab) and sensitization of anti-AChR CD4$^+$ T helper cells.[1] The AChR is formed by four subunits: α, β, γ (or ε), and δ.[1] The anti-AChR CD4$^+$ cells of MG patients have been the focus of several studies because they may be the prime movers in the pathogenesis of MG, and specific immunosuppressive treatments of the autoimmune CD4$^+$ cells have been successful in experimental animals.[1] They recognize primarily the AChR α subunit.[1] CD4$^+$ T cells comprise different subpopulations: Th1 cells secrete interleukin-2 (IL-2) and interferon-γ (IFN-γ), provide helper function for particular immunoglobulin classes and subclasses, and have cytolytic activity; Th2 cells secrete IL-4 and IL-5 and may provide help for all immunoglobulin classes.[2] Th1 cells may be involved in MG pathogenesis since CD4$^+$ lines specific for different AChR epitopes comprised Th1 cells.[1]

We sought identification of the sequence regions of the human muscle AChR α subunit recognized by the blood Th1 cells from MG patients, under circumstances where no bias clonal propagation or loss might have occurred. We challenged the blood CD4$^+$ Th1 cells from 12 MG patients and 3 healthy controls, using overlapping

[a]This work was supported by NINCDS Grant No. NS23919 and a research grant from the Muscular Dystrophy Association (to B. M. Conti-Fine).
[c]Z-Y. Wang was a recipient of a Muscular Disease Research Fellowship from the Muscular Dystrophy Association.
[e]Previously known as B. M. Conti-Tronconi.

synthetic peptides screening the AChR α subunit sequence and an ELISPOT assay that detects antigen-induced IFN-γ secretion of individual Th1 cells.

MATERIALS AND METHODS

We tested 12 MG patients and 4 healthy subjects. The salient characteristics of the patients are reported in TABLE 1. Patients 3, 9, and 12 were tested twice. Peripheral blood mononuclear cells (PBMC) were isolated by Ficoll density gradient centrifugation and depleted of $CD8^+$ T cells using mouse anti-human CD8 mAb and paramagnetic beads coated with goat anti-mouse IgG Ab.[3] They are referred to as $CD4^+$-enriched PBMC. The AChR-reactive Th1 cells were counted by an ELISPOT assay that detects antigen-induced IFN-γ secretion of individual Th1 cells.[4] As antigens, we used 32 synthetic peptides, 14–20 residues long, spanning the sequence of the human muscle AChR α subunit, synthesized and characterized as we described previously.[3] The $CD4^+$-enriched PBMC were seeded in 96-well plates with nitrocellulose bottoms, coated with anti-human IFN-γ mAb, and cultured in the presence or absence of antigenic stimulus. The plates were incubated with rabbit anti-human IFN-γ Ab, biotinylated anti-rabbit IgG, and avidin-biotin peroxidase complex, sequentially. After staining, we counted the red-brown spots corresponding to individual cells that had secreted IFN-γ. The data were expressed as numbers of spots/10^5 cells. The significance of the responses was determined using Student's two-tailed t test.

TABLE 1. Clinical Characteristics of the MG Patients Studied

Patient No.	Age, Sex	DR Type[a]	Experiment Code[b]	Serum Anti-AChR Ab[c]	Disease Class[d]
1	59, F	ND	NA	++	IV
2	22, F	ND	NA	+	II
3	62, M	DRw17(3), DR4	a	−	II
			b	−	I
4	53, M	ND	NA	+	IV
5	16, F	ND	NA	++	IV
6	28, F	DRw15(2), DR4	NA	++	IV
7	27, F	DR9, DRw8	NA	+	IV
8	45, F	DR2, DR6	a	+++	II
9	62, M	DRw17(3), DR7	a	+	II
			b	+	II
10	63, F	ND	NA	+++	IV
11	50, F	DRw15(2), DR4	NA	ND	II
12	56, F	DR5, DRw6	a	+	IV
			b	+	II

[a]ND, not determined.
[b]As indicated in FIGURE 1. NA, not applicable.
[c]Terms: −, 0 mM; +, 0–10 mM; ++, 10–20 mM; +++, >20 mM; ND, not determined.
[d]At the time of the experiment.

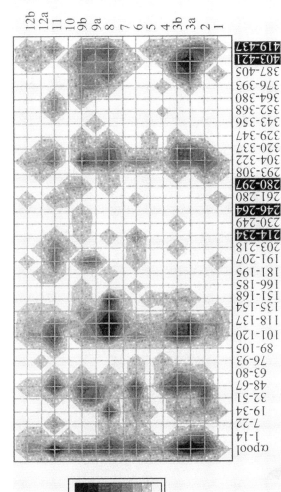

α subunit peptides

FIGURE 1. Summary representation of the significant responses of the CD4$^+$-enriched PBMC from 12 MG patients to the α pool and to the individual α subunit peptide sequences. The data are represented as a contour map: each horizontal strip represents the results obtained with the CD4$^+$-enriched PBMC of one patient in one experiment, as indicated on the right. The response to the α pool is followed by that to the individual peptides (one peptide for each vertical line), starting with the amino-terminal peptide sequence. The average ($n = 3$) number of cells/culture of 10^5 CD4$^+$-enriched PBMC that responded significantly to the presence of the individual peptide antigens is indicated using the gray scale depicted on the left. The background values, that is, the average number of cells that in a given patient and in a given experiment secreted IFN-γ spontaneously, were subtracted from the data reported here. The boxed peptides represent transmembrane sequence segments (M1, M2, M3, and M4). Reprinted with permission from WANG, Z-Y. *et al.* 1997. Neurology **48**: 1643–1653.

RESULTS AND DISCUSSION

All patients recognized the pool of the α subunit peptides. All but one patient recognized numerous peptides. FIGURE 1 is a summary of the results obtained, represented as a contour map, as described in the legend. Each patient recognized several peptides and had an individual pattern of peptide recognition. However, most or all patients recognized four sequences (residues 48–67, 101–137, 304–322, and 403–437) that stimulated relative large numbers of Th1 cells. They include previously identified "immunodominant" sequences recognized by AChR-specific CD4[+] T cell lines from myasthenic patients.[3] Peptide 1–14 was also recognized frequently. The controls recognized, with a low precursor frequency, the peptide pool and a few peptides that frequently included the immunodominant sequences described above.

These results demonstrate that Th1 cells are involved in the anti-AChR response in MG and that their epitope repertoire is very complex. This indicates that, when MG is clinically evident, the AChR itself is the sensitizing antigen and the target of the autoimmune Th1 cells; however, it does not exclude that molecular mimicry between one AChR epitope and a microbial structure triggers the autoimmune response since it has been shown that, once the CD4[+] cell tolerance is broken for one epitope, the autoimmune response can spread to other epitopes within the same or other nearby autoantigens.[1]

These data demonstrate that Th1 cells are involved in the anti-AChR response in MG. Th1 cells secrete cytokines involved in the stimulation of inflammatory responses, while Th2 cells secrete anti-inflammatory cytokines. In multiple sclerosis and experimental autoimmune encephalomyelitis, the pathogenic CD4[+] cells are Th1, which are very active in the acute phases of these diseases, while remission of the symptoms correlates with high activity of the Th2 subset.[5] Other observations implicate IFN-γ in the development of MG and experimental MG (EMG). MG patients have high levels of AChR-reactive blood T cells that secrete IFN-γ and express IFN-γ mRNA. EMG in Lewis rats is associated with elevated levels of lymphoid cells that secrete IFN-γ and express IFN-γ mRNA in response to AChR stimulation.[6] IFN-γ transgenic mice that produce IFN-γ at the neuromuscular junction develop functional disruption of the junction and muscular weakness reminiscent of MG.[7]

Although the complexity of the anti-AChR Th1 repertoire in MG patients suggests that development of immunosuppressive treatments targeted on epitope-specific autoimmune T cells will be difficult, the existence of immunodominant T epitope sequences might facilitate that task.

REFERENCES

1. CONTI-FINE, B. M. et al. 1997. Myasthenia Gravis: The Immunobiology of an Autoimmune Disease. R. G. Landes/Chapman & Hall. Austin/London.
2. ROMAGNANI, S. 1995. Biology of Th1 and Th2 cells. J. Clin. Immunol. **15:** 121–129.
3. PROTTI, M. P. et al. 1990. Immunodominant regions for T helper sensitization on the human nicotinic receptor subunit in myasthenia gravis. Proc. Natl. Acad. Sci. U.S.A. **87:** 7792–7796.
4. CZERKINSKY, C. C. et al. 1988. Reverse ELISPOT assay for clonal analysis of cytokine pro-

duction. I. Enumeration of gamma-interferon-secreting cells. J. Immunol. Methods **110:** 29–36.

5. OLSSON, T. 1995. Cytokine-producing cells in experimental autoimmune encephalomyelitis and multiple sclerosis. Neurology **45**(suppl. 6): S11–S15.

6. WANG, Z-Y. *et al.* 1994. Induction of interferon-γ, interleukin-4, and transforming factor-β in rats orally tolerized against experimental myasthenia gravis. Cell. Immunol. **157:** 353–368.

7. GU, D. *et al.* 1995. Myasthenia gravis–like syndrome induced by expression of interferon-γ in the neuromuscular junction. J. Exp. Med. **181:** 547–557.

CD4+ Epitope Spreading and Differential T Cell Recognition of Muscle Acetylcholine Receptor Subunits in Myasthenia Gravis[a]

ZENG-YU WANG,[b,c] DAVID K. OKITA,[b] JAMES F. HOWARD, JR.,[d]
AND BIANCA M. CONTI-FINE[b,e]

[b]Department of Biochemistry
College of Biological Sciences
and
Department of Pharmacology
School of Medicine
University of Minnesota
Twin Cities Campus, Minnesota 55108

[d]Department of Neurology
University of North Carolina at Chapel Hill
Chapel Hill, North Carolina 27599

INTRODUCTION

In myasthenia gravis (MG), the antimuscle acetylcholine receptor (AChR) antibodies directly cause the symptoms, but anti-AChR CD4+ T helper (Th) cells are required for their synthesis.[1] The AChR is formed by four homologous subunits and exists in two isoforms. Embryonic muscle AChR contains α, β, γ, and δ subunits. After innervation, the γ subunit is replaced by the ε subunit.[2] Adult extrinsic ocular muscles (EOM) still express the γ subunit.[3] The α subunit has an important role in the MG pathogenesis because it is recognized by most anti-AChR antibodies and CD4+ T cells.[1] Little is known about the role of non-α subunits in the anti-AChR response in MG. Also, the distribution of myasthenic weakness in ocular MG (oMG) and generalized MG (gMG) might be related to differential immune recognition of the AChR subunits and to a preferential response to the γ subunit in oMG.

We investigated whether the CD4+ T cells in MG recognize muscle AChR subunits other than the α, whether T cells in gMG and oMG recognize the AChR subunits differently, and how the CD4+ recognition of different AChR subunits evolves, as gMG progresses.[4]

[a]This work was supported by NINCDS Grant No. NS23919 and by a research grant from the Muscular Dystrophy Association (to B. M. Conti-Fine).

[c]Z-Y. Wang was a recipient of a Neuromuscular Disease Research Fellowship from the Muscular Dystrophy Association.

[e]Previously known as B. M. Conti-Tronconi.

MATERIALS AND METHODS

We tested 25 gMG patients whose MG symptoms had started from 1 month to 30 years prior to the test, 4 oMG patients, and 6 healthy controls. We determined the proliferative response *in vitro* of their blood CD4⁺ T cells to pools of overlapping synthetic peptides, 14–23 residues long, spanning the sequences of the α, β, γ, δ, and ε human AChR subunits.[4–8] We used the peptide pools as equimolar solutions of each of the peptides spanning the sequence of an AChR subunit (α, β, γ, δ, and ε pool). Peripheral blood mononuclear cells (PBMC) were isolated by Ficoll density gradient centrifugation and depleted of CD8⁺ T cells using mouse anti-human CD8 mAb and paramagnetic beads coated with goat anti-mouse IgG Ab.[9] They are referred to as CD4⁺-enriched PBMC. For most experiments, we used the CD4⁺-enriched PBMC. In a few patients, the low hematocrit did not allow us to draw an amount of blood sufficient for the CD8⁺ depletion: in those cases, we used the total PBMC. Comparable results were obtained with either cell population. The cells were cultured for 4 days

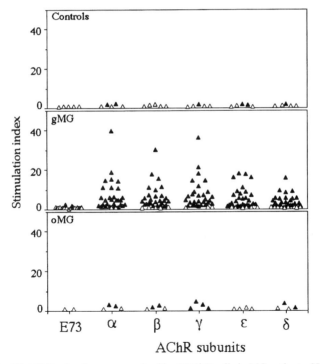

FIGURE 1. All AChR subunits are recognized by CD4⁺ T cells in MG patients. SI's obtained by testing in proliferation assays CD4⁺-enriched PBMC or PBMC from controls and patients with gMG or oMG, with the AChR subunit peptide pools and with a control peptide E73 (a 20-residue synthetic peptide unrelated to the AChR sequence), as indicated below the plots. The SI's that reflect a significant proliferative response, as compared to the spontaneous cell proliferation in the absence of antigenic stimuli, are indicated with black symbols.

in the presence or absence of antigenic stimulus and pulsed for 16 h with ^{3}H-thymidine. Data are expressed as a stimulation index (SI: the ratio between the ^{3}H-thymidine incorporation in the presence of a stimulus and that of the same cells in the absence of any stimulus).

RESULTS AND DISCUSSION

In gMG patients, the CD4[+] cells recognized all AChR subunits to comparable extents (FIGURE 1). The T cells from oMG patients had much lower *in vitro* responses to the AChR subunits than the gMG patients and did not recognize the AChR ε subunit, while they always recognized the γ subunit significantly (FIGURE 1). The other AChR subunits were not recognized by all oMG patients. The differential recognition of the γ and the ε subunits in oMG patients might be related to the preferential involvement of EOM, which express AChR containing the γ subunit.

In gMG patients, the severity of the symptoms did not correlate with the intensity of the T cell response (data not shown). On the other hand, gMG patients whose disease has lasted 4 years or less had lower responses to the AChR subunits than patients whose disease had lasted for 5–18 years, and some did not recognize some AChR subunits significantly, while gMG patients that have had clinical symptoms for longer periods of time (5–18 years) responded always to all AChR subunits (FIGURE 2).

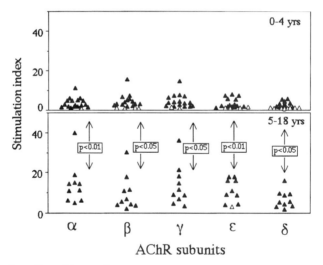

FIGURE 2. Spreading of the T cell response to all AChR subunits during the course of gMG. The results of a proliferation assay using PBMC or CD4[+]-enriched PBMC from gMG patients are compared with the years elapsed between the first appearance of the symptoms and the time of the assay. The SI's that reflect a significant proliferative response, as compared to the spontaneous cell proliferation in the absence of antigenic stimuli, are indicated with black symbols. gMG patients are separated into two groups, according to the duration of their symptoms. The significance of the difference in the responses to different AChR subunits between the two groups is indicated in the boxes.

The present data indicate that the autoimmune CD4⁺ response in MG ultimately involves the whole AChR molecule, and they support the possibility that this complex response results from the spreading of CD4⁺ sensitization to increasing larger parts of the AChR molecule as the disease progresses, with recognition of an increasing number of AChR subunits. It is likely that an increasing number of AChR epitopes are recognized within each subunit as the disease and the anti-AChR immune response evolve since the extent of the T cell response to the peptide pools was higher in the patients whose disease had lasted for 5 years or longer than in those whose symptoms had appeared less than 4 years prior to the test (FIGURE 2).

These findings indicate that, when MG is clinically evident, the AChR itself is the target and the sensitizing antigen of the autoimmune CD4⁺ T cells; however, they do not exclude that molecular mimicry between one AChR epitope and a microbial structure might trigger the anti-AChR response.[10] Once the CD4⁺ cell tolerance is broken for one epitope, the autoimmune response can spread to other epitopes within the same[11] or other nearby autoantigens.[11,12]

REFERENCES

1. CONTI-FINE, B. M. *et al.* 1997. Myasthenia Gravis: The Immunobiology of an Autoimmune Disease. R. G. Landes/Chapman & Hall. Austin/London.
2. GU, Y. & Z. W. HALL. 1988. Immunological evidence for a change in subunits of the acetylcholine receptor in developing and denervated rat muscle. Neuron **1:** 117–125.
3. HORTON, R. H. *et al.* 1993. The "embryonic" γ subunit of the nicotinic acetylcholine receptor is expressed in adult extrinsic ocular muscles. Neurology **43:** 983–986.
4. WANG, Z-Y. *et al.* 1998. T cell recognition of the muscle acetylcholine receptor subunits in generalized and ocular myasthenia gravis. Neurology. In Press.
5. PROTTI, M. P. *et al.* 1990. Immunodominant regions for T helper sensitization on the human nicotinic acetylcholine receptor α subunit in myasthenia gravis. Proc. Natl. Acad. Sci. U.S.A. **87:** 7792–7796.
6. PROTTI, M. P. *et al.* 1991. Myasthenia gravis: T epitopes of the δ subunit of human muscle acetylcholine receptor. J. Immunol. **146:** 2253–2261.
7. PROTTI, M. P. *et al.* 1992. Myasthenia gravis: CD4⁺ epitopes on the embryonic γ subunit of human muscle acetylcholine receptor. J. Clin. Invest. **90:** 1558–1567.
8. MOIOLA, L. *et al.* 1994. Epitopes on the β subunit of human muscle acetylcholine receptor recognized by CD4⁺ cells of myasthenia gravis patients and healthy subjects. J. Clin. Invest. **93:** 1020–1028.
9. MANFREDI, A. A. *et al.* 1993. Myasthenia gravis: T helper repertoire on the γ and δ subunits of human muscle acetylcholine receptor. J. Clin. Invest. **92:** 1055–1067.
10. OLDSTONE, M. B. A. 1987. Molecular mimicry and autoimmune disease. Cell **50:** 819–820.
11. LEHMANN, P. V. *et al.* 1992. Spreading of T-cell autoimmunity to cryptic determinants of an autoantigen. Nature **358:** 155–157.
12. MILLER, S. D. *et al.* 1995. Evolution of the T cell repertoire during the course of experimental immuno-mediated demyelinating diseases. Immunol. Rev. **144:** 225–244.

Coimmunization of MHC Class II Competitor Peptides during Experimental Autoimmune Myasthenia Gravis Induction Resulted Not Only in a Suppressed, but Also in an Altered Immune Response[a]

MARCA H. M. WAUBEN,[b] ASTRID C. W. E. HOEDEMAEKERS,[c]
YVO M. F. GRAUS,[c] JOSEE P. A. WAGENAAR,[b] WILLEM VAN EDEN,[b]
AND MARC H. DE BAETS[c]

[b]Institute of Infectious Diseases and Immunology
Faculty of Veterinary Medicine
Utrecht University
3584 CL Utrecht, the Netherlands

[c]Department of Immunology
Faculty of Medicine
University of Limburg
6229 ER Maastricht, the Netherlands

Coimmunization of an antigenic peptide together with an unrelated peptide, which binds to the same MHC class II molecule, has been shown to prevent induction of antigen-specific T cell responses by blockade of the MHC peptide binding site.[1] Furthermore, inhibition of experimental autoimmune diseases by disease nonrelated MHC class II competitor peptides has been demonstrated in several animal models.[2-6] In all these models, disease was mediated by $CD4^+$ T cells that could passively transfer the disease into naive recipient animals.

To address the question of whether MHC class II blocking peptides could also be used to interfere in a disease model mediated by autoantibodies, we studied the experimental autoimmune myasthenia gravis (EAMG) model in Lewis rats. Both EAMG and human myasthenia gravis (MG) are T cell–dependent autoimmune disorders mediated by antibodies against the acetylcholine receptor (AChR).[7-9] The binding of anti-AChR autoantibodies to AChR at the neuromuscular junction causes impairment of neuromuscular transmission, by reducing the amount of AChR via complement-mediated lysis[10] and antibody-modulated internalization.[11] In Lewis rats, EAMG can be induced by immunization with purified AChR from the electric organs of *Torpedo californica* (tAChR) in CFA.[12] Although there is an 80% sequence homology between the *Torpedo* and mammalian AChR α-subunit,[13] only about 1% of

[a]The research of M. H. M. Wauben was supported by the Netherlands Organization for Scientific Research (NWO) (Grant No. 900-509-214). The research of Y. M. F. Graus, A. C. W. E. Hoedemaekers, and J. P. A. Wagenaar was supported by "Het Prinses Beatrixfonds". A. C. W. E. Hoedemaekers and Y. M. F. Graus contributed equally to this study.

338

anti-tAChR antibodies cross-react with syngeneic AChR.[14] Most of the pathogenic cross-reactive antibodies are directed to the AChR main immunogenic region, sequence 67–76 of the α-subunit.[15] Also, T cell recognition of tAChR is predominantly focused on the α-subunit of the pentameric AChR.[16] The major T cell epitope involved in tAChR-induced EAMG in Lewis rats is the 97–112 sequence of the α-subunit of tAChR.[17,18] This epitope is recognized by specific CD4[+] T cells in an MHC class II RT1.B[L]-restricted fashion.[18]

We have found that coimmunization of a strong RT1.B[L]-binding ovalbumin peptide (OVA323–339) along with tAChR efficiently inhibited EAMG induction.[19] Although it has been shown previously that analogues of immunodominant myasthenogenic T cell epitopes can inhibit both *in vitro* T cell proliferation as well as *in vivo* priming of lymph node cells by these epitopes,[20] this is the first time that an MHC competitor peptide has been shown to be effective *in vivo* in the inhibition of an antibody-mediated autoimmune disease process. To investigate whether the inhibition of EAMG was due to blockade of the immunodominant RT1.B[L]-restricted T cell response, we evaluated whether the tAChR97–112-specific T cell response was decreased. Time course experiments showed a clear change in the kinetics of the tAChR-specific proliferative LN cell responses of OVA323–339-coimmunized rats. The fact that, at days 14 and 21 after tAChR/CFA immunization in the presence of OVA323–339, the T cell response was strongly decreased as compared to the control groups could well be due to a partial MHC blockade of RT1.B[L] molecules. However, at day 40 after coimmunization of OVA323–339 together with tAChR/CFA, both the magnitude of the tAChR and the immunodominance of the tAChR97–112-specific proliferative LN cell responses were not changed as compared to the control groups. This indicates that addition of OVA323–339 did not result in changes in the immunodominance hierarchy of T cell epitopes in tAChR.

Previously, it has been shown that administration of MHC class II competitor peptides can inhibit the induction of T cell–dependent primary and secondary antibody responses.[21] Also, in our experiments, the antirat AChR antibody response was not detectable in rats immunized with tAChR/CFA in the presence of OVA323–339. However, although the anti-tAChR antibody response, of which about 1% cross-reacts with rat AChR,[14] was also significantly lowered in OVA323–339-coimmunized rats, serum anti-tAChR antibodies could still be detected in these rats, indicating that the antibody response was not fully inhibited. In addition to the pronounced decrease of the anti-tAChR antibody response, we observed a change in the isotype distribution of the anti-tAChR antibody response. OVA323–339-coimmunized rats showed significantly higher IgG1 responses as compared to the tAChR/CFA-immunized rats. Similar to mice,[22] it has been shown in rats that the preferential production of IgG1 antibodies reflects the preferential activation of Th2-like cells.[23] Thus, the isotype shift observed in OVA323–339-coimmunized rats is compatible with a shift from Th1 towards a more Th2-dominated Ig isotype. Interestingly, it has been shown that selective generation of Th1 or Th2 responses can be influenced by the presentation of different densities of the same peptide-MHC complex on the APC surface.[24–26] High MHC class II peptide densities favored Th1-like responses, while low densities favored Th2-like responses. In our experiments, it could well be that OVA323–339 did not fully block all RT1.B[L] molecules on the APC, but did lower the tAChR97–112/RT1.B^L density, thereby affecting the T cell response not only quantitatively, but also qualitatively. Although the EAMG inhibition in our experiments is most likely primarily due to the drastically decreased anti-tAChR antibody titer, changes in the isotypes of the serum anti-tAChR antibody response could have contributed as well.

In general, if ligand density is an immunoregulatory determinant, the quality of MHC competitor peptides to change the ligand concentration on APC, and thereby alter the immune response not only in a quantitative, but also in a qualitative sense, offers renewed possibilities for the competitor peptide approach.

REFERENCES

1. ADORINI, L., S. MULLER, F. CARDINAUX, P. V. LEHMANN, F. FALCIONI & Z. A. NAGY. 1988. Nature **334:** 623.
2. GAUTAM, A. M., C. I. PEARSON, A. A. SINHA, D. E. SMILEK, L. STEINMAN & H. O. McDEVITT. 1992. J. Immunol. **148:** 3049.
3. LAMONT, A. G., A. SETTE, R. FUJINAMI, S. M. COLON, C. MILES & H. M. GREY. 1990. J. Immunol. **145:** 1687.
4. SMITH, S. C. & P. M. ALLEN. 1991. J. Immunol. **147:** 2141.
5. WAUBEN, M. H. M., I. JOOSTEN, A. SCHLIEF, R. VAN DER ZEE, C. J. P. BOOG & W. VAN EDEN. 1994. J. Immunol. **152:** 4211.
6. WAUBEN, M. H. M., A. KOZHICH, I. JOOSTEN, A. SCHLIEF, C. J. P. BOOG & W. VAN EDEN. 1994. Eur. J. Immunol. **24:** 1053.
7. COMPSTON, D. A. S., A. VINCENT, J. NEWSOM-DAVIS & J. R. BATCHELOR. 1980. Brain **103:** 579.
8. BELL, J., S. SMOOT, C. NEWBY, K. TOYKA, L. RASSENTI, K. SMIT, R. HOHLFELD, H. O. McDEVITT & L. STEINMAN. 1986. Lancet **ii:** 1058.
9. KAUL, R., M. SHENOY, E. GOLUSZKO & P. CHRISTADOSS. 1994. J. Immunol. **152:** 3152.
10. LENNON, V. A., M. E. SEYBOLD, J. M. LINDSTROM, C. COCHRANE & R. ULEVITCH. 1978. J. Exp. Med. **147:** 973.
11. HEINEMANN, S., J. MERLIE & J. M. LINDSTROM. 1978. Nature **274:** 65.
12. LINDSTROM, J. M., B. EINARSON, V. A. LENNON & M. E. SEYBOLD. 1976. J. Exp. Med. **144:** 726.
13. NODA, M., Y. FURUTANI, H. TAKAHASHI, M. TOYOSATO, T. TANABE, S. SHIMIZU, S. KIKYOTANI, T. KAYANO, T. HIROSE, S. INAYAMA & S. NUMA. 1983. Nature **305:** 818.
14. DE BAETS, M. H., B. EINARSON, J. M. LINDSTROM & W. O. WEIGLE. 1982. J. Immunol. **128:** 2228.
15. LINDSTROM, J., B. EINARSON & J. MERLIE. 1978. Proc. Natl. Acad. Sci. U.S.A. **75:** 769.
16. KROLICK, K. & O. URSO. 1978. Cell. Immunol. **105:** 75.
17. FUJII, Y. & J. LINDSTROM. 1988. J. Immunol. **140:** 1830.
18. ZHANG, Y., T. BARKAS, M. JUILLERAT, B. SCHWENDIMANN & H. WEKERLE. 1988. Eur. J. Immunol. **18:** 551.
19. WAUBEN, M. H. M., A. C. W. E. HOEDEMAEKERS, Y. M. F. GRAUS, J. P. A. WAGENAAR, W. VAN EDEN & M. H. DE BAETS. 1996. Eur. J. Immunol. **26:** 2866.
20. KATZ-LEVY, Y., S. KIRSCHNER, M. SELA & E. MOZES. 1993. Proc. Natl. Acad. Sci. U.S.A. **90:** 7000.
21. GUERY, J., M. NEAGU, G. RODRIGUEZ-TARDUCHY & L. ADORINI. 1993. J. Exp. Med. **177:** 1461.
22. SNAPPER, C. M., F. D. FINKELMAN & W. E. PAUL. 1988. Immunol. Rev. **102:** 51.

23. SAOUDI, A., J. KUHN, K. HUYGEN, Y. DE KOZAK, T. VELU, M. GOLDMAN, P. DRUET & B. BELLON. 1993. Eur. J. Immunol. **23:** 3096.

24. MURRAY, J. S., D. FERRANDIS-EDWARDS, C. WOLFE & T. SCHOUNTZ. 1994. Eur. J. Immunol. **24:** 2337.

25. SECRIST, H., R. H. DEKRUYFF & D. T. UMETSU. 1995. J. Exp. Med. **181:** 1081.

26. PFEIFFER, C., J. STEIN, S. SOUTHWOOD, H. KETELAAR, A. SETTE & K. BOTTOMLY. 1995. J. Exp. Med. **181:** 1569.

Low Level of TGF-β in Early Stages of Myasthenia Gravis

A. P. BATOCCHI, A. EVOLI, M. LINO, L. MAJOLINI,
C. MINISCI, AND P. TONALI

Institute of Neurology
Catholic University
00168 Rome, Italy

INTRODUCTION

It is well known that human Th cells are classified into Th1 and Th2 subtypes depending on their cytokine secretion profiles and that the two subtypes reciprocally regulate each other through the cytokines they secrete.

IL-2, IFN-γ, and TNF-β are produced by Th1 cells and are involved in delayed-type hypersensitivity. IL-4 and IL-5 (together with IL-10, IL-6, and IL-13) are produced by Th2 cells and are related to humoral immunity.[1]

TGF-β is produced by activated T lymphocytes, B cells, and macrophages. This strong anti-inflammatory cytokine suppresses the proliferative response of CD4[+] or CD8[+] T cell clones to IL-2 and inhibits the IL-12-induced Th1 cytokine (IFN-γ, TNF-α) production by naive human CD4[+] T cells. TGF-β is also inhibitory on several levels of B cell function and it enhances isotype switching to IgA.[2]

Recently, it has become clear that an imbalance between Th1 and Th2 responses is associated with many diseases, such as multiple sclerosis, rheumatoid arthritis, and systemic sclerosis. It is not yet clear if Th1- or Th2-mediated response (or both) is involved in pathogenesis of MG.

In order to investigate the role of cytokines in MG, we studied *in vitro* production of IFN-γ, IL-4, and TGF-β in patients and controls matched for age and sex.

PATIENTS AND METHODS

Eighteen patients with generalized MG and 18 healthy subjects matched for age (±2 years) and sex were included in the study. All patients were studied in the early stage and active phase of the disease, before the thymectomy and immunosuppressive therapy. None of the patients or controls were affected by other autoimmune diseases.

TGF-β and IFN-γ were measured in 18 patients and 18 controls, and IL-4 was measured in 11 patients and 8 controls. Clinical data of the patients and controls are shown in TABLE 1.

Peripheral blood mononuclear cells (PBMCs) (4×10^6) from healthy and MG subjects were cultured in RPMI serum with 10% FCS in the absence (spontaneous pro-

TABLE 1. Clinical Data of Patients and Controls Matched for Age and Sex

Donor	Sex	Current Age (Years)	DT[a] (Months)	Osserman Classification	Thymic Pathology	AChR-Ab (nM/L)
MG patients						
P1	m	42	12	2B	thymoma	>10
P2	m	45	24	2B	thymoma	5
P3	m	48	2	2B	thymoma	7
P4	f	36	5	2B	thymoma	>12
P5	f	18	3	3	hyperplasia	>40
P6	f	13	3	2B	thymoma	>12
P7	f	35	24	2A	hyperplasia	>10
P8	f	22	12	2B	hyperplasia	>12
P9	f	21	8	2A	hyperplasia	>12
P10	f	40	9	2B	hyperplasia	>50
P11	f	23	5	2B	hyperplasia	>20
P12	f	32	24	2A	hyperplasia	9.02
P13	f	30	13	2A	hyperplasia	8.06
P14	m	11	7	3	hyperplasia	>16
P15	m	62	3	2B	NT[b]	3
P16	f	68	12	2A	NT	>10
P17	f	30	6	2B	hyperplasia	>20
P18	f	26	24	2B	hyperplasia	5.4
Healthy controls						
C1	m	40				
C2	m	43				
C3	m	49				
C4	f	36				
C5	f	20				
C6	f	13				
C7	f	34				
C8	f	24				
C9	f	23				
C10	f	42				
C11	f	25				
C12	f	32				
C13	f	32				
C14	m	11				
C15	m	62				
C16	f	69				
C17	f	30				
C18	f	28				

[a]DT: corrected ΔT (time interval from onset of disease).
[b]NT: not thymectomized.

duction) or presence of 10 ng/mL phorbol 12-myristate 13-acetate (PMA) and 0.5 mg/mL ionomycin (mitogen-induced production). After 24 hours, culture supernatant was collected and stored at –70 °C until used. All cytokines (IL-4, IFN-γ, TGF-β) were detected in supernatant by commercial ELISA (Genzyme). Statistical analysis of cytokine levels was performed by either Wilcoxon's test or Student's t test ($p < 0.05$).

RESULTS

Spontaneous production of IL-4, IFN-γ, and TGF-β was determined in culture with only medium. There were no differences between MG patients and healthy subjects in IFN-γ (FIGURE 1A) and IL-4 (FIGURE 1C) levels. Spontaneous production of TGF-β was significantly lower ($p < 0.01$) in MG patients than in healthy subjects (FIGURE 1B). There were no differences between patients and controls in mitogen-induced production of IFN-γ, IL-4, and TGF-β (data not shown). Spontaneous production of IFN-γ was significantly higher ($p < 0.05$) in MG patients with thymic hyperplasia than in healthy controls (FIGURE 1D). There was no correlation between cytokine levels, severity of disease, and anti-AChR titer.

DISCUSSION

Anti-AChR antibody production in MG is induced by CD4[+] Th cells reactive against AChR epitopes and it is not yet clear if Th1- and/or Th2-mediated responses are involved in the pathogenesis of the disease. The mechanism of peripheral tolerance could be impaired in MG since AChR-reactive lymphocytes are present in both MG patients and controls. Peripheral tolerance can be related to two mechanisms: anergy and cytokine-mediated suppression of autoreactive clones. Active suppression requires specifically activated Th cells that suppress the cellular immune response in an antigen-nonspecific fashion by the release of cytokines such as TGF-β.[3]

Previous reports have shown no differences in the number of peripheral blood cells that spontaneously secrete IL-4 and IFN-γ between MG patients and controls,[4] while an increased number of IFN-γ, IL-4, and TGF-β mRNA–expressing cells has been found in the peripheral blood of MG patients.[5]

We found no differences in spontaneous and mitogen-induced productions of IFN-γ and IL-4 between MG patients and controls, while a significant difference ($p < 0.01$) in PBMC spontaneous TGF-β production was present.

There may not be a parallel between synthesis of this cytokine, expressed by mRNA positive cells, and secretion since the induction of TGF-β secretion is most likely posttranscriptionally controlled.[6]

Moreover, the previous studies were based on an unselected MG population, while all of our patients were affected by generalized MG and were in both an early stage and an active phase of the disease, before thymectomy and immunosuppressive therapy.

The low TGF-β level that we found in the early stage of the disease suggests that mechanisms involved in peripheral tolerance to AChR can play an important role in

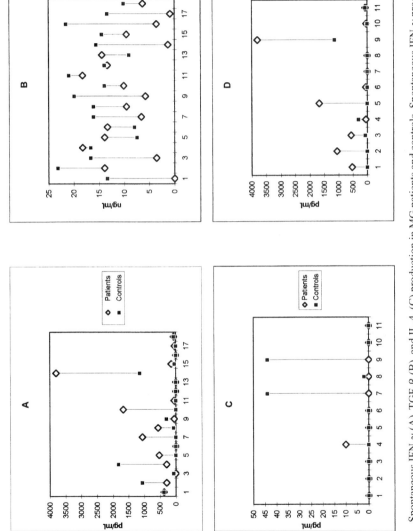

FIGURE 1. Spontaneous IFN-γ (A), TGF-β (B), and IL-4 (C) production in MG patients and controls. Spontaneous IFN-γ production and thymic hyperplasia in MG (D). Spontaneous TGF-β production is significantly lower in MG patients ($p < 0.01$) (B). Spontaneous IFN-γ production is significantly higher in MG with thymic hyperplasia ($p < 0.05$) (D).

the pathogenesis of MG. These data are also in accordance with the upregulation of TGF-β mRNA–expressing cells observed in thymectomized patients as compared with nonthymectomized patients;[5] this fact implies a possible role of this cytokine in the recovery from the disease.

REFERENCES

1. ROMAGNANI, S. 1991. Human Th1 and Th2 subsets: doubt no more. Immunol. Today **12**(8): 256.
2. MASSAGUE, J. 1990. The transforming growth factor-beta family. Annu. Rev. Cell Biol. **6**: 597–641.
3. KHOURY, S. J., W. W. HANCOCH & H. L. WEINER. 1992. Oral tolerance to myelin basic protein and natural recovery from experimental autoimmune encephalomyelitis associated with down-regulation of inflammatory cytokines and differential up-regulation of TGF-β, IL-4, and PGE expression in the brain. J. Exp. Med. **176**: 1355–1364.
4. QING, Y. *et al.* 1994. Acetylcholine receptor–reactive T cells in myasthenia gravis: evidence for the involvement of different subpopulations of T helper cells. J. Neuroimmunol. **50**: 177–186.
5. LINK, J. *et al.* 1994. Augmented IFN-γ, IL-4, and TGF-β mRNA expression in blood mononuclear cells in myasthenia gravis. J. Neuroimmunol. **51**: 185–192.
6. WAHL, S. M., N. MCCARTNEY-FRANCIS & S. E. MEGENHAUGEN. 1989. Inflammatory and immunomodulatory roles of TGF-β. Immunol. Today **10**: 258.

Secretion of TH-2-type Cytokines by Acetylcholine Receptor (AChR)–stimulated Mononuclear Cells

SAMIA RAGHEB AND ROBERT P. LISAK

Department of Neurology
Division of Neuroimmunology
Wayne State University School of Medicine
and
Detroit Medical Center
Detroit, Michigan 48201

Autoimmune myasthenia gravis (MG)[1] is an antibody-mediated disease in which the nicotinic AChR is the target antigen. Pathogenic AChR-specific antibodies are present in the circulation of 85–90% of patients with generalized MG and the presence of these antibodies leads to deficits in neuromuscular transmission. The majority of AChR-specific antibodies are directed against the α-subunit, although antibodies with specificities to other AChR subunits may also be present. The production of anti-AChR antibodies *in vitro* is T cell–dependent. Peripheral blood T cells from MG patients are stimulated *in vitro* by epitopes on the α-subunit of the AChR; likewise, T cells from normal nonmyasthenic controls are also stimulated by α-subunit epitopes. However, B cells from normal controls do not produce detectable amounts of AChR-specific antibodies; therefore, peripheral tolerance to the AChR is maintained in nonmyasthenics.

B cell activation, proliferation, and differentiation are known to be regulated in part by cognate interactions with T cells and by soluble cytokine signals.[2] Furthermore, inflammatory (TH-1) and helper (TH-2) CD4[+] T cell subsets are known to regulate each other's growth, differentiation, and effector function through soluble cytokines.[3,4] Therefore, T cell cross-regulation with resultant cytokine shifts can profoundly affect B cell function. To characterize and compare the soluble cytokine signals that are provided by AChR-stimulated T cells, we investigated cytokine production and secretion *in vitro* by mononuclear cells in MG patients versus normal controls. TABLE 1 highlights the important pleiotropic functions of the cytokines of interest.

Peripheral blood mononuclear cells (PBMC) were isolated from patients with MG (*n* = 9) and from normal healthy nonmyasthenic controls (*n* = 4) by Ficoll Hypaque centrifugation. Cell viability was consistently >95% as determined by dye exclusion. PBMC were cultured with synthetic peptides corresponding to segments of the α-, γ-, and ε-subunits of the AChR to examine cytokine secretion following autoantigen stimulation. Cytokine secretion by peptide-stimulated PBMC was compared to cytokine secretion by cells stimulated with the exogenous antigen, tetanus toxoid (TT). PBMC were also cultured with medium alone to determine constitutive cytokine se-

TABLE 1. Summary of the Notable Functions of Cytokines

IFN-γ: TH-1-type
- antiviral activity
- induces/upregulates MHC class II expression
- activates macrophages and NK cells

IL-2: TH-1-type
- T cell growth factor (TCGF)
- supports growth of B cells, NK cells, and LAK cells

IL-4: TH-2-type
- B cell growth factor (BCGF)
- induces CD23 expression on B cells
- enhances IgG1 and IgE production by B cells

IL-6: TH-2-type
- B cell stimulating factor (BCSF-2)
- induces proliferation and differentiation of B cells
- expansion of activated T cells
- induces acute-phase reactions

IL-10: TH-2-type
- cytokine synthesis inhibitory factor (CSIF)
- downregulation of MHC class II expression
- inhibits cytokine synthesis by TH-1 cells
- potent growth and differentiation factor for activated B cells

cretion. In preliminary experiments, we determined that four days of culture was optimal for interleukin-2 (IL-2) secretion (data not shown). Therefore, after four days, culture supernatants were collected. Levels of interferon-γ (IFN-γ), IL-2, IL-4, IL-6, and IL-10 were determined by ELISA.

FIGURE 1 shows the mean results for PBMC obtained from MG patients. Secretion of all the cytokines tested was inducible, although there was minimal IL-6 secretion by unstimulated PBMC cultures. TT-stimulated PBMC secreted IFN-γ, IL-2, and IL-6. By contrast, α-synthetic peptide–stimulated PBMC did not secrete appreciable amounts of IFN-γ or IL-2 when compared to unstimulated cultures. Instead, they secreted high levels of IL-6 and IL-10 (reaching ng/mL concentrations) and some IL-4. In a few limited preliminary experiments, PBMC that were stimulated with γ- and ε-synthetic peptides also produced predominantly IL-6 and IL-10 (data not shown).

In addition to examining cytokine secretion by synthetic peptide–stimulated PBMC, replicate cultures were set up to measure ^{3}H-thymidine incorporation by 2×10^5 cells (data not shown). Interestingly, when the responses of individual patients to each peptide were examined, there was no obvious correlation between PBMC proliferation and cytokine secretion. In some cases, there was not a peptide-induced proliferative response (defined as a stimulation index of <3), yet there was significant cytokine secretion. When there was a correlation between peptide-induced PBMC proliferation and cytokine secretion, the proliferative response appeared to correlate

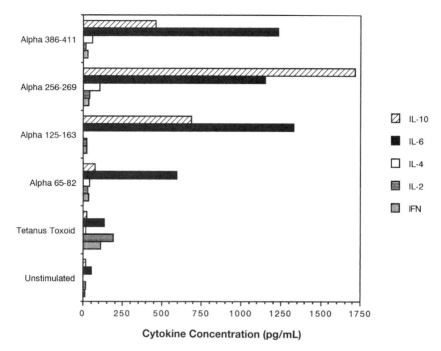

FIGURE 1. *In vitro* cytokine secretion by peripheral blood mononuclear cells (PBMC). PBMC were cultured at a concentration of 5×10^6 cells per mL in RPMI 1640 medium supplemented with 2% heat-inactivated normal human serum (type AB). PBMC were stimulated with synthetic peptides of the AChR or with tetanus toxoid. Unstimulated cells were cultured with medium alone to determine constitutive cytokine secretion. After four days, culture supernatants were collected and frozen at $-70\ ^{\circ}$C. Levels of IFN-γ, IL-2, IL-4, IL-6, and IL-10 were measured by sandwich ELISA using commercially available kits. Mean values are shown for nine patients with MG.

with IL-6 rather than IL-2 secretion. IL-6 is known to support the expansion of activated T cells.

Similar experiments with PBMC isolated from normal nonmyasthenic controls showed that the cytokine secretion patterns of TT-stimulated and synthetic peptide–stimulated cells were similar to those of MG patients. It has been previously shown by several groups that patients with MG and nonmyasthenic controls also have similar *in vitro* proliferative responses to α-subunit epitopes (reviewed in reference 1), although the frequency of responding cells may be higher in MG patients. These results demonstrate that epitopes on the AChR preferentially lead to production and secretion of TH-2-type cytokines. While some cytokine production may be monocyte-derived, the results suggest that AChR-responsive T cells produce primarily IL-4, IL-6, and IL-10; these are cytokines that are important for, and can upregulate, B cell growth and differentiation.

REFERENCES

1. RAGHEB, S. & R. P. LISAK. 1994. The immunopathogenesis of acquired (autoimmune) myasthenia gravis. *In* Handbook of Myasthenia Gravis and Myasthenic Syndromes, p. 239–276. Dekker. New York.
2. PARKER, D. C. 1993. T cell–dependent B cell activation. Annu. Rev. Immunol. **11:** 331–360.
3. STREET, N. E. & T. R. MOSMANN. 1991. Functional diversity of T lymphocytes due to secretion of different cytokine patterns. FASEB J. **5:** 171–177.
4. PAUL, W. E. & R. A. SEDER. 1994. Lymphocyte responses and cytokines. Cell **76:** 241–251.

In Vitro Production of Antiacetylcholine Receptor Antibody and IgG by Peripheral Blood Lymphocytes of Patients with Myasthenia Gravis

HIROAKI YOSHIKAWA, KATSUAKI SATOH, KAZUO IWASA, AND MASAHARU TAKAMORI

Department of Neurology
School of Medicine
Kanazawa University
Kanazawa, Ishikawa 920, Japan

INTRODUCTION

Myasthenia gravis (MG) is a prototypic organ-specific autoimmune disease targeting the nicotinic acetylcholine receptor (AChR) on the postsynaptic membrane of the neuromuscular junction.[1] The production of antiacetylcholine receptor antibody (AChR Ab) is dependent on the activation of helper T lymphocytes.[2] Although 90% of MG patients are seropositive for AChR Ab, their clinical grade does not always correlate to the clinical severity of their disease.[3] We have also found difficulties in the diagnosis of patients with seronegative MG. We therefore studied the production of AChR Ab and IgG *in vitro* using peripheral blood lymphocytes (PBL) from MG patients and paying special attention to serum AChR Ab values.

MATERIALS AND METHODS

Blood was obtained from 5 male and 26 female MG patients between the ages of 17 and 85 years under full informed consent. Clinical grade was classified according to Osserman.[4] Thirteen patients were classified as type I, 13 as IIa, 2 as IIb, 2 as III, and 1 as IV. Fifteen patients were first diagnosed with MG at our clinic, but had not yet received treatment. Sixteen patients had already received thymectomy, and 11 of the 15 newly diagnosed patients received thymectomy after PBL culturing. Twelve patients had prednisolone (PSL) treatment after thymectomy. Thymic pathology was follicular hyperplasia in 10 patients, thymoma in 9, normal in 7, and unknown in 1. Thirteen patients were negative for serum AChR Ab. Peripheral blood lymphocytes (PBL) were separated by Ficoll-Hypaque density gradient and cultured in RPMI 1640/5% CBS for 7 days. Culture medium was collected for determinations of AChR Ab and IgG. The volume of AChR Ab in culture medium was measured by immunoprecipitation assay (IPA) using AChR labeled with $[^{125}I]$-α-bungarotoxin. AChR was derived from TE671 cell lines.[5] The volume of AChR Ab in serum was determined with an IPA kit (Cosmic Corporation) using TE671 as the source of AChR. The volume of IgG in culture medium was determined by ELISA. The volume of IgG in sera was determined with a Behring nephelometer.

RESULTS

Twelve MG PBL (38.7%) produced a significant amount of AChR Ab in culture medium (>2.38 fmol/mL, mean + 3 SD of normal control). Five patients were receiving immunosuppressants and 7 were not. There was no difference in the amount of supernatant AChR Ab between patients with and without PSL. No correlation was found between thymic histology and AChR Ab value in either serum or supernatant. Three seronegative patients produced a significant volume of AChR Ab in culture medium. One patient, classified as IIa, had received thymectomy and had been treated with PSL. The other 2 patients had received no prior therapy and were classified as being of ocular type. There was no correlation between clinical severity and AChR Ab volume in culture supernatant (FIGURE 1). Ocular- or generalized-type classifications had no effect on AChR Ab production *in vitro*. The volume of AChR Ab in culture medium was significantly correlated with that in serum ($\rho_S = 0.479$; $p = 0.0087$, Spearman's rank correlation test). Also, the volume of AChR Ab in culture medium significantly correlated with that of IgG in culture medium ($\rho_S = 0.689$; $p = 0.0002$, Spearman's rank correlation test) (FIGURE 2). Normal PBL produced an extremely small volume of IgG in culture medium (mean ± SD = 1.56 ± 0.57 µg/mL, $n = 10$).

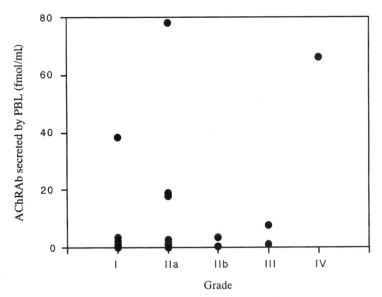

FIGURE 1. AChR Ab in supernatant of PBL culture from patients with MG. Each value of AChR Ab secreted by PBL was plotted as a classification of the patient's clinical grade according to Osserman.

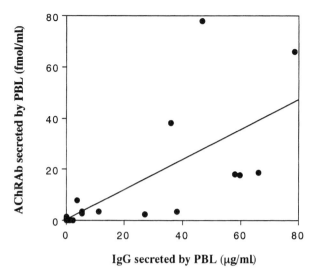

FIGURE 2. AChR Ab secreted by PBL was plotted in correlation with IgG secreted by PBL. AChR Ab production in culture medium was significantly correlated to IgG production in culture medium ($\rho_S = 0.689$; $p = 0.0002$, Spearman's rank correlation test).

DISCUSSION

As previously reported, the volume of AChR Ab produced by PBL of MG patients was significantly correlated with that produced in serum.[6] The large volume of AChR Ab in serum may be responsible for the production by PBL; otherwise, B lymphocytes in MG patients are equally activated to produce AChR Ab. The significant correlation between AChR Ab and IgG produced by PBL *in vitro* suggests polyclonal activation of B lymphocytes in MG patients. High IgG secretion in culture medium is a characteristic feature for patients with MG whose PBL produced a high AChR Ab volume *in vitro*. We found that PBL from selected seronegative MG patients produced AChR Ab *in vitro*. Although the positive result is not remarkable (3 of 13 patients; 23.1%), some seronegative patients may be served by culturing this PBL for detection of AChR Ab production.

REFERENCES

1. DRACHMAN, D. B. 1994. Myasthenia gravis. N. Engl. J. Med. **330:** 1797–1810.
2. NEWSOM-DAVIS, J. *et al.* 1981. Thymus cells in myasthenia gravis selectively enhance production of anti-acetylcholine-receptor antibody by autologous blood lymphocytes. N. Engl. J. Med. **305:** 1313–1318.
3. LENNON, V. A. 1997. Serological profile of myasthenia gravis and distinction from the Lambert-Eaton myasthenic syndrome. Neurology **48**(suppl. 5): S23–S27.

4. OSSERMAN, K. E. & G. GENKINS. 1966. Studies in myasthenia gravis: short-term massive corticotropin therapy. JAMA **198:** 699–702.
5. SOMNIER, F. E. 1994. Anti-acetylcholine receptor (AChR) antibodies measurement in myasthenia gravis: the use of cell line TE671 as a source of AChR antigen. J. Neuroimmunol. **51:** 63–68.
6. LISAK, R. P. *et al.* 1983. *In vitro* synthesis of antibodies to acetylcholine receptor by peripheral blood mononuclear cells of patients with myasthenia gravis. Neurology **33:** 604–608.

Identification of a Novel HLA Class II Association with DQB1*0502 in an Italian Myasthenic Population

FULVIO BAGGI,[a] CARLO ANTOZZI,[a] FRANCESCA ANDREETTA,[a]
PAOLO CONFALONIERI,[a] EMILIO CIUSANI,[b] ANN B. BEGOVICH,[c]
HENRY A. ERLICH,[c] FERDINANDO CORNELIO,[a]
AND RENATO MANTEGAZZA[a]

[a]Department of Neuromuscular Diseases
[b]Laboratorio Analisi
National Neurological Institute "C. Besta"
20133 Milan, Italy

[c]Roche Molecular System Incorporated
Alameda, California

INTRODUCTION

Different studies have investigated the association of HLA antigen with myasthenia gravis (MG). HLA was initially analyzed by conventional serological methods and different associations with MG were described: HLA-A1, B8, and DRw3 alleles were found in Caucasian MG patients without thymoma with early-onset disease and intermediate titers of AChR Ab, whereas increased frequencies of HLA-A3, B7, and DRw2 have been demonstrated in older MG patients with low AChR Ab levels.[1,2] Genetic susceptibility to the disease has also been investigated by molecular typing, and associations between HLA class II alleles and MG are known. However, the observed associations were weak, the numbers of patients studied were small, and the antigen correlations differed between ethnically distinct populations of myasthenics. We studied the distribution of HLA class II alleles in a population of Italian MG patients using the polymerase chain reaction (PCR) followed by dot-blot hybridization with sequence-specific oligonucleotide (SSO) probes.

MATERIALS AND METHODS

Patients

One hundred thirty-four unrelated generalized MG patients (diagnosed by clinical, electrophysiological, and immunological criteria) were studied. Thirty-three patients (24.6%) were classified as Osserman grade I at onset, but became generalized during follow-up. A limit of 40 years of age was chosen to distinguish early-onset from late-onset patients. The main clinical and immunological features of the patients are reported in TABLE 1. Anti-AChR antibody levels were grouped as negative,

355

TABLE 1. Main Clinical and Immunological Characteristics of MG Patients

	Females	Males
MG patients ($n = 134$)	99	35
Disease onset		
<40 years ($n = 88$)	65	23
>40 years ($n = 46$)	34	12
Osserman grade at disease onset		
1 ($n = 33$)	26	7
2A ($n = 37$)	25	12
2B ($n = 62$)	47	15
3 ($n = 2$)	1	1
Anti-AChR Ab titer		
negative ($n = 22$)	16	6
low ($n = 44$)	33	11
intermediate ($n = 64$)	47	17
high ($n = 4$)	3	1
Pharmacological treatments		
steroid ($n = 49$)	32	17
azathioprine ($n = 9$)	7	2
steroid + aza ($n = 42$)	32	10
none ($n = 34$)	28	6

Thymectomized MG Patients ($n = 85$)

	Sex		Disease Onset	
	Females	Males	<40 Years	>40 Years
Thymic pathology	62	23	63	22
thymoma ($n = 31$)	18	13	14	17
hyper./inv.[a] ($n = 54$)	44	10	49	5

[a]Hyperplasia or involuted thymus.

low (>0–10 pmol/mL), intermediate (>10–100 pmol/mL), and high (>100 pmol/mL). Ninety-eight healthy subjects, representative of the Italian population, were recruited as controls.

HLA Typing

Genetic typing of DRB1, DPB1, and DQB1 was performed by the sequence-specific oligonucleotide (SSO) technique. DQA1 typing was performed with a commercially available reverse dot-blot assay (AmpliType® HLA-DQα, Perkin Elmer, Norwalk, Connecticut). Genomic DNA (0.5 µg) was amplified using primers flanking the second exons coding for the polymorphic domains of DRB1, DQA1, DQB1, and DPB1. Five µL of the PCR product was denatured in 45 µL of 0.4 N NaOH/25 mM EDTA and spotted onto nylon membranes. Hybridization was performed with HRP-labeled oligonucleotide probes. Negative control (no DNA) and control DNAs (homozygous cell lines) were included on each membrane.

Statistical Analysis

Relative risk (*RR*) was estimated according to Wolf's formula with Haldane's correction. Statistical significance was tested by the χ^2 test or by Fisher's exact test when the criteria of the χ^2 test were not fulfilled. *P* values were corrected for the number of alleles identified (*Pc*) at each locus [$Pc = 1 - (1 - P)^n$]. The significance level was taken as *P* < 0.05.

RESULTS

No association with any HLA DRB1 antigen was identified in the entire MG population. However, the DRB1*0301 antigen was present in 30 early-onset MG patients (34.1%) and in 3 late-onset MG patients (6.5%), with *RR* = 6.48 and *Pc* = 0.005. In the group of MG women with disease onset of <40 years, the *0301 allele was present in 38.5%, with an associated *RR* = 2.93 and *Pc* = 0.047. DRB1*0701 was found in only 6.2% of this group (*RR* = 0.21, *Pc* = 0.022) (TABLE 2). HLA DQA1 antigen frequencies in MG patients did not differ significantly from controls. The DQA2 (DQA1*0201) frequency was reduced in early-onset MG patients (*RR* = 0.35, *Pc* = 0.018). In the combined group of MG females with disease onset of <40 years, the DQA2 allele was present in 7.7% of the subjects (*RR* = 0.24, *Pc* = 0.0056) (TABLE 2). The DQB1*0502 allele was positively associated with disease in the whole myasthenic group: 24.6% versus 7.1% of controls (*RR* = 4.03, *Pc* = 0.0084). This association was also observed when MG patients were grouped according to sex: in MG women, the antigen frequency was increased (23.2%, *RR* = 3.75, *Pc* = 0.013); the association was significant also in MG men (28.6%, *RR* = 5.02, *Pc* = 0.026). The DQB1*0502 antigen was present in 29.5% of early-onset MG patients (*RR* = 5.17, *Pc* = 0.0006) and in early-onset MG women (29.2%, *RR* = 5.12, *Pc* = 0.0022) (TABLE 2). No significant associations with any of the DPB1 alleles were found either in the whole MG group or in any of the subgroups. Eighty-five of 134 MG patients underwent therapeutical thymectomy and, in 31 cases, thymoma was diagnosed. Twenty-four of 54 thymoma-negative MG patients (44.4%) were DRB1*0301 (*RR* = 3.74, *Pc* = 0.009); when compared to the thymoma-positive group, the difference was more striking (*RR* = 9.48, *Pc* = 0.004) (TABLE 2). DQB1*0502 was present in 13 of 54 MG patients (24.1%, *RR* = 3.97, *Pc* = 0.041) (TABLE 2). When thymectomized MG patients were subgrouped according to sex, age at disease onset, Osserman grade at onset, and anti-AChR titer, no significant associations were found.

CONCLUSIONS

We have identified a new association with the DQB1*0502 allele in our Italian MG patients. We confirmed the association of MG with DRB1*0301, and the protec-

TABLE 2. Distribution of DRB1*0301, *0701, DQA2, and DQB1*0502 in Italian MG Patients according to Clinical and Histological Parameters

	DRB1 *0301	DRB1 *0701	DQA2 (*0201)	DQB1 *0502
Controls (n = 98)	17.3%	25.5%	27.6%	7.1%
MG (n = 134)	24.6%	17.2%	18.7%	24.6%, RR 4.03
MG Subgroups:				
Sex				
females (n = 99)	28.3%	16.2%	18.2%	23.2%, RR 3.75
males (n = 35)	14.3%	20.0%	20.0%	28.6%, RR 5.02
Disease onset				
early-onset (n = 88)	34.1%[b]	10.2%	11.4%, RR 0.35	29.5%, RR 5.17
late-onset (n = 46)	6.5%	30.4%	32.6%	15.2%
Thymectomized MG				
thymoma (n = 31)	6.5%	32.3%	32.3%	22.6%, RR 3.73
hyper./inv.[a] (n = 54)	44.4%,[c] RR 3.74	11.1%	11.1%	24.1%, RR 3.97
Combined group				
females, early-onset (n = 65)	38.5%, RR 2.93	6.2%, RR 0.21	7.7%, RR 0.24	29.2%, RR 5.12
early-onset, no thymoma (n = 49)	49.0%, RR 4.47	12.2%	12.2%	22.4%, RR 3.64

[a]Hyperplasia or involuted thymus.
[b]Early-onset versus late-onset: RR 6.48, Pc 0.005.
[c]MG patients with thymic hyperplasia or involuted thymus versus MG patients with thymoma: RR 9.48, Pc 0.004.

tive effect of the DRB1*0701 allele in female MG patients with disease onset under 40 years. The DRB1*0301 allele was also found in early-onset MG with a relatively high risk (RR = 6.48) when compared to late-onset MG. We noted a negative association of the DRB1*0701 allele in early-onset MG women versus controls (RR = 0.21, Pc = 0.022). Linkage disequilibrium among the alleles, DRB1*1601, DQA1*0102, and DQB1*0502, is known; in this regard, some DQB1*0502+ MG patients were also positive for DRB1*1601 (22 of 33) and for DQA1.2 (26 of 33), but neither of these two alleles was associated with MG. We did not find an association with DR2 (previously reported for Italian MG patients); our data suggest that, within DR2-positive individuals, only the DRB1*1601-DQA1*0102-DQB1*0502 haplotypes are at increased risk for MG. No significant HLA associations were observed when we considered anti-AChR antibody level or response to immunosuppressive therapy. Thymic abnormalities, such as hyperplasia or thymomas (cortical or medullary), are frequently found in MG patients. The increased DRB1*0301 frequency observed in thymectomized MG patients without thymoma is in keeping with previous reports. Our data further define the immunogenetics of MG, which is not linked to a single allele, consistent with previous studies. The distribution of HLA antigens in our patients underlines the biological and clinical heterogeneity of MG.

REFERENCES

1. COMPSTON, D. A. S., A. VINCENT, J. NEWSOM-DAVIS & J. R. BATCHELOR. 1980. Clinical, pathological, HLA antigen, and immunological evidence for disease heterogeneity in myasthenia gravis. Brain **103:** 579–601.
2. TOURNIER-LASSERVE, E. & J. F. BACH. 1993. The immunogenetics of myasthenia gravis, multiple sclerosis, and their animal models. J. Neuroimmunol. **47:** 103–114.

Susceptibility of HLA DR3 Transgenic Mice to Experimental Autoimmune Myasthenia Gravis[a]

R. RAJU,[b,c] W-Z. ZHAN,[d] P. KARACHUNSKI,[e] G. C. SIECK,[d]
B. M. CONTI-FINE,[e] AND C. S. DAVID[b]

[b]Department of Immunology
[d]Department of Anesthesiology Research
Mayo Clinic
Rochester, Minnesota 55905

[e]Department of Biochemistry
University of Minnesota
St. Paul, Minnesota 55108

INTRODUCTION

MHC class II susceptibility genes have been described in different autoimmune diseases like type I diabetes (HLA DR4, DR3, DQ8), rheumatoid arthritis (HLA DR4), pemphigus vulgaris (HLA DR4, DR6), etc.[1] Studies on the HLA association of MG, although not extensive, are also described.[2] In Caucasians, B8 and/or DR3 haplotypes have been found to be associated with young MG patients, mainly women without thymoma and with high levels of AChR antibodies.[3] MG was also found to be positively associated with the DQB1*0604 allele, particularly in patients with thymoma.[4] The strongest association of MG in Jamaicans was found to be with HLA B8, HLA B13, and DQw4 and was negatively associated with HLA A2.[5] A significantly higher frequency of DQB1*03, which includes *0301, *0302, and *0303, was found in female patients less than 30 years in age at onset of disease as compared with healthy controls. In the mouse, it has been shown that the H2[b] haplotype is strongly susceptible to experimental autoimmune myasthenia gravis (EAMG).[6] In this paper, we address the role of HLA DRA1*0101/DRB1*0301 (DR3) in EAMG by using mice transgenic to this HLA class II molecule.

[a]This work was supported by NIH Grant Nos. AI-14764 (to C. S. David), NS-23919 (to B. M. Conti-Fine), and HL-37680 (to G. C. Sieck).
[c]Recipient of an Osserman Postdoctoral Fellowship of the Myasthenia Gravis Foundation of America.

MATERIALS AND METHODS

Mice

HLA DR3 (DRA1*0101/DRB1*0301) transgenic mice were obtained from Gunther Hammerling[7] and DR3.Ab° mice were generated as previously described.[8] In Ab° mice, the Ab gene is nonfunctional and these mice do not express an H2A molecule.[9] DR3.q/q mice were generated by repeated backcrossing of B10.DR3.f/f to B10.Q.

TAChR Purification and Disease Induction

TAChR was purified from *Torpedo californica* (Aquatic Research Consultants, California) electric organ by the method of Lindstrom *et al.*[10] Mice were given three injections (sc) of TAChR (20 μg/mouse) separated by 1 month. The first injection was given in Freund's complete adjuvant and subsequently in incomplete adjuvant. After 12 weeks, mice were sacrificed. Anti-AChR antibodies in the sera were assayed by a radioimmunoprecipitation assay using ^{125}I-labeled α-bungarotoxin.[10]

Disease Assessment

Clinical Assessment

Muscle weakness was assessed every week in a blind study as described in reference 11. Briefly, mice were allowed to grip their paws on cage-top grids and pulled off the grid by their tail consecutively for 25 times for forced exercise. They were scored as given in the legend to FIGURE 1. Grade 1 weakness was ascertained using pancuronium (0.03 mg/kg-ip)–induced forced exercise, whereby the weakness is exaggerated.

Electrophysiology

Neuromuscular junction failure in TAChR-injected and uninjected mice was studied as previously described in reference 12. Briefly, the diaphragm muscle bundles from anesthetized mice were stimulated repetitively via phrenic nerve for 2 min, with a direct muscle stimulation superimposed for 2 s every 15 s. The ratio (N/M) of the initial tetanic force produced by nerve stimulation (N) to the initial force produced by muscle stimulation (M) was estimated. The contribution of neuromuscular transmission failure (NMTF) to the total force decline was determined from the following equation: $NMTF = (NS - MS)/(1 - MS)$, where NS is the force loss during nerve stimulation and MS is the force loss during muscle stimulation.

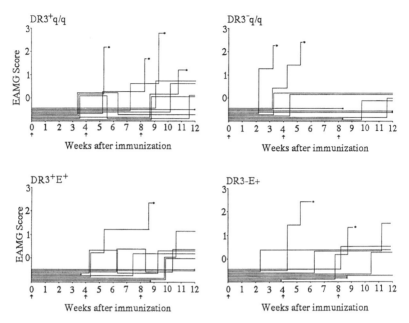

FIGURE 1. EAMG in mice immunized with TAChR. Arrows on the x-axis show the days immunized. Score—grade 0 = no weakness at rest or after exercise (25 consecutive paw grips on cage-top steel grids); grade 1 = normal strength at rest, but weak with chin on the floor and inability to raise the head after exercise; grade 2 = grade 1 weakness at rest; grade 3 = morbidity, dehydration, or quadriplegia; * = the mouse was killed or died. A horizontal line ending with a blunt end denotes death of the mouse due to reasons other than EAMG.

RESULTS AND DISCUSSION

The presentation of pathogenic epitopes to CD4+ T cells is important in the manifestation and perpetuation of myasthenia gravis, through generation of high-affinity antibodies. The influence of a human class II molecule, DR3, in EAMG pathogenesis is examined in this study.[13] We had five groups of mice, DR3+q/q, DR3−q/q, DR3+E+.Ab°, DR3-E+.Ab°, and DR3-E−.Ab°, and the results are shown in FIGURE 1. The DR3.Ab° mice express H2E molecules due to the pairing of DRα with mouse Eβ. We found that both DR3+q/q (n = 10) as well as DR3−q/q (n = 8) develop EAMG subsequent to TAChR immunization. This confirms the previous studies showing H2q as a susceptible strain. Two mice scored grade 3 in each group. The majority of the mice that showed EAMG signs clinically remained grade 1. Hence, there is only a marginal increase in severity and incidence of EAMG in DR3 transgenic mice. In the DR3+E+.Ab° and DR3-E+.Ab° groups, only one mouse in each group had an EAMG score of 3. At 12 weeks, the DR3+E+.Ab° and DR3-E+.Ab° groups had one and two mice, respectively, scoring grade 2. None of the DR3−E−.Ab° developed clinical signs of EAMG as expected (data not shown). It is evident from the electrophysiological studies (FIGURE 2) that all three mice tested in each group had significant neuromus-

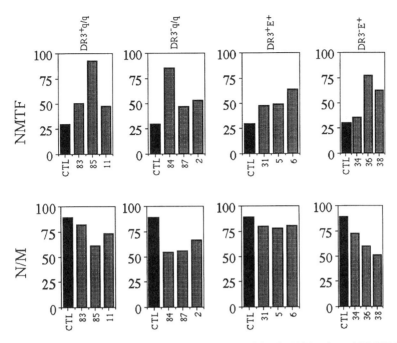

FIGURE 2. Neuromuscular junction failure as represented by the N/M ratio and NMTF for each group. CTL denotes the value of uninjected normal control and is the mean of three observations.

cular junction failure as assessed from the N/M ratio or NMTF. The mean titers of anti-TAChR antibodies in these mice after three immunizations were 5.1 ± 1.7, 6.3 ± 2.9, 4.8 ± 1.9, and 4.4 ± 0.8 (μM of α-BgTx binding sites) in the DR3⁺q/q, DR3⁻q/q, DR3⁺E⁺.Ab°, and DR3⁻E⁺.Ab° groups, respectively, demonstrating the development of significant anti-TAChR antibody titers in the mice. These results show that the H2E molecule is also a susceptibility allele for EAMG. Since the DR3⁺ mice also express the H2E molecule, we cannot determine the role played by the DR3 molecule. Currently, we are developing a line that is DR3⁺E⁻.Ab°, which will be used in future studies to determine the specific role of the DR3 molecule. The role of HLA DQ genes on extended DQ-DR haplotypes in the pathogenesis of MG will also be determined.

REFERENCES

1. NEPOM, G. T. 1991. Annu. Rev. Immunol. **9:** 493–525.
2. KAUL, R., M. SHENOY & P. CHRISTADOSS. 1994. Adv. Neurol. Immunol. **4:** 387–402.
3. TOLA, M. R., L. M. CANIATTI, I. CASETTA *et al.* 1994. Acta Neurol. Scand. **90:** 318–323.
4. VIEIRA, M. L., S. CAILLAT-ZUCMAN, P. GAJDOS *et al.* 1993. J. Neuroimmunol. **47:** 115–122.

5. BARTON, E. N., M. SMIKLE & O. S. MORGAN. 1992. South. Med. J. **85:** 904–906.
6. CHRISTADOSS, P. 1987. Ann. N.Y. Acad. Sci. **505:** 901–902.
7. STRAUB, G., D. A. A. VIGNALI, G. SCHONRICH *et al.* 1994. Immunogenetics **40:** 104–108.
8. KONG, Y. M., L. C. LOMO, R. W. MOTTE *et al.* 1996. J. Exp. Med. **184:** 1167–1172.
9. COSGROVE, D., D. GRAY, A. DIERICH *et al.* 1991. Cell **66:** 1051–1066.
10. LINDSTROM, J., B. EINARSON & S. TZARTOS. 1981. Methods Enzymol. **74:** 432–460.
11. CHRISTADOSS, P., C. S. DAVID & S. KEVE. 1992. Clin. Immunol. Immunopathol. **62:** 235–239.
12. KUEI, J. H., R. SHADMEHR & G. C. SIECK. 1990. J. Appl. Physiol. **68:** 174–180.
13. PROTTI, M. P., A. A. MANFREDI, R. M. HORTON *et al.* 1993. Immunol. Today **14:** 363–368.

Epitope Spreading in Experimental Autoimmune Myasthenia Gravis

MARK A. AGIUS,[a] GEORGE M. TWADDLE,[b]
AND ROBERT H. FAIRCLOUGH[a]

[a]Department of Neurology
University of California at Davis
Davis, California 95615

[b]Department of Cell Biology
Evanston Hospital
Evanston, Illinois

INTRODUCTION

The phenomenon of epitope (determinant) spreading has been documented in immune responses to self antigens.[1] In this process, immune responses develop to endogenous epitopes generated as a consequence of processing of self antigens during the course of an ongoing inflammatory or autoimmune reaction. An autoimmune response may be initially directed against only a single immunogenic determinant. This may occur, perhaps, as a consequence of a misdirected immune response, as in a cross-reactive one, or as a result of loss of tolerance to changes in the structure of the self molecule, perhaps as a consequence of chemical modification. In the case of patients with acquired myasthenia gravis (MG), the humoral response to the acetylcholine receptor (AChR) is often dominated by antibodies to a region, namely, the main immunogenic region or MIR, located on the extrasynaptic portion of the alpha subunit. In addition, however, antibodies to multiple other epitopes on the AChR often occur in MG, including those to ones located on the cytoplasmic surface. The mechanism of epitope spreading suggests that AChRs, damaged by the initial autoimmune attack directed at an extrasynaptic epitope, are processed by antigen-presenting cells and results in the generation of novel immunogenic determinants.

MATERIALS AND METHODS

Rat Immunization and Screening of Serum Reactivity

Female Lewis rats were immunized with 50–150 μg of peptide alone (MC fusion) or peptides conjugated to keyhole-limpet hemocyanin (ML and KM fusions) by glutaraldehyde. Initial immunization in complete Freund's adjuvant was followed by 2–3 weekly immunizations in incomplete Freund's adjuvant. Serum was screened for binding to both peptide and membrane-bound AChR in ELISA. Serum reactivity to peptide and AChR was detected at a serum dilution of $1:10^3$–$1:10^4$. There was no reactivity of serum to control unrelated proteins, including bovine serum albumin, bovine hemoglobin, and dry milk proteins, nor to ACTH peptide hormone, unrelated α *Torpedo* peptide (α127–145), and murine AChR peptide (α185–197). Animals did not develop experimental myasthenia.

Hybridoma Production and Screening

B cell hybridomas were produced in three polyethylene glycol–mediated fusions between immune rat splenocytes and the immunoglobulin nonsecreting mouse myeloma Sp2/0-Ag14 five days after the rats received an intraperitoneal injection of 150 μg of peptide or peptide conjugate in saline. Hybridomas were screened for AChR binding in ELISA. Cell lines were cloned twice by limiting dilution. mAb 37C was generated from the MC fusion and mAb 65GC was generated from the KM fusion.

RESULTS

Immunized animals remained healthy and did not develop signs of experimental autoimmune myasthenia gravis. Animals demonstrated anti-AChR reactivity in their serum. In addition, serum revealed reactivity to the immunizing peptide. mAb 37C was produced from a fusion between mouse myeloma cell line Sp2/0 and splenic lymphocytes from a Lewis rat immunized with alpha peptide 192–212. The synthesized peptide corresponded to sequences for *Torpedo* AChR implicated in the binding of acetylcholine. Hybridoma screening involved immunoblotting to intact AChR in ELISA. Cloned anti-AChR hybridomas were further tested for binding to immunoblots of denatured AChR. mAb 37C bound to the beta subunit, but not to the alpha subunit of *Torpedo* AChR. The specificity of this mAb for the beta subunit was confirmed by the use of control alpha chain–specific and beta chain–specific mAbs.

The peptide used in the KM animal corresponding to alpha 127–145 of *Torpedo californica* included the disulfide-bonded cys128-cys142 and the N-linked oligosaccharide attachment site at Asn 141. Immunization with this alpha peptide resulted in the generation of an mAb, namely, mAb 65GC, directed to the gamma subunit. Similar to the ML fusion, subunit reactivity was determined by immunoblotting to separated, denatured *Torpedo* AChR subunits. The gamma chain mAb showed no cross-reactivity with the alpha chain.

DISCUSSION

In both instances, for mAb 37C and 65GC, the immunization with synthetic alpha chain peptides resulted in the production of antibodies directed at sequences on AChR subunits that were not present in the immunogen and that were not identified in the alpha chain. These monoclonals generated in the animals in the course of an ongoing autoimmune reaction did not cross-react with the alpha subunit nor with synthetic peptides used in the immunization. The production of antibodies to these non-cross-reactive epitopes is likely to be mediated by the process of epitope spreading. This process represents one mechanism explaining the generation of antibodies to intracellular antigens in MG.

REFERENCE

1. VANDERLUGT, C. J. & S. D. MILLER. 1996. Epitope spreading. Curr. Opin. Immunol. **8:** 831–836.

Myasthenia Gravis with Thymic Hyperplasia Is Associated with Polymorphisms in the Tumor Necrosis Factor Region

P. HJELMSTRÖM,[a,b,c] C. S. PEACOCK,[d] R. GISCOMBE,[a] R. PIRSKANEN,[e]
A. K. LEFVERT,[a] J. M. BLACKWELL,[d] AND C. B. SANJEEVI[b]

[a]Department of Medicine
[b]Department of Molecular Medicine
Karolinska Institute
Karolinska Hospital
S-171 76 Stockholm, Sweden

[d]Department of Medicine
University of Cambridge Clinical School
Addenbrooke's Hospital
Cambridge CB2 2QQ, United Kingdom

[e]Department of Neurology
Karolinska Institute
Söder Hospital
S-118 83 Stockholm, Sweden

Myasthenia gravis (MG) has a complex pattern of inheritance, and several genetic and environmental factors are important in conferring susceptibility to the disease. As in many other autoimmune diseases, an increased risk for development of MG is conferred by genetic factors in the human leukocyte antigen (HLA) region on the short arm of chromosome 6. MG is a heterogeneous disease and it is possible to divide the patients into different subgroups depending on the age at onset, gender, clinical features, and HLA associations.[1] In Caucasian patients with generalized MG, an early disease onset (below 30 years), and thymic hyperplasia, there is an increased frequency of alleles on the extended DR3 haplotype (A1, B8, TNFB*1, DR3, DQ2, TAP2*0101).[1–4] The alleles on the extended DR3 haplotype are in strong linkage disequilibrium (LD) and it has been difficult to determine which of the alleles display the strongest association with MG. Stratification analysis has shown that the associations between MG and alleles in the centromeric TAP loci are due to linkage.[5] Degli-Esposti and coworkers proposed after mapping of recombinant haplotypes that two markers on the extended DR3 haplotype may confer susceptibility to MG: one of them is located in the HLA class II region and the other between the HLA-B and tumor necrosis factor (TNF) loci.[2] The aims of our study were to analyze (i) the associations between polymorphisms in the TNF region and generalized MG with thymic

[c]Present address: Department of Epidemiology and Public Health, Yale University School of Medicine, New Haven, Connecticut 06520-8034.

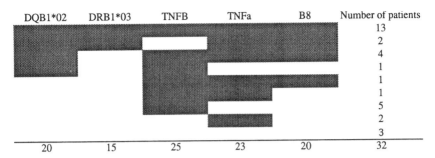

FIGURE 1. Presence or absence of different parts of the extended DR3 haplotype. Shaded areas denote presence of the alleles on the extended DR3 haplotype.

hyperplasia and (ii) if the associations are independent or secondary to LD with other alleles on the extended DR3 haplotype.

Thirty-two thymectomized Swedish Caucasian patients with generalized MG and thymic hyperplasia were included in the study and compared with 155 healthy, unrelated, population-based controls. Twenty-four (75%) of the patients were females and the mean age of onset was 26.0 (13.2–38.9) years. The HLA-DQ, DR, and TAP genotypes of the patients and controls have previously been reported.[4,5] Typing for a biallelic NcoI RFLP polymorphism located at the first intron of the TNF-β (lymphotoxin alpha [LT-α]) gene was done as previously described.[6] Restriction digests generated fragments of 555 bp and 185 bp for the TNFB*1 allele (5.5-kb allele) and 740 bp for the TNFB*2 allele (10-kb allele). Analysis of the TNFa microsatellite polymorphism, located 3.5 kb upstream of the LT-α gene, was done as described by Nedospasov and coworkers.[7] HLA-B8 typing was performed in the patients with standard serological typing methods. Due to the paucity of DNA in the control material, typing could be performed only in 73 controls for NcoI RFLP LT-α alleles and in 90 controls for TNFa microsatellite alleles. Statistical analysis was done using chi-square test with Yates correction or Fisher's exact test when any of the expected frequencies were less than five. Odds ratios (OR) were calculated as cross products of 2×2 contingency tables to determine the strength of the associations. Probability (p) values were corrected for the number of comparisons made.

The frequencies of different alleles on the extended DR3 haplotype in the patients and controls are shown in TABLE 1. The strongest associations are found with the TNFa2 microsatellite allele and with DQB1*02 (DQ2). The associations with the TAP2*0101 allele and the TNFB*1 allele are not significant after correction for multiple comparisons, which could be due to the low polymorphism of the TAP2 and TNFB loci. The association is stronger with DQB1*02 (DQ2) than with DRB1*03 (DR3) and this is interesting as DQ2 also is in LD with DR7. Stratification analysis of the associations (data not shown) suggests that the TNFa2 association indeed could be independent from the DQ2 and DR3 associations. However, the LD in the extended DR3 haplotype is very strong and further studies are indicated to determine whether there are two factors on this haplotype associated with MG and thymic hyperplasia, as suggested by Degli-Esposti and coworkers.[2] FIGURE 1 shows the pres-

TABLE 1. Associations between MG with Thymic Hyperplasia and Different Alleles on the Extended DR3 Haplotype[a]

	TAP2*0101	DQB1*02	DRB1*03	TNFB*1	TNFa2
patients	26/32 (81%)	20/32 (63%)	15/32 (47%)	25/32 (78%)	23/32 (72%)
controls	51/70 (73%)	43/152 (28%)	27/145 (19%)	42/73 (58%)	33/90 (37%)
odds ratio	1.61	4.22	3.86	2.64	4.41
95% CI	0.58–4.51	1.97–9.05	1.77–8.39	1.03–6.75	1.89–10.3
p value	ns	<0.001	<0.005	<0.05	<0.001
p corrected	ns	<0.01	<0.01	ns	<0.01

[a]ns denotes nonsignificant. The results for TAP2, DQB1, and DRB1 typing have been reported previously.[4,5]

ence or absence of different parts of the extended DR3 haplotype in the patients. It is notable that DQ2 was found as frequent as B8 in the patients and that the highest frequencies were found for the TNFB*1 and TNFa2 alleles. This further indicates that MG with thymic lymphoid follicular hyperplasia is associated with polymorphisms in the TNF region. It is tempting to speculate that this association might be due to an increased secretion of the proinflammatory cytokines, TNF-α and LT-α, which is known to cause formation of lymphoid follicular structures in chronic inflammatory autoimmune diseases.[8] In conclusion, MG with thymic hyperplasia is associated with polymorphisms in the TNF region.

REFERENCES

1. COMPSTON, D. A. et al. 1980. Clinical, pathological, HLA antigen, and immunological evidence for disease heterogeneity in myasthenia gravis. Brain **103**: 579–601.
2. DEGLI-ESPOSTI, M. A. et al. 1992. An approach to the localization of the susceptibility genes for generalized myasthenia gravis by mapping recombinant ancestral haplotypes. Immunogenetics **35**: 355–364.
3. VIEIRA, M. L. et al. 1993. Identification by genomic typing of non-DR3 HLA class II genes associated with myasthenia gravis. J. Neuroimmunol. **47**: 115–122.
4. HJELMSTRÖM, P. et al. 1995. Different HLA-DQ are positively and negatively associated in Swedish patients with myasthenia gravis. Autoimmunity **22**: 59–65.
5. HJELMSTRÖM, P. et al. 1997. TAP polymorphisms in Swedish myasthenia gravis patients. Tissue Antigens **49**: 176–179.
6. MESSER, G. et al. 1991. Polymorphic structure of the tumor necrosis factor (TNF) locus: an NcoI polymorphism in the first intron of the human TNF-β gene correlates with a variant amino acid in position 26 and a reduced level of TNF-β production. J. Exp. Med. **173**: 209–219.
7. NEDOSPASOV, S. A. et al. 1991. DNA sequence polymorphism at the human tumor necrosis factor (TNF) locus: numerous TNF/lymphotoxin alleles tagged by two closely linked microsatellites in the upstream region of the lymphotoxin (TNF-β) gene. J. Immunol. **147**: 1053–1059.
8. KRATZ, A. et al. 1996. Chronic inflammation caused by lymphotoxin is lymphoid neogenesis. J. Exp. Med. **183**: 1461–1472.

Thymus, Thymoma, and Specific T Cells in Myasthenia Gravis[a]

D. BEESON,[b] A. P. BOND,[b] L. CORLETT,[b] S. J. CURNOW,[b] M. E. HILL,[b]
L. W. JACOBSON,[b] C. MACLENNAN,[b] A. MEAGER,[c] A-M. MOODY,[b]
P. MOSS,[d] N. NAGVEKAR,[b] J. NEWSOM-DAVIS,[b] N. PANTIC,[b]
I. ROXANIS,[b] E. G. SPACK,[e] A. VINCENT,[b] AND N. WILLCOX[b,f]

[b]Neurosciences Group
Institute of Molecular Medicine
University of Oxford
Oxford OX3 9DS, United Kingdom

[c]National Institute for Biological Standards and Control
South Mimms EN6 3QG, United Kingdom

[d]Department of Molecular Immunology
Institute of Molecular Medicine
University of Oxford
Oxford OX3 9DS, United Kingdom

[e]Anergen Incorporated
Redwood City, California 94063

INTRODUCTION

The initiation of autoimmune responses is very difficult to study in humans, but myasthenia gravis (MG) offers invaluable opportunities. For example, it seems more than coincidence that there are thymic abnormalities in two subgroups of MG patients; about 10% have a thymoma[1] and, in the 40% with early-onset MG (EOMG; <40 years of age), there is medullary hyperplasia[2] (see below). The muscle weakness in these patients is clearly mediated by IgG autoantibodies to the acetylcholine receptor (AChR, reviewed in reference 3), an exceptionally well-characterized autoantigen.[4] The antibodies are very heterogeneous, have a high affinity for conformational epitopes, and almost certainly depend on helper T cells (Th).[3]

Our main research aims are to understand the basis of predisposition and autoimmunization and to identify potential targets for selective immunotherapy in the responding cells. Our strategies have therefore been both to search for expression of AChR subunits in the MG thymus and thymoma and to characterize AChR-specific T cells in patients and controls. We hope that their dominant epitopes, presenting class II molecules, or the T cell receptor (TCR) genes that they use to recognize them may suggest promising immunotherapeutic approaches. Since purified human AChR is so

[a]This work was supported by the Medical Research Council and Myasthenia Gravis Association/Muscular Dystrophy Group of Great Britain and by the Sir Jules Thorn Charitable Trust.
[f]To whom all correspondence should be addressed.

scarce and the pathogenic Th are probably rare, very limited information can be gleaned from the responses of fresh T cells *ex vivo*. Their specificities can only be precisely defined after T cell lines and clones have been established by restimulation *in vitro* with antigen in some more plentiful and convenient form.

Methodological Options

When mice or rats are immunized with whole AChR, the α subunit is thought to be immunodominant.[5,6] Even with the evolutionarily distant *Torpedo* AChR, the responder Th recognize a very limited range of epitopes;[5,6] in autologous AChR, they may be even more restricted. Since T cells respond to unfolded antigens, we and others[7–9] have used isolated recombinant human AChR subunits to select a series of T cell lines from patients (and controls). These are proving to recognize recurring epitopes (see TABLE 1) and also respond to native human AChR at remarkably high sensitivity. However, until recently, our success rate in selecting these T cells has been low, partly because the rare AChR-specific precursors are often outnumbered by other T cells reactive to *E. coli* contaminants in the recombinant antigen preparations.[7,8]

Other groups have selected with pooled synthetic AChR subunit peptides instead and find a much greater heterogeneity.[10] Because of this striking contrast, we reinvestigated this synthetic approach; most of the T cells that we now raised against peptides proved to be specific for contaminants/sequence errors.[8,11] Only 1 of 20 sublines recognized any lengthier recombinant antigen (although many different preparations were tested), and even this was specific for a cryptic epitope requiring artificial unmasking, for example, by trypsinization.[11] Previous work in other laboratories may well be beset by the same difficulties; their prevalence may result partly from prior tolerance to the correct sequence and/or from unnatural loading of class II molecules at the high peptide molarities used *in vitro*.[8,11] In our view, the synthetic approach has created an exaggerated impression of heterogeneity, and the truly patho-

TABLE 1. Summary of AChR-specific Clones Isolated from MG Patients

T Cell Clone	Source	Epitope Core	Presenting Class II	Th Type
AChR α Subunit				
PM-A1	MG hyperplastic thymus	149–156	DR4	Th1
GD-B4	MG PBL	P3A insert + 59–65	DQw5	Th1
MB-1D3	MG thymoma	75–90	DP14	Th0
KB-D1	MG thymoma	149–156	DR52a	Th0
AChR ε Subunit				
RF-F0	MG PBL	202–219	DR52a	Th1
LH-F9	MG PBL	202–219	DR52a	Th1
MW-C3	MG PBL	202–219	DR52a	ND

genic T cells that respond to physiological amounts of AChR *in vivo* may be much more restricted,[8,11] as implied by our results with recombinant antigen.

RESULTS AND DISCUSSION

Thymoma in MG; Specific T Cells and AChR Expression

The tumors so regularly associated with certain autoimmune disorders must hold vital clues to their initiation. The Lambert-Eaton myasthenic syndrome is a telling example where small cell lung cancers occur in about 60% of patients.[12] The neoplastic cells express calcium channels, and these apparently provoke the production of autoantibodies that attack similar channels in nerve terminals.[13] If the tumor can be removed, the autoantibodies and clinical signs usually decline.[14]

In thymoma-associated MG, the evidence is more confusing. On the one hand, these tumors typically resemble disorganized thymic cortex and often generate numerous maturing thymocytes.[3,15] Thus, in theory, they might merely export a wide range of autoreactive T cells that they have failed to tolerize against self antigens[16] and that then begin responding in the periphery. Indeed, the weakness (and anti-AChR antibody titers) can often increase after thymomectomy and may even begin postoperatively,[17] suggesting a rather indirect link with the tumor. On the other hand, these patients show no signs of generalized autoreactivity. Rather, their autoantibodies are mainly muscle-specific, characteristically recognizing internal striational antigens such as actin, myosin, and titin,[18,19] in addition to AChR. Thus, it seems likelier that thymomas actively immunize specific Th; a particularly attractive suggestion is that these react to an epitope shared by these muscle antigens[19] and subsequently induce a variety of distinct autoantibodies as determinants spread.

The Search for Autoimmunizing Epitopes and Cell Types

Whereas some muscle epitopes may be present in the thymoma epithelial cells,[20] whole AChR has never been detected there. While mRNA for the AChR α subunit has been found in several studies by very sensitive PCR assays,[21,22] as yet there is no clear evidence for any AChR polypeptide product in thymomas. Indeed, only a single related epitope has been reported[23,24] and it is present in a 153-kDa polypeptide, possibly of neurofilament origin,[25] that clearly does not correspond to any known AChR subunit. This epitope resembles the 373–380 sequence in the cytoplasmic domain of the AChRα, which is very immunogenic in experimental animals.[26] Its expression is apparently MG-related, as it is seen in most thymomas from MG patients, but in few from nonmyasthenics.[23,24] If it is involved in autoimmunization, as suggested previously, one might expect the patients' T cells or autoantibodies to recognize it. However, we have found no sign of either possibility, despite carefully checking for autoantibodies in 11 cases[27a] and for T cell responses in 28 patients (see below).

We first screened for responses to PPD (of tuberculin) and full-length AChR α subunit (FIGURE 1). Thymoma suspensions (enriched for mature T cells) responded to full-length AChR α subunit somewhat more frequently than those from the adjacent thymic remnant ("thymus") or the PBL. Stimulation by purified *Torpedo* AChR was

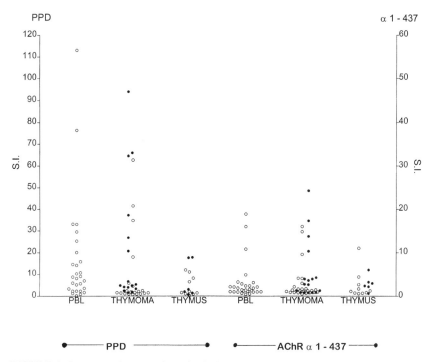

FIGURE 1. Responses (expressed as stimulation indices, SI) of T cells from PBL and thymoma and from the adjacent uninvolved thymus (where available, "Thymus") to AChR α1–437 and PPD of tuberculin (on different scales). Mature thymoma T cells were enriched either by density separation or by corticosteroid pretreatment of the donor patient. An equal number of fresh irradiated PBL was included when APC were rare (solid symbols), as in cryostored thymus suspensions; the consequently improved responses are shown here (where available). In six early cases, α37–429 was used instead of α1–437.

also detected in 9 of the 13 thymomas tested (SI's ranging from 2.1 to 12). By contrast, responses to PPD were more consistent with PBL, although significant with some thymoma suspensions, suggesting some colonization by recirculating T cells (FIGURE 1).

When we next checked systematically with recombinant polypeptides and synthetic peptides covering the α370–380 region, we found no significant recognition.[27a] Instead, as with the patients' serum antibodies, the T cell epitopes mapped so far all appear to reside in the extracellular domain (FIGURE 2, see below). These results thus question the proposed initiating role of the α370–380 region in thymomas.

To check for other autoimmunogenic elements, we reinvestigated the expression of AChR subunit mRNA, initially screening by RT-PCR and then attempting to quantitate by less-sensitive RNase protection assays. By RT-PCR, we found some expression of α, β, γ, δ, and ε mRNAs in many of the thymoma samples, although with considerable variation. By RNase protection, only ε mRNA was detected, in about

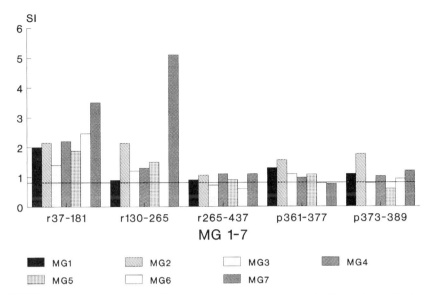

FIGURE 2. Responses to extracellular versus cytoplasmic epitopes by T cells from MG thymomas in the seven MG cases tested systematically with the AChR α antigens shown: r, recombinant polypeptide; p, synthetic peptide.

half of the samples, and at variable levels.[28] We were also able to test thymic tumors from two patients with MG plus autoimmune neuromyotonia.[29] Interestingly, they were almost entirely epithelial, without detectable immature thymocytes, but with strong labeling for chromogranin, thus resembling atypical thymic carcinoids.[29] They again expressed AChR ε mRNA, which was also seen very strongly in a similar tumor from a patient without MG or neuromyotonia.

We are now testing for T cell and antibody responses to this subunit/adult AChR in patients with or without this unexpected ε subunit expression. We hope thus to distinguish between active immunization of mature T cells and a failure to tolerize nascent thymocytes developing in these tumors. We favor the former because of (i) the narrow spectrum of autoantibodies in these patients[18–20] and (ii) the striking absence of immature thymocytes in occasional thymomas even from MG patients with no corticosteroid pretreatment.

After previously stimulating thymoma T cells with recombinant α subunit, we eventually selected two clones whose epitopes could be mapped with synthetic peptides (TABLE 1). Clone I responded to α75–90, presented by HLA-DP14. The other clone is specific for α148–159 plus DR52a (FIGURE 3); almost exactly the same sequence is recognized by the PM-A1 Th clone previously selected from a hyperplastic MG thymus and restricted to HLA-DR4.[7,8] None of these T cells responds to the corresponding *Torpedo* sequence (e.g., FIGURE 3), which illustrates the need to use human antigen. However, all three clones respond strikingly well to minute amounts of whole AChR (especially when presented on immunomagnetic beads), which is con-

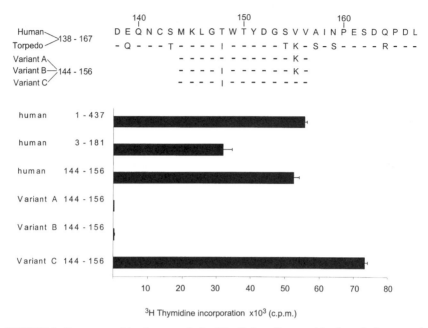

FIGURE 3. Responses of the thymoma-derived T cell clone II to peptides from the human and *Torpedo* α subunit sequences. Whereas stimulations were maximal with recombinant human α1–437 or α3–181, they were undetectable with *Torpedo* AChR (10 μg/mL; not shown).

sistent with a potential for *in vivo* pathogenicity. We suggest that the natural α148–160 epitope is processed particularly well from whole AChR, perhaps because of the nearby glycosylation at [141]Asn or the [128]Cys-[142]Cys disulfide loop.

The restricting HLA-DP14 allele for clone I is rare. However, it is very similar to the more-common HLA-DP3 that does not present antigens to this clone,[27b] even though it differs only by [23]Gln→Met, [50]Arg→Gln, and [83]Ala→Thr in DPα and by [9]His→Tyr in DPβ.[30] We suggest possible alignments of DP-restricted epitopes in FIGURE 4.[31–37] Both DPβ0301 and 1401 have very distinctive acidic residues at either end of their α helices[30] and, interestingly, there appear to be complementary basic residues at the ends of the peptides that they present (FIGURE 4). By contrast, these are less evident near the N-terminus of other peptides presented by DPβ0401, possibly because it has hydrophobic instead of basic amino acids at positions 84–87. The preferences of DR52a are discussed briefly below and detailed elsewhere.[39]

As discussed below, it may be significant that both HLA-DP and DRB3 (including DR52a) isotypes are expressed at low levels on peripheral APC. This might also help to explain two other unexpected findings. First, for both clones, we initially found that Mabs to HLA-DR, -DP, and -DQ blocked their responses almost equally strongly (e.g., see reference 7). Perhaps this was a result of incidental depletion of these sparse bystander molecules below the required threshold by each of these Mabs. Second, with clone II, we found extraordinarily variable presentation (from 0 to 100%) of recombi-

DPβ Allele 87 84	1 5 7 9 10	DPβ 57 55	EPITOPE	Ref
0401 **M P G G**	N F T V S F W L R V P K V S A S H	E A A	Tet.tox 949 - 965	31
	N S G L E P G V V A E K V V R N L		Hsp 65 454 - 470	32
	A Q R F G I S N Y C Q I Y P P N A		Der p I 108 - 124	33
0402 **M P G G**	Q A G F F L L T R I L T I P Q S L	E E D	Hep B 16 - 32	34
	V R Q I R S G E R F L K I W S Q T		Rabies Ns 105 - 121	35
	Q A R I L A V E R Y L K D Q		HIVgp 41 582 - 595	36
0301 **V A E D**	E Q K R G R V D N Y C R H N Y G V	D E D	DR3 β 69 - 85	37
1401 **V A E D**	K K I H I P S E K I W R P D L V L	D E D	hu AChR α 76 - 92	This Paper
	- - - R L - - D D V - L - - - - -		Torpedo α	

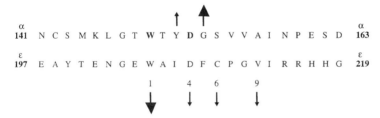

α
141 N C S M K L G T W T Y D G S V V A I N P E S D 163

ε
197 E A Y T E N G E W A I D F C P G V I R R H H G 219

FIGURE 4. **(Top)** Proposed alignment of selected HLA-DP-restricted epitopes. Key sequence differences in the α helix of the DPβ alleles are shown at either side **in the order in which they would contact the peptide.** As discussed in the text, DPβ residues 84–87 line a hydrophobic pocket in which the side chain of peptide p1 might be accommodated: the acidic residues at 84 and 85 in DP3 and DP14 might explain the apparent preference for basic residues at p1 in the corresponding peptides. Similarly, in these alleles, there is a smaller D at position 57 than the E of DP4, which might be compensated by the larger R (than K) at peptide p9. Rammensee *et al.*[38] have found hydrophobic residues at p1, p7, and p10 in peptides eluted from DP0401, and Hammond *et al.*[36] noted the acidic residues at p5 and the K at p9 in DP0402-restricted epitopes. **(Bottom)** Proposed alignment of DR52a-restricted epitopes from AChR α and ε. In the α, [141]N is glycosylated and there is a disulfide loop from [128]C→[142]C. In the ε, position 229 is just external to the first transmembrane segment. For α148–159, the arrows pointing upwards indicate TCR contact residues and those pointing down have class II–binding side chains.[39] HLA-DR52a is HLA-DRB3*0101.

nant and peptide antigens by irradiated PBL from one healthy DR52a$^+$ donor on different occasions, perhaps implying a fluctuating expression of DR52a, for example, on activated APC. Alternatively, this clone may require some limiting type of accessory molecule or APC such as B cells or dendritic cells. Remarkably, in view of this, both isotypes are evidently expressed (like other class II molecules) by the T cells themselves because they can clearly present specific peptides to each other at high concentrations, giving substantial "autopresentation" (not shown).

We searched for likely autosensitizing microenvironments in the second thymoma, taking advantage of the Mabs to the Vβ2 and DR52a/DR3 used by clone II.[27b] Because of prior corticosteroid therapy, lymphocytes were sparse and were mostly CD3$^+$. The abundant epithelial cells labeled minimally for class II, which was expressed much more strongly on scattered CD68$^+$ macrophages and rare foci of B cells in the perivascular spaces. Because both of these seemed to be contacted more frequently by Vβ2$^+$ than Vβ5.2$^+$ T cells, these professional APC seemed the likeliest autoimmunizing cell type.[27b] Possibly, however, the epithelial cells might have been more clearly class II$^+$ before the steroid therapy.

The choice of "minority" presenting class II isotypes by both clones is intriguing; if they are expressed unusually strongly in thymomas, these might, in theory, activate T cells that are not fully tolerant to the epitopes that they present. In view of their totally different peptide- and class II–specificity, the very similar Vα1.2-Jα17.2 usage by these clones is also very surprising;[27b] it might reflect some restriction in Vα rearrangements in T cells developing in thymomas. If it proves to be widespread, TCR targeting might be an appropriate selective therapeutic approach.

Anticytokine Antibodies, Infections, and Metastases

An even more surprising finding is that about 90% of MG/thymoma patients have antibodies to interferon-α (IFN-α) and about 60% to IL-12, but not to IFN-β or IFN-γ, IL-1α or β, TNFα or β, or TGFβ1 or 2.[40] Most positive sera neutralize IFN-α and/or IL-12 activity in bioassays, often at very high titer. Similar antibodies occur in up to 30% of late-onset MG patients without thymoma and in about 30% of thymoma patients without MG, but rarely in early-onset MG (EOMG), seronegative MG, or LEMS cases.[40] The high prevalence is particularly striking in MG/thymoma cases because most of their other autoantibodies are against muscle antigens.

These antibodies might have important practical consequences for the patients. In two informative cases, both antibodies increased strikingly around the time of tumor recurrence/metastasis, suggesting that their production is provoked or enhanced by the tumor[40] (see also FIGURE 5). However, in other cases without recurrence, they can clearly persist for years, often in spite of prolonged immunosuppressive therapy (FIGURE 5). When they do, they may be associated with intractable infections; one patient developed persistent lung infections after removal of her recurrence and eventually died of cryptococcal meningitis.[40] A further patient with antibodies to IFN-α contracted an AIDS-like syndrome and died of Pneumocystis pneumonia. Clearly, immunosuppressive therapy requires careful monitoring in these cases. Furthermore, these antibodies may be relevant to the immunodeficiency sometimes associated with thymoma;[41] they might also interfere in cytokine therapy.

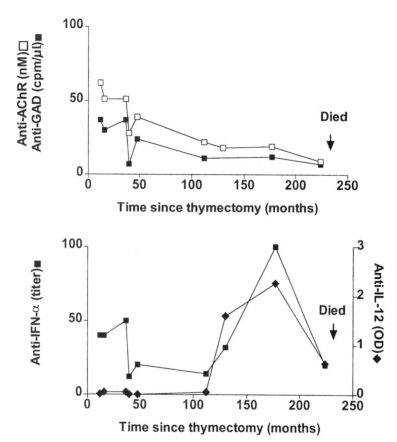

FIGURE 5. Serum antibodies against AChR and glutamic acid decarboxylase (GAD) (top) and against IFN-α (neutralization titers) and IL-12 (ELISA) (bottom) measured serially in an MG/thymoma patient. A thymoma was removed at time 0 from a man at age 46 with a 2.7-year history of MG (and 4 years of diabetes mellitus). Three years later, intensive plasma exchange sharply reduced all of his autoantibodies. Those against AChR and GAD (top) remained low during his subsequent 12 years of maintenance on azathioprine, which was then replaced by corticosteroids. Pleural metastases were found 8 years postthymectomy and were successfully treated with chemotherapy; around this time, his anticytokine antibodies rose strikingly (bottom). About 17.5 years postoperatively, he developed the stiff-man syndrome shortly before dying of bronchopneumonia at age 65.

These antibodies may also have etiological significance. Interestingly, both cytokines are normally produced by professional APC, which we have already implicated in autoimmunization against AChR in MG thymomas (see above). We propose that these APC also immunize against the IFN-α and/or IL-12 that they themselves produce, possibly because of the potent adjuvant activity of IL-12 or perhaps for other microenvironmental reasons. Second, both cytokines, especially IL-12, normally create a bias towards Th1 responses, and one might expect this to be counteracted by the neutralizing antibodies. This, in turn, may contribute to the intractable infections, as well as to the Th0 phenotype of our thymoma-derived T cell clones (TABLE 1) that contrasts so sharply with the uniformly Th1 profiles of those that we have selected from EOMG patients.

Thymic Hyperplasia in MG

Hyperplastic changes have long been recognized in the MG thymus, especially in early-onset cases,[2] and include medullary infiltration by germinal centers (GC) and T cell areas very similar to those in peripheral lymph nodes.[42] The AChR-specific plasma cells here are proving to be a rich source of mRNA for cloning combinatorial antibodies.[43,44] However, it remains controversial as to whether the changes are causative or are an effect of the responses in MG. They are positively implicated (a) by the presence of rare myoid cells expressing fetal AChR[45] that (b) these patients' autoantibodies often prefer[3] and (c) by the beneficial effects of thymectomy on their myasthenia.[3] On the other hand, (d) the degree of hyperplasia is very variable, ranging from almost pure lymph node appearances at one extreme to nearly normal thymus at the other.[46] Furthermore, (e) "hyperplastic indices" correlate very poorly with MG duration, clinical severity, and response to surgery.[46] Moreover, (f) hyperplasia is not unique to MG and has been observed in humans and mice with systemic lupus erythematosus for example,[3,46] suggesting that it could be an effect of circulating immune complexes or activated T cells or, indeed, of anti-AChR antibodies attacking the myoid cells. Finally, (g) it is still not clear whether these latter are *agents provocateurs* or innocent victims, or even whether they are under any immune attack in MG.[45,46]

Typically, the hyperplastic abnormalities are almost entirely in the thymic medulla and there are few resemblances to the thymomas (where both epithelial and lymphoid cells are usually mainly cortical in phenotype). The infiltrating GC and T cell zones often compress the true epithelial areas into bands and arches (FIGURE 6). The latter usually include the few myoid cells; while these are positive for AChR and other muscle antigens,[45] we have never seen expression of HLA–class II or the accessory molecules ICAM-1, LFA-3, or B7.1 on or in them. Thus, if they are *agents provocateurs*, then presumably HLA–class I–restricted cytotoxic T cells, professional APC, and/or some "inflammatory" process must be involved too. It may be relevant that IFN-γ readily induces *de novo* class II expression on cultured human myoblasts (which myoid cells resemble in several ways). If these are HLA-DR4-matched, they can then present their endogenous AChR α149–160 epitope to the PM-A1 Th clone (S. J. Curnow *et al.*, in preparation), just as HLA-DR4-transfected TE-671 cells can do;[47] the latter are then specifically killed by this Th1 clone.

The epithelial bands are surrounded by a laminin[+] border that may be fenestrated focally near the GC.[42] Even in this "epicenter" of hyperplasia, the myoid cells do not appear to congregate consistently (see legend to FIGURE 6). However, the epithelial cells seem especially hyperplastic here; they are particularly densely packed, with few "dendritic" processes, and may even spread into the T cell areas towards the GC (FIGURE 6). Furthermore, they show more labeling for EGF receptor and α2, α3, and α6 integrins here than in other more normal areas (FIGURE 6). Again, however, it is

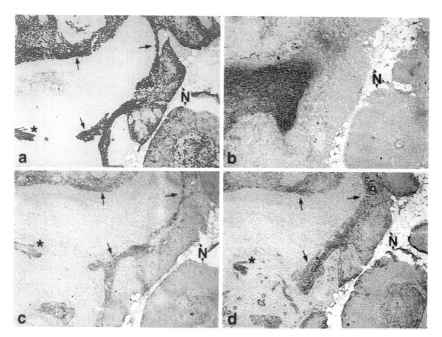

FIGURE 6. Thymic hyperplasia in a patient with EOMG. The same area has been immuno-stained for cytokeratin (a, Mab LP34), B cells and germinal centers (GC) (b, Mab RFB6), epidermal growth factor receptor (EGFR) (c), and $\alpha 3$ integrin (d). To the right are two small relatively normal thymic lobules (N) with cortex partially surrounding islets of medulla (including a Hassall body in the lower corner). To the left is a large keratin-negative area of extra-parenchymal infiltrate including a large GC (b) with a T cell zone around it. Partially surrounding the T cell zone are medullary epithelial bands (arrows) (a), which label more strongly for EGFR (c) than the relatively normal medulla to the right. They also express more $\alpha 3$ integrin (d), which forms a continuous border separating them from the normal area, whereas there is no obvious barrier to communication with the T cell zone; indeed, there is an isolated patch of medullary epithelium within it (asterisk) (a). Integrin $\alpha 3$ is also expressed on endothelium. In adjacent sections, we found no myoid cells in this entire region.

not yet clear whether this epithelial hyperplasia could be attracting the nearby infiltrate or is merely an effect of it.

Autoimmunization by Thymic AChR ε Subunits?

On screening hyperplastic thymus for AChR mRNAs by RT-PCR, we found expression of those encoding the α–ε subunits, as expected. By RNase protection, however, we were again only able to detect ε mRNA, in about half of the samples, and not γ mRNA, even though myoid cells are known to contain fetal AChR.[45] While these rare cells may be the source of the α–δ signals in RT-PCR, the ε might derive from some other cell type—possibly epithelial. This would be surprising because, in general, its expression is strictly localized to the end plate region in adult/maturing muscle. However, some workers believe that autoantigen expression in the thymus may be necessary to prevent autoimmune responses and that defects in this screening process may be one of their causes.[48,49] If, instead, the AChR ε proves to be in some potent antigen-presenting cell type, then this might be a significant "missing link" with the changes in MG thymomas.

To distinguish between these possibilities of a failure to induce tolerance or of active autoimmunization, we have screened for responses to AChR α, γ, and ε subunits by both blood and thymic T cells from EOMG patients. So far, we have had greater success with PBL, perhaps for technical reasons or possibly because many responding cells have emigrated from the thymus by the time of diagnosis. In three of four potential responders, we obtained clones specific for the ε rather than the γ or α subunits. Moreover, they clearly recognize adult rather than fetal AChR.[50] Strikingly, they all respond to the same synthetic ε202–219 peptide (FIGURE 7), which is again

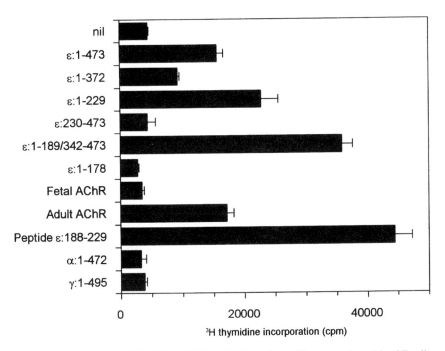

FIGURE 7. Responses of T cell line CAM to AChR ε polypeptide preparations. Blood T cells from an EOMG patient were stimulated with recombinant human AChR ε subunit; after expansion in IL-2, they were restimulated with AChR ε at limiting numbers (30 cells per 20-μL well) and expanded in IL-2. One of the resulting lines shows a clear response to adult AChR, but not fetal AChR (absorbed to immunomagnetic beads[50]), as well as to a synthetic 189–229 peptide from the ε sequence. However, an additional response to another ε polypeptide from which this region is deleted (1–189/342–473) may well prove to be against an *E. coli* contaminant. This illustrates the need to confirm specificity with independent AChR antigen preparations and synthetic peptides.

presented by DR52a (TABLE 1); another similar clone from an older HLA-DR1$^+$/DR52a$^+$ patient with D(−)penicillamine-induced MG behaved very similarly.[51] Inevitably, with these small numbers, we cannot prove that there is a higher success rate with the ε versus the α or γ subunits in these patients; on the other hand, it is no easier to explain by differences in antigen concentration or purity. To test whether responsiveness correlates with strong or weak ε expression in the thymus is clearly a high priority. Presumably, in either case, this may be a recurring epitope partly because of efficient processing from full-length ε and whole AChR.

The preference for HLA-DR52a is intriguing for three reasons:

(a) If DR52a is expressed weakly, it might, in theory, induce self-tolerance less efficiently in the thymus.

(b) DR52a is a member of the HLA-DQ2-DR3-B8 haplotype that is prevalent in EOMG patients, but is not found in DQ2-DR3-B18, which is rare (M. Janer *et al.*, in preparation). Thus, it could explain the consistently stronger association with B8 than with DR3 in EOMG,[52] something we are now pursuing.

(c) DR52a is very similar to DR3; they share a unique ^{71}Lys-^{73}Gly^{74}Arg--^{77}Asn motif in DRβ; the ^{74}Arg imposes a preference for Asp at position 4 in the peptides that either allele presents.[39,53] However, the key differences at each end of their peptide-binding grooves may serve to broaden the repertoire of epitopes that they collectively present when they occur together. The smaller ^{86}Gly of DR52a allows more binding of bulkier anchor residues in the first hydrophobic pocket than does the less permissive ^{86}Val of DR3.[39] Thus, if the ^{149}Trp in AChR α is changed to Phe, the resulting peptide can now be presented by DR3 as well as by DR52a to clone II, exactly as for clone PM-A1 by DR4 subtypes with ^{86}Val.[54] In the center of the ε202–219 sequence, there is a potential DR52a motif (FIGURE 4, bottom) and we hope to test for presentation of analogous ^{205}Trp→Phe substituents by DR3 to our new T cell clones. If there was a Phe instead of the Trp in the natural sequence of either epitope, they might be presented by a considerably broader range of class II alleles. Perhaps, fortunately, ^{149}Trp is apparently essential for ACh binding. DR52a and DR3 also differ by their ^{57}Val and ^{57}Asp, respectively.[30]

Towards Selective Immunotherapy

If these patients' Th do prove to recognize a limited number of dominant epitopes in the AChR, selective immunotherapy might be more widely applicable in EOMG. Specific unresponsiveness can be induced by directly engaging the TCR without optimal costimulation (reviewed in reference 55). To do this, we have compared three methods, testing clone PM-A1 as a prototype. We have used an Mab to its TCR Vβ5.1, soluble DR4 complexed with the α145–163 peptide, or excess free peptide that these strongly class II$^+$ T cells can present to each other (with minimal costimulation).[56] As summarized in TABLE 2, pretreatment with each of these agents in the absence of APC greatly inhibits the response to a potent challenge stimulus, and each is highly specific.[55] However, their long-term effects differ greatly. Thus, the appropriate anti-Vβ Mab causes a rapid short-term TCR blockade, but the T cells begin to

TABLE 2. Summary of Effects of Preincubation of PM-A1 T Cells with DR4:Peptide Complex, Free Peptide, and Anti-Vβ5.1 Mab

	Preincubation[a]		
	DR4:Peptide Complex	Free Peptide	Anti-Vβ5.1 Mab
% Inhibition of Response[b]	46–99% (27)	30–94% (20)	25–96% (22)
Induction Time	>6 hours, 37 °C	>6 hours, 37 °C	<10 min, 37 °C
IC_{50}[c]	$1–8 \times 10^{-10}$ M (5)	$2–7 \times 10^{-8}$ M (3)	$1–2 \times 10^{-9}$ M (5)
Duration of Effect	>96 hours	<24 hours	<24 hours
% Cell Loss	35–87% (9)	13–87% (6)	(−62)–(−7)% (9)[d]
Surface IL-2 Receptor	increase	increase	increase
Cell Size	increase	increase	increase
Surface T Cell Receptor	decrease	decrease	decrease

[a]The standard conditions involved a preincubation of 18 hours (except for the measurement of induction time) with DR4:peptide α145–163 (F149) complex [2.8×10^{-10} M], free peptide α145–163 (F149) [1×10^{-7} M], or anti-Vβ5.1 Mab [6.2×10^{-8} M]. Proliferative responses were then determined following challenge with APC and Ag (optimal dose of AChR α130–265). The number of experiments is shown in parentheses.

[b]Percent inhibition was determined as the percentage decrease from the control response to APC and Ag.

[c]IC_{50} was the concentration required for a 50% reduction in the response.

[d]These negative values indicate an increase in cell number following preincubation.

recover within 24–48 hours and actually show enhanced survival by day 4 (relative to untreated cells). With the soluble complexes, several hours (>6) of preincubation are required, but after that a profound and almost permanent unresponsiveness ensues. This reflects apoptosis in around 30–80% of the cells and anergy in the survivors. With free peptide, higher molarities are required (probably to achieve similar class II occupancy) and the effects are more variable and less dramatic. Again, there may be apoptosis in up to 40% of the cells, but responsiveness recovers more rapidly in the remainder, which may then show enhanced survival.[56]

These strikingly contrasting effects after directly engaging the same TCR may reflect differences in the duration or the valency of these interactions that could, in turn, then lead to different internal signaling. Alternatively, T cell–T cell presentation of excess peptide may also allow some weak costimulation and/or greater CD4 recruitment that may partially counteract the tolerogenic effects and increase their variability. In any case, this is unlikely to be an important mechanism *in vivo* because it depends on improbably high concentrations of both peptide and class II[+] specific T cells. By contrast, soluble peptide:class II complexes have already given encouraging results in animal models of MG,[57] as well as of multiple sclerosis.

Before application in patients, many further key issues need to be addressed: which Th cell subsets are most pathogenic and most susceptible to these treatments, especially in their natural state in the patients; the importance of the valency of the interactions and whether oligomeric complexes might be even more effective; how to enhance the apoptosis and prevent Th cells from escaping it. Nevertheless, agents that can circulate widely and enter tissues freely may prove to be essential in anti-body-mediated autoimmune (or allergic) diseases such as MG, in which the pathogenic T cells are not concentrated in a target organ where they would be especially amenable to bystander immunosuppression. Both for this reason and because they mimic the least diverse facet of the response, specific peptide:class II complexes offer great promise, especially if our evidence of recurring recognition of the same T cell epitopes is confirmed and extended.

ACKNOWLEDGMENTS

We thank our many previous colleagues who helped to lay the foundations for the present studies.

REFERENCES

1. SOUADJIAN, J. V. *et al.* 1974. The spectrum of diseases associated with thymoma. Arch. Intern. Med. **134:** 373–379.
2. CASTLEMAN, B. & E. H. NORRIS. 1949. The pathology of the thymus gland in myasthenia gravis: a study of 35 cases. Medicine **28:** 27–58.
3. WILLCOX, N. & A. VINCENT. 1988. Myasthenia gravis as an example of organ-specific autoimmune disease. *In* B Lymphocytes in Human Disease, p. 469–506. Oxford University Press. London/New York.
4. BEESON, D. *et al.* 1993. Primary structure of the human muscle acetylcholine receptor: cDNA cloning of the gamma and epsilon subunits. Eur. J. Biochem. **215:** 229–238.
5. FUJII, Y. & J. LINDSTROM. 1988. Specificity of the T cell immune response to acetylcholine receptor in experimental autoimmune myasthenia gravis. J. Immunol. **140:** 1830–1837.
6. BELLONE, M. *et al.* 1991. Experimental myasthenia gravis in congenic mice: sequence mapping and H-2 restriction of T helper epitopes on the α subunits of *Torpedo californica* and murine acetylcholine receptors. Eur. J. Immunol. **21:** 2303–2310.
7. WILLCOX, N. *et al.* 1993. Approaches for studying the pathogenic T cells in autoimmune patients. Ann. N.Y. Acad. Sci. **681:** 219–237.
8. HAWKE, S. *et al.* 1996. Autoimmune T cells in myasthenia gravis: heterogeneity and potential for specific immunotargeting. Immunol. Today **17:** 307–311.
9. MELMS, A. *et al.* 1992. T cells from normal and myasthenic individuals recognize the human acetylcholine receptor: heterogeneity of antigenic sites on the α-subunit. Ann. Neurol. **31:** 311–318.
10. PROTTI, M. P. *et al.* 1993. Myasthenia gravis: recognition of a human autoantigen at the molecular level. Immunol. Today **14:** 363–368.
11. MATSUO, H. *et al.* 1995. Recognition of unnatural epitopes by peptide-selected T cell lines in myasthenia gravis patients and controls. J. Immunol. **155:** 3683–3692.
12. O'NEILL, J. H., N. M. MURRAY & J. NEWSOM-DAVIS. 1988. The Lambert-Eaton myasthenic syndrome: a review of 50 cases. Brain **111:** 577–596.
13. LANG, B. *et al.* 1981. Autoimmune aetiology for myasthenic (Eaton-Lambert) syndrome. Lancet **ii:** 224–226.
14. CHALK, C. *et al.* 1990. Response of the Lambert-Eaton myasthenic syndrome to treatment of associated small-cell lung carcinoma. Neurology **40:** 1552–1556.
15. WILLCOX, N. 1993. Myasthenia gravis. Curr. Opin. Immunol. **5:** 910–917.
16. CHILOSI, M. *et al.* 1986. Myasthenia gravis: immunohistological heterogeneity in microenvironmental organization of hyperplastic and neoplastic thymuses suggesting different mechanisms of tolerance breakdown. J. Neuroimmunol. **11:** 191–204.

17. NAMBA, T., N. G. BRUNNER & D. GROB. 1978. Myasthenia gravis in patients with thymoma, with particular reference to onset after thymectomy. Medicine **57:** 411–433.
18. AARLI, J. A. *et al.* 1990. Patients with myasthenia gravis and thymoma have in their sera IgG autoantibodies against titin. Clin. Exp. Immunol. **82:** 284–288.
19. WILLIAMS, C. L. & V. A. LENNON. 1986. Thymic B lymphocyte clones from patients with myasthenia gravis secrete monoclonal striational antibodies reacting with myosin, alpha-actinin, or actin. J. Exp. Med. **164:** 1043–1059.
20. GILHUS, N-E. *et al.* 1984. Rabbit antiserum to a citric acid extract of human skeletal muscle staining thymomas from myasthenia gravis patients. J. Neuroimmunol. **7:** 55–64.
21. HARA, Y. *et al.* 1991. Neoplastic epithelial cells express α-subunit of muscle nicotinic acetylcholine receptor in thymoma from patients with myasthenia gravis. FEBS Lett. **279:** 137–140.
22. WHEATLEY, L. M. *et al.* 1992. Molecular evidence for the expression of nicotinic acetylcholine receptor α-chain in mouse thymus. J. Immunol. **148:** 3105–3109.
23. KIRCHNER, T. *et al.* 1988. Pathogenesis of myasthenia gravis: acetylcholine receptor–related antigenic determinants in tumor-free thymuses and thymic epithelial tumors. Am. J. Pathol. **130:** 268–280.
24. MARX, A. *et al.* 1990. Characterization of a protein with an acetylcholine receptor epitope from myasthenia gravis–associated thymomas. Lab. Invest. **62:** 279–286.
25. MARX, A. *et al.* 1996. Expression of neurofilaments and of a titin epitope in thymic epithelial tumors. Am. J. Pathol. **148:** 1839–1850.
26. TZARTOS, S. J. & M. S. REMOUNDOS. 1992. Precise epitope mapping of monoclonal antibodies to the cytoplasmic side of the acetylcholine receptor α subunit: dissecting a potentially myasthenogenic epitope. Eur. J. Biochem. **207:** 915–922.
27. (a) NAGVEKAR, N. *et al.* 1997. Epitopes expressed in myasthenia gravis thymomas are not recognized by patients' T cells or autoantibodies. Submitted; (b) NAGVEKAR, N. *et al.* 1997. A pathogenetic role for the thymoma in myasthenia gravis; autosensitization of IL4-producing T cell clones recognizing extracellular acetylcholine receptor epitopes presented by minority class II isotypes. Submitted.
28. MACLENNAN, C. *et al.* Expression levels of mRNAs encoding acetylcholine receptor subunits in MG thymus and thymoma. In preparation.
29. MACLENNAN, C. *et al.* 1997. Expression of muscle acetylcholine receptor mRNA in atypical carcinoid tumors of the thymus. In preparation.
30. MARSH, S. G. E., J. E. MOSES & J. G. BODMER. 1992. HLA class II sequence polymorphism detectable by serology. *In* HLA 1991, p. 610–620. Oxford University Press. London/New York.
31. MELLINS, E. *et al.* 1991. A gene required for class II–restricted antigen presentation maps to the major histocompatibility complex. J. Exp. Med. **174:** 1607–1615.
32. HENWOOD, J. *et al.* 1993. Restricted T cell receptor expression by human T cell clones specific for mycobacterial 65-kDa heat-shock protein: selective *in vivo* expansion of T cells bearing defined receptors. Eur. J. Immunol. **23:** 1256–1265.
33. HIGGINS, J. A. *et al.* 1994. Overlapping T cell epitopes in the group I allergen of *Dermatophagoides* species restricted by HLA-DP and HLA-DR class II molecules. J. Allergy Clin. Immunol. **93:** 891–899.
34. CELIS, E., D. OU & L. OTVOS. 1988. Recognition of hepatitis B surface antigen by human T lymphocytes. J. Immunol. **140:** 1808–1815.
35. CELIS, E. *et al.* 1990. Identification of a rabies virus T cell epitope on the basis of its similarity with hepatitis B surface antigen peptide presented to T cells by the same MHC molecule (DPw4). J. Immunol. **145:** 305–310.
36. HAMMOND, S. A. *et al.* 1991. Characterization of a conserved T cell epitope in HIV-1 gp41 recognized by vaccine-induced human cytolytic T cells. J. Immunol. **146:** 1470–1477.

37. DE KOSTER, S., D. C. ANDERSON & A. TERMIJTELEN. 1989. T cells sensitized to synthetic HLA-DR3 peptide give evidence of continuous presentation of denatured HLA-DR3 molecules by HLA-DP. J. Exp. Med. **169:** 1191–1196.
38. RAMMENSEE, H-G., T. FRIEDE & S. STEVANOVIC. 1995. MHC ligands and peptide motifs: first listing. Immunogenetics **41:** 178–228.
39. NAGVEKAR, N. *et al.* 1997. Mapping an HLA-DR52a-restricted epitope from the human acetylcholine receptor: comparison of natural and artificial epitopes. In preparation.
40. MEAGER, A. *et al.* 1997. Spontaneous neutralising antibodies to interferon-α and inter-leukin-12 in thymoma-associated myasthenia gravis. Lancet. In press.
41. ASHERSON, G. L. & A. D. B. WEBSTER. 1980. Thymoma and immunodeficiency. *In* Diagnosis and Treatment of Immunodeficiency, p. 78–98. Blackwell. Oxford.
42. JANOSSY, G. *et al.* 1986. Cellular differentiation of lymphoid subpopulations and their microenvironments in the human thymus. Curr. Top. Pathol. **75:** 89–125.
43. GRAUS, Y. *et al.* 1997. Human anti-nicotinic acetylcholine receptor recombinant Fab fragments isolated from thymus-derived phage display libraries from myasthenia gravis patients reflect predominant specificities in serum and block the action of pathogenic serum antibodies. J. Immunol. **158:** 1919–1929.
44. FARRAR, J. *et al.* 1997. Diverse Fabs specific for acetylcholine receptor epitopes from a myasthenia gravis thymus combinatorial library. Int. Immunol. **9:** 1311–1318.
45. SCHLUEP, M. *et al.* 1987. Acetylcholine receptors in human thymic myoid cells *in situ*: an immunohistological study. Ann. Neurol. **22:** 212–222.
46. SCHLUEP, M. *et al.* 1988. Myasthenia gravis thymus: clinical, histological, and culture correlations. J. Autoimmun. **1:** 445–467.
47. BAGGI, F. M. *et al.* 1993. Presentation of endogenous acetylcholine receptor epitope by an MHC class II–transfected human muscle cell line to a specific CD4+ T cell clone from a myasthenia gravis patient. J. Neuroimmunol. **46:** 57–66.
48. ALDERUCCIO, F. *et al.* 1993. An autoimmune disease with multiple molecular targets abrogated by the transgenic expression of a single autoantigen in the thymus. J. Exp. Med. **178:** 419–426.
49. VAFIADIS, P. *et al.* 1997. Insulin expression in human thymus is modulated by INS VNTR alleles at the IDDM2 locus. Nat. Genet. **15:** 289–292.
50. HILL, M. *et al.* 1997. T cell responses to the ε subunit of the acetylcholine receptor in myasthenia gravis. In preparation.
51. HILL, M. *et al.* 1997. Specific T cell responses to D(–)penicillamine in patients with and without myasthenic complications. In preparation.
52. DEGLI-ESPOSTI, M. A. *et al.* 1992. An approach to the localization of the susceptibility genes for generalized myasthenia gravis by mapping recombinant ancestral haplotypes. Immunogenetics **35:** 355–364.
53. STERN, L. J. *et al.* 1994. Crystal structure of the human class II MHC protein HLA-DR1 complexed with an influenza virus peptide. Nature **368:** 215–221.
54. HAWKE, S. *et al.* 1997. Cross-restriction of a T cell clone to HLA-DR alleles associated with rheumatoid arthritis; clues to arthritogenic peptide motifs. In preparation.
55. NICOLLE, M. W. *et al.* 1994. Specific tolerance to an acetylcholine receptor epitope induced *in vitro* in myasthenia gravis CD4+ lymphocytes by soluble major histocompatibility complex class II–peptide complexes. J. Clin. Invest. **93:** 1361–1369.
56. BOND, A. *et al.* 1997. Diverse patterns of unresponsiveness in an acetylcholine receptor–specific T cell clone from a myasthenia gravis patient after engaging the T cell receptor with three different ligands. J. Neuroimmunol. In press.
57. SPACK, E. G. *et al.* 1995. Induction of tolerance in experimental autoimmune myasthenia gravis with solubilized MHC class II:acetylcholine receptor peptide complexes. J. Autoimmun. **8:** 787–807.

Thymocytes and Cultured Thymic Epithelial Cells Express Transcripts Encoding α-3, α-5, and β-4 Subunits of Neuronal Nicotinic Acetylcholine Receptors

Preferential Transcription of the α-3 and β-4 Genes by Immature CD4+8+ Thymocytes and Evidence for Response to Nicotine in Thymocytes[a]

MIRTA MIHOVILOVIC,[b] STEPHEN DENNING,[c] YUN MAI,[b]
CLARE M. FISHER,[b] LEONA P. WHICHARD,[d]
DHAVALKUMAR D. PATEL,[d,e] AND ALLEN D. ROSES[b,f]

[b]Department of Medicine
Division of Neurology
Duke University Medical Center
Durham, North Carolina 27710

[c]Ohio Heart Care
Canton, Ohio 44718

[d]Department of Medicine
Division of Rheumatology, Allergy, and Clinical Immunology
[e]Department of Immunology
[f]Department of Neurobiology
Duke University Medical Center
Durham, North Carolina 27710

INTRODUCTION

Normal thymus, hypertrophic thymus from myasthenia gravis (MG) patients, and thymomas from MG and non-MG patients express transcripts encoding the α-3, α-5, and β-4 subunits of nicotinic neuronal acetylcholine receptors (AChRs).[1–3] This pattern of transcription suggests that neuronal AChRs similar to those expressed in ganglia are expressed in thymus and that these receptors may be of importance in transducing signals delivered through the autonomic nervous system or may be responsive to local production of ACh.

Thymocytes express α-3 AChR transcripts, while peripheral blood lymphocytes (PBL) do not express these transcripts,[2] suggesting that there is a relationship between AChR subunit gene expression and T cell development. To investigate this possibility, we analyzed the transcription of α-5 and β-4 subunit genes in thymocytes and PBL as well as the transcription of the α-3, α-5, and β-4 neuronal AChR subunit

[a]This work was supported by a clinical grant from the Muscular Dystrophy Association.

genes in thymocyte populations at different stages of their intrathymic maturation pathway: immature double-positive (DP) CD4+CD8+, and single-positive (SP) CD4+8– and CD4–8+ subsets.

Both thymic lymphoid cells and epithelial cells could be directly innervated by fibers of the autonomic nervous system[4] and/or could respond to local production of ACh. In this context, we also investigated the transcription of AChR subunit genes in thymic epithelial cells.

Cholinergic agonists, under conditions that measure nicotinic influences on thymic cell metabolism, stimulate thymic epithelial cell growth,[5] modulate thymocyte apoptosis,[6] and inhibit thymocyte calcium ionophore A23187–induced apoptosis.[7] To investigate functional responses to nicotine, we have studied the effect of nicotine on the bioreductive capacity of short-term thymocyte cultures.

MATERIALS AND METHODS

Purification and characterization of PBL, thymocytes, and thymocyte subsets as well as growth and characterization of epithelial cell cultures have been described previously.[2,8,9] Total RNA from thymocyte subsets and cultured thymic cells was isolated using a phenol chloroform–based method and a minimum of 125,000 cells (STAT-60, TEL-TEST "B" Incorporated, Friendswood, Texas). RT-PCR assays were done using total RNA and either rTth reverse transcriptase/DNA polymerase (Perkin Elmer Cetus, Norwalk, Connecticut) (α-3 and β-4 protocols) or reverse transcriptase (M-MLV reverse transcriptase, GIBCO-BRL, Gaithersburg, Maryland) followed by PCR in the presence of Taq DNA polymerase (Boehringer Mannheim, Indianapolis, Indiana) (α-5 and amyloid precursor protein [APP] protocols);[2,10] when indicated, the β-4 RT-PCR product was reamplified using a nested PCR.[10]

Thymic fibroblast cultures were established as indicated for the epithelial cell cultures,[9] but omitting EGF from the media. Short-term thymocyte cultures were maintained in RPMI 1640 supplemented with 10% FCS and 10 μg/mL of gentamicin (GIBCO-BRL) at 37 °C in an atmosphere with 5% CO_2.[10]

The effect of nicotine on thymocyte bioreductive capacity was assessed using short-term cultures of thymocytes and the Cell Titer 96 AQ kit (Promega, Madison, Wisconsin).

Unless otherwise stated, thymic cells used in the study were derived from normal donors.

RESULTS AND CONCLUSIONS

Thymocytes and thymic epithelial cells express transcripts encoding the α-3, α-5, and β-4 subunits of nicotinic neuronal AChRs, suggesting that neuronal AChRs similar to those expressed in ganglia are expressed in these thymic cells (FIGURE 1, I and II). It is important, however, to point out that while α-3 and β-4 gene transcription is restricted to thymocytes and thymic epithelial cells, α-5 gene transcription occurs in all cells tested, including thymic fibroblasts (FIGURE 1, II).

RT-PCR analyses of thymocyte subsets indicate that immature CD4+8+ thymo-

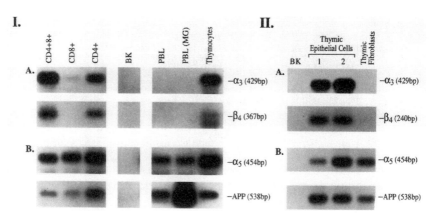

FIGURE 1. (I) Expression of α-3, α-5, and β-4 AChR subunit transcripts in total thymocytes and thymocyte subsets. RT-PCR for the α-3 and β-4 AChR subunit transcripts is shown in part A and for the α-5 AChR subunit and APP transcripts in part B. RT-PCRs were done as indicated in the text using total RNA derived from either 250,000 sorted CD4+8−, CD4−8+, and CD4+8+ cells (0.40 μg of RNA/assay based on RNA yield obtained from total thymocyte populations) or as follows: non-MG PBL, 1.5 μg; MG PBL, 0.75 μg; thymocytes, 0.5 μg (α-3 protocol) and 1.5 μg (α-5, β-4, and APP protocols). Note that the APP transcript level for the MG PBL preparation shown is atypically elevated and that the RT-PCR-generated doublet seen in the β-4 panel produces the expected β-4 product upon reamplification (nested PCR). The MG patient from which PBL were prepared presented with an atrophic thymus and an anti-AChR titer of 6.9 nM at the time of thymectomy; 3 years after thymectomy, the titer was 5.4 nM. PBL were obtained 3.5 years postthymectomy when the titer had fallen below 2.6 nM after plasma exchange therapy. (II) Expression of α-3, α-5, and β-4 AChR subunit transcripts in cultured thymic epithelial cells. RT-PCR for the α-3 and β-4 AChR subunit transcripts is shown in part A and for the α-5 AChR subunit and APP transcripts in part B. Total RNA was obtained from independent thymic epithelial cell cultures and one thymic fibroblast culture grown as indicated in the text. RT-PCR was done using 0.5 μg of total RNA. The β-4 RT-PCR product was reamplified using a nested PCR.

cytes express higher levels of the α-3 and β-4 transcripts than more mature thymocytes. Representative results (three independent thymocyte sets have been analyzed for α-3 transcription and two for β-4 transcription) are shown in FIGURE 1, IA. Compared to freshly isolated thymocytes, PBL do not express α-3 and β-4 AChR subunit transcripts (FIGURE 1, IA). These results expand previous observations[2] and indicate that there is transcriptional regulation of neuronal α-3 and β-4 AChR subunit genes during the process of thymocyte maturation. In addition, the fact that both α-3 and β-4 AChR subunit transcripts are preferentially downregulated in SP CD4−8+ thymocytes (FIGURE 1, IA) argues in favor of an active role for putative neuronal nicotinic AChRs at the time of intrathymic differentiation between cells of CD4+8− and CD4−8+ lineage.

Expression of nicotinic neuronal AChR subunit genes in thymocytes and their transcriptional regulation during thymocyte maturation suggest that neuronal nicotinic AChRs are expressed in these cells. Strengthening this notion, nicotine (0.1–10

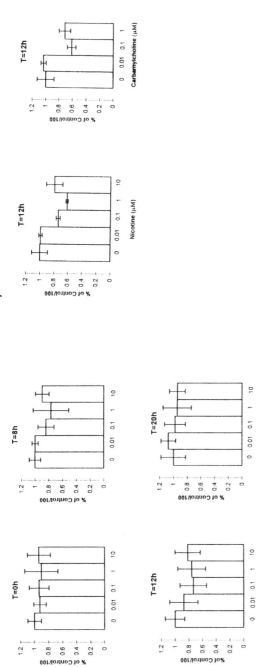

FIGURE 2. Effect of nicotine and carbamylcholine on the bioreductive capacity of short-term thymocyte cultures. Freshly isolated thymocytes were maintained in culture as indicated in the text for 4 h at 37 °C and plated in 96-well plates at a density of 400,000 to 600,000 cells/well. Wells received ligands at the indicated concentrations; then, at the indicated times, bioreductive capacity of the cultures was measured using the Promega Cell Titer 96 AQ kit as indicated by the manufacturer. Each data point was run in triplicate. Data are normalized by assigning 100% activity to control cultures that received buffer instead of the cholinergic ligand. The average response of eight preparations is shown in part A and a typical significant response in part B. Note that it is not clear why different human thymocyte preparations differ in their responses (see RESULTS AND CONCLUSIONS). It is possible that tissue and thymocyte handling and/or instability of cholinergic ligand binding by thymocytes in culture could influence their response. In this context, it is important to indicate that we have observed that α-3 and β-4 AChR subunit transcripts are rapidly downregulated in short-term thymocyte cultures by a process that is not reversed by stimulation with phytohemagglutinin and IL-2.[10] This observation indicates that factors within the thymic microenvironment influence expression of the α-3 and β-4 AChR subunit genes by developing T cells.

μM) reduces the metabolic activity associated with apoptosis in cultured thymocytes (FIGURE 2). Decreases in bioreductive capacity of the cultures are best observed at 8 and 12 h after incubation with the ligand. FIGURE 2A shows the average response of eight preparations (four responding significantly, three showing an inhibitory trend, and one presenting no response; see legend of FIGURE 2), while FIGURE 2B shows a typical significant response to both nicotine and carbamylcholine.

In conclusion, we have shown that (1) thymocytes and thymic epithelial cells express α-3, α-5, and β-4 subunit transcripts, (2) α-3 and β-4 AChR subunit transcripts are expressed at the highest levels in immature CD4+CD8+ thymocytes, and (3) nicotine appears to accelerate apoptosis in cultured thymocytes. By analogy to the role played by neuronal nicotinic receptors in neurosecretory cells, putative thymic neuronal nicotinic AChRs could modulate the neurosecretory activity of thymic cells, affect thymocyte maturation, and influence the outcome of thymic-mediated immune responses.

REFERENCES

1. MIHOVILOVIC, M. & A. D. ROSES. 1991. Expression of mRNAs in human thymus coding for the α-3 subunit of a neuronal acetylcholine receptor. Exp. Neurol. **111:** 175–180.
2. MIHOVILOVIC, M. & A. D. ROSES. 1993. Expression of α-3, α-5, and β-4 neuronal acetylcholine receptor subunit transcripts in normal and myasthenia gravis thymus: identification of thymocytes expressing α-3 transcripts. J. Immunol. **151:** 6517–6524.
3. MIHOVILOVIC, M., C. HULETTE, J. MITTELSTAEDT, C. AUSTIN & A. D. ROSES. 1993. Nicotinic neuronal acetylcholine receptor α-3 subunit transcription in normal and myasthenic thymus. Ann. N.Y. Acad. Sci. **681:** 83–96.
4. KENDALL, M. D. & A. A. AL-SHAWAF. 1991. Innervation of the rat thymus gland. Brain Behav. Immun. **5:** 9–28.
5. TOMINAGA, K., Y. KINOSHITA, F. HATO, A. MASUDA & M. MATSUYAMA. 1989. Effect of cholinergic agonists on the proliferation and protein synthesis in a culture thymic epithelial cell line. Cell. Mol. Biol. **35:** 679–686.
6. RINNER, I., T. KUKULANSKY, P. FELSNER, E. SKREINER, A. GLOBERSON, M. KASAI, K. HIROKAWA, W. KORSATKO & K. SCHUAENSTEIN. 1994. Cholinergic stimulation modulates apoptosis and differentiation of murine thymocytes via a nicotinic effect on thymic epithelium. Biochem. Biophys. Res. Commun. **203:** 1057–1062.
7. WRIGHT, S., J. ZHONG, H. ZHENG & J. K. LARRICK. 1993. Nicotine inhibition of apoptosis suggests a role in tumor promotion. FASEB J. **7:** 1045–1051.
8. KURTZBERG, J., S. M. DENNING, L. M. NYCUM, K. H. SINGER & B. F. HAYNES. 1989. Immature thymocytes can be driven to differentiate into non-lymphoid lineages by cytokines from thymic epithelial cells. Proc. Natl. Acad. Sci. U.S.A. **86:** 7575–7579.
9. SINGER, K. H., E. A. HARDEN, A. L. ROBERTSON, D. F. LOBACH & B. F. HAYNES. 1985. *In vitro* growth and phenotypic characterization of mesodermal-derived and epithelial components of normal and abnormal human thymus. Hum. Immunol. **13:** 161–176.
10. MIHOVILOVIC, M., S. DENNING, Y. MAI, L. P. WHICHARD, D. D. PATEL & A. D. ROSES. 1997. Thymocytes and cultured thymic epithelial cells express transcripts encoding α-3, α-5, and β-4 subunits of neuronal nicotinic acetylcholine receptors: preferential transcription of the α-3 and β-4 genes by immature CD4+8+ thymocytes. J. Neuroimmunol. **79:** 176–184.

Regulation of Acetylcholine Receptor Alpha Subunit mRNA Expression in Myasthenic Thymus

Y. ZHENG, L. M. WHEATLEY, T. LIU, AND A. I. LEVINSON[a]

Allergy/Immunology Division
University of Pennsylvania School of Medicine
Philadelphia, Pennsylvania 19104-6144

INTRODUCTION

Based on clinical, pathological, and immunologic lines of investigation, the thymus is considered to play a primary role in the pathogenesis of the autoimmune disease, myasthenia gravis (MG). It has been known for some time that the autoantigen, muscle acetylcholine receptor (AChR), is expressed on thymic myoid cells (reviewed in reference 1). We and others have provided evidence that the muscle AChR is also expressed on other thymic stromal cell populations, including epithelial cells derived from both MG and normal thymuses.[1–3] These observations have reinforced the hypothesis that the thymus represents a key site for autosensitization. The objectives of the present experiments were to determine (1) the relationship between the expression of the two major isoforms of the muscle alpha subunit (AChRα) in the thymus and a thymic epithelial cell line derived from normal human thymic epithelial cells (TEC) (kindly provided by Hergen Spits, the Netherlands), (2) if the expression of AChRα is increased in MG versus normal thymus, and (3) if the expression of AChRα in TEC is modulated by cytokines.

RESULTS AND DISCUSSION

Relative Expression of P3A– and P3A+ Isoforms

Two major isoforms of the nAChRα chain, denoted P3A– and P3A+, are expressed in human muscle.[4] P3A+ exceeds P3A– in length by 25 amino acids due to the insertion of a 75-bp exon (3A) between exons 3 and 4 (see FIGURE 1). We observed expression of both isoforms in the thymus and TEC, confirming our earlier reports.[1] Of interest, the smaller P3A– isoform was present in a 5-fold excess over the larger isoform in both MG ($n = 14$) and control ($n = 7$) thymus and at a 2.5-fold excess in TEC. This contrasts with the relationship of these isoforms in normal and MG muscle, where they are produced in equivalent amounts.[4,5] Wakkach *et al.* recently reported finding the expression of mRNAs encoding both isoforms in MG and human thymus and thymic epithelial cells.[3] However, they concluded that both isoforms

---

[a]To whom all correspondence should be addressed.

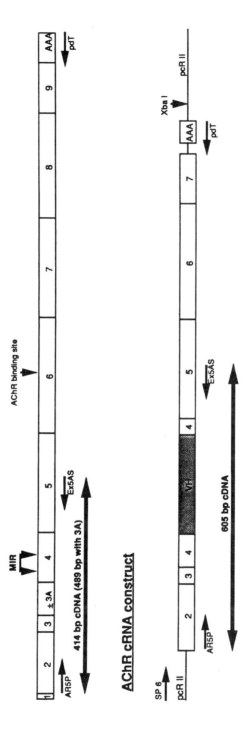

FIGURE 1. Semiquantitative RT-PCR. To quantitate the expression of muscle AChRα isoforms in tissue or cells, we developed a semiquantitative RT-PCR for which we engineered an AChRα cRNA construct. This construct was derived from an AChRα cDNA clone isolated by us from the human TE671 rhabdomyosarcoma cell line. Into this cDNA, we ligated a cDNA fragment that encoded part of human VH3 cDNA. To facilitate purification of full-length cRNA, a poly-A tail was ligated into the polylinker of the vector. We then added graded amounts of cRNA to total RNA prepared from the various tissues or cells of interest, prepared cDNA using oligo-dt, and amplified the cDNAs encoding the AChRα isoforms using a 5′ primer that anneals to exon 2 and a 3′ primer that anneals to exon 5. The template mRNA yields cDNA bands of 489 bp and 414 bp, indicative of the P3A+ and P3A− isoforms, respectively. The cRNA yields a cDNA band of 605 bp.

were present in equal proportions in TEC and thymus, even though several of the Southern blots shown in their publication demonstrate that P3A– is the dominant species. Our findings indicate that there is differential expression of the AChRα isoforms in the thymus and TEC relative to skeletal muscle. The significance of this finding to the development of MG remains to be determined.

Relative Expression of AChRα in MG versus Control Thymus

Using our semiquantitative nAChRα RT-PCR (FIGURE 1), we next determined the relative amounts of mRNAs encoding AChRα isoforms in thymus and TEC. We observed that P3A– mRNA expression was 2.5-fold greater in MG thymus than in control thymus, whereas P3A+ expression was 2.8-fold greater in MG thymus than in control thymus (FIGURE 2). These results parallel findings in skeletal muscle where mRNA expression was found to be greater in MG muscle than in control muscle.[5] In a subsequent study, the same investigative group reported that there was no quantitative difference in the AChRα mRNA expression of MG and control TEC, but the authors did not perform a quantitative analysis of AChRα in whole thymic extracts. Our results for whole thymic extracts likely reflect the expression of muscle AChRα mRNAs by myoid cells as well as epithelial cells. Therefore, it is possible that much of the increased AChRα expression observed by us is derived from contributions made by the myoid cells. Alternatively, it is possible that *in vivo* differences in AChR expression by epithelial cells are obscured when the cells are cultured *in vitro*.

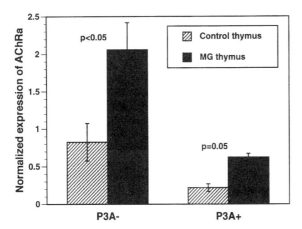

FIGURE 2. Relative expression of AChRα in MG versus control thymus. Compilation of semiquantitative RT-PCR results from 14 MG thymuses and 7 control thymuses. The signal intensity of the AChRα bands generated from control or MG thymus specimens, as determined by phosphor-imaging, is normalized to the signal intensity of the AChRα standard. The normalized values shown on the y-axis were determined by calculating the mean ratio of thymic AChRα/AChRα standard. Error bars represent ± 1 SD. The expression of P3A– and P3A+ isoforms in MG thymus is 2.5- and 2.8-fold greater, respectively, than that in control thymus.

Notwithstanding these considerations, our finding of increased AChRα mRNA expression in MG thymus may reflect the antecedent action of local environmental factors, including anti-AChRα antibodies and cytokines.

Effect of Cytokines on the Expression of Muscle AChRα by TEC

We next addressed the effect of several cytokines on the expression of AChRα mRNA by our normal TEC line. Using our semiquantitative RT-PCR, we compared the expression of both AChRα isoforms in cultures of untreated TEC to that of TEC incubated for six hours in the presence of varying concentrations of IL-1, IL-4, IL-6, and interferon-γ (IFN-γ). In 12 experiments, we observed that IFN-γ increased expression of the P3A− and P3A+ isoforms by factors of 2.7 and 2.8, respectively, whereas none of the other cytokines had a discernible effect. It is known that IFN-γ also upregulates the expression of MHC antigens on TEC.[6]

This finding raises the possibility that IFN-γ may alter expression of thymic AChRα *in vivo* in a manner that leads to the development or perpetuation of MG. Accordingly, low-affinity autoreactive T cells that have escaped central deletion might encounter TEC that have upregulated both AChRα and MHC antigens as a consequence of local IFN-γ production. Such an encounter in the context of costimulatory signals could lead to abrogation of self-tolerance and activation of AChRα-reactive helper T cells. T cells responding to an inflammatory stimulus, for example, a viral infection, in the thymus may provide a source of local IFN-γ production. Studies are currently under way to test this hypothesis.

REFERENCES

1. WHEATLEY, L. M. *et al.* 1993. Molecular analysis of intrathymic nicotinic acetylcholine receptor. Ann. N.Y. Acad. Sci. **681:** 74.
2. WHEATLEY, L. *et al.* 1992. Molecular characterization of the nicotinic acetylcholine receptor alpha chain in mouse thymus. J. Immunol. **148:** 3105.
3. WAKKACH, A. *et al.* 1996. Expression of acetylcholine receptor genes in human thymic epithelial cells: implications for myasthenia gravis. J. Immunol. **157:** 37524.
4. BEESON, D. *et al.* 1990. The human muscle acetylcholine receptor alpha-subunit exists as two isoforms: a novel exon. EMBO J. **9:** 2101.
5. GUYON, T. *et al.* 1994. Regulation of acetylcholine receptor α-subunit variants in human myasthenia gravis: quantification of steady state levels of messenger RNA in muscle biopsy using the polymerase chain reaction. J. Clin. Invest. **94:** 16.
6. GALY, A. H. M. & H. SPITS. 1991. IL-1, IL-4, and IFN-γ differentially regulate cytokine production and cell surface molecule expression in cultured human thymic epithelial cells. J. Immunol. **147:** 3823.

Respective Role of Thymus and Muscle in Autoimmune Myasthenia Gravis[a]

N. MOULIAN,[b] A. WAKKACH,[b,c] T. GUYON,[b] S. POËA,[b] A. AÏSSAOUI,[b,c]
P. LEVASSEUR,[d] S. COHEN-KAMINSKY,[b] AND S. BERRIH-AKNIN[b,e]

[b]CNRS ERS-566
[d]Département de Chirurgie Thoracique
Hôpital Marie Lannelongue
92350 Le Plessis-Robinson, France

INTRODUCTION

Myasthenia gravis (MG) is characterized clinically by muscle weakness enhanced by physical effort. Although acetylcholine receptor (AChR) expressed on muscle is the main target of the disease, the thymus also plays an important role. TABLE 1 summarizes the numerous arguments indicating a relationship between MG, the anti-AChR antibodies, and the thymus.[1–12] In addition, no alteration of thymus structure or function is observed in induced experimental models of MG,[13] suggesting that the thymus is probably the site where the autoimmune anti-AChR response is initiated, triggered, and maintained, likely in response to the intrathymic AChR.

Since the 1970s, when the thymus was found to contain binding sites for α-bungarotoxin,[14] there has been speculation about whether the thymus expresses muscle AChR or AChR-like proteins. Various cells have been reported to contain AChR-like proteins, including epithelial cells, thymocytes, and myoid cells. Attempts to identify intrathymic AChR expression at the molecular level have yielded controversial results (reviewed in reference 15). Since thymic epithelial cells (TEC) are involved in selection processes and express class II antigens, these cells could be considered good candidates for antigen presentation. Thus, we analyzed the expression of AChR genes in human TEC enriched in cultures.

Anti-AChR antibodies are found in about 85% of MG patients and their presence is diagnostic for acquired myasthenia gravis.[16] However, several studies have failed to show a correlation between severity of the disease (i.e., the loss of receptor) and anti-AChR antibody titer, whereas the reduced AChR number at the end plates correlates with the disease grade.[17,18] Thus, severity of MG disease seems to be related not only to the absence or presence of antibodies against AChR, but also to other individual factors. Among these factors, we wondered whether a compensatory mechanism could take place after the autoimmune attack and whether it could be variable from one patient to another.

[a]This research was supported by grants from AFM (Association Française contre les Myopathies), CNRS (Centre National de la Recherche Scientifique), and CNAMTS (Caisse Nationale d'Assurance Maladie des Travailleurs Salariés).
[c]Recipient of a doctoral grant from AFM.
[e]To whom all correspondence should be addressed.

TABLE 1. Myasthenia Gravis, Thymus, and Anti-AChR Antibodies

Frequent morphological thymus abnormalities (thymoma and hyperplasia)[1]
Thymic abnormalities only in seropositive patients[2]
Beneficial effect of thymectomy[3,4]
After thymectomy, decrease of:
—anti-AChR antibody titers[5]
—*in vitro* production of anti-AChR antibodies from stimulated PBL[6]
Spontaneous production of anti-AChR antibodies by thymocytes from MG hyperplasia[7]
Presence of AChR-reactive T cells[8,9]
Activation state of T and B lymphocytes[10,11]
Transfer by MG thymic explants of pathogenic parameters in SCID mice[12]

To define the respective role of thymus and muscle in the physiopathology of MG disease, we analyzed the presence of the main partners of the autoimmune response in the thymus. In muscle, in order to explore the compensatory mechanism that could take place after the autoimmune attack, we analyzed the α-subunit AChR mRNA levels by quantitative RT-PCR, using an internal standard constructed by mutagenesis.

ALL THE PARTNERS OF THE AUTOIMMUNE RESPONSE ARE PRESENT IN THE THYMUS

The arguments in favor of the thymus as the site for initiation of anti-AChR antibody production are summarized in TABLE 1. The classical immune response leading to antibody synthesis is shown in FIGURE 1. Recognition of peptides along with co-stimulatory molecules results in T cell activation. Effector cytokines instruct the acti-

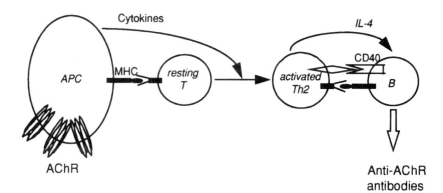

FIGURE 1. The different partners involved in the humoral response are present in the thymus. Hypothetical immune response scheme leading to anti-AChR antibody production in the thymus. According to our results, the epithelial cells could serve as APC. The Th2 activated cells could be Fas-overexpressing cells.

vated T helper cells to differentiate into a particular effector cell type (Th1 or Th2). The activation of B cells is dependent upon interactions with Th2 activated cells and IL-4 production.[19] Th2 activated cells result from resting T cells that have encountered antigen-presenting cells (APC). Since the anti-AChR antibody production is T helper cell–dependent, we wondered whether it was possible to identify the thymic activated T cells.

FAS, THE FIRST MARKER TO BE ASSOCIATED WITH THE ANTI-ACHR ANTIBODY TITER

The presence of activated T cells in the thymus has been previously shown by some groups,[20] but not by others.[21] Thymic cells from hyperplastic thymus have a higher response to r-IL-2 as compared to normal thymic cells, although the expression of CD25 is not significantly higher.[11] Fas molecule is a receptor inducing death signaling;[22] its expression is increased during T cell activation.[23] We recently explored the expression of Fas among total cells from MG versus normal thymuses (FIGURE 2). In age-matched control thymuses, a small proportion of thymocytes (0.4–2.8%) showed strong Fas expression (Fas^{hi}). In thymuses from patients with negative or borderline anti-AChR antibody titer (<1 nM), the proportion of Fas^{hi} thymocytes was not significantly different from control values (1.3 ± 0.2% versus 1.5 ± 0.3% in controls). By contrast, MG patients with positive titers (1 nM) had far higher proportions of Fas^{hi} thymocytes and this increase is correlated with the autoantibody

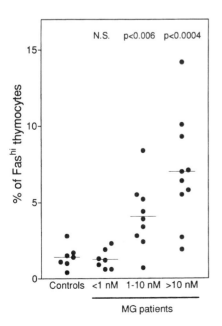

FIGURE 2. The number of Fas-overexpressing cells in MG thymus is related to the serum anti-AChR antibody titer. The proportion of Fas^{hi} thymocytes was determined in 26 MG patients and 7 age-matched control subjects. Three groups of patients (anti-AChR antibody titer: <1 nM, 1–10 nM, and >10 nM) are distinguished and compared with controls using the Mann-Whitney test. The bar represents the mean value. Only the two groups of patients with positive anti-AChR antibody titers differed from the controls.

titer (4.1 ± 0.7% in thymuses from MG patients with an intermediate titer, $p < 0.006$ compared to controls; and 7.0 ± 1.1% in thymuses from MG patients with a high titer, $p < 0.0004$ compared to controls) (FIGURE 2).

We then explored the possible involvement of Fas[hi] thymocytes in the proliferative response to peptides from the AChR. CD8-depleted and CD8- and Fas[hi]-depleted cells were obtained by separation on magnetic beads. These cells were cultured in the absence or in the presence of p169–181 (from the AChR α-subunit), which was previously shown to stimulate the proliferative response in MG patient, but not control subject lymphocytes.[24] In these experiments, CD4–CD8– cells constituted a source of antigen-presenting cells. As shown in FIGURE 3, p169–181 induced a significant proliferation response in CD8-depleted cells. This response was abrogated when

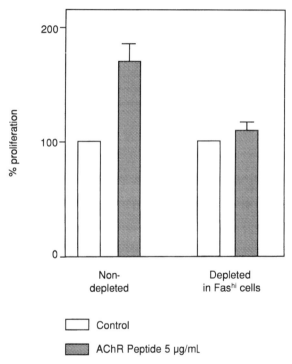

FIGURE 3. Depletion of Fas[hi] cells abrogates T cell proliferative response to AChR peptides. Thymocytes from three patients were first depleted of CD8+ cells using anti-CD8 magnetic beads; they underwent an additional depletion of Fas[hi] cells using goat anti-mouse–coated magnetic beads on which anti-Fas antibody was fixed. After a 6-day period of culture in the presence of p169–181 from the AChR α-subunit (5 μg/mL), the incorporation of ³H-thymidine (1 μCi for 0.2 × 10⁶ cells during 20 hours) was analyzed. It is expressed as a proportion of the proliferative response in the absence of peptide (mean ± SEM from three patients; four to eight determinations for each patient). When Fas[hi] cells are depleted, the proliferative response to p169–181 is abolished.

Fas[hi] cells were depleted. These experiments indicate that cells involved in the prolif-erative response to p169–181 from the AChR are Fas[hi] cells.

These findings thus suggest that Fas[hi] thymocytes, that is, activated thymocytes, comprise autoreactive T cells that induce the autoimmune response against the AChR in the MG thymus. To identify any peripheral event associated with Fas[hi] thymocyte accumulation, we analyzed Fas expression in peripheral lymphocytes from the same MG patients collected at the time of thymectomy. We did not observe any significant modification in CD4+Fas[hi] or CD8+Fas[hi] peripheral cell proportion.[25] Therefore, Fas expression modification in MG patients was observed in the thymic compartment, but not in the peripheral compartment; Fas could be considered as a thymic marker associated with the anti-AChR antibody titer.

EVIDENCE OF AChR EXPRESSED IN HUMAN CULTURED TEC

To determine whether muscle α-subunit mRNA was expressed in TEC, we exam-ined its expression by RT-PCR. Total RNA was purified from TEC highly enriched in culture and from thymic extracts. In TEC cultures, the percentage of epithelial cells was consistently higher than 95%, and fibroblasts represented about 5% of cultured cells. Myoid cells, identified with an antidesmin antibody, represented less than 0.1%. FIGURE 4 shows representative data for thymic extracts and TEC from three different normal thymuses. We found that α-subunit mRNA was clearly present in both the thymic extracts and TEC. The cDNAs coding for the two isoforms were con-sistently amplified (704 and 629 bp). However, the two isoforms were present in

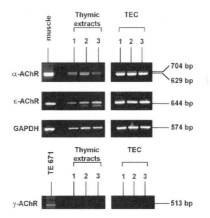

FIGURE 4. Analysis of AChR mRNA expression in human TEC. The two isoforms of α-AChR are expressed in thymic epithelial cells as well as in thymic extracts, but the P3A– iso-form is much more expressed in TEC as compared to thymic extracts. The ε-chain, but not the γ-chain, is expressed in cultured TEC, similar to thymic extracts. Muscle cells were used as positive control for the ε-subunit and TE671 cells were used as positive control for the γ-sub-unit.

equal proportions in muscle as well as in thymic extracts, while in TEC the P3A– isoform was much more expressed than the P3A+ isoform (FIGURE 4). Amplification products of GAPDH mRNA, used as a control, were observed in all mRNA extracts.

To explore whether the adult and/or fetal forms are present in TEC, we analyzed the expression of mRNA coding for γ- and ε-subunits by RT-PCR. The ε-subunit was amplified in all samples, while the γ was not (FIGURE 4). To confirm that a γ PCR product was totally absent, we performed a Southern blot of the PCR amplification product using the γ-specific primer labeled with ^{32}P-γdATP as a probe, which was negative in TEC as well as thymic extracts (not shown).

These results obtained from normal thymuses were also compared to those from MG thymuses. Very similar results were obtained, suggesting that there is no qualitative differential expression of AChR between MG and normal thymuses.[26] In addition, by quantitative RT-PCR, we could not detect any difference between MG and normal expression in TEC.[26]

Thus, our data indicate no qualitative nor quantitative differences in transcript expression between normal and MG thymuses. The presence of AChR in the thymus by itself is not sufficient to induce the autoimmune disease. However, we could not exclude quantitative differences at the protein level between MG patients and controls and/or at early stages of the disease. Alternatively, the autoimmune response could emerge from abnormal antigen presentation, related to the increased activation state already shown in hyperplastic thymuses.[27]

IS THERE A MECHANISM OF COMPENSATION AFTER THE AUTOIMMUNE ATTACK?

We asked whether the muscle is only a passive target or if there is a possible regulation of AChR genes after the autoimmune attack. Thus, we analyzed the mechanisms that control AChR gene expression in human MG. We developed a quantitative reverse transcription–polymerase chain reaction technique (RT-PCR) to evaluate the mRNA levels of the two α-subunit AChR isoforms in muscle biopsy samples from myasthenic patients relative to controls, by using an internal standard constructed by site-directed mutagenesis. We examined 7 control biopsies and 26 muscle samples from MG patients, 7 with a mild form of the disease (3 seronegative and 4 seropositive) and 19 with a severe form (6 seronegative and 13 seropositive). FIGURE 5 shows the results expressed as the total number of molecules of α-subunit mRNA per μg of total RNA. The mean number of AChR α-subunit molecules was $30 \times 10^5/\mu$g of mRNA in control samples versus $23.6 \times 10^5/\mu$g of mRNA for patients with the moderate form of the disease ($26.8 \times 10^5/\mu$g of mRNA and $21.2 \times 10^5/\mu$g of mRNA for seronegative and seropositive patients, respectively) and $114.2 \times 10^5/\mu$g of mRNA in patients with the severe form of the disease ($128 \times 10^5/\mu$g of mRNA and $108 \times 10^5/\mu$g of mRNA for seronegative and seropositive patients, respectively). The mean increase in AChR α-subunit mRNA variants in patients with severe forms was about 4.5-fold ($p < 0.003$ versus controls), whereas levels were normal in patients with moderate forms. It thus appeared that the increase in α-subunit mRNA correlates with MG severity, but not with the anti-AChR antibody titer. The differential expres-

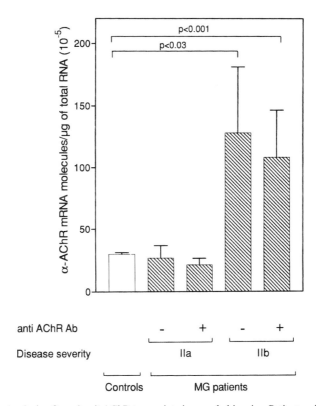

FIGURE 5. Analysis of α-subunit AChR transcripts in muscle biopsies. Patients with or without anti-AChR antibodies show a similar increase in total α-subunit transcripts as correlated with severity of the disease: a striking increase in total α-subunit transcripts is observed in all severely affected patients, whereas no modification of messenger RNA levels is observed in moderately affected patients as compared to controls. Results are expressed as the mean ± SEM.

sion of the P3A exon was calculated in the four groups of MG patients and the controls and was very similar in the four groups of patients (ranging from 49.6% to 53.7%) and in controls (48.5%).

Our data point to a compensatory mechanism for the loss of AChR expression and indicate a higher mean value of α-subunit mRNA in severely affected patients than in moderately affected patients. Since loss of AChR is greater in the former group of patients,[17,18] the most likely explanation is that a transcriptional regulation exists in patients showing a high rate of degradation. Our investigations concerning α-subunit mRNA precursors indicate that, in severely affected patients, pre-mRNA level, in addition to mature mRNA level, is enhanced compared to controls.[28] These results are in accordance with data shown by Asher *et al.*, who demonstrated an increase of

AChR α-subunit transcripts associated with an increase of transcriptional factors such as myogenin and MRF4 in rat muscles after passive transfer of EAMG by anti-AChR antibodies.[29] Thus, these data suggest that an accelerated rate of transcription of the message coding for the α-subunit causes an increased message content and increases receptor synthesis, in response to the attack by autoantibodies.

It is noticeable that the patients with undetectable anti-AChR antibodies had the same levels of mRNA as seropositive patients, suggesting that AChR undergoes similar degradation in the two subgroups of patients. Possible explanations are a very high pathogenicity of anti-AChR antibodies present at a very low titer (undetectable) in seronegative patients or an indirect effect on other synaptic proteins that could in turn induce a loss of AChR expression. This last hypothesis is supported by reports of antibodies bound to end plates in these patients[30] and evidence of antibodies to structures other than AChR.[31] Alternatively, increased mRNA levels could be due to attack by antibodies directed against a target involved in muscle activity or in the transduction of the electrical signal. Klarsfeld and Changeux have shown that blocking of the spontaneous electrical activity of cultured chick myotubes with tetrodotoxin greatly increased the levels of mRNA coding for the α-subunit of AChR.[32]

CONCLUDING REMARKS

First, our data on thymic Fas expression indicate that activated Fas++ cells are present only in the thymus of patients presenting anti-AChR antibodies, suggesting that they are likely engaged in anti-AChR response. The autoreactive role of these cells has been demonstrated in experiments indicating that depletion of Fas-expressing cells reduces significantly the proliferative response to the p169–181 (from the α-subunit) that we previously showed to be a T cell antigenic site.[24] Thus, the Fas-expressing cells are possibly T helper cells, producing IL-4 and giving help for antibody production. In this respect, Th2 murine high IL-4 producer clones were shown to express a high Fas level, while Th1 clones were rather high producers of Fas ligand.[33,34]

Second, our results on AChR gene expression by TEC indicate clearly that these cells do express the adult form of the AChR. Of note, the relative proportion of the P3A+ isoform is different between TEC and thymic extracts. The consequence of this distinct ratio remains to be investigated. The compared analysis between MG and normal samples did not indicate any quantitative nor qualitative differences.

Third and last, our analysis of AChR mRNA in muscle indicates a compensatory mechanism only in severely affected patients, regardless of their anti-AChR antibody titer.

Altogether, our data are compatible with the hypothesis that the thymus is the main site of activation and of anti-AChR antibody production. The thymus represents the effector site in seropositive myasthenia gravis. Muscle, by its ability to compensate for the loss of AChR after the autoimmune attack, could play an additional individual role in the disease severity, especially if this ability to compensate varies from one patient to another.

REFERENCES

1. LEVINE, G. & J. ROSAI. 1978. Thymic hyperplasia and neoplasia: a review of current concepts. Hum. Pathol. **9:** 495–515.
2. BERRIH, S., E. MOREL, C. GAUD, F. RAIMOND, H. LE BRIGAND & J. F. BACH. 1984. Anti-AChR antibodies, thymic histology, and T cell subsets in myasthenia gravis. Neurology **34:** 66–71.
3. MULDER, D. G., M. GRAVES & C. HERRMANN. 1989. Thymectomy for myasthenia gravis: recent observations and comparisons with past experience. Ann. Thorac. Surg. **48:** 551–555.
4. MOLNAR, J. & A. SZOBOR. 1990. Myasthenia gravis: effect of thymectomy in 425 patients; a 15-year experience. Eur. J. Cardiothorac. Surg. **4:** 8–14.
5. KUKS, J. B., H. J. OOSTERHUIS, P. C. LIMBURG & TH. THE. 1991. Anti-acetylcholine receptor antibodies decrease after thymectomy in patients with myasthenia gravis: clinical correlations. J. Autoimmun. **4:** 197–211.
6. KUKS, J. B., H. J. OOSTERHUIS, P. C. LIMBURG & TH. THE. 1992. Antibodies to acetylcholine receptors in myasthenia gravis: *in vitro* synthesis by peripheral blood lymphocytes before and after thymectomy. Clin. Exp. Immunol. **87:** 246–250.
7. WILLCOX, N., J. NEWSOM-DAVIS & L. R. CALDER. 1984. Cell types for anti-acetylcholine receptor antibody by cultured thymocytes and blood lymphocytes in myasthenia gravis. Clin. Exp. Immunol. **58:** 97–106.
8. MELMS, A. S., B. C. G. CHRESTEL, H. SCHALKE, H. WEKERLE, A. MAURON, M. BALLIVET & T. BARKAS. 1989. Autoimmune T lymphocytes in myasthenia gravis: determination of target epitopes using T lines and recombinant products of the mouse nicotinic acetylcholine receptor gene. J. Clin. Invest. **83:** 785–790.
9. SOMMER, N., N. WILLCOX, G. C. HARCOURT & J. NEWSOM-DAVIS. 1990. Myasthenic thymus and thymoma are selectively enriched in acetylcholine receptor–reactive T cells. Ann. Neurol. **28:** 312–319.
10. COHEN-KAMINSKY, S., P. LEVASSEUR, J. P. BINET & S. BERRIH-AKNIN. 1989. Evidence of enhanced recombinant interleukin-2 sensitivity in thymic lymphocytes from patients with myasthenia gravis: possible role in autoimmune pathogenesis. J. Neuroimmunol. **24:** 75–85.
11. LEPRINCE, C., S. COHEN-KAMINSKY, S. BERRIH-AKNIN, B. VERNET DER GARABEDIAN, D. TRETON, P. GALANAUD & Y. RICHARD. 1990. Thymic B cells from myasthenia gravis patients are activated B cells: phenotypic and functional analysis. J. Immunol. **145:** 2115–2122.
12. SCHÖNBECK, S., F. PADBERG, R. HOHFELD & H. WEKERLE. 1992. Transplantation of thymic autoimmune microenvironment to severe combined immunodeficiency mice. J. Clin. Invest. **90:** 245–250.
13. MEINL, E., W. E. KLINKERT & H. WEKERLE. 1991. The thymus in myasthenia gravis: changes typical for the human disease are absent in experimental autoimmune myasthenia gravis of the Lewis rat. Am. J. Pathol. **139:** 995–1008.
14. ENGEL, W. K., J. L. TROTTER, D. E. MCFARLIN & C. L. MCINTOSH. 1977. Thymic epithelial cell contains acetylcholine receptor. Lancet **1:** 1310–1311.
15. WHEATLEY, L. M., D. URSO, Y. ZHENG, E. LOH & A. I. LEVINSON. 1993. Molecular analysis of intrathymic nicotinic acetylcholine receptor. Ann. N.Y. Acad. Sci. **681:** 74–82.
16. LINDSTROM, J. M., M. L. SEYBOLD, V. A. LENNON, S. WHITTINGHAM & D. D. DUANE. 1976. Antibody to acetylcholine receptor in myasthenia gravis: prevalence, clinical correlates, and diagnostic value. Neurology **26:** 1054–1059.
17. LINDSTROM, J. M. & E. H. LAMBERT. 1978. Content of acetylcholine receptor and antibod-

ies bound to receptor in myasthenia gravis, experimental autoimmune myasthenia gravis, and Eaton-Lambert syndrome. Neurology **28**: 130–138.

18. PESTRONK, A., D. B. DRACHMAN & S. G. SELF. 1985. Measurement of junctional acetylcholine receptors in myasthenia gravis: clinical correlates. Muscle Nerve **8**: 245–251.

19. LANE, P. 1996. Development of B-cell memory and effector function. Curr. Opin. Immunol. **8**: 331–335.

20. ICHIKAWA, Y., H. SHIMIZU, M. YOSHIDA & S. ARIMORI. 1992. Two-color flow cytometric analysis of thymic lymphocytes from patients with myasthenia gravis and/or thymoma. Clin. Immunol. Immunopathol. **62**: 91–96.

21. FUJII, N., Y. ITOYAMA & I. GOTO. 1990. Increase in differentiated type of T lineage cells in the myasthenic thymus: two-color fluorocytometric analysis. Ann. Neurol. **27**: 642–646.

22. VAN PARIJS, L. & A. K. ABBAS. 1996. Role of Fas-mediated cell death in the regulation of immune responses. Curr. Opin. Immunol. **8**: 355–361.

23. MIYAWAKI, T., T. UEHARA, R. NIBU, T. TSUJI, A. YACHIE, S. YONEHARA & N. TANIGUCHI. 1992. Differential expression of apoptosis-related Fas antigen on lymphocyte subpopulations in human peripheral blood. J. Immunol. **149**: 3753–3758.

24. BERRIH-AKNIN, S., S. COHEN-KAMINSKY, V. LEPAGE, D. NEUMANN, J. F. BACH & S. FUCHS. 1991. T cell antigenic sites involved in myasthenia gravis: correlations with antibody titer and disease severity. J. Autoimmun. **4**: 137–153.

25. MOULIAN, N., J. BIDAULT, A. M. YAMAMOTO & S. BERRIH-AKNIN. 1997. Thymocyte Fas expression is dysregulated in myasthenia gravis patients with anti-acetylcholine receptor antibody. Blood **89**: 3287–3295.

26. WAKKACH, A., T. GUYON, C. BRUAND, S. TZARTOS, S. COHEN-KAMINSKY & S. BERRIH-AKNIN. 1996. Expression of acetylcholine receptor genes in the human thymic epithelial cells. J. Immunol. **157**: 3752–3760.

27. EMILIE, D., M. C. CREVON, S. COHEN-KAMINSKY, M. PEUCHMAUR, O. DEVERGNE, S. BERRIH-AKNIN & P. GALANAUD. 1991. *In situ* production of interleukins in hyperplastic thymus from myasthenia gravis patients. Hum. Pathol. **22**: 461–468.

28. GUYON, T., P. LEVASSEUR, F. TRUFFAULT, C. COTTIN, C. GAUD & S. BERRIH-AKNIN. 1994. Regulation of acetylcholine receptor α-subunit variants in human myasthenia gravis: quantification of steady state levels of messenger RNA in muscle biopsy using polymerase chain reaction. J. Clin. Invest. **94**: 16–24.

29. ASHER, O., W. A. KUES, V. WITZEMANN, S. J. TZARTOS, S. FUCHS & M. C. SOUROUJON. 1993. Increased gene expression of acetylcholine receptor and myogenic factors in passively transferred experimental autoimmune myasthenia gravis. J. Immunol. **151**: 6442–6450.

30. LU, C. Z., L. LU, Z. S. HAO, D. G. XIA, J. QAIN & B. G. W. ARNASON. 1993. Antibody-secreting cells to acetylcholine receptor and to presynaptic membrane receptor in seronegative myasthenia gravis. J. Neuroimmunol. **43**: 145–149.

31. YAMAMOTO, T., T. SATO & H. SUGITA. 1987. Antifilamin, antivinculin, and antitropomyosin antibodies in myasthenia gravis. Neurology **37**: 1329–1333.

32. KLARSFELD, A. & J. P. CHANGEUX. 1985. Activity regulates the level of acetylcholine receptor alpha-subunit mRNA in cultured chick myotubes. Proc. Natl. Acad. Sci. U.S.A. **82**: 4558–4562.

33. HAHN, S., T. STALDER, M. WERNLI, D. BURGIN, J. TSCHOPP, S. NAGATA & P. ERB. 1995. Down-modulation of CD4+ T helper type 2 and type 0 cells by T helper type 1 cells via Fas/Fas-ligand interaction. Eur. J. Immunol. **25**: 2679–2685.

34. NAKANISHI, K., K. MATSUI, S. KASHIWAMURA, Y. NISHIOKA, J. NOMURA, Y. NISHIMURA, N. SAKAGUCHI, S. YONEHARA, K. HIGASHINO & S. SHINKA. 1996. IL-4 and anti-CD40 protect against Fas-mediated B cell apoptosis and induce B cell growth and differentiation. Int. Immunol. **8**: 791–798.

Muscle Nicotinic Acetylcholine Receptor mRNA Expression in Hyperplastic and Neoplastic Myasthenia Gravis Thymus[a]

C. A. MacLENNAN, D. BEESON, N. WILLCOX, A. VINCENT, AND J. NEWSOM-DAVIS

Neurosciences Group
Institute of Molecular Medicine
John Radcliffe Hospital
Headington, Oxford OX3 9DS, United Kingdom

INTRODUCTION AND METHODS

There are well-recognized associations between thymic abnormalities and the autoimmune disease, myasthenia gravis (MG). About 50–70% of MG patients have hyperplastic thymuses and 10% have thymomas. Interestingly, we have also seen tumors resembling atypical thymic carcinoids in rare patients with MG and neuromyotonia. B cells and T cells that are reactive to the acetylcholine receptor (AChR) can be isolated from the hyperplastic MG thymus, and thymectomy often produces clinical improvement.[1] It may be that abnormal expression of AChR or an AChR-like protein in the thymus is involved in the pathogenesis of MG by affecting the selection of developing T cells or by activating mature AChR-responsive T cells. Rare musclelike myoid cells bearing AChR exist,[2] but these are present in both normal and MG thymus. Several RT-PCR studies have demonstrated the presence of mRNA encoding the five different AChR subunit genes (α, β, δ, ε, and γ) in thymus and thymoma.[3–5] The significance of these results is uncertain. They imply low-level AChR subunit expression in thymic epithelial cells, although some of the signal detected could be attributable to myoid cells or even illegitimate transcription.

To help resolve these problems, we used the less sensitive, but more quantitative RNase protection assay (RPA) technique to investigate the levels of AChR subunit gene expression in thymic extracts from MG patients and control subjects. ^{32}P-labeled RNA probes generated from cDNAs encoding the five AChR subunit mRNAs[6] were used as described previously.[7] RPA findings were compared to the results of RT-PCR amplification using paired oligonucleotide primers derived from the five AChR subunit cDNAs.

RESULTS

The integrity of the RNA was confirmed by performing assays to detect β-actin (FIGURES 1A and 2A). Using RPA, we detected mRNA encoding the ε-subunit in ap-

[a]This work was supported by the Wellcome Trust and the MGA/MDG of Great Britain.

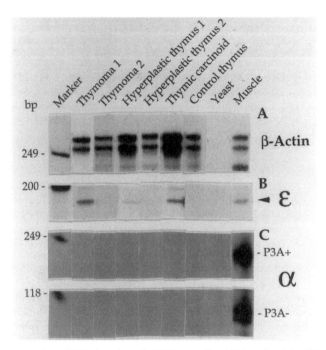

FIGURE 1. Examples of RPA detection of mRNA encoding **(A)** β-actin, **(B)** AChR ε-subunit, and **(C)** AChR α-subunit, in thymoma, hyperplastic thymus, atypical thymic carcinoid (all with MG), and control thymus. The autoradiograph from β-actin RPA was exposed for 4 hours at room temperature. Autoradiographs from ε- and α-subunit RPA were exposed for 2 weeks at −70 °C.

proximately 50% of thymomas and hyperplastic thymuses from MG patients, in two thymic carcinoids, but not in three control thymuses (FIGURE 1B). Using this assay, α-, β-, δ-, and γ-subunit mRNAs were not found in any thymic tissue (FIGURE 1C), although all five AChR subunit mRNAs could be clearly detected in partially dener-vated muscle. In contrast, when using RT-PCR, we were able to detect mRNA encod-ing all the AChR subunits including ε (FIGURE 2B). RT-PCR of thymoma identified mRNA encoding both P3A+ and P3A− α-subunit isoforms, with the P3A− form pre-dominating (FIGURE 2C). This is at variance with a previous report in which the P3A+ form was not seen.[8]

DISCUSSION

Our results show that abnormal transcription levels of the ε-subunit mRNA can occur in thymic tumors and in thymic hyperplasia. High-level transcription of ε-sub-unit mRNA is usually restricted to subsynaptic nuclei at the neuromuscular junction,[9] where replacement of the γ-subunit by the ε switches the AChR from fetal subtype

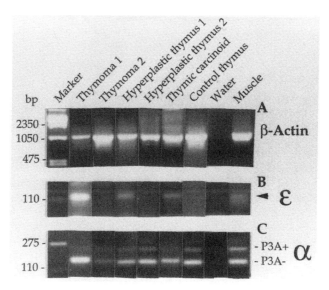

FIGURE 2. Examples of RT-PCR amplification from RNA isolated from thymic tissues as in FIGURE 1 for **(A)** β-actin, **(B)** AChR ε-subunit, and **(C)** AChR α-subunit. Products were run on 2% agarose gels and visualized under ultraviolet light after staining with ethidium bromide.

($\alpha_2\beta\gamma\delta$) to adult subtype ($\alpha_2\beta\epsilon\delta$). Myoid cells express complete fetal and possibly adult AChR.[2] Results from RT-PCR analysis are probably detecting mRNA synthesized by myoid cells and a low level of transcripts in some other cell type, possibly thymic epithelial cells. These cells may also be expressing the higher level of ε-subunit mRNA that we saw with RPA in certain thymoma, thymic carcinoid tumors, and hyperplastic thymuses, but not in normal thymus. Several key questions remain to be addressed: whether and in which cell types the ε-subunit mRNA is translated into protein and whether its overexpression correlates with autoimmunization or self-tolerance to the AChR.

REFERENCES

1. WHEATLEY, L. M., D. URSO *et al.* 1993. Molecular analysis of intrathymic nicotinic acetylcholine receptor. Ann. N.Y. Acad. Sci. **681**: 74–82.
2. SCHLUEP, M., N. WILLCOX *et al.* 1987. Acetylcholine receptors in human thymic myoid cells *in situ*: an immunohistological study. Ann. Neurol. **22**: 212–222.
3. HARA, H., K. HAYASHI *et al.* 1993. Nicotinic acetylcholine receptor mRNAs in myasthenic thymuses: association with intrathymic pathogenesis of myasthenia gravis. Biochem. Biophys. Res. Commun. **194**: 1269–1275.
4. KAMINSKI, H. J., R. A. FENSTERMAKER *et al.* 1993. Acetylcholine receptor subunit gene expression in thymic tissue. Muscle Nerve **16**: 1332–1337.
5. WAKKACH, A., T. GUYON *et al.* 1996. Expression of acetylcholine receptor genes in human thymic epithelial cells. J. Immunol. **157**: 3752–3760.

6. BEESON, D., M. BRYDSON *et al.* 1993. Primary structure of the human muscle acetylcholine receptor: cDNA cloning of the γ and ε subunits. Eur. J. Biochem. **215:** 229–238.

7. MACLENNAN, C., D. BEESON *et al.* 1997. Acetylcholine receptor expression in human extraocular muscles and their susceptibility to myasthenia gravis. Ann. Neurol. **41:** 423–431.

8. ANDREETTA, F., F. BAGGI *et al.* 1997. Acetylcholine receptor α-subunit isoforms are differentially expressed in thymuses from myasthenic patients. Am. J. Pathol. **150:** 341–348.

9. SANES, J., Y. JOHNSON *et al.* 1991. Selective expression of an acetylcholine receptor–lacZ transgene in synaptic nuclei of adult muscle fibres. Development **113:** 1181–1191.

Expression of Muscle Proteins in Thymomas of Patients with Myasthenia Gravis[a]

YOHAN LIYANAGE, MICHELLE TEO, CAL MacLENNAN,
ALEX BUCKEL, DAVID BEESON, NICK WILLCOX,
JOHN NEWSOM-DAVIS, AND ANGELA VINCENT

Neurosciences Group
Institute of Molecular Medicine
John Radcliffe Hospital
University of Oxford
Headington, Oxford OX3 9DS, United Kingdom

Thymomas occur in 10–15% of patients with myasthenia gravis (MG) and are associated with antibodies to skeletal muscle proteins, such as ryanodine receptor and titin, as well as antibodies to the muscle acetylcholine receptor (AChR).[1,2] A few patients with thymoma have acquired neuromyotonia, with or without coexistent myasthenia gravis (see Vincent *et al.* in this volume). Expression in thymomas of proteins normally present in muscle tissue, for instance, AChR, myogenin, and titin, has been reported previously and has been implicated in the initiation of autoimmunization[1,2] (see MacLennan *et al.* in this volume and in preparation). Here, we have looked for the presence of other muscle proteins, including agrin, a component of the extracellular matrix that is synthesized by both nerve and muscle and that triggers the clustering of AChRs on the muscle surface; erbB3, a tyrosine kinase that forms part of the receptor for the nerve-derived acetylcholine receptor–inducing agent (ARIA; heregulin β1), which plays a role in the control of AChR synthesis; β2-laminin, a component of the basal lamina protein s-laminin; rapsyn, part of the cytoskeleton in muscle cells that is required for AChR clustering and the assembly of the postsynaptic apparatus; *Shaker*-type voltage-gated potassium channels (VGKCs) that might be implicated in acquired neuromyotonia; and utrophin, a dystrophin-related protein expressed in many tissues that, in muscle, is thought to link F-actin in the cytoskeleton to a transmembrane protein complex at the neuromuscular junction.

Thymic tissue was obtained at thymectomy from 20 patients: 16 had thymomas, including 1 without MG; 2 had hyperplastic thymuses, both with MG; and 2 had normal thymuses. Two of the patients had symptoms of acquired neuromyotonia (see Vincent *et al.* in this volume). Myoblasts from primary human muscle cell cultures were used as a positive control for the expression of the muscle proteins. Total RNA was isolated from the tissue by the guanidium isothiocyanate method of extraction. First-strand cDNA was synthesized using an oligo-dT primer and MMLV reverse transcriptase, and this was subsequently used in PCR. Oligonucleotide primers used for the amplification of each mRNA are shown in TABLE 1. The cycling conditions for the amplification reactions were 94 °C for 1 min, 55 °C for 1 min, and 72 °C for

[a]This work was supported by the Muscular Dystrophy Group of Great Britain and the Wellcome Trust.

TABLE 1. PCR Primers and Results of PCR Analysis of 16 Thymomas

Protein	PCR Primers	Size of Band	No. of Thymoma Cases Positive
erbB3	5′ GATACATGCCCATGAACCAGGGTAATC 3′ 5′ GAGGTGTGTATCTGGCATGACATAAC 3′	341 bp	16/16
utrophin	5′ GCCTCCACCACAGGAAGTGTGGAAG 3′ 5′ CTGCAGCCCCTTGGAAGTGGCG 3′	656 bp	16/16
VGKC	5′ TTCCAGCGCCAGGTGTGGC 3′ 5′ CTGCAGCCCCTTGGAGTGGCG 3′	511 bp	12/16
rapsyn	5′ CTGAGCCAGCTCAAGCTGCAC 3′ 5′ GCCAGGGGAGCACGCCCTCGG 3′	620 bp	8/16
agrin	5′ GGCCTGCACACCTTTGCACGGGACC 3′ 5′ GAGCCGGTCACAGGGGCCTCATTG 3′	985 bp	6/16
β2-laminin	5′ GCGGGATCCGGCTGTGTGCCGC 3′ 5′ CAGGCTCAAGGCAGACAG 3′	852 bp	3/16

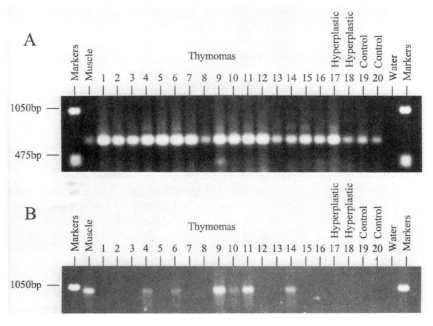

FIGURE 1. PCRs on patient thymoma and thymus cDNA: (A) utrophin; (B) agrin.

1.5 min for 35 cycles. The products were analyzed by electrophoresis on agarose gels and visualized with ethidium bromide.

mRNAs encoding all six proteins were detected in the cDNA from cultured muscle, indicating that the cycling conditions were sufficient for the amplification of all fragments. Utrophin mRNA was detected in all thymuses and thymomas examined (FIGURE 1A), as was erbB3 (data not shown), suggesting that the expression of these proteins in MG thymic tissue is probably not of pathological significance. However, mRNAs of the other four proteins were not detected in the control or hyperplastic thymuses, but were found in some, but not all, of the thymomas: VGKC mRNAs were the most common, followed by rapsyn, agrin (FIGURE 1B), and β2-laminin. The results are summarized in TABLE 1. Two thymomas were found to contain all six mRNAs, but no correlation could be made between the expression of the mRNAs and the histopathology of the thymomas (not shown). However, these results suggest new candidate proteins involved in the etiology of thymoma-associated myasthenia gravis, and both T cell responses and antibody responses to these proteins may be informative.

REFERENCES

1. KORNSTEIN, M. J., O. ASHER & S. FUCHS. 1995. Acetylcholine receptor alpha-subunit and myogenin mRNAs in thymus and thymoma. Am. J. Pathol. **146(6):** 1320–1324.
2. MARX, A., A. WILISCH, A. SCHULTZ *et al.* 1996. Expression of neurofilaments and of a titin epitope in thymic epithelial tumors: implications for the pathogenesis of myasthenia gravis. Am. J. Pathol. **148(6):** 1839–1850.

Antiacetylcholine Receptor Fab Fragments Isolated from Thymus-derived Phage Display Libraries from Myasthenia Gravis Patients Reflect Predominant Specificities in Serum and Block the Action of Pathogenic Serum Antibodies

YVO F. GRAUS,[a,b] MARC H. DE BAETS,[b] AND DENNIS R. BURTON[a]

[a]Department of Immunology
Scripps Research Institute
La Jolla, California 92037

[b]Department of Immunology
University of Maastricht
Maastricht, the Netherlands

Myasthenia gravis (MG) is a prototype antibody-mediated autoimmune disease because clinical symptoms can be induced by passive transfer of antibody alone. To investigate the individual contribution of antihuman AChR (huAChR) antibody specificities in MG, it is necessary to dissect the polyclonal anti-huAChR response into monoclonal specificities. A hyperplastic thymus is frequently associated with MG and contains abundant anti-huAChR-producing B cells in germinal centers. Thymic lymphocytes are therefore an ideal source of B cells to construct a combinatorial antibody phage display library to analyze individual members of the anti-huAChR response in MG patients. We have recently described[1] the first recombinant antibodies from thymus tissue from two MG patients; this considerably expands the number of human anti-huAChR antibodies available since only one such IgG antibody has been previously described from an EBV-transformed cell line.[2]

Four different Fab clones, namely, 66, 70, 587, and 637, were identified by sequence analysis and their specificity for huAChR was extensively demonstrated in several assays, including solid-phase RIA, immunoprecipitation RIA, and binding to AChR–expressing TE671 cells and to AChRs at the neuromuscular junction in monkey intercostal muscle sections by immunofluorescence. Moreover, epitope mapping studies using competitive inhibition showed that all four Fabs recognize determinants associated with the MIR on the AChR α-subunit since all are inhibited to some extent by rodent anti-MIR antibodies. It appears that the Fabs recognize two distinct determinants since three of the Fabs are mutually inhibitory (Fabs 66, 70, and 587), but do not inhibit binding of the fourth (Fab 637). Furthermore, inhibition between anti-huAChR Fabs and serum anti-huAChR demonstrated that the Fabs comprise a considerable fraction of the polyclonal anti-huAChR response, up to 90% even in unrelated MG patients.

It was further demonstrated that the anti-huAChR Fab fragments can induce AChR loss by antigenic modulation *in vitro* when cross-linked with a secondary antibody. AChR loss by antigenic modulation was measured *in vitro* by incubation of huAChR-expressing TE671 cultures with increasing amounts of Fab 637, Fab 587, or control Fab 495 and subsequent incubation with goat-antihuman F(ab')$_2$ antibody to cross-link bound Fab. Cross-linked Fabs 637 and 587 were able to induce 60% and 30% AChR loss, respectively, whereas no AChR loss was observed with irrelevant Fab 495 (FIGURE 1). Moreover, AChR loss by antigenic modulation induced by cross-linked Fab 637 was comparable to AChR loss induced by intact mAb 35. In contrast, binding of monovalent Fab fragments did not result in any AChR loss. This finding indicates that these antibody specificities probably have pathogenic potential as intact divalent IgG molecules *in vivo*. Similar observations have been made for Fab fragments prepared from serum IgG from MG patients.[3]

Since the recombinant anti-huAChR Fabs do not interfere with receptor function, are unable to activate complement, and compete with serum antibodies for binding to huAChR, it is feasible that they may be used to prevent binding of serum antibodies and to protect the AChR against degradation by intact antibody *in vivo*, for example, during a myasthenic crisis. This concept was verified *in vitro* by protecting TE671 cells from AChR loss induced by MG serum antibodies using a combination of two recombinant Fabs. Serum of a typical MG patient with associated thymic hyperplasia

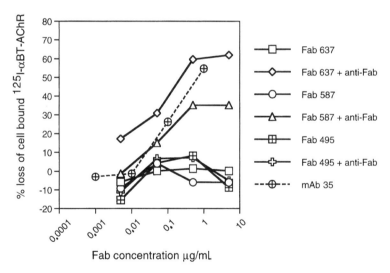

FIGURE 1. Divalently linked anti-huAChR Fabs induce AChR loss by antigenic modulation. AChR loss by means of antigenic modulation was determined for anti-huAChR Fabs alone or divalently linked with goat-antihuman F(ab')$_2$ IgG using cultured TE671 cells. Anti-huAChR Fabs 637 and 587 alone did not result in loss of surface AChR on cultured TE671 cells labeled with ^{125}I-αBT. Cross-linking of Fab bound to AChR with a second antibody resulted in a significant loss of surface ^{125}I-αBT-AChR from TE671 cells due to an increased internalization of AChR molecules. The AChR loss induced by divalently linked Fab 637 was comparable to the AChR loss induced by intact mAb 35. Divalently linked control Fab 495 did not induce AChR loss.

was able to decrease the AChR concentration to 40% of the maximum concentration in the presence of 2 μg/mL of control Fab 495. In contrast, a combination of Fabs 637 and 587 (2 μg/mL) was able to limit AChR loss and to maintain the AChR concentration at 80% (FIGURE 2A). Fabs 637/587 were also able to protect against AChR loss induced by serum anti-huAChR from a patient with thymoma-associated MG (FIGURE 2B).

A similar observation has been made previously using the Fab fragment of a rat

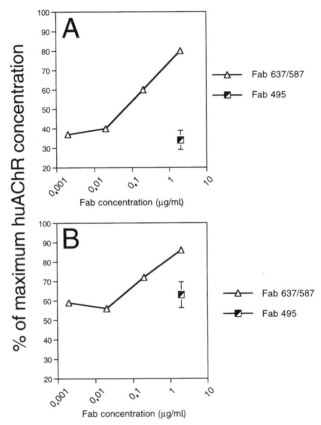

FIGURE 2. Anti-huAChR Fabs protect against AChR loss by antigenic modulation induced by MG serum antibodies. Cultured TE671 cells were incubated with anti-huAChR Fabs 637 and 587 or control Fab 495 prior to incubation with serum anti-huAChR antibodies. The capacity of Fab to protect against AChR loss by antigenic modulation was determined at an MG serum dilution giving submaximal AChR loss. (A) Protection against AChR loss by serum of an MG patient with thymic hyperplasia. A combination of Fabs 637 and 587 protected against AChR loss, leaving 80% of the AChR intact at 2 μg/mL. Control Fab 495 at 2 μg/mL did not protect AChR against antigenic modulation by MG 12, leaving only 40% of the AChR intact. (B) Protection against AChR loss by serum of an MG patient with associated thymoma.

anti-AChR mAb.[4] However, the use of human Fab fragments is preferable in any *in vivo* application to avoid antirodent responses.[5] Furthermore, the recombinant human Fabs could be improved in affinity by several orders of magnitude using an established mutagenesis/selection strategy[6] allowing for extremely efficient competition with serum anti-huAChR antibodies. The major drawback in the suggested strategy is the rapid clearance of Fab fragments from the circulation. This could be circumvented by coupling Fabs to a long-lived serum protein such as serum albumin or to an Fc with point mutations to eliminate complement and Fc receptor activation,[7] that is, an Fab-Fc molecule. Alternatively, an extremely high-affinity ($K_a > 10^{11}$ M^{-1}) *in vitro* evolved anti-huAChR Fab would bind essentially irreversibly to AChR and would thus be cleared very slowly. Further such Fabs might form lead compounds for the design of reagents capable of inhibiting autoantibody binding to AChR without disrupting receptor function. In any case, the overall strategy would be to rapidly reverse a myasthenic crisis by an initial plasmapheresis to remove excess anti-huAChR antibodies and subsequently use competitor Fab or Fab-based molecules to shield epitopes on newly synthesized AChR molecules, thus allowing rapid reestablishment of functional AChR molecules.

REFERENCES

1. GRAUS, Y., M. DE BAETS, P. PARREN, S. BERRIH-AKNIN, J. WOKKE, P. VAN BREDA VRIESMAN & D. BURTON. 1997. Human anti-nicotinic acetylcholine receptor recombinant Fab fragments isolated from thymus-derived phage display libraries from myasthenia gravis patients reflect predominant specificities in serum and block the action of pathogenic serum antibodies. J. Immunol. **158:** 1919–1929.

2. KAMO, I., S. FURUKAWA, A. TADA, Y. MANO, Y. IWASAKI, T. FURUSE, N. ITO, K. HAYASHI & E. SATOYOSHI. 1982. Monoclonal antibody to acetylcholine receptor: cell line established from thymus of patient with myasthenia gravis. Science **215:** 995.

3. DRACHMAN, D., C. ANGUS, R. ADAMS, J. MICHELSON & G. HOFMAN. 1978. Myasthenic antibodies cross-link acetylcholine receptors to accelerate degradation. N. Engl. J. Med. **298:** 1116.

4. SOPHIANOS, D. & S. TZARTOS. 1989. Fab fragments of monoclonal antibodies protect the human acetylcholine receptor against antigenic modulation caused by myasthenic sera. J. Autoimmun. **2:** 777.

5. MAMALAKI, A., N. TRAKAS & S. J. TZARTOS. 1993. Bacterial expression of a single-chain Fv fragment which efficiently protects the acetylcholine receptor against antigenic modulation caused by myasthenic antibodies. Eur. J. Immunol. **23:** 1839.

6. YANG, W-P., K. GREEN, S. PINZ-SWEENEY, A. BRIONES, D. BURTON & C. BARBAS III. 1995. CDR walking mutagenesis for the affinity maturation of a potent human anti-HIV-1 antibody into the picomolar range. J. Mol. Biol. **254:** 392.

7. BURTON, D. & J. WOOF. 1992. Human antibody effector function. Adv. Immunol. **51:** 1.

Production of Fab Fragments against the Human Acetylcholine Receptor from Myasthenia Gravis Thymus Lambda and Kappa Phage Libraries[a]

I. MATTHEWS,[b] J. FARRAR,[b] S. McLACHLAN,[c] B. RAPOPORT,[c]
J. NEWSOM-DAVIS,[b] N. WILLCOX,[b] AND A. VINCENT[b]

[b]Neurosciences Group
Institute of Molecular Medicine
University of Oxford
Oxford OX3 9DU, United Kingdom

[c]Thyroid Molecular Biology Unit
Veterans Administration Medical Center
San Francisco, California

INTRODUCTION

Myasthenia gravis (MG) is an antibody-mediated autoimmune disease, evidenced by the induction of the disease on passive transfer of antibody alone. These autoantibodies to the AChR lead to a loss of receptor and to muscle weakness, but the severity of the disease does not correlate with the anti-AChR antibody titer in MG patients. This discrepancy could be the result of variable proportions of AChR autoantibodies, in individual patients, that recognize different epitopes on the receptor. AChR autoantibodies are heterogeneous in light-chain type, IgG subclass, and binding sites on different subunits.[1,2] Attempts to dissect this polyclonal antibody response to the AChR have included making human AChR antibodies by immortalizing blood B cells by cell fusion or with EBV.[3,4] However, the monoclonal antibodies produced were mainly IgM class and did not bind the human AChR, and some bound equally well to *Torpedo* AChR. By contrast, the antihuman AChR antibody response is predominantly IgG and shows little cross-reactivity with *Torpedo* AChR.

Our aim was to clone pathogenic antibodies representative of those in the serum of MG patients. Results of the kappa Fabs have been described elsewhere.[5]

METHODS

The donor patient was a 22-year-old female (AB) with a 4-year history of MG with high serum anti-AChR titer (500 nmoles/L). From thymus cell suspensions, immunoglobulin genes were amplified and used to create two combinatorial libraries of

[a]This work was supported by the Association Française contre les Myopathies and the Medical Research Council of Great Britain.

418

IgG1 heavy/kappa light chains and IgG1 heavy/lambda light chains in the Im-munoZap vector (Stratagene). The libraries were screened with human muscle AChR labeled with 2 nM ^{125}I-α-BuTx (>2000 Ci/mmol). Positive plaques were cloned and the Fabs were expressed as soluble proteins, concentrated 50-fold, and used in this form or after protein G purification.

AChR extracts were prepared in 0.1% Triton X100 and labeled with 2 nM ^{125}I-α-BuTx. Fabs were tested by immunoprecipitation for binding to AChR from human, mouse, and rat muscle and *Torpedo* electric organ using conventional immunoprecip-itation techniques. Epitope specificity of the Fabs was determined by competition with murine monoclonal antibodies (mAbs) that have been mapped to different sub-units (see Vincent *et al.* in this volume). Assay details have been described else-where.[5]

RESULTS AND DISCUSSION

Screening of 4×10^5 recombinant clones identified 4 positives from the kappa li-brary and 22 from the lambda library. All Fabs immunoprecipitated ^{125}I-α-BuTx-la-beled AChR from human muscle extracts in a dose-dependent manner. Although pro-tein G–purified Fab was used for the kappa clones, it was found unnecessary for the lambda clones since *E. coli* extracts, containing expressed Fab, efficiently precipitat-ed the AChR. None of the Fabs bound *Torpedo* AChR, consistent with the lack of binding of AB serum and MG sera generally. AB serum was able to bind rat and mouse AChR to 50% of the reactivity with human AChR. The kappa Fabs also showed binding of varying degrees to rat and mouse muscle AChR.[5] Surprisingly, none of the lambda Fabs bound to mouse or rat AChR (data not shown).

The binding specificities of the patient's serum and Fabs were investigated by competition with mAbs against known sites. About 50–70% of the anti-AChR anti-body in serum was inhibited by mAb D6α or C3α (FIGURE 1A) and about 30% was inhibited by mAb C2γ. No inhibition was found with B3β. Fabs ABK1 and 3 showed clear specificity for the MIR, while ABK5 preferred binding to the γ-subunit; this subunit is specific to fetal-type AChR and many MG antibodies show a preference for fetal rather than adult AChR. Only 4 out of 22 lambda Fabs significantly inhibited binding of the mAbs; 3 bound to the MIR and 1 to the γ-subunit (FIGURE 1B). Re-cently, Graus *et al.*[6] used the phage display pComb3H system to isolate 4 Fabs on mAb-immobilized human AChR. These Fabs also bound the MIR and may indicate bias of this method against other antibody specificities.

CONCLUSIONS

Fab fragments, produced by *in vitro* combination of heavy and light chains, im-munoprecipitate human AChR from muscle and show similar specificities to anti-bodies found in the donor's serum. The Fabs bound AChR of other species (except *Torpedo*); some bound fetal rather than adult AChR and most competed with mAbs against the receptor. Differences in reactivity between the kappa library and lambda

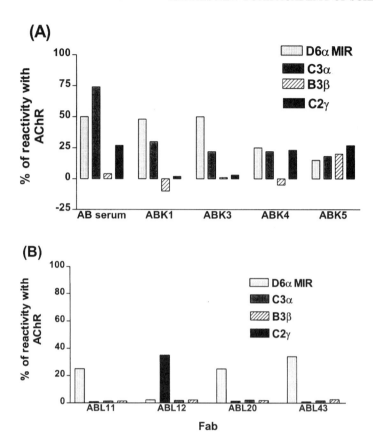

FIGURE 1. Inhibition of mAb binding to AChR by Fabs. The mAbs include D6α against the MIR, C3α against an overlapping α-subunit epitope, B3β against the β-subunit, and C2γ against the γ-subunit. Preincubation of 50 μL of AChR with a saturating amount of Fab for 2 h at room temperature was followed by similar incubation with 0.1 μL of ascites of each mAb. The mAbs were precipitated with 2 μL of normal mouse serum as carrier and 20 μL of goat antimouse IgG. Inhibition of mAb binding by each Fab is expressed as 100 × (cpm precipitated by mAb in the absence of Fab – cpm precipitated by mAb in the presence of Fab)/(cpm precipitated by mAb in the absence of Fab – cpm precipitated by carrier serum only). **(A)** Competition with kappa Fabs. **(B)** Competition with lambda Fabs (only 4 of the Fabs produced a significant result).

library clones may be due to gene usage. The kappa Fabs use 4 different V_H genes (DP-42, 65, 7, and 58) and 3 different V_K genes (DPK-22, 9, and 23),[5] and DNA sequencing of the lambda Fabs is under way. The availability of human anti-AChR antibodies representative of those in serum should produce insights into pathogenicity and new therapeutic strategies.

REFERENCES

1. VINCENT, A. *et al.* 1987. Antibody heterogeneity and specificity in MG. Ann. N.Y. Acad. Sci. **505:** 106.
2. TZARTOS, S. J. *et al.* 1982. Specificities of antibodies to acetylcholine receptor in sera of MG patients measured by monoclonal antibodies. Proc. Natl. Acad. Sci. U.S.A. **79:** 188.
3. CARDONA, A. *et al.* 1995. Evidence for an antigen-driven selection process in human autoantibodies against acetylcholine receptor. Mol. Immunol. **32:** 1215.
4. KAMO, I. *et al.* 1982. Monoclonal antibody to acetylcholine receptor: cell line established from thymus of patient with MG. Science **215:** 995.
5. FARRAR, J. *et al.* 1997. Diverse Fabs specific for acetylcholine receptor epitopes from a MG thymus combinatorial library. Int. Immunol. **9:** 1311.
6. GRAUS, Y. F. *et al.* 1997. Human anti-nicotinic acetylcholine receptor recombinant Fab fragments isolated from thymus-derived phage display libraries from MG patients block the action of pathogenic serum antibodies. J. Immunol. **158:** 1919.

Titin Transcripts in Thymomas

GEIR OLVE SKEIE,[a] ALEXANDRA FREIBURG,[b]
BERNHARD KOLMERER,[b] SIEGFRIED LABEIT,[b]
JOHAN A. AARLI,[a] AND NILS ERIK GILHUS[a]

[a]Department of Neurology
Haukeland University Hospital
5021 Bergen, Norway

[b]European Molecular Biology Laboratory
Heidelberg, Germany

INTRODUCTION

Thymoma patients with myasthenia gravis (MG) typically have antibodies against a number of muscle proteins in addition to AChR, including titin,[1] a myofibrillar protein that plays an important role in the elastic recoil of striated muscle.[2] The main immunogenic region (MIR) on titin for MG antibodies is located near the A/I-junction. We have recently identified a second titin epitope for MG patients' antibodies centrally in the I-band near the N2-line of titin.[3]

The initiation of paraneoplastic MG is thought to involve positive selection of autoreactive T cells to aberrantly expressed peptides within the thymoma.[4] The aim of this study was to investigate if titin mRNAs that code for the regions of titin to which the autoimmune responses are directed are expressed in thymomas from MG/thymoma patients.

MATERIALS AND METHODS

Thymoma tissue was obtained from four patients. Thymus tissue was obtained from one late-onset and one young-onset MG patient and three control children aged 2–3 years. Tonsillar tissue and a colon carcinoma were used as controls. The tissue was snap-frozen in liquid nitrogen and stored at –80 °C. An isolated membrane fraction was prepared from one thymoma (from an MG patient), one normal thymus, and one tonsil by differential centrifugation.[5]

RT-PCR

The RNA was extracted and purified using the protocol of the Qiagen total RNA Maxi kit (Qiagen GmbH, Hilden, Germany). Ten μg of total RNA was reverse-transcribed into cDNA with M-MLV-Reverse Transcriptase as specified by the supplier (Promega, Heidelberg, Germany). The cDNA samples were PCR-tested with a human calmodulin primer pair. From all six thymus/thymoma cDNA samples, a PCR fragment was generated that was visible on an ethidium bromide agarose gel.

The titin MIR and titin N2-A primer pairs were derived from the human titin cDNA sequence.[2] MIR—x99a: ttt ctcgagc CCA ACA ATG GAT TTA AGT GCA; x100: ttt acgcgt ta TGG GGC CTC TTG TGT GTC C (expression primers, capital letters match the human titin sequence). N2-A—sp961: GTA TCA GAG TCG TAG AAA AAA CCA CTG C; sp962: TCA GTT CTG TTG GTC CTT TGT ACC ATG TT. Amplifications were carried out at 40 s at 95 °C, 90 s at 64 °C, and 45 s at 74 °C for 35 cycles for the MIR primers and at 30 s at 95 °C and 4 min at 68 °C for the N2-A primers.

Two μL of the PCR reactions was separated on 1% agarose gels, transferred to nylon membranes, cross-linked by UV light, and hybridized to randomly labeled MIR and N2-A probes.

Immunohistochemistry and Western Blots

Immunostaining (ABC technique) was used. The titin antibodies used were T12 (a mouse monoclonal IgG antibody directed against the Z-disk titin) and 9D10 (a mouse monoclonal IgM antibody directed against the PEVK fragment of titin). The thymoma, thymus, and tonsil membrane preparations were electrophoresed on 7.5% SDS-polyacrylamide gels and transblotted onto nitrocellulose. The T12 and 9D10 anti-titin antibodies were used in dilutions of 1:25, 1:50, and 1:100.

RESULTS

Transcription of Titin Genes in Thymomas

Titin mRNAs for MIR and N2-line titin were strongly expressed in three out of the four thymomas examined (FIGURE 1). The hyperplastic thymus from the young-onset MG patient showed strong mRNA expression for both MIR and N2-line titin (FIGURE 1, lane 6).

In the thymus from the late-onset MG patient with thymic atrophy, mRNAs for the MIR and the N2-line titin regions were not detectable (FIGURE 1, lane 3).

Expression of Titin in Thymomas

The 9D10 anti-titin antibody stained the surface of epithelial thymoma cells (FIGURE 2). Staining of myoid cells was seen in normal and hyperplastic thymus. Weak staining of epithelial cells around Hassall's corpuscles was seen in sections from one normal thymus and the hyperplastic thymus. The 9D10 antibody did not stain cells in the normal tonsil or colon carcinoma. The 9D10 anti-titin antibody stained a protein of approximately 220 kDa in the thymoma membrane extract not present in the normal thymus or the tonsil extracts. The T12 anti-titin antibody stained myoid cells in tissue sections, but was otherwise negative.

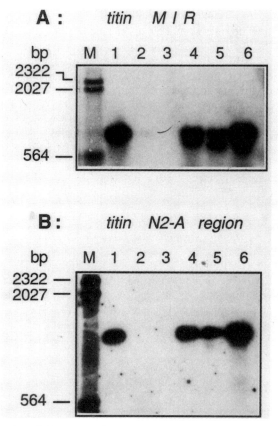

FIGURE 1. Detection of titin mRNAs for **(A)** MIR titin transcripts and **(B)** N2-A region titin transcripts, by RT-PCR and Southern blot analysis. Terms—M: marker; bp: base pairs; lane 1: thymoma 1; lane 2: thymoma 2; lane 3: atrophic thymus; lane 4: thymoma 3; lane 5: thymoma 4; lane 6: hyperplastic thymus.

DISCUSSION

This study shows that thymomas express titin mRNAs coding for the MIR and the central I-band titin, which are regions of titin to which autoantibodies are circulating in thymoma MG patients. The titin antibody 9D10 stained neoplastic thymoma epithelial cells in tissue sections as well as a peptide in a thymoma extract, indicating that titin is translated in amounts sufficient to be detected by immunohistochemistry and Western blots.

Epitopes from or cross-reactive with skeletal muscle antigens reactive with thymoma MG patients' autoantibodies such as AChR and ryanodine receptor[5] have pre-

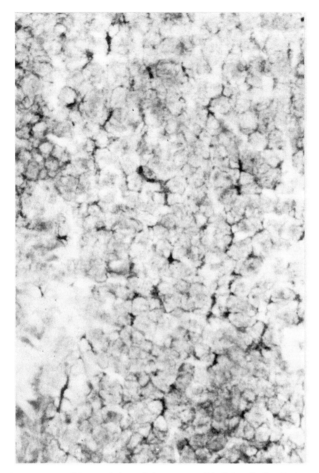

FIGURE 2. Immunoperoxidase staining of thymoma epithelial cells by the 9D10 titin antibody. Magnification: ×560.

viously been identified in thymomas. Thymoma epithelial cells in culture can present AChR peptides to relevant T cell lines.[6] Thus, the neoplastic cells are able to present their neoantigens for developing T cells. We have previously shown that peripheral blood T cells from MG patients are reactive with epitopes contained in the MIR titin fragment.[7] As 90% of thymoma patients have titin antibodies and the thymoma titin mRNAs contain the main immunogenic region for both T cells and B cells, it is most likely that aberrant positive selection of titin-reactive T cells within the thymoma is the initiating event for titin autoreactivity in thymoma MG.

REFERENCES

1. AARLI, J. A. *et al.* 1990. Patients with myasthenia gravis and thymoma have in their sera IgG autoantibodies against titin. Clin. Exp. Immunol. **82:** 284–288.
2. LABEIT, S. & B. KOLMERER. 1995. Titins: giant proteins in charge of muscle ultrastructure and elasticity. Science **270:** 293–296.
3. LUEBKE, E. *et al.* 1998. Striational autoantibodies in myasthenia gravis: evidence for titin epitope spreading. Submitted.
4. WILLCOX, N. 1993. Myasthenia gravis. Curr. Opin. Immunol. **5:** 910–917.
5. MYGLAND, Å. *et al.* 1995. Thymomas express epitopes shared by the ryanodine receptor. J. Neuroimmunol. **62:** 79–83.
6. GILHUS, N. E. *et al.* 1995. Antigen presentation by thymoma epithelial cells from myasthenia gravis patients to potentially pathogenic T cells. J. Neuroimmunol. **56:** 65–76.
7. SKEIE, G. O. *et al.* 1997. Titin antibody positive myasthenia gravis patients have a cellular immune response against the main immunogenic region of titin. Eur. J. Neurol. **4:** 131–137.

Using Histochemical Methods to Study Pathological Features of Hyperplastic Thymus and Thymoma in Patients with Myasthenia Gravis

L. H. TU, G. Y. CAI, X. M. ZHU, AND R. Q. ZHANG

Department of Neurology
Changhai Hospital
Shanghai 200433, China

INTRODUCTION

Abnormalities of thymus gland are always accompanied with myasthenia gravis (MG). The pathological changes are closely related to clinical condition, effect of treatment, and prognosis.

Clinically, we expect to distinguish the pathological feature of the thymus, but in fact it is more difficult to differentiate nonneoplastic thymus from thymoma (including benign and malignant).[1–5]

CLINICOEXPERIMENTAL RESEARCH: PART I

Clinical Materials and Methods

Ten patients with hyperplastic thymus and 13 patients with thymoma in myasthenia gravis were studied by routine and immunohistochemical methods on paraffin sections using monoclonal antibodies against thymic epithelial cells (UCHLI), myoid cells (antidesmin antibody), and rabbit antihuman citric acid extract of skeletal muscle antibody (CAE-Ab), in order to determine the hyperplastic thymus and thymoma.

Results

In the nonneoplastic group, lymphoid follicular hyperplasia (LFH) (6 cases) and B cells with diffuse infiltration (4 cases) were found. All of them had medullary hyperplasia and B cell infiltration.

In the thymoma group, corticoepithelial type (6 cases) with round or ovary nucleus and prominent central nucleoli as well as medullo-corticomedullary mixed type (7 cases) were found, but medullary type with only fusiform cells was not found. The epithelial cells of both thymoma and hyperplastic thymus were labeled with antikeratin monoclonal antibodies, but only epithelial cells of the thymoma were stained by the antiserum antibodies of rabbit to the citric acid extract of human skeletal muscle (CAE-Ab).

Conclusions

The germinal center, which arises from B cells, is the most remarkable change in hyperplastic thymus. Enlargement of the epithelial perivascular space (PVS) of the thymus and disruption of the epithelial cell barrel at the medullary boundary are more liable to occur with B cell infiltration. Those B cells and T cells immunized by the antigen of the myoid cell induce the immune response to nAChR. Therefore, it is suggested that thymectomy, radiation therapy, or immunosuppressive drugs should be adapted towards the thymus gland.

Thymoma arises from the epithelial cells of the thymus. The corticoepithelial cell is prone to be invasive to pericardium and will metastasize and relapse. Citric acid extract of human skeletal muscle (CAE) is a sarcolemma antigen. Most patients with thymoma have CAE-Ab in their sera. Thymoma can usually be labeled by CAE-Ab.

CLINICOEXPERIMENTAL RESEARCH: PART II

Clinical Materials and Methods

Fifty-one surgicopathologic samples of thymus (35 thymoma and 16 hyperplastic) in 44 cases with MG (31 thymoma and 13 hyperplastic thymus) were obtained by means of argyrophilic stain of nucleolar organizer regions (AgNORs) and immuno-histochemical stain of proliferating cell nuclear antigen (PCNA). The main purpose was to distinguish a thymoma between benign and malignant.

Results

Comparison of the results of these two histochemical tests with regard to the difference between thymoma (malignant and benign) and hyperplastic thymus is shown in TABLE 1.

TABLE 1. Results of the Two Histochemical Tests

Cases	Means of AgNORs per Nucleus of Epithelial Cell	Mean Percentages of PCNA-positive Epithelial Cells
Malignant thymoma ($n = 13$)	4.3 ± 0.8	$23.9 \pm 6.5\%$
Benign thymoma ($n = 32$)	2.8 ± 0.6	$11.1 \pm 4.1\%$
Hyperplastic thymus ($n = 16$)	2.4 ± 0.5	$8.2 \pm 2.6\%$

Conclusions

The results suggest that using histochemical stain and calculating AgNORs and PCNA for thymus epithelial cells to analyze the activity of cell proliferation can help to distinguish between the benign and malignant thymoma and to determine a patient's prognosis. The results of these two histochemical stain tests are reliable and consistent, but the staining method of AgNORs is easier.

AgNORs may be regarded as the marker of rDNA and its transcription, and PCNA as the specific marker of the S period in the cycle of cell proliferation. Both of them reflect the activity of cell proliferation. Furthermore, knowledge of the clinical condition of a patient and combining with the tumor biological behavior may contribute to the confirmation of the pathological diagnosis.

REFERENCES

1. ROSAI, J. & G. D. LEVINE. 1976. Tumors of the thymus. *In* Atlas of Tumor Pathology. Armed Forces Institute of Pathology. Washington, District of Columbia.
2. KIRCHNER, T., B. SCHALKE, A. MELUS *et al.* 1986. Immunohistological patterns of non-neoplastic changes in the thymus in myasthenia gravis. Virchows Arch. **B52:** 237.
3. MÜLLER-HERMELINK, H. K., G. P. MARINO, U. SCHUMACHER *et al.* 1985. Immunohistological evidences of cortical medullary differentiation in thymoma. Virchows Arch. Pathol. Anat. **408:** 143.
4. TATEYAMA, H., T. MIZUNO, J. TADA *et al.* 1993. Thymic epithelial tumours: evaluation of malignant grade by quantification of proliferating cell nuclear antigen and nuclear organizer regions. Virchows Arch. A: Pathol. Anat. Histopathol. **422:** 265.
5. PICH, A., R. CHIARLE, L. CHIUSA *et al.* 1994. Argyrophilic nucleolar organizer region counts predict survival in thymoma. Cancer **74:** 1568.

Percutaneous Paracentesis into Thymus Gland for Intervention Treatment of Myasthenia Gravis

Report of Ten Cases

L. H. TU,[a] J. M. JIANG,[a] R. Q. ZHANG,[a] Q. L. XIE,[b] W. XU,[b] Y. CHEN,[b]
T. H. ZHANG,[c] J. J. DING,[c] Z. Y. ZHANG,[c] S. Y. WANG,[c] X. Y. SUN,[d]
P. J. WANG,[e] AND T. Z. LU[e]

aDepartment of Neurology
bDepartment of Physical Therapy
cDepartment of Cardiology
dDepartment of Ultrasonics
eCT Room
Changhai Hospital
Shanghai 200433, China

INTRODUCTION

Thymus in the pathogenesis and treatment of myasthenia gravis (MG) has great important significance.

Guided by ultrasonography or CT scanning, the effect of percutaneous paracentesis into thymus gland for intervention treatment with microwave heat radiation and dexamethasone injected locally has been found to be very significant.[1–4] The results of this treatment are reported below.

CLINICAL MATERIALS

Ten patients with MG (M4, F6) were 9–50 years old. The courses of disease were 2 months to 11 years. The types of Osserman's classification included 4 cases of type I, 2 cases of type II, 1 case of type III, and 3 cases of type IV. The thymus pathologic changes included 9 cases with hyperplasia and 1 case with thymoma.

Apparatus and needles: A microwave therapeutor was made by our hospital. Percutaneous paracentesis needles included liver puncture needle (20 gauge) for percutaneous centesis, kidney puncture needle (18 gauge) for biopsy of thymus, and microwave antenna needle for heat radiation treatment.

METHODS OF TREATMENT

Operating Procedures

Patient's position: Both shoulders supinated on a pillow in a bed; head extended posteriorly to expose upper chest.

Survey of thymus: The position, figure, and size of the thymus were detected by ultrasonoscope probe or CT scanner from the upper margin to the lower part of the sternum.

Centesis point and pathway: The centesis point was selected just above the upper margin of the sternum, as called "Tian-Tu puncture point" by Chinese traditional medicine. With local anesthesia, using a liver puncture needle to make a hole in the skin, it extended along the posterior board at the medium line of the sternum into the thymus gland. The end of the needle was shown by scanning as a bright point. Finally, a microwave antenna needle was extended into the thymus gland at a certain depth.

Although the position and size of the thymus gland varied from patient to patient, the needle could be slightly deviated from the medium line; it should be limited within the mediastinum as close to its anterio-upper part as possible.

Heat radiation of 2450 mHz microwaves with 60–80 W was used for 5–10 s at each point, for 4–6 points per treatment. Ten mg of dexamethasone was injected locally as well. To prevent infection, norfloxacin was taken. This treatment was adopted 1–2 times per week, for 2–3 times of treatment overall in general.

Thymus aspiration biopsy by percutaneous paracentesis: Before microwave treatment, a kidney needle connected with a rubber tube to a 50-mL syringe was used for centesis into the thymus gland, to aspirate the thymus tissue, and then it was put on a glass slide.

Using May-Grünwald-Giemsa stain and immunohistologic stain of monoantibodies of B cells, T cells, epithelial cells, or antiserum of CAE-Ab (thymoma-associated antibody), the thymus was observed under microscope.

RESULTS

Image changes of thymus after microwave treatment—Ultrasonography: In 8 cases before treatment, the lengths of the thymus measured from upper to lower, left to

TABLE 1. Effects of Treatment

	Cases Followed Up	
Treatment Effects	1 Year	3 Years
cured completely	1	2
cured essentially	3	2
improved significantly	3	4
improved	3	1

right, and anterior to posterior were 2–3.7 cm, 1.1–2.3 cm, and 0.9–1.8 cm, respectively; after treatment, their shrink rates were 31.6–44.2%. The resounds of coagulated tissue increased.

CT scanning: In 2 cases before microwave treatment, the thymus images were shown to be of high density; after treatment, the densities decreased.

Some effects could appear as soon as within 1 week (see TABLE 1). For example:

Case 1: male, 15 years old. Both of his eyes opened with difficulty for 2 mm, which improved in the morning and worsened in the afternoon. Widths of palpebral fissures when narrowed were only 3 mm, and both eyeballs were almost fixed completely. Hyperplastic thymus was shown by CT scanning. After percutaneous paracentesis intervention treatment (PPIT) for the first time, both eyes opened remarkably. After the sixth time of treatment, he was completely cured.

Case 2: male, 43 years old. He had generalized weakness with difficulty in swallowing for 4 years. A thymoma of 9 × 6 × 3 cm was shown by CT scanning. Even with right thoracic exploratory cooperation, the thymoma could not be removed because of metastasis to superior vena cava and pericardium. Malignant thymoma of epithelial cells presented with microcystic degeneration. After PPIT of the thymus, he became better. One year later, he returned to work and pyridostigmine was withdrawn.

CONCLUSIONS

This therapy (PPIT) is indicated for MG patients accompanied with hyperplastic thymus or thymoma, without intention to perform thymectomy or in those incapable of being operated upon. They were better at an age of not less than 12 years old and were capable of cooperating with this treatment.

One must be strict to control the indication and familiar with the anatomy of the mediastinum to prevent complications. TV-monitored image amplification fluoroscopy is most suitable for puncture needle placement, to take a biopsy, and for microwave treatment within the thymus lesion.

REFERENCES

1. WEIBRED, G. L., D. J. LYONS, L. C. TAO et al. 1984. Percutaneous fine-needle aspiration biopsy of mediastinal lesions. AJR **143:** 525.
2. ZHANG, Z. Y., C. F. SUN, L. T. XU et al. 1985. Percutaneous puncture biopsy for diagnosis of intrathoracic and intramediastinal lesions. Surg. J. Thorax Cardiovasc. (Chin.) **1:** 227.
3. SCANDDLING, G. K. 1979. Role of the thymus in myasthenia gravis. In Clinical Immunology, p. 137. Blackwell. Oxford.
4. XIE, Q. L. 1994. Prospects of microwaves in medical applications. Chin. Photo. Electr. **3:** 4.

Drug-induced Autoimmune Myasthenia Gravis[a]

AUDREY S. PENN,[b,c,d] BARBARA W. LOW,[e] ISRAELI A. JAFFE,[f]
LIANG LUO,[b] AND JEFFREY J. JACQUES[b]

[b]Department of Neurology
Columbia University College of Physicians and Surgeons
New York, New York

[c]National Institute of Neurological Disorders and Stroke
Bethesda, Maryland

[e]Department of Biochemistry and Molecular Biophysics
[f]Department of Medicine
Columbia University College of Physicians and Surgeons
New York, New York

Myasthenia gravis (MG) may be induced, aggravated, or exposed by certain classes of drugs. These include quinoline derivatives that function as anti-arrhythmics, including quinine, quinidine, procainamide, and disopyramide, and antimalarials such as chloroquine and hydroxychloroquine. The quinoline drugs act directly on neuromuscular transmission to alter both presynaptic and postsynaptic components and thereby exacerbate MG.[1,2] Antibiotics of certain types also may worsen or exacerbate MG, especially aminoglycosides such as streptomycin and kanamycin and carbapenems such as imipenem.[3,4] Two early case reports of MG associated with trimethadione have been cited regularly, but no new cases have been reported.[5,6]

Therapy of rheumatoid arthritis, scleroderma, primary biliary cirrhosis, Wilson's disease, and cystinuria with D-penicillamine (D-P) has been associated with the development of a variety of autoimmune diseases and serologies including MG, systemic lupus erythematosus, pemphigus, thyroiditis, and Goodpasture's syndrome.[7–9] Similarly, antinuclear antibodies, antibodies to insulin, and antinuclear cytoplasmic antibodies have been detected with and without clinical disease.[10–13] D-P-induced myasthenia gravis (D-P-MG) is indistinguishable from spontaneous MG in clinical presentation, altered electrophysiology, pharmacological responses, and presence of antibodies to acetylcholine receptor (anti-AChR).[14–17] In contrast to spontaneous MG, D-P-MG is reversible upon drug withdrawal and anti-AChR titers fall gradually.

D-P, captopril, and α-methylpropionylglycine (thiopronine), which induce MG by autoimmune mechanisms, are exclusively sulfhydryl reducing agents with free thiol groups.[18,19] Pyrithioxine and thiopyridoxine, both disulfides, are also effective as drug therapies for rheumatoid arthritis (FIGURE 1). Neither disulfide-containing drug

[a]This work was supported in part by NIH Grant No. NS17904.
[d]Address for correspondence: National Institutes of Health, National Institute of Neurological Disorders and Stroke, 31 Center Drive, Bethesda, Maryland 20892-2540.

433

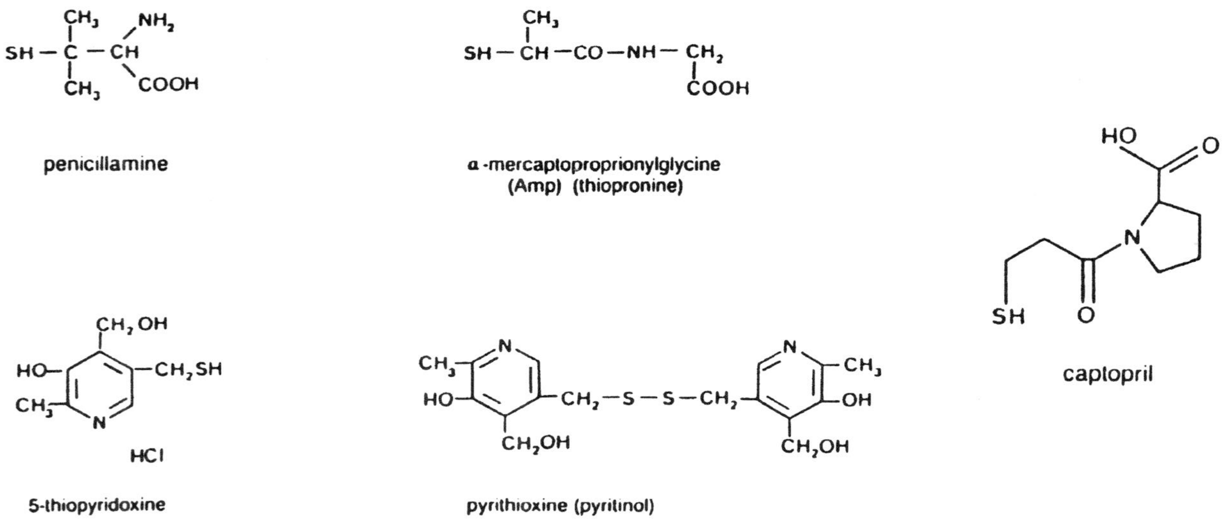

FIGURE 1. Chemical formulas of penicillamine and other sulfhydryl compounds used as drugs in rheumatoid arthritis (after reference 18, with permission).

has been reported to induce MG. D-P is highly chemically reactive. It will reduce cystine, providing therapy for cystinuria,[20] and will form a mixed disulfide with the cysteine produced. Because it is less reactive than either dithiothreitol or mercaptoethanol, it tends to form mixed disulfides with other thiols as it does with cysteine. We have shown previously that it will bind covalently to acetylcholine receptor (AChR) alpha and gamma subunits and have hypothesized that it binds to one or both alpha subunit cysteines 192 or 193 after reducing the readily reducible disulfide bond formed from these cysteines.[21] This bond is located at about 1 nm from the ligand-binding site on the alpha subunit of AChR.[22] Xu and colleagues have confirmed that D-P acts near the ligand-binding site since they showed that D-P blocked the binding of monoclonal antibodies to *Torpedo* AChR, which themselves blocked the action of agonists.[23] The D-P effect was abolished by pretreatment with *N*-ethylmaleimide. D-P may similarly reduce disulfide bonds and bind to thiols on the insulin molecule. It will also bind to various plasma proteins and this property has been used to investigate its pharmacokinetics.[24] Nearly all is bound irreversibly at 3 hours after iv administration to rats. Although D-P will be present long enough to be presented to immune cells, immune responses to D-P and its derivatized proteins depend heavily on species and strain differences and thus on genetic predisposition.

Animal models of immune disorders that have developed after D-P administration vary in type and severity. Brown-Norway rats developed antinuclear antibodies, circulating immune complexes, and disseminated intravascular coagulation with granulomatous lesions and IgG deposits in the kidneys after about 8 weeks of oral D-P.[25] Lewis and Sprague-Dawley varieties did not.[26] Mice of the C57BL/KsJ (H-2d) and C3H/HeJ (H-2k) strains, but not Balb/c (H-2d) or C57BL/6 (H-2b), developed antibodies against insulin.[10] The mice were not clinically ill. Similarly, A.SW (H-2s) mice developed antinuclear antibodies specific for either DNA or histone-DNA complexes after receiving D-P or quinidine.[27] We have studied mice treated chronically with D-P by daily (5 of 7) injections of 40 mg/kg (approximately 1 mg per mouse per day). None of these developed clinical signs after 6 months. However, when mice were treated and then exposed to a single inoculating dose of *Torpedo* AChR, strain A (IAk) mice showed clinical and electrophysiological evidence of myasthenia at 9 weeks after the injection.[28,38] Antibody titers in C57BL/6 (IAb) and C3H/HeJ (IAk) were significantly higher than in matched animals who received only saline followed by the single injection of AChR. In a similar study of guinea pigs, no antibodies to AChR were found in D-P-treated animals, but there was evidence of proliferative responses to AChR by their spleen cells.[29]

D-P ELICITS IMMUNE RESPONSES TO ITSELF AS MEASURED AS DELAYED HYPERSENSITIVITY AND IN MIXED LYMPHOCYTE REACTIONS (MLRs)

Immune responses to D-P depend upon its chemical reactivity and ability to bind to and derivatize proteins. It is also able to generate immune responses to itself by derivatizing immune cells.[30–33] After immunization of various murine strains with D-P in complete Freund's adjuvant (CFA), C3H/He, B10.AM, and A.TI mice, all IAk, showed delayed hypersensitivity to D-P.[31] T cell proliferative responses to D-P-de-rivatized spleen cells were found after Balb/c mice were treated with D-P hydrochlo-ride.[32] This response differentiated between D-P and L-P, indicating that specificity was also related to chemical structure. D-P disulfide was not effective.[32] There was also a relatively restricted derivatization dose for cells at about 1.35 mM and a treat-ment dose for animals of 1 mg per mouse per day (40 mg/kg). An extension of this work demonstrated that the responding T cells were helper (CD4+) phenotype and that generation of the antigenic moiety did not require intracellular processing, sug-gesting that D-P may bind directly to surface molecules.[33] We have shown that T cells from IAk mice exposed chronically to D-P will proliferate to a greater extent to syn-geneic spleen cells highly enriched in dendritic cells (DC) that were exposed to 1.35 mM D-P overnight than to untreated DC.[34] Since this is a version of an MLR, known to reflect reactions of T cells to MHC class II molecules, we suspect that D-P may bind to surface MHC molecules and be presented directly, thus amplifying the re-sponse to the DC. We hypothesized that the ability of D-P to be presented by the most proficient antigen-presenting cells, which function to drive naive T cells, could be the initiating event in a sequence culminating in immune responses to D-P-derivatized cells or proteins. Indeed, D-P has the capacity to function as a hapten. Immunization of rabbits with D-P KLH induced specific IgG anti-D-P responses detected using D-P-conjugated human serum albumin[35] and a similar strategy has been used to pro-duce antibodies to captopril.[36]

We have hypothesized that derivatization of AChR by D-P via formation of a mixed disulfide could trigger the immune response to AChR culminating in myasthe-nia.[21] Since D-P also alters the equilibrium binding properties of acetylcholine to both purified and membrane-bound AChR, it is also possible that this effect reflects an altered conformation that is antigenic.[21] We proceeded to examine rabbits, mice, and humans, treated with D-P, for immune responses to D-P and to AChR. Rabbits and humans were tested for the presence of antibodies to the D-P group using D-P-modified albumins. We also compared reactions to AChR and to AChR modified by D-P as described in our previous studies[21] to assess possible differences that could be related to the presence of the D-P group. Because of possible contributions of regions of AChR contiguous to or surrounding the putative binding site for D-P at cysteine-cysteine 192–193 on the alpha subunit, we also studied reactions to the calf alpha se-quence peptide 179–191 (Lys-Glu-Ser-Arg-Gly-TRP-Lys-His-TRP-Val-Phe-Tyr-Ala) and the human sequence in which Trp 184 has been reversed to position 187 (Lys-Glu-Ser-Arg-Gly-SER-Lys-His-TRP-Val-Phe-Tyr-Ala). The transfer of a tryp-tophan residue at 184 in the human sequence to position 187 produces a sequence that could be expected to show alpha-neurotoxin binding properties similar to the calf sequence.[37] We also used the calf sequence 179–196 (Lys-Glu-Ser-Arg-Gly-Trp-Lys-His-Trp-Val-Phe-Tyr-Ala-Cys-Cys-Ser-Pro-Asp-Thr) modified by an ac-etamidomethyl group on one cysteine residue for some studies in mice.

Mice of IAk H-2 haplotype were treated with D-P as described[38] and tested for cell-mediated reactions to AChR, D-P-AChR, and peptides. For cell studies, we em-ployed a preparation of AChR in which CHAPS detergent was used. This allowed re-moval of detergent by dialysis just prior to addition to cells and produced a prepara-tion with a specific activity of 8 nmoles/mg after affinity chromatography.[39]

ANTIBODIES TO D-P, TO AChR, AND TO
AChR PEPTIDE IN RABBITS TREATED WITH D-P

Rabbits develop significant clinical myasthenia when immunized with AChR.[40] First, we studied two groups of rabbits hyperimmunized with D-P-modified AChR (D-P-AChR) for development of EAMG. They developed myasthenic weakness entirely similar to the experimental myasthenia induced by AChR. We then evaluated rabbits to which D-P was administered for up to 6 months. Rabbits given 40 mg/kg D-P daily showed no suggestion of weakness when tested weekly by repetitive hind-leg extension after hopping several room lengths on rough floor matting. Two died suddenly for unknown reasons at 1.5 and 6 months after the initiation of injections; a third died after 3 months and was found to have extensive intrathoracic hemorrhage, which suggested that collagen may have been disaggregated because of documented lathyrogenic effects of D-P.[41] Four others were terminated under ketamine and butabarbital anesthesia after 5 to 6 months.

Antibodies to AChR

Antibody titers to D-P-AChR were compared to those against AChR using ELISA and radioimmunoassay (RIA). The AChR preparations used in the RIAs were treated with ^{125}I-α-bungarotoxin as described.[40,42] ELISA was achieved by plating 1.5 mg/mL of purified AChR or D-P-AChR (0.3 mg/well) as described.[43] Peroxidase-conjugated antibodies, raised in goats, to IgG and IgM were used at 1:6000 and at 1:10,000, respectively. Sera from rabbits immunized with D-P-AChR reacted to a greater degree with D-P-AChR than with AChR when examined by ELISA or RIA, which suggests a reaction to epitopes present on D-P-AChR and not on AChR (FIGURES 2A and 2B, TABLE 1). Binding curves generated by varying the amounts of antigen confirmed higher recognition of the D-P-modified AChR at all antigen doses studied (FIGURE 2C). No differences were found when antisera raised to unmodified AChR[40] were tested.

We also detected antibodies to both modified and unmodified *Torpedo* AChR in serum from 4 of the 5 surviving rabbits that had only been given D-P. Antibodies were measured using RIA and ELISA. IgG titers rose steadily and were sustained to termination at the sixth month.

Low antibody titers to D-P-modified *Torpedo* AChR and unmodified AChR were also detected by RIA in a range similar to D-P-treated human patients (TABLE 1). Titers derived from binding curves of the samples starting with those obtained during the second month of D-P treatment (TABLE 1) were significantly elevated over controls. Full binding curves against D-P-AChR and AChR showed higher binding of D-P-AChR at higher serum concentrations, but became superimposable as sera were diluted out (FIGURE 3). Therefore, D-P-AChR bore additional reactive determinants as compared to AChR, which could be detected with less dilute serum from rabbits treated only with D-P containing relatively uncommon antibody species present in low titers.

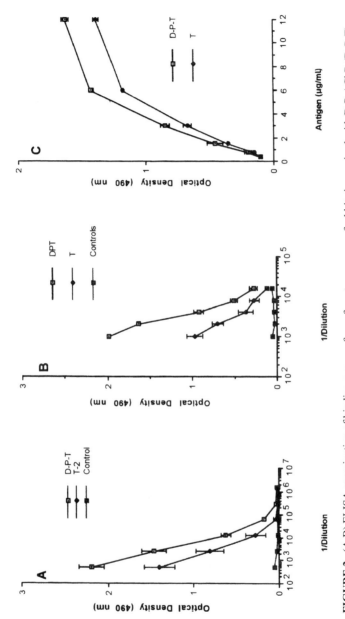

FIGURE 2. (A,B) ELISA examination of binding curves of sera from two groups of rabbits immunized with D-P-AChR (D-P-T) as compared to reactions with AChR (T). Data points are means of triplicates. Error bars represent two standard deviations. (C) Binding curve of group A rabbits against D-P-AChR and AChR generated by plating increasing doses of antigen.

TABLE 1. Antibody Responses of D-P-treated Rabbits

Rabbit No.	Anti-AChR[a]		Anti-AChR[b]	D-P-RSA		Peptide	
	DPT	T	DPT/T	Titer[c]	OD Ratio[d]	Titer[e]	OD Ratio[d]
6207 (A)	12.4	7.0	625/625	80	4.7	3125	11.6
3973 (B)	9.7	9.3	625/625	160	6.1	625	11.3
4137 (D)	6.0	5.0	125/125	80	2.3	n.d.[g]	n.d.
4104 (C)	2.0	4.0	125/125	640	11.0	15,625	13.2
D-P-AChR[f]	14.3 μM	13.9 μM	64,000/16,000	6250/1250	7.7	625/125	
controls	0.5	0.5	25/25	5	1	25	

[a]pmoles/mL precipitated in RIA versus *Torpedo* AChR (T) and D-P-treated AChR (DPT).

[b]Titers from the linear portion of ELISA binding curves of serum versus DPT and T expressed as the reciprocal of dilution at which the experimental-matched control value is at 1:25 dilution (control OD: 0.060±0.001/0.052±0.006).

[c]Titers from the linear portion of ELISA binding curves of serum versus D-P-derivatized rabbit albumin expressed as the reciprocal of dilution at which the experimental-matched control value is at 1:10 dilution (control OD: 0.044±0.009).

[d]Ratios of optical densities of experimental and mean control sera at 1:10 dilution.

[e]Titers from the linear portion of ELISA binding curves of serum versus alpha 179–191, human sequence with Trp at position 187, expressed as the reciprocal of dilution at which the experimental-matched control value is at 1:25 dilution (OD: 0.070±0.008).

[f]Pooled samples from rabbits after boosting with D-P-AChR.

[g]n.d. = not determined.

Antibodies to D-P-modified Albumins

Rabbit albumin was used in order to minimize reactions against foreign determinants. It was derivatized by two methods that produced D-P attached to lysine residues either via propionyl or via disulfide bonds.[44,45] Serum samples from the 4 rabbits that had detectable antibodies to modified and unmodified *Torpedo* AChR after prolonged D-P administration (see above) also showed low, but measurable reactions with the D-P-modified rabbit albumin (D-P-RSA) (TABLE 1). These were measured by ELISA-plating 25 μg/mL (5 μg/well) of rabbit albumin (RSA) or D-P-RSA in 0.06 M carbonate buffer, pH 9.4, by incubation in a humidified atmosphere at 4 °C overnight. Wells were washed with phosphate-buffered saline (PBS) containing 0.05% Tween 20 (PBS/T). Uncoated sites were blocked by incubation with nonfat milk in PBS/T for 1 hour at room temperature. Following three more washes with PBS/T, the serum to be analyzed was added to every other well in every other row in serial fivefold dilutions starting at 1:5. After 2 hours at room temperature, wells were washed as described above. The optimal working dilution of second antibody was determined by a preliminary titration against control rabbit serum and antigen and by assay of the peroxidase activity of the conjugate against *o*-phenylenediamine at 490 nm. Bound conjugate was visualized by addition of a freshly prepared solution containing 2 mM *o*-phenylenediamine in citrate-phosphate buffer, pH 5.0, mixed with

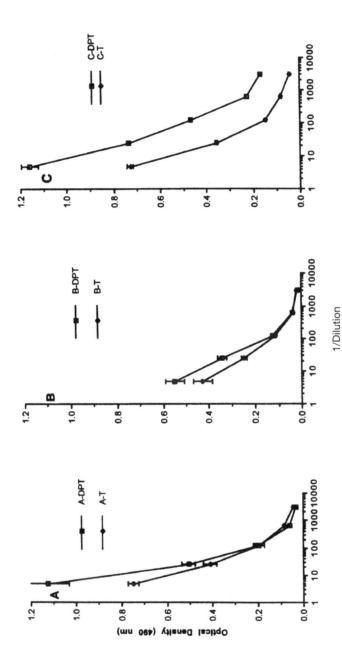

FIGURE 3. ELISA examination of binding of serum from individual rabbits (A, B, C) treated with D-P at peak response (45–60 days) to D-P-AChR (D-P-T) as compared to AChR (T). Data points are means of triplicates. Error bars represent two standard deviations. Control sera, <0.1 OD at 1:5 dilution.

50% H_2O_2. The reaction was terminated after 10 minutes with H_2SO_4 and each well was read at 490 nm on an ELISA reader (Biotek, Winooski, Vermont).

There was no apparent correlation between titers of anti-AChR and reactions with D-P-RSA. The 2 rabbits with no anti-AChR also showed no reaction with D-P-RSA. We also found antibodies to D-P, as presented on RSA, in sera from rabbits immunized with D-P-modified *Torpedo* AChR (TABLE 1), but no reactivity to unmodified RSA. Sera from rabbits immunized with unmodified *Torpedo* AChR with comparable titers to AChR did not react with either D-P-RSA or RSA (data not shown). Together, these findings provide evidence that rabbits treated chronically with D-P or immunized with D-P-AChR had antibodies recognizing the D-P group.

Antibodies to α Subunit Sequence 179–191 with Trp at 187

Calf sequence peptide α179–191 and human sequence α179–191 (Trp 187/Ser 184) were synthesized using an Applied Biosystems 430A automated synthesizer and purified by ion exchange chromatography (Pharmacia FPLC mono-Q) followed by reverse-phase HPLC. Identity and purity of the peptides were established by both amino acid composition and sequence analysis. We have shown that the calf sequence is immunogenic in IAk mice.[46] When we tested the D-P-treated rabbits for the presence of antibodies to these peptides by ELISA, significant titers were found (FIGURE 4, TABLE 1). Indeed, titers were higher than those to AChR, D-P-derivatized albumin, or D-P-AChR.

Lower, but detectable titers were also found in sera from rabbits immunized with D-P-AChR (TABLE 1). No antibodies to this peptide were detected in sera from rabbits immunized with unmodified AChR or from control rabbits. The presence of antibodies to this sequence in D-P-treated rabbits supports our hypothesis that regions contiguous to the proposed D-P binding site could contribute to the *in vivo* immunogenicity.

DO MICE TREATED WITH D-P DEVELOP
CELLULAR RESPONSES TO AChR?

We have shown that IAk mice, both strain C3H/eb (H-2k) and A (H-2a), develop augmented antibody responses to a single inoculum of AChR after D-P treatment as compared to antibody titers in saline-treated, AChR-primed syngeneic mice.[28] Initiation of an immune response to AChR should involve helper T cell activity against epitopes on AChR, or to an AChR peptide involved in D-P binding or to a cross-reacting antigen targeted by D-P. We therefore examined mice treated chronically with D-P for up to 6 months as well as mice immunized with D-P emulsified in CFA.

Mice were injected into the peritoneum (IP) with freshly prepared D-P hydrochloride (40 mg/kg) for 5 of 7 days for up to 6 months. Controls received saline. They were then injected with saline/CFA emulsion in one hind footpad and IP. Other groups were hyperimmunized with D-P in Freund's adjuvant using a priming dose in

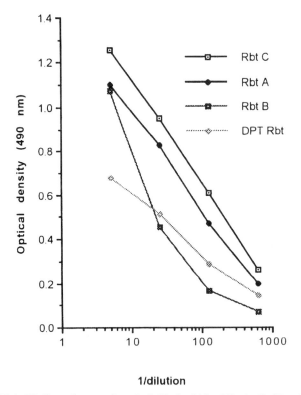

FIGURE 4. Binding of serum from individual rabbits (Rbt A, B, C) and from D-P-AChR (DPT)–immunized rabbits to human alpha subunit sequence peptide 179–191 (Trp 187/Ser 184) examined by ELISA. Data points are means of triplicates.

CFA and two boosts in incomplete Freund's adjuvant. Popliteal lymph nodes (PLN) and spleens were removed 9 days after the adjuvant injections.[47] Single cell suspensions were prepared in Click's medium supplemented with Hepes buffer, 15 mM, pH 7.0, and 10% horse serum.[48] Cells (5×10^6/mL, 0.1 mL) were plated into wells of microtiter plates in triplicate. Peptide, in 0.1 mL, was added in varying doses; AChR was added at 0.5 to 1 mg/mL as previously determined. Cultures were allowed to incubate for a total of 96 hours in an atmosphere of 95% air/5% CO_2. Tritiated (^{3}H) thymidine, 1 μCi, was added for the final 16 hours. Cells were then harvested onto glass fiber paper using a cell harvester (Mini-mash automated sample harvester, Whitaker M.A. Bioproducts, Walkersville, Maryland). ^{3}H-Thymidine, incorporated into DNA, was counted, after the paper strips dried, in a liquid scintillation counter.

We found significant responses (stimulation index > 2.0) of PLN cells from mice treated with D-P for 4 to 6 months to the alpha subunit peptide 179–196, whereas controls did not react (FIGURE 5). Responses to AChR were not significantly different from controls. In contrast, PLN cells from mice immunized and boosted with D-P in

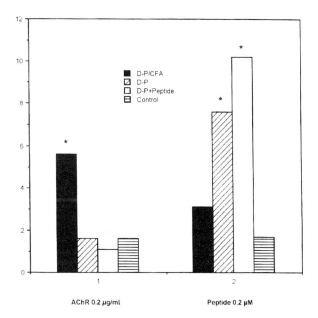

AChR 0.2 µg/mL   Peptide 0.2 µM

FIGURE 5. Responses of popliteal lymph node cells from C3Heb/FeJ mice against AChR and peptide calf sequence alpha 179–196-Acm. Terms—D-P/CFA: mice were primed with D-P/CFA; D-P: mice were treated with D-P and then injected with CFA in saline; D-P + peptide: mice were primed with D-P/CFA and boosted with peptide/CFA; control: mice were primed with saline and boosted with CFA in saline. Final injections were given 9 days before cells were obtained. Stimulation index (SI): cpm experimental/cpm control. Media cpm: D-P/CFA 320; D-P 376; D-P + peptide 520. An asterisk indicates a significant SI over normal control at ≤2.0.

adjuvant showed significant responses to AChR and low, but significant, responses to peptide. Spleen cell responses failed to reach significance in either treatment paradigm.

We found very low antibody titers in 4 of 60 mice treated for at least 4 months (data not shown); they did not show any clinical signs.

It has been shown that D-P derivatizes spleen cells that are likely to be dendritic cells, B cells, or both.[32–34] Helper T cells from mice of the H-2k strain will respond to D-P-derivatized spleen cells.[32,33] It is therefore possible that the immune system will also respond to D-P derivatives of other cells or proteins. The presence of D-P-AChR in treated mice of specific H-2 strains, especially those bearing IAk, would then generate immune reactions against AChR. Our data suggest that indeed reactions develop against an alpha subunit sequence in the immediate vicinity of the most likely binding site for D-P. It is intriguing that actual priming with D-P in CFA into footpads produced responses to AChR, while chronic exposure to D-P followed by intradermal CFA generated response to the peptide sequence. Neither protocol resulted in antibody responses to AChR. The reactive T cells may be of the TH1 type since D-P in CFA has been shown to generate delayed hypersensitivity associated with LY1, CD4 T cell phenotypes.

RESPONSES OF PATIENTS TREATED WITH D-P

We have studied 6 patients with D-P-MG (TABLE 2) and serum samples from another 29 patients treated with D-P, but without clinical symptoms that warranted further evaluation. All, but one, had been treated for rheumatoid arthritis; the other for scleroderma. The anti-AChR titers in serial samples from 3 of the 6 D-P-MG patients fell toward the normal range over 6 to 12 months. Serial samples were not available in the other 29 patients. Although information on histocompatibility testing was not available on all 35 patients, 4 of the 6 with D-P-MG showed HLA haplotypes reported to occur with increased frequency in D-P-MG (2 Bw35, 2 DR7, 2 DR1).[17] Control samples came from patients with spontaneous MG, who were matched roughly for age, sex, and anti-AChR titer; from patients with polymyositis, rheumatoid arthritis with rheumatoid factor not receiving D-P [3 with MG, 6 without], Lambert-Eaton syndrome,[2] and neuropathies; and from normal individuals (control bank) reported previously.[42] All samples were obtained by venipuncture and were stored, in aliquots, at −70 °C until use. Informed consent was obtained from all patients.

Antibodies to AChR

Antibody titers against both human and *Torpedo* AChR were assessed by RIA as described previously[40,42] and by ELISA as described above for rabbit serum. Patients with D-P-MG all showed significantly elevated titers of anti-AChR, measured by the standard RIA against AChR-enriched human muscle extract (TABLE 2). Therefore, AChR also contributed epitopes that generate antibodies when AChR alone is the antigen, a conclusion also reached by a study of D-P-MG antibodies using competing monoclonal antibodies of defined specificity.[15]

Serum from all 6 patients also reacted with *Torpedo* AChR when tested by RIA or ELISA (TABLE 2). This allowed comparisons with *Torpedo* AChR modified by D-P. Reactions with D-P-AChR were significantly greater than those against unmodified AChR at the more concentrated regions of the ELISA binding curves in 3/4 patients (data not shown). Slightly higher titers against D-P-AChR, measured by RIA, were significant in only 2 patients of these 4. Both IgM and IgG anti-AChR were detected. Three had higher IgG titers, but anti-AChR were exclusively IgM in 1 patient.

Antibodies to D-P Presented on Albumin

ELISAs on D-P-modified human albumin were performed as for rabbit sera with the following modifications. The coating concentration for modified and unmodified human albumin (HSA) was 25 μg/mL (5 μg/well) in borate buffer, pH 8.4. Uncoated

TABLE 2. D-P Myasthenia Gravis

Patient	Duration of D-P Rx (Months)	Severity of MG[a]	Antibodies to				HLA			Peptide
			AChR-H[b]	DPT/T[b]	DPT/T[c]	D-P-HSA[d]	A	B	DR	
G	5	II	6.0	1.0/0.8	160/160	1560	2, w30	17, 18	1, 7	25
K	6	II	14.5	7.8/11	320/160	625	w24, 11	27, w35	n.d.	125
M	12	II	7.5	3/4	80/80	1560	28, 36	5, w35	2, 7	625
Mr	10	III	46.0	11.7/9.3	80/40	10,240	3, w24	7, 27	1, 6	n.d.[e]
P	24	III	250.0	3.7/3.3	320/320	250	n.d.	n.d.	n.d.	125
T	4	III	100.0	7.0/4.0	160/160	1560	n.d.	n.d.	n.d.	125

[a]II: Mild generalized disease sparing oropharyngeal muscles. III: Moderate generalized disease with mild or moderate oropharyngeal muscles or wheelchair-bound.

[b]H: Human AChR preparations; control values < 0.5 pmoles/mL. Affinity-purified *Torpedo* AChR (T) or D-P-modified *Torpedo* AChR (DPT); controls subtracted.

[c]Titers from ELISA binding curves of serum versus D-P-AChR (DPT) and *Torpedo* AChR (T) expressed as the reciprocal of dilution at which the experimental-matched mean control value is at 1:10 dilution (OD: 0.100 ± 0.009).

[d]Titers from ELISA binding curves of serum versus D-P-derivatized human albumin (D-P-HSA) expressed as the reciprocal of dilution at which the experimental-matched mean control is at 1:12.5 dilution (OD: 0.075 ± 0.012).

[e]n.d. = not determined.

sites were blocked with 2.5% chicken serum. Horseradish peroxidase–conjugated antibodies raised in goats was used. Anti-IgG was at a dilution of 1:2500; anti-IgM at 1:8000.

Sera from patients with generalized D-P-MG recognized D-P presented on human albumin (D-P-HSA), but did not react with HSA alone above controls (TABLE 2). Background reactivity with unmodified HSA, quenched by blocking with 2.5% chicken serum in borate buffer, was similar to that found with control sera. Control samples including the 12 from patients matched for age, sex, and titer of anti-AChR and 6 with rheumatoid arthritis did not. These experiments establish that, in subjects with reactions to D-P-AChR, the D-P group is recognized as presented on another carrier, to which it has been linked by disulfide bonds.

Antibodies to α179–191

Among D-P-MG patients, there was an IgM response of modest titer in patient M and a primarily IgG response in patients T and K (TABLE 2).

We conclude that treatment with D-P and the development of D-P-MG are associated with the development of immune responses to D-P itself. D-P triggers immune responses that can be measured using D-P-AChR, unmodified AChR, or D-P-conjugated albumins. In addition, D-P triggers responses to AChR. These occur in relationship to specific genetic backgrounds as shown by response of humans and mice. Antibodies to a peptide segment that constitutes most of the prime alpha toxin-binding site and is contiguous to the D-P reducible disulfide bond within 1 nm of the ligand-binding site can be measured. These were found in those treated with D-P on a chronic basis, especially rabbits. Therefore, B cells are involved in the immune responses to both peptide and drug. Although D-P treatment alters the equilibrium binding of ACh and thus may induce a conformational change, the absence of weakness in rabbits suggests that this alteration does not produce the conformational epitope responsible for experimental myasthenia in rabbits; however, it may in humans. Nevertheless, we hypothesize that the immunogenicity of this region of the alpha subunit is potentiated by the presence of D-P covalently bound by a disulfide. This could alter MHC binding to this epitope or influence T cell responses. There are precedents for both. Substitution of critical residues in a subdominant peptide from rat interphotoreceptor retinoid protein with corresponding residues from the defined bovine immunogenic peptide resulted in increased binding of the substituted peptide to MHC and increased induction of uveoretinitis.[49] In addition, derivatization of lysozyme with a hapten, phosphorylcholine, converted low antibody responder mice into high responders by generating more efficient T cell stimulation.[50] This may explain the development of antibodies to AChR as well as experimental myasthenia in strain A mice.[28] A third possibility involves epitope spreading, with the derivatized peptide serving to initiate additional T helper cell responses to other critical epitopes that trigger antibody production.[51,52] Another possibility would simply involve direct triggering of B cells by the presence of the hapten, D-P, resulting in binding to B cells of critical conformational determinants.

In this example of drug-induced autoimmunity, the alteration of a self protein by an external influence plays a critical role. We have shown that this sulfhydryl reducing agent can act at multiple sites in the sequence of initiation of immune responses and we suspect that different sites are important in different species. Clearly, in humans of specific genetic backgrounds, D-P also acts to trigger production of pathogenic antibodies that cause MG, but that will disappear along with clinical MG after the drug is discontinued. We suspect that very similar immune responses are involved in triggering MG by captopril and thiopronine. It is probable that derivatization of other proteins by D-P during therapy results in a similar sequence of immune response, although different histocompatibility antigens will bind to different D-P-modified peptides.

REFERENCES

1. SHY, M. E., D. J. LANGE, J. W. HOWARD, A. P. GOLD, R. E. LOVELACE & A. S. PENN. 1985. Quinidine exacerbating myasthenia gravis: a case report and intracellular recordings. Ann. Neurol. **19:** 120.
2. SIEB, J. P., M. MILONE & A. G. ENGEL. 1996. Effects of the quinoline derivatives quinine, quinidine, and chloroquine on neuromuscular transmission. Brain Res. **712:** 179–189.
3. ALVAN, G. & C. E. NORD. 1995. Adverse effects of monobactams and carbapenems. Drug Saf. **12:** 305–312.
4. ARGOV, Z., L. NICHOLSON, P. R. FAWCETT, F. L. MASTAGLIA & M. HALL. 1980. Neuromuscular transmission and acetylcholine receptor antibodies in rheumatoid arthritis patients on D-penicillamine [letter]. Lancet **1:** 203.
5. BOOKER, H. E., R. W. CHUN & M. SANGUINO. 1968. Myasthenia gravis syndrome associated with trimethadione. JAMA **212:** 2262–2263.
6. PETERSON, H. 1968. Association of trimethadione therapy and myasthenia gravis. N. Engl. J. Med. **274:** 506–507.
7. JAFFE, I. A. 1981. Induction of auto-immune syndromes by penicillamine therapy in rheumatoid arthritis and other diseases. Springer Semin. Immunopathol. **4:** 193–207.
8. KORMAN, N. J., R. W. EYRE, J. ZONE & J. R. STANLEY. 1991. Drug-induced pemphigus: autoantibodies directed against the pemphigus antigen complexes are present in penicillamine and captopril-induced pemphigus. J. Invest. Dermatol. **96:** 273–276.
9. MARCUS, S. N., D. CHADWICK & R. J. WALKER. 1984. D-Penicillamine-induced myasthenia gravis in primary biliary cirrhosis. Gastroenterology **86:** 166–168.
10. BRIK, R., G. TENENBAUM, M. BLANK, Y. SHOENFELD, D. BARZILAI, K. BLOCH & P. VARDI. 1995. D-Penicillamine-induced autoantibodies in a mouse model. Clin. Exp. Rheumatol. **13:** 483–488.
11. VARDI, P., R. BRIK, D. BARZILAI, M. LORBER & Y. SCHARF. 1992. Frequent induction of insulin autoantibodies by D-penicillamine in patients with rheumatoid arthritis. J. Rheumatol. **19:** 1527–1530.
12. MACH, P. S., H. BROUILHET & B. AMOR. 1986. The induction of human antinuclear antibodies by D-penicillamine: activation of inducer helper T cells in the absence of irradiation sensitive suppressor T cells. Clin. Exp. Immunol. **63:** 408–413.
13. MATHIESON, P. W., D. S. PEAT, A. SHORT & R. A. WATTS. 1986. Coexistent membranous nephropathy and ANCA-positive crescentic glomerulonephritis in association with penicillamine. Nephrol. Dial. Transplant. **11:** 863–866.
14. KUNCL, R. W., A. PESTRONK, D. B. DRACHMAN & E. RECHTHAND. 1986. The pathophysiology of penicillamine-induced myasthenia gravis. Ann. Neurol. **20:** 740–744.
15. TZARTOS, S. J., E. MOREL, A. EFHIMIADIS, A. F. BUSTARRET, J. D'ANGLEJAN, A. A. DROSOS

& H. A. MOUTSOPOULOS. 1988. Fine antigenic specificities of antibodies in sera from patients with D-penicillamine-induced myasthenia gravis. Clin. Exp. Immunol. **74:** 80–86.

16. DROSOS, A. A., L. CHRISTOU, V. GALANOPOULOU, A. G. TZIOUFAS & E. K. TSIAKOU. 1993. D-Penicillamine induced myasthenia gravis: clinical, serological, and genetic findings. Clin. Exp. Rheumatol. **11:** 387–391.

17. GARLEPP, M. J., R. L. DAWKINS & F. T. CHRISTIANSEN. 1983. HLA antigens and acetylcholine receptor antibodies in penicillamine induced myasthenia gravis. Br. Med. J. Clin. Res. **286:** 338–340.

18. JAFFE, I. A. 1986. Adverse effects profile of sulfhydryl compounds in man. Am. J. Med. **80:** 471–476.

19. SUDA, M., J. KUBOTA, Y. YAMAGUCHI, Y. FUJIOKA, Y. SAITO & T. AOKI. 1993. A study of trientine therapy in Wilson's disease with neurological symptoms. Brain Dev. **25:** 429–434.

20. TABACHNIK, M., H. N. EISEN & B. LEVIN. 1954. A new mixed disulfide: penicillamine-cysteine. Nature **174:** 701–702.

21. BEVER, C. T., JR., H. W. CHANG, A. S. PENN, I. A. JAFFE & E. BOCK. 1982. Penicillamine-induced myasthenia gravis: effects of penicillamine on acetylcholine receptor. Neurology **32:** 1077–1082.

22. KAO, P. N. & A. KARLIN. 1986. Acetylcholine receptor binding site contains a disulfide cross-link between adjacent half-cystinyl residues. J. Biol. Chem. **261:** 8085–8088.

23. XU, Q., R. H. FAIRCLOUGH & D. P. RICHMAN. 1993. Effects of D-penicillamine on multiple immunogenic epitopes of the acetylcholine receptor. Ann. N.Y. Acad. Sci. **681:** 335–338.

24. COLEMAN, J. W., A. L. FOSTER, J. H. YEUNG & B. K. PARK. 1988. Drug-protein conjugates—XV. A study of the disposition of D-penicillamine in the rat and its relationship to immunogenicity. Biochem. Pharmacol. **37:** 737–742.

25. DONKER, A. J., R. C. VENUTO, A. O. VLADUTIU, J. R. BRENTJENS & G. A. ADRES. 1984. Effects of prolonged administration of D-penicillamine or captopril in various strains of rats. Clin. Immunol. Immunopathol. **30:** 142–155.

26. TOURNADE, H., L. PELLETIER, R. PASQUIER, M. C. VIAL, C. MANDET & P. DRUET. 1990. D-Penicillamine-induced autoimmunity in Brown-Norway rats: similarities with $HgCl_2$-induced autoimmunity. J. Immunol. **144:** 2985–2991.

27. MONESTIER, M., K. E. NOVICK & M. J. LOSMAN. 1994. D-Penicillamine- and quinidine-induced antinuclear antibodies in A.SW (H-2s) mice: similarities with autoantibodies in spontaneous and heavy metal–induced autoimmunity. Eur. J. Immunol. **24:** 723–730.

28. BEVER, C. T., JR., K. L. DRETCHEN, G. J. BLAKE, H. W. CHANG, A. S. PENN & R. ASOFSKY. 1984. Augmented anti-acetylcholine receptor response following long-term penicillamine administration. Ann. Neurol. **16:** 9–13.

29. BURRES, S. A., M. E. KANTER, D. P. RICHMAN & B. G. ARNASON. 1981. Studies on the pathophysiology of chronic D-penicillamine-induced myasthenia. Ann. N.Y. Acad. Sci. **377:** 640–651.

30. HURTENBACH, U., H. GLEICHMANN, N. NAGATA & E. GLEICHMANN. 1987. Immunity to D-penicillamine: genetic, cellular, and chemical requirements for induction of popliteal lymph node enlargement in the mouse. J. Immunol. **139:** 411–416.

31. ISHII, N. 1988. Genetic control of delayed-type hypersensitivity to D-penicillamine antigen. Int. Arch. Allergy Appl. Immunol. **85:** 150–153.

32. NAGATA, N., U. HURTENBACH & E. GLEICHMANN. 1986. Specific sensitization of Lyt-1+2– T cells to spleen cells modified by the drug D-penicillamine or a stereoisomer. J. Immunol. **136:** 136–142.

33. O'DONNELL, C. A. & J. W. COLEMAN. 1992. A T-cell response to the anti-arthritic drug penicillamine in the mouse: requirements for generation of the drug-derived antigen. Immunology **76:** 604–609.

34. PENN, A. S. & J. J. JACQUES. 1993. Cells from mice exposed chronically to D-penicillamine show proliferative responses to D-penicillamine-treated self (macrophage/dendritic cells): a graft-versus-host response? Ann. N.Y. Acad. Sci. **681:** 319–322.

35. FOSTER, A. L., B. K. PARK & J. W. COLEMAN. 1987. A specific enzyme-linked immunosorbent assay for definition of the IgG antibody response to disulphide-conjugated D-penicillamine in the rabbit. Int. Arch. Allergy Appl. Immunol. **84:** 271–276.

36. YEUNG, J. H., J. W. COLEMAN & B. K. PARK. 1985. Drug-protein conjugates—IX. Immunogenicity of captopril-protein conjugates. Biochem. Pharmacol. **34:** 4005–4012.

37. LOW, B. & P. CORFIELD. 1985. Alpha-toxin binding site—theoretical and model studies. Asia Pac. J. Pharmacol. **2:** 115–127.

38. BEVER, C. T., JR. & R. ASOFSKY. 1985. Augmented IgG anti-acetylcholine receptor response following chronic penicillamine administration. J. Neuroimmunol. **35:** 131–137.

39. CHANG, H. & E. BOCK. 1979. Structural stabilization of isolated acetylcholine receptor: specific interaction with phospholipids. Biochemistry **18:** 172–179.

40. PENN, A., H. CHANG, R. LOVELACE, W. NIEMI & A. MIRANDA. 1976. Antibodies to acetylcholine receptor in rabbits: immunological and electrophysiological studies. Ann. N.Y. Acad. Sci. **274:** 354–396.

41. NIMNI, M. E. 1977. Mechanism of inhibition of collagen crosslinking by penicillamine. Proc. R. Soc. Med. **70:** 65–72.

42. SOLIVAN, B. C., D. J. LANGE, A. S. PENN, D. YOUNGER, A. JARETZKI III, R. E. LOVELACE & L. P. ROWLAND. 1988. Seronegative myasthenia gravis. Neurology **38:** 514–517.

43. WASSERMAN, N., A. PENN, P. FREIMUTH, N. TREPTOW, S. WENTZEL, W. CLEVELAND & B. ERLANGER. 1982. Anti-idiotypic route to antiacetylcholine receptor antibodies and experimental myasthenia gravis. Proc. Natl. Acad. Sci. U.S.A. **79:** 4810–4814.

44. SHEEHAN, J. C. & D. D. H. YANG. 1958. The use of *N*-formylamino acids in peptide synthesis. J. Am. Chem. Soc. **80:** 1154.

45. CARLSSON, J., H. DREVIN & R. AXEN. 1978. Protein thiolation and reversible protein-protein conjugation: succinimidyl 3-(2-pyridyldithio)propionate, a new bifunctional reagent. Biochem. J. **173:** 723–737.

46. PENN, A. S., R. MITTLER, L. S. LEVINSOHN & B. W. LOW. 1988. T-cell epitope recognized in acetylcholine receptor alpha-toxin binding site. Ann. Neurol. **24:** 162–163.

47. CORRADIN, G., H. M. ETLINGER & J. M. CHILLER. 1977. Lymphocyte specificity to protein antigens. I. Characterization of the antigen-induced *in vitro* T cell–dependent proliferative response with lymph node cells from primed mice. J. Immunol. **119:** 1048–1053.

48. CLICK, R., L. BENCK & B. ALTER. 1972. Immune responses *in vitro*. I. Culture conditions for antibody synthesis. Cell. Immunol. **3:** 264–276.

49. KOZHICH, A. T., R. R. CASPI, J. A. BERZOFSKY & I. GERY. 1997. Immunogenicity and immunopathogenicity of an autoimmune epitope are potentiated by increasing MHC binding through residue substitution. J. Immunol. **158:** 4145–4151.

50. MIKSZTA, J. A. & B. S. KIM. 1996. Conversion of low antibody responders into high responders by up-regulating the T cell response to a selective epitope. J. Immunol. **157:** 2883–2890.

51. LEHMANN, P. V., T. FORSTHUBER, A. MILLER & E. E. SERCARZ. 1992. Spreading of T cell autoimmunity to cryptic determinants of an autoantigen. Nature **358:** 155–157.

52. MILICH, D. R., A. MCLACHLAN, A. MORIARTY & G. B. THORNTON. 1987. A single 10-residue pre-S(1) peptide can prime T cell help for antibody production to multiple epitopes within the pre-S(1), pre-S(2), and S regions of HBsAg. J. Immunol. **138:** 4457–4465.

Antibody Effector Mechanisms in Myasthenia Gravis

The Complement Hypothesis[a]

DAVID P. RICHMAN,[b] MARK A. AGIUS,[b] CHRISTINE A. KIRVAN,[b,c]
CHRISTOPHER M. GOMEZ,[d] ROBERT H. FAIRCLOUGH,[b]
BONITA L. DUPONT,[b,e] AND RICARDO A. MASELLI[b]

[b]Department of Neurology
and
Center for Neuroscience
University of California, Davis
Davis, California 95616

[d]Department of Neurology
University of Minnesota
Minneapolis, Minnesota 55455

Myasthenia gravis (MG) and experimental autoimmune myasthenia gravis (EAMG) are autoimmune diseases in which disordered neuromuscular transmission is the result of autoantibody-induced damage to the acetylcholine receptor (AChR)–containing postsynaptic end plate membrane. While an anti-AChR T cell response (primarily CD4+ cells) is crucial in MG and EAMG, the role of these cells appears to be solely to provide help to the antibody-producing B cells. We have used monoclonal antibodies (mAbs) to study the antibody effector mechanisms involved in disease pathogenesis. A wide array of data suggests that the major mechanism involves very efficient complement activation as a result of antibodies bound to the very densely packed (almost crystalline) AChR molecules normally present in the peaks of the end plate synaptic folds. To test the predominant role of complement activation in the pathogenesis of MG and EAMG, we have examined a number of model systems in which complement activation is absent or reduced. Because these systems involve a number of possibly confounding variables, we have engineered recombinant/hybrid antibodies with modified C_H regions that poorly fix complement, with the goal of testing the ability of these antibodies to induce EAMG or to prevent the disease induced by antibodies that are effective in activating complement.

IMMUNOPATHOGENESIS OF MYASTHENIA GRAVIS

Myasthenia gravis (MG) is an acquired autoimmune disease of neuromuscular transmission in which the postsynaptic nicotinic acetylcholine receptor (AChR) is

[a]This work was supported in part by grants from the National Institutes of Health (Nos. NS15462, NS19779, NS24304, and NS01226) and the Muscular Dystrophy Association.
[c]Recipient of a Viets Fellowship from the Myasthenia Gravis Foundation.
[e]Recipient of an Osserman Fellowship from the Myasthenia Gravis Foundation.

the target of the immune attack. Crucial to the identification of this pathogenic process was the serendipitous observation of Patrick and Lindstrom[1] that rabbits immunized with AChR purified from the electric organ of the electric eel developed a disease similar to MG. In fact, subsequent analysis demonstrated that the experimental disease is identical to human MG in nearly every aspect examined.[2,3] The immunized animals produce high levels of antibodies against the fish electric organ AChR, as well as somewhat lower levels of antibodies directed against their own muscle AChRs. The animal disease, which is inducible in many mammalian species, was later named experimental autoimmune myasthenia gravis (EAMG) by Lennon and colleagues.[4] This model of MG has yielded extremely useful information concerning the precise pathogenic mechanisms operative in the human disease and has provided an efficient means of testing new treatments.

In addition to the antibody response noted above, circulating T cells reactive with AChR are present in both human MG and EAMG.[5–8] Remarkably, whereas there is considerable destruction of the AChR-containing postsynaptic membrane of the neuromuscular junction, along with macrophage infiltration (see below), T cells have only rarely been identified at this site.[9] The circulating autoimmune T cells, primarily of the CD4 phenotype,[8,10–12] are crucial for the autoimmune response in MG and EAMG, but appear to exer. their effects only by providing help to the autoimmune B cells.[9–12]

AChR, the target antigen, is a classical allosteric protein. Its function is to translate the binding energy of two molecules of acetylcholine (ACh) into a conformational change in the AChR that results in the opening of a cationic channel. Hence, the tertiary structure of the AChR is crucial to its function. It is a transmembrane glycoprotein comprising five subunits, $\alpha_2\beta\gamma\delta$ or $\alpha_2\beta\gamma\varepsilon$. Each subunit spans the membrane, with the majority of its mass in the extracellular (synaptic) environment, along with a small cytoplasmic tail. The two ACh binding sites are each located on the synaptic portions of each α-subunit.[13]

In both the human and animal diseases, immunodominant AChR epitopes play the major role in pathogenesis. In humans and in inbred rats and mice—the most highly studied hosts for EAMG—these epitopes are primarily located on the extracellular portion of the AChR. Most involve the α-subunits, but at sites distinct from the ACh-binding sites.

It is noteworthy that the immunodominant epitopes for B cells (antibody-binding epitopes) and for T cells are distinct. Those for B cells appear to be more restricted than those for T cells. They are identified by the binding of autoantibody and are, therefore, conformational; that is, the three-dimensional structure of the epitope within the native AChR molecule defines the site's antigenicity. This situation contrasts with T cell epitopes, which in the course of the immune response are processed within antigen-presenting cells into small linear peptide segments bound to major histocompatibility complex (MHC) molecules. The primary immunodominant epitope for antibody, the so-called main immunogenic region (MIR) identified originally by Tzartos and Lindstrom,[14,15] comprises α67–76. In both human and rodent myasthenia, about 50% of anti-AChR antibodies appear to bind to this extracellular region (see references 14 and 16) of the α-subunit. Other epitopes on the extracellular surface of the AChR also appear to play varying roles as targets of the autoantibodies.

The dominant T cell epitopes have been studied in both human MG and a number of animal models. In inbred C57BL6 mice, which have been most carefully studied, the epitopes involved are α111–126, α146–162, α182–198, and α360–378.[17–19] In humans, segments α48–67, α101–137, α304–322, and α403–437 appear to be strongly recognized by T cells from most patients with MG, regardless of their MHC (HLA) expression.[10,20]

ANTIBODIES AS IMMUNE EFFECTORS

The antibody molecule may be considered as a bridge between the target antigen molecule and the effector machinery of the immune system (FIGURE 1). One side of the bridge, the front end (Fab fragment) of the molecule, precisely identifies the corresponding three-dimensional epitope. This exquisite sensitivity is encoded in the variable regions of the light and heavy chains of the antibody molecule. The three-dimensional antigenic structures targeted by the tertiary structure of this combined variable region define the B cell epitopes. Even minor modifications of this front end of the antibody molecule are likely to have significant effects on the autoimmune at-

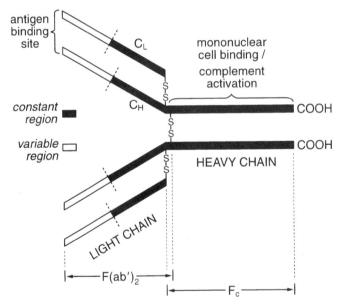

FIGURE 1. An antibody molecule (IgG) can be considered as a bridge between the target antigen and the inflammatory components of the immune system. It comprises two heavy and two light chains joined by disulfide bonds. Antigen binding occurs in the variable region and binding to the inflammatory components occurs through the constant region of the heavy chain.

tack and the resulting disease. In MG, a significant proportion of the autoantibodies are directed against the MIR. The role of the T cell–dominant epitopes in targeting the MIR is unknown, especially in the situation that occurs in MG and EAMG in which T cells are not present at the site of the antibody attack.

The present analysis will primarily focus on the other side of the "bridge", the back end of the antibody molecule consisting of the constant region of the heavy chain (Fc region). This so-called effector region of the molecule induces its effects through the binding of inflammatory elements of the immune system: complement and inflammatory cells. Activation of the classical complement cascade is initiated by binding of complement component Clq to its receptor in the Fc portion of the antibody molecule. This occurs at residues 231–238, 279–295, and 318–331 of the heavy chain (FIGURE 1).[21–28] Fc interaction with inflammatory cells occurs through the direct binding of Fc to Fc receptors (FcR) in the plasma membrane. The FcR binding regions of the Fc are relatively well defined. For example, the macrophage FcR binding site involves primarily residues 234–237 and 331.[29,30]

Clq binding by Fc leads to activation of the classical complement pathway cascade with resultant production of chemoattractants for macrophages and the eventual production of membrane attack complexes (MAC). The latter molecules, released in the vicinity of the membrane-bound antigen, result in destruction of the membrane and, if the membrane attack is strong enough, cell lysis. Binding of the attracted macrophages to the Fc portion of bound antibody leads to their activation, to release of cytokines, and subsequently to target cell lysis, cell death, and phagocytosis.[31]

MONOCLONAL ANTIBODIES AS MODELS OF ANTI-AChR ANTIBODY EFFECTOR ACTIVITY IN MG AND EAMG

We have made use of monoclonal antibodies (mAbs) as model antibody systems. Each mAb is a single antibody molecule with a single set of front-end and back-end functions (FIGURE 1). Our goal has been to use these molecules to elucidate the sequence of events that occurs in MG and EAMG. The mAbs can be selected or modified to express various combinations of characteristics, and the ability of each characteristic to effect complement binding or macrophage binding and activation can be determined *in vitro*. With that information, mAbs can then be used *in vivo* to analyze the effect of individual antibody characteristics on disease development.

In MG and EAMG, a number of investigators have identified three major effector mechanisms by which anti-AChR antibodies appear to induce altered neuromuscular transmission.[32–35] The first mechanism involves solely front-end function of the anti-AChR antibodies. In this instance, the antibodies function as chemical inhibitors (competitive or noncompetitive) of ACh binding. Those antibodies with variable regions directed against the ACh-binding sites on the α-subunits, or to other sites that otherwise effect ACh binding, or to sites involved in the chain of events in the AChR molecule leading from ACh binding to channel opening, may all have the similar result of blocking AChR function and thereby blocking neuromuscular transmission.[36–40] The second mechanism, referred to as AChR modulation, also involves front-end function alone. It is a consequence of the bivalent nature of the $F(ab')_2$ portion of the antibody molecule (FIGURE 1). Antibody molecules, at conditions of antigen excess, are able to cross-link adjacent AChR molecules in the muscle end plate membrane. The cross-linking has been demonstrated to increase the rate of AChR turnover in the membrane, resulting in a lowered steady-state concentration of AChR.[32,36,38,41] The third mechanism involves back-end function, that is, complement fixation leading to end plate membrane lysis. A large number of studies in MG and EAMG have demonstrated an important role for this effector mechanism.[33,35,42–52] The associated role of macrophages in this inflammatory process has been more controversial.[42–45,47,48,53]

A considerable body of information analyzing each of these mechanisms has accumulated making use of mAbs. For mAbs directed against the ACh-binding site, inhibition of ACh binding has been of both the competitive and noncompetitive type.[40] These mAbs block ACh-induced opening of the AChR ion channel *in vitro*.[40] *In vivo*, these mAbs produce an extremely severe form of EAMG, coming on within an hour of injection of the mAb (FIGURE 2).[37] Hence, antibodies directed against functionally important sites on the AChR are capable of inducing severe MG. In the human disease, and to some extent in the form of EAMG induced by active immunization with antigen, the proportion of the circulating antibodies directed against these sites is relatively low.[38,39]

A number of investigators have demonstrated *in vitro* that anti-AChR antibodies induce antigenic modulation. Most have made use of polyclonal anti-AChR serum and have observed a 2–3-fold increase in the rate of AChR turnover in the mem-

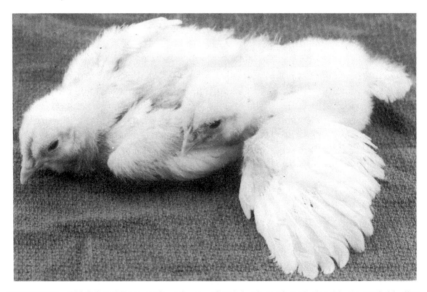

FIGURE 2. Chick hatchlings at three hours after injection of mAb that blocks ACh binding. Both animals were extremely weak and unable to right themselves. Both eventually died. (Reprinted from reference 37 with permission of the authors.)

branes of cultured myotubes and in muscle cell lines.[36,38,41] In one previous *in vivo* study[54] in which only clinical weakness was assessed, injection of bivalent $F(ab')_2$ fragments of an mAb directed against the MIR portion of the α-subunit induced a mild form of EAMG. In contrast, injections of intact mAb caused severe passive transfer EAMG.

The third pathogenic mechanism also has been studied through the use of syngeneic mAbs to induce the passive transfer form of EAMG.[47,55,56] When most intact mAbs directed against the extracellular portion of the AChR are injected into syngeneic animals, weakness develops about 48 hours after injection and peaks at 72 hours. Electrophysiologic analysis demonstrates disordered neuromuscular transmission typical of MG. Histologically, there is destruction of muscle end plate membrane with frank necrosis of the entire end plate. The membrane debris in the synaptic cleft contains IgG and complement components, including MAC,[34] and the end plate is infiltrated with activated macrophages. After 72 hours, the clinical disease gradually improves, along with clearing of the inflammation at the end plates and re-formation of the synapses, but with simplified end plate membranes.[48] In animals either deficient in[50] or depleted of[49,51] complement, the passive transfer disease cannot be induced. It should be noted that, in this situation, intact anti-AChR mAb is injected and, hence, its ability to increase AChR turnover should remain intact. The explanation for the conflicting results concerning the role of AChR turnover in these two systems, ineffective complement cascade components versus inability of the $F(ab')_2$ fragments to initiate activation of the cascade, is unclear. In addition, the efficacy of an antibody for complement fixation appears to be crucial to its potential to induce the passive transfer form of EAMG. We have previously studied a group of mAbs that bind AChR with equal affinity. These mAbs varied in their potency in inducing EAMG, with strong correlation with their ability to fix complement (FIGURE 3).[52]

As noted above, the passive transfer form of EAMG is associated with a considerable degree of macrophage infiltration of the neuromuscular junction.[47,48] In the human disease, such infiltration has been more difficult to demonstrate. However, focal inflammatory infiltrates in muscle have been observed in MG as early as 1905 by Buzzard. He referred to these lesions as "lymphorrhages", but the nature of the mononuclear infiltrating cells was not determined.[57] Such collections of cells have been reported a number of times since Buzzard's original observation,[58,59] but the relationship of these lesions to neuromuscular junctions remained unknown.

More recently, Pascuzzi and colleagues[60] have been able to examine a lymphorrhage lesion in more detail. Cholinesterase staining determined that the inflammatory cell collections were in fact at neuromuscular junctions. In a more extensive study of the neuromuscular junction in MG patients, making use of material from anconeus muscle biopsies, we have been able to observe cellular infiltration at about 30% of neuromuscular junctions. However, the number of infiltrating cells was considerably less than those seen in passive transfer EAMG or in a typical lymphorrhage. Analogous to the lesions in EAMG, we were able to identify the cells infiltrating the neuromuscular junctions as macrophages.[53]

In passive transfer EAMG, during the period of recovery from the acute phase of the disease, the animals are refractory to a second episode of the acute disease, whether they are injected with the same mAb or a different mAb directed against a

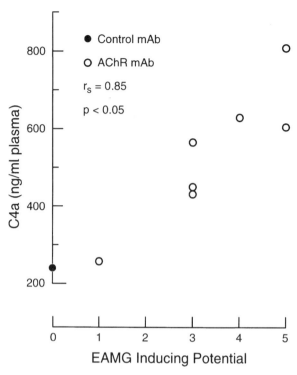

FIGURE 3. Correlation of ability of anti-AChR mAbs to fix complement with their potency for inducing passive transfer EAMG. Generation of complement component C4a by various mAb/AChR complexes was assessed[52] for a series of anti-AChR mAbs of varying disease-inducing potencies determined by the clinical severity of EAMG, as defined in TABLE 2, induced by a standard dose of mAb.[52]

site in the AChR molecule distant from the target of the first mAb.[61] This refractory state correlates with a simplified end plate membrane and with the associated reduction in density of packing of the AChRs in the end plate membrane.[62] In the normal neuromuscular junction, AChR molecules are concentrated at the peaks of the end plate folds, which are in apposition to the active zones (sites of ACh release) in the nerve terminal. The AChRs in the peaks of the folds are packed at a nearly crystalline density of 10^4 per μm^2. It is a reasonable hypothesis that the binding of anti-AChR antibody to the tightly packed AChRs in this location results in very high density of bound antibody and, hence, very tightly packed Fc ends of these antibodies.[49,61–63] The hypothesis proposes that the very high density of bound Fc segments results in highly efficient activation of complement and, hence, the production of large concentrations of both chemoattractants and MAC. It is the high concentration of these two products that causes the severe end plate membrane damage and the macrophage infiltration characteristic of the acute phase of the passive transfer disease. In the recovery from the acute phase, the AChR density lags behind. When these recovering end plates with lower densities of AChR are reexposed to anti-AChR antibodies, the bound antibody fails to lead to a sufficiently high concentration of Fc segments to produce the highly efficient complement activation required for the acute form of the disease.

THE COMPLEMENT HYPOTHESIS IN MG

Our current hypothesis is that anti-AChR antibodies in MG and EAMG induce their major effects on neuromuscular transmission through complement-induced end plate membrane damage and the induced infiltration of macrophages. Support for this hypothesis has been derived from a number of studies of the form of passive transfer EAMG induced by injection of mAbs or modified mAbs. All of these studies have made use of mAbs derived from Lewis rats immunized with AChR purified from fish electric organ. Many of the mAbs cross-react with chicken muscle AChR.[64] When these particular rat mAbs are injected into chickens, only those that block AChR function induce clinical signs of EAMG (FIGURE 2) or disordered neuromuscular transmission.[37] Because of species differences, none of the rat mAbs is capable of binding chicken complement or inducing host macrophage infiltration.[37] However, these intact mAbs are capable of cross-linking chicken AChRs and inducing AChR turnover. Hence, in the case of rat mAbs injected into chickens, increased AChR turnover is not sufficient to produce the clinical, electrophysiologic, or histologic findings of EAMG.

A similar set of passive transfer experiments were carried out using the rat mAbs injected into guinea pigs. We and others have determined that rat IgG2a antibody does not fix guinea pig complement, whereas it is quite potent in fixing rat complement (TABLE 1). Rat IgG2b fixes guinea pig complement as well as it fixes rat complement. We made use of an anti-MIR rat mAb, 132A, of the IgG2a subclass, that

TABLE 1. Ability of Various mAbs Complexed to Membrane-bound AChR to Fix Guinea Pig Complement

Ig Subclass	Anti-AChR mAb	% Hemolysis of Indicator Cells[a]
IgG2a	132A	80 ± 4[b]
IgG2a	152A	84 ± 7
IgG2a	249E	84 ± 6
IgG2a	370	82 ± 9
IgG2b	371A	6 ± 1
IgG2b	421H	6 ± 1
IgG2b	387D	7 ± 0
—	none (AChR alone)	87 ± 4

[a]In this CH_{50} assay, immune complexes are incubated for 1 h at room temperature with guinea pig plasma to deplete complement. The amount of complement remaining is determined by the addition of indicator RBCs, and the quantitation of RBC lysis by OD_{410} reading of the supernatant. The % hemolysis is relative to the total lysis obtained with addition of distilled water to the RBCs.

[b]Mean ± SD of triplicate determinations.

vigorously activates rat complement and induces very severe passive transfer EAMG in rats. This mAb, which cross-reacts with guinea pig AChR, in doses as high as 20 mg/kg, was incapable of inducing EAMG in guinea pigs, as determined clinically and electrophysiologically and by biochemical and histologic analysis of AChR content and AChR density. In contrast, an IgG2b anti-MIR mAb of equal potency in inducing rat EAMG induced very severe disease in guinea pigs at doses of 6 mg/kg.

A third study was carried out in Lewis rats,[65] comparing the ability of F(ab')$_2$ fragments of mAb 132A to induce passive transfer EAMG with the ability of intact mAb 132A to induce disease. Two groups of animals were analyzed clinically, electrophysiologically, and histologically (TABLE 2). The first group received intact mAb 132A. The second group received an equal dose of 132A F(ab')$_2$ fragments. All the animals injected with intact 132A mAb developed moderate to severe EAMG. None of the animals injected with F(ab')$_2$ fragments of mAb 132A developed any evidence of EAMG. Hence, in this experimental system, F(ab')$_2$ fragments of mAb 132A, which are capable of inducing increased AChR turnover, did not induce clinical, electrophysiological, or histological evidence of EAMG.

In a second experiment, one group of animals received intact mAb 132A alone, while a second group received a simultaneous injection of 132A F(ab')$_2$ fragments (FIGURE 4). In threefold excess, the F(ab')$_2$ fragments completely blocked the induc-

TABLE 2. Inability of 132A F(ab')$_2$ to Induce Acute Passive Transfer EAMG

Rat Number	Weight (g)	Dose of F(ab')$_2$ (nmol/kg)	Dose of Intact 132A (nmol/kg)	Clinical Score[a]	EMG (% Decrement)	End Plate Inflammation[b]
1	156	20	0	0	0	−
2	156	20	0	0	0	−
3	177	20	0	0	0	−
4	178	20	0	0	0	−
5	144	33	0	0	0	−
6	154	33	0	0	0	−
7	159	33	0	0	0	−
8	171	60	0	0	0	−
9	175	80	0	0	0	−
10	150	0	20	3	34	+
11	152	0	20	4	59	+
13	156	0	20	5	ND	+
14	162	0	20	4	44	+
15	170	0	20	4	46	+
16	176	0	20	4	50	+
17	180	0	20	3	71	+
18	161	0	26.6	5	ND	+
19	170	0	26.6	3	65	+
20	170	0	26.6	3	46	+
21	176	0	26.6	3	31	+

[a]1 = weak grip, 2 = abnormal gait, 3 = inability to walk, 4 = inability to stand, 5 = death within the first 48 h.
[b]+ = present; − = absent.

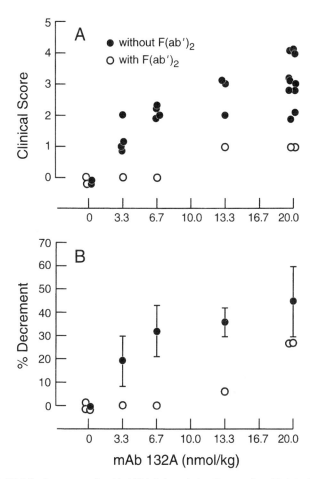

FIGURE 4. $F(ab')_2$ fragments of mAb 132A injected simultaneously with intact mAb 132A block development of passive transfer EAMG when given in at least threefold excess. Development of disease was determined by (A) clinical score (see TABLE 2) and (B) decremental response to repetitive nerve stimulation (see reference 47). Female Lewis rats, 180–220 g, injected simultaneously (open circles) with 20 nmol/kg of $F(ab')_2$ fragments and various doses of intact mAb, were assessed at 48 h after injection. Control animals (filled circles) were injected only with intact 132A mAb.

tion of EAMG by intact mAb. The latter results suggest that $F(ab')_2$ fragments of mAb 132A are not only unable to induce EAMG, but are capable of blocking the binding of intact mAb 132A and preventing the disease induced by the intact antibody. If the complement hypothesis holds, then anti-AChR antibodies, modified to eliminate the ability to fix complements, may be effective in treating EAMG and perhaps human MG.

The results described above contrast with those of Loutrari *et al.*[54] in which F(ab')$_2$ derived from an anti-MIR mAb was injected into Lewis rats. One distinction between this study and the one described above was the means of analyzing the EAMG induced. The Loutrari study[54] made use solely of the clinical findings in the injected animals, whereas the study described above assessed histologic and electrophysiologic parameters as well. One difficulty common to both studies is the short half-life, about 5–6 hours, of the injected F(ab')$_2$ fragments.[52,54] The discrepancy between the results of the two studies, along with the confounding variable of the rapid clearance of the F(ab')$_2$ fragments from the circulation, has led us to focus on intact antibody molecules in which the ability to activate complement has been modified. The studies described above using IgG2a and IgG2b rat mAbs injected into guinea pigs, as well as the multiple studies involving animals depleted of complement components or deficient in individual components,[49–51] are examples of this type of experiment. Since these studies all make use of intact anti-AChR antibodies, the question of rapid antibody clearance is eliminated. On the other hand, each of them involves changes in the host (recipient animals) that raise the possibility of other confounding variables.

To most directly address these questions, we have embarked on a study using modified, but intact, syngeneic anti-AChR mAbs. We are developing recombinant/ hybrid antibodies by genetically engineering the heavy chain of the anti-MIR rat mAb, 132A (see reference 66; also Kirvan, Richman, and Agius, manuscript in preparation). The strategy is to exchange the γ2a constant region of the heavy chain of this mAb, which fixes rat complement very effectively, with a γ1 rat heavy chain constant region, which fixes complement poorly. This effort makes use of our previously cloned and sequenced heavy and light chain cDNAs[67] of mAb 132A and a genomic clone of the rat γ1 heavy chain constant region. We have successfully constructed both the hybrid 132A-γ1 heavy chain gene and the wild-type 132A-γ2a heavy chain gene, cloned into heavy chain rat expression vectors, for example, pAH3504 and pBK-RSV.[66] The intact mAb 132A light chain cDNA has also been cloned into a rat light chain expression vector, pBK-pZeoSV.[66] The heavy and light chain vectors in various combinations have been doubly transfected into lymphoblastoid cell lines, which then express either unmodified "wild-type" mAb 132A of IgG2a subclass or the recombinant/hybrid 132A mAb of IgG1 subclass. The intact mAbs produced by these transfected lines have the *in vitro* properties predicted (TABLE 3) and should enable us to definitively test the complement hypothesis and

TABLE 3. *In Vitro* Characteristics of Recombinant/Hybrid 132A Antibodies[66]

Cell Line	AChR Binding	Anti-Id Binding	Heavy Chain Subclass[a]	Light Chain
132A hybridoma	+	+	IgG2a	κ
Control hybrid (132A-γ2a)	+	+	IgG2a	κ
Hybrid (132A-γ1)	+	+	IgG1	κ

[a]Determined using a panel of subclass-specific goat anti-rat antisera.

the ability of the recombinant/hybrid mAb to block the disease-inducing wild-type antibody.

CONCLUSIONS

The anti-AChR mAbs have been quite useful in dissecting the individual pathogenic mechanisms in MG and EAMG by which these antibody-induced diseases occur. It is the single set of characteristics that each mAb possesses that has permitted these analyses. The mAbs available in our library have been essentially randomly selected. We have chosen mAbs to study from the library that have a set of front-end and back-end characteristics that will be useful to address particular questions concerning MG pathogenesis. The recombinant technology now allows us to go beyond the limitations of using randomly produced mAbs. Rather, we can rationally produce mAbs with the required characteristics to address individual questions. In spite of the limitations of these transfected cell lines in producing large quantities of the recombinant/hybrid mAbs, the precision of analysis that they permit represents a significant advance in the ability to identify the crucial steps in the antibody pathogenesis of MG and to better treat the disease by rationally blocking those steps.

The data from a number of studies from our group and from other investigators suggest that the major pathogenic mechanisms active in MG depend on vigorous complement activation, which is a consequence of autoantibody binding to the very densely packed antigen (AChR) at the peaks of the folds of the postsynaptic membrane.

REFERENCES

1. PATRICK, J. & J. LINDSTROM. 1973. Autoimmune response to acetylcholine receptor. Science **180:** 871–872.
2. DRACHMAN, D. B. 1994. Myasthenia gravis. N. Engl. J. Med. **330:** 1797–1810.
3. RICHMAN, D. P. & M. A. AGIUS. 1994. Acquired myasthenia gravis: immunopathology. Neurol. Clin. North Am. **12:** 273–284.
4. LENNON, V. A., J. M. LINDSTROM & M. E. SEYBOLD. 1975. Experimental autoimmune myasthenia gravis (EAMG): a model of myasthenia gravis in rats and guinea pigs. J. Exp. Med. **141:** 1365–1375.
5. ABRAMSKY, O., A. AHARONOV, D. TEITELBAUM *et al.* 1975. Myasthenia gravis and acetylcholine receptor: effect of steroids in clinical course and cellular immune response to acetylcholine receptor. Arch. Neurol. **32:** 684–687.
6. RICHMAN, D. P., J. PATRICK & B. G. W. ARNASON. 1976. Cellular immunity in myasthenia gravis: response to purified acetylcholine receptor and autologous thymocytes. N. Engl. J. Med. **294:** 694–698.
7. HOHLFELD, R., I. KALIES, B. KOHLEISEN, K. HEININGER, B. CONTI-TRONCONI & K. TOYKA. 1986. Myasthenia gravis: stimulation of antireceptor autoantibodies by autoreactive T cell lines. Neurology **36:** 618–621.
8. PROTTI, M. P., A. A. MANFREDI, C. STRAUB, J. F. J. HOWARD & B. M. CONTI-TRONCONI.

1990. CD4+ T cell response to the human acetylcholine receptor alpha subunit in myasthenia gravis: a study with synthetic peptides. J. Immunol. **144:** 1276–1281.

9. NAKANO, S. & A. G. ENGEL. 1993. Myasthenia gravis: quantitative immunocytochemical analysis of inflammatory cells and detection of membrane attack complex at the endplate in 30 patients. Neurology **43:** 1167–1172.

10. CONTI-TRONCONI, B. M. *et al.* 1994. The nicotinic acetylcholine receptor: structure and autoimmune pathology. Crit. Rev. Biochem. Mol. Biol. **29:** 69–123.

11. ZHENG, G., B. XIAO, M. BAKHIET, P. MEIDE, H. WIGZELL, H. LINK & T. OLSSON. 1996. Both CD4$^+$ and CD8$^+$ T cells are essential to induce experimental autoimmune myasthenia gravis. J. Exp. Med. **184:** 349.

12. AHLBERG, R. *et al.* 1994. Treatment of myasthenia gravis with anti-CD4$^+$ antibody: improvement correlates to decreased T-cell autoreactivity. Neurology **44:** 1732–1737.

13. KARLIN, A. & M. AKABAS. 1995. Toward a structural basis for the function of nicotinic acetylcholine receptors and their cousins. Neuron **15:** 1231–1244.

14. TZARTOS, S., M. SEYBOLD & J. LINDSTROM. 1982. Specificity of antibodies to acetylcholine receptors in sera from myasthenia gravis patients measured by monoclonal antibodies. Proc. Natl. Acad. Sci. U.S.A. **79:** 188–192.

15. TZARTOS, S., M. CUNG, P. DEMANGE, H. LOUTRARI, A. MAMALAKI, M. MARRAUD, I. PAPADOUII, C. SAKARELLOS & V. TSIKARIS. 1991. The main immunogenic region (MIR) of the nicotinic acetylcholine receptor and the anti-MIR antibodies. Mol. Neurobiol. **5:** 1–29.

16. LENNON, V. A. & G. E. GRIESMANN. 1989. Evidence against acetylcholine receptor having a main immunogenic region as target for autoantibodies in myasthenia gravis. Neurology **39:** 1069–1076.

17. YOKOI, T., B. MULAC-JERICEVIC, J. KURISAKI & M. Z. ATASSI. 1987. T lymphocyte recognition of acetylcholine receptor: localization of the full T cell recognition profile on the extracellular part of the α chain of *Torpedo californica* acetylcholine receptor. Eur. J. Immunol. **17:** 1697.

18. BELLONE, M., N. OSTLIE, S. LEI & B. M. CONTI-TRONCONI. 1991. Experimental myasthenia gravis in congenic mice: sequence mapping and H-2 restriction of T helper epitopes on the α subunits of *Torpedo californica* and murine acetylcholine receptors. Eur. J. Immunol. **21:** 2303.

19. SHENOY, M., E. GOLUSZKO & P. CHRISTADOSS. 1994. The pathogenic role of acetylcholine receptor alpha chain epitope within alpha 146–162 in the development of experimental autoimmune myasthenia gravis in C57BL6 mice. Clin. Immunol. Immunopathol. **73:** 338–343.

20. PROTTI, M. P. *et al.* 1993. Myasthenia gravis: recognition of a human autoantigen at the molecular level. Immunol. Today **14:** 363–368.

21. DORRINGTON, K. J. 1985. The functional differentiation of the Fc region of immunoglobulin G. Ann. Inst. Pasteur Immunol. **136C:** 260–263.

22. DUNCAN, A. R. & G. WINTER. 1988. The binding site for Clq on IgG. Nature **332:** 738–740.

23. CANFIELD, S. M. & S. L. MORRISON. 1991. The binding affinity of human IgG for its high affinity Fc receptor is determined by multiple amino acids in the C_H2 domain and is modulated by the hinge region. J. Exp. Med. **173:** 1483–1491.

24. LUND, J., J. D. POUND, P. T. JONES, A. R. DUNCAN, T. BENTLEY, M. GOODALL, B. A. LEVINE, R. JEFFERIS & G. WINTER. 1992. Multiple binding sites on the C_H2 domain of IgG for mouse FcγRII. Mol. Immunol. **29:** 53–59.

25. XU, Y., R. OOMEN & M. H. KLEIN. 1994. Residue at position 331 in the IgG1 and IgG4 CH2 domains contributes to their differential ability to bind and activate complement. J. Biol. Chem. **269:** 3469–3474.

26. Morgan, A., N. D. Jones, A. M. Nesbitt, L. Chaplin, M. W. Bodmer & J. S. Emtage. 1995. The N-terminal end of the CH2 domain of chimeric human IgG1 anti-HLA-DR is necessary for Clq, Fc gamma RI, and Fc gamma RIII binding. Immunology **86:** 319–324.

27. Ward, E. S. & V. Ghetie. 1995. The effector functions of immunoglobulins: implications for therapy. Ther. Immunol. **2:** 77–94.

28. Miletic, V. D. & M. M. Frank. 1995. Complement-immunoglobulin interactions. Curr. Opin. Immunol. **7:** 41–47.

29. Lund, J., G. Winter, P. T. Jones, J. D. Pound, T. Tanaka, M. R. Walker, P. J. Artymiuk, Y. Arata, D. R. Burton, R. Jefferis & J. J. Woof. 1991. Human FcγRI and FcγRII interact with distinct but overlapping sites on human IgG1. J. Immunol. **147:** 2657–2662.

30. Michaelsen, T. E., A. Aase, L. Norderhaug & I. Sandlie. 1992. Antibody dependent cell-mediated cytotoxicity induced by chimeric mouse-human IgG subclasses and IgG3 antibodies with altered hinge region. Mol. Immunol. **29:** 319–326.

31. Van Goor, H., G. Ding, D. Kees-Folts, J. Grond, G. F. Schreiner & J. R. Diamond. 1994. Macrophages and renal disease. Lab. Invest. **71:** 456–464.

32. Lindstrom, J., D. Shelton & Y. Fujii. 1988. Myasthenia gravis. Adv. Immunol. **12:** 233–284.

33. Engel, A. G. & G. Fumagalli. 1982. Mechanisms of acetylcholine receptor loss from the neuromuscular junction. Ciba Found. Symp. **90:** 197–224.

34. Engel, A. G. 1980. Morphological and immunopathological findings in myasthenia gravis and congenital myasthenic syndromes. J. Neurol. Neurosurg. Psychiatry **43:** 577.

35. Lindstrom, J. M., A. G. Engel, M. E. Seybold, V. A. Lennon & E. Lambert. 1976. Pathological mechanisms in experimental autoimmune myasthenia in rats with anti-acetylcholine receptor antibodies. J. Exp. Med. **144:** 739.

36. Bevan, S., R. W. Kuhlberg & S. F. Heinemann. 1977. Human myasthenia sera reduce acetylcholine sensitivity of human muscle cells in tissue culture. Nature **276:** 262.

37. Gomez, C. M. & D. P. Richman. 1983. Anti-acetylcholine receptor antibodies directed against the α-bungarotoxin binding site induce a unique form of experimental myasthenia. Proc. Natl. Acad. Sci. U.S.A. **80:** 4089–4093.

38. Drachman, D. B., R. N. Adams, L. F. Josifek & S. G. Self. 1982. Functional activities of auto-antibodies to acetylcholine receptors and the clinical severity of myasthenia gravis. N. Engl. J. Med. **307:** 769.

39. Pachner, A. R. 1989. Anti-acetylcholine receptor antibodies block bungarotoxin binding to native human acetylcholine receptor on the surface of TE671 cells. Neurology **39:** 1057–1061.

40. Mihovilovic, M., D. Donnelly-Roberts, D. P. Richman & M. Martinez-Carrion. 1994. Pathogenesis of hyperacute experimental autoimmune myasthenia gravis. J. Immunol. **152:** 5997–6002.

41. Kao, I. & D. Drachman. 1977. Myasthenic immunoglobulin accelerates acetylcholine receptor degradation. Science **196:** 526.

42. Lennon, V. A. *et al.* 1975. Experimental autoimmune myasthenia gravis (EAMG): a model of myasthenia gravis in rats and guinea pigs. J. Exp. Med. **141:** 1365.

43. Sohashi, K., A. Engel, J. Lindstrom & E. Lambert. 1978. Ultrastructural localization of immune complexes at the endplate in experimental autoimmune myasthenia gravis. J. Neuropathol. **37:** 212.

44. Gomez, C. M., D. P. Richman, P. W. Berman *et al.* 1979. Monoclonal antibodies against purified nicotinic acetylcholine receptor. Biochem. Biophys. Res. Commun. **88:** 575–582.

45. LENNON, V. A. & E. H. LAMBERT. 1980. Myasthenia gravis induced by monoclonal antibodies to acetylcholine receptors. Nature **285:** 238.
46. MOSHLY-ROSEN, D., S. FUCHS & Z. ESBHAR. 1979. Monoclonal antibodies against defined determinants of acetylcholine receptor. FEBS Lett. **106:** 389.
47. RICHMAN, D. P., C. M. GOMEZ, P. W. BERMAN *et al.* 1980. Monoclonal anti-acetylcholine receptor antibodies can cause experimental myasthenia. Nature **286:** 738.
48. GOMEZ, C. M., R. L. WOLLMANN & D. P. RICHMAN. 1984. Induction of the morphologic changes of both acute and chronic experimental myasthenia by monoclonal antibody directed against acetylcholine receptor. Acta Neuropathol. **63:** 131–143.
49. LENNON, V., M. SEYBOLD, J. LINDSTROM *et al.* 1978. Role of complement in the pathogenesis of experimental autoimmune myasthenia gravis. J. Exp. Med. **147:** 973–983.
50. CHRISTADOSS, P. 1988. C5 gene influences the development of murine myasthenia gravis. J. Immunol. **140:** 2589–2592.
51. BIESECKER, G. & C. M. GOMEZ. 1989. Inhibition of acute passive transfer experimental autoimmune myasthenia gravis with Fab antibody to complement C6. J. Immunol. **142:** 2654–2659.
52. DuPONT, B. L. & D. P. RICHMAN. 1987. Complement activation by anti-acetylcholine receptor monoclonal antibody *in vitro* correlates with potency of EAMG response *in vivo*. Ann. N.Y. Acad. Sci. **505:** 725–727.
53. MASELLI, R. A., D. P. RICHMAN & R. L. WOLLMANN. 1991. Inflammation at the neuromuscular junction in myasthenia gravis. Neurology **41:** 1497–1504.
54. LOUTRARI, H., A. KOKLA & S. J. TZARTOS. 1992. Passive transfer of experimental myasthenia gravis via antigenic modulation of acetylcholine receptor. Eur. J. Immunol. **22:** 2449–2452.
55. TZARTOS, S. J. & J. M. LINDSTROM. 1980. Monoclonal antibodies used to probe acetylcholine receptor structure: localization of the main immunogenic region and detection of similarities between subunits. Proc. Natl. Acad. Sci. U.S.A. **77:** 755.
56. LENNON, V. A. & E. H. LAMBERT. 1980. Myasthenia gravis induced by monoclonal antibodies to acetylcholine receptors. Nature **285:** 238.
57. BUZZARD, E. F. 1905. The clinical history and post-mortem examination of five cases of myasthenia gravis. Brain **28:** 438.
58. LISAK, R. P. & R. L. BARCHI. 1982. *In* Myasthenia Gravis, p. 97–98. Saunders. Philadelphia.
59. RUSSELL, D. S. 1953. Histological changes in the stripped muscles in myasthenia gravis. J. Pathol. Bacteriol. **65:** 279–289.
60. PASCUZZI, R. M. & J. F. CAMPA. 1988. Lymphorrhage localized to the muscle end-plate in myasthenia gravis. Arch. Pathol. Lab. Med. **112:** 934–937.
61. COREY, A. L., D. P. RICHMAN, C. A. SCHUMAN, C. M. GOMEZ & B. G. W. ARNASON. 1985. Use of monoclonal antiacetylcholine receptor antibodies to investigate the macrophage inflammation of acute experimental myasthenia gravis: refractoriness to a second episode of acute disease. Neurology **35:** 1455–1460.
62. COREY, A. L., D. P. RICHMAN, R. L. WOLLMANN & M. A. AGIUS. 1987. Refractoriness to a second episode of experimental myasthenia gravis: correlation with acetylcholine receptor concentration and morphologic appearance of the post-synaptic membrane. J. Immunol. **138:** 3269–3275.
63. RICHMAN, D. P., R. L. WOLLMANN, R. A. MASELLI, C. M. GOMEZ, A. L. COREY, M. A. AGIUS & R. H. FAIRCLOUGH. 1993. Effector mechanisms of myasthenic antibodies. Ann. N.Y. Acad. Sci. **681:** 264–273.
64. GOMEZ, C. M., D. P. RICHMAN, S. A. BURRES & B. G. W. ARNASON. 1981. Monoclonal hybridoma anti-acetylcholine receptor antibodies: antibody specificity and effect of passive transfer. Ann. N.Y. Acad. Sci. **377:** 97–109.

65. DuPont, B. L., G. M. Twaddle & D. P. Richman. 1987. Suppression of passive transfer acute experimental myasthenia by F(ab')₂ fragments. J. Neuroimmunol. **16:** 47.

66. Kirvan, C. A., S. Zhu, D. P. Richman & M. A. Agius. 1998. Expression and initial characterization of recombinant antiacetylcholine receptor antibodies in experimental autoimmune myasthenia gravis. This volume.

67. Agius, M. A., B. Sanyal & D. P. Richman. 1993. Molecular structure of a monoclonal antiacetylcholine receptor antibody and of a corresponding monoclonal antiidiotopic antibody. Ann. N.Y. Acad. Sci. **681:** 274–275.

Expression and Initial Characterization of Recombinant Antiacetylcholine Receptor Antibodies in Experimental Autoimmune Myasthenia Gravis[a]

CHRISTINE A. KIRVAN, SHAN ZHU, DAVID P. RICHMAN,
AND MARK A. AGIUS[b]

Department of Neurology
University of California at Davis
Davis, California 95616

INTRODUCTION

Experimental autoimmune myasthenia gravis (EAMG) can be induced by passive transfer of monoclonal antibody (mAb) directed against the acetylcholine receptor (AChR). The anti-AChR mAb 132A (γ2a, κ) is a main immunogenic region (MIR) antibody that causes severe EAMG. One possible mechanism by which anti-AChR antibodies mediate pathogenicity is by complement activation. Complement activation is controlled through the heavy-chain constant region of the antibody and is IgG subclass variable. To directly evaluate the role of antibody-mediated complement activation in the pathogenesis of myasthenia, we have generated a recombinant 132A mAb by replacing the wild-type heavy-chain constant region, γ2a, which is a good activator of complement, with a γ1 heavy-chain constant (C_H) region. The rat γ1 constant region is a poor activator of complement.[1]

MATERIALS AND METHODS

Rapid amplification of cDNA ends (5'RACE) was used to rescue 132A V_H and V_L sequences from total RNA extracted from the 132A hybridoma. Reverse transcription (RT) and antisense primers corresponded to C_H1 sequences of γ2a for mAb 132A V_H and 5'-kappa sequences for V_L. Four 132A V_H clones and five V_L clones generated from polymerase chain reaction (PCR) amplification were sequenced. The heavy chain of 132A and a kappa light-chain constant region were also obtained from a cDNA library. PCR site-directed mutagenesis was utilized to introduce a novel *SacII* restriction enzyme site into the 3' end of the 132A V_H and the 5' end of the γ1 heavy-chain sequence (gift of M. Bruggemann[1]). V_H and γ1 clones were digested and spliced together and then cloned into the mammalian transfection vector

[a]This work was supported by grants from the National Institutes of Health (Nos. NS19779 and NS01226) and by the Viets Fellowship of the Myasthenia Gravis Foundation.
[b]To whom all correspondence should be addressed.

TABLE 1. Binding Characteristics of Wild-type and Hybrid 132A Antibodies

mAb	AChR	Anti-id[a]	Anti-γ1	Anti-γ2a	Anti-κ
132A hybridoma[b]	+	+	−	+	+
132A-γ2a mAb[c]	+	+	−	+	+
132A-γ1 mAb	+	+	+	−	+

[a]Anti-id binding and class and subclass identity were determined in ELISA using anti-id mAb HC4A[2] and class and subclass specific antisera.
[b]Wild-type 132A mAb secreted by hybridoma.
[c]Engineered wild-type 132A.

pAH3504 (gift of S. Morrison). 132A light chain was constructed by splicing 132A V_L and kappa fragments at a common *DsaI* site. The intact light chain was cloned into the mammalian transfection vector pBK-RSV. The light chain and a 3′ intron were subsequently cloned into the pZeo-SV mammalian transfection vector. The wild-type 132A heavy chain obtained from the 132A cDNA library was cloned into the pBK-RSV transfection vector. The heavy- and light-chain clones were sequentially transfected by electroporation into the nonsecretory rat myeloma cell line YB2/0. Clones were selected and screened for antibody production. Subclass specificity, AChR, and anti-idiotopic (anti-id) binding were tested in ELISA as previously described.[2,3]

RESULTS AND CONCLUSIONS

A hybrid mAb 132AV$_H$-γ1 was generated and wild-type 132A heavy chain and light chain were also produced by genetic engineering. PCR site-directed mutagenesis was used to generate compatible 132A V_H and γ1 constant region cDNA fragments that were subsequently ligated into a mammalian transfection vector to produce the intact 132A-γ1 hybrid heavy chain. The wild-type 132A-γ2a heavy chain was obtained from a cDNA library. The chains were then cloned into appropriate transfection vectors and introduced into the YB2/0 cell line. Positive clones were screened for the production of rat IgG (TABLE 1). Both recombinant mAbs, 132A-γ2a wild type and the 132A-γ1 hybrid, bind to the AChR and the anti-id mAb HC4A. In addition, IgG subclass analysis shows that each recombinant mAb has the appropriate heavy-chain subclass.

REFERENCES

1. BRUGGEMANN, M., C. TEALE, M. CLARK, C. BINDON & H. WALDMANN. 1989. A matched set of rat/mouse chimeric antibodies: identification and biological properties of rat H chain constant regions mu, gamma 1, gamma 2a, gamma 2b, gamma 2c, epsilon, and alpha. J. Immunol. **142:** 3145–3150.
2. AGIUS, M. A., C. J. GEANNOPOULOS, R. H. FAIRCLOUGH & D. P. RICHMAN. 1988. Monoclonal

antiidiotopic antibodies against myasthenia-inducing anti-acetylcholine receptor monoclonal antibodies: preponderance of nonparatope-directed antibodies affecting antigen binding. J. Immunol. **140:** 62–68.

3. BLAIR, D. A., M. MIHOVILOVIC, M. A. AGIUS, R. H. FAIRCLOUGH & D. P. RICHMAN. 1987. Human × human hybridomas from patients with myasthenia gravis: possible tools for idiotypic therapy for myasthenia. Ann. N.Y. Acad. Sci. **505:** 155–167.

Homology of an Antiacetylcholine Receptor Monoclonal Antibody with a Monoclonal Antibody to Campath-1 Antigen Suggests Usage of the Same V_H Genes[a]

MARK A. AGIUS,[b] CHRISTINE A. KIRVAN,[b] AND BHARATI SANYAL[c]

[b]Department of Neurology
University of California at Davis
Davis, California 95616

[c]Department of Neurology
University of Chicago
Chicago, Illinois 60637

INTRODUCTION

The pathogenic potential of individual antiacetylcholine receptor (anti-AChR) antibodies varies considerably and it appears that the fine antigenic specificity of these antibodies may be important for disease induction. The Lewis rat anti-AChR monoclonal antibody (mAb) 132A (γ2a, κ) is a representative complement-activating, anti-AChR antibody. mAb 132A binds to the main immunogenic region (MIR) of the α subunit of the AChR and causes severe experimental autoimmune myasthenia gravis (EAMG) on passive transfer. The cDNA sequences corresponding to heavy and light chains of mAb 132A were analyzed for gene usage and homology with other rat antibodies.

MATERIALS AND METHODS

Library synthesis[1] and rapid amplification of cDNA ends (5′RACE) methodology were utilized to generate cDNA clones. For 5′RACE, reverse transcription and antisense primers corresponded to the constant heavy-chain (C_H) 1 sequences of γ2a. The sense primers used corresponded to the mAb 132A leader sequence and a poly-dTTP primer. For library synthesis, mRNA was isolated from an mAb 132A hybridoma cell line. Double-stranded cDNA obtained by reverse transcription and second-strand synthesis was ligated to EcoRI linkers and cloned into a lambda ZapII vector. Plaques were screened using a ^{32}P-γ[ATP]-labeled γ2a 5′-oligonucleotide fragment. Sequencing was performed using the dideoxy-chain termination method. Homology searching of V_H, D_H, and J_H gene segments as well as with the intact mAb 132A variable region was performed using the EMBL and GenBank nucleotide and amino-acid databases utilizing the GCG Wisconsin software package.

[a]This work was supported by NIH Grant Nos. NS01226 and NS19779.

RESULTS

The 132A heavy-chain sequence has been cloned and sequenced by both 5'RACE and cDNA library methods. The 5'RACE amplification generated four separate mAb 132A V_H clones. Both methods produced clones with identical variable region nucleotide and deduced amino-acid sequences. The accession number of the 132A heavy chain is L22652. mAb 132A V_H gene usage differs from that of the few other anti-AChR mAbs whose sequences are known. The overall homology of nucleotide and amino-acid sequences of V_H between 132A and the Lewis rat mAb YTH34.5HL is 97.1%. The V_H gene encodes for the leader sequence, FR1, CDR1, FR2, CDR2, FR3, and the 5' end of CDR3. The leader, CDR1, FR2, and FR3 sequences of the heavy chains of the two antibodies are identical. The FR1 region has only two nucleotide substitutions, one of which is an A substituted for a G. The second substitution in FR1 still codes for leucine. There are two amino-acid differences in CDR2, N for D and N for K. There is no significant homology between CDR3 or FR4 (encoded by D_H and J_H genes) or between the light-chain variable regions of these mAbs.

CONCLUSIONS

Not many rat antibodies have been sequenced and only a few that have are pathogenic autoantibodies. Furthermore, the knowledge of rat V_H genes is limited. mAb YTH34.5HL[2] is a Lewis rat–derived γ2a mAb directed against the Campath-1 antigen (CD52) present on all human lymphocytes and monocytes.[3] On the basis of the almost complete identity of V_H gene regions, it is likely that the two antibodies use the same V_H germline gene with few substitutions.

REFERENCES

1. AGIUS, M. A., B. SANYAL & D. P. RICHMAN. 1993. Molecular structure of a monoclonal anti-acetylcholine receptor antibody and of a corresponding monoclonal antiidiotopic antibody. Ann. N.Y. Acad. Sci. **681:** 274–275.
2. DYER, M. J., G. HALE, F. G. HAYHOE & H. WALDMANN. 1989. Effects of CAMPATH-1 antibodies *in vivo* in patients with lymphoid malignancies: influence of antibody isotype. Blood **73:** 1431–1439.
3. ROWAN, W. C., G. HALE, J. P. TITE & S. J. BRETT. 1995. Cross-linking of the CAMPATH-1 antigen (CD52) triggers activation of normal human T lymphocytes. Int. Immunol. **7:** 69–77.

Acetylcholine Receptor Antibody Measurements in Acquired Myasthenia Gravis

Diagnostic Sensitivity and Predictive Value for Thymoma

AATIF M. HUSAIN,[a] JANICE M. MASSEY,[a] JAMES F. HOWARD,[b]
AND DONALD B. SANDERS[a]

[a]Department of Medicine (Neurology)
Duke University Medical Center
Durham, North Carolina 27710

[b]Department of Neurology
University of North Carolina
Chapel Hill, North Carolina 27599

Acquired myasthenia gravis (AMG) is an autoimmune disorder that results in a decrease in the number of acetylcholine receptors (AChR) at the neuromuscular junction.[1] The diagnosis of AMG is based on clinical presentation, electromyographic (EMG) evaluation, laboratory testing, and response to immunotherapy.

Electromyographic techniques can be used to confirm a diagnosis of AMG.[2] The most-sensitive electrodiagnostic technique is single-fiber EMG (SFEMG). Circulating antibodies against the AChR, known as AChR antibodies (ARA), can be measured and they constitute the basis for the laboratory diagnosis of AMG. Three types of ARA can be measured: binding, modulating, and blocking ARA. Each of these has specific interactions with the AChR. Several laboratories have reported sensitivities of the various ARA subtypes.[3–7] Some have reported that certain ARA profiles are specific for patients with thymoma.[3]

We undertook this study to review our experience with ARA and to determine if any ARA pattern was specific for predicting the presence of thymoma.

METHODS

Since 1980, the MG clinics at Duke University Medical Center and University of North Carolina Memorial Hospital at Chapel Hill have maintained a common database that contains clinical, electromyographic, and laboratory data of all patients with MG seen at these institutions. This database was reviewed to identify patients appropriate for analysis.

To determine the sensitivity of ARA in our patients, we reviewed the ARA results of all AMG patients who were tested before beginning immunosuppression or thymectomy. We also noted whether these patients had thymoma. Patients with elevated binding ARA were classified as seropositive.

Patients identified for analysis were divided into three groups based on clinical characteristics at the time that ARA measurements were performed to facilitate comparison with other reports. Patients with only ocular symptoms and signs at the time of antibody testing were classified as ocular myasthenia; those with mild generalized weakness were classified as mild generalized myasthenia; and those with bulbar symptoms and signs or significant generalized weakness were classified as moderate/severe myasthenia. Seropositivity and frequency of elevated modulating and blocking ARA values were determined for each of these groups. We also compared the frequency of elevation of the various ARA subtypes in patients with thymoma and in those without thymoma.

RESULTS

A total of 655 patients with AMG had ARA determinations performed before immunosuppression and thymectomy. Of these, 56 had thymoma. For the initial analysis, we excluded those with thymoma. Of the 102 nonthymoma patients with ocular myasthenia, 60 (59%) were seropositive; of the 232 nonthymoma patients with mild generalized myasthenia, 161 (69%) were seropositive; and of the 265 nonthymoma patients with moderate/severe myasthenia, 218 (82%) were seropositive (see TABLE 1).

Binding, modulating, and blocking ARA values were determined before immunosuppression and thymectomy in 125 nonthymoma patients and 13 patients with thymoma. In the nonthymoma patients, at least one ARA subtype was elevated in 91 (73%); binding ARA value was elevated in 88 (70%); modulating ARA value was elevated in 70 (56%); and blocking ARA value was elevated in 25 (20%). The ARA modulating value was $\geq 90\%$ in 47 (38%) of nonthymoma patients (see TABLE 2).

In the 13 patients with thymoma, all had elevated binding, 9 (69%) had elevated modulating, and 7 (54%) had elevated blocking ARA values. The ARA modulating value was $\geq 90\%$ in 5 (38%) of the patients with thymoma.

DISCUSSION

It has been 20 years since Lindstrom et al. first reported the results of binding ARA measurements in AMG. In that time, there have been many reports discussing the sensitivity of binding ARA determinations in AMG.[8] These have been reviewed elsewhere.[9] The reported seropositivity has ranged between 74% and 93% in patients with AMG; we have previously reported 75% seropositivity.[9] Most of these reports have only analyzed results of binding ARA, the most readily available assay tech-

TABLE 1. Binding Antibody Findings in 599 Patients without Thymoma

	No. of Patients	No. Seropositive (%)
Ocular	102	60 (59)
Mild generalized	232	161 (69)
Moderate/severe	265	218 (82)

TABLE 2. Elevated Values of ARA Subtypes in 138 Patients

ARA Subtype (Abnormal Range)	Patients without Thymoma ($n = 125$)	Patients with Thymoma ($n = 13$)
Binding ARA (>0.02 nmol/L)	88 (70%)	13 (100%)
Modulating ARA (>20%)	70 (56%)	9 (69%)
Modulating ARA (≥90%)	47 (38%)	5 (38%)
Blocking ARA (>25%)	25 (20%)	7 (54%)
At least one ARA elevated	91 (73%)	13 (100%)

nique. In our analysis of all AMG patients who had binding ARA measurements, we found a seropositivity rate of 73%. As in previous reports, the proportion of seropositivity increased with disease severity.[3–5,7] Thus, whereas only 59% of patients with ocular myasthenia were seropositive, 82% with moderate/severe AMG were seropositive.

We suspect that the sensitivity of ARA measurement is lower in our series than in others because of a difference in diagnostic technique. In our MG clinics, the diagnosis of AMG is based on the overall clinical course, including response to immunotherapy, and extensive physiologic testing, including SFEMG. This makes it possible to arrive at a more definite diagnosis in many patients with mild disease who might otherwise be classified differently. Sensitivity of SFEMG has been reported elsewhere and is 99% in patients with generalized MG.[10] Thus, we are likely to have a greater percentage of seronegative AMG patients than clinics in which ARA measurements are the cornerstone of diagnosis. Referral patterns also may affect our results since seronegative patients are more likely to be referred to our academic centers for confirmation of the diagnosis, and seropositive patients with mild or easily managed disease are less likely to be referred.

Howard, Lennon, and colleagues have reported the sensitivity of binding, modulating, and blocking ARA subtypes in ocular, mild generalized, and moderate/severe generalized myasthenia.[3,11] Overall, they found elevated binding and modulating ARA in 86% of patients and elevated blocking ARA in 52%. They also noted that, in patients with thymoma, modulating ARA values are often ≥90%. In our patient population, binding, modulating, and blocking ARA measurements were less sensitive than those reported by Howard, Lennon, and colleagues.[3,11] The reasons are likely the same as those mentioned above. Also, modulating ARA levels did not differentiate our patients with thymoma from those without thymoma: of 38% of each group had modulating ARA values ≥90%. Our data indicate that the modulating ARA values cannot be used to indicate which patients have thymoma and which do not.

CONCLUSIONS

In our patient population, the sensitivity of binding, modulating, and blocking ARA measurements is lower than reported elsewhere, possibly because of techniques that we use in diagnosing AMG (i.e., long-term follow-up and SFEMG). We have not found any patterns of ARA values that predict the presence of thymoma.

REFERENCES

1. FAMBROUGH, D. M., D. B. DRACHMAN & S. SATYAMURTI. 1973. Neuromuscular junction in myasthenia gravis: decreased acetylcholine receptors. Science **182:** 293–295.
2. SANDERS, D. B. 1987. The electrodiagnosis of myasthenia gravis. Ann. N.Y. Acad. Sci. **505:** 539–555.
3. HOWARD, F. M., V. A. LENNON, J. FINLEY, J. MATSUMOTO & L. R. ELVEBACK. 1987. Clinical correlations of antibodies that bind, block, or modulate human acetylcholine receptors in myasthenia gravis. Ann. N.Y. Acad. Sci. **505:** 526–538.
4. VINCENT, A. & J. NEWSOM-DAVIS. 1982. Anti-acetylcholine receptor antibodies. J. Neurol. Neurosurg. Psychiatry **43:** 590–600.
5. KORNFELD, P., J. NALL, B. SMITH, T. W. MITTAG, A. N. BENDER, E. P. AMBINDER, S. H. HOROWITZ, A. E. PAPATESTAS, H. GROSS & G. GENKINS. 1981. Acetylcholine receptor antibodies in myasthenia gravis. Muscle Nerve **4:** 413–419.
6. LIMBURG, P. C., T. H. THE, E. HUMMEL-TAPPEL & H. J. G. H. OOSTERHUIS. 1983. Anti-acetylcholine receptor antibodies in myasthenia gravis: Part 1—Relation to clinical parameters in 250 patients. J. Neurol. Sci. **58:** 357–370.
7. SOMNIER, F. E. 1993. Clinical implementation of anti-acetylcholine receptor antibodies. J. Neurol. Neurosurg. Psychiatry **56:** 496–504.
8. LINDSTROM, J. M., M. E. SEYBOLD, V. A. LENNON, S. WHITTINGHAM & D. D. DUANE. 1976. Antibody to acetylcholine receptor in myasthenia gravis: prevalence, clinical correlates, and diagnostic value. Neurology **26:** 1054–1059.
9. SANDERS, D. B., P. I. ANDREWS, J. F. HOWARD & J. M. MASSEY. 1997. Seronegative myasthenia gravis. Neurology **48**(suppl. 5): S40–S45.
10. SANDERS, D. B. & E. V. STALBERG. 1996. AAEM minimonograph #25: single-fiber electromyography. Muscle Nerve **19:** 1069–1083.
11. LENNON, V. A. 1997. Serologic profile of myasthenia gravis and distinction from the Lambert-Eaton myasthenic syndrome. Neurology **48**(suppl. 5): S23–S27.

Construction of Single-Chain Fv Fragments of Anti-MIR Monoclonal Antibodies[a]

S. J. TZARTOS, P. TSANTILI, D. PAPANASTASIOU, AND A. MAMALAKI

Hellenic Pasteur Institute
Athens 11521, Greece

Many monoclonal antibodies (mAbs) against the acetylcholine receptor (AChR) bind to the main immunogenic region (MIR), located at the extracellular side of the AChR α-subunit.[1] Univalent fragments of anti-MIR mAbs, like Fab or scFv (the latter consists of only the variable regions of the heavy, VH, and light, VL, chains expressed as a single polypeptide chain), efficiently protect the AChR against the destructive activity of intact mAbs and sera from myasthenic patients.[2,3] In order to apply this observation to the clinic, humanized or human antibody fragments of very high affinity have to be designed.

We had earlier constructed the anti-MIR scFv198 with *in vitro* protective activity for human AChR.[3] We now present the construction of another anti-MIR scFv (no. 195) with much higher affinity for human AChR. In parallel, the first scFv (no. 198) was subjected to humanization by the replacement of the CDRs of the variable chains of a human immunoglobulin by those of scFv198. The very low affinity of the produced humanized fragment was subsequently enhanced by site-directed mutagenesis.

scFv195

The anti-MIR mAb195 was derived from rats immunized with human muscle AChR.[4] Specific first-strand VH and VL cDNAs from hybridoma mRNA were synthesized by using primers from the 5' end of the CH1 or Cκ regions. Subsequently, PCR was performed by using primers designed according to the 5' end and 3' end sequences of each V region of the parental mAb. The PCR products were linked in a second PCR step (PCR assembly) by the linker $(Gly_4-Ser)_3$ in the order VH-linker-VL; the assembled scFv195 was cloned into pHEN1 phagemid vector, which was further used to transform the HB2151 *E. coli* strain.

Most *E. coli* supernatants of the scFv195 clones did not bind ^{125}I-αBgt-labeled human AChR. Only 2 out of 16 clones tested were positive: 1 producing a high-affinity scFv (no. 6) for the human AChR and another producing a very low affinity scFv (no. 22). These 2 clones and 1 of the negative clones were used for further study.

The 3 clones had identical VH chains, but different VL_K. The VL_K amino-acid sequence of the negative clone was identical with the VL_K of the parental mouse myeloma fusion partner (S194/5.xxO.BU.1). The VL_K of the negative and high-affinity clones differed from each other by 28%. The VL_K of the low-affinity clone was

[a]This work was supported by grants from the Association Française contre les Myopathies and by Project Nos. BMH1-CT93-1100 and ERBCHRXCT940547 of the European Union.

identical to the high-affinity clone for the most part, but its CDR3 and a part of framework-3 were almost identical to those of the myeloma. The difference of 12 amino acids was apparently responsible for the dramatic difference in the affinity between the low-affinity and the high-affinity clones.

Competition experiments between intact anti-MIR mAbs and scFv195 (clone no. 6) for binding to the human AChR showed that the scFv195 inhibited binding of the anti-MIR mAbs, but not of an mAb that binds to the cytoplasmic side of the AChR. Therefore, scFv195 has the same specificity with the parental mAb.

TABLE 1 shows that the functional scFv195 has two orders of magnitude higher affinity (K_d= 0.8 nM) for human AChR than that of the earlier constructed scFv198. Yet, its affinity is much lower than that of the parental antibody.

HUMANIZED scFv198

For the humanization of the scFv of the rat mAb198, the CDRs of its VH and VL chains were grafted into the variable regions of the human immunoglobulin by replacing the corresponding human CDRs. To achieve the minimum distortion of the conformation of the antigen binding site, human immunoglobulins, H1G1 for VH and Human Daudi for VL, with the most homologous framework regions to those of the rodent mAb, were selected. The humanized scFv198 was constructed by PCR. The produced protein exhibited very low binding to *Torpedo* AChR and did not bind to human AChR.

Molecular modeling was then performed using ABGene software.[5] Four VH residues were identified that needed to be changed from human to murine: VH27(G→F), VH29(F→L), VH30(S→T), and VH71(L→R). Three mutants were constructed by site-directed mutagenesis: mutant A contained the VH71 mutation, mutant B contained the VH27, 29, and 30 mutations, and mutant C contained all four mutations. Mutant C revealed a very good recovery of AChR binding activity; mutant A also exhibited very significant, although lower, enhancement of AChR binding activity.

CONCLUSIONS

A recombinant scFv of an anti-MIR mAb (no. 195) was constructed with high affinity for human AChR (K_d = 0.8 nM). Its VL CDR3 plays a very important role in AChR recognition.

TABLE 1. Binding Affinities of scFv and the Original mAbs to ^{125}I-αBgt-labeled Human AChR Measured by Scatchard Plots

Antibody	Dissociation Constants (K_d) for Human AChR (nM)	
	Intact mAb	scFv
mAb 198	21.6	80.7
mAb 195	0.04	0.8

The humanization of an earlier constructed scFv (no. 198) was also obtained. Although its binding to the AChR was dramatically reduced, site-directed mutations at four selected residues of its VH chain caused very significant recovery of its binding activity.

These results may form significant steps towards the construction of a very high affinity humanized antibody fragment capable of *in vivo* protecting human AChR.

ACKNOWLEDGMENTS

We thank E. Eliopoulos, C. Poulas, and Ch. Liolitsas for valuable help in the molecular modeling.

REFERENCES

1. MAMALAKI, A. & S. J. TZARTOS. 1994. Nicotinic acetylcholine receptor: structure, function, and main immunogenic region. Adv. Neuroimmunol. **4:** 339–354.
2. SOPHIANOS, D. & S. J. TZARTOS. 1989. Fab fragments of monoclonal antibodies protect the human acetylcholine receptor against antigenic modulation caused by myasthenic sera. J. Autoimmun. **2:** 777–789.
3. MAMALAKI, A., N. TRAKAS & S. J. TZARTOS. 1993. Bacterial expression of a single-chain Fv fragment which efficiently protects the acetylcholine receptor against antigenic modulation caused by myasthenic antibodies. Eur. J. Immunol. **23:** 1839–1845.
4. TZARTOS, S., L. LANGEBERG, S. HOCHSCHWENDER & J. LINDSTROM. 1983. Demonstration of a main immunogenic region on acetylcholine receptors from human muscle using monoclonal antibodies to human receptor. FEBS Lett. **158:** 116–118.
5. MANDAL, C., B. D. KINGERY, J. M. ANCHIN, S. SUBRAMANIAM & D. S. LINTHICUM. 1996. ABGEN: a knowledge based automated approach for antibody structure modeling. Nat. Biotechnol. **14:** 323–328.

Epitope Analysis of AChR Ab in Patients with Myasthenia Gravis Using Sensitive Enzyme Immunoassay

MASATOSHI HAYASHI,[a,b] TAKEYUKI KOHNO,[c]
JUNJI YOSHINAGA,[d] AND KAICHI KIDA[a]

[a]Department of Pediatrics
Ehime University School of Medicine
Ehime 791-02, Japan

[b]Department of Pediatrics
Uwajima City Hospital
Uwajima, Ehime 798, Japan

[c]Faculty of Pharmaceutical Sciences
Setsunan University
Osaka 573-01, Japan

[d]Department of Neurology
Hiroshima City Hospital
Hiroshima 730, Japan

Acetylcholine receptor antibody (AChR Ab), which is the pathogenic autoantibody in myasthenia gravis (MG), is available in the diagnosis and judgment of clinical effectiveness in MG. However, there is a rate of about 10% of "seronegative MG" and we sometimes see patients with mild symptoms compared to high AChR Ab titer, although AChR Ab titer is relatively associated with severity. MG is known to be heterogeneous and has a subtype of "low responder MG" as a peculiar clinical entity.[1,2] Ocular MG, which is predominant in juvenile Japanese patients, has low AChR Ab titer (i.e., seronegative), which seems to be "low responder MG".[2,3] It is important to explain the pathogenesis of MG, especially "low responder MG". We have reported the possibility that heterogeneity of MG might be due to the specificity of involved muscles or different genetic background, such as HLA or Gm allotype.[4–6] In this study, we analyzed specific epitopes for myasthenogenicity, by examining Ab to fragmented peptides using sensitive enzyme immunoassay.

SUBJECTS AND METHODS

Fifty-one MG patients (18 ocular, 29 generalized, and 4 juvenile) before immunotherapy were participants in this study. AChR Ab was measured using a double precipitation method with human AChR as an antigen, purified from rhabdomyosarcoma cell line TE-671.[7] Antipeptide antibody was measured using ELISA and sensitive enzyme immunoassay (immune complex transfer enzyme immunoassay), which was established by Kohno and Ishikawa,[8] with 12 kinds of fragmented synthetic peptides coinciding with the extracellular domain and 1 with the intracellular domain of the AChR α subunit as antigens. Ten healthy controls participated in this study for antipeptide antibody, and the measured values were assessed by the ratio with the cutoff index, which was the mean + 2SD of the values in healthy controls.

RESULTS

Of 46 MG patients who were examined for AChR Ab, AChR Ab was detected in 72% (67% of ocular MG and 74% of generalized MG). Antibodies against all 12 peptides were detected in a relatively high incidence (11–64%) when assayed by sensitive enzyme immunoassay, whereas 5 of the 12 antipeptide antibodies were detected in a small number of patients (less than 5% incidence) when assayed by ELISA (FIGURE 1). We especially observed a high incidence of antipeptide antibodies in

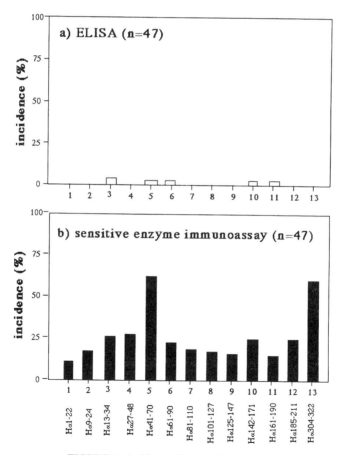

FIGURE 1. Incidence of antipeptide antibody.

Hα41–70 (64%) and Hα304–322 (62%) using sensitive enzyme immunoassay (FIG-URE 2). A combination of antipeptide antibodies to Hα41–70 and Hα304–322 measured by sensitive enzyme assay gave a high probability of MG, showing that 40 of 47 MG patients (85%) had either of them. Furthermore, 10 of 13 MG patients (77%) who had no detectable AChR Ab had either of the two antipeptide antibodies. When analyzed by a combination of AChR Ab titer and two antipeptide antibodies (Hα41–70 and Hα304–322) by sensitive immunoassay, 43 of 46 MG patients (93%) had at least one of them. However, we could not recognize any specific association of antipeptide antibody with clinical type or severity.

DISCUSSION

B cell epitopes have been studied by using ELISA assay or B cell clones that have been established by stimulating with specific antigen. However, these methods have tough problems: limitation of detectable level for ELISA assay and artificial modification of culture for the cloning method. Our method of sensitive enzyme immunoassay (immune complex transfer enzyme immunoassay), which needs a small amount of serum, made it possible to study directly the pathophysiology in individual pa-

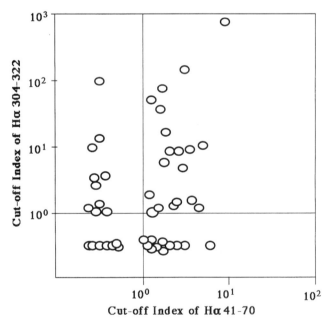

FIGURE 2. High incidence of Ab in MG patients to Hα41–70 and Hα304–322. Each value (O) was designated to be the Ab titer, which was divided by the cutoff index value. Cutoff index (—): Designated as 1 (10^0), which was determined to be the mean + 2SD of the measured values in healthy controls.

tients and was more sensitive than conventional ELISA. It is the reason why we could detect antipeptide antibody in MG patients who had no detectable AChR Ab. We showed directly polyclonality of AChR Ab in MG by showing a high incidence of antipeptide antibody in MG patients and that of various kinds of antipeptide antibodies in an individual MG patient. Furthermore, we indirectly proved heterogeneity in MG by showing that autoantibody to AChR or its fragmented peptide cannot explain the clinical type of MG.

REFERENCES

1. Mossman, S., A. Vincent & J. Newsom-Davis. 1986. Myasthenia gravis without acetylcholine receptor antibody: a distinct disease entity. Lancet **i:** 116–118.
2. Hayashi, M., J. Yoshinaga & K. Kida. 1996. Possible distinct pathogenesis in low responder myasthenia gravis: association of soluble interleukin-2 receptor with acetylcholine receptor antibody titer or abnormal thymus. J. Neurol. Neurosurg. Psychiatry **61:** 207–208.
3. Hayashi, M., K. Kida, I. Yamada *et al.* 1986. Anti-acetylcholine receptor antibody in juvenile and adult myasthenia gravis. Acta Paediatr. Jpn. **28:** 781–787.
4. Kida, K., M. Hayashi, I. Yamada *et al.* 1987. Heterogeneity in myasthenia gravis: HLA phenotypes and autoantibody responses in ocular and generalized types. Ann. Neurol. **21:** 274–278.
5. Hayashi, M., K. Kida, I. Yamada *et al.* 1989. Differences between ocular and generalized myasthenia gravis: binding characteristics of anti-acetylcholine receptor antibody against bovine muscles. J. Neuroimmunol. **21:** 227–233.
6. Hayashi, M. 1994. Pathogenesis of ocular myasthenia gravis. Muscle Nerve **17** (suppl. 1): S64.
7. Hayashi, M., T. Takaoka, K. Manabe *et al.* 1995. Comparison of antibody titer to human and rat acetylcholine receptor in myasthenia gravis. Brain Dev. **17:** 38–41.
8. Kohno, T., T. Mitsukawa, E. Ishikawa *et al.* 1989. More sensitive and simpler immune complex transfer enzyme immunoassay for antithyroglobulin IgG in serum. J. Clin. Lab. Anal. **3:** 163–168.

Antibodies Affecting Ion Channel Function in Acquired Neuromyotonia, in Seropositive and Seronegative Myasthenia Gravis, and in Antibody-mediated Arthrogryposis Multiplex Congenita

ANGELA VINCENT, LESLIE JACOBSON, PAUL PLESTED,
AGATA POLIZZI, TERESA TANG, SIETSKE RIEMERSMA,
CLAIRE NEWLAND, SARA GHORAZIAN, JEREMY FARRAR,
CAL MACLENNAN, NICHOLAS WILLCOX, DAVID BEESON,
AND JOHN NEWSOM-DAVIS

Neurosciences Group
Institute of Molecular Medicine
John Radcliffe Hospital
University of Oxford
Headington, Oxford OX3 9DS, United Kingdom

INTRODUCTION

Three autoimmune ion channel disorders are now recognized that affect neuromuscular transmission. Antibodies to acetylcholine receptors (AChR) are well recognized as causative in myasthenia gravis, but much remains to be understood concerning the etiology and pathology of the different forms of the disease. The Lambert-Eaton myasthenic syndrome is caused by antibodies to voltage-gated calcium channels and is the subject of several other contributions in this volume. Acquired neuromyotonia is associated with antibodies to voltage-gated potassium channels (VGKC) that are thought to be pathogenic. This chapter first summarizes the role of anti-VGKC antibodies in neuromyotonia and then discusses findings from our laboratory that relate to antibody specificity in myasthenia gravis (MG), seronegative myasthenia, and a related fetal/neonatal disorder, arthrogryposis multiplex congenita.

AUTOIMMUNITY IN ACQUIRED NEUROMYOTONIA
(ISAACS' SYNDROME)

Acquired neuromyotonia or Isaacs' syndrome is a disorder that usually presents in adult life and consists of spontaneous muscle activity with twitching, painful cramps, and increased sweating. An autoimmune basis for neuromyotonia was suggested by the association with other autoimmune disorders or with tumors such as thymoma and small cell lung cancer that are frequently associated with immune-mediated neurological diseases, by induction in rare cases by penicillamine treatment, and by the presence of oligoclonal bands in cerebrospinal fluid from some patients. For a review, see reference 1. Proof of the autoimmune nature of the disease came from the same approaches that had earlier demonstrated the role of antibodies in myasthenia gravis and the Lambert-Eaton myasthenic syndrome. Some patients improve temporarily following plasma exchange[2-4] and, in a few cases, immunosuppression or intravenous immunoglobulin has been found effective.[1] Injection of neuromyotonia IgG into mice did not produce spontaneous muscle activity, but increased the resistance to curare-induced paralysis,[2] increased the number of packets of ACh released per nerve impulse, increased the duration of sensory action potentials, and induced spontaneous activity in dorsal root ganglia cell cultures.[5] The latter effects were similar to those resulting from application of low doses of the potassium channel blocker, 3,4-diaminopyridine, suggesting that antibodies to VGKC expressed by the motor nerve might be involved. Because VGKC are responsible for resetting the membrane potential after each nerve impulse, reduced VGKC activity would lead to neuronal hyperexcitability.

Antibodies to VGKC were first detected in a proportion of neuromyotonia patients using ^{125}I-α-dendrotoxin-labeled VGKC extracted from human frontal cortex.[5] This assay is now in routine use, although only about 65% of patients are positive, and the titers are low (FIGURE 1).

A novel immunohistochemical method has also been used to detect anti-VGKC

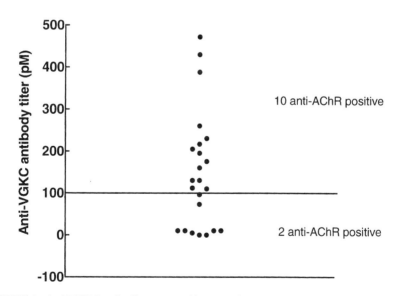

FIGURE 1. Anti-VGKC antibodies measured in serum from patients with acquired neuromyotonia by immunoprecipitation of ^{125}I-α-dendrotoxin-labeled voltage-gated potassium channels extracted from human frontal cortex.[5,6] The dotted line denotes the cutoff based on the mean ± 2SD of results from healthy and other neurological controls. Sera were also tested for anti-AChR antibodies; positive values were found in 12 of 23 sera and did not correlate with anti-VGKC antibody levels. Eight of these patients had a thymoma.

antibodies.[6] In this technique, VGKC subunit cRNAs are expressed in *Xenopus* oocytes; frozen sections of the oocytes are tested for binding of patients' antibodies by immunohistochemistry. Using this approach, anti-VGKC antibodies were found in all neuromyotonia patients. The discrepancy between the two assays may relate to differing sensitivity or to the fact that, in the immunohistochemical assay, relatively high concentrations of individual VGKC subunits can be tested.

It has been recognized that neuromyotonia may occur in association with myasthenia gravis and thymoma (e.g., see reference 7). Interestingly, several neuromyotonia patients with or without thymoma proved to have anti-AChR antibodies (FIGURE 1). There is no clear correlation between the presence of the two antibodies, but both VGKC and AChR subunits can be detected in thymoma tissue by PCR (see Liyanage *et al.* and MacLennan *et al.* elsewhere in this volume).

ANTI-AChR ANTIBODY REACTIVITY WITH ADULT AND FETAL AChR

It has long been recognized that antibodies to AChR in MG sera are heterogeneous in their immunochemistry and in their specificity for different epitopes on the AChR. In particular, several studies have demonstrated variability in the competition between monoclonal anti-AChR antibodies and anti-AChR antibodies in MG sera.[8,9] In addition, there is evidence for antibodies that react differentially with fetal or adult AChR.[10]

It has, however, been difficult to compare antibody specificity for human adult and fetal AChR because of the small amounts of the former in human muscle. To overcome this problem and to provide a better source of adult AChR for diagnostic assays, we have stably transfected the TE671 cells, which normally produce fetal AChR, with cDNA for the ε subunit. These cells, called TE671-ε to distinguish them from TE671-γ or wild type, produce large amounts of AChR, of which >70% is of the adult form.[11] Use of the TE671-γ and TE671-ε cells has allowed us to compare the binding of patients' sera to the two forms. Sera from some low-titer patients show a preference for the adult AChR or fetal AChR,[11] and a few cases have antibodies that are specific for adult AChR (FIGURE 2). In most cases with moderate or high titers of anti-AChR, the sera recognize each form (presumably because most of the antibodies are directed equally to the γ and ε subunits, or to the other subunits), although it is common for antibodies to bind slightly better to the fetal form (see below).

THYMOMA-ASSOCIATED MG

In thymoma-associated MG, the thymic tumor does not appear to express the intact AChR,[12,13] but individual AChR subunits have been identified by RNase protection assays (MacLennan *et al.*, in preparation). Although all the subunits can be detected by PCR techniques, in a high proportion of thymomas the ε subunit predominates when the less sensitive, but more quantitative technique of RNase protection is employed. This suggests that the ε subunit may be involved in the initiation of the au-

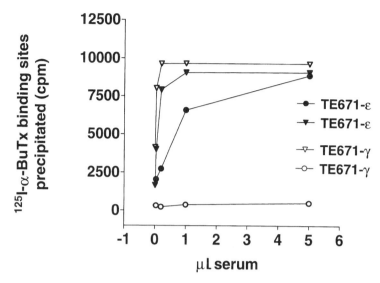

FIGURE 2. Immunoprecipitation by an MG serum (circles) of ^{125}I-α-BuTx-labeled AChR extracted from TE671-γ (open symbols) and TE671-ε (closed symbols) cells. This serum, unusually, binds quite strongly to adult AChR and does not show any binding to fetal AChR. This male patient had generalized MG. For comparison, results are shown from a typical female patient (triangles) whose antibodies recognized both forms equally.

toimmunity (see also Willcox *et al.* elsewhere in this volume). Thus, it was of interest to see whether thymoma/MG patients' antibodies bound preferentially to the adult form of the AChR. The reverse was found in most thymoma cases; only two sera bound more strongly to adult than to fetal AChR, and these displayed high ε subunit expression and low total anti-AChR titers (MacLennan *et al.*, in preparation).

OCULAR MG

Ocular weakness predominates in many patients at presentation and purely ocular symptoms may persist after other symptoms have responded to treatment. It has been demonstrated that multiply innervated muscle fibers, which represent about 20% of the fibers in ocular muscle, express the γ subunit, suggesting that antibodies specific for fetal AChR might be an important cause of ocular muscle weakness[14,15] (see also Kaminski elsewhere in this volume). However, by RNase protection, we found a far greater amount of ε subunit than γ subunit overall in ocular muscle.[16] Thus, although the multiply innervated slow-twitch fibers contain γ subunit, they probably also contain ε subunit and the extent to which antibodies that are fetal AChR–specific are responsible for ocular muscle weakness is debatable (see also reference 17 and comments below).

It was noteworthy that about 50% of sera from ocular MG patients had higher titers of antibody against adult AChR than against fetal AChR and that inclusion of adult AChR improved the yield of positive results in diagnostic assays.[16,18] However, it should be noted that when total anti-AChR levels are very low, as in many cases of ocular MG, the pathogenic antibodies may be underrepresented in the serum as a result of their absorption by the muscle AChR (see reference 19).

DEFINITION OF BINDING SITES FOR MONOCLONAL ANTIBODIES ON HUMAN AChR

Ten mAbs raised against human AChR were shown to bind to five regions (Table 1; see also Jacobson et al. elsewhere in this volume), none of which overlapped the α-bungarotoxin (α-BuTx) binding site.[8,20] One region was specific for fetal AChR and was therefore presumed to lie on the γ subunit. Two regions appeared to overlap the main immunogenic region, originally defined by Tzartos and Lindstrom,[21] and one of the mAbs (D6) showed very similar binding characteristics to anti-MIR mAb 35.[22] However, we were unable to demonstrate binding of any of the mAbs to synthetic peptides of the AChR α subunit (Jacobson and Vincent, unpublished data).

Now, each of the mAbs has been mapped by Western blotting of recombinant AChR subunits expressed in *E. coli*. The results confirm the α subunit binding of mAbs D6, C3, and G10 and the γ subunit binding of C2, C9, B8, and F8, which are fetal-specific. We have also found that B3 binds the β subunit and that C7 and G3 bind the δ subunit (Jacobson et al., in preparation). Thus, there are binding sites on each of the four subunits of fetal AChR, and the subunit specificities correspond remarkably well to the regions defined in our previous studies, which suggested that region 1 was close to the α-BuTx binding site near the α/γ interface, whereas region 5 was close to the site near the α/δ interface[22] (Table 1).

TABLE 1. AChR Subunit Binding Sites for Monoclonal Antibodies Raised against Human AChR

	Monoclonal Antibody				
	B8, C2, C9, F8	B3	C3, G10	D6	C7, G3
Binding site defined by competition studies[22]	1	2	3	4	5
Specificity	Fetal AChR α/γ interface		Overlapping MIR	MIR	α/δ interface
Binding site defined by immunoblotting on recombinant AChR subunits (Jacobson et al., in preparation)	γ1–174	β1–161	α3–181	α3–181	δ1–194

CLONING OF ANTI-AChR ANTIBODIES FROM
A COMBINATORIAL LIBRARY

It would clearly be useful to obtain monoclonal antibodies representative of the MG patients' repertoires in order to study the specificity and pathogenicity of individual human anti-AChR antibodies. We have cloned 4 Fabs using a kappa light chain/IgG1 heavy chain library created from mRNA obtained from the thymus of one early-onset female patient.[23] Two of the Fabs (e.g., ABk1) compete with anti-MIR mAbs and bind to both $\alpha\varepsilon$ and $\alpha\gamma$ dimers, whereas another (ABk5) binds only to $\alpha\gamma$ dimers (FIGURE 3) and is specific for the fetal isoform (see also Matthews *et al.* elsewhere in this volume). Because anti-MIR and fetal-specific antibodies were seen in the patient's serum,[23] these results suggest that combinatorial libraries may be a useful approach to studying individual human autoantibodies. Over 20 Fabs have been obtained from the lambda light chain/IgG1 library from this patient and are being characterized (Matthews *et al.*, this volume). Graus and colleagues have also cloned specific Fabs from MG thymus samples.[24]

ANTIBODIES SPECIFIC FOR FETAL AChR CAUSING
ARTHROGRYPOSIS MULTIPLEX CONGENITA

Antibodies binding preferentially to fetal forms of the AChR could be particularly damaging to the fetus *in utero*. Recently, antibodies that specifically inhibit the function of fetal AChR have been found to associate with a severe developmental abnor-

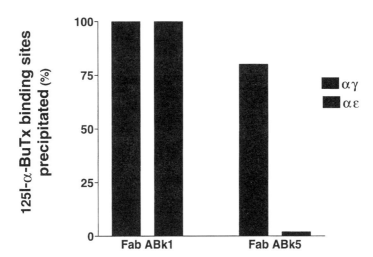

FIGURE 3. Immunoprecipitation of AChR subunit dimers by Fabs cloned from a combinatorial library. Fab ABk1 binds equally to $\alpha\gamma$ and $\alpha\varepsilon$ dimers, consistent with its specificity for the MIR.[23] By contrast, Fab ABk5 binds to $\alpha\gamma$, but not to $\alpha\varepsilon$ dimers, and was inhibited by monoclonal antibodies specific for the γ subunit.[23]

mality, arthrogryposis multiplex congenita (AMC). AMC is a syndrome consisting of joint contractures at birth or detected *in utero*, often associated with hydramnios, lung hypoplasia, and micrognathia. These features appear to result from lack of fetal movement *in utero* and, in some cases, they can be severe enough to cause fetal death or stillbirth. AMC sometimes reflects a genetic disorder of muscle or the central nervous system, but most often the cause is unknown, or environmental factors are implicated. For instance, joint contractures were demonstrated in chick embryos injected with curare.[25] Arthrogryposis has also been reported in association with typical maternal myasthenia gravis with transient neonatal MG.[26] For a review of arthrogryposis, see reference 27.

We studied two women with histories of severe AMC in their offspring.[28–30] One woman was completely asymptomatic despite high levels of anti-AChR antibodies,[29] and the other was only diagnosed as having MG after the stillbirth of her fourth affected child.[28] The severe fetal paralysis (demonstrated by complete lack of fetal movement on ultrasound), combined with the relative lack of maternal involvement, suggested that placental transfer of antibodies specific for fetal AChR might be involved in causing the fetal damage.

There were no differences in reactivity with adult or fetal AChR when sera from these two mothers were titrated in standard immunoprecipitation assays.[30] However, the sera inhibited α-BuTx binding to about 50% of its binding sites on fetal AChR (FIGURE 4a). Moreover, when the sera were tested for their ability to inhibit the func-

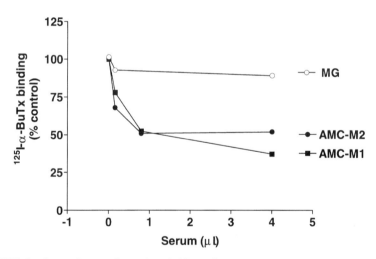

FIGURE 4a. Serum from mothers whose babies suffer from severe arthrogryposis multiplex congenita contains antibodies that specifically inhibit the function of fetal AChR. Inhibition of α-BuTx binding to AChR in human muscle extracts (predominantly of fetal type) by sera from two mothers (AMC-M) of AMC babies. In each case, the inhibition plateaus at about 50%, presumably because the antibodies bind to only one of the two α-BuTx binding sites (see FIGURE 4d).

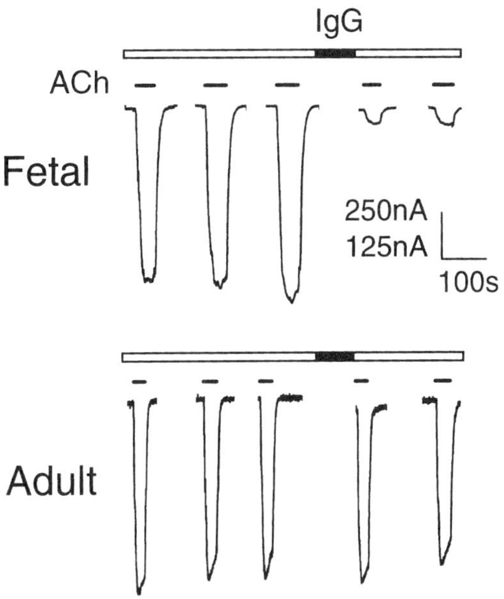

FIGURE 4b. Inhibition of ACh-induced currents of fetal AChR expressed in *Xenopus* oocytes by IgG purified from AMC-M sera. No effect was seen when the IgG was tested on adult AChR. Taken, with permission, from reference 30.

tion of the AChRs, a striking difference was observed (FIGURE 4b). IgG from the two patients was applied to fetal and adult AChRs expressed in *Xenopus* oocytes. IgG diluted 1:50 markedly inhibited the ACh responses of fetal AChR, but had no effect on those of adult AChR.[28,30] In addition, the two sera, and three others kindly donated by Beatrice Vernet der Garabedian and Bruno Eymard, inhibited carbchhol-induced Na$^+$ influx through fetal AChRs in TE671 cells, even when diluted 1:100, and had little or no effect on adult AChRs in TE671-ε cells.[30]

Further confirmation of the fetal specificity of these antibodies was shown by the protection of fetal AChR function by preincubation with the mAbs that bind to the γ subunit (FIGURE 4c), but not by one that binds to the β subunit. Thus, we hypothesize that antibodies from AMC mothers bind to a site on the γ subunit that partially overlaps the ACh-binding site on the adjacent α subunit (FIGURE 4d).

These results indicate a role for antibodies against fetal AChR in causing some cases of AMC. It is noteworthy that neither mother had clear signs of ocular muscle weakness in spite of high levels of serum antibodies to fetal AChR (see ocular myasthenia, above). To confirm the role of these antibodies in AMC, and to establish a model that can be used to investigate other putative antibody-mediated conditions, we have injected serum from mothers of AMC babies into pregnant mice. When 0.5 mL of plasma was injected daily from E13 till E20, the pups were stillborn and showed signs of lack of fetal movement such as fixed limbs and muscle atrophy (see Jacobson *et al.* elsewhere in this volume). This model can now be employed to investigate the effects of sera from other neurological disorders.

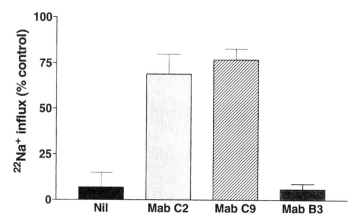

FIGURE 4c. The inhibition of AChR function seen in TE671-γ cells was prevented by preincubation of the cells in monoclonal antibodies that bind to the γ subunit (mAb C2 and C9), but not by a monoclonal antibody to the β subunit (B3).

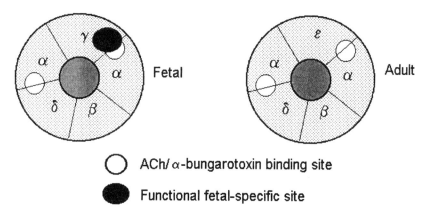

FIGURE 4d. Proposed binding site for antibodies from AMC-M sera. The antibodies bind to the γ subunit, but in such a way that ACh binding, or ACh-induced channel opening, is blocked.

CHARACTERIZING SERUM FACTORS IN SERONEGATIVE MG (SNMG)

At least 10–15% of patients with typical signs of generalized MG do not have detectable antibody by standard tests, including those that look at "blocking" or "modulating" antibodies.[31] We have previously reviewed the evidence for the existence of immunological factors, possibly IgM, in plasma from SNMG patients.[32] Briefly, SNMG patients responded to plasma exchange and immunosuppression,[33] and *in vivo* injection of their Ig fractions induced changes in neuromuscular transmission in the mouse hemidiaphragm preparation.[33,34] SNMG plasmas inhibited the function of AChR in TE671 cells, and the active factor was in the non-IgG fraction and copurified with IgM;[35] the effect was partially dependent on intracellular calcium,[36] suggesting that the antibodies might act indirectly by altering intracellular signaling.[37] Moreover, attempts to demonstrate that SNMG plasma antibodies bound directly to the AChR were unsuccessful.[33,35,36]

We have now found additional evidence consistent with an indirect effect of SNMG plasmas. We used TE671-ε cells to ensure that the effects seen are applicable to the neuromuscular junction where adult AChR is expressed. SNMG plasmas transiently reduced AChR function (as measured by carbachol-induced ^{22}Na$^+$ influx) by up to 85% at 1:20 dilution. The inhibition of function was greatest after about 10 min of incubation and thereafter reversed even in the continuing presence of the plasma (see Plested *et al.* elsewhere in this volume). Control plasma showed little or no inhibition. The effects of SNMG plasmas varied between individuals, but overall were highly significant (FIGURE 5a).

One possibility is that the SNMG plasma factor may act to stimulate an intracellular pathway (perhaps calcium-dependent) that leads to AChR phosphorylation and reduced function. It is well accepted, for instance, that AChR phosphorylation by cAMP-dependent protein kinase (PKA) or tyrosine kinases leads to increased AChR desensitization.[38] The effect would be expected to be rapid (as seen in TE671-ε cells) and would probably be transient because many of the metabotropic receptors themselves desensitize over a period of minutes.

These results led us to measure PKA activity in TE671 cells and to investigate the results of stimulating PKA activity on AChR function. PKA activity is low endogenously in TE671 cells, but can be stimulated by CGRP, salbutamol, dibutyryl cAMP, and cholera toxin. Each of these compounds applied for 30–60 min moderately re-

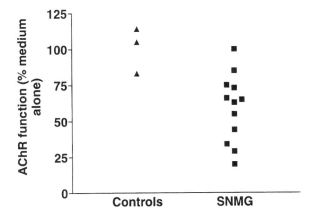

FIGURE 5a. SNMG plasmas transiently inhibit AChR function in TE671-ε cells. Carbachol-induced ^{22}Na$^+$ flux was measured after 10 min of incubation in SNMG plasmas at 1:20 dilution. The mean values, 59.1 ± 23.7 (SD; $n = 12$), were significantly different from controls, 100.7 ± 15.9 (SD; $n = 3$, $p < 0.005$).

duces AChR function in TE671 cells,[37] and CGRP shows a marked transient inhibition similar to that found with SNMG plasma (Plested *et al.*, in preparation). However, SNMG plasmas did not have any demonstrable effect on PKA activity in TE671-ε cells, suggesting that the putative target for the SNMG plasma factor acts via another pathway.

If SNMG plasma contains a factor that transiently affects AChR function, it might be possible to see this during short incubations of the mouse hemidiaphragm. Application of SNMG plasmas at room temperature reduced the twitch tension of the mouse hemidiaphragm when a low concentration of *d*-tubocurarine was included in the bath (FIGURE 5b), whereas control plasmas under the same conditions had no demonstrable effect. To see if there was a transient effect on AChR function, MEPP amplitudes were measured before and after application of SNMG plasmas and control plasma (diluted 1:2 in Krebs solution; coded samples). SNMG plasmas produced a small reduction in MEPP amplitudes that tended to reverse over a period of 15 min (FIGURE 5c), whereas the control plasma–treated muscles showed a small increase in MEPP amplitude (FIGURE 5c). However, these results were not significant because of the wide interfiber variation in MEPP amplitudes. To overcome this problem, the plasmas were applied (coded) to strips of hemidiaphragm during impalement of single muscle fibers; in this case, although the changes were small, the MEPP amplitudes were significantly reduced by two SNMG plasmas compared to control (Tang *et al.*, in preparation).

In conclusion, SNMG plasma appears to contain a factor that is not IgG (and may be IgM[35]) and that causes a rapid reduction in AChR function both in TE671-ε and TE671-γ cells and at the mouse neuromuscular junction; there may also be longer-term effects as seen in FIGURE 5b. However, the target or targets for these actions of

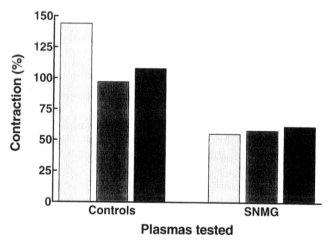

FIGURE 5b. SNMG plasmas reduce nerve-evoked twitch tension in mouse hemidiaphragm preparations. The twitch tension was measured before and after a 3-hour application of three control and three SNMG plasmas in the presence of curarized Krebs solution with 0.6 μg/mL of *d*-tubocurarine (see also reference 33).

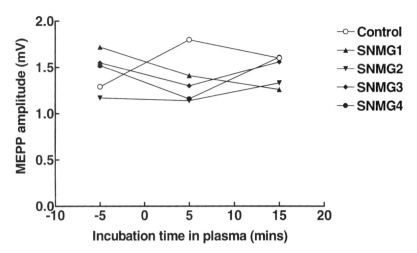

FIGURE 5c. SNMG plasmas transiently reduce AChR function at the mouse neuromuscular junction. MEPP amplitudes (a measure of AChR function) were measured before and following application of four SNMG plasmas and one control plasma. The results for each 10-min time period were pooled. There was an apparent rapid, but slight, inhibitory effect of SNMG plasmas; however, because of the relatively large interfiber variation in the MEPP amplitudes, the values were not statistically different.

SNMG plasmas are still unknown. Further studies are in progress to investigate other second messenger systems that might be involved in the SNMG action.

SUMMARY AND CONCLUSIONS

A new autoimmune disease affecting the neuromuscular junction has been defined. Acquired neuromyotonia is associated with antibodies to voltage-gated potassium channels that act, at least in part, by reducing potassium channel function with resulting neuronal hyperactivity. This condition is quite frequently associated with thymoma and, in many cases, antibodies to acetylcholine receptors are present as well as antibodies to VGKC.

Improvements in techniques and the availability of cloned DNA and recombinant forms of the AChR subunits have led to new observations concerning the specificity and roles of antibodies in myasthenia gravis. The transfection of a cell line with the ε subunit means that we can now accurately compare antibodies reactive with adult and fetal human AChR. This may help to determine the relationship between AChR subunit expression in different tissues and the induction of antibodies that bind specifically to the two forms, as well as to clarify the role of antibodies to fetal or adult AChR in causing ocular muscle symptoms. Serum antibodies from a few mothers with obstetric histories of recurrent arthrogryposis multiplex congenita in their babies specifically inhibit the function of fetal AChR. These observations not only explain the cause of some cases of arthrogryposis multiplex congenita, but also suggest that other fetal-specific antibodies might be responsible for other fetal or neonatal conditions. An animal model has been established to enable us to investigate the role of maternal serum factors in causing such disorders.

Seronegative MG has been the subject of many studies from our laboratory over the last ten years. The transience of the effects of SNMG plasmas on AChR function strongly suggests that the plasma antibodies do not bind directly to the AChR, but inhibit function by some indirect mechanism. They do not appear to act via the cAMP-dependent protein kinase pathway, and studies are in progress to investigate the involvement of other second messenger systems.

REFERENCES

1. NEWSOM-DAVIS, J. & K. R. MILLS. 1993. Immunological associations of acquired neuromyotonia (Isaacs' syndrome): report of five cases and literature review. Brain 116: 453–469.
2. SINHA, S., J. NEWSOM-DAVIS, K. MILLS et al. 1991. Autoimmune aetiology for acquired neuromyotonia (Isaacs' syndrome). Lancet 338: 75–77.
3. BADY, B., G. CHAUPLANNAZ, C. VIAL et al. 1991. Autoimmune aetiology for acquired neuromyotonia. Lancet 338: 1330.
4. WINTZEN, A. R., J. G. VAN DIJK & A. BRAND. 1994. Neuromyotonia with early response to plasmapheresis associated with proximal action myoclonus with late response to plasmapheresis. Muscle Nerve 17(suppl. 1): S221.
5. SHILLITO, P., P. C. MOLENAAR, A. VINCENT et al. 1995. Acquired neuromyotonia: evidence for autoantibodies against K+ channels of peripheral nerves. Ann. Neurol. 38: 714–722.
6. HART, I. K., C. WATERS, A. VINCENT et al. 1997. Autoantibodies detected to expressed K+ channels are implicated in neuromyotonia (Isaacs' syndrome). Ann. Neurol. 41: 238–246.
7. HALBACH, M., V. HOMBERG & H-J. FREUND. 1987. Neuromuscular, autonomic, and central cholinergic hyperactivity associated with thymoma and acetylcholine receptor–binding antibody. J. Neurol. 234: 433–436.
8. VINCENT, A., P. J. WHITING, M. SCHLUEP et al. 1987. Antibody heterogeneity and specificity in myasthenia gravis. Ann. N.Y. Acad. Sci. 505: 106–120.
9. TZARTOS, S. J., T. BARKAS, M. T. CUNG et al. 1991. The main immunogenic region of the acetylcholine receptor: structure and role in myasthenia gravis. Autoimmunity 8: 259–270.
10. VINCENT, A. & J. NEWSOM-DAVIS. 1982. Acetylcholine receptor antibody characteristics in myasthenia gravis. 1. Patients with generalized myasthenia or disease restricted to ocular muscles. Clin. Exp. Immunol. 49: 257–265.
11. BEESON, D., M. AMAR, I. BERMUDEZ et al. 1996. Stable high level expression of the adult subtype of human muscle acetylcholine receptor in the TE671 cell line following transfection with cDNA encoding the ε subunit. Neurosci. Lett. 207: 57–60.
12. GEUDER, K. I., A. MARX, V. WITZEMANN et al. 1992. Genomic organization and lack of transcription of the nicotinic acetylcholine receptor subunit genes in myasthenia gravis–associated thymoma. Lab. Invest. 66: 452–458.
13. KAMINSKI, H. J., R. A. FENSTERMAKER, F. W. ABDUL KARIM et al. 1993. Acetylcholine receptor subunit gene expression in thymic tissue. Muscle Nerve 16: 1332–1337.

14. HORTON, R. M., A. A. MANFREDI & B. M. CONTI-TRONCONI. 1993. The "embryonic" gamma subunit of the nicotinic acetylcholine receptor is expressed in adult extraocular muscle. Neurology **43(5):** 983–985.

15. KAMINSKI, H., L. KUSNER & C. BLOCK. 1996. Expression of acetylcholine receptor isoforms at extraocular endplates. Invest. Ophthalmol. Visual Sci. **321:** 406–411.

16. MACLENNAN, C., D. BEESON, A-M. BUIJS *et al.* 1997. Acetylcholine receptor expression in human extraocular muscles and their susceptibility to myasthenia gravis. Ann. Neurol. **41:** 423–431.

17. KAMINSKI, H. J. & U. L. RUFF. 1997. Ocular muscle involvement by myasthenia gravis. Editorial. Ann. Neurol. **41:** 419–420.

18. BEESON, D., L. JACOBSON, J. NEWSOM-DAVIS *et al.* 1996. A transfected human muscle cell line expressing the adult subtype of the human muscle acetylcholine receptor for diagnostic assays in myasthenia gravis. Neurology **47:** 1552–1555.

19. VINCENT, A. 1980. Immunology of acetylcholine receptors in relation to myasthenia gravis. Physiol. Rev. **60:** 756–824.

20. WHITING, P. J., A. VINCENT & J. NEWSOM-DAVIS. 1986. Myasthenia gravis: monoclonal antihuman acetylcholine receptor antibodies used to analyze antibody specificities and responses to treatment. Neurology **36:** 612–617.

21. TZARTOS, S. J. & J. L. LINDSTROM. 1980. Monoclonal antibodies to probe acetylcholine receptor structure: localization of the main immunogenic region and detection of similarities between subunits. Proc. Natl. Acad. Sci. U.S.A. **77:** 755–759.

22. HEIDENREICH, F., A. VINCENT, A. ROBERTS *et al.* 1988. Epitopes on human acetylcholine receptor defined by monoclonal antibodies and myasthenia gravis sera. Autoimmunity **1:** 285–297.

23. FARRAR, J., S. PORTOLANO, N. WILLCOX *et al.* 1997. Diverse Fabs specific for acetylcholine receptor epitopes from a myasthenia gravis thymus combinatorial library. Int. Immunol. In press.

24. GRAUS, Y. F., M. H. DE BAETS, P. W. H. PARREN *et al.* 1997. Human anti-nicotinic acetylcholine receptor recombinant Fab fragments isolated from thymus-derived phage display libraries from myasthenia gravis patients reflect predominant specificities in serum and block the action of pathogenic serum antibodies. J. Immunol. **158:** 1919–1929.

25. DRACHMAN, D. B. & A. J. COULOMBRE. 1961. Experimental clubfoot and arthrogryposis multiplex congenita. Lancet **ii:** 523.

26. VERNET DER GARABEDIAN, B., M. LACOKOVA, B. EYMARD *et al.* 1994. Association of neonatal myasthenia gravis with antibodies against the fetal acetylcholine receptor. J. Clin. Invest. **94:** 555–559.

27. HALL, J. G. 1990. Arthrogryposes (multiple congenital contractures). *In* Principles and Practice of Medical Genetics. Churchill Livingstone. New York.

28. VINCENT, A., C. NEWLAND, L. BRUETON *et al.* 1995. Arthrogryposis multiplex congenita with maternal autoantibodies specific for a fetal antigen. Lancet **346:** 24–25.

29. BARNES, P., D. KANABAR, L. BRUETON *et al.* 1994. Recurrent congenital arthrogryposis leading to a diagnosis of myasthenia gravis in an initially asymptomatic mother. Neuromusc. Dis. **5:** 59–65.

30. RIEMERSMA, S., A. VINCENT, D. BEESON *et al.* 1996. Association of arthrogryposis multiplex congenita with maternal antibodies inhibiting fetal acetylcholine receptor function. J. Clin. Invest. **98:** 2358–2363.

31. SANDERS, D. B., I. ANDREWS, J. F. HOWARD *et al.* 1997. Seronegative myasthenia gravis. Neurology **48**(suppl. 5): S40–S45.

32. VINCENT, A., Z. LI, A. HART *et al.* 1993. Seronegative myasthenia gravis: evidence for plasma factor(s) interfering with acetylcholine receptor function. Ann. N.Y. Acad. Sci. **681:** 529–538.

33. MOSSMAN, S., A. VINCENT & J. NEWSOM-DAVIS. 1986. Myasthenia gravis without acetyl-choline-receptor antibody: a distinct disease entity. Lancet **i:** 116–119.

34. BURGES, J., D. W. WRAY, S. PIZZIGHELLA *et al.* 1990. A myasthenia gravis plasma im-munoglobulin reduces miniature endplate potentials at human endplates *in vitro.* Muscle Nerve **13:** 407–413.

35. YAMAMOTO, T., A. VINCENT, T. A. CIULLA *et al.* 1991. Seronegative myasthenia gravis: a plasma factor inhibiting agonist-induced acetylcholine receptor function copurifies with IgM. Ann. Neurol. **30:** 550–557.

36. BARRETT-JOLLEY, R., N. BYRNE, A. VINCENT *et al.* 1994. Seronegative myasthenia gravis plasmas reduce acetylcholine-induced currents in TE671 cells. Pflügers Arch. **428:** 492–498.

37. LI, Z., N. FORESTER & A. VINCENT. Modulation of acetylcholine receptor function in TE671 (rhabdomyosarcoma) cells by non-AChR ligands; a role in seronegative myasthe-nia gravis? J. Neuroimmunol. **64:** 179–184.

38. HUGANIR, R. L. & K. MILES. 1989. Protein phosphorylation of nicotinic acetylcholine re-ceptors. Crit. Rev. Biochem. **24:** 183–215.

Morvan's Fibrillary Chorea

Electrodiagnostic and In Vitro *Microelectrode Findings*

R. A. MASELLI, M. AGIUS, E-K. LEE, N. BAKSHI,
R. N. MANDLER, AND W. ELLIS

Department of Neurology
University of California at Davis
Davis, California 95616

Morvan's fibrillary chorea is a disease that comprises (1) continuous muscle activity with electromyographic features of neuromyotonia, (2) autonomic dysfunction with intense hyperhidrosis, and (3) central nervous system abnormalities with insomnia and changes of personality. The complete syndrome has been observed in association with gold, mercury, and manganese intoxication.[1] On the other hand, continuous muscle activity and autonomic and central nervous system hyperactivity have also been reported in a patient with thymoma and positive acetylcholine receptor (AChR)–binding antibodies.[2] Recently, autoantibodies against potassium channels have been shown to be involved in neuromyotonia.[3]

We are here describing a case showing all the components of Morvan's syndrome in association with a thymoma and positive AChR antibodies. The patient was a 48-year-old right-handed man who first developed a vesicular rash over his legs and thighs. A few months after, he started to experience progressive weakness involving legs, thighs, and forearms. This was associated with intermittent jerking movements of limbs, muscle twitching, and muscle cramping on exertion. One year prior to admission, he developed left ptosis and diplopia. He also suffered symptoms of autonomic dysfunction, including bowel and bladder incontinence and hyperhidrosis. During six months prior to admission, he showed changes of personality, including insomnia and irritability. Two weeks prior to admission, he developed agitation and hallucinations. On examination, he was confused and agitated. He had paresis of the left medial rectus muscle and the external rectus muscle on both sides. He had left ptosis and bilateral facial paresis. He had generalized weakness, multifocal fasciculations, and myokymia in muscles of the limbs and trunk. Reflexes were symmetric and diminished in the lower extremities. Plantar responses were flexor.

ELECTRODIAGNOSTIC STUDIES

Motor conduction velocities in the right peroneal, right tibial, and right median serves were normal. However, the compound muscle action potentials (CMAPs) were followed by multiple repetitive after-discharges that obliterated the silent period and the F-wave responses. The sensory conduction velocity in the right sural nerve was normal. Repetitive stimulation of the right ulnar, right axillary, and right facial nerves at 2 Hz revealed no significant decrement. However, repetitive stimulation of the right ulnar nerve at 30 Hz resulted in a 42% increment of the CMAP area. Needle EMG showed spontaneous bursts of doublets, multiplets, and long runs of repetitive motor unit potentials with an intraburst frequency of up to 160 Hz and this was resistant to nerve block (FIGURE 1).

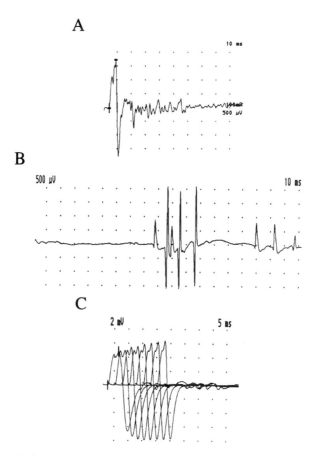

FIGURE 1. (A) Compound muscle action potential recorded from the abductor hallucis muscle in response to electrical stimulation of the right tibial nerve. The compound muscle action potential is followed by repetitive after-discharges that obliterate the silent period and the F-wave responses. (B) Spontaneous bursts of repetitive motor unit potentials with an intraburst frequency of 100 Hz. This spontaneous activity recorded from the right tibialis anterior muscle persisted after nerve block. (C) Moderate incremental response to stimulation of the right ulnar nerve at 20 Hz.

IN VITRO MICROELECTRODE STUDIES

Spontaneous miniature end plate potential amplitudes were reduced in amplitude and frequency. In addition, the mean end plate potential quantal content was also markedly reduced (FIGURE 2).

HOSPITAL COURSE

The patient required admission to ICU intubation and mechanical ventilation. After treatment with sedatives, Dilantin, and plasmapheresis, there was partial improve-

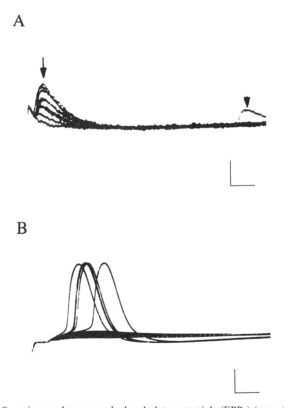

FIGURE 2. (A) Superimposed nerve-evoked end plate potentials (EPPs) (arrow) and spontaneous miniature end plate potentials (MEPPs) (arrowhead) recorded *in vitro* from the left anconeus muscle. MEPP amplitudes are reduced and EPP amplitudes fluctuate in a stepwise manner consistent with a combined postsynaptic and presynaptic failure. The calibration bars are 1 mV and 5 ms. (B) Superimposed EPPs and action potentials recorded *in vitro*. The EPP amplitudes are small and the action potentials showed marked "jitter" and impulse blocking due to impaired neuromuscular transmission. The calibration bars are 20 mV and 2 ms.

ment. He was found to have a thymoma by chest CT and he experienced further improvement after thymectomy.

CONCLUSIONS

First, Morvan's fibrillary chorea is associated with involvement of the peripheral, autonomic, and central nervous system. Second, the EMG findings are characterized by neuromyotonia. Third, in our patient, repetitive nerve stimulation and *in vitro* studies demonstrated both presynaptic and postsynaptic failure of neuromuscular transmission. Fourth, the most likely etiology of this syndrome is heavy-metal intoxication or underlying malignancy, especially thymoma. Fifth, the treatment includes Dilantin, plasmapheresis, and thymectomy. Sixth and last, the most likely pathogenesis of this syndrome is the generation of autoantibodies directed against multiple targets in the peripheral, autonomic, and central nervous system. The physiologic abnormalities reported in this patient are most probably accounted for by an immunologic attack of ligand- and voltage-activated channels, especially end plate acetylcholine receptor channels, presynaptic voltage-gated calcium channels, and nerve potassium channels.

REFERENCES

1. SERRATRICE, G. & J. AZULAY. 1994. Que reste-t-il de la Chorée fibrillaire de Morvan. Rev. Neurol. (Paris) **150**(4): 257–265.
2. PERINI, M., A. GHEZZI, P. BASSE & R. MONTAMINI. 1994. Association of neuromyotonia with peripheral neuropathy, myasthenia gravis, and thymoma: a case report. Ital. J. Neurol. Sci. **15**: 307–310.
3. HART, I. K., C. WATERS, A. VINCENT, C. NEWLAND, D. BEESON, O. PONGS, C. MORRIS & J. NEWSOM-DAVIS. 1997. Autoantibodies detected to expressed K^+ channels are implicated in neuromyotonia. Ann. Neurol. **41**(2): 238–246.

Seronegative Myasthenia Plasmas and Non-IgG Fractions Transiently Inhibit nAChR Function[a]

C. PAUL PLESTED, JOHN NEWSOM-DAVIS,
AND ANGELA VINCENT

Neurosciences Group
Institute of Molecular Medicine
John Radcliffe Hospital
University of Oxford
Headington, Oxford OX3 9DS, United Kingdom

About 10–15% of myasthenia gravis (MG) patients with typical clinical features of MG do not have detectable serum antiacetylcholine receptor (AChR) antibodies (seronegative MG, SNMG), as determined by the immunoprecipitation of ^{125}I-α-bungarotoxin (BuTx)–labeled human AChR. However, both clinical and experimental evidence suggest the presence of pathogenic humoral factors (for reviews, see references 1 and 2): babies born to SNMG mothers present with transient neonatal MG;[3] patients respond to plasma exchange and immunosuppressive therapy;[4] and mice injected with SNMG plasma show a defect in neuromuscular transmission.[4,5] Moreover, SNMG plasmas and non-IgG fractions inhibit nAChR function in TE671 cells that express fetal-type AChR,[6] and this effect may be dependent on intracellular calcium.[7] Importantly, though, attempts to demonstrate binding of Ig to AChR were uniformly unsuccessful[2,4,6] and the target for the humoral factor(s) remains unknown.

The nAChR is a neurotransmitter-activated ion channel composed of five homologous protein subunits ($\alpha_2\beta\delta\gamma$ or $\alpha_2\beta\delta\varepsilon$). The receptor has been shown to be modulated by changes in its state of phosphorylation[8] and agents that increase cAMP have been shown to desensitize the nAChR by increasing the phosphorylation of the γ and δ subunits. Indeed, such agents were found to reduce AChR function in TE671 cells.[9]

Here, we have further investigated the effects of SNMG plasma and non-IgG fractions on AChR function. We used ε-subunit-transfected TE671 cells that express the adult form of AChR[10] and used carbachol-induced ^{22}Na$^+$ flux to examine AChR function. We looked at the time course of the SNMG effects, investigated the activity of cAMP-dependent protein kinase A (PKA), and looked at the effect of SNMG plasma on this activity. All plasmas were heat-inactivated and dialyzed against HEPES-Locke buffer. Cultures of TE671-ε cells were performed as described previously.[10] The cAMP-dependent protein kinase A assay was carried out using the pseudosubstrate, Kemptide (Sigma).[11]

SNMG plasma (1/20) transiently inhibited carbachol-induced ^{22}Na$^+$ flux (FIGURE 1). This effect was rapid (maximal inhibition after 10 minutes) and, even in the con-

[a]This work was supported by Action Research and the Medical Research Council of Great Britain.

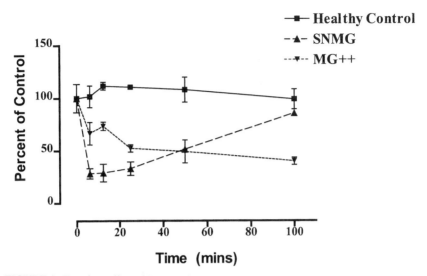

FIGURE 1. Transient effect of SNMG plasmas on AChR function in TE671-ε cells. The cells were treated with SNMG plasma for various time intervals before the AChR function was measured by carbachol-induced Na flux as described previously. Results are expressed as the % of cells treated with medium alone. A seropositive MG plasma (MG++) showed slow onset and persistent inhibition of AChR function, whereas the effect of the SNMG plasma was faster and transient; by 100 minutes, the AChR function had returned to normal values.

tinued presence of SNMG plasma, reversed within 80 minutes. This result contrasts with that of the anti-AChR positive MG plasma, which only gradually reduced AChR function and showed no transience in its effect (FIGURE 1). Furthermore, non-IgG fractions from SNMG patients also transiently inhibited $^{22}Na^+$ flux (data not shown).

To confirm that activation of PKA reduced AChR function in TE671-ε cells, we tested calcitonin gene–related peptide (CGRP: 1 μM). This caused a rapid inhibition of AChR function (FIGURE 2), which was greatest within 10 minutes of application, and the effect was inhibited by a 30-minute preincubation of the cells with the PKA inhibitor, H89 (500 nM).

CGRP and dibutyryl cAMP (a nonhydrolyzable analogue of cAMP) increased PKA activity, and H89 inhibited CGRP and dibutyryl cAMP–induced PKA activity (data not shown). Therefore, we investigated whether activation of the cAMP/PKA pathway was involved in the mechanism of SNMG by (1) direct measurement of PKA activity and (2) modulation by H89. Of seven SNMG plasmas tested, none increased PKA activity (data not shown). Furthermore, H89, which blocked CGRP-induced inhibition of $^{22}Na^+$ flux, had no effect on SNMG-induced inhibition of AChR function (FIGURE 2).

This study has demonstrated a previously unrecognized transient effect of SNMG plasmas on AChR function. We had already proposed that SNMG plasmas act indirectly to reduce AChR function; the transience suggests that the mechanism by which

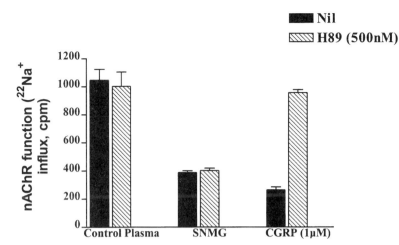

FIGURE 2. Effect of the protein kinase A inhibitor, H89, on the inhibition of AChR function by SNMG plasma and CGRP. The TE671 cells were pretreated with H89 (500 nM) before application of SNMG plasma (1:20 dilution) or CGRP (1 μM) for 10 minutes. AChR function was measured as in FIGURE 1. H89 had no direct effect on AChR function nor did it prevent the inhibition by SNMG plasma. However, it effectively prevented the action of CGRP.

SNMG plasmas act may itself become desensitized. Many substances increase cAMP-dependent kinase activity, and agents that activate this activity would be expected to affect AChR function. Indeed, CGRP and dibutyryl cAMP both increased PKA activity and reduced AChR function. However, we could not demonstrate that the effect of SNMG plasmas on AChR function involves PKA.

Other potential signal transduction systems in muscle are currently being investigated to elucidate the mechanism of action of SNMG. Indeed, signal transduction systems and modification of such pathways in pathological states may be important in the pathogenesis and as potential targets for therapy in other autoimmune diseases.

REFERENCES

1. SANDERS, D. B., I. ANDREWS, J. F. HOWARD *et al.* 1997. Seronegative myasthenia gravis. Neurology **48(suppl. 5):** S40–S45.
2. VINCENT, A., Z. LI, A. HART *et al.* 1993. Seronegative myasthenia gravis: evidence for plasma factor(s) interfering with acetylcholine receptor function. Ann. N.Y. Acad. Sci. **681:** 529–538.
3. MIER, A. K. & J. N. HAVARD. 1985. Diaphragmatic myasthenia in mother and child. Postgrad. Med. J. **61:** 725–727.
4. MOSSMAN, S., A. VINCENT & J. NEWSOM-DAVIS. 1986. Myasthenia gravis without acetylcholine-receptor antibody: a distinct disease entity. Lancet **i:** 116–119.
5. BURGES, J., D. W. WRAY, S. PIZZIGHELLA *et al.* 1990. A myasthenia gravis plasma im-

munoglobulin reduces miniature endplate potentials at human endplates *in vitro*. Muscle Nerve **13:** 407–413.

6. YAMAMOTO, T., A. VINCENT, T. A. CIULLA *et al.* 1991. Seronegative myasthenia gravis: a plasma factor inhibiting agonist-induced acetylcholine receptor function copurifies with IgM. Ann. Neurol. **30:** 550–557.

7. BARRETT-JOLLEY, R., N. BYRNE, A. VINCENT *et al.* 1994. Seronegative myasthenia gravis plasmas reduce acetylcholine-induced currents in TE671 cells. Pflügers Arch. **428:** 492–498.

8. HUGANIR, R. L. & K. MILES. 1989. Protein phosphorylation of nicotinic acetylcholine receptors. Crit. Rev. Biochem. **24:** 183–215.

9. LI, Z., N. FORESTER & A. VINCENT. 1996. Modulation of acetylcholine receptor function in TE671 (rhabdomyosarcoma) cells by non-AChR ligands: a role in seronegative myasthenia gravis? J. Neuroimmunol. **64:** 179–184.

10. BEESON, D., M. AMAR, I. BERMUDEZ *et al.* 1996. Stable high level expression of the adult subtype of human muscle acetylcholine receptor in the TE671 cell line following transfection with cDNA encoding the ε subunit. Neurosci. Lett. **207:** 57–60.

11. HEASLEY, L. E. & G. L. JOHNSON. 1989. Detection of NGF and EGF-regulated protein kinases in PC12 cells with synthetic peptide substrates. Mol. Pharmacol. **35:** 331–338.

Muscle Striation Antibodies in Myasthenia Gravis

Diagnostic and Functional Significance

JOHAN A. AARLI, GEIR OLVE SKEIE, ÅSE MYGLAND,
AND NILS ERIK GILHUS

Department of Neurology
Haukeland Hospital
University of Bergen
N-5021 Bergen, Norway

In 1960, Strauss and coworkers demonstrated that the globulin fraction from a pool of sera from patients with myasthenia gravis (MG) contained complement-fixing antibodies that reacted with the cross-striations of skeletal muscle.[1] Beutner *et al.* confirmed the observation and demonstrated the autoantibody nature of the antibodies. They also reported that sera from some MG patients react with skeletal muscle only, while others react with both skeletal and heart tissue.[2] These antibodies are frequently found in the sera of patients with MG and thymoma, and van der Geld and Strauss demonstrated that the muscle striational antibodies also react with the myoid cells of the thymus.[3]

While Strauss and coworkers interpreted their data as an antibody reaction with the A-bands of skeletal muscle,[1] Vetters reported that some MG sera also contain antibodies that bind to the I-bands.[4,5] These observations were followed by a dispute on the nature and localization of the antigen and by the demonstration that even normal IgG could bind to the cross-striations by the Fc part, thus giving rise to false-positive reactions.[6] After Lindstrom and Patrick's paper in 1973,[7] most investigators turned their attention to the acetylcholine receptor (AChR) antibodies, which are more relevant for the muscle fatigability in MG. However, muscle striation antibodies can be demonstrated in most cases of MG associated with thymoma and also in some cases of MG with thymus atrophy, although they are not present in the early-onset form of MG with hyperplasia of the thymus. Muscle striation antibodies may therefore be of a special significance for the understanding of disease mechanisms in thymomatous MG and late-onset MG with thymus involution.

These antibodies have been called antistriated muscle antibodies, striational antibodies, muscle striation antibodies, CA antibodies, and nonreceptor muscle antibodies. They were first described using indirect immunofluorescence, but can be demonstrated using a variety of immunological techniques (FIGURE 1). Several attempts at identifying the skeletal muscle antigen(s) reacting with muscle striation antibodies yielded conflicting results. It soon became clear that the morphological techniques applied, such as indirect immunofluorescence on sections of striated muscle tissue, were too crude to allow the identification of the target antigen.

In an attempt to isolate such antigens, Aarli showed that the skeletal and heart muscle antibodies react with a citric acid (CA) extract of skeletal and heart muscle.[8]

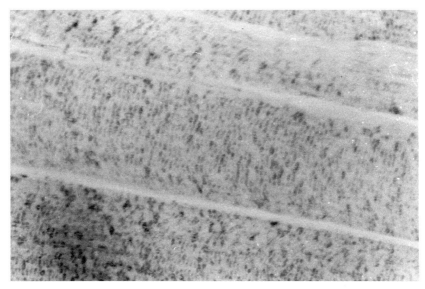

FIGURE 1. Section of rat striated muscle stained with antibodies from a myasthenia gravis patient with thymoma. The serum is affinity-purified on titin immobilized on nitrocellulose. Intense staining with cross-striational pattern.

They were therefore called CA antibodies. IgG CA antibodies were demonstrated in approximately 85% of MG patients with thymoma and in only 8% of sera from non-thymoma MG patients.[9] The CA extract was too crude for further analysis of the antigen(s) reacting with the muscle striational antibodies.

Williams and coworkers found that thymic B-lymphocyte clones from MG patients secreted autoantibodies that reacted with myosin, α-actinin, and actin.[10] Ohta *et al.* reported that some MG patients with thymoma had low levels of antibodies to tropomyosin, α-actinin, and actin, but they found that the titers were low and did not correlate with the titers of antimuscle striation antibodies as examined by immunofluorescence.[11] Only two non-AChR muscle antigens have been identified as being of major importance in MG and have been studied in further detail: titin and ryanodine receptor. This discussion will therefore concentrate on the immunological aspects of titin and ryanodine receptor antibodies in MG.

TITIN ANTIBODIES

In 1990, Aarli *et al.* demonstrated that sera from some MG patients with thymoma react *in vitro* with a large muscle polypeptide. This antigen is present in heart and skeletal muscle and has the same electrophoretic mobility as titin (FIGURE 2). In addition, it shares antigenic determinants with titin. Using immunoelectromicroscopy, Aarli *et al.* showed that affinity-purified antibodies to the large polypeptide produced

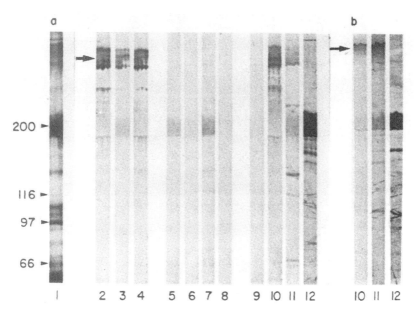

FIGURE 2. Binding of IgG from patients with MG and thymoma to a large muscle protein corresponding to titin. (a) A homogenate of rat skeletal muscle was solubilized, separated on 4.5% polyacrylamide gels, and (lane 1) stained for Coomassie blue, or the proteins were transferred to nitrocellulose for immunochemical staining. The relative mobilities of molecular-mass markers are indicated in kDa. Lanes 2–4 were exposed to sera from patients with myasthenia gravis and thymoma; lanes 5 and 6, myasthenia without thymoma; lane 7, amyotrophic lateral sclerosis; and lane 8, a healthy individual. All sera were used at a dilution of 1/500 and bound IgG was detected using a peroxidase-conjugated secondary antibody. The arrow indicates the staining of a large protein only seen with the sera of MG patients with thymoma. Lane 10, staining with antibody affinity-purified from serum of a MG thymoma patient, by elution from the high-molecular-weight region; and lane 9, antibody eluted from a control region. The same large protein is stained with (lane 11) a polyclonal antibody against titin, while there is no staining of this area with (lane 12) an antimyosin monoclonal antibody. (b) Purified myofibrillary proteins from rabbit skeletal muscle were blotted and stained as in part a. The affinity-purified IgG from the thymoma patient stains the band corresponding to titin (arrow). Reprinted courtesy of reference 12.

a distinct staining at the edge of the A/I-band junction[12] (FIGURE 3). The staining pattern obtained was compared with the localization of already-described titin epitopes. Earlier, Fürst *et al.* had prepared monoclonal antibodies specific for titin and showed that such antibodies identified repetitive and nonrepetitive epitopes, one of them apparently with a localization corresponding exactly to the binding now demonstrated with the MG sera.[13,14] Aarli *et al.* therefore concluded, on the basis of the results of immunoblotting and immunoelectromicroscopy, that most MG patients with thymoma have antibodies that react with titin.[12]

Titin (also referred to as connectin[15]) is a giant filamentous protein of striated

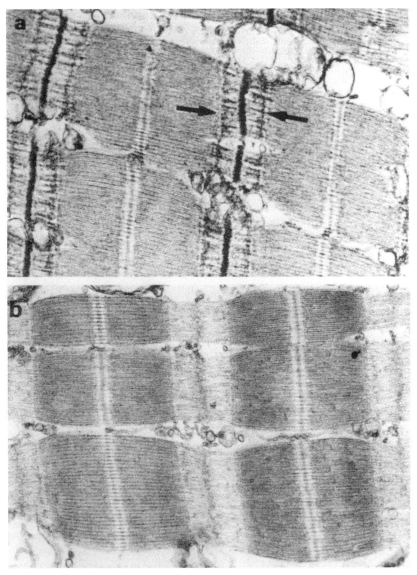

FIGURE 3. (a) Electron micrograph of rat skeletal muscle stained with the same antibodies as in FIGURE 2. There are intense staining lines near the edge of the A/I-junctions (arrow). Magnification: ×9000. (b) The same kind of section as in part a, but stained with control antibodies. Reprinted courtesy of reference 12.

muscle with a molecular weight near 3 kDa. It constitutes approximately 10% of the total protein mass of striated muscle. Single titin molecules span half-sarcomeres in striated muscles, from the Z-disk to the M-line, and are longer than 1 micrometer. The titin filaments contribute to muscle assembly and to the ability of the muscles to spring back after they are stretched. The change of length during stretching and contraction is mainly in the I-band, while the A-band part of titin is functionally stiff and highly ordered.[16]

In immunoelectromicroscopy, titin antibody–containing MG sera give a distinct staining of the muscle fibers close to the A/I-band junction. Animals immunized with whole titin develop antibodies preferentially in the same region.[17] This region was therefore designated the MIR (main immunogenic region) of titin, corresponding to the MIR seen in AChR in MG.[18] The MIR has been mapped by immunoscreening human cardiac titin cDNA expression libraries with MG sera. The MIR epitope is included in the recombinantly obtained MGT-30 (myasthenia gravis thymoma 30-kDa) protein.[18]

The molecular weight of MGT-30 is approximately 1% of that of whole titin. Its sequence is small enough to be expressed efficiently in *E. coli.* The expressed recombinant antigen MGT-30 protein has thus been applied in a sensitive ELISA assay for the detection of muscle striational antibodies.[18]

Recent investigations using immunofluorescence microscopy on single, stretched myofibrils have shown that the MIR epitope, which is contained in the MGT-30 peptide, is located within the functionally stiff titin region.[19,20] Lübke *et al.* have adapted a method that allows mechanical manipulation of isolated, single myofibrils. Using this technique, they found that a few MG sera contain, in addition to titin MIR antibodies reacting at the A/I-band junction, titin antibodies that react with another titin epitope, which covers an I-band titin segment that spans from the N1-line to the N2-line of the half-sarcomere.[21] This region is known to be differentially spliced dependent on muscle type.

Thus, some MG sera label only one single site on the titin filament at the A-band edge, the MIR of titin (group I sera). Others (group II sera) stain both the MIR and an I-band epitope.[21] The observation of epitope spreading in MG, as described by Lübke *et al.*, [21] may explain the occurrence of antibodies to various muscle antigens found in sera from some MG patients with thymoma. It is possible that the immune response in the initial phase of the disease is restricted to the MIR region of titin, and the additional immunoreactivity to other I-band epitopes may develop during the course of the disease. This has been interpreted as evidence of epitope spreading.

There is no evidence that MG patients with group II sera have a more severe disease than patients with group I sera. There is, therefore, in thymoma patients, no statistically significant correlation between an immune response characterized by epitope spreading and the severity of MG.[21]

TITIN EPITOPES IN THE THYMUS

Marx and coworkers demonstrated that the monoclonal antibody mAb155 stained neoplastic epithelial cells of MG-associated thymoma. In addition, this antibody reacted with an acetylcholine receptor (AChR) epitope[22] and gave a striational immunoreactivity with skeletal muscle type II fibers. The autoimmune process in thymomatous MG may be initiated by the tumor epithelial cells that express the AChR epitope.

Why do some patients with MG produce, in addition to the AChR antibodies, antibodies to titin? Can titin epitopes be demonstrated in thymomas? There are some earlier data that indicate that neoplastic epithelial cells can express a muscle antigen on their surface. Gilhus *et al.* demonstrated that antigen(s) in a CA extract of skeletal muscle shares epitopes with neoplastic thymic epithelial cells.[23] This was later confirmed by Dardenne, Savino, and Bach.[24] However, it was not until titin was identified as a major antigen in thymoma MG that it became possible to clarify the association between a non-AChR muscle protein and the immunological effects of thymic epithelial cell neoplasia.

It is not unexpected that the myoid cells of the thymus, which have similarities with skeletal muscle cells, contain both titin mRNA and titin itself. There are myoid cells in the hyperplastic thymus. Titin can therefore be detected in hyperplastic MG thymus. However, patients with early-onset MG and thymus hyperplasia do not develop titin antibodies and neither can such antibodies be detected in the sera of healthy controls.[18]

A thymoma is an epithelial tumor and does not contain myoid cells. Intact titin has not been demonstrated in thymoma tissue.[25,26] However, Skeie and coworkers recently demonstrated titin mRNA in thymoma tissue.[27] The tissue was taken from the center of the tumor in order to avoid contamination with myoid cells from the surrounding thymus tissue. The mRNAs identified in thymoma tissue code for the MIR and for the central I-band titin (N2-line), which are the regions of titin to which autoantibodies can be detected.[21]

A thymoma (lymphoepithelioma) contains abundant cortical and maturing thymocytes in a microenvironment that might allow aberrant positive or negative selection of nascent T lymphocytes.[28,29] If negative selection were defective, a broad-spectered autoreactivity should be expected. Many patients with early-onset MG and thymus hyperplasia exhibit clinical or serological evidence of other autoimmune disorders. In contrast, patients with MG and thymoma do not show any global autoreactivity.[30]

Gilhus and coworkers have shown that thymoma epithelial cells in culture are able to present AChR peptides to relevant T-lymphocyte lines.[31] Thymomas from MG patients also express accessory molecules crucial for antigen presentation.[28] Although native titin is not present in thymomas, both MIR and the N2-line epitopes are transcribed in such tumors. Because the neoplastic thymic epithelial cells are able to present their neoantigens for developing T lymphocytes, and peripheral blood T lymphocytes from some MG patients are reactive with titin epitopes, it is most likely that aberrant positive selection of titin reactive T lymphocytes within the thymoma is the initiating event for anti-titin autoreactivity in thymoma MG.[27,32]

Some patients with late-onset MG and thymus involution, but no evidence of thymus neoplasia, also have antibodies to titin. Why such patients produce titin autoantibodies is less clear. Pescamona *et al.* have reported histological evidence of microscopic thymoma of multifocal cortical and medullary origin in some of these patients.[33] Titin mRNA expression has so far not been demonstrated in atrophic thymus from MG patients.[27] The mechanisms leading to MG and to titin antibody production in these patients must therefore be different from those observed in thymoma MG.

DIAGNOSTIC VALUE OF TITIN ANTIBODIES

Muscle striation antibodies, whether demonstrated by immunofluorescence as CA antibodies or as titin or MGT-30 antibodies, are demonstrated in 80–90% of all MG patients with thymoma. They are almost never detected in the sera of MG patients with early-onset MG and thymus hyperplasia. The demonstration of such antibodies in a young MG patient (<40 years) is therefore, for clinical purpose, diagnostic of a thymoma.[18,34] Although titin antibodies represent a sensitive marker for the presence of a thymoma in MG patients, the specificity is low in patients with onset of MG after the age of 40 because some patients with MG and thymus involution also have such antibodies.[35]

McFarlin, Barlow, and Strauss reported that some nonmyasthenic patients with thymoma also have muscle striation antibodies. Using immunofluorescent technique, they detected such antibodies in the sera of 6 out of 12 patients who had been operated for a thymoma and who did not have clinical or electrophysiological features of MG.[36] The thymomas in these 6 patients did not differ pathologically from those that accompany MG. MG, however, may appear many years after thymectomy in patients who have been operated for a thymoma.[37]

Gilhus *et al.* showed that antibodies to striated muscle (CA antibodies) are also found in high concentrations in sera from some non-MG patients with thymic tumors with nonepithelial histology.[38] These patients have antibodies to AChR. Their tumors may lack the AChR-related epitope, which may explain why these patients never developed MG.

It has been claimed that antibodies to titin and to other non-AChR antigens of skeletal muscle may develop secondary to titin release from muscle damaged by antibodies to AChR. However, such antibodies have not been demonstrated even in cases of long-standing, severe disease in early-onset, nonthymoma MG. Neither have titin antibodies been detected in the sera of patients with muscle cell damage of other causes.

Titin antibodies are also found in nearly half of the sera of older, nonthymoma MG patients. This is not a consequence of age because similar antibodies are not detected among age-matched controls; nor is it an effect of long-standing MG because there is no relation between muscle antibody titer and disease duration.[39] These patients all have an atrophy of the thymus that morphologically does not differ from the normal, age-related thymus involution.[40] The titin antibody-positive late-onset MG patients thus have a similar immunological profile to thymoma MG patients. Skeie and coworkers compared the clinical severity of the disease in nonthymoma MG patients and found that patients who had circulating antibodies against MGT-30 had a more severe form of the disease.[35]

Keynes, Oosterhuis, and others have commented that thymoma MG patients have a more severe, brittle, and aggressive form of the disease and that they do less well than nonthymoma patients. This is not necessarily related to the size of the tumor. Even patients with very small thymomas may develop a fulminant neuromuscular disorder.[41,42] It has been speculated, but never documented, that the severe MG found in thymoma patients may be caused by a more widespread autoimmune myopathy.[35] Patients with late-onset MG and MGT-30 titin antibodies have the same humoral immune response as those with thymoma, and the diagnostic value of titin antibodies in nonthymoma late-onset MG may therefore lie in the evaluation of the prognosis.[43]

Titin is an intracellular antigen. There is increasing evidence that autoantibodies against some intracellular antigens can have functional effects, either by passing the cell membrane or through the expression of the epitope on the surface of the cell.[44,45] There is, however, so far no direct evidence that the titin antibodies are inducing pathological effects. They may as well represent indicators of a pathological process that, in addition to the AChR antibody–mediated neuromuscular transmission defect, influences the muscle cell function of the patient. The negative effect of titin antibodies on the prognosis is related to the simultaneous presence of antibodies to the ryanodine receptor, first described by Mygland et al.[46] Such antibodies have so far only been detected in sera of patients who also have MGT-30 antibodies.

RYANODINE RECEPTOR ANTIBODIES

The ryanodine receptor (RyR) is a Ca^{2+}-release channel located in the sarcoplasmic reticulum of striated muscle. It plays an essential role in muscle contraction by responding to sarcolemma depolarization with opening of the ion channel and release of Ca^{2+} from the sarcoplasmic reticulum to the contractile proteins.[47] Mendell et al., using immunoelectromicroscopy, first demonstrated that Fab fragments of muscle antibodies bound to the microsomal fraction of skeletal homogenates and that the principal site of binding was the sarcoplasmic reticulum surrounding the I-band of the sarcomere. They speculated whether an autoantibody attaching to the sarcoplasmic reticulum might seriously impair muscle function, but found no evidence that such antibodies could interfere with the neuromuscular transmission.[48]

Mygland et al. examined a suspension of purified vesicles from the sarcoplasmic reticulum of skeletal muscle and found that it bound IgG from some MG patients. Immunoblotting revealed that the MG antibodies reacted with a 320-kDa protein that was stained by an antiserum to RyR.[46] The MG antibodies were also shown to react with purified RyR.[49] RyR antibodies are detected in about one-half of MG patients with thymoma. Thymoma patients with RyR antibodies, especially those with high antibody levels, do significantly less well than RyR antibody-negative thymoma patients.[50] Whether the association between RyR antibodies and MG severity is due to pathogenic effects of antibodies on muscle function or reflects a stronger immune response involving cytotoxic T lymphocytes and inflammatory muscle damage in antibody-positive patients is not known.

Skeie et al. have examined if such antibodies can influence the RyR function in vitro. They found that sera from most MG patients with RyR antibodies inhibited [^{3}H]-ryanodine binding to the sarcoplasmic reticulum. These patients had a more severe MG than those with noninhibiting antibodies.[51] Ryanodine is used as a conformational probe to indicate the gating state of the Ca^{2+}-release channel. The results show that RyR antibodies in the sera of MG patients have a high affinity and that the binding of such antibodies may affect Ca^{2+} release by locking the RyR ion channel in a closed position. This will again increase the susceptibility of skeletal muscle cells to fatigability in a way that is not ameliorated by acetylcholine esterase inhibitors.

CONCLUSIONS

Approximately 85% of MG patients with thymoma have muscle striation antibodies. The major autoantigen is titin and the principal epitope is located in its main immunogenic region. Some patients have evidence of epitope spreading with antibody activity against a second titin epitope, localized between the N1-line and the N2-line of the half-sarcomere. Neoplastic thymomatous epithelial cells from MG patients do not contain intact titin, but express mRNA coding for both titin epitopes. Nearly half of older, nonthymoma MG patients also have titin antibodies. Titin antibody-positive late-onset MG patients have a more severe disease than MG patients without such antibodies.

About 50% of MG patients with thymoma also have antibodies against ryanodine receptor. These antibodies have a high affinity to the receptor and inhibit binding of ryanodine to the sarcoplasmic reticulum.

The immune reactivity to titin and ryanodine receptor, observed in some MG patients, is probably an element of the pathogenesis of the disease. This immune response is part of the immune disturbances seen in MG and is important for the understanding of the heterogeneity of the disease.

REFERENCES

1. STRAUSS, A. J. L., B. SEEGAL, J. C. HSU, P. M. BURKHOLDER, W. NASTUK & K. E. OSSERMAN. 1960. Immunofluorescence demonstration of a muscle binding, complement fixing serum globulin fraction in myasthenia gravis. Proc. Soc. Exp. Biol. **1195:** 184–191.
2. BEUTNER, E. H., E. WITEBSKY, D. RICKEN & R. H. ADLER. 1962. Studies on autoantibodies in myasthenia gravis. JAMA **182:** 46–58.
3. VAN DER GELD, H. & A. J. L. STRAUSS. 1966. Myasthenia gravis: immunological relationship between striated muscle and thymus. Lancet **i:** 57–60.
4. VETTERS, J. M. 1965. Immunofluorescence staining patterns in skeletal muscle using the serum of myasthenic patients and normal controls. Immunology **9:** 93–95.
5. VETTERS, J. M. 1967. Muscle antibodies in myasthenia gravis. Immunology **13:** 275–280.
6. AARLI, J. A. & O. CLOSS. 1972. Myasthenia gravis: cross-striational fluorescence of muscle fibers mediated by Fc fragments. J. Immunol. **109:** 271–274.
7. PATRICK, J. & J. LINDSTROM. 1973. Autoimmune response to acetylcholine receptors. Science **180:** 871–872.
8. AARLI, J. A. 1972. Myasthenia gravis: antibodies to an acid-soluble muscle antigen reacting with antibodies in myasthenia gravis sera. Acta Pathol. Microbiol. Scand. Sect. B **80:** 453–459.
9. AARLI, J. A., N. E. GILHUS & H. HOFSTAD. 1987. CA-antibody: an immunological marker of thymic neoplasia in myasthenia gravis? Acta Neurol. Scand. **63:** 55–57.
10. WILLIAMS, C. L. & V. A. LENNON. 1986. Thymic B-lymphocyte clones from patients with myasthenia gravis secrete monoclonal striational autoantibodies reacting with myosin, α-actinin, or actin. J. Exp. Med. **164:** 1043–1059.
11. OHTA, M., K. OHTA, N. ITOH, M. KUROBE, K. HAYASHI & H. NISHITANI. 1990. Anti-skeletal muscle antibodies in the sera from myasthenic patients with thymoma: identification of anti-myosin, actomyosin, actin, and α-actinin antibodies by a solid-phase radioimmunoassay and a Western blotting analysis. Clin. Chim. Acta **187:** 255–264.
12. AARLI, J. A., K. STEFANSSON, L. S. G. MARTON & R. WOLLMANN. 1990. Patients with myasthenia gravis and thymoma have in their sera IgG autoantibodies against titin. Clin. Exp. Immunol. **82:** 284–288.

13. FÜRST, D. O., R. NAVE, M. OSBORN & K. WEBER. 1989. Repetitive titin epitopes with a 42-nm spacing coincide in relative major myosin-associated proteins: an immunoelectron-microscopical study on myofibrils. J. Cell Sci. **94:** 119–125.

14. FÜRST, D. O., M. OSBORN, R. NAVE & K. WEBER. 1988. The organization of titin filaments in the half-sarcomere revealed by monoclonal antibodies in immunoelectron microscopy: a map of ten nonrepetitive epitopes starting at the Z line extends close to the M line. J. Cell Biol. **106:** 1563–1572.

15. MARUYAMA, K., S. MATSUBARA, R. NATORI, Y. NONOMURA, S. KIMURA, K. OHASHI, F. MURAKAMI, S. HANDA & G. EGUCHI. 1977. Connectin, an elastic protein of muscle: characterization and function. J. Biochem. (Tokyo) **82:** 317–337.

16. LABEIT, S. & B. KOLMERER. 1995. Titins: giant proteins in charge of muscle ultrastructure and elasticity. Science **270:** 293–296.

17. FULTON, A. B. & W. B. ISAACS. 1991. Titin, a huge, elastic sarcomeric protein with a probable role in morphogenesis. Bioessays **13:** 157–161.

18. GAUTEL, M., A. LAKEY, D. P. BARLOW, Z. HOLMES, S. SCALES, K. LEONARD, S. LABEIT, Å. MYGLAND, N. E. GILHUS & J. A. AARLI. 1993. Titin antibodies in myasthenia gravis: identification of a major immunogenic region of titin. Neurology **43:** 1581–1585.

19. LABEIT, S., B. KOLMERER & W. A. LINKE. 1997. The giant protein titin: emerging roles in physiology and pathophysiology. Circ. Res. **80:** 290–294.

20. LINKE, W. A., M. IVEMEYER, N. OLIVIERI, B. KOLMERER, J. C. RÜEGG & S. LABEIT. 1996. Towards a molecular understanding of the elasticity of titin. J. Mol. Biol. **261:** 62–71.

21. LÜBKE, E., A. FREIBURG, G. O. SKEIE, B. KOLMERER, S. LABEIT, J. A. AARLI, N. E. GILHUS, R. WOLLMANN, M. WÜSSLING, J. RÜEGG & W. A. LINKE. 1997. Striational autoantibodies in myasthenia gravis: evidence for titin epitope spreading. Submitted.

22. MARX, A., M. OSBORN, S. TZARTOS, K. I. GEUDER, B. SCHALKE, W. NIX, T. KIRCHNER & H. K. MÜLLER-HERMELINK. 1992. A striational muscle antigen and myasthenia gravis associated thymomas share an acetylcholine-receptor epitope. Dev. Immunol. **2:** 77–84.

23. GILHUS, N. E., J. A. AARLI, B. CHRISTENSSON & R. MATRE. 1984. Rabbit antiserum to a citric acid extract of human skeletal muscle staining thymoma from myasthenia gravis patients. J. Neuroimmunol. **7:** 55–64.

24. DARDENNE, M., W. SAVINO & J. F. BACH. 1987. Thymomatous epithelial cells and skeletal muscle share a common epitope defined by a monoclonal antibody. Am. J. Pathol. **126:** 194–198.

25. KIRCHNER, T., S. TZARTOS, F. HOPPE, B. SCHALKE, H. WEKERLE & H. K. MÜLLER-HERMELINK. 1988. Pathogenesis of myasthenia gravis: acetylcholine receptor–related antigenic determinants in tumor-free thymuses and thymic epithelial tumors. Am. J. Pathol. **130:** 268–280.

26. MARX, A., A. WILISCH, A. SCHULTZ, A. GREINER, B. MAGI, V. PALLINI, B. SCHALKE, K. TOYKA, W. NIX, T. KIRCHNER & H. K. MÜLLER-HERMELINK. 1996. Expression of neurofilaments and of a titin epitope in thymic epithelial tumors. Am. J. Pathol. **148:** 1839–1850.

27. SKEIE, G. O., A. FREIBURG, B. KOLMERER, S. LABEIT, J. A. AARLI, S. A. APPIAH-BOADU & N. E. GILHUS. 1997. Titin transcripts in thymomas. Submitted.

28. WILLCOX, N. 1993. Myasthenia gravis. Curr. Opin. Immunol. **5:** 910–917.

29. MARX, A., D. SCHOMIG, A. SCHULTZ, S. GATTENLOHNER, A. JUNG, A. MELMS & H. K. MÜLLER-HERMELINK. 1994. Distribution of molecules mediating thymocyte-stroma-interactions in human thymus, thymitis, and thymic epithelial tumors. Thymus **23:** 83–89.

30. AARLI, J. A., N. E. GILHUS & R. MATRE. 1992. Myasthenia gravis with thymoma is not associated with an increase of other autoimmune disorders. Autoimmunity **11:** 159–162.

31. GILHUS, N. E., N. WILLCOX, G. HARCOURT, N. NAGVEJAR, D. BEESON, A. VINCENT & J. NEWSOM-DAVIS. 1995. Antigen presentation by thymoma epithelial cells from myasthenia gravis patients to potentially pathogenic T cells. J. Neuroimmunol. **56:** 65–76.

32. Skeie, G. O., J. A. Aarli, R. Matre, A. Freiburg & N. E. Gilhus. 1997. Titin antibody positive myasthenia gravis patients have a cellular immune response against the main immunogenic region of titin. Eur. J. Neurol. **4:** 1–7.

33. Pescarmona, E., S. Rosati, A. Pisacane, E. A. Rendina, F. Venuta & C. D. Baroni. 1992. Microscopic thymoma: histological evidence of multifocal cortical and medullary origin. Histopathology **20:** 263–266.

34. Lanska, D. J. 1991. Diagnosis of thymoma in myasthenics using anti-striated muscle antibodies: predictive value and gain in diagnostic certainty. Neurology **41:** 520–524.

35. Skeie, G. O., Å. Mygland, J. A. Aarli & N. E. Gilhus. 1995. Titin antibodies in patients with late onset myasthenia gravis: clinical correlations. Autoimmunity **20:** 99–104.

36. McFarlin, D. E., M. Barlow & A. J. L. Strauss. 1966. Antibodies to muscle and thymus in nonmyasthenic patients with thymoma. N. Engl. J. Med. **275:** 1321–1326.

37. Rowland, L. P., H. Aranow, Jr. & P. F. A. Hoefer. 1957. Myasthenia gravis appearing after removal of a thymoma. Neurology **7:** 584–588.

38. Gilhus, N. E., J. A. Aarli, R. W. C. Janzen & R. Matre. 1985. Skeletal muscle antibodies in patients with a thymoma, but without myasthenia gravis, J. Neuroimmunol. **8:** 69–78.

39. Kuks, J. B. M. 1992. The Thymus and Myasthenia Gravis. Drukkerij Regenboog. Groningen.

40. Perlo, V. P., B. Arnason & B. Castleman. 1975. The thymus gland in elderly patients with myasthenia gravis. Neurology **25:** 294–295.

41. Keynes, G. 1946. The surgery of the thymus gland. Br. J. Surg. **33:** 201–214.

42. Oosterhuis, H. J. 1981. Observations of the natural history of myasthenia gravis and effect of therapeutic measures. Ann. N.Y. Acad. Sci. **377:** 678–689.

43. Somnier, F. & W. Trojaburg. 1993. Neurophysiological evaluation in myasthenia gravis: a comprehensive study of a complete patient population. Electroencephalogr. Clin. Neurophysiol. **89:** 73–87.

44. Gross, W. L., W. H. Schmitt & E. Csernok. 1992. ANCA and associated diseases: immunodiagnostic and pathogenetic aspects. Clin. Exp. Immunol. **91:** 1–12.

45. Ma, J., N. King, C. L. Chen, R. Penny & S. N. Breit. 1993. Antibody penetration of viable human cells. II. Anti-RNP antibodies binding to RNP antigen expressed on cell surface, which may mediate the antibody internalization. Clin. Exp. Immunol. **93:** 396–404.

46. Mygland, Å., O. B. Tysnes, J. A. Aarli, P. R. Flood & N. E. Gilhus. 1992. Myasthenia gravis patients with a thymoma have antibodies against a high molecular weight protein in sarcoplasmic reticulum. J. Neuroimmunol. **37:** 1–7.

47. Takeshima, H., I. Masamitsu, H. Takekura, N. Miyuki, J. Kunu, O. Minowa, H. Takano & T. Noda. 1994. Excitation-contraction uncoupling in mice lacking functional skeletal muscle ryanodine-receptor gene. Nature **369:** 556–559.

48. Mendell, J. R., J. N. Whitaker & W. K. Engel. 1973. The skeletal muscle binding site of antistriated muscle antibody in myasthenia gravis: an electron microscopic immunohistochemical study using peroxidase conjugated antibody fragments. J. Immunol. **111:** 847–856.

49. Mygland, Å., O. B. Tysnes, R. Matre, P. Volpe, J. A. Aarli & N. E. Gilhus. 1992. Ryanodine receptor autoantibodies in myasthenia gravis patients with a thymoma. Ann. Neurol. **32:** 589–591.

50. Mygland, Å., J. A. Aarli, R. Matre & N. E. Gilhus. 1994. Ryanodine receptor autoantibodies related to the severity of thymoma associated myasthenia gravis. J. Neurol. Neurosurg. Psychiatry **57:** 843–846.

51. Skeie, G. O., P. K. Lunde, O. M. Sejersted, Å. Mygland, J. A. Aarli & N. E. Gilhus. 1997. Myasthenia gravis sera containing anti-ryanodine receptor antibodies inhibit binding of [^{3}H]-ryanodine to sarcoplasmic reticulum. Submitted.

Rapsyn Antibodies in Myasthenia Gravis[a]

MARK A. AGIUS,[b] SHAN ZHU,[b] CHRISTINE A. KIRVAN,[b]
ANNE L. SCHAFER,[b] MIKE Y. LIN,[b] ROBERT H. FAIRCLOUGH,[b]
JOEL J-F. OGER,[c] TARIQ AZIZ,[c] AND JOHAN A. AARLI[d]

[b]Department of Neurology
University of California at Davis
Davis, California 95616

[c]University of British Columbia
Vancouver, British Columbia, Canada

[d]Department of Neurology
University of Bergen
Bergen, Norway

INTRODUCTION

Rapsyn is required for acetylcholine receptor (AChR) clustering, which in turn is required for normal neuromuscular transmission. Rapsyn is a cytoplasmic 43-kDa protein present on the inner aspect of the cell membrane. Rapsyn localizes to the end plates, binding noncovalently with the beta subunit of the AChR. There is a one-to-one stoichiometry of rapsyn with AChRs. Animals genetically deficient in rapsyn synthesize AChRs, but these fail to cluster at the neuromuscular junction and the animals die soon after birth.[1] Preparation of AChR-enriched membranes from the electric organ of *Torpedo californica* is achieved by 1 M salt wash of homogenized electric organ followed by differential centrifugation. This produces membranes enriched in AChRs, the 43-kDa, as well as the 58-kDa, 87-kDa, and higher-molecular-weight synapse organizing proteins. Preparations enriched for rapsyn can be prepared from the pH 11 extract of the AChR-enriched membranes. The close association of rapsyn with AChR and the role of rapsyn in establishing AChR density at end plates prompted us to investigate the possibility of an antirapsyn immune attack in patients with acquired myasthenia gravis (MG).

MATERIALS AND METHODS

AChR and Rapsyn

Electric organ of *Torpedo californica* was dissected, homogenized in salt, subjected to differential centrifugation, and extracted in water at pH 11 as previously described.[2] The predominant component of this extract is rapsyn. AChR is undetected in polyacrylamide gel electrophoresis of this extract.

[a]This work was supported by the Myasthenia Gravis Foundation Viets Fellowship.

Serum

Serum was obtained by informed consent from patients with MG as well as from control individuals. Antirapsyn antibodies were detected on immunoblots prepared by standard methodology.[3]

Animal Experiments

Female Lewis rats were immunized with 50 μg of the pH 11 extract of *Torpedo* enriched membranes in complete Freund's adjuvant (CFA). Animals were monitored for weakness and weight. Serum was obtained from tail bleeding. Serum anti-AChR antibody titer was obtained by a radioimmunoassay using solubilized *Torpedo* AChR. Serum antirapsyn and anti-AChR antibody reactivity was also tested by immunoblots.

Muscle AChR Density

Muscle AChR density was measured in the diaphragm at four months. The assay involved a modification of the standard AChR density measurement, involving a measurement of α-bungarotoxin (α-bgtx) binding sites per end plate. Measurements were performed in triplicate on serially consecutive muscle fiber bundles of freshly dissected rat diaphragm of equivalent size and weight. Analysis of specific α-bgtx binding sites was done on two of the consecutive serial sections. Total gamma counts were determined by incubating one bundle with ^{125}I-labeled α-bgtx, whereas nonspecific counts were determined by incubating a second bundle with ^{125}I-labeled α-bgtx after first incubating with unlabeled α-bgtx. The number of end plates per muscle fiber bundle was determined under fluorescence microscopy by incubating a consecutive serial muscle fiber bundle with rhodamine-labeled α-bgtx. Nonspecific rhodamine-labeled α-bgtx binding was assessed by preincubating a fourth muscle fiber bundle with unlabeled α-bgtx. Microscopic analysis was performed without the need for embedding or fixing. Statistical analysis was undertaken using Student's two-tailed *t* test.

RESULTS

Rapsyn Antibodies in Patients with MG

We initially screened the sera from 15 patients with acquired MG and pooled human normal serum. We detected antibodies to the 43-kDa protein in 2 of the 15 (15%) myasthenic patients, but not in pooled normal human serum. The 43-kDa band corresponded to the molecular weight protein recognized by a specific antirapsyn antibody (gift of Stanley Froehner). One of these patients also demonstrated reactivity with proteins of 58-kDa and 87-kDa molecular weights as well as to proteins of lower molecular weights. There did not appear to be any correlation in rapsyn anti-body–positive patients with clinical characteristics.

To further investigate a possible pathogenic role for antirapsyn antibodies in some patients with acquired myasthenia, we undertook an analysis of sera from patients with MG and controls obtained from Vancouver, Canada, and Bergen, Norway. This analysis was performed by immunoblotting in a coded and blinded fashion and was done in collaboration with J. Oger and J. Aarli, who provided the sera.

We detected antirapsyn antibodies in a subpopulation of MG patients (TABLE 1). These included 1 of 10 patients with high positive AChR antibody titers, 1 of 10 with borderline titers, 3 of 17 with seronegative myasthenia, and 2 of 17 with thymoma and anti-AChR antibodies. Overall, the incidence of antirapsyn antibodies was low; they were present in 7 of 54 or 13% of patients tested. They were not present in healthy controls. They were not specific to myasthenia, however, and were present in 1 of 10 patients with autoimmune neurological disease. This patient carried a diagnosis of possible multiple sclerosis. Most interesting was the detection of antirapsyn antibodies in 7 of 9 patients tested with systemic lupus (TABLE 1).

Rapsyn Antibodies in Morvan's Fibrillary Chorea

A patient in whom antirapsyn antibodies were detected had a thymoma, myasthenia gravis with anti-AChR antibodies, a severe presynaptic defect, neuromyotonia, and central and autonomic dysfunction consistent with Morvan's fibrillary chorea.

Rapsyn Antibodies in Chronic Procainamide-associated Myopathy (CPAM)

A patient in whom antirapsyn antibodies were detected developed ptosis and severe dysphagia after taking oral procainamide for a few years. He had evidence for serological lupus with a high serum antinuclear antibody titer (1:1280) without anti-

TABLE 1. Serum Antirapsyn Antibodies in MG Patients and Controls

Diagnosis	Anti-AChR Antibodies	No. of Patients Tested	No. of Patients Positive for Rapsyn Antibodies
Vancouver, Canada			
myasthenia gravis	high positive titer	10	1
	borderline positive titer	10	1
	seronegative titer	9	2
other neurological illnesses	negative	10	1
healthy controls	negative	10	0
Bergen, Norway			
myasthenia gravis	seronegative titer	8	1
thymoma	positive titer	17	2
SLE	negative titer	9	7

double-stranded DNA antibodies. This patient did not have evidence for MG. Serum AChR antibodies were negative for precipitating, binding, and blocking antibodies. In addition, single muscle fiber electromyography revealed normal fiber density and jitter. This patient improved dramatically after procainamide was discontinued.

Active Immunization with Rapsyn Results in Weakness and Loss of AChR Density

To further investigate if an antirapsyn immune attack has the potential to be pathogenic, we immunized four 6-week-old female Lewis rats with the pH 11 extract of the membranes derived from *Torpedo* electric organ. Two received 50 μg of extract in CFA and two received 200 μg of extract in CFA. Five rats served as controls, three of which received injections of normal saline and two received equivalent amounts of CFA. One of the animals immunized with 200 μg of the pH 11 extract developed moderately severe weakness three weeks after immunization. This weakness persisted until the animal was sacrificed. At the time of the development of weakness, the rats had detectable antirapsyn activity as determined by immunoblotting. The antirapsyn activity increased up through the fourth and fifth weeks. Furthermore, the pattern of serum reactivity to the *Torpedo* pH 11 extracted proteins at the neuromuscular junction demonstrated by this particular rat overlapped that observed in MG patients. The rats failed to demonstrate detectable anti-AChR antibodies as tested in a radioimmunoassay with solubilized *Torpedo* AChR at this time. Trace binding to *Torpedo* AChR subunits was noted on immunoblots at five weeks after immunization with pH 11 extract. This reactivity developed two weeks subsequent to the onset of weakness. The animals were sacrificed at four months after immunization and AChR density was measured in skeletal muscle. Consecutive serial sections of intact muscle fibers from rat diaphragms were used in the analysis. The number of AChRs in intact muscle fibers was determined by gamma counting after incubation with ^{125}I-labeled α-bgtx. This is a modification of the more-conventional method of determining AChR density that utilizes staining for cholinesterase to allow the counting of end plates. The mean AChR density of normal rat diaphragm was 75 million α-bgtx binding sites per end plate with a standard deviation of 17 million. Whereas all control animals had AChR densities that were above 50 million α-bgtx binding sites per end plate, the animals that were immunized with rapsyn had a mean of 30 million sites per end plate. The difference in AChR density in rapsyn-immunized animals and controls was significant, with a p value of less than 0.01 (TABLE 2).

DISCUSSION AND CONCLUSIONS

We have detected antirapsyn antibodies as well as antibodies to other synapse organizing proteins in a subpopulation of patients with MG. These antibodies are not specific to MG as they have been detected in the serum of patients with other immune diseases. However, the close association of rapsyn with the AChR raises the possibility of a secondary antirapsyn immune attack in patients with acquired MG who have antibodies to the AChR. Furthermore, the colocalization of rapsyn with the beta subunit of the AChR suggests that antirapsyn antibodies in myasthenia may arise

TABLE 2. AChR Density of Rapsyn-immunized Rats and Controls

Lewis Rat	Immunization Schedule	AChR Density (Molecules of α-bgtx Binding Sites/End Plate × 10^7)
1	control: normal saline	8.40
2	control: normal saline	5.66
3	control: normal saline	9.83
4	control: CFA alone	6.10
5	control: CFA alone	7.48
Total control animals ($n = 5$)		7.49 ± 1.70 (mean ± SD)
6	50 μg rapsyn in CFA	3.10
7	50 μg rapsyn in CFA	4.15
8	200 μg rapsyn in CFA	3.69
9	200 μg rapsyn in CFA	1.14
Total rapsyn-immunized animals		3.02 ± 1.33 (mean ± SD) ($p < 0.01$)

as a consequence of epitope spreading. The critical role that rapsyn plays in promoting the high density concentration of AChRs at the neuromuscular junction suggests the possibility that an antirapsyn immune attack may contribute to the pathogenicity in MG. Consequently, in patients with detectable anti-AChR antibodies, coexisting antirapsyn antibodies may, in part, explain the poor correlation between anti-AChR antibody titers and disease severity. Similarly, antirapsyn antibodies may generate dysfunction of neuromuscular transmission and weakness in some patients with seronegative MG.

The significance of antirapsyn reactivity in the majority of lupus patients tested is unclear. In this context, the lupuslike syndromes associated with procainamide may provide some insight. Procainamide is known to bind to rapsyn at the neuromuscular junction.[4] The presence of antirapsyn antibodies in a patient with procainamide-induced myopathy and serologic lupus suggests that, in this context, chemical interaction of procainamide with rapsyn may induce an immunogenic response.

Immunization of Lewis rats with rapsyn resulted in production of antirapsyn antibodies with overt weakness prior to the detection of anti-AChR antibodies on immunoblots. The animals subsequently develop biochemical evidence for experimental MG with loss of AChR density. However, these animals do not demonstrate anti-AChR serum titers in a radioimmunoassay with solubilized AChR. These animal data support the hypothesis that an antirapsyn immune response has the potential to be pathogenic.

REFERENCES

1. GAUTAM, M., P. G. NOAKES, J. MUDD, M. NICHOL, G. C. CHU, J. R. SANES & J. P. MERLIE. 1995. Failure of postsynaptic specialization to develop at neuromuscular junctions of rapsyn-deficient mice. Nature 377: 232–236.

2. ELLIOTT, J., S. G. BLANCHARD, W. WU, J. MILLER, C. D. STRADER, P. HARTIG, H-P. MOORE, J. RACS & M. A. RAFTERY. 1980. Purification of *Torpedo californica* post-synaptic membranes and fractionation of their constituent proteins. Biochem. J. **185:** 667–677.

3. BLAIR, D. A., M. MIHOVILOVIC, M. A. AGIUS, R. H. FAIRCLOUGH & D. P. RICHMAN. 1987. Human × human hybridomas from patients with myasthenia gravis: possible tools for idiotypic therapy for myasthenia. Ann. N.Y. Acad. Sci. **505:** 155–167.

4. ZHU, S., R. H. FAIRCLOUGH & M. A. AGIUS. 1996. Anti-rapsyn antibodies may contribute to pathogenicity in myasthenia gravis. FASEB J. **10:** 4163.

Antibodies to AChR, Synapse-organizing Proteins, Titin, and Other Muscle Proteins in Morvan's Fibrillary Chorea[a]

MARK A. AGIUS, SHAN ZHU, EUN-KYU LEE, JOHAN A. AARLI,
CHRISTINE KIRVAN, ROBERT H. FAIRCLOUGH,
AND RICARDO MASELLI

Department of Neurology
University of California at Davis
Davis, California 95615

INTRODUCTION

Morvan's description of fibrillary chorea (MFC) included multiple, irregular contractions of the long muscle, hyperhidrosis, skin lesions, insomnia, and morbid delusions.[1] The muscle twitching is characterized on electromyography (EMG) by neuromyotonia with repetitive motor unit potentials firing in irregular bursts and with a high intraburst frequency. Two patients reported by Halbach *et al.* had acetylcholine receptor (AChR) antibodies and thymoma, without clinical myasthenia gravis (MG).[2] An autoimmune etiology for neuromyotonia has been postulated based on its association with MG, humorally mediated peripheral neuropathies, its response to plasmapheresis, and the recent detection in some patients of antibodies against voltage-gated potassium channels.

CASE REPORT

A 49-year-old male developed progressive generalized weakness over several months associated with muscle twitching at rest and exertional cramping. He developed ptosis, diplopia, severe constipation, urinary incontinence, anorexia and weight loss, excessive sweating, tachycardia, angina, paroxysmal syncope, anxiety, and insomnia. He also developed confusion, with delirium. On examination, he was hypertensive with sinus tachycardia and fever. He had ptosis, with weakness of lateral recti and left medial rectus. He had continuous generalized muscle twitches with moderate muscle atrophy and symmetric generalized weakness. Sensory and cerebellar testing was normal. Ankle reflexes were absent and plantar reflexes were flexor. He had elevated serum anti-AChR and striated muscle antibodies. In addition, N-type calcium channel antibodies, but not P/Q-type calcium channel antibodies, were present in serum. EMG demonstrated the presence of neuromyotonia with doublets, triplets, and multiplets and continuous neuromyotonic discharges of a frequency close to 200 Hz without evidence of denervation. Conduction block of the right common peroneal

[a]This work was supported by the Viets Fellowship of the Myasthenia Gravis Foundation.

nerve with 1% Xylocaine failed to eliminate neuromyotonia in the right tibialis anterior. *In vitro* microelectrode studies showed the presence of severe postsynaptic and presynaptic defects. Muscle biopsy showed muscle fiber necrosis replaced by macrophages in severely involved areas. The neuromyotonia improved on phenytoin, whereas confusion decreased and strength improved with plasmapheresis. A CT scan of the chest revealed a thymoma, which was treated surgically. Sustained, marked improvement coincided with the introduction of high-dosage oral prednisone.

MATERIALS AND METHODS

Synapse-organizing proteins (SOPs) including rapsyn, syntrophin (58-kDa protein), and dystrobrevin (87-kDa protein) were purified from *Torpedo californica* electric organ by differential centrifugation followed by alkali extraction. Serum antibodies to SOPs were detected by immunoblotting using standard methodology. Monoclonal antibodies to calsequestrin, SERCA, troponin, calmodulin, myosin, and actin were obtained from Affinity Bioreagents, Incorporated (Golden, Colorado). Serum antibodies were determined by immunoblotting. Rat muscle extracts were prepared by SDS digestion, followed by polyacrylamide gradient gel electrophoresis of skeletal muscle from Lewis rats. Serum antibodies to titin were determined in ELISA and to ryanodine receptor (RyR) by immunoblotting. Measurements of serum antibodies to striated muscle antibodies, AChR, and P/Q- and N-type calcium channels were determined at the Mayo clinical laboratories.

RESULTS

Immunoblotting showed reactivity of serum with rapsyn (43 kDa) as well as syntrophin (58 kDa) derived from *Torpedo californica*. Specific reactivity for rapsyn was confirmed with the use of a monoclonal antibody specific for rapsyn (gift of Stanley Froehner). In addition, reactivity was detected for several rat muscle-extracted proteins. These included proteins of molecular weights corresponding to about 200 kDa, 110 kDa, 95 kDa, 63 kDa, and 38 kDa. Monoclonal antibodies to myosin (200 kDa), SERCA (sarcoplasmic and endoplasmic reticulum calcium ATPase) (110 kDa), triadin (95 kDa), calsequestrin (63 kDa), and troponin T (38 kDa) identified protein bands in the muscle extract corresponding to similar molecular weights as the muscle proteins bound by the MFC serum. Serum from four patients with noninflammatory myopathy did not show reactivity with the muscle proteins that are bound by the MFC serum. In addition, there was a lack of reactivity to these proteins in muscle extract by sera from four additional healthy individuals.

DISCUSSION

In the reported patient, MFC was associated with thymoma and MG and was characterized by a confusional state, autonomic dysfunction, neuromyotonia, and myopathy. The patient was found to have autoantibodies to several muscle antigens.

These autoantibodies included antibodies against the nicotinic AChR, as well as to postsynaptic, cytoskeletal proteins at the neuromuscular junction and to titin and several additional intracellular proteins. The presence of a myopathy pathologically in this patient suggests that these antibodies may have contributed to pathogenicity.

Antibodies to N-type calcium channels were also present. The detection of anti-AChR and anti-calcium channel antibodies in this patient correlates with the presence electrophysiologically of postsynaptic and presynaptic defects, respectively. The central nervous system manifestations and dysautonomia and their course in this patient suggest the likely presence of also antineuronal antibodies. The persistence of neuromyotonia after nerve block suggests that the muscle activity is generated at the distal nerve terminals or in the muscle itself. Antibodies to other tissue-specific antigens were not detected. The presence of a thymoma in this patient suggests that the muscle and neuromuscular junction antibodies that he demonstrates may have arisen as a paraneoplastic phenomenon, possibly as a consequence of a cross-reactive immune response.

REFERENCES

1. MORVAN, A. 1890. De la choree fibrillaire. Gaz. Hebdomadaire Med. Chir. **27:** 173–200.
2. HALBACH, M., V. HOMBERG & H. J. FREUND. 1987. Neuromuscular, autonomic, and central cholinergic hyperactivity associated with thymoma and acetylcholine receptor–binding antibody. J. Neurol. **234:** 433–436.

Antirapsyn Antibodies Occur Commonly in Patients with Lupus[a]

MARK A. AGIUS,[b] SHAN ZHU,[b] AND JOHAN A. AARLI[c]

[b]Department of Neurology
University of California at Davis
Davis, California 95615

[c]Department of Neurology
University of Bergen
Bergen, Norway

INTRODUCTION

Rapsyn is a 43-kDa protein that noncovalently binds the beta subunit of the acetylcholine receptor (AChR). It is found on the cytoplasmic side of the neuromuscular junction and is required for the clustering of AChRs at high density at the synaptic folds. The primary structure of rapsyn is characterized by several cysteine residues that are likely to be important functionally and that contribute to the protein's high reactivity. We have observed antirapsyn antibodies in a patient receiving procainamide for several years who developed a chronic myopathy with bulbar weakness (chronic procainamide-associated myopathy, CPAM). The presence of antirapsyn antibodies in this patient suggested that chronic therapy with procainamide may result in immunogenicity of nonstandard proteins at the neuromuscular junction. Procainamide is a well-established pharmacologic cause of lupus and this patient also demonstrated serological evidence of procainamide-induced lupus with an ANA titer of 1280. Here, we have screened patients with MG as well as lupus for antibodies to rapsyn in a blinded, coded fashion and have found antirapsyn antibodies in a majority of patients with lupus.

MATERIALS AND METHODS

Rapsyn-enriched preparations were generated by differential centrifugation followed by alkali extraction of membranes from *Torpedo californica*. Antirapsyn antibodies are detected by immunoblotting using standard methodology.[1] Sera were tested in a coded, blinded fashion. Sera from 9 patients with lupus, 8 patients with seronegative myasthenia gravis, 17 patients with thymoma, and 10 healthy individuals were tested. The lupus sera and the sera from thymoma patients and myasthenia gravis patients were provided by the University of Bergen, Norway. The coded sera from healthy controls were also tested in a blinded fashion with other sera and were derived from Joel Oger, University of British Columbia, Vancouver, Canada.

[a]This work was supported by the Viets Fellowship of the Myasthenia Gravis Foundation.

RESULTS

Sera from patients with lupus and myasthenia gravis, as well as from healthy individuals, were tested for antirapsyn reactivity. This analysis was done in a coded and blinded fashion. Serum antirapsyn antibodies were detected in 7 out of the 9 patients with lupus tested. All 9 patients had anti-dsDNA antibodies. In addition, serum rheumatoid factor was present in all patients in the absence of clinical evidence of rheumatoid arthritis. Eight patients with seronegative myasthenia gravis were tested. Of these, only 1 was positive for antirapsyn antibodies. Of 17 additional patients with thymoma and anti-AChR antibodies, 2 were positive for antirapsyn antibodies. In addition, antirapsyn antibodies were not detected in the 10 healthy controls tested.

DISCUSSION

Antirapsyn antibodies were detected in the serum of 7 out of the 9 (78%) lupus patients tested and in none of the normal controls. Thus, rapsyn is added to the list of intracellular autoantigens detected in systemic lupus erythematosus. Whereas antirapsyn antibodies are not specific for lupus, the high sensitivity that they appear to possess in lupus suggests that they may have a diagnostic role in this disease. The pathogenesis and the possible pathogenic role for these autoantibodies in lupus are unclear. The presence of antirapsyn antibodies in a patient with chronic procainamide-associated myopathy (CPAM) also suggests a possible association of antirapsyn reactivity in lupus.[2] Procainamide is a cause of drug-induced lupus and also is known to bind rapsyn. It is possible that this noncovalent binding may result in haptenization of rapsyn, leading to the generation of an antirapsyn immune attack.

REFERENCES

1. BLAIR, D. A., M. MIHOVILOVIC, M. A. AGIUS, R. H. FAIRCLOUGH & D. P. RICHMAN. 1987. Human × human hybridomas from patients with myasthenia gravis: possible tools for idiotypic therapy for myasthenia. Ann. N.Y. Acad. Sci. **505:** 155–166.
2. ZHU, S., R. H. FAIRCLOUGH & M. A. AGIUS. 1996. Anti-rapsyn antibodies may contribute to pathogenicity in myasthenia gravis. FASEB J. **10:** 4163.

Antirapsyn Antibodies in Chronic Procainamide-associated Myopathy (CPAM)

MARK A. AGIUS, SHAN ZHU, AND ROBERT H. FAIRCLOUGH

Department of Neurology
University of California at Davis
Davis, California 95615

INTRODUCTION

The antiarrhythmic agent, procainamide, is associated with the development of a lupuslike syndrome. Procainamide binds the 43-kDa protein, rapsyn, and the 87-kDa protein at the postsynaptic membrane[1] and this may explain its membrane-stabilizing effect. Procainamide aggravates the disorder of neuromuscular transmission in patients with myasthenia gravis (MG). The cause of this weakness has been attributed to both presynaptic and postsynaptic effects. However, the postsynaptic effects appear to be more significant.[2] In addition, short-term administration of procainamide has also been associated with the development of an acute myopathy that may mimic MG[3] and that in some cases has been necrotizing. We present a patient with chronic procainamide-associated myopathy (CPAM) and serologic evidence of procainamide-induced lupus and propose an autoimmune mechanism for development of the chronic myopathy.

CASE REPORT

An 84-year-old male had been receiving oral procainamide for several years. He presented with a 2-year history of dysphagia, hoarseness, dysarthria, and drooling. Cranial nerve examination revealed mild ptosis without fatigability, and extraocular movements were restricted. The nasolabial folds were flattened bilaterally, but orbicularis oculi and oris muscles had normal strength. Voice was dysphonic. Palate movement was sluggish. Neck flexion, extension, tongue strength, and motor strength were normal. Deep tendon reflexes were present throughout and brisk at the knees and ankles without clonus. Plantar reflexes were flexor. Mental status, cerebellar, sensory, and Romberg testings were normal. General medical examination was unremarkable. Serum antiacetylcholine receptor (AChR) antibodies were not present. Repetitive stimulation was negative for decrement, and single muscle fiber electromyography showed normal fiber density and no increased jitter. Swallowing studies confirmed oropharyngeal weakness. Serum antinuclear antibodies were detected at a titer of 1:1280 with a homogeneous pattern, whereas double-stranded DNA antibodies were not present. Rheumatoid factor was positive at 117 IU/mL. Serum creatine kinase, alkaline phosphatase, AST, and lactic dehydrogenase were all within normal range. Dysphagia and hoarseness improved markedly within two months of discontinuing procainamide. Progressive improvement also continued over several subsequent months and has persisted two years later.

MATERIALS AND METHODS

An antirapsyn ELISA was developed utilizing pH 11 extract of *Torpedo californica* enriched for AChR. Immunoblotting was done using standard methodology.

RESULTS

A monoclonal antirapsyn antibody (gift of Stanley Froehner) was used to develop an ELISA for detection of antirapsyn antibody (FIGURE 1). Serum from the patient presented here titrated membranes enriched for 43 kDa (FIGURE 2). In addition, the serum immunoblotted to the 43-kDa protein, but not to AChR. Representative normal human sera and serum from a patient with an unrelated neurological disease do not bind AChR nor the 43-kDa protein.

DISCUSSION

Procainamide binds peripheral membrane proteins including the 43-kDa postsynaptic protein, rapsyn. Rapsyn is noncovalently attached to the AChR and is essential for clustering of AChRs at the peaks of the folds of the postsynaptic membrane. The marked inhibition of postsynaptic transmission by procainamide is likely due, at least

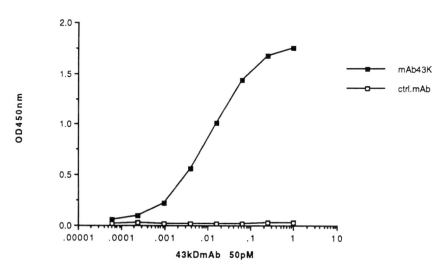

FIGURE 1. Binding of anti–43-kDa mAb to membranes containing 43 kDa.

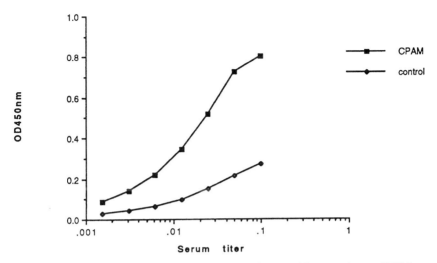

FIGURE 2. Titration of crude *Torpedo*-enriched membranes with serum from a CPAM patient. CPAM serum binding to membranes containing 43 kDa.

in part, to an affect on the 43-kDa protein and other peripheral membrane proteins. Furthermore, procainamide-induced worsening in MG and procainamide-induced acute myopathy may be explained by similar direct mechanisms. However, chronic procainamide administration also results in the development of lupus antibodies in 90% of individuals and in clinical evidence of lupus in 30%. The patient reported here presented with a chronic myopathy affecting bulbar muscles, without electrophysiological evidence of MG, in the context of serological evidence of procainamide-induced lupus. Moreover, immunoblots identify the presence of anti–43-kDa antibodies in the absence of antibodies to other neuromuscular junction proteins. We postulate that the binding of procainamide to the 43-kDa protein results in haptenization of this protein and in generation of a chronic autoimmune myopathy (chronic procainamide-associated myopathy or CPAM) distinct from MG.

REFERENCES

1. BLANCHARD, S. G. & M. A. RAFTERY. 1979. Identification of the polypeptide chains in *Torpedo californica* electroplax membranes that interact with a local anesthetic analog. Proc. Natl. Acad. Sci. U.S.A. **76:** 81–85.
2. LEE, D. C., Y. I. KIM, H. H. LIU & T. R. JOHNS. 1983. Presynaptic and postsynaptic actions of procainamide on neuromuscular transmission. Muscle Nerve **6:** 442–447.
3. MILLER, C. D., M. A. OLESHANSKY, K. F. GIBSON & L. R. CANTILENA. 1993. Case report: procainamide-induced myasthenia-like weakness and dysphagia. Ther. Drug Monit. **15:** 251–254.

Myasthenia Gravis–associated Ryanodine Receptor Antibodies Inhibit Binding of Ryanodine to Sarcoplasmic Reticulum

G. O. SKEIE,[a] P. K. LUNDE,[b] O. M. SEJERSTED,[b] Å. MYGLAND,[a]
J. A. AARLI,[a] AND N. E. GILHUS[a]

[a]Department of Neurology
University of Bergen
5021 Bergen, Norway

[b]Institute for Experimental Medical Research
University of Oslo
Oslo, Norway

INTRODUCTION

Myasthenia gravis (MG) is characterized by an increased fatigability of skeletal muscle.[1] Antibodies (Ab) against the nicotinic acetylcholine receptor (AChR) impair the neuromuscular transmission. However, MG patients with a thymoma have Ab to non-AChR antigens of striated muscle as well.[2,3]

The ryanodine receptor (RyR) is the sarcoplasmic reticulum (SR) Ca^{2+}-release channel and plays an essential role in muscle contraction. Ca^{2+} release can be affected by various endogenous and exogenous agents that modulate the opening state of the ion channel. Ryanodine is a plant alkaloid that binds selectively and with high affinity to the Ca^{2+}-release channel. The degree of binding depends on the conformational state of the ion channel and reflects the Ca^{2+}-release activity.[4]

In the present study, we investigated whether RyR antibodies from MG thymoma patients have functional effects on Ca^{2+}-release activity by examining the capacity of RyR Ab–positive MG sera to interfere with [^{3}H]-ryanodine binding to SR.

MATERIALS AND METHODS

Fourteen sera from thymoma MG patients with RyR Ab were examined. Control sera were collected from 7 RyR Ab–negative MG patients and 6 healthy blood donors. The patients were classified according to the MG severity at the peak of illness—1: minor symptoms; 2: mild generalized symptoms; 3: moderate generalized symptoms; 4: severe generalized symptoms; 5: MG death.

Sera were tested for the presence of RyR Ab in Western blot.[3] In some RyR Ab assays, the SR preparation was preincubated with ryanodine for 45 min before it was mixed with sample buffer and run into the SDS-gel.

Inhibition of [³H]-Ryanodine Binding

SR-membranes were isolated and purified from skeletal muscle as previously described.[5] Patient and control sera were preincubated for 45 min with SR-membrane protein, and [³H]-ryanodine was added for another 45 min of incubation at 37 °C. Bound and free [³H]-ryanodine were then separated by filtration. The filters containing the SR-bound [³H]-ryanodine were washed and [³H]-ryanodine was measured in counts per minute (cpm) by liquid scintillation counting. Inhibition in the [³H]-ryanodine binding experiments is given as a percentage calculated for each serum: inhibition (%) = (mean cpm for all control sera – cpm for actual MG patient) × 100/mean cpm in blood donors.

RESULTS

Inhibition of [³H]-Ryanodine Binding

Sera from 9 out of 14 RyR Ab–positive MG patients gave a 15–54% inhibition of ryanodine binding at a dilution of 1:10 (FIGURE 1). Control sera from MG patients with AChR and titin Ab, but no RyR Ab, gave no inhibition ($p < 0.01$, $\chi^2 = 9.8$). When optimizing conditions for [³H]-ryanodine binding by increasing pH, by increasing concentrations of [³H]-ryanodine, by using higher dilution of sera, or by increasing the amount of SR protein, the inhibiting effect of the RyR Ab–positive sera was no longer detected.

Inhibition of MG Autoantibody Binding

In blots where the SR preparation had been preincubated with ryanodine, the bands representing RyR became weaker (FIGURE 2), indicating that less RyR was free to bind RyR Ab.

Association with Clinical Parameters

MG patients with RyR Ab inhibiting [³H]-ryanodine binding had a more severe MG than patients without inhibiting Ab; disability score of 4.6 ± 0.5 as compared to 3.6 ± 0.5 in RyR Ab–positive MG patients with no inhibiting antibodies ($p = 0.006$).

DISCUSSION

This study shows that RyR antibodies circulating in MG patients with thymoma inhibit ryanodine binding to the RyR. The inhibition was concentration-dependent as the effect disappeared at increasing serum dilutions and also at increasing concentrations of ryanodine. There was a reciprocal competition between the RyR Ab and

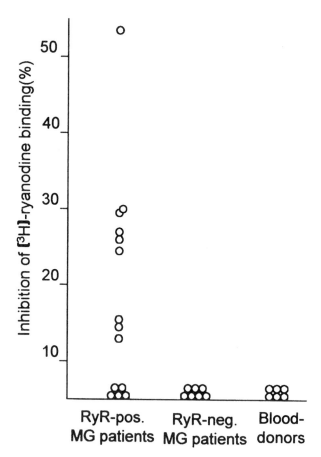

FIGURE 1. The capacity of sera from RyR antibody–positive and RyR antibody–negative MG patients and blood donors to inhibit [³H]-ryanodine binding to an SR-membrane preparation.

ryanodine for binding to the RyR as preincubation of SR with ryanodine inhibited staining by RyR Ab in Western blots.

[³H]-Ryanodine binds to sites within a conformational-sensitive area of the channel. Conditions that open the channel enhance [³H]-ryanodine binding, whereas conditions that close the channel inhibit [³H]-ryanodine binding.[4] [³H]-Ryanodine binding is therefore used as a conformational probe to indicate the gating state of the RyR. Thus, the inhibition of [³H]-ryanodine binding by RyR Ab from MG patients indicates that the antibodies affect Ca^{2+} release from the SR by causing conformational changes that close the RyR ion channel.

The RyR may have a role in physiological muscle fatigability because the RyR channel function is modified by ligands that are generated during exercise. In MG

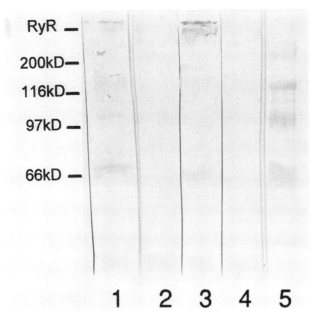

FIGURE 2. Western blot showing staining of the RyR by various MG sera. Lanes 1 and 3: ryanodine-preincubated and pure SR preparations stained by the same RyR-positive MG serum. The preincubated SR (lane 1) shows a much weaker staining. Lanes 2 and 4: the preincubated and pure SR preparations reacted with an RyR-negative serum. Lane 5: markers.

patients, RyR Ab may increase the susceptibility of muscle cells to such physiological fatigability. Patients with RyR Ab that inhibited [^{3}H]-ryanodine binding had the most severe disease. This adds support to the hypothesis that the RyR antibodies have functional effects *in vivo*.

REFERENCES

1. LINDSTROM, J. 1985. Immunobiology of myasthenia gravis, experimental autoimmune myasthenia gravis, and Lambert-Eaton syndrome. Annu. Rev. Immunol. **3:** 109–131.
2. AARLI, J. A. *et al.* 1990. Patients with myasthenia gravis and thymoma have in their sera IgG autoantibodies against titin. Clin. Exp. Immunol. **82:** 284–288.
3. MYGLAND, Å. *et al.* 1992. Ryanodine receptor autoantibodies in myasthenia gravis patients with a thymoma. Ann. Neurol. **32:** 589–591.
4. CORONADO, R. *et al.* 1994. Structure and function of ryanodine receptors. Am. J. Physiol. **266:** c1485–c1504.
5. LUNDE, P. K. & O. M. SEJERSTED. 1997. [^{3}H]-Ryanodine binding to small samples of skeletal muscle. Scand. J. Clin. Lab. Invest. In press.

Sera from Myasthenia Gravis Patients Recognize the PEVK Domain of Titin

MIRTA MIHOVILOVIC,[a] YUN MAI,[a] CAROL AUSTIN,[a] AND ALLEN D. ROSES[a,b]

[a]Division of Neurology
[b]Department of Neurobiology
Duke University Medical Center
Durham, North Carolina 27710

INTRODUCTION

Most myasthenia gravis (MG) patients have circulating anti-AChR antibodies, while a smaller number also carry antiskeletal muscle antibodies. Within this population, antibodies directed to the titin main immunogenic region (MIR) are detected in 97% of patients that present with thymic neoplasia[1] and in a smaller percentage of patients that present with thymic atrophy[1] or late-onset nonthymoma MG.[2]

Screening of an expression cDNA cardiac muscle library with MG sera led to the description of the MIR of titin[1] located downstream from its PEVK domain.[3] Here, we report that screening of an expression skeletal muscle library with MG sera resulted in the isolation of three cDNA clones derived from the PEVK domain of skeletal muscle titin. In addition, using a recombinant peptide encoded by 381 bp common to the 5' end of the isolated clones, we show that MG patients have antirecombinant peptide antibodies and that there is no particular association between antirecombinant peptide antibody titers and the histopathological characteristics of MG thymi.

METHODS

Production and screening of the cDNA skeletal muscle library were done using standard procedures[4-6] and detection of MG antibody binding using antihuman peroxidase conjugates as secondary antibody and diaminobenzidine as the redox acceptor.

cDNA sequencing was done after subcloning the restricted cDNA fragments into the Bluescript SK+ vector (Stratagene, La Jolla, California).[4] In-frame subcloning into the NdeI/XhoI-restricted pET21a vector (Novagen, Madison, Wisconsin) was done using PCR-amplified products. After sequence verification (automated sequencing using an Applied Biosystem 373A DNA Sequencer), the His-tagged peptide was produced and purified as recommended by the supplier (Novagen).

ELISAs were done as previously described[7] using donor sera diluted 1/200.

RESULTS AND CONCLUSIONS

Screening of a human skeletal muscle expression cDNA library with pooled sera from MG patients known to stain skeletal muscle cross-striations[6] resulted in the isolation of three immunoreactive clones representing two variants of the PEVK (proline, glutamic acid, valine, lysine) domain of skeletal muscle titin. The cDNA clones encode for peptides of 461 and 487 amino acids (PEVK molar content of 66% and 78%, respectively). In addition, the two PEVK domain variants share 143 amino acids at their 5′ end that are encoded by positions 19081 to 19510 of skeletal muscle titin cDNA (GenBank accession no. X90569), suggesting that this sequence represents a PEVK domain immunogenic region. To further investigate this possibility, we

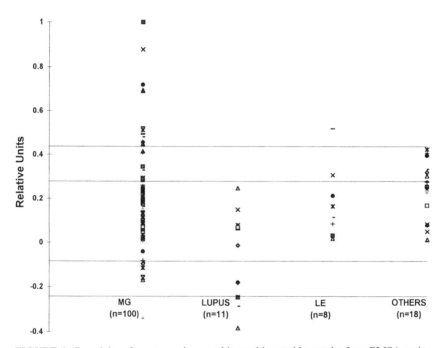

FIGURE 1. Reactivity of sera towards recombinant titin peptide: results from ELISAs using as antigen the recombinant PEVK domain titin peptide encoded by positions 19081 to 19461 of skeletal muscle titin cDNA (GenBank accession no. X90569). Here, 100 MG, 11 lupus erythematosus (Lupus), 8 Lambert-Eaton syndrome (LE), and 18 normal samples (Others) have been tested. OD readings are normalized against the MG sample that has the highest titer towards the peptide. The blank corresponds to a normal human serum that shows an average titer of 0.10 relative units. The upper bar in the graph represents the value of the blank ± 2SD. Positive samples are seen above this bar. Eight percent of the MG patients have titers higher than the value of the blank ± 3SD. None of the non-MG samples show reactivity above the blank ± 3SD. MG samples are derived from 70 patients; all other samples correspond to 1 sample per donor. Note that, in the graph, some of the data points overlap, giving the impression that a lower number of MG samples are positive for antititin peptide activity.

have cloned a 127-amino-acid 5′-end sequence shared by the titin clones in the pET21a vector and have used the expressed recombinant peptide as antigen in ELISAs. Analyses of 100 MG, 11 lupus erythematosus, 8 Lambert-Eaton syndrome, and 18 normal samples have shown that 18% of the MG samples reacted with the antigen, none of the lupus and normal samples showed immunoreactivity, and 1 of the Lambert-Eaton samples showed antititin peptide activity higher than our cutoff value of 2 standard deviations above the blank (FIGURE 1). The 100 MG samples tested are derived from 70 patients seen at the Duke University Medical Center. Normalizing the data by the number of tested patients, we observed that 21% of the patients have anti-PEVK domain peptide antibodies. Six of the 18 positive samples shown in

TABLE 1. Relationship between Titers for Antititin Recombinant Peptide Antibodies, Anti-AChR Antibodies, and Thymectomy[a]

Sample No.	Thymectomy	Thymic Histological Characteristics	Sampling (Months from Thymectomy)	Antititin (Units)	Anti-AChR (nM)
1	not done			1.00	0.75–1.00
2		atrophy	pre (2)	0.88	0.25
3		not known	pre (1)	0.73	7.12
4		normal	post (98)	0.72	10.4 (T)[e]
5		hyperplasia	pre (6)	0.71	46.50
6[b]		atrophy	pre (1.5)	0.70	0.08
7		not known	pre (38)	0.69	0.28
8	not done			0.69	14.60[f]
9		atrophy	post (56)	0.53	0.20–0.34
10		hyperplasia	pre (2)	0.51	30.80
11		hyperplasia	post (18)	0.51	32.10 (T)
12[c]		hyperplasia	post (31)	0.50	42.60
13[c]		hyperplasia	at thymectomy	0.49	103.00
14		hyperplasia	post (0.5)	0.49	1.09
15[d]		thymoma	post (47)	0.48	8.09[g]
16[d]		thymoma	at thymectomy	0.46	0.90
17		not known	pre (1.5)	0.46	0.18
18[b]		atrophy	post (58)	0.45	0.08 (T)

[a]The table gives some of the characteristics associated with positive MG samples. The 8 samples with the highest antirecombinant peptide titers (i.e., antititin titer higher than that of the blank ± 3SD) are associated with normal, atrophic, or hyperplastic thymi. No correlation is found between antirecombinant peptide and anti-AChR titers. One of the 4 thymoma-associated MG patients showed circulating anti-PEVK domain peptide antibodies. Prethymectomy and postthymectomy follow-ups in 18 patients (3 shown in this table) indicate that thymectomy is not always associated with a decrease in antititin PEVK domain peptide titer (work in progress).
[b]Samples derived from the same patient (L.G.).
[c]Samples derived from the same patient (D.W.).
[d]Samples derived from the same patient (J.P.).
[e](T) indicates that the titer was measured at the time of thymectomy.
[f]Anti-AChR titer tested 60 months prior to antititin antibody testing.
[g]Anti-AChR titer tested 36 months prior to antititin antibody testing.

FIGURE 1 and TABLE 1 correspond to 3 sample pairs, each representing 1 prethymectomy/at thymectomy sampling and 1 postthymectomy sampling. In contrast to the strong association reported between the immune response to the titin main immunogenic region and thymoma-associated MG,[1] the MG anti-PEVK domain response was detected in 5 out of 15 patients that presented with thymic hyperplasia-associated MG, 2 out of 16 patients that presented with thymic atrophy-associated MG, 1 out of 7 patients that presented with normal thymic histology-associated MG, and 1 out of 4 patients that presented with thymoma-associated MG. In conclusion, the PEVK domain of skeletal muscle titin can be involved in the breakdown of tolerance observed in MG, but further studies are necessary to establish any correlation that may exist between the responses to different immunodominant epitopes within titin and the course of autoimmune responses in MG.

REFERENCES

1. GAUTEL, M. *et al.* 1993. Titin antibodies in myasthenia gravis: identification of a major immunogenic region of titin. Neurology **43:** 1581–1585.
2. AARLI, J. *et al.* 1998. Muscle striation antibodies in myasthenia gravis: diagnostic and functional significance. This volume.
3. LINKE, W. A. *et al.* 1996. Towards a molecular understanding of the elasticity of titin. J. Mol. Biol. **261:** 62–71.
4. MIHOVILOVIC, M. & A. D. ROSES. 1991. Expression of mRNAs in human thymus coding for the α-3 subunit of a neuronal acetylcholine receptor. Exp. Neurol. **111:** 175–180.
5. HUYNH, T. V. *et al.* 1985. Constructing and screening cDNA libraries in λgt10 and λgt11. *In* DNA Cloning. Volume 1, p. 49–78. IRL Press. Oxford/Washington, District of Columbia.
6. MIHOVILOVIC, M. *et al.* 1990. Analysis of self-antigens in myasthenia gravis employing cDNA cloning techniques. E.O.S. J. Immunol. Immunopharmacol. **10:** 190–191.
7. MIHOVILOVIC, M. & D. P. RICHMAN. 1987. Monoclonal antibodies as probes of the α-bungarotoxin and cholinergic binding regions of the acetylcholine receptor. J. Biol. Chem. **262:** 4978–4986.

Anti-titin and Antiryanodine Receptor Antibodies in Myasthenia Gravis Patients with Thymoma

FULVIO BAGGI,[a] FRANCESCA ANDREETTA,[a] CARLO ANTOZZI,[a]
ORNELLA SIMONCINI,[a] PAOLO CONFALONIERI,[a] SIEGFRIED LABEIT,[b]
FERDINANDO CORNELIO,[a] AND RENATO MANTEGAZZA[a]

[a]Department of Neuromuscular Diseases
National Neurological Institute "C. Besta"
20133 Milan, Italy

[b]European Molecular Biology Laboratory
Heidelberg, Germany

INTRODUCTION

Most myasthenia gravis (MG) patients with thymic abnormalities have autoantibodies not only to the nicotinic acetylcholine receptor (AChR), but also to components of striated muscle such as titin and ryanodine receptor (RyR). Titin is a 2800-kDa protein that comprises 10% of the myofibrillar mass and is involved in the elastic recoil of muscle. RyR is the calcium release channel of the sarcoplasmic reticulum involved in the mechanism of excitation-contraction coupling in striated muscle. Antibodies (Abs) against titin and RyR are more frequently found in MG patients with thymic neoplasia and might be considered as specific markers in these patients. We studied the presence of anti-titin and anti-RyR Abs in a group of 106 thymectomized MG patients.

METHODS

One hundred six myasthenic patients—78 females (73.5%) and 28 males (26.5%)—underwent therapeutical thymectomy by VATET (video-assisted trans-sternal extended thymectomy) at Policlinico "S. Marco", Zingonia, Italy. MG diagnosis was established according to clinical, pharmacological, and electrophysiological criteria; anti-AChR Ab titer was measured using either fetal calf or human AChR. Anti-titin Abs were assayed by the ELISA method using the MGT-30 recombinant fragment of titin.[1] All sera were diluted 1:200 in PBS. To determine the cutoff value, 58 control sera were tested in a single experiment. The mean optical density (at 450 nm) was 0.251 (SD 0.121), with a resulting cutoff of 0.614 (mean + 3SD) (FIGURE 1). Antiryanodine receptor Abs were assayed by Western blot analysis.[2] RyR was isolated from rabbit skeletal muscle, run on SDS-PAGE, and transferred to nitrocellulose sheets. The membranes were incubated for 2 hours with sera diluted 1:50, washed with TBS-Tween 20 (0.05%), and incubated with peroxidase-conjugated rabbit anti-

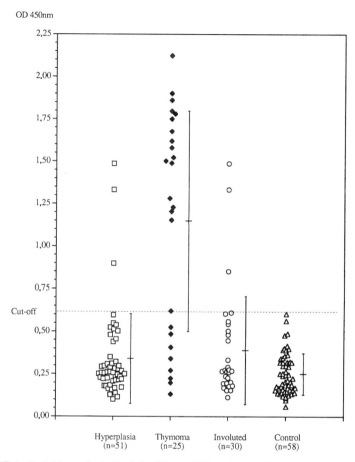

FIGURE 1. Anti-titin antibody levels in different MG patients and controls. The cutoff value corresponds to the mean OD value of controls + 3SD.

human IgG (1:500). In each experiment, positive and negative control sera were included. Sera from 8 patients (one with thymic hyperplasia) were available for anti-titin Ab follow-up of at least one year after thymectomy. Statistical analysis was performed using a chi-square test, with a *p* value < 0.05.

RESULTS

The OD values corresponding to anti-titin Ab levels in thymectomized MG patients are plotted in FIGURE 1, grouped according to thymic pathology. Anti-titin Abs were detected in 22 MG patients and antiryanodine receptor Abs in 33 MG patients. Their presence was well correlated with thymic histology: anti-MGT-30 Abs were detected in 16 of 25 (64%) MG patients with thymoma, but were also found in 3 of 51 (6%) hyperplastic and 3 of 30 (10%) involuted thymuses (TABLE 1). Anti-RyR Abs were found in 20 of 25 (80%) thymomas, as well as in 7 of 51 (14%) hyperplastic and 6 of 30 (20%) involuted thymuses (TABLE 1). Anti-AChR Abs were present in 92/106 patients: 23/30 hyperplastic, 44/51 involuted, and 25/25 thymoma. All patients positive for anti-titin were also positive for anti-AChR Abs; all patients positive for anti-RyR Abs (but 1) were also positive for anti-AChR Abs. Both autoantibodies were detected in 15 of 25 (60%) patients with thymoma, as compared to 3 cases in the involuted group and only 1 case in the hyperplastic group. No specific correlation was found between the presence of any of the two autoantibodies and classification of thymoma. Removal of thymoma was not associated with a disappearance of anti-titin Abs; random fluctuations were observed in certain patients (as well as in the hyperplastic patient included).

CONCLUSIONS

Myasthenia gravis is considered to be more severe and associated with a higher mortality in patients with thymoma as compared to nonneoplastic MG. The presence of anti-titin and anti-RyR Abs in MG with thymoma suggests that these antigens may have a pathogenetic role in association with neoplastic transformation of the thymus. Therefore, we evaluated the presence of anti-titin and anti-RyR antibodies in our group of thymectomized MG patients. Anti-RyR Abs were identified in 80% of MG patients with thymoma, as compared to 64% of patients positive for anti-titin Abs. On the contrary, anti-RyR Abs were present in 20% of involuted and 14% of hyperplastic thymuses, as compared to anti-titin Abs, present in 10% of involuted and 6% of hyperplastic samples. Hence, anti-titin Abs appeared to be more specific for MG with thymoma. Only 15 of the thymomas (60%) were positive for both antibodies, but did not improve specificity. Anti-titin and anti-RyR Abs were always observed in association with anti-AChR Abs, except for 1 MG patient with involuted thymus, positive for anti-RyR Abs only. Removal of thymoma (and of hyperplastic thymus) was not associated with a disappearance of anti-titin Abs as well as anti-AChR Abs, after one-year follow-up. These patients need to be evaluated further to correlate the presence of anti-titin and anti-RyR Abs with the clinical outcome. Evaluation of autoimmunity to titin and RyR might help in the presurgical screening of MG patients.

TABLE 1. Presence of Anti-titin and Anti-RyR Antibodies in Thymectomized MG Patients Related to Their Thymic Histology[a]

	Anti-titin Abs Positive	Anti-RyR Abs Positive
Involuted ($n = 30$)	3 (10%)	6 (20%)
Hyperplasia ($n = 51$)	3 (6%)	7 (14%)
Thymoma ($n = 25$)	16 (64%)	20 (80%)

[a]Involuted versus thymoma group: $p = 0.0001$. Hyperplasia versus thymoma group: $p = 0.0001$.

REFERENCES

1. GAUTEL, M., A. LAKEY, D. P. BARLOW, Z. HOLMES, S. SCALES, K. LEONARD, S. LABEIT, Å. MYGLAND, N. E. GILHUS & J. A. AARLI. 1993. Titin autoantibodies in myasthenia gravis: identification of a major immunogenic region of titin. Neurology **43:** 1581–1585.
2. MYGLAND, Å., O. B. TYSNES, J. A. AARLI, P. R. FLOOD & N. E. GILHUS. 1992. Myasthenia gravis patients with a thymoma have antibodies against a high molecular weight protein in sarcoplasmic reticulum. J. Neuroimmunol. **37:** 1–7.

Motor Dysfunction and Autoantibodies in Spontaneous Thymoma Buffalo/Mna Rats

KAZUO IWASA, KIYONOBU KOMAI, TOMOYA ASAKA,
EISHUN NITTA, AND MASAHARU TAKAMORI

Department of Neurology
Kanazawa University School of Medicine
Kanazawa 920, Japan

Many patients of myasthenia gravis (MG) with thymoma have both antiacetylcholine receptor (AChR) antibodies and antibodies that react with some components of skeletal muscle. Ryanodine receptor (RyR), which is related to excitation-contraction coupling (E-C coupling) and functions as a calcium-induced calcium-release channel, was recently discovered as one of the targets of striational antibodies,[1] and the RyR epitope was detected in thymoma epithelial cells from MG patients.[2] In consonance with the report that demonstrated a defect of E-C coupling and contractility in myasthenic muscles,[3] we showed that the sera from MG patients with anti-RyR antibody inhibit the release of Ca^{2+} from the sarcoplasmic reticulum in response to caffeine in cultured cells. In view of these facts, we focused attention on Buffalo/Mna (Buf/Mna) rats, characterized by spontaneous thymoma and contractile fatigue.[4]

METHODS

Antibodies Assay

Male Buf/Mna rats over 12 weeks old were studied. Antirat AChR antibodies were measured by immunoprecipitation assay using ^{125}I-α-bungarotoxin. Anti-RyR antibody was determined by immunoblotting.[1] The RyR1 antigen for immunoblots was prepared from rabbit skeletal muscle. Separated proteins in the SDS–7.5% polyacrylamide gel were electrophoretically transblotted onto polyvinylidene difluoride (PVDF) membranes. After blocking, the membranes (strips) were incubated overnight with a 1:20 dilution of the test serum and with mouse anti-RyR monoclonal antibody in PBS with Tween 20. Specific antibodies used by us were directed against the rabbit RyR1. After incubation with a horseradish peroxidase (HRP)–conjugated second antibody, the strips were reacted with diaminobenzidine (DAB) in H_2O_2 for 5–10 min.

Immunohistochemistry of Thymoma

Cryostat sections of thymoma (12 μm) were thoroughly dried and incubated with 0.5% H_2O_2 in methanol for 10 min. The materials were incubated overnight at 4 °C with rabbit anti-RyR polyclonal antibody, mouse anticytokeratin monoclonal antibody, and mouse antidesmin monoclonal antibody, followed by the incubation with HRP-conjugated goat antirabbit IgG antibody or HRP-conjugated goat antimouse IgG antibody for 30 min at room temperature.

Electrophysiological Study

The muscle samples were massively stimulated by platinum-plate electrodes under curarization to record twitch and tetanus isometrically. Properties of the neuromuscular transmission were measured by conventional intracellular microelectrodes.

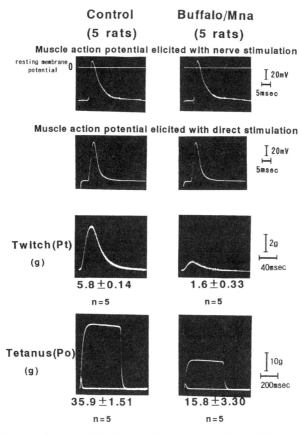

FIGURE 1. Muscle action potentials elicited with nerve stimulation and direct stimulation did not change in control rats and Buf/Mna rats. The phrenic-diaphragma from Buf/Mna rats showed a selective block of muscle contraction as evidenced by decreased twitch and tetanic force without alteration in parameters of presynaptic and postsynaptic components of neuromuscular transmission and membrane properties.

The muscle action potential elicited by direct or nerve stimulation was recorded in Ringer solution containing dantrolene sodium (20 mg/mL).

RESULTS AND DISCUSSION

In Buf/Mna rats studied by us, lymphocytic thymomas develop spontaneously after 8 weeks of age, along with progressive fatigability of hindlimb muscles without any microscopical abnormalities. When sacrificed at 6 months after birth, the elec-

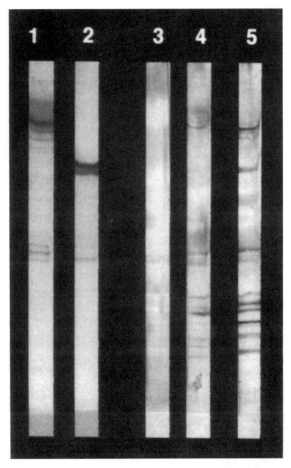

FIGURE 2. Immunoblots of ryanodine receptor (RyR) with sera from Buf/Mna rats. Lane 1: anti-RyR monoclonal antibody. Lane 2: antimyosin monoclonal antibody. Lane 3: serum from a control rat. Lane 4: serum from a Buf/Mna rat at 3 months after birth. Lane 5: serum from a Buf/Mna rat at 6 months after birth.

trophysiological study showed a selective block of muscle contraction as evidenced by decreased twitch and tetanus without alteration in neuromuscular transmission and membrane properties (FIGURE 1). In the serum, antibodies to RyR were detected, but not to AChR (FIGURE 2). The immunohistochemical study showed the presence of RyR in thymoma epithelial cells of Buf/Mna rats.

The results from Buf/Mna rats suggest that the anti-RyR antibody raises against the RyR expressed in the thymus and plays a role in impairing E-C coupling and contractility in the muscle. This finding may be a counterpart of the feature seen in MG patients with thymoma in whom E-C coupling is blocked together with the neuromuscular transmission block.

ACKNOWLEDGMENTS

We thank T. Ezaki for advice concerning this research, and H. Takeshima and G. Kuwajima for donating antibodies against the ryanodine receptor.

REFERENCES

1. IWASA, K. 1997. Muscle Nerve **20:** 753–756.
2. MYGLAND, Å., G. KUWAJIMA, K. MIKOSHIBA, O. TYSNES, J. A. AARLI & N. E. GILHUS. 1995. J. Neuroimmunol. **62:** 79–83.
3. PAGALA, M. K. D., N. V. NANDAKUMAR, S. A. T. VENKATACHARI, K. RAVINDRAN, T. NAMBA & D. GROB. 1990. Muscle Nerve **13:** 1012–1022.
4. KATO, F. & M. WATANABE. 1982. J. Pharm. Dyn. **5:** 1005–1011.

Agrin-induced Aggregation of Acetylcholine Receptors in Muscles of Rats with Experimental Autoimmune Myasthenia Gravis[a]

MENDELL RIMER[b]

Department of Neurobiology
Stanford University School of Medicine
Stanford, California 94305

INTRODUCTION

Myasthenia gravis (MG) is a human autoimmune disease whose main feature is the failure in muscle contraction that results from the reduction in concentration of acetylcholine receptors (AChRs) on the surface of muscle fibers at neuromuscular junctions (NMJs).[1] Agrin is secreted by motor neurons at normal NMJs to induce muscle fibers to form and maintain the high concentration of AChRs.[2] Thus, one way to reverse the loss of AChRs at myasthenic NMJs may be to increase levels of agrin secreted by motor neurons and/or levels of its receptors expressed in the muscle fiber's plasma membrane. As a first step towards learning whether an increase in agrin-mediated AChR aggregation could reverse the effects of MG, I determined whether the application of neural agrin to muscle fibers of rats undergoing experimental autoimmune MG (EAMG) could induce the formation of AChR aggregates *in vivo*.

MATERIALS AND METHODS

AChR was purified from *T. californica* electric organ as described by Chak and Karlin.[3] EAMG was induced in 8–10-week-old female Lewis rats by injection (sc) of 50–100 µg of purified AChR emulsified in an equal volume of CFA. Monthly boosts with 50 µg of AChR in IFA were done as needed. Uninjected animals and animals injected with CFA diluted in PBS were used as controls. Rats were observed and weighed every other day. Signs of muscle weakness were scored on a scale ranging from 0 for normal, + for weak grip and cry, ++ for hunched posture with head down, to +++ for generalized weakness with tremor. Blood was collected by retina/orbital bleeding under anesthesia (Metofane, Pitman-Moore) and serum samples were stored at –80 °C until used. Anti-AChR antibody titer was measured by a standard ELISA assay. When chronic myasthenic symptoms were observed at least in two

[a]This work was supported by a postdoctoral fellowship from the MG Foundation.
[b]Present address: National Biotechnology Information Facility, New Mexico State University, Las Cruces, New Mexico 88003.

consecutive weighing days, left legs of EAMG and control rats were denervated by cutting a segment of the sciatic nerve in the thigh and, 3 days later, 50–100 μg of a CMV expression vector carrying the full-length rat agrin cDNA (Y4Z8) was injected into the proximal extrajunctional regions of denervated and contralateral normal soleus muscles. One week after injection, muscles were removed, frozen in liquid-N_2-cooled isopentane, and stored at –80 °C. Frozen cross sections were cut from the injected region of each muscle, and sections were costained with a commercial monoclonal antibody specific to rat neural agrin (Agrin-86, StressGen) visualized with fluorescein-conjugated secondary antibody (Cappel Organon Teknika Corporation) and with Texas Red–α-bungarotoxin (Molecular Probes) to label AChRs. Sections were examined under epifluorescence.

RESULTS AND DISCUSSION

Soleus muscles of EAMG rats were transfected after they reached +++ symptoms and chronic weight loss. By this time, rats were 14–18 weeks old. All EAMG rats developed a high titer of antibodies to AChR as measured by ELISA (data not shown). FIGURE 1 shows cross sections from the transfected region for denervated and innervated soleus muscles from an EAMG rat. AChR aggregates were found on muscle fibers in the immediate vicinity of transfected cells, identified by their distinctive sarcoplasmic staining for neural agrin. As expected, more AChR aggregates were observed in denervated than in innervated muscles. No AChR aggregates were seen in muscles where agrin-transfected cells were not detected. The mean number of agrin-transfected cells per cross section was not statistically different between EAMG (3.0 ± 1.7, mean ± SEM, $n = 4$) and control (1.6 ± 0.4, $n = 3$) denervated muscles. However, it was much lower than that for denervated muscles of younger male Wistar rats (12.3 ± 3.25, $n = 7$).[4] This is in agreement with previous findings in which much higher activity levels of a muscle-injected CAT (chloramphenicol acetyltransferase) reporter plasmid were observed in male mice of 4–6 weeks of age than in females of the same age or animals older than 10 weeks.[5] I determined the mean number of

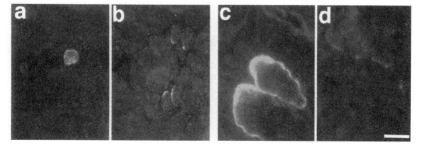

FIGURE 1. Agrin-induced AChR aggregates in denervated (a, b) and innervated (c, d) soleus muscles of EAMG rats. AChR aggregates, labeled with Texas Red–α-bungarotoxin (b, d), were observed on fibers in the vicinity of agrin-transfected fibers, recognized by their strong sarcoplasmic staining for neural agrin (a, c). Scale bar: 45 μm (a, b); 30 μm (c, d).

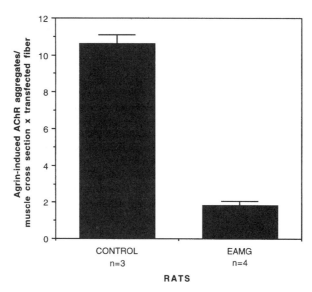

FIGURE 2. Denervated soleus muscles from EAMG rats showed 5-fold less agrin-induced AChR aggregates than denervated soleus muscles from control animals. Cross sections from transfected EAMG and control denervated muscles were stained as in FIGURE 1, and AChR aggregates and agrin-transfected cells were counted in at least five cross sections per muscle. Values expressed as the mean ± SEM.

agrin-induced AChR aggregates per cross section per agrin-transfected cell for several EAMG and control denervated soleus muscles. FIGURE 2 shows that EAMG muscles had about 5-fold less agrin-induced AChR aggregates than muscles from control animals. Interestingly, the latter number (10.6 ± 0.5, $n = 3$) was very close to that obtained in a previous study[4] for younger male Wistar rats (7.9 ± 1.4, $n = 3$). Thus, while age, sex, and strain type had a significant decreasing effect on the transfection efficiency with the agrin-encoding plasmid, these variables did not seem to affect neural agrin's aggregating activity. This could mean that in both, muscle fibers from young male Wistar rats and from older female control Lewis rats, saturating amounts of neural agrin were produced. Lower levels of neural agrin expression and/or secretion per transfected fiber could account for the reduced number of agrin-induced AChR aggregates in EAMG muscles. Alternatively or in addition, an increased rate of AChR degradation known to occur in EAMG muscles[1] could explain the results. Lastly, deficiencies in EAMG muscles in the expression levels of proteins that mediate the agrin-induced AChR aggregation such as the tyrosine kinase MuSK[6] or the protein rapsyn[7] should be further investigated.

ACKNOWLEDGMENTS

I am grateful to U. J. McMahan, in whose laboratory this work was carried out.

REFERENCES

1. DRACHMAN, D. B. 1994. Myasthenia gravis. N. Engl. J. Med. **330:** 1797–1810.
2. MCMAHAN, U. J. 1990. The agrin hypothesis. Cold Spring Harbor Symp. Quant. Biol. **50:** 407–418.
3. CHAK, A. & A. KARLIN. 1992. Purification and reconstitution of nicotinic acetylcholine receptor. *In* Methods in Enzymology. Vol. 207, p. 546.
4. COHEN, I. *et al.* 1997. Agrin-induced postsynaptic-like apparatus in skeletal muscle fibers *in vivo.* Mol. Cell. Neurosci. **9:** 237–253.
5. WELLS, D. J. & G. GOLDSPINK. 1992. Age and sex influence expression of plasmid DNA directly injected into mouse skeletal muscle. FEBS Lett. **306:** 203–205.
6. VALENZUELA, D. M. *et al.* 1995. Receptor tyrosine kinase specific for the skeletal muscle lineage: expression in embryonic muscle, at the neuromuscular junction, and after injury. Neuron **15:** 573–584.
7. GAUTAM, M. *et al.* 1995. Failure of postsynaptic specialization to develop at neuromuscular junctions of rapsyn-deficient mice. Nature **377:** 232–236.

Differential Susceptibility of Young and Old Rat Neuromuscular Junctions to Antibody-mediated AChR Degradation in Experimental Autoimmune Myasthenia Gravis

A. HOEDEMAEKERS,[a] J-L. BESSEREAU,[b] Y. GRAUS,[a,c]
T. GUYON,[d] J-P. CHANGEUX,[b] S. BERRIH-AKNIN,[d]
P. VAN BREDA VRIESMAN,[a] AND M. DE BAETS[a,e]

[a]Department of Immunology
Maastricht University
6200 MD Maastricht, the Netherlands

[b]CNRS-UAD-1284
Institut Pasteur
Unité de Neurobiologie Moléculaire
75724 Paris Cedex 15, France

[d]CNRS-URA-1159
Hôpital Marie Lannelongue
92350 Le Plessis-Robinson, France

Myasthenia gravis (MG) is an autoimmune disease in which autoantibodies cause loss of functional acetylcholine receptor (AChR) and destruction of the postsynaptic membrane. Although the pathogenesis of MG is entirely antibody-mediated, anti-AChR antibody titer or the amount of AChR complexed with antibody correlates poorly with the severity of neuromuscular dysfunction.[1–3] However, it has been shown previously that certain AChR α-subunit gene haplotypes are associated with a higher susceptibility for MG.[4] Furthermore, analysis of AChR α-subunit mRNA concentrations in muscle biopsies from MG patients revealed increased levels in the amounts of α-subunit mRNA in severely affected MG patients, whereas no increase was found in moderately ill MG patients, independent of the anti-AChR antibody titers.[5] It therefore seems likely that the autoantigen itself influences susceptibility and clinical course of MG.

Passive transfer experimental autoimmune myasthenia gravis (EAMG) is a good model in which to analyze the response of the target organ to the antibody-mediated immune attack in MG. It is induced by passive transfer of polyclonal or monoclonal [anti–Main Immunogenic Region (MIR)] antibodies.[6,7] In susceptible rats, clinical signs of disease and AChR loss develop within 24–48 hours. Impairment of neuromuscular transmission in these rats triggers a cascade of events, resulting in in-

[c]Present address: The Netherlands Cancer Institute, Division of Immunology, 1066 CX Amsterdam, the Netherlands.
[e]To whom all correspondence should be addressed.

creased levels of mRNA coding for the different subunits of the AChR.[8,9] Aged BN rats, in contrast to young BN rats, are resistant to induction of EAMG.[10,11] Passive transfer of anti-MIR mAb does not induce muscular weakness nor clinical signs of disease in aged rats. This resistance could not be attributed to deficient antibody uptake, increased antibody clearance, inaccessibility of the AChR for antibody, absence of infiltrating macrophages, or deficient complement activation.[10–12] Therefore, it is most likely that resistance to EAMG in aged rats resides at the level of the target organ.

The mechanisms that could account for this age-related resistance include different AChR gene expression in aged rats, resulting in more efficient AChR neosynthesis. EAMG has been shown to result in increased AChR mRNA levels.[13] We measured the amount of AChR α-subunit mRNA in young and aged rats by competitive RT-PCR, using RNA transcribed from a mutant P3A+ cDNA fragment as internal control.[5] The number of α-subunit mRNA molecules measured in aged control rats was comparable to that in young control rats (FIGURE 1). Injection of anti-MIR mAb did not result in an increase in the number of α-subunit mRNA molecules in resistant aged rats. In contrast, the mean number of α-subunit mRNA molecules increased significantly in young rats, from $4.1 \pm 0.5 \times 10^8/\mu g$ RNA in young control rats to $12.1 \pm 1.6 \times 10^8/\mu g$ RNA in susceptible young rats at 48 hours after injection of anti-MIR mAb ($p < 0.05$). Upon denervation, however, young and aged rats showed a comparable increase in AChR α-subunit mRNA, indicating that aged rats are potentially capable of increasing AChR α-subunit mRNA synthesis to a similar level as young rats.

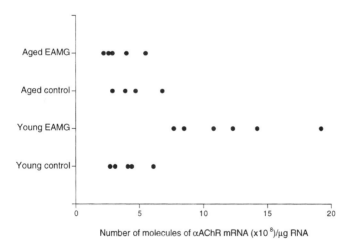

Number of molecules of αAChR mRNA ($\times 10^8$)/μg RNA

FIGURE 1. Resistance to EAMG in aged rats is not a result of increased AChR α-subunit mRNA synthesis. In EAMG-resistant aged rats, no increase in the number of α-subunit mRNA molecules was found compared to age-matched control rats. In young rats, however, a significant increase in the mean number of α-subunit mRNA molecules was measured ($p < 0.05$). The amount of α-subunit mRNA is expressed as the number of molecules per μg total RNA extracted. Points represent individual rats.

In normal innervated muscle, AChR genes are preferentially expressed in the subjunctional regions of the muscle fiber. Yet, synaptic domains represent less than 1% of the fibers.[14] Variations in AChR mRNA levels, quantified in total muscle RNA by mass techniques, mainly represent variations in extrasynaptic regions of the myofiber. This implies that synaptic compensatory mechanisms would have remained unnoticed in the RT-PCR experiments described above. Therefore, α- and ε-subunit mRNA expression was analyzed by means of *in situ* hybridization experiments. In aged control rats, both α- and ε-subunit transcripts were densely accumulated at the end plate regions. Injection of anti-MIR mAb in aged rats did not result in any apparent changes in the distribution or density of the clusters of grains at the level of the end plates. In contrast, injection of anti-MIR mAb in young rats elicited a dramatic reduction of the size and density of the synaptic clusters of grains for both the α- and ε-subunit mRNA transcripts ($p < 0.001$). Altogether, these results indicate that injection of monoclonal anti-AChR antibodies in aged rats does not induce AChR neosynthesis to compensate for AChR loss.

In vivo AChR protein degradation rates were measured in young and aged rats upon induction of passive transfer EAMG. Twenty-four hours after injection of anti-

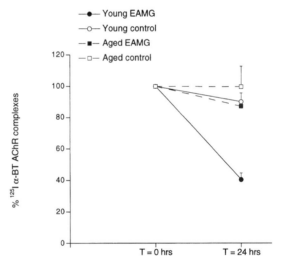

FIGURE 2. Aged rats are resistant to antibody-mediated AChR degradation. *In vivo* AChR degradation rates were measured in young and aged rats after induction of passive transfer EAMG. AChR was labeled with ^{125}I-α-BT at 24 hours prior to induction of EAMG. At 24 hours after induction of EAMG, no significant decrease in the amount of ^{125}I-α-BT-labeled AChR was found in aged rats ($12.8 \pm 8.6\%$ decrease compared to age-matched control rats), whereas young rats showed a significant decrease of $59.5 \pm 4.2\%$ in the amount of ^{125}I-α-BT-labeled AChR. Results are expressed as % loss of ^{125}I-α-BT-labeled AChR. The fraction of AChR labeled at the time point of EAMG induction was considered 100% (actual fraction of ^{125}I-α-BT-labeled AChR was $29.6 \pm 1.8\%$ and $28.7 \pm 1.0\%$ in young and aged rats, respectively). Points represent the mean ± SD of at least 5 rats per group.

MIR mAb, aged rats showed no significant decrease in the amount of ^{125}I-α-BT-labeled AChR as compared to age-matched PBS-treated rats (FIGURE 2). Anti-MIR mAb–injected susceptible young rats, however, showed a significant decrease in ^{125}I-α-BT-labeled AChR of 59.5 ± 4.2% ($p < 0.05$). These experiments indicate that in aged rats the AChR in the postsynaptic membrane is resistant against the antibody-mediated autoimmune attack.

Proteins of the basal lamina and the postsynaptic cytoskeleton are known to play an important role in clustering and anchoring of AChR in the postsynaptic membrane.[15] Age-related changes in the concentrations of these proteins may increase the rigidity of the postsynaptic membrane, which may result in resistance to antigenic modulation and subsequent internalization. The relative amounts of s-laminin, agrin, 43K, and utrophin were analyzed semiquantitatively in muscle biopsies of young and aged rats by confocal laser microscopy. The amount of s-laminin and 43K protein was significantly increased in normal old versus normal young rats. The amount of agrin significantly decreased with aging. The amount of utrophin was comparable in young and aged rats.

The results of this study show that the age-related resistance to EAMG is determined by resistance of the AChR to degradation, which may be related to differences in composition of the postsynaptic membrane in aged rats. Furthermore, these results suggest that susceptibility and clinical course of MG are determined not only by the immune attack towards the neuromuscular junction, but also by the target organ.

REFERENCES

1. LINDSTROM, J. 1976. Antibody to acetylcholine receptor in myasthenia gravis: prevalence, clinical correlates, and diagnostic value. Neurology **26:** 1054–1059.
2. ROSES, A. 1981. No direct correlation between serum antiacetylcholine receptor antibody levels and clinical state of individual patients with myasthenia gravis. Neurology **31:** 220–224.
3. VERSCHUUREN, J. 1992. Role of acetylcholine receptor antibody complexes in muscle in experimental autoimmune myasthenia gravis. J. Neuroimmunol. **36:** 117–125.
4. GARCHON, H-J. 1994. Involvement of human muscle acetylcholine receptor α-subunit gene (CHRNA) in susceptibility to myasthenia gravis. Proc. Natl. Acad. Sci. U.S.A. **91:** 4668–4672.
5. GUYON, T. 1994. Regulation of acetylcholine receptor α subunit variant RNA in human myasthenia gravis: quantification of steady-state levels of messenger RNA in muscle biopsy using the polymerase chain reaction. J. Clin. Invest. **94:** 16–24.
6. TOYKA, K. 1975. Myasthenia gravis: passive transfer from man to mouse. Science **190:** 397–399.
7. TZARTOS, S. 1987. Passive transfer of experimental autoimmune myasthenia gravis by monoclonal antibodies to the main immunogenic region of the acetylcholine receptor. J. Neuroimmunol. **15:** 185–194.
8. ASHER, O. 1988. Increased levels of acetylcholine receptor α-subunit mRNA in experimental autoimmune myasthenia gravis. FEBS Lett. **233:** 277–281.
9. ASHER, O. 1990. Acetylcholine receptor gene expression in experimental autoimmune myasthenia gravis. FEBS Lett. **267:** 231–235.
10. GRAUS, Y. 1993. Age-related resistance to experimental autoimmune myasthenia gravis in rats. J. Immunol. **150:** 4093–4103.

11. HOEDEMAEKERS, A. 1997. Age- and sex-related resistance to experimental autoimmune myasthenia gravis in Brown Norway rats. Clin. Exp. Immunol. **107:** 189–197.
12. HOEDEMAEKERS, A. *et al.* 1997. Macrophage infiltration at the neuromuscular junction does not contribute to AChR loss and age-related resistance to EAMG. J. Neuroimmunol. **75:** 147–155.
13. ASHER, O. 1993. Increased gene expression of acetylcholine receptor and myogenic factors in passively transferred experimental autoimmune myasthenia gravis. J. Immunol. **151:** 6442–6450.
14. HALL, Z. & J. SANES. 1993. Synaptic structure and development: the neuromuscular junction. Cell **72:** 99–121.
15. SANES, J. 1995. The synaptic cleft of the neuromuscular junction. Dev. Biol. **6:** 163–173.

Immunization of bm12 Mice with High Doses of Acetylcholine Receptor Overcomes Their Resistance to Experimental Autoimmune Myasthenia Gravis[a]

PETER I. KARACHUNSKI,[b] NORMA S. OSTLIE,[b] SIJIN LEI,[b]
DAVID K. OKITA,[b] JON M. LINDSTROM,[c] AND
BIANCA M. CONTI-FINE[b,d]

[b]Department of Biochemistry
College of Biological Sciences
University of Minnesota
St. Paul, Minnesota 55108
and
Department of Pharmacology
School of Medicine
University of Minnesota
Minneapolis, Minnesota 55455

[c]Department of Neuroscience
University of Pennsylvania Medical Center
Philadelphia, Pennsylvania 19104

The I-A^{bm12} mutation in C57BL/6 (B6) mice yields the bm12 strain, which is resistant to experimental autoimmune myasthenia gravis (EAMG) induced by immunization with conventional low doses of *Torpedo* acetylcholine receptor (TAChR), while the parental B6 strain is highly susceptible to EAMG induction.[1]

We demonstrated previously[2,3] that after immunization with low doses of TAChR (20–30 μg/injection) both bm12 and B6 mice had an intense CD4$^+$ response to the TAChR, developed comparable serum concentrations of anti-TAChR antibodies (Ab), and had Ab bound to muscle acetylcholine receptor (AChR). However, anti-TAChR CD4$^+$ cells from B6 mice recognized primarily three epitopes formed by the TAChR α subunit (within the sequences Tα150–169, Tα181–200, and Tα360–378), while those from bm12 mice did not respond to the TAChR α subunit and used different TCR Vβ genes than the B6 strain.[3,4] Thus, EAMG resistance of bm12 mice is due to a subtle shift in the anti-AChR Ab repertoire and to an absence of highly path-

[a]This work was supported by a research grant from the Council for Tobacco Research and by NINCDS Grant No. NS 23919 (to B. M. Conti-Fine). Research in the laboratory of J. Lindstrom was supported by grants from the NIH (No. NS 11323) and the Muscular Dystrophy Association.

[d]Previously known as Bianca M. Conti-Tronconi.

ogenic Abs. This is likely related to the absence of $CD4^+$ cells sensitized to epitopes within the sequence $T\alpha150–160$, due to the inability of the $I-A^{bm12}$ molecule to present this sequence.[2,3]

In this study, we further investigated the mechanisms of the apparent resistance of bm12 mice to EAMG induction. We found that resistance to EAMG of bm12 mice was not due to unique properties of their muscle AChR because bm12 and B6 mice had the same muscle AChR content and curare sensitivity. Also, bm12 mice had the same susceptibility as B6 mice to passively transferred EAMG, induced by injection of a highly pathogenic[5] anti-AChR monoclonal Ab, mAb 35, that binds to the main immunogenic region (MIR) of the AChR.[5]

We immunized bm12 mice with increasingly larger amounts of TAChR (10–100 μg/injection; three injections, four weeks apart), using a protocol that we described previously.[2,3] We tested the strength of the mice at one month after the third TAChR immunization, with a pancuronium-sensitized inverted grid test:[3] the muscle strength is expressed as holding time, which in normal mice is 12 minutes or more. Mice with EAMG have a holding time of 8 minutes or less: after treatment with the anti-cholinesterase drug edrophonium chloride, their holding time returns to normal values. Only one of the eight mice immunized with low doses of TAChR (10–25 μg) developed very mild myasthenic weakness (FIGURE 1A). Immunization with higher doses of TAChR overcame the resistance of bm12 to EAMG induction: 50–75% of the mice immunized with 50 μg of TAChR and 75% of those immunized with 100 μg developed EAMG (FIGURE 1). After immunization with 50 μg of TAChR, bm12 and B6 mice developed EAMG with the same incidence (FIGURE 1B).

The bm12 mice immunized with different doses of TAChR developed comparable serum concentrations of anti-TAChR Ab, suggesting that a qualitative rather than a quantitative difference in the anti-TAChR Ab produced by this mutant strain caused their different susceptibility to EAMG as compared to the parental B6 strain. Analysis of the Ab repertoire using a competition assay and the anti-MIR mAb 35 showed that the sera of bm12 mice had significantly less anti-MIR Abs, which are highly pathogenic.[5]

Spleen T cells from bm12 mice immunized with high doses (50 μg) of TAChR were tested in a proliferation assay in vitro that we described previously.[2,3] They responded well to both the native TAChR and the TAChR α subunit. They recognized significantly several TAChR α subunit peptides (FIGURE 2): of them, the peptide sequence $T\alpha91–110$ was recognized most strongly (FIGURE 2) and consistently in all mice. This TAChR sequence region sensitizes highly pathogenic $CD4^+$ cells in Lewis rats.[6,7]

The present findings confirm that $CD4^+$ cells specific for AChR α subunit epitopes are especially effective in driving the synthesis of pathogenic anti-AChR Ab. This may be related to the high pathogenic potential of anti-AChR Ab recognizing AChR epitopes formed by the α subunit—and the MIR in particular—and to the described preferential collaboration between B cells making Ab against epitopes formed by a particular surface domain of the antigen and $CD4^+$ T cells specific for sequence regions of the antigen in spatial proximity to those forming the Ab epitope domain.[8–10]

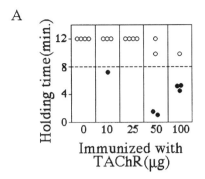

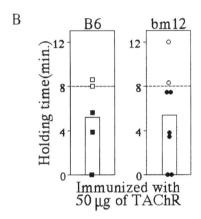

FIGURE 1. (A) Muscle strength of bm12 mice immunized with different doses of TAChR. The mice were injected subcutaneously three times with the amounts of TAChR indicated, and emulsified in complete Freund's adjuvant for the first injection and incomplete Freund's adjuvant for the other injections. Control mice (plot "0 mg") received PBS in the proper adjuvant. The panels report the results obtained at one month after the third immunization, testing the muscle strength of individual mice with the pancuronium-sensitized "inverted grid" test:[3] the strength is measured as holding time. Mice with a holding time below 8 minutes were considered to have EAMG weakness, which was reversed by administration of the acetylcholinesterase inhibitor, edrophonium chloride. (B) Muscle strength of bm12 and B6 mice immunized with 50 μg of TAChR. The mice were injected subcutaneously three times with 50 μg of TAChR, and emulsified in complete Freund's adjuvant for the first injection and incomplete Freund's adjuvant for the second and third injections. The muscle strength of individual mice was tested at one month after the third TAChR injection with the pancuronium-sensitized "inverted grid" test.

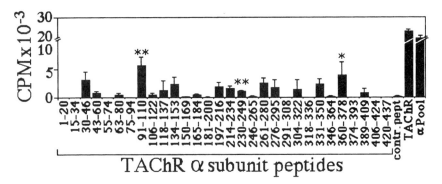

FIGURE 2. T cells from bm12 mice immunized with 50 μg of TAChR are sensitized to α subunit epitopes and they recognize primarily the sequence region α91–110. T cells purified from the spleen of a bm12 mouse were tested in five-day proliferation assays[3] for their ability to recognize purified TAChR (5 μg/mL); a pool of overlapping synthetic peptides, 20 residues long, spanning the complete TAChR α subunit sequence (α pool, 5 μg/mL); the individual peptides screening the α subunit sequence (10 μg/mL); and a control 20-residue peptide unrelated to the TAChR sequence, as indicated along the abscissa. Each column represents the average ^{3}H-thymidine incorporation ± SD of triplicate cultures. The significance of the response, as compared to the ^{3}H-thymidine incorporation of T cells cultured in the presence of a 20-residue synthetic peptide unrelated to the TAChR sequence, was determined using a two-tailed Student's t test (**$p < 0.01$, * $p < 0.05$). The T cells recognized the TAChR and the α pool strongly. They recognized significantly several α subunit peptides: peptide α91–110 was recognized most strongly and consistently in different mice.

REFERENCES

1. CHRISTADOSS, P. *et al.* 1985. Mutation at I-A beta chain prevents experimental autoimmune myasthenia gravis. Immunogenetics **21:** 33–38.
2. BELLONE, M. *et al.* 1991. The I-A[bm12] mutation, which confers resistance to experimental myasthenia gravis, drastically affects the epitope repertoire of murine CD4[+] cells sensitized to nicotinic acetylcholine receptor. J. Immunol. **147:** 1484–1491.
3. KARACHUNSKI, P. I. *et al.* 1995. Mechanisms by which the I-A[bm12] mutation influences susceptibility to experimental myasthenia gravis: a study in homozygous and heterozygous mice. Scand. J. Immunol. **42:** 215–225.
4. INFANTE, A. J. *et al.* 1992. Preferential use of a T cell Vβ gene by acetylcholine receptor reactive T cells from myasthenia gravis susceptible mice. J. Immunol. **148:** 3385–3390.
5. LINDSTROM, J. M. *et al.* 1988. Myasthenia gravis. Adv. Immunol. **42:** 233–284.
6. FUJII, Y. & J. LINDSTROM. 1988. Regulation of antibody production by helper T cell clones in experimental autoimmune myasthenia gravis. J. Immunol. **141:** 3361–3369.
7. ZODA, T. E. & K. A. KROLICK. 1993. Antigen presentation and T cell specificity repertoire in determining responsiveness to an epitope important in experimental autoimmune myasthenia gravis. J. Neuroimmunol. **43:** 131–138.
8. MYERS, C. D. 1991. Role of B cell antigen processing and presentation in the humoral immune response. FASEB J. **5:** 2547–2553.
9. BARNETT, B. C. *et al.* 1989. The immune response of BALB/c mice to influenza hemagglu-

tinin: commonality of the B cell and T cell repertoires and their relevance to antigenic drift. Eur. J. Immunol. **19:** 515–521.

10. TINDLE, R. W. *et al.* 1991. A "public" T-helper epitope of the E7 transforming protein of human papillomavirus 16 provides cognate help for several E7 B-cell epitopes from cervical cancer–associated human papillomavirus genotypes. Proc. Natl. Acad. Sci. U.S.A. **88:** 5887–5891.

Nasal Administration of Synthetic Acetylcholine Receptor T Epitopes Affects the Immune Response to the Acetylcholine Receptor and Prevents Experimental Myasthenia Gravis[a]

PETER I. KARACHUNSKI, NORMA S. OSTLIE, DAVID K. OKITA, AND BIANCA M. CONTI-FINE[b]

Department of Biochemistry
College of Biological Sciences
University of Minnesota
St. Paul, Minnesota 55108
and
Department of Pharmacology
School of Medicine
University of Minnesota
Minneapolis, Minnesota 55455

Management of myasthenia gravis (MG) is based on the use of anticholinesterase drugs, nonspecific immunosuppressants, and repeated plasma exchanges.[1] Those treatments have different shortcomings: ideal treatments would specifically turn off or control the autoimmune response against muscle acetylcholine receptor (AChR) that causes MG symptoms.

T cells can be specifically tolerized by giving the antigen (Ag) through routes that downregulate CD4[+] responses, such as by oral, nasal, and intraperitoneal administration.[2] Those procedures can prevent and/or treat CD4[+] T cell–mediated autoimmune diseases.[3–6] It is not clear if they could be used for antibody (Ab)–mediated diseases like MG because those procedures do not directly downregulate the autoimmune B cells and, in fact, they may stimulate the B cell specific for the administered Ag[2,7] and exacerbate Ab-mediated autoimmune diseases.[6] Synthetic T epitope sequences may be safer for T cell tolerance procedures than the whole Ag molecule since peptide-specific Abs very seldom cross-react with the cognate native Ag.[8] Short peptides cross epithelia more easily than large proteins: thus, synthetic CD4[+] epitope sequences may be more effective than the whole Ag for tolerance induction.[3] However, they are not suitable for oral tolerance procedures because they are easily digested by the gastrointestinal proteases.[7]

We investigated if nasal administration of synthetic AChR sequences forming CD4[+] epitopes induced specific immunological tolerance, and prevented experimen-

[a]This work was supported by a research grant from the Council for Tobacco Research and by NINCDS Grant No. NS 23919 (to B. M. Conti-Fine).
[b]Previously known as Bianca M. Conti-Tronconi.

tal autoimmune MG (EMG), caused in C57BL/6 (B6) mice by immunization with purified *Torpedo* AChR (TAChR).[9] The anti-TAChR CD4[+] T cells of B6 mice recognize primarily epitopes within residues 146–169, 181–200, and 360–378 of the TAChR α subunit: the sequence α146–169 is the most immunogenic and it is recognized by highly pathogenic CD4[+] cells.[10]

T cells of mice that received nasal administration of synthetic peptides corresponding to the TAChR α subunit residues, α150–169, α181–200, and α360–378, and that were immunized to those peptides, did not respond *in vitro* to those epitopes.

Nasal administration of an equimolar pool of those three CD4[+] epitope peptides (α pool) or of peptide α150–169 alone, given before and during immunization with TAChR, prevented EMG induction (FIGURE 1). B6 mice are very susceptible to EMG after TAChR immunization, with variable frequency (20–70%).[1] We tested the mice strength with a pancuronium-sensitized inverted grid test:[9] their muscle strength is expressed as holding time, which in normal mice is 12 minutes or more. Mice with EMG have a holding time of 8 minutes or less: after treatment with the anti-cholinesterase drug edrophonium chloride, their holding time returns to normal val-

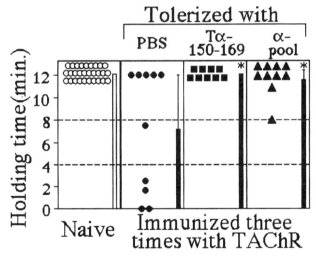

FIGURE 1. Nasal administration of TAChR CD4[+] epitope peptides protects against EMG. Peptide α150–169, α pool, or peptide-free PBS was administered weekly, starting two weeks before immunization with TAChR. Mice were immunized with 50 μg of purified TAChR[9] for three times, at four-week intervals. Their muscle strength was measured two weeks after the third TAChR injection, using a curare-sensitized holding test.[9] Mice with a holding time of 8 minutes are normal, those with a holding time of 4–8 minutes are moderately sick, and those with a holding time of less than 4 minutes are severely sick. The 4- and 8-minute levels are indicated by dashed horizontal lines. The plot "Naive" reports the values obtained for the mice used in these experiments prior to immunization with TAChR. The other plots report the results obtained for the mice sham-tolerized with PBS or tolerized with peptide Tα150–169 or with α pool, as indicated above the plots. The average holding times ± SD of the different groups are reported: an asterisk indicates a significant difference as compared to the sham-tolerized group ($p < 0.02$).

TABLE 1. Spleen T Cell Response to TAChR and TAChR Epitopes, and Serum Anti-TAChR Ab Concentration at 10 Weeks after Beginning of the TAChR Immunization, in B6 Mice Tolerized to Peptide Tα150–169 and to α Pool and in Mice Sham-Tolerized with PBS[a]

Tolerizing Treatment	T Cell Response to S.I.[b]					Concentration of Anti-AChR Ab (μM)[c]
	AChR	Tα150–169	Tα181–200	Tα360–378		
PBS (n = 10)	16 ± 7.5	3.7 ± 1.9	2.1 ± 1.1	2.2 ± 1		7.2 ± 1.8
Tα150–169 (n = 9)	10.9 ± 7.8	1.7 ± 0.6 (p < 0.01)[d]	1.7 ± 0.8	1.8 ± 0.5		5.5 ± 1.5 (p < 0.009)[d]
α pool (n = 10)	8.8 ± 6.6 (p < 0.03)[d]	2.2 ± 1.7 (p < 0.01)[d]	1.4 ± 0.7	2.2 ± 1.9		4.3 ± 1.6 (p < 0.0001)[d]

[a]Mice (9–10 for each group) inhaled equal volumes (25 μL) of PBS containing peptide Tα150–169 (50 μg) or α pool (50 μg of each peptide), or peptide-free PBS weekly, starting two weeks prior to the beginning of the immunization with TAChR. The mice were immunized three times, at one-month intervals, with TAChR.

[b]Spleen T cells were tested in proliferation assays *in vitro* in the presence of TAChR or the epitope peptides. The T cell response is expressed as S.I. (i.e., the ratio of the cpm obtained in the presence of a given antigen and those of nonstimulated cultures). The values are the averages of the S.I.'s obtained in triplicate cultures for the individual mice of each group.

[c]Determined by radioimmunoprecipitation assay[9] and expressed as μM of precipitable TAChR/[125I]-α-BTX complexes.

[d]Significance of the difference between this average and that of the PBS-treated group, determined in a two-tailed Student's *t* test.

ues. Five of 10 sham-tolerized mice, treated with peptide-free PBS, developed myasthenic weakness. None of the mice that received the tolerizing treatment with α pool or with α150–169 developed EMG.

The nasal peptide treatment affected both anti-TAChR T cell and Ab responses (TABLE 1). Spleen T cells from mice tolerized with the sequence α150–169 or the α pool had reduced responses in proliferation assays *in vitro* to the TAChR and to α150–169 as compared to the sham-tolerized mice. The difference in T cell responsiveness to TAChR was statistically significant only for the α pool–treated mice: this is likely due to the T cell responses to other TAChR epitopes. In agreement with previous reports, the proliferative responses to α181–200 and α360–378 were very low, even in the sham-tolerized mice, making it impossible to evaluate the tolerizing effect of nasal administration for those epitopes. Mice tolerized with peptide α150–169 or the α pool had significantly lower levels of anti-AChR Ab than sham-tolerized mice.

In conclusion, these data demonstrate that nasal administration of synthetic TAChR sequences forming CD4$^+$ epitopes effectively prevents EMG in mice, and this can be obtained even by administering a single immunodominant CD4$^+$ epitope sequence. Different mechanisms may be involved in the protective effects of this treatment, including (*i*) specific activation of modulatory Th2 cells, which may downregulate anti-AChR Th1 cells that drive the synthesis of pathogenic Ab by B cells, and (*ii*) induction of anergy of pathogenic CD4$^+$ T cells specific for the epitopes administered. Although the procedure described here affects the anti-AChR Ab-secreting B cells indirectly, it could be a viable candidate for MG management if associated with plasmapheresis and azathioprine, which eliminate the circulating anti-AChR Ab and suppress the activated B cells. The combined effects of these approaches might result in a long-lasting downregulation of the anti-AChR response, in both the CD4$^+$ and the B cell compartments.

REFERENCES

1. CONTI-FINE, B. M. *et al.* 1997. Myasthenia Gravis: The Immunobiology of an Autoimmune Disease. R. G. Landes Company. Austin.
2. NOSSAL, G. 1995. Choices following antigen entry: antibody formation or immunologic tolerance? Annu. Rev. Immunol. **13:** 1–27.
3. METZLER, B. & D. C. WRAITH. 1993. Inhibition of experimental autoimmune encephalomyelitis by inhalation, but not oral administration of the encephalitogenic peptide: influence of MHC binding affinity. Int. Immunol. **5:** 1159–1169.
4. CHEN, Y. *et al.* 1996. Oral tolerance in myelin basic protein T-cell receptor transgenic mice: suppression of autoimmune encephalomyelitis and dose-dependent induction of regulatory cells. Proc. Natl. Acad. Sci. U.S.A. **93:** 388–391.
5. AL-SABBAGH, A. *et al.* 1996. Antigen-driven peripheral immune tolerance—suppression of experimental autoimmune encephalomyelitis and collagen-induced arthritis by aerosol administration of myelin basic protein or type II collagen. Cell. Immunol. **171:** 111–119.
6. GENAIN, C. P. *et al.* 1996. Late complications of immune deviation therapy in a nonhuman primate. Science **274:** 2054–2057.
7. NEUTRA, M. *et al.* 1996. Antigen sampling across epithelial barriers and induction of mucosal immune response. Annu. Rev. Immunol. **14:** 275–300.

8. CONTI-FINE, B. M. *et al.* 1996. Antibodies as tools to study the structure of membrane proteins: the case of the nicotinic acetylcholine receptor. Annu. Rev. Biophys. Biomol. Struct. **25:** 197–229.

9. KARACHUNSKI, P. *et al.* 1997. Protection from experimental myasthenia gravis in C57Bl/6 mice by sniffing of synthetic CD4$^+$ T cell epitopes. J. Clin. Invest. **100:** 3027–3035.

10. KARACHUNSKI, P. *et al.* 1995. Mechanisms by which the I-A^{bm12} mutation influences susceptibility to experimental myasthenia gravis: a study in homozygous and heterozygous mice. Scand. J. Immunol. **42:** 215–225.

An Animal Model of Maternal Antibody-mediated Arthrogryposis Multiplex Congenita (AMC)[a]

LESLIE JACOBSON, AGATA POLIZZI, AND ANGELA VINCENT

Neurosciences Group
Institute of Molecular Medicine
John Radcliffe Hospital
University of Oxford
Headington, Oxford OX3 9DS, United Kingdom

Arthrogryposis multiplex congenita (AMC) is a nonprogressive condition characterized by multiple joint contractures in two or more body regions.[1] Most cases are sporadic and result from lack of fetal movement *in utero*. AMC is often associated with hypotonia, micrognathia, lung hypoplasia, intrauterine growth retardation, and perinatal death. Some cases may have a genetic basis, but in many environmental factors may be involved.

AMC is sometimes associated with maternal myasthenia gravis (MG).[2] AMC-M1 is an asymptomatic woman who has one surviving firstborn son, but subsequently had a 35-week intrauterine death and five terminations for AMC. AMC-M2 has one surviving daughter (second child) and had a total of three stillborn babies before myasthenia was eventually diagnosed.[3,4] She has since been treated for her MG and has had a fifth pregnancy with a successful outcome (unpublished observations). Both these women had high levels of serum anti-AChR antibodies, and their plasmas and IgG preparations were shown to inhibit the function of fetal AChR[4,5] with no effect on adult AChR. Thus, antibodies specific for a functional site on fetal AChR appear to be responsible for causing AMC in these women (see also Vincent *et al.* in this volume).

These observations suggest that maternal antibodies might be a cause of other developmental abnormalities, even in the absence of maternal disease. To investigate this possibility, an animal model is required. We have therefore developed an experimental animal model of AMC by injecting human anti-AChR antibodies into pregnant mice and looking at the effects on the mouse fetuses.

To look at placental transfer of human IgG, plasma (0.5 mL) from AMC-M2 was injected into pregnant dams daily from E11 to E18 and one dam was sacrificed daily. The anti-AChR antibody levels in the dam's serum, in amniotic fluid, and in a fetal body extract were measured at each time point. There was evidence of substantial placental transfer of antibody beginning at around E15 (FIGURE 1).

To see the effects of transfer of the anti-AChR antibodies on fetal development, plasmas (0.5 mL) from both AMC-M1 and AMC-M2 were injected into pregnant mice from E11 to E18 (three separate dams for each AMC-M plasma and two control

[a]This work was supported by the Medical Research Council and the Myasthenia Gravis Association/Muscular Dystrophy Group of Great Britain and Northern Ireland.

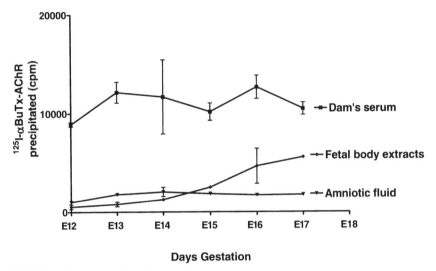

FIGURE 1. Passive transfer of human IgG across the mouse placenta. Plasma (0.5 mL) from AMC-M2 was injected into pregnant mice from day E11 to day E18. At daily intervals thereafter, one dam was killed under anesthesia, and the anti-AChR antibody in the dam's serum, in amniotic fluid, and in an extract of the fetal carcasses was measured. Placental transfer of antibody began around E15.

plasma–injected dams). On E20, before spontaneous delivery, the dams were killed under anesthesia, the fetuses were observed for movement, and then they were removed and weighed. For each dam, anti-AChR antibodies were assayed in the serum, in amniotic fluid, and in a body extract of the pooled fetuses. The total AChR was also measured.

The offspring from the dams injected with AMC-M plasma showed no signs of life *in utero* and there was no evidence of spontaneous movement. By contrast, the dams injected with control plasma moved *in utero* (FIGURE 2). The weights of fetuses dissected out of dams injected with AMC-M and control plasma were not significantly different. This suggests that the anti-AChR antibody did not interfere with weight gain during development.

The AChR content of the dams' muscles was not reduced. By contrast, the ^{125}I-α-BuTx binding in the fetal extracts from the animals injected with AMC-M plasma was reduced by more than 30% in comparison with values from fetuses of control plasma–injected dams. This compares well with the >40% reduction of ^{125}I-α-BuTx binding to fetal AChR that was found in denervated muscle extracts.[5]

The animal model that we have established for the transfer of pathogenic antibodies across the mouse placenta can be used to investigate not only arthrogryposis, but also other conditions. The model will enable us to test whether antibodies specific for fetal antigens, or those antigens inaccessible in adult life, play a role in inducing birth defects. Demonstration of a pathogenic effect of antibodies using this model could

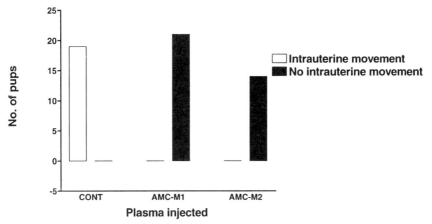

FIGURE 2. Effects on mouse pups of injections of control and AMC-M plasmas into dams from day E11 to day E18. All the pups of the dams injected with control plasma moved *in utero*, whereas the dams injected with AMC plasma showed no signs of movement *in utero*. Results are pooled from three AMC-M1, three AMC-M2, and two controls. Similar results were obtained when the pregnancies were allowed to proceed naturally; in this case, the pups of the AMC-M-injected dams were stillborn and did not survive, whereas the control-injected dams had normal pups.

lead to treatment of mothers with immunotherapy such as plasma exchange and intravenous IgG, which have been shown to be an effective short-term treatment for MG and other autoimmune disorders and which resulted in a successful outcome in AMC-M2's fifth pregnancy.

REFERENCES

1. HALL, J. G., S. D. REED & G. GREENE. 1982. The distal arthrogryposes: delineation of new entities—review and nosologic discussion. Am. J. Med. Genet. **11:** 185–239.
2. VERNET–DER GARABEDIAN, B., M. LACOKOVA, B. EYMARD *et al.* 1994. Association of neonatal myasthenia gravis with antibodies against the fetal acetylcholine receptor. J. Clin. Invest. **94:** 555–559.
3. BARNES, P., D. KANABAR, L. BRUETON *et al.* 1994. Recurrent congenital arthrogryposis leading to a diagnosis of myasthenia gravis in an initially asymptomatic mother. Neuromusc. Dis. **5:** 59–65.
4. VINCENT, A., C. NEWLAND, L. BRUETON *et al.* 1995. Arthrogryposis multiplex congenita with maternal autoantibodies specific for a fetal antigen. Lancet **346:** 24–25.
5. RIEMERSMA, S., A. VINCENT, D. BEESON *et al.* 1996. Association of arthrogryposis multiplex congenita with maternal antibodies inhibiting fetal acetylcholine receptor function. J. Clin. Invest. **98:** 2358–2363.

Oral Administration of an Immunodominant TAChR Epitope Modulates Antigen-specific T Cell Responses in Mice

C. ANTOZZI,[a] F. BAGGI,[a] F. ANDREETTA,[a] O. SIMONCINI,[a] R. LONGHI,[b]
F. CORNELIO,[a] AND R. MANTEGAZZA[a]

[a]Department of Neuromuscular Diseases
National Neurological Institute "C. Besta"
20133 Milan, Italy

[b]Istituto di Chimica degli Ormoni
CNR
Milan, Italy

INTRODUCTION

Myasthenia gravis (MG) and its animal model (experimental autoimmune myasthenia gravis, EAMG) are T cell–dependent autoimmune disorders in which autoantibodies to the acetylcholine receptor (anti-AChR Ab) are produced, leading to muscle weakness.[1] Treatment of human MG relies upon generalized immunosuppression, which is clinically effective, but nonspecific in its interaction with the immune system and a source of potentially severe side effects.[2] The ideal treatment for MG should specifically eliminate the autoimmune response to the AChR. Several immunomodulating approaches have been studied in EAMG and other experimental animal models; among these, the oral administration of the antigen has been proposed as a tool to induce a condition of suppression or anergy.[3] In EAMG, oral and nasal administration of *Torpedo* AChR (TAChR) was effective in reducing T cell responses, anti-AChR Ab titers, and clinical signs of EAMG in Lewis rats.[4–6]

The administration of immunodominant T cell epitopes of the AChR could be an alternative to the use of the intact antigen. T cells from B6 mice susceptible to EAMG proliferate maximally to epitopes corresponding to amino acids 111–126, 146–162, and 182–198 of the α-chain of the AChR.[7] We investigated the effect of the oral administration of the synthetic peptide α146–162 on specific T cell responses in C57BL/6 mice immunized with α146–162 peptide or TAChR.

METHODS

TAChR was affinity-purified from *Torpedo californica* electroplax tissue (Aquatic Research Consultants, California) as reported[5] and used for animal immunization, oral feeding, and *in vitro* proliferation assays.

TAChR α146–162 peptide was synthesized by F-moc chemistry and corresponds to the sequence LGIWTYDGTKVSISPES.

C57BL/6 mice, 6–8 weeks old, were purchased from Charles River, Italia.

Oral feeding protocols: (a) Mice, gently anesthetized with ether, received 1 mg of TAChR (in 0.4 mL, without soybean trypsin inhibitor) by gavage; four feedings were administered over an 8-day period. Control animals were given PBS. (b) Mice, gently anesthetized with ether, received 0.5 mg or 1 mg of the synthetic peptide α146–162 (in 0.4 mL, without soybean trypsin inhibitor) by gavage; four feedings were administered over an 8-day period. Control animals were given PBS.

Immunization: Two days after the last feeding, mice were immunized by injection in the hind footpads with 20 μg of TAChR or 50 μg of peptide α146–162 emulsified in complete Freund's adjuvant.

Lymphoproliferation studies: Animals were sacrificed at 10 days after immunization with TAChR or peptide; draining lymph nodes were removed, processed into single-cell suspensions, and cultured in 96-well microtiter plates. Lymph node cells (LNC) were cultured at 2×10^5 cells and stimulated with various concentrations of TAChR (0.025, 0.25, and 2.5 μg/mL) or peptide (1, 10, and 50 μg/mL). Cultures were pulsed overnight with [^{3}H]thymidine (1 μCi/well) at the end of a 4-day culture period.

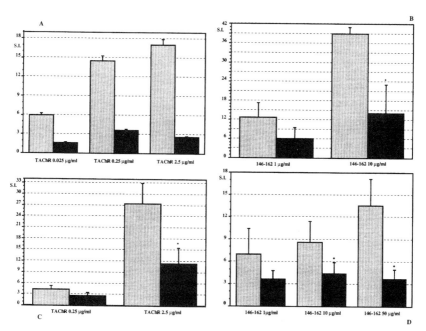

FIGURE 1. (A–D) Effect of TAChR and α146–162 peptide administration on T cell responses in mice (see text for details).

RESULTS

In vitro T cell responses to the TAChR were significantly reduced by four feedings of 1 mg of the receptor (FIGURE 1A).

The oral administration of 0.5 mg of peptide (four feedings over 8 days) reduced the following:

(a) T cell proliferation to α146–162 peptide in mice treated and immunized with the same peptide (FIGURE 1B);

(b) T cell proliferation to TAChR in mice treated and immunized with α146–162 peptide (FIGURE 1C, TAChR concentration of 2.5 µg/mL);

(c) T cell proliferation to α146–162 peptide in mice treated with the peptide and immunized with TAChR (FIGURE 1D);

(d) T cell proliferation to TAChR in mice treated with α146–162 peptide and immunized with TAChR (FIGURE 2A, TAChR concentration of 2.5 µg/mL);

Also, the effect of α146–162 peptide feeding on T cell responses to TAChR in TAChR-immunized mice was significant at all concentrations of receptor when each dose of peptide was increased to 1 mg (FIGURE 2B).

CONCLUSIONS

Oral tolerance has been proposed as an antigen-specific therapy in several experimental models of autoimmune disease.[3] Oral and nasal administration of *Torpedo* AChR was effective in EAMG induced in Lewis rats. As an alternative to the intact antigen, we evaluated the modulating effect of the oral administration of an immunodominant T cell epitope of the α-subunit of the acetylcholine receptor (peptide α146–162) on T cell responses in C57BL/6 mice. The oral administration of peptide α146–162 reduced proliferative T cell responses not only to the peptide itself, but also to the TAChR in mice immunized with either the peptide or the TAChR. This observation suggests that peptides containing T cell epitope(s) might be exploited as

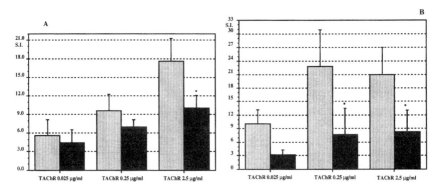

FIGURE 2. (A, B) Effect of different oral doses of α146–162 peptide on T cell responses in mice immunized with TAChR.

potential substitutes of the intact antigen to induce a state of reduced responsiveness. Further studies are needed to investigate (a) whether treatment with peptides is able to modulate the synthesis of anti-AChR Abs and reduce the acetylcholine receptor loss at motor end plates and (b) the immunological mechanisms associated with the oral administration of peptides.

REFERENCES

1. LINDSTROM, J. M., D. SHELTON & Y. FUJII. 1988. Myasthenia gravis. Adv. Immunol. **42:** 233–284.
2. DRACHMAN, D. B. 1996. Immunotherapy in neuromuscular disorders: current and future strategies. Muscle Nerve **19:** 1239–1251.
3. WEINER, H. L. *et al.* 1994. Oral tolerance: immunologic mechanisms and treatment of animal and human organ-specific autoimmune diseases by oral administration of autoantigens. Annu. Rev. Immunol. **121:** 809–837.
4. WHANG, Z-Y., J. ZIAO & H. LINK. 1993. Suppression of experimental autoimmune myasthenia gravis by oral administration of acetylcholine receptor. J. Neuroimmunol. **44:** 209–214.
5. OKUMURA, S., K. McINTOSH & D. B. DRACHMAN. 1994. Oral administration of acetylcholine receptor: effects on experimental myasthenia gravis. Ann. Neurol. **36:** 704–713.
6. MA, C-G., G-X. ZHANG, B-G. XIAO, J. LINK, T. OLSSON & H. LINK. 1995. Suppression of experimental autoimmune myasthenia gravis by nasal administration of acetylcholine receptor. J. Neuroimmunol. **58:** 51–60.
7. SHENOY, M., M. OSHIMA, M. Z. ATASSI & P. CHRISTADOSS. 1993. Suppression of experimental autoimmune myasthenia gravis by epitope-specific neonatal tolerance to synthetic region of α146–162 of acetylcholine receptor. Clin. Immunol. Immunopathol. **66:** 230–238.

Modulation of Experimental Autoimmune Myasthenia Gravis by Recombinant Fragments of the Human Acetylcholine Receptor[a]

MIRIAM C. SOUROUJON,[b,c] DORA BARCHAN,[b] AND SARA FUCHS[b]

[b]Department of Immunology
The Weizmann Institute of Science
Rehovot 76100, Israel

[c]The Open University
Tel Aviv, Israel

Recombinant fragments corresponding to immunopathological regions of the human acetylcholine receptor (AChR) were employed in order to affect the anti-AChR response in experimental autoimmune myasthenia gravis (EAMG). A large portion of the autoantibodies in myasthenia are directed to the extracellular domain of the AChR α-subunit and, within it, primarily to the main immunogenic region (MIR). We have therefore employed fragments corresponding to the entire extracellular domain of the human AChR α-subunit (Hα1–210) and to segments of it that encompass either the MIR (Hα1–121) or the ACh-binding site (Hα122–210). The immunomodulatory potential of the recombinant fragments was tested *in vitro* in TE671 cells and in EAMG passively transferred by an anti-AChR monoclonal antibody (mAb), as well as in EAMG induced by immunization with *Torpedo* AChR.

RESULTS AND DISCUSSION

The recombinant fragments were synthesized by PCR on cDNA from TE671 cells, which are known to express the human muscle-type AChR, and subcloned into the expression vector pGEX-2T in which the expressed proteins are fused to the glutathione S-transferase (GST). The immunochemical specificities of the recombinant fragments were assessed by their reactivity in ELISA and in Western blot, with anti-AChR mAbs directed either to the MIR (mAb 198)[1] or to the ACh-binding site (mAb 5.5).[2]

The ability of the recombinant proteins to interfere with the antigenic modulation of AChR by anti-AChR antibodies was tested in TE671 cells. The effect of fragment Hα1–121 on the antigenic modulation caused by mAb 198 is shown in FIGURE 1. Preincubation with increasing concentrations of fragment Hα1–121 had a dose-dependent protective activity (FIGURE 1A, hatched columns). At a concentration of 100 μg/mL, the accelerated degradation of AChR in TE671 by mAb 198 was completely

[a]This work was supported in part by the Muscular Dystrophy Association of America, the Association Française contre les Myopathies, and the Robert Koch-Minerva Center in Autoimmune Diseases at the Weizmann Institute of Science.

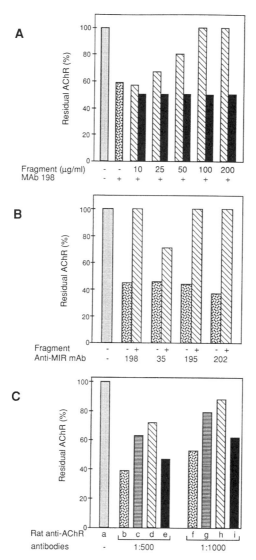

FIGURE 1. Effect of recombinant fragments on AChR degradation in TE671 cells induced by mAb 198 (A), various anti-MIR mAbs (B), and polyclonal rat anti-AChR antibodies (C). **A:** TE671 cells were incubated with medium (left column), with 1 μg/mL of mAb 198 alone (dotted column), or with mAb 198 preincubated with either Hα1–121 (hatched columns) or Hα122–210 (black columns) at concentrations of 10–200 μg/mL. **B:** TE671 cells were incubated with medium (left column) or with mAbs 198 (1 μg/mL), 35 (1 μg/mL), 195 (5 μg/mL), and 202 (5 μg/mL), either alone (dotted columns) or preincubated with Hα1–121 (hatched columns). **C:** TE671 cells were incubated with medium (a, left column) or with polyclonal anti-AChR rat serum at a 1:500 dilution (b–e) and at a 1:1000 dilution (f–i), in the presence of medium (b, f), 400 μg/mL of fragment Hα1–210 (c, g), 300 μg/mL of fragment Hα1–121 (d, h), or 300 μg/mL of fragment Hα122–210 (e, i).

abolished. The entire extracellular fragment Hα1–210 had the same effect as the shorter fragment Hα1–121. However, preincubation of mAb 198 with fragment Hα122–210, which does not contain the MIR, did not affect the antigenic modulation induced by mAb 198 (FIGURE 1A, black columns). As shown for mAb 198, fragment Hα1–121 had a similar protective effect against antigenic modulation induced by two other anti-MIR mAbs (FIGURE 1B; mAb 195 and mAb 202) and a smaller effect on the modulation caused by mAb 35, possibly because the recombinant fragments hardly bind to this antibody in solution. Moreover, these fragments protected AChR in TE671 cells against antigenic modulation induced by polyclonal anti-AChR sera from myasthenic rats (FIGURE 1C). In the absence of any fragment, the residual AChR content following incubation with a 1:1000 dilution of serum was 50%, whereas in the presence of Hα1–210 or Hα1–121 it was raised to 80% and 88%, respectively. Fragment Hα122–210 affected the antigenic modulation induced by polyclonal anti-AChR serum to a much lower extent, in agreement with the notion that a large portion of the antibodies, responsible for AChR loss in myasthenia, are directed to the MIR-containing region.

The recombinant fragments were employed in an attempt to modulate *in vivo* the course of EAMG induced by passive transfer of mAb 198. Myasthenic symptoms were observed 24–48 h following antibody administration and were accompanied by a reduction in the muscle AChR content (48% of normal controls; TABLE 1). As shown in TABLE 1, preincubation of mAb 198 with fragment Hα1–121 prevented the appearance of myasthenic symptoms and the reduction in the muscle AChR content (97% of control). Similar results were obtained with the Hα1–210 recombinant fragment (data not shown), but not with Hα122–210, GST, or BSA. Administration of the recombinant fragments alone did not result in any myasthenic symptoms in the rats.

The immunomodulatory potential of the recombinant fragments was tested also by their ability to modulate EAMG that was actively induced by *Torpedo* AChR. Nasal administration of the recombinant fragments prior to the immunization with *Torpedo* AChR turned out to be a promising approach. Successful attempts to modu-

TABLE 1. Recombinant Fragments Modulate Experimental Myasthenia Passively Transferred by a Monoclonal Anti-AChR Antibody

| | | | AChR Content[a] | |
Treatment	Anti-AChR mAb 198	Myasthenic Symptoms	fmoles/mg Protein	% of Control
–	–	–	39.9 ± 6.3	100
–	+	+	19.2 ± 3.5	48
Hα1–121	+	–	38.8 ± 6.9	97
Hα122–210	+	+	24.5 ± 2.4	61
GST	+	+	19.2 ± 4.5	48
BSA	+	+	21.4 ± 2.4	53

[a]Muscle AChR content was determined by α-bungarotoxin binding to AChR present in Triton X-100 extracts from rat leg muscles, 48 h after Ig administration. The values (mean ± SEM) are averages derived from at least three different animals.

late experimental models of autoimmune diseases including EAMG, by oral or nasal administration of the autoantigen, have been reported.[3,4] However, safe and effective suppression of human myasthenia may require the administration of nonmyasthenogenic, homologous proteins, such as recombinant fragments corresponding to appropriate regions of the AChR molecule. The tested fragments were given nasally to rats over a period of 10 consecutive days and, 3 days later, the rats were immunized with *Torpedo* AChR. Control rats received GST instead of the recombinant fragments. Five weeks after the immunization with AChR, 9 out of 10 control rats developed clear symptoms of EAMG, whereas only 4 out of 36 rats that received the different recombinant fragments developed clinical symptoms of the disease. There were no significant differences between the groups that were pretreated with Hα1–210, Hα1–121, or Hα122–210. The pretreated rats had a reduced proliferative T cell response to AChR, as measured by ^{3}H-thymidine incorporation, and reduced levels of IL-2 and IFN-γ, as compared to control, GST-treated myasthenic rats.

Our results suggest that recombinant fragments, corresponding to selected portions of the human AChR, affect the autoimmune response to AChR in a manner that may be employed for antigen-specific immunotherapy of MG. This has been demonstrated for EAMG that has been induced by an anti-MIR mAb, as well as by active immunization with AChR, in which the immunopathological response is polyclonal. Nasal administration of low concentrations of the recombinant fragments has been effective and thus could provide a convenient therapeutic modality in humans.

REFERENCES

1. SOPHIANOS, D. & S. J. TZARTOS. 1989. Fab fragments of monoclonal antibodies protect the human acetylcholine receptor against antigenic modulation caused by myasthenic sera. J. Autoimmun. **2**(6): 777–789.
2. MOCHLY-ROSEN, D. & S. FUCHS. 1981. Monoclonal anti-acetylcholine receptor directed against the cholinergic binding site. Biochemistry **20**: 5920–5924.
3. DRACHMAN, D. B., S. OKUMURA, R. N. ADAMS & K. R. McINTOSH. 1996. Oral tolerance in myasthenia gravis. Ann. N.Y. Acad. Sci. **778**: 258–272.
4. MA, C. G., G. X. ZHANG, B. G. XIAO, Z. Y. WANG, J. LINK, T. OLSSON & H. LINK. 1996. Mucosal tolerance to experimental autoimmune myasthenia gravis is associated with down-regulation of AChR-specific IFN-gamma-expressing Th1-like cells and up-regulation of TGF-beta mRNA in mononuclear cells. Ann. N.Y. Acad. Sci. **778**: 273–287.

IFN-γ Is Required to Induce Experimental Autoimmune Myasthenia Gravis

G-X. ZHANG,[a] B-G. XIAO,[a] X-F. BAI,[a] A. ÖRN,[b] P. H. VAN DER MEIDE,[c]
AND H. LINK[a]

[a]Division of Neurology
Huddinge University Hospital
[b]Microbiology and Tumor Biology Center (MTC)
Karolinska Institute
Stockholm, Sweden

[c]BPRC
Rijswijk, the Netherlands

Interferon-gamma (IFN-γ) has been considered to play a crucial disease-promoting role in cell- and antibody-mediated autoimmunity.[1] However, IFN-γ may also exert immunosuppressive activity.[2] To further study the systemic immune response mediated by IFN-γ in autoantibody-mediated experimental autoimmune myasthenia gravis (EAMG), which is an animal model for human myasthenia gravis,[3] IFN-γ receptor knockout (IFN-γR–/–) mice and wild-type littermates were inoculated with *Torpedo* acetylcholine receptor (AChR) emulsified in Freund's complete adjuvant (FCA). They were evaluated with regard to clinical muscle weakness, AChR-induced T and B cell responses, and cytokine profiles.

MATERIALS AND METHODS

IFN-γR–/– (129/Sv/Ev × C57BL/6) mice and wild-type mice were obtained from M. Aguet (Genentech, San Francisco, California). All mice used were female, 8–12 weeks of age, weighing 20–30 g. Mice were immunized with 20 μg AChR in FCA and boosted on days 30 and 60 after the primary immunization (p.i.). The disease symptoms were graded (0–3 grades) every other day in a blinded fashion and confirmed by ip injection of neostigmine. Assays were performed for anti-AChR antibody level, isotype, and affinity in serum, for AChR-specific IgG antibody secreting cells, for AChR-reactive IFN-γ secreting cells, and for lymphocyte proliferative responses in mononuclear cells (MNC) from the lymph nodes at 100 days p.i. The numbers of cytokine mRNA expressing cells were determined by *in situ* hybridization.

RESULTS

Seven out of 15 wild-type mice developed severe to mild muscle weakness after immunization with AChR + FCA. In contrast, IFN-γR–/– mice exhibited less severe

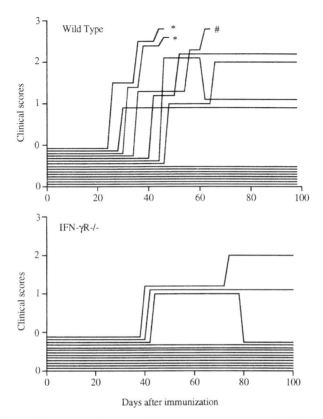

FIGURE 1. Clinical course of EAMG in IFN-γR–/– mice (*n* = 13) and wild-type mice (*n* = 15). Mice were immunized with AChR + FCA and boosted twice monthly. Symbols: (*) died; (#) humanely sacrificed.

clinical disease than the wild-type mice ($p < 0.05$) (FIGURE 1). IFN-γR–/– mice had significantly lower levels of serum anti-AChR antibodies at 4 and 10 weeks p.i. (FIGURE 2A), lower relative affinity of anti-AChR at weeks 6, 8, and 10 p.i. (FIGURE 2B), and lower numbers of AChR-specific IgG antibody secreting cells. The decrease of antibody to AChR was mainly due to a decrease of IgG2a. There were no differences for lymphocyte proliferative responses between IFN-γR–/– mice and wild-type mice. AChR-reactive IFN-γ secreting cells and AChR-reactive IFN-γ mRNA expressing cells were dramatically elevated in the IFN-γR–/– mice compared to wild-type mice, probably reflecting failure of a negative feedback loop due to a blockade of signal transduction pathways normally activated via IFN-γR. The numbers of AChR-reactive TNF-α and IL-1β mRNA expressing cells in IFN-γR–/– mice were lower than those in wild-type mice. There were no differences for AChR-reactive IL-4, IL-10, or TGF-β mRNA expressing cells.

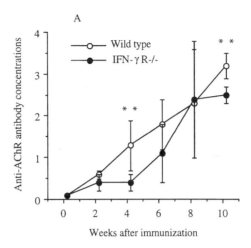

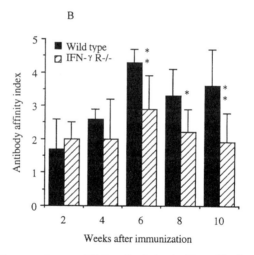

FIGURE 2. (A) Serum antimouse AChR antibody levels. The antibody concentrations were measured weekly by RIA and expressed as moles of α-bungarotoxin binding sites bound per liter of serum. (B) Relative affinity of serum anti-AChR IgG antibodies at different time points after immunization with AChR + CFA. Symbols refer to mean values and bars to SD; (*) $p <$ 0.05, (**) $p < 0.01$.

DISCUSSION

The production of IFN-γ is mostly of benefit for the host in the defense against microorganisms. However, many of the activities of IFN-γ may throw the normal immune response "off balance" and cause profound changes that may lead to autoimmunity. Elevated levels of circulating cells secreting IFN-γ or expressing IFN-γ mRNA in response to AChR could reflect strong AChR-specific Th1 responses. After expressing IFN-γ within the neuromuscular junction (NMJ) by the transgenic technique, EAMG-resistant BALB/c mice exhibit clinical weakness, accompanied by infiltration of MNC and autoantibody deposition at motor end plates, implying that IFN-γ in the milieu of the muscle tissue induces humoral autoimmunity without circulating anti-AChR antibodies.[4] IFN-γ is an important cytokine to induce B cell memory and affinity maturation.[5] Blocking the signal of IFN-γ in IFN-γ receptor–deficient mice might lead to a change in the quantity and quality of antibodies. Our data imply the effects of IFN-γ on B cell memory, isotype switching, and affinity maturation.

In the cytokine network, IFN-γ promotes the differentiation of Th1 cells, which produce IFN-γ, IL-2, and lymphotoxin. These cytokines together with IL-1β were associated with myasthenia gravis. Decreased levels of these proinflammatory cytokines might be responsible for the low susceptibility to EAMG in IFN-γR–/– mice. In the present study, the lack of IFN-γ receptor did not influence the expression of IL-4, IL-10, or TGF-β. Taken together, our results indicate that IFN-γ is critically involved in the systemic humoral responses in EAMG by upregulating the production and affinity of autoantibody against AChR. Decreased levels of proinflammatory cytokines might also contribute to the low susceptibility to EAMG in IFN-γR–/– mice.

REFERENCES

1. BILLIAU, A. 1996. Interferon-γ in autoimmunity. Cytok. Growth Fact. Rev. **7:** 25–34.
2. KRAKOWSKI, M. & T. OWENS. 1996. Interferon-γ confers resistance to experimental allergic encephalomyelitis. Eur. J. Immunol. **26:** 1641–1646.
3. LINDSTROM, J. *et al.* 1988. Myasthenia gravis. Adv. Immunol. **42:** 233–285.
4. GU, D. *et al.* 1995. Myasthenia gravis–like syndrome induced by expression of interferon-γ in the neuromuscular junction. J. Exp. Med. **181:** 547–557.
5. RIZZO, L. V. *et al.* 1992. Generation of B cell memory and affinity maturation: induction with Th1 and Th2 T cell clones. J. Immunol. **148:** 3733–3739.

Cytokine Profiles of Experimental Autoimmune Myasthenia Gravis after Treatment by the Synthetic Immunomodulator Linomide

G-X. ZHANG,[a] L-Y. YU,[a] F-D. SHI,[a] B-G. XIAO,[a] J. BJÖRK,[b]
G. HEDLUND,[b,c] AND H. LINK[a]

[a]Division of Neurology
Huddinge University Hospital
Karolinska Institute
Stockholm, Sweden

[b]Pharmacia & Upjohn
Lund Research Center
Lund, Sweden

[c]The Wallenberg Laboratory
Lund University
Lund, Sweden

Myasthenia gravis (MG) and its animal model, experimental autoimmune myasthenia gravis (EAMG), are antibody-mediated autoimmune diseases.[1] The production of anti-AChR antibodies is regulated by AChR-specific type-1 and -2 T helper cells of cytokines.[2,3] Linomide, a quinoline-3-carboxamide compound, effectively suppresses certain experimental autoimmune diseases.[4] Here, we report that Linomide suppresses EAMG and affects the profiles of Th1 and Th2 cytokines.

MATERIALS AND METHODS

Twenty female Lewis rats were immunized by injection sc with 50 μg of *Torpedo* acetylcholine receptor (AChR) emulsified in complete Freund's adjuvant (CFA). Linomide (Pharmacia Leo Therapeutics AB, Helsingborg, Sweden) was dissolved in 0.9% saline and injected sc at a single daily dose from day 0 to 49 postimmunization (p.i.). Five rats received Linomide at 1.6, 5 rats received 16, and 5 rats received 160 mg/kg/day. Five control rats received PBS daily. Clinical weakness, serum anti-AChR IgG antibodies, anti-AChR IgG antibody secreting cells, and AChR-reactive IFN-γ secreting cells were evaluated. To examine the involvement of immunoregulatory cytokines and the underlying mechanisms involved in the suppression of EAMG by Linomide, *in situ* hybridization with radiolabeled synthetic oligonucleotide probes was adopted to enumerate mononuclear cells expressing mRNA for the Th1 cytokines, IFN-γ, IL-12, TNF-α, and TNF-β; the Th2 cytokines, IL-4, 6, and 10, as well as IL-1β; and the Th3 cytokine, TGF-β, in mononuclear cells (MNC) at 49 days p.i.

RESULTS

The major, second phase of weakness characteristic for EAMG in rats treated with Linomide at doses of 16 or 160 mg/kg/day had a later onset and lower clinical score than in the PBS-injected EAMG rats ($p < 0.01$; FIGURE 1). Levels of serum anti-AChR antibodies were lower in rats treated with Linomide at a dose of 160 mg/kg/day, and at 3 and 7 weeks p.i. after treatment with 16 mg/kg/day ($p < 0.01$). Linomide at doses of 160 or 16 mg/kg/day also suppressed the number of anti-AChR IgG antibody secreting cells among lymph node MNC ($p < 0.05$). After *in vitro* stimulation with AChR, lower values of AChR-reactive IFN-γ secreting Th1-like cells were found in rats treated with Linomide at doses of 160 and 16 mg/kg/day when compared to control rats ($p < 0.05$ and $p < 0.01$).

Cytokine profiles were evaluated in lymph node cells of rats receiving the most effective dose (160 mg/kg/day) of Linomide versus PBS-injected EAMG rats. For Th1 cytokines, Linomide-treated rats had lower numbers of AChR-reactive IFN-γ, IL-12, and TNF-α mRNA expressing cells when compared to control rats ($p < 0.05$ or 0.01) (FIGURE 2). For Th2 cytokines, the levels of AChR-induced IL-4 and IL-10 mRNA expressing cells in lymph nodes of Linomide-treated rats were lower than the

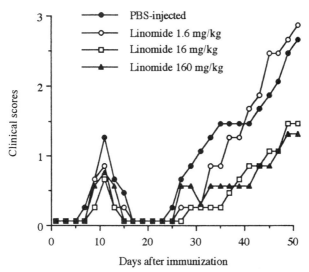

FIGURE 1. Clinical course of EAMG in control rats receiving PBS and rats receiving Linomide at 1.6, 16, and 160 mg/kg/day. Symbols indicate the mean clinical scores of each group on the indicated day.

levels of PBS-injected rats. There was no significant difference for the numbers of AChR-reactive IL-1β or TGF-β between Linomide-treated and PBS-injected control EAMG rats (FIGURE 2).

DISCUSSION

The present study confirmed that Linomide suppresses clinical signs of actively induced EAMG when administered at doses of 16 or 160 mg/kg/day in daily injections. The suppression is accompanied by decreased B and T cell responses, as well as by decreased Th1 and Th2 cytokine mRNA expression inducible by AChR.

Abnormal T cell responses to AChR and its four subunits are characteristic for both EAMG and human MG. MG patients have high numbers of AChR-reactive IFN-γ, TNF-α, TNF-β, and IL-12 mRNA expressing cells. Here, we provide evidence for a potent effect of Linomide on AChR-reactive TNF-α and IL-12 mRNA expression, which could contribute to the suppression of EAMG. The involvement of the Th2 cytokines, IL-4, 6, and 10, in MG and EAMG is expected on the basis of the strong B cell response found in these diseases. The suppressed IL-4 and IL-10 production is probably one reason for the suppressed clinical EAMG and B cell responses after administration of Linomide.

It is hypothesized that Linomide may amplify the naturally existing suppressor/regulatory network. To elucidate this possibility, we evaluated in the present study the mRNA expression of the endogenous immunosuppressive cytokine TGF-β, which is important in downregulating MG and EAMG. We did not find any

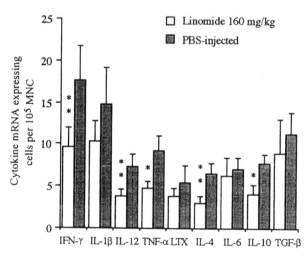

FIGURE 2. Mean numbers of AChR-reactive cytokine mRNA expressing cells per 10^5 MNC isolated from popliteal and inguinal lymph nodes of EAMG rats receiving Linomide at a dose of 160 mg/kg/day and of control rats receiving PBS. Rats were sacrificed on day 49 p.i. Symbols refer to mean values and bars to SD; (*) $p < 0.05$, (**) $p < 0.01$.

correlation between TGF-β mRNA expressing cell levels and the improvement of EAMG induced by Linomide. Whether Linomide can amplify the suppressor/regulatory network by inducing some other immunosuppressive cytokines (e.g., IFN-α) is not known. Taken together, we now present evidence that the suppression of clinical EAMG by Linomide is associated with the downregulation of autoantigen-induced Th1 and Th2 cytokines. These observations make Linomide a candidate for treatment of human myasthenia gravis.

REFERENCES

1. DRACHMAN, D. B. 1994. Myasthenia gravis. N. Engl. J. Med. **330:** 1797–1810.
2. ZHANG, G-X., V. NAVIKAS & H. LINK. 1997. Cytokines and the pathogenesis of myasthenia gravis. Muscle Nerve **22:** 543–551.
3. ASTHANA, D. *et al.* 1993. Regulation of antibody production by helper T cell clones in experimental autoimmune myasthenia gravis is mediated by IL-4 and antigen-specific T cell factors. Clin. Immunol. Immunopathol. **67:** 240–248.
4. KARUSSIS, D. M. *et al.* 1993. Treatment of chronic-relapsing experimental autoimmune encephalomyelitis with the synthetic immunomodulator Linomide (quinoline-3-carboxamide). Proc. Natl. Acad. Sci. U.S.A. **90:** 6400–6404.

Effect of Anti-idiotopic Antibody on the Course of Experimental Autoimmune Myasthenia Gravis[a]

MARK A. AGIUS AND ERIC YUEN

Department of Neurology
University of California at Davis
Davis, California 95615

INTRODUCTION

We have previously demonstrated that physiological doses of anti-idiotope (anti-id) suppress the production of the corresponding idiotope and the total antiacetylcholine receptor (AChR) antibody response in Lewis rats.[1] This effect was demonstrated when anti-idiotope was injected 2 weeks prior to active immunization with AChR. Here, we have investigated the role of various factors that may influence the anti-id-induced effect, including the dosage and timing of the anti-idiotope dose.

MATERIALS AND METHODS

Two experiments were performed. An initial experiment involved 32 female Lewis rats. In this experiment, two doses (physiological low dose of 0.5 mg/kg and physiological high dose of 5.0 mg/kg) were used at day 1, 8, 20, and 35 after active immunization with AChR as well as weekly from day 23. At 7 weeks of age, 30 rats were actively immunized with 50 μg of *Torpedo californica* AChR intradermally in the dorsal footpads in 300 μL of complete Freund's adjuvant (CFA) containing human mycobacterium. The animals were tested for weight gain, weakness, and serum anti-AChR titer. Muscle AChR content was measured at day 79 of immunization. Serum anti-AChR antibody titer and muscle AChR content were measured by radioimmunoassay as previously described.[2]

A second experiment with 32 Lewis rats investigated the role of 0.5 mg/kg of anti-id at day 1 and day 8 of active immunization. Ten-week-old female Lewis rats were immunized with 36 μg of AChR in CFA. At day 1 or day 8 of immunization, they were treated with intraperitoneal administration of anti-id HC4A, Lewis rat immunoglobulin (Ig) prepared by ammonium sulfate precipitation, or normal saline. Rats were weighed every 2 weeks and muscle AChR content was measured at week 16 of immunization.

[a]This work was funded by NIH Grant No. NS01226.

TABLE 1. AChR Content in EAMG Animals Treated with Anti-id: Experiment 1

Animal Group (n)	Anti-id Dose	Anti-id Timing	Muscle AChR Content[a]
1. (8)	control IgG	day 1, 8, 20, 35, weekly	14.3
2. (2)	0.5 mg/kg	day 1	12.9
3. (2)	5.0 mg/kg	day 1	11.9
4. (2)	0.5 mg/kg	day 8	16.5
5. (2)	5.0 mg/kg	day 8	13.8
6. (2)	0.5 mg/kg	day 20	9.1
7. (2)	5.0 mg/kg	day 20	10.2
8. (2)	0.5 mg/kg	weekly from day 23	12.7
9. (2)	5.0 mg/kg	weekly from day 23	11.8
10. (2)	0.5 mg/kg	day 35	12.7
11. (2)	5.0 mg/kg	day 35	12.4
12. (2)	normal healthy controls	normal healthy controls	26.4

[a]Measured in pmol/g of extracted membrane muscle protein.

RESULTS

Animals immunized with AChR developed EAMG with detectable weakness, decreased muscle AChR content, and elevated anti-AChR antibody titer. Control immunized animals were also actively immunized with AChR, but were treated with normal rat Ig or normal saline, whereas test animals received anti-id. There was no difference between anti-id-treated and control animals in muscle strength, serum anti-AChR antibody titer, and muscle AChR content when anti-id was administered with or after immunization with AChR (TABLES 1 and 2). Control normal healthy animals that had not been immunized with AChR had normal strength and muscle AChR content and undetectable anti-AChR antibodies.

TABLE 2. AChR Content in EAMG Animals Treated with Anti-id: Experiment 2

Animal Group (n)	Anti-id Dose	Anti-id Timing	Muscle AChR Content (pmol/g) (Mean ± SD)
EAMG rats			
1. (7)	0.5 mg/kg anti-id	day 1	13.46 ± 6.24
2. (4)	0.5 mg/kg control Ig	day 1	14.58 ± 1.38
3. (4)	normal saline	day 1	12.28 ± 5.22
4. (7)	0.5 mg/kg anti-id	day 8	10.69 ± 2.79
5. (4)	0.5 mg/kg control Ig	day 8	11.33 ± 3.76
6. (4)	normal saline	day 8	18.40 ± 7.58
Normal rats			
7. (2)	—	—	23.75 ± 3.89

DISCUSSION

A suppressive effect on idiotope levels and on serum anti-AChR antibody levels has been previously documented with large physiologic doses of anti-id given 2 weeks prior to active immunization with AChR. In contrast, the suppression effect of anti-id is not detected when anti-id is given with immunization and after immunization with AChR. The anti-id-mediated effect is also abrogated with a large immunogen dose. These findings suggest that the timing of administration of anti-id, the dose of anti-id, as well as the immunogen dose are important factors in determining the modulatory effect of anti-id on autoimmune processes.

REFERENCES

1. AGIUS, M. A. & D. P. RICHMAN. 1987. Antiidiotopic modification of the anti-acetylcholine receptor immune response and of experimental autoimmune myasthenia gravis in Lewis rats. Ann. N. Y. Acad. Sci. **505:** 896–897.
2. AGIUS, M. A. & D. P. RICHMAN. 1986. Suppression of development of experimental autoimmune myasthenia gravis with isogeneic monoclonal antiidiotopic antibody. J. Immunol. **137:** 2195–2198.

Analysis of Risk Factors for Acquired Myasthenia in Dogs

G. DIANE SHELTON,[a] ALAN SCHULE,[a] AND PHILIP H. KASS[b]

[a]Department of Pathology
University of California, San Diego
La Jolla, California 92093

[b]Department of Population Health and Reproduction
School of Veterinary Medicine
University of California, Davis
Davis, California 95616

Acquired canine myasthenia gravis (CMG) is a naturally occurring disorder in the dog and has been shown to be similar to the human disorder in many important ways. Several clinical presentations are described, including focal forms with weakness limited to the pharyngeal, esophageal, and/or facial musculature; a "classical" presentation associated with exercise-related weakness; and also an acute fulminating form with generalized collapse.[1–9] Acquired CMG may be associated with other immune-mediated disorders including hypothyroidism[7] and is a paraneoplastic disorder associated with thymoma and other neoplasias.[8] The diagnosis of CMG is confirmed by the demonstration of circulating AChR antibodies using ^{125}I-labeled α-bungarotoxin–canine AChR in a radioimmunoassay.

During the years 1991–1995, 8330 canine serum samples were submitted by veterinarians throughout the United States to the Comparative Neuromuscular Laboratory at the University of California, San Diego, and tested for the presence of acetylcholine receptor antibodies by immunoprecipitation radioimmunoassay. All dogs tested had various forms of muscle weakness, exercise intolerance, and/or acquired megaesophagus, and 1154 of these dogs had acetylcholine receptor antibody titers > 0.6 nmol/L (canine reference < 0.6 nmol/L). The database generated from this large population of dogs was used to determine the most frequent presenting clinical signs and the relative risks associated with acquired CMG relating to breed, sex, age, state of origin, and month of clinical presentation. Proportionate changes in the risk of acquired CMG were evaluated using unconditional logistic regression. Mixed-breed dogs were used as a reference breed for comparison, and California was used as a reference state for comparison. Results are presented as odds ratios (OR) and 95% confidence intervals (95% CI). Because MG incidence was <5% within all levels of covariates, the OR value was used to estimate the relative risk.

Clinical presentations consistent with generalized MG were described in 57% of the positive submissions, and localized bulbar weakness without clinically detectable limb muscle weakness was described in 43% of the samples (TABLE 1). Of dogs with generalized MG, 13.1% did not show clinical signs of esophageal or pharyngeal dysfunction. An anterior mediastinal mass was found in 3.4% of the cases.

Relative risk for acquired CMG was calculated for 61 breeds of dogs. Several breeds of dogs were at a higher relative risk when compared to the mixed-breed dog. The five breeds with the highest relative risk of MG were the Akita, terrier, Scottish terrier, German shorthair pointer, and Chihuahua (TABLE 2). While these dogs were at higher risk, they accounted for only 7.5% of the total morbidity. The Rottweiler, Doberman, Dalmatian, and Jack Russell terrier had lower relative risks. The five breeds of dogs accounting for the highest total morbidity (49.9%) included the German shepherd dog, golden retriever, mixed-breed dogs, Labrador retriever, and the dachshund. Dogs in the 1–15 years of age group had a 55% increase in the risk of MG (OR = 1.6, 95% CI = 1.1–2.2) and dogs in the 16+ years of age group had a 4.09-fold increase in the risk of MG (OR = 4.1, 95% CI = 1.7–9.7) as compared to dogs in the <1 age group. There was some protection for intact males (OR = 0.8, 95% CI = 0.7–1.01) over intact or spayed females and neutered males. No meaningful differences in risk by state of origin or month of sample submission were found.

As shown in this study, an increased relative risk for acquired CMG was found in several breeds of purebred dogs when compared to mixed-breed dogs. Since a clear genetic predisposition to autoimmune disease has been demonstrated in humans, breed predispositions for acquired CMG support a genetic basis in dogs. As in human MG, there was also some influence of age and sex, with dogs greater than 1 year having an increased risk and some hormonal protection for intact males.

ACKNOWLEDGMENTS

We would like to thank Jon Lindstrom for the generous gift of iodinated bungarotoxin.

TABLE 1. Clinical Presentations in 1154 Dogs with Acquired Myasthenia Gravis[a]

Focal Myasthenia Gravis			Generalized Myasthenia Gravis		
Clinical Sign	No. of Dogs	% Total Cases	Clinical Sign	No. of Dogs	% Total Cases
M	367	31.8	G, M	440	38.1
M, P	7	<1	G, M, P	7	<1
M, LP, B	3	<1	G, M, B	34	2.9
M, P, B	3	<1	G, M, LP	3	<1
M, LP	6	<1	G, no M	77	6.7
M, B	14	1.2	G, no M, LP	1	<1
M, CMM	16	1.3	G, no M, B	5	<1
P	13	1.1	G, M, CMM	15	1.3
P, LP	2	<1	G, M, B, CMM	2	<1
MISC	7	<1	MISC	10	<1

[a]M = megaesophagus; P = pharyngeal weakness; LP = laryngeal paralysis; B = poor or absent blink; CMM = cranial mediastinal mass; G = generalized weakness; MISC = poor esophageal motility (3), chronic pneumonia (1), cranial mediastinal mass only (2), extraocular muscle weakness only (1), generalized weakness and third-degree heart block (3). Information was not available for 122 cases. Reprinted with permission from *J. Am. Vet. Med. Assoc.* 1997. **211:** 1428–1431.

TABLE 2. Relative Risk of Various Breeds of Dogs for Acquired Myasthenia Gravis[a]

Breed	No. of Cases	No. of Controls	OR	95% CI	Breed	No. of Cases	No. of Controls	OR	95% CI
Mixed	129	1005	1		Irish setter	3	59	0.4	0.1–1.3
Golden retriever	146	746	1.5	1.2–2.0	Keeshond	8	38	1.6	0.7–3.6
Labrador retriever	103	668	1.2	0.9–1.6	Malamute	10	62	1.3	0.6–2.5
Dachshund	36	112	2.5	1.7–3.8	Maltese	5	35	1.6	0.6–4.1
Cocker spaniel	31	207	1.17	0.8–1.8	Bullmastiff	7	54	1	0.4–2.3
Akita	29	39	5.8	3.5–9.7	Miniature schnauzer	14	110	1	0.6–1.8
Collie	27	108	2	1.2–3.1	German shepherd dog	159	448	2.8	2.1–3.6
Sheltie	25	82	2.4	1.5–3.9	Old English sheepdog	7	41	1.3	0.6–3.0
Poodle	23	166	1.1	0.7–1.7	Pitbull	14	42	2.6	1.4–4.9
Scottish terrier	19	31	4.8	2.6–8.7	Samoyed	3	28	0.8	0.3–2.8
Australian shepherd	19	45	3.3	1.9–5.8	Welsh corgi	4	39	0.8	0.3–2.3
Rottweiler	15	265	0.4	0.3–0.8	Pomeranian	7	36	1.5	0.7–3.5
Newfoundland	17	65	2	1.2–3.6	Chinese shar pei	5	42	0.9	0.4–2.4
Beagle	14	57	1.9	1.0–3.5	Shih tzu	10	40	2	1.0–4.0
Airedale	4	40	0.8	0.3–2.2	Husky	17	56	2.4	1.3–4.2
Bassett hound	6	48	1	0.4–2.3	Springer spaniel	17	82	1.6	0.9–2.8
Border collie	6	25	1.9	0.8–4.6	Terrier group	16	23	5.4	2.8–10.5
Boston terrier	2	29	0.5	0.1–2.3	Weimaraner	2	39	0.4	0.0–1.7
Boxer	18	92	1.5	0.9–2.6	Yorkshire terrier	5	53	0.7	0.3–1.9
Brittany spaniel	4	37	0.8	0.3–2.4	German shorthair	13	22	4.6	2.3–9.4
Bulldog	3	52	0.4	0.1–1.5	Pekinese	1	12	0.6	0.0–5.0

(continued)

TABLE 2 (*continued*)

Breed	No. of Cases	No. of Controls	OR	95% CI	Breed	No. of Cases	No. of Controls	OR	95% CI
Chesapeake Bay ret.	5	28	1.4	0.5–3.7	Bichon frise	1	25	0.3	0.0–2.3
Chow chow	6	41	1.1	0.5–2.7	Cairn terrier	5	15	2.6	0.9–7.3
Chihuahua	9	16	4.4	1.9–10.1	English setter	3	19	1.2	0.3–4.2
Pug	3	28	0.8	0.3–2.8	Jack Russell terrier	4	236	0.1	0.0–0.4
Lhasa apso	5	37	1.1	0.4–2.7	Rhodesian Ridgeback	1	21	0.4	0.0–2.8
West Highland white ter.	6	31	1.5	0.6–3.7	Giant schnauzer	8	19	3.3	1.4–7.7
Dalmatian	3	104	0.2	0.0–0.7	Vizsla	6	14	3.3	1.3–8.8
Doberman	13	223	0.5	0.3–0.8	Bernese mountain dog	3	24	1	0.3–3.3
Great Dane	6	108	0.4	0.2–1.0	Wirehair fox terrier	11	25	3.4	1.7–7.1
Greyhound	3	31	0.8	0.2–2.5	Other purebreds	43	281	1.2	0.8–1.7
					Missing information	7	580		

[a]OR = odds ratio. CI = confidence interval. Reprinted with permission from *J. Am. Vet. Med. Assoc.* 1997. **211:** 1428–1431.

REFERENCES

1. PALMER, A. C. 1974. Myasthenia in the dog. Vet. Rec. **16:** 452–454.
2. LENNON, V. A., E. H. LAMBERT, A. C. PALMER *et al.* 1981. Acquired and Congenital Myasthenia Gravis in Dogs: A Study of 20 Cases, p. 41–54. University of Tokyo Press. Tokyo.
3. GARLEP, M. J., P. H. KAY, B. R. FARROW *et al.* 1984. Autoimmunity in spontaneous myasthenia gravis in dogs. Clin. Immunol. Immunopathol. **31:** 301–306.
4. SHELTON, G. D., G. H. CARDINET III & J. M. LINDSTROM. 1988. Canine and human myasthenia gravis autoantibodies recognize similar regions on the acetylcholine receptor. Neurology **38:** 1417–1423.
5. GARLEP, M., B. FARROW, P. KAY *et al.* 1989. Antibodies to the acetylcholine receptor in myasthenic dogs. Immunology **37:** 807–810.
6. SHELTON, G. D., M. D. WILLARD, G. H. CARDINET III *et al.* 1990. Acquired myasthenia gravis: selective involvement of esophageal, pharyngeal, and facial muscles. J. Vet. Intern. Med. **4:** 281–284.
7. DEWEY, C. W., G. D. SHELTON, C. S. BAILEY *et al.* 1995. Neuromuscular dysfunction in five dogs with acquired myasthenia gravis and presumptive hypothyroidism. Prog. Vet. Neurol. **6:** 117–123.
8. KLEBANOW, E. R. 1992. Thymoma and acquired myasthenia gravis in the dog: a case report and review of 13 additional cases. J. Am. Anim. Hosp. Assoc. **28:** 63–69.
9. DEWEY, C. W., C. S. BAILEY, G. D. SHELTON *et al.* 1997. Clinical forms of acquired myasthenia gravis in dogs: 25 cases (1988–1995). J. Vet. Intern. Med. **11:** 50–57.

Apolipoprotein E in Myasthenia Gravis

M. ŠOŠTARKO,[a] J. SERTIĆ,[b] N. GREGURIĆ,[c]
A. STAVLJENIĆ-RUKAVINA,[b] Z. BRZOVIĆ,[a] AND V. MATIĆ[a]

[a]Department of Neurology
[b]Clinical Institute of Laboratory Diagnosis
[c]Institute of Nuclear Medicine
University Hospital Rebro
10000 Zagreb, Croatia

INTRODUCTION

Apolipoprotein E (apo E) is an important protein comprising 299 amino acids. It is mostly found in chylomicrons, but it is synthesized in different tissues and the liver is one of its primary sources. It plays a crucial role in the metabolism of lipids, which is reflected in the plasma lipid level. It has a very special role in atherogenesis. It is also related to the metabolism of the central nervous system and has a special role in the development of Alzheimer's disease. It also is involved in different biological processes such as cytoskeletal stability, nerve regeneration, proliferation of smooth muscles, and skeletal muscle metabolism. It is believed that apo E modulates T lymphocytes by acting on mitogens and antigens, also having an influence on the immune response.[1]

The apo E gene is located on chromosome 19q13.2 and it consists of four exons and three introns spanning 3597 nucleotides. It is genetically polymorphic, showing three common isoforms designated as apo E2, apo E3, and apo E4 with cysteine-arginine interchanges determining the codon positions 112 and 158. As every individual inherits two alleles, one from each parent, there are six possible genotypes.[2]

Since there is a possibility that apo E modulates T lymphocytes, which have a very important role in autoimmune disorders, we tried to find any possible correlation between myasthenia gravis phenotypes and apo E genotypes.

MATERIALS AND METHODS

Apo E genotypes were analyzed in two groups. One group had 56 myasthenia gravis patients and another 50 healthy examinees.

The diagnosis of myasthenia gravis was confirmed according to anamnesis, clinical signs and symptoms, electrophysiological and pharmacological tests, and detection of anti-AChR antibodies by radioimmunoassay.

The frequency of apo E genotypes due to allelic variation at amino acids 112 and 158 was analyzed by restriction isotyping and the ARMS method.[3]

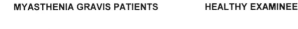

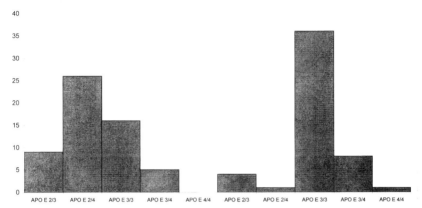

FIGURE 1. The distribution of apo E genotypes in myasthenia gravis patients and healthy examinees obtained by polymerase chain reaction.

RESULTS AND DISCUSSION

The distribution of apo E genotypes in myasthenia gravis patients and healthy examinees obtained by polymerase chain reaction is shown in FIGURE 1. Apo E2/4 genotype is the most frequent, with 26 patients or 46.43%. It is followed by apo E3/3 genotype, with 28.57% or 16 patients, and then there are apo E2/3 (16.07% or 9 patients) and apo E3/4 (8.93% or 5 patients). There was no patient with apo E4/4 genotype in the myasthenia gravis group.

The following genotypes were found in the group of healthy examinees: apo E3/3, with 72% or 36 examinees, was the most frequent; the others were apo E3/4 (16% or 8 examinees), apo E2/3 (8% or 4 examinees), apo E2/4 (2% or 1 examinee), and apo E4/4 (2% or 1 examinee).

It is obvious that apo E2/4 genotype is the most frequent in myasthenia gravis patients. The apo E3/3 genotype is the most frequent among the healthy examinees.

TABLE 1. Correlation between Apo E Genotype and Myasthenia Gravis (MG) Phenotype[a]

	Genotype Apo E2/3 (%)	Genotype Apo E2/4 (%)	Genotype Apo E3/3 (%)	Genotype Apo E3/4 (%)	Total (%)
MG severe form	3.57	32.14*	0*	0	35.71
MG moderate form	3.57	14.29	10.71	8.93*	37.5
MG mild form	8.93*	0*	17.86*	0	26.79
Total	16.07	46.43	28.57	8.93	

[a]An asterisk indicates a significant difference.

Otherwise, the frequency of the allele E3 is the highest among the white population in America and Europe.

The correlation between apo E genotype and myasthenia gravis phenotype shows the following features (see TABLE 1):

(a) Twenty patients or 35.71% in the group with myasthenia gravis developed the severe form of the disease. There are 18 patients or 32.14% with apo E2/4 genotype and there are also 2 patients or 3.57% with apo E2/3 genotype. The mean value of the anti-AChR antibody titers in the group with the severe form of myasthenia gravis is 15.20 nmol/L with SD = 1.51.

(b) Twenty-one patients developed the moderate form of myasthenia gravis and their mean value of anti-AChR antibody titers was 4.34 nmol/L with SD = 1.54. The correlation to apo E genotypes is as follows: apo E2/4, 8 patients or 14.29%; apo E3/3, 6 patients or 10.71%; apo E3/4, 5 patients or 8.93%; and apo E2/3, 2 patients or 3.57%.

(c) Fifteen patients developed the mild form of myasthenia gravis and the mean value of anti-AChR antibody titers was 1.81 nmol/L with SD = 0.54. Ten of them or 17.86% have apo E3/3 genotype and 5 patients or 8.93% have apo E2/3 genotype.

The intensity of clinical signs and symptoms of myasthenia gravis has a positive correlation with anti-AChR antibody titers. It is obvious that the severe form of myasthenia gravis developed in patients with apo E2/4 and, with this genotype, their is no patient with the mild form of the disease. Also, among the severe form of myasthenia gravis, there is no patient with genotype apo E3/3, which is the most frequent in the normal population. There are genotypes apo E2/3, apo E2/4, apo E3/3, and apo E3/4 among the patients with the moderate form of myasthenia gravis, but only the genotype apo E3/4 shows a significant difference among the others. The patients with the mild form of myasthenia gravis have genotypes apo E2/3 and apo E3/3, with the last one being the most frequent in the normal population. There is a significant difference between development of the form of myasthenia gravis and apo E genotypes ($\chi^2 = 40.923$, $p = 0.0000$, df = 6).

CONCLUSIONS

It is believed that apo E may moderate T lymphocytes by activation of mitogens or antigens. In that way, it has an influence on immune processes and it is reasonable to study the relationship between apo E genotypes and myasthenia gravis phenotypes. We tried to find any feature connected to the development of a different intensity of myasthenia gravis. The obtained results show that 46.43% of the observed patients have apo E2/4 genotype; in this group, most patients, namely, 18 patients or 32.14%, have the severe form of myasthenia gravis and there is no patient with the mild form of myasthenia gravis. Ten patients or 17.86% with the mild form of myasthenia gravis have apo E3/3 genotype. Otherwise, apo E3/3 genotype is the most numerous in the healthy population. The obtained results show a significant difference between the intensity of myasthenia gravis patients' signs and symptoms and their apo E genotypes. The anti-AChR antibody titers show a positive correlation with the intensity of clinical signs and symptoms of myasthenia gravis.

The obtained results may add to the possibility that apolipoprotein E, especially with genotype apo E2/4, might influence the intensity of the immune response in myasthenia gravis patients.

REFERENCES

1. GARLEP, M. J. *et al.* 1995. Apolipoprotein E ε4 in inclusion body myositis. Ann. Neurol. **38:** 957–959.
2. CONTOIS, J. H. *et al.* 1996. The underlying molecular mechanism of apolipoprotein E. Clin. Lab. Med. **16:** 105–123.
3. STAVLJENIĆ-RUKAVINA, A. *et al.* 1993. Apolipoprotein E phenotypes and genotypes as determined by polymerase chain reaction using allele-specific oligonucleotide probes and the amplification refractory mutation system in children with insulin-dependent diabetes mellitus. Clin. Chem. Acta **216:** 191–198.

The Role of Autoantibodies in Lambert-Eaton Myasthenic Syndrome[a]

BETHAN LANG,[b] SALLY WATERMAN,[b] ASHWIN PINTO,[b]
DOMINIC JONES,[b] FRASER MOSS,[c] JOHN BOOT,[c] PAUL BRUST,[d]
MARK WILLIAMS,[d] KENNETH STAUDERMAN,[d] MICHAEL HARPOLD,[d]
MASAKATSU MOTOMURA,[e] J. WIBE MOLL,[f] ANGELA VINCENT,[b]
AND JOHN NEWSOM-DAVIS[b]

[b]Neurosciences Group
Institute of Molecular Medicine
University of Oxford
Oxford OX3 9DU, United Kingdom

[c]Lilly Research Center Limited
Windlesham, Surrey, United Kingdom

[d]SIBIA Neurosciences Incorporated
La Jolla, California 92037

[e]First Department of Internal Medicine
Nagasaki University School of Medicine
Nagasaki 852, Japan

[f]Department of Neuro-Oncology
Dr. Daniel den Hoed Cancer Center
3075 EA Rotterdam, the Netherlands

The Lambert-Eaton myasthenic syndrome (LEMS) is an autoimmune disorder of neuromuscular transmission that causes fatigable muscle weakness, loss of tendon reflexes, and autonomic dysfunction.[1–3] LEMS antibodies bind to and induce a downregulation of voltage-gated channels (VGCCs),[4,5] resulting in a reduction in the nerve-evoked, Ca^{2+}-dependent release of acetylcholine from motor nerve terminals. Approximately 60% of patients have an associated small cell lung carcinoma (SCLC),[6] a tumor that is thought to be neuroendocrine in origin. This strong association with cancer makes LEMS a member of the group of paraneoplastic disorders. SCLC cells have been shown to express functional VGCCs[7,8] and preincubation in LEMS sera or IgG reduces the K^+-stimulated $^{45}Ca^{2+}$ flux into these cells.[8–10]

[a]This work was supported by the Medical Research Council (United Kingdom), the Myasthenia Gravis Association (United Kingdom), the Queen's Trust of Australia, the Leopold Muller Estate, the Sir Jules Thorne Charitable Trust, the Nuffield Foundation, and Jesus College, Oxford. A. Pinto is a recipient of a Wellcome Trust Research Fellowship and M. Motomura held a Wellcome Trust Research Travelling Fellowship.

DETECTION OF ANTIBODIES TO THE N- AND P-/Q-SUBTYPES OF VGCCs USING RADIOIMMUNOASSAYS

Neurons have been shown to express multiple types of VGCCs, which may be characterized by their electrophysiological and pharmacological profile.[11–13] The L-type VGCC, characterized by its long-lasting conductance, is found in excitable cells and in the cardiovascular system and is sensitive to dihydropyridines. By contrast, the N-, P-, and Q-type VGCCs appear to be confined to neuronal/neuroendocrine cells. The N-type VGCCs are involved in neurotransmitter release in amphibian neuromuscular junctions and mammalian brain, but the P-/Q-type VGCCs mediate transmitter release at the mammalian neuromuscular junction.[14,15] N-, P-, and Q-type VGCCs have been demonstrated in SCLC cells by biochemical, electrophysiological, and molecular biological techniques.[16–18]

The presence of serum antibodies to the VGCC subtypes have been detected in LEMS patients using specific neurotoxins. Initially, ω-conotoxin GVIA (ω-CgTx) derived from the fish-eating snail, *Conus geographus*, which binds specifically and essentially irreversibly to N-type VGCCs, was used as a basis for a radioimmunoassay (see FIGURE 1). Although initially a high number of patients were reported as having antibodies against ^{125}I-ω-CgTx-labeled (N-type) VGCCs,[19] subsequent reports in the literature have put this figure at 44–52%.[20,21]

Greater positivity has been obtained using a different *Conus* snail toxin, ω-conotoxin MVIIC (ω-CmTx), which binds to both P- and Q-type VGCCs.[22–24] Using ^{125}I-ω-CmTx to label digitonin extracts of human cerebellum, we have detected antibodies in greater than 92% of clinically definite LEMS patients ($n = 72$).[23] In our initial study, we also looked for the presence of these antibodies in control patients (see FIGURE 1). Only 1 of 66 was positive, an amyotrophic lateral sclerosis (ALS) patient with a very low titer. We have subsequently investigated larger numbers of controls (TABLE 1). In 90 patients with SCLC, but no neurological symptoms, we found anti-^{125}I-ω-CmTx-labeled VGCC antibodies in 3.3%. Also, 15% of patients ($n = 88$) with paraneoplastic encephalomyelitis or subacute sensory neuronopathy, who were positive for antineuronal nuclear antibody (anti-Hu or ANNA-1), had anti-P-/Q-type VGCC antibodies. Interestingly, a higher association was seen in patients with paraneoplastic encephalomyelitis or subacute sensory neuronopathy without associated antineuronal antibodies.[25]

Immunohistochemical staining has demonstrated that some typical LEMS patients, with or without cerebellar symptoms, do have antineuronal antibodies of as yet unknown specificity in their sera (see Polizzi *et al.* elsewhere in this volume).

ROLE OF AUTOANTIBODIES IN THE AUTONOMIC DYSFUNCTION OF LEMS PATIENTS

In addition to muscle weakness, around 80% of LEMS patients have some autonomic dysfunction such as dry mouth, constipation, impaired sweating, poor bladder control, and (in men) sexual impotence.[6] The neuronal basis of the autonomic symptoms has not been previously investigated. N-, P-, and Q-type VGCCs subserve trans-

A   [125I]ω-Conotoxin GVIA Assay

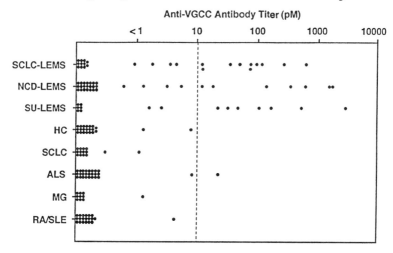

B   [125I]ω-Conotoxin MVIIC Assay

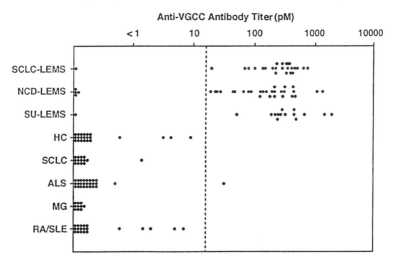

FIGURE 1. Serum antibodies in LEMS and control patients measured by immunoprecipitation of solubilized human cerebellar VGCCs labeled with [125I]-ω-CgTx GVIA (A) or [125I]-ω-CmTx MVIIC (B). Antibody titers were considered positive if greater than 10 pM (A) or 18 pM (B) (mean titer + 3 SD above mean for healthy controls). Terms: LEMS, Lambert-Eaton myasthenic syndrome; SCLC, small cell lung carcinoma; NCD, no cancer detected; SU, status uncertain; HC, healthy control; ALS, amyotrophic lateral sclerosis; MG, myasthenia gravis; RA/SLE, rheumatoid arthritis/systemic lupus erythematosus.

TABLE 1. Anti-ω-CmTx-labeled (P-/Q-type) VGCC Antibodies in Control Sera

Group	n	No. of Positives (>20 pM)	Positive (%)
SCLC (without neurological signs)	90	3	3.3
Paraneoplastic (subacute sensory neuronopathy, paraneoplastic encephalomyelitis, paraneoplastic cerebellar degeneration)	94	13	14
ANNA1+ (SCLC)	88	13	15
ANNA2+ (breast)	2	0	0
PCA+ (breast/gynecol.)	4	0	0
Other autoimmune diseases[a]	36	0	0
Healthy controls	40	0	0

[a]Other autoimmune disease controls: Guillain-Barré syndrome (3), myasthenia gravis (15), acquired neuromyotonia (3), polymyositis (1), systemic lupus erythematosus (10), and insulin-dependent diabetes mellitus (4).

mitter release from autonomic neurons,[26,27] and we present evidence here that antibodies to P- and Q-type VGCCs are responsible for the autonomic dysfunction.

We used the passive transfer model of LEMS, previously developed to investigate skeletal neuromuscular function, to study the effects on transmitter release from postganglionic parasympathetic neurons in the bladder and from postganglionic sympathetic neurons in the vas deferens.[28] Plasma was obtained from patients undergoing therapeutic plasmapheresis. IgG was prepared by the rivanol-ammonium sulfate method as previously described.[28] Control IgG was prepared from patients with other neurological disorders [Guillain-Barré syndrome (GBS), myasthenia gravis (MG), polymyositis (PM), and acquired neuromyotonia (NMT)], from patients with SCLC, but without neurological signs, and also from healthy volunteers.

Male albino mice were injected ip with IgG (10 mg in 1 mL per day) for eight days. On day 9, the mice were killed. The urinary bladder and vas deferentia were excised and mounted in organ baths in Krebs solution (see references 26 and 27). Electrically evoked contractions were recorded as described previously. Capsaicin (10 μM), guanethidine (3 μM), and hexamethonium (500 μM) were added to bladder preparations to inactivate functionally sensory neurons, block transmitter release from sympathetic neurons, and block nicotinic ganglionic transmission, respectively. Calcium-dependent, tetrodotoxin-sensitive contractions could thus be attributed to transmitter release from postganglionic parasympathetic neurons. Similarly, postganglionic sympathetic responses in vas deferens preparations were pharmacologically isolated using capsaicin and hexamethonium. Yohimbine (0.3 μM) was also added to vas deferens preparations to block presynaptic inhibition mediated by α_2 adrenoceptors. Preparations were stimulated at frequencies of 1–50 Hz in the absence and presence of calcium-channel neurotoxins. ω-CgTx GVIA (30 nM) was used to block N-type VGCCs. In the continued presence of ω-CgTx, ω-agatoxin IVA (ω-AgaTx) (300 nM), a toxin that specifically blocks P-type VGCCs, was added. ω-CmTx MVIIC (300 nM) was then added to block Q-type VGCCs.

FIGURE 2 shows the VGCC subtypes required for transmitter release from the parasympathetic neurons of the bladder of mice injected with control IgG. ω-CgTx GVIA reduced the contraction amplitude by approximately 50%, demonstrating the important role of N-type VGCCs in transmitter release at this site. Subsequent addition of ω-AgaTx IVA and ω-CmTx MVIIC also produced significant inhibition, indicating roles for P- and Q-type channels, respectively, in transmitter release. The remaining contraction was abolished by tetrodotoxin. Similar neurotoxin profiles were constructed for the vas deferens.

Mice passively transferred with LEMS IgG for eight days showed a marked difference (FIGURE 3) in both preparations. ω-CgTx GVIA abolished transmitter release, but ω-AgaTx IVA and ω-CmTx MVIIC had no further effect. Thus, we conclude that P- and Q-type VGCCs had already been downregulated by the LEMS antibodies and that transmitter release was solely dependent on calcium influx through N-type channels. Similar results were obtained in postganglionic sympathetic neurons in the vas deferens of mice injected with LEMS IgG. Injection of IgG from 9 patients caused a functional inhibition of P-type VGCCs. Eight of the 9 caused an inhibition of Q-type VGCCs and only 1 patient caused an inhibition of the N-type VGCCs. None of the controls produced any effect (TABLE 2).

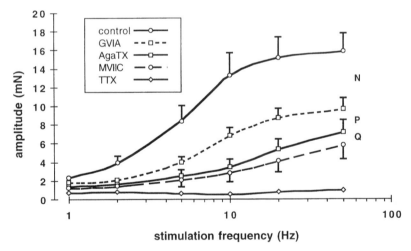

FIGURE 2. Subtypes of VGCCs required for transmitter release from parasympathetic neurons in the mouse bladder. Mice were injected with IgG from pooled healthy control serum ($n = 4$). ω-CgTx GVIA (30 nM) reduced contraction amplitude by approximately 50%, demonstrating the important role of N-type channels in transmitter release. Subsequent addition of ω-AgaTx IVA (300 nM) and ω-CmTx MVIIC (300 nM) also produced significant inhibition, indicating roles for P- and Q-type channels, respectively. The remaining contraction was abolished by tetrodotoxin (0.3 μM).

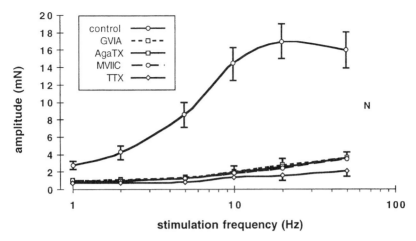

FIGURE 3. Effect of LEMS IgG on transmitter release from parasympathetic neurons in the bladder. ω-CgTx GVIA abolished transmitter release, but ω-AgaTx IVA and ω-CmTx MVIIC had no effect. Thus, P- and Q-type VGCCs had been downregulated by the LEMS antibodies and transmitter release was solely dependent on calcium influx through N-type channels (*n* = 4).

EFFECT OF LEMS IgG ON CLONED NEURONAL VGCCs

Neuronal VGCCs are multimeric proteins that consist of an α_1 subunit (which is thought to possess both channel function and drug binding sites), a β subunit (which is thought to be intracellular), and disulfide bridge–linked α_2/δ subunits. Six genes encoding the α_1 subunit have been reported (α_{1A}, α_{1B}, α_{1C}, α_{1D}, α_{1E}, and α_{1S}). α_{1C}, α_{1D}, and α_{1S} encode for L-type (dihydropyridine-sensitive) VGCCs, while the channel phenotype encoded for by the α_{1E} is as yet unknown. The α_{1B} gene has been shown to code for the ω-CgTx GVIA–labeled (N-type) VGCCs. The exact nature of

TABLE 2. Effect of LEMS IgG on Transmitter Release in Autonomic Neurons

	Functional Inhibition of P-type Channels	Functional Inhibition of Q-type Channels	Functional Inhibition of N-type Channels	Antibody Titer	Autonomic Symptoms
LEMS	9/9	8/9	1/9	9/9 P/Q+ 2/9 N+	9/9
Disease controls[a]	0/6	0/6	0/6	0/6	1/6 (GBS)
Healthy controls	0/2	0/2	0/2	0/2	0/2

[a]Disease controls: Guillain-Barré syndrome (GBS) (2), myasthenia gravis (1), acquired neuromyotonia (1), polymyositis (1), and small cell lung carcinoma without neurological symptoms (1).

the channel encoded for by the α_{1A} gene is uncertain and its expression with different isoforms of the other subunits appears to determine whether the channel exhibits P- or Q-type characteristics.

Human neuronal VGCC subunits have now been cloned and transfected into human embryonic kidney (HEK) cells. Four lines were studied: 10-13 (α_{1A-2}, β_{4a}, α_2/δ), which is potently blocked by ω-AgaTx IVA; G1A1 (α_{1B-1}, β_{1b}, α_2/δ) blocked by ω-CgTx GVIA; 5D12-20 (α_{1D}, α_2/δ, β_{3a}) blocked by dihydropyridines; and the resistant cell line E52-3 (α_{1E-3}, β_{1b}, α_2/δ) (for further methodology, see Pinto *et al.* elsewhere in this volume).

Transfected cells were incubated overnight in IgG prepared from patients with LEMS or from controls. The cells were loaded the following day with the fluorescent calcium-sensitive dye Fluo-3AM for one hour and then depolarized by exposure to a high concentration of KC1. The fluorescence change, which relates to the influx of calcium into the cells, was measured in real time using the Ascent Fluoroscan II. FIG-URE 4 shows the effect on calcium flux of preincubation of the cell lines in LEMS or control IgG as compared to cells grown in media alone. LEMS IgG causes a reduction in the K^+-stimulated calcium flux into cell line 10-13 by 75% ($p < 0.01$) as compared to control IgG. In the three other cell lines (G1A1, 5D12-20, E52-3), preincu-

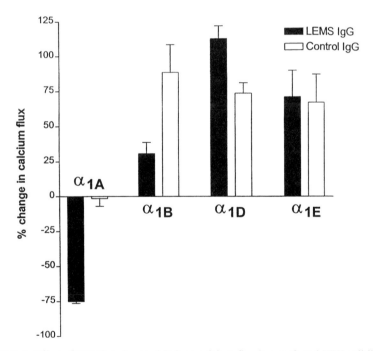

FIGURE 4. Effect of LEMS and control IgG on calcium flux in transfected HEK cell lines. Results are expressed as the percentage change in K^+-stimulated calcium flux as compared to cells grown in media alone. Incubation with LEMS IgG leads to a reduction in calcium flux in the α_{1A-2} (10-13) cell line only.

bation in both LEMS and control IgG causes a rise in calcium flux. Further experiments have shown that, within each of these three cell lines, there is no significant difference in K^+-stimulated calcium influx between LEMS and control treated cells (data not shown). These results show that, in an intact cell system, LEMS antibodies affect the function of P-/Q-type VGCCs, but not N-, L-, or R-type VGCCs.

CONCLUSIONS

We have used three different methods to investigate the target of autoantibodies from patients with LEMS. Using a standard radioimmunoassay, we have shown that more than 90% of patients have antibodies against the ^{125}I-ω-CmTx MVIIC–labeled (P-/Q-type) VGCCs, but less than 40% have them against the ^{125}I-ω-CgTx GVIA–labeled (N-type) VGCCs. We have investigated the role of these antibodies in the autonomic system using the mouse passive transfer model. These results demonstrated that 9/9 and 8/9 patients' IgG respectively block transmission through P-type and Q-type VGCCs, whereas only 1 of the 9 has any effect on N-type VGCCs. Finally, using HEK cells transfected with the genes for subunits of human VGCC subtypes, calcium influx through the 10-13 line that expresses the α_{1A} gene was affected by LEMS IgG, while the other VGCC subtypes were not affected. Thus, antibodies against the P-/Q-type VGCCs are the main pathogenic target in the majority of LEMS patients.

ACKNOWLEDGMENTS

We are grateful to P. Busby and H. McMath for technical assistance and to Pfizer for the kind gift of the ω-AgaTx IVA.

REFERENCES

1. ANDERSON, H. J., H. C. CHURCHILL-DAVIDSON & A. T. RICHARDSON. 1983. Bronchial neoplasm with myasthenia. Lancet **ii:** 1291.
2. LAMBERT, E. H., L. M. EATON & E. D. ROOKE. 1956. Defect of neuromuscular conduction associated with malignant neoplasma. Am. J. Physiol. **187:** 612–613.
3. LAMBERT, E. H. & D. ELMQVIST. 1971. Quantal components of end-plate potentials in the myasthenic syndrome. Ann. N.Y. Acad. Sci. **183:** 183–199.
4. LANG, B., J. NEWSOM-DAVIS, C. PEERS, C. PRIOR & D. W. WRAY. 1987. The effect of myasthenic syndrome antibody on presynaptic calcium channels in the mouse. J. Physiol. (Lond.) **390:** 257–270.
5. FUKUNAGA, H., A. G. ENGEL, B. LANG, J. NEWSOM-DAVIS & A. VINCENT. 1983. Passive transfer of Lambert-Eaton myasthenic syndrome with IgG from man to mouse depletes the presynaptic membrane active zones. Proc. Natl. Acad. Sci. U.S.A. **80:** 7636–7640.
6. O'NEILL, J. H., N. M. MURRAY & J. NEWSOM-DAVIS. 1988. The Lambert-Eaton myasthenic syndrome: a review of 50 cases. Brain **111:** 577–596.
7. MCCANN, F. V., O. S. PETTENGILL, J. J. COLE, J. A. G. RUSSELL & G. D. SORENSON. 1981. Calcium spike electrogenesis and other electrical activity in continuously cultured small cell carcinoma of the lung. Science **212:** 1155–1157.

8. ROBERTS, A., S. PERERA, B. LANG, A. VINCENT & J. NEWSOM-DAVIS. 1985. Paraneoplastic myasthenic syndrome IgG inhibits $^{45}Ca^{2+}$ flux in a human small cell carcinoma line. Nature **317:** 737–739.

9. JOHNSTON, I., B. LANG, K. LEYS & J. NEWSOM-DAVIS. 1994. Heterogeneity of calcium channel autoantibodies detected using a small-cell lung cancer line derived from a Lambert-Eaton myasthenic syndrome patient. Neurology **44:** 334–338.

10. DE AIZPURUA, H. J., E. H. LAMBERT, G. E. GRIESMANN, B. M. OLIVERA & V. A. LENNON. 1988. Antagonism of voltage-gated calcium channels in small cell carcinomas of patients with and without Lambert-Eaton myasthenic syndrome by autoantibodies, omega-conotoxin, and adenosine. Cancer Res. **48:** 4719–4724.

11. TSIEN, R. W., D. LIPSCOMBE, D. V. MADISON, K. R. BLEY & A. P. FOX. 1988. Multiple types of neuronal calcium channels and their selective modulation. Trends Neurosci. **11:** 431–438.

12. UCHITEL, O. D., D. A. PROTTI, V. SANCHEZ, B. D. CHERSKEY, M. SUGIMORI & R. LLINAS. 1992. P-type voltage-dependent calcium channel mediates presynaptic calcium influx and transmitter release in mammalian synapses. Proc. Natl. Acad. Sci. U.S.A. **89:** 3330–3333.

13. WHEELER, D. B., A. RANDALL & R. W. TSIEN. 1994. Roles of N-type and Q-type Ca^{2+} channels in supporting hippocampal synaptic transmission. Science **264:** 107–111.

14. HONG, S. J. & C. C. CHANG. 1995. Inhibition of acetylcholine release from mouse motor nerve by a P-type calcium channel blocker ω-agatoxin IVA. J. Physiol. (Lond.) **482**(2): 283–290.

15. BOWERSOX, S. S., G. P. MILJANICH, Y. SUGIURA, L. NADASDI, B. B. HOFFMAN, J. RAMACHANDRAN & C. P. KO. 1995. Differential blockade of voltage-sensitive calcium channels at the mouse neuromuscular junction by novel ω-cono peptides and Aga IVA. J. Pharmacol. Exp. Ther. **273:** 248–256.

16. LANG, B., A. VINCENT, N. M. MURRAY & J. NEWSOM-DAVIS. 1989. Lambert-Eaton myasthenic syndrome: immunoglobulin G inhibition of Ca^{2+} flux in tumor cells correlates with disease severity. Ann. Neurol. **25:** 265–271.

17. OGURO-OKANO, M., G. E. GRIESMANN, E. D. WIEBEN, S. J. SLAYMAKER, T. P. SNUTCH & V. A. LENNON. 1992. Molecular diversity of neuronal-type calcium channels identified in small cell lung carcinoma. Mayo Clin. Proc. **67:** 1150–1159.

18. PANCRAZIO, J. J., H. K. OIE & Y. I. KIM. 1992. Voltage-sensitive calcium channels in human small-cell lung cancer cell line. Acta Physiol. Scand. **144:** 463.

19. SHER, E., N. CANAL, G. PICCOLO, C. GOTTI, C. SCOPPETTA, A. EVOLI & F. CLEMENTI. 1989. Specificity of calcium channel autoantibodies in Lambert-Eaton myasthenic syndrome. Lancet **ii:** 640–643.

20. LEYS, K., B. LANG, A. VINCENT & J. NEWSOM-DAVIS. 1989. Calcium channel antibodies in Lambert-Eaton myasthenic syndrome. Lancet **ii:** 1107.

21. LENNON, V. A. & E. H. LAMBERT. 1989. Autoantibodies bind solubilized calcium channel–omega-conotoxin complexes from small cell lung carcinoma: a diagnostic aid for Lambert-Eaton myasthenic syndrome. Mayo Clin. Proc. **64:** 1498–1504.

22. MOTOMURA, M., I. JOHNSTON, B. LANG, A. VINCENT & J. NEWSOM-DAVIS. 1995. An improved diagnostic assay for Lambert-Eaton myasthenic syndrome. J. Neurol. Neurosurg. Psychiatry **58:** 85–87.

23. MOTOMURA, M., B. LANG, I. JOHNSTON, J. PALACE, A. VINCENT & J. NEWSOM-DAVIS. 1997. Incidence of serum anti-P/Q-type and anti-N-type calcium channel autoantibodies in Lambert-Eaton myasthenic syndrome. J. Neurol. Sci. **147:** 35–42.

24. LENNON, V. A., T. J. KRYZER, G. GRIESMANN, P. E. O'SUILLEABHAIN, A. J. WINDEBANK, A. WOPPMANN, G. P. MILJANICH & E. H. LAMBERT. 1995. Calcium channel antibodies in Lambert-Eaton syndrome and other neuroplastic syndromes. N. Engl. J. Med. **332:** 1467–1474.

25. MASON, W. P., F. GRAUS, B. LANG, J. HONNORAT, J-Y. DELATTRE, A. VALLDEORIOLA, J. C. ANTOINE, M. K. ROSENBLUM, M. R. ROSENFELD, J. NEWSOM-DAVIS, J. B. POSNER & J. DALMAU. 1997. Small-cell lung cancer, paraneoplastic cerebellar degeneration, and the Lambert-Eaton myasthenic syndrome. Brain. **120:** 1279–1300.
26. WATERMAN, S. A. 1996. Multiple types of voltage-gated calcium channel mediate transmitter release from parasympathetic neurons in the mouse bladder. J. Neurosci. **16:** 4155–4161.
27. WATERMAN, S. A. 1997. Role of N-, P-, and Q-type voltage-gated calcium channels in transmitter release from sympathetic neurones in the mouse isolated vas deferens. Br. J. Pharmacol. **120:** 393–398.
28. WATERMAN, S. A., B. LANG & J. NEWSOM-DAVIS. 1997. Effects of Lambert-Eaton myasthenic syndrome antibodies on autonomic neurons in the mouse. Ann. Neurol. In press.

Nicotinic Receptors and Calcium Channels in Small Cell Lung Carcinoma

Functional Role, Modulation, and Autoimmunity[a]

E. SHER,[b,c] A. CODIGNOLA,[b,d] M. PASSAFARO,[b,e] P. TARRONI,[b]
V. MAGNELLI,[f] E. CARBONE,[f] AND F. CLEMENTI[b]

[b]CNR Cellular and Molecular Pharmacology Center
Department of Medical Pharmacology
University of Milan
20129 Milan, Italy

[e]Institute of Biotechnologies Applied to Pharmacology
Roccelletta di Borgia, CZ, Italy

[f]Department of Neuroscience
University of Turin
Turin, Italy

INTRODUCTION

Small cell lung carcinoma (SCLC) is a very aggressive form of neuroendocrine lung tumor often associated with tobacco abuse. SCLC is composed of secretory cells that express a whole set of plasma membrane ion channels and receptors controlling cell excitability and the consequent Ca^{2+}-dependent release of several hormones and transmitters. Some of the released hormones, including serotonin (5HT), act as autocrine growth factors.[1,2] Therefore, the study of the properties of the ion channels and receptors expressed by these cells can lead to a possible pharmacological control of cell proliferation itself. Furthermore, the "inappropriate" expression of these membrane molecules on the growing SCLC causes an autoimmune response that, on the one hand, could be crucial for the inhibition of cell growth, but, on the other hand, could cause specific "paraneoplastic" disorders, caused by the cross-reactivity of these anti-SCLC antibodies with similar molecules expressed by the normal tissues, neurons in particular.

We will summarize in this paper some recent results that we obtained on the presence and function of nicotinic acetylcholine receptors (nAChRs) and voltage-operated calcium channels (VOCCs) in SCLC cells; we will describe some forms of modulation of these ion channels and their involvement as autoantigens in "paraneoplastic" disorders such as the Lambert-Eaton myasthenic syndrome (LEMS).

[a]This work was supported by a Telethon-Italia grant to E. Sher (No. 858).
[c]Present address: Lilly Research Centre, Erl Wood Manor, Windlesham, Surrey GU20 6PH, United Kingdom
[d]A. Codignola is a recipient of an AIRC (Italian Association for Cancer Research) fellowship.

RESULTS

Nicotinic Receptors in SCLC Cells

Despite its strict association with tobacco abuse, the demonstration of the presence of nicotinic receptors in SCLC is a relatively recent event. In 1985, Lennon and coworkers reported that only muscarinic, but not nicotinic, acetylcholine receptors were present in SCLC.[3] Since then, we[1,2,4,5] and others[6,7] have clearly demonstrated that nicotinic receptors are indeed present in SCLC. We described the presence in SCLC cells of $[^{125}I]$-α-bungarotoxin ($[^{125}I]$-α-Bgtx) binding sites,[4] as well as $[^3H]$-TPMP[5] and $[^{125}I]$-κ-bungarotoxin ($[^{125}I]$-κ-Bgtx) binding sites.[1] $[^3H]$-Nicotine and $[^{125}I]$-α-Bgtx binding sites in SCLC cells have been described also by Minna and collaborators[6] and by Quik and collaborators.[7] Immunological[4] and molecular[2,4,5] evidence clarified that the nicotinic receptors of SCLC are mainly of the "neuronal" type. In particular, the $[^{125}I]$-α-Bgtx binding sites were not recognized by mAb35, a monoclonal antibody recognizing the muscle-type $[^{125}I]$-α-Bgtx receptors.[4] Furthermore, Northern blotting and RT-PCR revealed the presence in SCLC cells of α_3, α_5, α_7, β_2, and β_4 "neuronal" nicotinic subunits, but not the presence of the α_1 muscular subunit.[2,4,5]

We can conclude that SCLC cells express neuronal-type nicotinic receptors, a fact that is not surprising in light of the large number of "neuronal" markers already described in these cells. We cannot exclude, however, that selective SCLC cell lines might not express nicotinic receptors or might even express muscle-type receptors.

Nicotinic Receptors and Hormone Release from SCLC

In neurons and chromaffin cells, the activation of presynaptic or postsynaptic nicotinic receptors stimulates Ca^{2+} influx and neurotransmitter release.[8,9] We found that nicotinic receptor activation by nicotine or cytisine stimulates the Ca^{2+}-dependent release of $[^3H]$-5HT from SCLC cells.[1,2] This stimulated release is antagonized by nonselective nicotinic antagonists such as mecamylamine,[1] but also by a number of peptide toxins acting selectively on the α-Bgtx-sensitive, α_7-containing nicotinic receptor.[2,10] As shown in Figure 1, nicotine-induced (as well as cytisine-induced, not shown) $[^3H]$-5HT release is antagonized by mecamylamine, α-Bgtx, κ-Bgtx, and the two *Conus* peptides, α-conotoxin MI and α-conotoxin ImI. The effects of all these toxins are dose-dependent (not shown; see references 2 and 10). κ-Bgtx could antagonize both α_7- and α_3-containing nicotinic receptors, both expressed by SCLC cells (see above). However, we believe that most of the κ-Bgtx effects here described are mediated by its binding to the α_7-containing receptor. This is suggested by the fact that most of the specific $[^{125}I]$-κ-Bgtx binding to SCLC cells is antagonized by α-Bgtx (α_7) and very little of the binding is on the α-Bgtx-insensitive (α_3) nicotinic receptor (Figure 2).

The antagonism by α-conotoxin ImI is particularly interesting because this toxin has been shown to be rather selective for α_7-containing neuronal nicotinic receptors.[11,12] The availability, in the future, of selective α_3 antagonists will help in defining if also these receptors participate in the control of secretion from SCLC cells. An

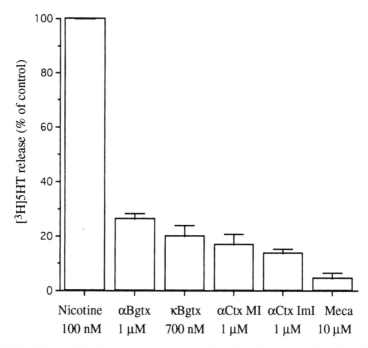

FIGURE 1. Effects of nicotinic antagonists on nicotine-induced hormone release from SCLC cells. Nicotine induces a dose- and calcium-dependent [³H]-5HT secretion from GLC8 human SCLC cells (see references 1, 2, and 10). Maximal secretion, obtained with 100 nM nicotine (23.7 ± 0.8% over basal), is blocked by 1 μM α-bungarotoxin (α-Bgtx) (73.7 ± 2% of inhibition); by 700 nM κ-bungarotoxin (κ-Bgtx) (80 ± 4% of inhibition); by the two *Conus* toxins, α-conotoxin MI (α-Ctx MI) and ImI (α-Ctx ImI), both at 1 μM (83 ± 4% and 86.3 ± 1.4% of inhibition, respectively); and by 10 μM mecamylamine (Meca) (95.5 ± 2% of inhibition). Each column represents the average of 3–5 experiments, each performed in quadruplicate as described in reference 1. Similar results were obtained with two other human SCLC cell lines, NCI-H69 and NCI-N592 (not shown).

antisense ($α_7$, $α_3$) approach is also in progress in our laboratory in order to address this topic.

Nicotinic Receptors and SCLC Cell Proliferation

We found that nicotine and cytisine are mitogenic for SCLC cells *in vitro*.[1,2,10] The dose response of this effect as well as its stereoselectivity and Ca^{2+} dependency are parallel to the drugs' effects on hormone release. Furthermore, both nicotine- and cytisine-induced cell proliferation are antagonized by the same drugs and peptide toxins (FIGURE 3) blocking nicotine- and cytisine-induced hormone release (see above). These results suggest that the same receptors dominating nicotine's effects on

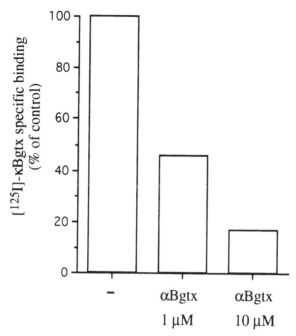

FIGURE 2. α-Bungarotoxin competition of [^{125}I]-κ-bungarotoxin binding in SCLC cells. Specific [^{125}I]-κ-bungarotoxin binding to GLC8 cells is antagonized by two different doses of α-bungarotoxin (α-Bgtx) (1 and 10 μM) (54% and 83% of inhibition, respectively). The data shown here are from one representative experiment performed in triplicate as described in reference 4.

release (α$_7$) are also dominating cell proliferation. However, activation of the nicotinic receptor, and the subsequent Ca^{2+} influx, can stimulate the two processes (secretion and cell proliferation) either "in parallel" or "in series," or in a combined manner. We found that the 5HT$_1$ serotonin receptor antagonist methiotepine significantly, although not completely, reduces nicotine-induced cell proliferation.[1] Since methiotepine did not affect nicotine-induced serotonin release, we suggested that nicotine could be mitogenic for SCLC cells because it stimulates the release of serotonin, which then acts as an autocrine growth factor.[1] We are still investigating the possibility that the nicotine-induced Ca^{2+} influx could represent a mitogenic signal *by itself*, independently from, or synergistically with, the Ca^{2+}-dependent release that it also stimulates.

Calcium Channels in SCLC

Some basic electrical properties of SCLC cells have been reported by McCann and collaborators.[13,14] KC1-induced $^{45}Ca^{2+}$ influx was then shown by Roberts *et al.*[15]

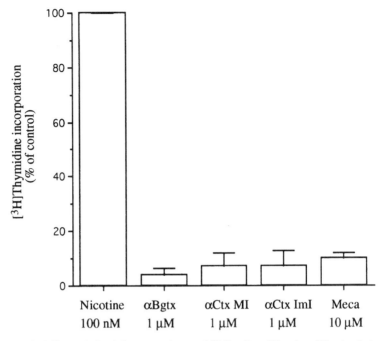

FIGURE 3. Effects of nicotinic antagonists on SCLC cell proliferation. Nicotine induces a dose-dependent stimulation of *in vitro* GLC8 cell proliferation, measured as [³H]-thymidine incorporation (see references 1, 2, and 10). Maximal stimulation, obtained with 100 nM nicotine, is antagonized by 1 μM α-bungarotoxin (α-Bgtx) (96 ± 2.4% of inhibition); by 1 μM of the two *Conus* toxins, α-conotoxin MI (α-Ctx MI) and ImI (α-Ctx ImI) (93 ± 5% and 94 ± 6% of inhibition, respectively); and by 10 μM mecamylamine (Meca) (90 ± 2% of inhibition). Each column represents the average of 3–5 experiments, each performed in quadruplicate as described in reference 1. Similar results were obtained with two other human SCLC cell lines, NCI-H69 and NCI-N592 (not shown).

and de Aizpurua *et al.*,[16] while KCl-induced increase in $[Ca^{2+}]_i$ was characterized by Sher *et al.*[17] Ca^{2+} (or Ba^{2+}) currents have been studied more recently with the patch-clamp technique by Pancrazio *et al.*,[18] Codignola *et al.*,[19] Viglione *et al.*,[20] Barry *et al.*,[21] Sher *et al.*,[22] and Meriney *et al.*[23]

The first papers on SCLC VOCCs concluded that only L-type VOCCs were present in these cells.[15,16,18] By using more detailed approaches, both we[17,19,22] and others[21,23] have then shown that SCLC cells express multiple VOCC subtypes.

The presence of L-type VOCCs in SCLC cells was demonstrated by showing DHP's effects on KCl-induced $^{45}Ca^{2+}$ influx,[15,16] increase in $[Ca^{2+}]_i$[17] and Ca^{2+} currents,[18,19] [³H]-DHP binding,[15] and the presence of the α_{1D} mRNA.[19]

SCLC cells express also N-type VOCCs, as revealed by [¹²⁵I]-ω-Ctx GVIA binding assays,[17] ω-Ctx GVIA effects on KCl-induced $^{45}Ca^{2+}$ influx,[16] increase in $[Ca^{2+}]_i$[17] and Ca^{2+} currents,[19] and finally the presence of the α_{1B} mRNA.[19]

The presence of P/Q-type VOCCs was shown by studying ω-aga IVA and ω-Ctx MVIIC effects on KC1-induced $^{45}Ca^{2+}$ influx,[24] ω-aga IVA effects on Ca^{2+} currents,[19,21,23] [^{125}I]-ω-Ctx MVIIC binding sites,[24] and detection of the α_{1A} mRNA.[19,21]

SCLC cells also express α_2-δ VOCC subunits[25] and β VOCC subunits.[19] The latter are represented by at least an isoform of β_2 and a new member of the β gene family that was called MysB because it was first cloned from a human hippocampal cDNA library by means of LEMS serum.[26] SCLC might also express the muscle-type α_{1S} subunit.[25]

Calcium Channels and Hormone Release in SCLC

To our knowledge, only a few papers addressed the role of VOCCs in the control of hormone release from SCLC cells. We have shown that increasing concentrations of KC1 stimulate a dose-dependent release of [^{3}H]-5HT from SCLC cells, which is completely dependent on the influx of Ca^{2+} from the extracellular medium.[19] KC1-induced [^{3}H]-5HT release is antagonized dose-dependently by cadmium, DHPs, verapamil, ω-Ctx GVIA, and ω-aga IVA, implicating all VOCC subtypes in this process.[19] KC1-induced [H]-5HT release is also antagonized dose-dependently by DPDPE, a δ opioid agonist, which modulates N- and P/Q-type VOCCs in SCLC cells (see reference 22 and see below).

As an indirect measure of secretion, Kim and collaborators have measured the depolarization-induced increase in single-cell capacitance.[20] They also concluded that multiple types of VOCCs participate in this process, but revealed a dominant role of the L- and P/Q-type, at least in the cells they used.

Calcium Channels and SCLC Cell Proliferation

As discussed above, the nicotinic-induced Ca^{2+} influx "per se" and/or the Ca^{2+}-dependent release of mitogenic hormones can mediate the mitogenic effects of nicotine on SCLC cells. The opening of VOCCs, by causing the same two events, should also be effective in stimulating SCLC cell proliferation. We here report, for the first time, that KC1 is indeed an effective mitogen for SCLC cells *in vitro*. As shown in FIGURE 4, GLC8 SCLC cells exposed to KC1 incorporated significantly more [^{3}H]-thymidine than the control cells. KC1 effects were dose-dependent. Furthermore, KC1 effects on cell proliferation were potently antagonized by DPDPE (which antagonizes non-L-type VOCCs and hormone release in SCLC cells, see below) (FIGURE 4) and by DHPs, ω-Ctx GVIA, and ω-aga IVA (Sher *et al.*, manuscript in preparation).

Opioids and Nerve Growth Factor Inhibit SCLC Cell Proliferation

Opioids have been shown to participate in autocrine loops in SCLC cells.[27] Minna and coworkers have shown that μ, κ, and δ opioid agonists are all effective in inhibiting *in vitro* SCLC cell proliferation[6] by stimulating apoptosis.[28]

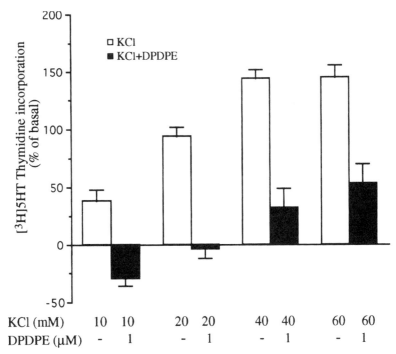

FIGURE 4. DPDPE inhibition of depolarization-induced SCLC cell proliferation. Depolarization induced by KCl causes a dose-dependent increase in *in vitro* GLC8 cell proliferation, determined as [³H]-thymidine incorporation (see reference 1). This increase is counteracted by the simultaneous presence of 1 μM DPDPE. At the two lowest KCl concentrations, 10 and 20 mM, which cause an increase of $38.2 \pm 9.7\%$ and $94 \pm 8\%$ over basal, respectively, DPDPE exhibits an inhibitory effect also on "basal" proliferation ($-30.5 \pm 5\%$ and $-3.5 \pm 9\%$, respectively). At 40 mM KCl, DPDPE inhibits the stimulation from $143.5 \pm 8.5\%$ to $32 \pm 17\%$ over basal. At 60 mM KCl, DPDPE inhibits the stimulation from $144.7 \pm 11\%$ to $53 \pm 17\%$ over basal. Each column represents the average of 3–5 experiments, each performed in quadruplicate as described in reference 1. Similar results were obtained with two other human SCLC cell lines, NCI-H69 and NCI-N592 (not shown).

By performing RT-PCR in the GLC8 SCLC cell line, we found that these cells express only δ opioid receptors.[22] We then found that the selective δ agonist DPDPE potently inhibits basal and stimulated SCLC cell proliferation (see also Codignola *et al.* elsewhere in this volume). Opioid effects are seen already after 4–5 days of treatment.

More recently, we found that SCLC cells express also NGF receptors (gp140*TrkA* and gp75[NGFR]), whose activation inhibits SCLC cell proliferation, both *in vitro* and *in vivo* in the "nude" mouse (Missale *et al.*, manuscript in preparation). NGF effects are more slow to develop, being fully effective after 15 days of treatment, and are slowly reversible upon removal of NGF. NGF effects are accompanied by an upregulation of

NGF receptors, by a stimulation of endogenous NGF production, by the acquirement of retinoic acid sensitivity, and by a downregulation of nicotinic responsiveness (see below).

Opioids Inhibit Calcium Channels and Hormone Release in SCLC

Lennon and coworkers first described a muscarinic modulation of KC1-induced $^{45}Ca^{2+}$ influx in SCLC cells.[29] In a recent patch-clamp study, we showed that VOCCs in GLC8 cells are potently antagonized by the δ opioid agonist DPDPE, but not by the μ agonist DAMGO or the κ agonist U50488.[22] DPDPE effects are dose-dependent (IC_{50} = 0.64 nM), reversible, antagonized by naloxone, mediated by a PTX-sensitive G protein, and typically voltage-dependent. The main target of this modulation is the N-type VOCC, with the P/Q-type VOCC being also partly inhibited, but the L-type VOCC is not affected at all. In line with these effects, DPDPE also inhibits KC1-induced hormone release from SCLC cells (see above).

However, we have found that DPDPE is able to antagonize also the release stimulated by the Ca^{2+} ionophore ionomycin and by the Ca^{2+}-mobilizing agent thapsigargin.[22] Also, these "distal" (with respect to the VOCCs) inhibitory effects are mediated by a PTX-sensitive G protein, but (at variance with VOCC modulation) they are counteracted by increasing cAMP levels. The exact target or targets of this "distal," G protein–mediated modulation of the secretory process are still unknown.

Nerve Growth Factor Downregulates Nicotinic Receptors in SCLC

As described above, SCLC cells express different nicotinic receptor subtypes, whose activation leads to hormone secretion and cell proliferation.

Among the several effects that NGF exerts on SCLC cells, we found that it causes a drastic reduction in the ability of the cells to respond to nicotine (see also Codignola *et al.* elsewhere in this volume). While the shape of the dose-response curve is not changed, the maximal effect of nicotine on cell proliferation is reduced by 77 ± 5% and by 77.5 ± 4.8% in NCI-N592 and GLC8 cells, respectively.

More importantly, this effect of NGF is probably caused by a downregulation of the nicotinic receptors (and not by an inability of the cells to proliferate) because (a) the cells continue to proliferate perfectly in response to serotonin and (b) there is a parallel downregulation of the ability of nicotine to stimulate hormone release. This latter effect is also specific because the cells continue to release normally in response to KC1. We are currently investigating if this downregulation of the nicotinic receptors is exerted at the mRNA or protein level.

LEMS Autoantibodies Recognize Multiple Subtypes of Calcium Channels

SCLC patients, like all cancer patients, mount an immune response against their growing tumor. Any membrane protein and, in case of tumor necrosis, any intracellular protein could represent a potential antigen. At least in some cases, these anti-

SCLC antibodies are likely to be effective in inhibiting SCLC growth. However, some antibodies produced against membrane proteins could recognize similar molecules on the normal tissues of the patients, giving rise to the so-called autoimmune paraneoplastic disorders. The best characterized of these disorders is the Lambert-Eaton myasthenic syndrome (LEMS), where antibodies are produced against SCLC VOCCs, but also recognize VOCCs on the patients' neurons, causing the neurological disease, characterized by a widespread deficit in neurotransmitter release.[30,31]

A presynaptic neuromuscular effect of LEMS antibodies, compatible with a reduction in functional VOCCs, was shown in humans and in passively transferred rodents;[30-33] recently, in a passive transfer study, a direct reduction of presynaptic neuromuscular Ca^{2+} currents, studied extracellularly, was reported.[34] LEMS antibodies also inhibit in vitro [^{3}H]-acetylcholine release from rat cortical synaptosomes.[35]

The recognition of VOCCs by LEMS antibodies, however, has been mainly demonstrated in cellular model systems. The first study in this direction was by Roberts et al.,[15] who showed that LEMS antibodies inhibited KC1-induced $^{45}Ca^{2+}$ influx in a human SCLC cell line. This first evidence was then confirmed by other studies utilizing the same technique.[36]

The effects of LEMS antibodies were also studied on the Ca^{2+} currents of patch-clamped cells (TABLE 1). LEMS antibodies have been reported to inhibit Ca^{2+} currents in bovine chromaffin cells,[37] NG108 rat glioma/mouse neuroblastoma cells,[38] thyroid C cells,[39] IMR32 human neuroblastoma cells,[40] murine DRG cells,[41] murine motoneurons,[42] SCLC cells,[20,23] and RINm5F rat insulinoma cells.[43]

Some of our results on the effects of LEMS antibodies in IMR32 and RINm5F cells are summarized below. IMR32 cells express mainly N-type VOCCs,[44] which are poorly represented in RINm5F cells.[45] On the other hand, RINm5F cells, but not IMR32 cells, express P/Q-type VOCCs, which also participate in the control of secretion (FIGURE 5). Both cell types express some L- and T-type VOCCs. For these reasons, the two cell types were chosen as good models for checking the selectivity of LEMS antibodies towards the different VOCC subtypes. Our results suggest that

TABLE 1. Electrophysiological Studies on the Downregulation of Ca^{2+} Currents by LEMS Antibodies

Author	Cell Type	VOCC Subtypes Affected
Peers et al.[38]	rodent NB × glioma	high threshold (L?); T spared
Kim & Neher[37]	bovine chromaffin	high threshold (?)
Kim et al.[39]	rat thyroid C cell line	high threshold
Grassi et al.[40]	human neuroblastoma	N, L, T
Smith et al.[34]	murine NMJ (extracellular)	non-L
Viglione et al.[20]	human SCLC	P/Q, L
Magnelli et al.[43]	rat insulinoma	P/Q, L
Meriney et al.[23]	human SCLC	N, L, P/Q
Garcia et al.[41]	murine DRG	T; high threshold
Garcia & Beam[42]	murine motoneuron	T; non-L, L spared
	murine cardiac myocytes	T and L spared
	murine skeletal myotubes	T and L spared

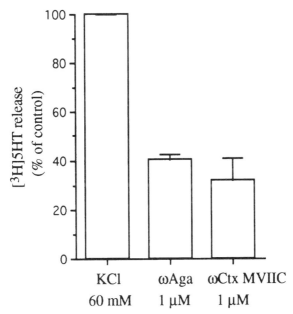

FIGURE 5. P/Q-type calcium channels in RINm5F insulinoma cells. KC1 induces a dose-dependent [³H]-5HT release from rat insulinoma RINm5F cells (see reference 62). Maximal [³H]-5HT release evoked by 60 mM KC1 is counteracted by both 1 μM ω-agatoxin IVA (ω-Aga IVA) and 1 μM ω-conotoxin MVIIC (ω-Ctx MVIIC) (59.7 ± 2% and 68 ± 8.7% of inhibition, respectively). Each column represents the average of 3–5 experiments, each performed in quadruplicate as described in reference 62.

both N- and P/Q-type VOCCs are downregulated by LEMS sera (FIGURE 6). Furthermore, significant inhibition of both T- and L-type VOCCs was also observed. These results, together with those of other groups,[23,36,42] indicate that LEMS antibodies broadly recognize many VOCC subtypes. At least in the case of our IgG samples, we can exclude the presence of a "contaminant" (Cd²⁺-like or protease-like) in the preparations that could "nonspecifically" block all VOCC types. When we tested the same identical LEMS IgGs on invertebrate VOCCs, absolutely no effects were found (Sher and Richmond, unpublished results). This is probably due to the species-specificity of human antibodies and to the presence in these invertebrate neurons of VOCCs that do not fit in the "vertebrate" classifications.[46] In any case, these results exclude "proteolytic" or "nonspecific" effects causing the broad VOCC downregulation discussed above.

However, there is evidence that P/Q-type VOCCs could represent the most-important target of LEMS antibodies. It seems, indeed, that a higher percentage of patients can immunoprecipitate P/Q-type VOCCs than N-type VOCCs (TABLE 2).

It should be recalled that the presynaptic VOCCs in both the human[55] and the rodent[56] neuromuscular junction are mainly of the P/Q-type, suggesting that the P/Q-type antibodies could be more relevant for the neuromuscular defects in LEMS.

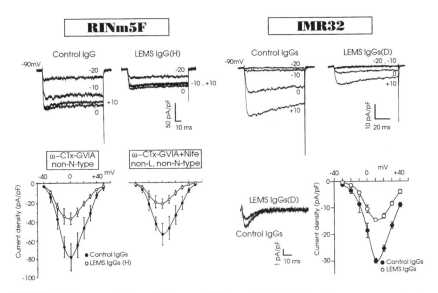

FIGURE 6. Downregulation of N-type and P/Q-type VOCCs by Lambert-Eaton myasthenic syndrome antibodies. (Left) Inhibition of Ba^{2+} currents in RINm5F rat insulinoma cells by LEMS IgG(s) (H). (Top) LEMS IgGs reduce the current densities at the different test potentials (V_h = –80 mV), without changing their activation-inactivation kinetics. (Bottom) I/V plots showing the average inhibition of non-N-type currents (L + P/Q) and the average inhibition of non-L, non-N (P/Q) currents by LEMS IgGs (H). No effect on single P/Q channel properties was found (see reference 43). (Right) Inhibition of Ba^{2+} currents in IMR32 human neuroblastoma cells by LEMS IgGs (D). (Top) LEMS IgGs reduce the current densities at the different test potentials, with no obvious changes in their kinetics. (Bottom) Inhibition of low-threshold (T-type) currents in IMR32 cells activated at –30 mV from a V_h = –80 mV, and I/V plots showing the average inhibition of both low-threshold (T-type) and high-threshold (N + L-type) Ca^{2+} channels. No changes in single N-type Ca^{2+} channels were observed (see reference 40).

However, not only in frog neuromuscular junctions,[57] but also in the more-studied rodent neuromuscular junctions, VOCCs other than the P/Q-type are likely to be coexpressed, including the N-type[34,58] and "resistant" types (see references 55 and 56; and Magnelli, Baldelli, and Carbone, unpublished results). This latter evidence leaves open the possibility that also autoantibodies with non-P/Q-type specificity could participate in the pathogenesis of LEMS *neuromuscular* defects. In any case, N-type VOCC antibodies are likely to be responsible for the typical autonomic dysfunctions of LEMS patients because, in sympathetic neurons, the N-type VOCC dominates.[59,60]

It is still a matter of investigation if this "broad" VOCC recognition is due to the presence of multiple antibodies against different channels or to cross-reacting antibodies. While both hypotheses are possible, and not mutually exclusive, it should be noted that neither we nor others have found T-type VOCCs in SCLC cells, while some patients do have antibodies recognizing these channels.

TABLE 2. Prevalence of Anti-VOCC Autoantibodies in LEMS Patients as Revealed by ω-Conotoxin(s) Labeling and Immunoprecipitation

Author	N-type VOCC (Labeled with [^{125}I]-ω-Ctx GVIA): % of Positive			P/Q-type VOCC (Labeled with [^{125}I]-ω-Ctx MVIIC): % of Positive		
	Total	Without Cancer	With Cancer	Total	Without Cancer	With Cancer
Sher et al.[47]	90.4	91.6	90	–	–	–
Lennon & Lambert[48]	52	30	76	–	–	–
Leys et al.[49]	44	61	28	–	–	–
Pelucchi et al.[50]	79	79	79	–	–	–
Motomura et al.[51]	55	55	55	–	–	–
Motomura et al.[52]	–	–	–	85	76	90
Lennon et al.[24]	49	36	73	95	91	100
Suenaga et al.[53]	62	42	75	74	57	85
Arsac et al.[54]	58	–	–	–	–	–

LEMS Autoantibodies Inhibit Hormone Release from Insulinoma and SCLC Cells

LEMS antibodies are clearly inhibiting neurotransmitter release at the human neuromuscular junctions and autonomic synapses, as well as in the same structures of passively transferred rodents. On the other hand, LEMS antibodies seem to leave muscle and cardiac VOCCs unaffected. Less characterized is the potential ability of LEMS antibodies to affect VOCCs and hormone release from endocrine glands, leading to clinical or subclinical endocrine dysfunctions.

Kim and coworkers showed that LEMS antibodies inhibit growth hormone and prolactin release from *in vitro* cultured rat pituitary cells.[61] They also showed that VOCCs are downregulated in adrenal chromaffin cells[37] and thyroid C cells,[39] although they did not check for effects on hormone release. It would be interesting to reevaluate if LEMS patients have defects of hormone release from these organs.

We have found that LEMS antibodies inhibit depolarization-induced hormone release from RINm5F insulinoma cells (FIGURE 7). This release is at least in part mediated by P/Q-type VOCCs (see above, FIGURE 5), and the same P/Q channels are downregulated by LEMS antibodies (see above). In light of these results, it is worth reinvestigating glucose tolerance in LEMS patients.

Kim and collaborators have shown that LEMS IgG can inhibit, in SCLC cells, the depolarization-induced increase in cell capacitance, which is a measure of exocytosis.[20]

We also found that LEMS antibodies inhibit depolarization-induced hormone release from SCLC cells (FIGURE 8). This latter result is interesting not only because SCLC is composed of endocrine cells, but also because release of mitogenic hormones from SCLC cells is crucially involved in the control of SCLC cell proliferation (see above). It is therefore possible that anti-VOCC antibodies could act in a

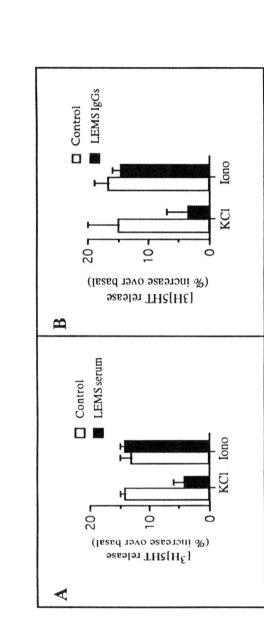

FIGURE 7. Lambert-Eaton myasthenic syndrome antibodies inhibit hormone release from RINm5F insulinoma cells. Both LEMS serum (A) and purified LEMS IgGs (B) strongly reduce KC1 (60 mM)–evoked [³H]-5HT release (71.4 ± 1% and 76.6 ± 3.5% of inhibition, respectively), while they do not affect the ionomycin (Iono) (1 μM)–evoked secretion (13 ± 2% over basal in control *versus* 14 ± 1% in LEMS serum, and 16.5 ± 2.5% over basal in control *versus* 14.5 ± 1.5% in LEMS IgGs, respectively). Control human serum did not influence either KC1- or ionomycin-stimulated [³H]-5HT release (not shown). Each column represents the average of 2 experiments performed in quadruplicate as described in reference 62.

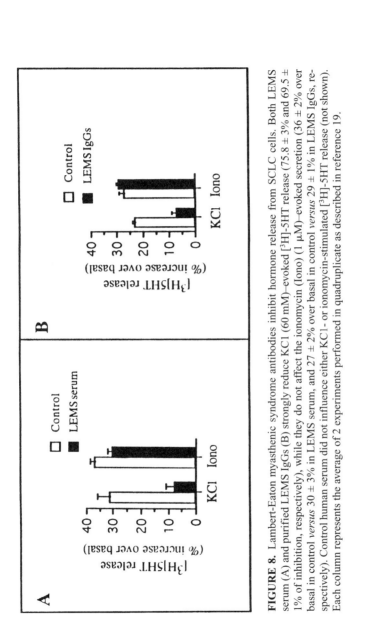

FIGURE 8. Lambert-Eaton myasthenic syndrome antibodies inhibit hormone release from SCLC cells. Both LEMS serum (A) and purified LEMS IgGs (B) strongly reduce KC1 (60 mM)–evoked [³H]-5HT release (75.8 ± 3% and 69.5 ± 1% of inhibition, respectively), while they do not affect the ionomycin (Iono) (1 μM)–evoked secretion (36 ± 2% over basal in control *versus* 30 ± 3% in LEMS serum, and 27 ± 2% over basal in control *versus* 29 ± 1% in LEMS IgGs, respectively). Control human serum did not influence either KC1- or ionomycin-stimulated [³H]-5HT release (not shown). Each column represents the average of 2 experiments performed in quadruplicate as described in reference 19.

similar way as the "calcium antagonists" described above that not only inhibit depolarization-induced release, but also cell proliferation. We have indeed preliminary results showing that LEMS antibodies, but not control sera, can inhibit both "basal" and depolarization-induced *in vitro* SCLC cell proliferation (Gasperi, Codignola, and Sher, unpublished results).

SUMMARY AND PERSPECTIVES

There has been growing interest in recent years in the biology of SCLC and, in particular, in the plasma membrane ion channels and receptors controlling cell excitability, hormone release, and cell proliferation ("stimulus–secretion–cell proliferation coupling"). We have here summarized the current knowledge on the presence, molecular properties, modulation, and functional role of "neuronal" nicotinic receptors and "neuronal" voltage-operated calcium channels in SCLC cells. These ion channels are involved in two major biological and clinical aspects of SCLC, that is, cell proliferation and paraneoplastic autoimmunity. A more-precise knowledge of the neuronal molecules targeted by the autoantibodies in SCLC patients could help in achieving a better clinical control of these paraneoplastic disorders by both selective immunological approaches and specifically targeted drugs (see the therapeutic section of this volume).

More importantly, we believe that drugs that directly inhibit these channels (nicotinic antagonists, calcium antagonists) or indirectly modulate them (opioids, NGF) could become new biological weapons against this still-uncurable cancer.

ACKNOWLEDGMENTS

We thank all the colleagues in the neurological and pneumological clinics that helped us in following the different patients under study. Particular thanks is extended to A. Pelucchi (Servizio di Fisiopatologia Respiratoria "G. Campari", Milan, Italy) for his continuous support.

REFERENCES

1. CATTANEO, M. G., A. CODIGNOLA, L. M. VICENTINI, F. CLEMENTI & E. SHER. 1993. Nicotine stimulates a serotonergic autocrine loop in human small cell lung carcinoma. Cancer Res. **53:** 5566–5568.
2. CODIGNOLA, A., P. TARRONI, M. G. CATTANEO, L. M. VICENTINI, F. CLEMENTI & SHER. 1994. Serotonin release and cell proliferation are under the control of α-bungarotoxin-sensitive nicotinic receptors in small cell lung carcinoma cell lines. FEBS Lett. **342:** 286–290.
3. CUNNINGHAM, J. M., V. A. LENNON, E. H. LAMBERT & B. SCHEITHAUER. 1985. Acetylcholine receptors in small cell lung carcinomas. J. Neurochem. **45:** 159–167.
4. CHINI, B., F. CLEMENTI, N. HUKOVIC & E. SHER. 1992. Neuronal-type α-bungarotoxin receptors and the α_5 nicotinic receptor subunit gene are expressed in neuronal and nonneuronal human cell lines. Proc. Natl. Acad. Sci. U.S.A. **89:** 1572–1576.
5. TARRONI, P., F. RUBBOLI, B. CHINI, R. ZWART, M. OORTGIESEN, E. SHER & F. CLEMENTI.

1992. Neuronal-type nicotinic receptors in human neuroblastoma and small-cell lung carcinoma cell lines. FEBS Lett. **312:** 66–70.

6. MANECKJEE, R. & J. D. MINNA. 1990. Opioid and nicotine receptors affect growth regulation of human small-cell lung cancer. Proc. Natl. Acad. Sci. U.S.A. **87:** 3294–3298.

7. QUIK, M., J. CHAN & J. PATRICK. 1994. Alpha-bungarotoxin blocks the nicotinic receptor mediated increase in cell number in a neuroendocrine cell line. Brain Res. **665:** 161–167.

8. GRAY, R., A. S. RAJAN, K. A. RADCLIFFE, M. YAKEHIRO & J. A. DANI. 1996. Hippocampal synaptic transmission enhanced by low concentrations of nicotine. Nature **383:** 713–716.

9. RATHOUZ, M. M., S. VIJAYARAGHAVAN & D. K. BERG. 1996. Elevation of intracellular calcium levels in neurons by nicotinic acetylcholine receptors. Mol. Neurobiol. **12:** 117–131.

10. CODIGNOLA, A., J. M. MCINTOSH, M. G. CATTANEO, L. M. VICENTINI, F. CLEMENTI & E. SHER. 1996. α-Conotoxin Imperialis I inhibits nicotine-evoked hormone release and cell proliferation in human neuroendocrine carcinoma cells. Neurosci. Lett. **206:** 53–56.

11. MCINTOSH, J. M., D. YOSHIKAMI, E. MAHE, D. B. NIELSEN, J. D. RIVIER & B. M. OLIVERA. 1994. A nicotinic acetylcholine receptor ligand of unique specificity, α-conotoxin ImI. J. Biol. Chem. **269:** 16733–16739.

12. JOHNSON, D. S., J. MARTINEZ, A. ELGOYHEN, S. F. HEINEMANN & J. M. MCINTOSH. 1995. α-Conotoxin ImI exhibits subtype-specific nicotinic acetylcholine receptor blockade: preferential inhibition of homomeric α_7 and α_9 receptors. Mol. Pharmacol. **48:** 194–199.

13. MCCANN, F. V., O. S. PETTENGILL, J. J. COLE, J. A. G. RUSSEL & G. D. SORENSON. 1981. Calcium spike electrogenesis and other electrical activity in continuously cultured small cell carcinoma of the lung. Science **212:** 1155–1157.

14. MCCANN, F. V., J. J. COLE, O. S. PETTENGILL, J. A. G. RUSSEL & G. D. SORENSON. 1985. *In* The Electrophysiology of the Secretory Cell, p. 241–266. Elsevier. Amsterdam/New York.

15. ROBERTS, S., B. PERERA, B. LANG, A. VINCENT & J. NEWSOM-DAVIS. 1985. Paraneoplastic myasthenic syndrome IgG inhibits $^{45}Ca^{2+}$ flux in a human small cell carcinoma line. Nature **317:** 737–739.

16. DE AIZPURUA, H. J., E. H. LAMBERT, G. E. GRIESMANN, B. M. OLIVERA & V. A. LENNON. 1988. Antagonism of voltage-gated calcium channels in small cell carcinoma of patients with and without Lambert-Eaton syndrome by autoantibodies ω-conotoxin and adenosine. Cancer Res. **48:** 4719–4724.

17. SHER, E., A. PANDIELLA & F. CLEMENTI. 1990. ω-Conotoxin-sensitive voltage-operated calcium channels in small-cell lung carcinoma cell lines: pharmacological, functional, and immunological properties. Cancer Res. **50:** 3892–3896.

18. PANCRAZIO, J. J., H. K. OIE & Y. I. KIM. 1989. Voltage-dependent ion channels in small cell lung cancer cell lines. Cancer Res. **49:** 5901–5906.

19. CODIGNOLA, A., P. TARRONI, F. CLEMENTI, A. POLLO, M. LOVALLO, E. CARBONE & E. SHER. 1993. Calcium channel subtypes controlling serotonin release from human small cell lung carcinoma cell lines. J. Biol. Chem. **268:** 26240–26247.

20. VIGLIONE, M. P., T. J. O'SHAUGHNESSY & Y. I. KIM. 1995. Inhibition of calcium currents and exocytosis by Lambert-Eaton syndrome antibodies in human lung cancer cells. J. Physiol. **488:** 303–317.

21. BARRY, E. L. R., M. P. VIGLIONE, Y. I. KIM & S. C. FROEHNER. 1995. Expression and antibody inhibition of P-type calcium channels in human small cell lung carcinoma cells. J. Neurosci. **15:** 274–283.

22. SHER, E., P. CESARE, A. CODIGNOLA, F. CLEMENTI, P. TARRONI, A. POLLO, V. MAGNELLI & E. CARBONE. 1996. Activation of δ-opioid receptors inhibits neuronal-like calcium channels and distal steps of Ca^{2+}-dependent secretion in human small-cell lung carcinoma cells. J. Neurosci. **16:** 3672–3684.

23. MERINEY, S. D., S. C. HULSIZER, V. A. LENNON & A. D. GRINNEL. 1996. Lambert-Eaton

myasthenic syndrome immunoglobulins react with multiple types of calcium channels in small-cell lung carcinoma. Ann. Neurol. **40:** 739–749.

24. LENNON, V. A., T. J. KRYZER, G. E. GRIESMANN, P. E. O'SUILLEABHAIN, A. J. WINDEBANK, A. WOPPMANN, G. P. MILJANICH & E. H. LAMBERT. 1995. Calcium-channel antibodies in the Lambert-Eaton syndrome and other paraneoplastic syndromes. N. Engl. J. Med. **332:** 1467–1474.

25. MORTON, M. E., T. N. CASSIDY, S. C. FROEHNER, B. P. GILMOUR & R. L. LAURENS. 1994. Alpha 1 and alpha 2 calcium channel subunit expression in human neuronal and small cell carcinoma cells. FASEB J. **8:** 884–888.

26. ROSENFELD, M. R., E. WONG, J. DALMAU, G. MANLEY, J. B. POSNER, E. SHER & H. M. FURNEAUX. 1993. The beta subunits of Ca^{2+} channel complexes are Lambert-Eaton myasthenic syndrome antigens. Ann. Neurol. **33:** 113–120.

27. ROTH, K. A. & J. D. BARCHAS. 1985. Small-cell lung carcinoma cell lines contain opioid peptides and receptors. Cancer Res. **45:** 769–773.

28. MANECKJEE, R. & J. D. MINNA. 1994. Opioids induce while nicotine suppresses apoptosis in human lung cancer cells. Cell Growth Differ. **5:** 1033–1040.

29. WILLIAMS, C. L. & V. A. LENNON. 1990. Activation of M_3 muscarinic acetylcholine receptors inhibits voltage-dependent calcium influx in small cell lung carcinoma. J. Biol. Chem. **265:** 1443–1447.

30. VINCENT, A., B. LANG & J. NEWSOM-DAVIS. 1989. Autoimmunity to the voltage-gated calcium channel underlies the Lambert-Eaton myasthenic syndrome, a paraneoplastic disorder. Trends Neurosci. **12:** 496–502.

31. SHER, E., E. BIANCARDI, M. PASSAFARO & F. CLEMENTI. 1991. Physiopathology of neuronal voltage-operated calcium channels. FASEB J. **5:** 2677–2683.

32. KIM, Y. I. 1986. Passively tranferred Lambert-Eaton syndrome in mice receiving purified IgG. Muscle Nerve **9:** 523–530.

33. LAMBERT, E. H. & V. A. LENNON. 1988. Selected IgGs rapidly induce Lambert-Eaton myasthenic syndrome in mice: complement independence and EMG abnormalities. Muscle Nerve **11:** 1133–1145.

34. SMITH, D. O., M. W. CONKIN, P. J. JENSEN & W. D. ATCHISON. 1995. Decreased calcium currents in motor nerve terminals of mice with Lambert-Eaton myasthenic syndrome. J. Physiol. **487:** 115–123.

35. MEYER, E. M., A. E. MOMOL, B. S. KRAMER, W. E. ROSS & G. SCOTT. 1986. Effects of serum fractions from patients with Eaton-Lambert syndrome on rat cortical synaptosomal [³H]acetylcholine release. Biochem. Pharmacol. **35:** 3412–3414.

36. JOHNSTON, I., B. LANG, K. LEYS & J. NEWSOM-DAVIS. 1994. Heterogeneity of calcium channel autoantibodies detected using a small cell lung cancer line derived from a Lambert-Eaton myasthenic syndrome patient. Neurology **44:** 334–338.

37. KIM, Y. I. & E. NEHER. 1988. IgG from patients with Lambert-Eaton syndrome blocks voltage-dependent calcium channels. Science **239:** 405–408.

38. PEERS, J., B. LANG, J. NEWSOM-DAVIS & D. W. WRAY. 1990. Selective action of myasthenic syndrome antibodies on calcium channels in a rodent neuroblastoma × glioma cell line. J. Physiol. **421:** 293–308.

39. KIM, Y. I., J. K. BLANDINO & T. J. O'SHAUGHNESSY. 1993. Inhibitory action of Lambert-Eaton syndrome IgG on calcium currents in a thyroid C-cell line. Ann. N.Y. Acad. Sci. **681:** 398–401.

40. GRASSI, C., V. MAGNELLI, V. CARABELLI, E. SHER & E. CARBONE. 1994. Inhibition of low- and high-threshold Ca^{2+} channels of human neuroblastoma IMR32 cells by Lambert-Eaton myasthenic syndrome (LEMS) IgGs. Neurosci. Lett. **181:** 50–56.

41. GARCIA, K. D., M. MYNLIEFF, D. B. SANDERS, K. G. BEAM & J. P. WALROND. 1996. Lam-

bert-Eaton sera reduce low-voltage and high-voltage activated Ca^{2+} currents in murine dorsal ganglion neurons. Proc. Natl. Acad. Sci. U.S.A. **93:** 9264–9269.

42. GARCIA, K. D. & K. G. BEAM. 1996. Reduction of calcium currents by Lambert-Eaton syndrome sera: motoneurons are preferentially affected and L-type currents are spared. J. Neurosci. **16:** 4903–4913.

43. MAGNELLI, V., E. PARLATORE, C. GRASSI, E. SHER & E. CARBONE. 1996. Down-regulation of non-L, non-N-type (Q-like) Ca^{2+} channels by Lambert-Eaton myasthenic syndrome (LEMS) antibodies in rat insulinoma RINm5F cells. FEBS Lett. **387:** 47–52.

44. CARBONE, E., E. SHER & F. CLEMENTI. 1990. Ca^{2+} currents in human neuroblastoma IMR32 cells: kinetics, permeability, and pharmacology. Pflügers Arch. **416:** 170–179.

45. SHER, E., E. BIANCARDI, A. POLLO, E. CARBONE, G. LI, C. B. WOLLHEIM & F. CLEMENTI. 1992. ω-Conotoxin-sensitive, voltage-operated Ca^{2+} channels in insulin-secreting cells. Eur. J. Pharmacol. **216:** 407–414.

46. RICHMOND, J. E., E. SHER & I. COOKE. 1995. Characterization of the calcium currents in freshly dissociated crustacean peptidergic neuronal somata. J. Neurophysiol. **73:** 2357–2368.

47. SHER, E., C. GOTTI, N. CANAL, C. SCOPPETTA, G. PICCOLO, A. EVOLI & F. CLEMENTI. 1989. Specificity of calcium channel autoantibodies in Lambert-Eaton myasthenic syndrome. Lancet **2:** 640–643.

48. LENNON, V. A. & E. H. LAMBERT. 1989. Autoantibodies bind solubilized calcium channel–ω-conotoxin complexes from small cell lung carcinoma: a diagnostic aid for Lambert-Eaton myasthenic syndrome. Mayo Clin. Proc. **64:** 1498–1504.

49. LEYS, K., B. LANG, I. JOHNSTON & J. NEWSOM-DAVIS. 1991. Calcium channel autoantibodies in the Lambert-Eaton myasthenic syndrome. Ann. Neurol. **29:** 307–314.

50. PELUCCHI, A., E. CICERI, F. CLEMENTI, L. MARAZZINI, A. FORESI & E. SHER. 1993. Calcium channel autoantibodies in myasthenic syndrome and small cell lung cancer. Am. Rev. Respir. Dis. **147:** 1229–1232.

51. MOTOMURA, M., A. SUENAGA, H. MATSUO, M. TSUJIHATA & S. NAGATAKI. 1994. Anti-voltage-gated calcium channel antibodies in the Lambert-Eaton myasthenic syndrome. Clin. Neurol. **34:** 980–984.

52. MOTOMURA, M., I. JOHNSTON, B. LANG, A. VINCENT & J. NEWSOM-DAVIS. 1995. An improved diagnostic assay for Lambert-Eaton myasthenic syndrome. J. Neurol. Neurosurg. Psychiatry **58:** 85–87.

53. SUENAGA, A., S. SHIRABE, T. NAKAMURA, M. MOTOMURA, M. TSUJIHATA, H. MATSUO, Y. KATAOKA, M. ITOH & S. NAGATAKI. 1996. Specificity of autoantibodies reactive with ω-conotoxin MVIIC–sensitive calcium channel in Lambert-Eaton myasthenic syndrome. Muscle Nerve **19:** 1166–1168.

54. ARSAC, C., C. RAYMOND, N. MARTIN-MOUTOT, B. DARGENT, G. COURAUD, J. POUGET & M. SEAGAR. 1996. Immunoassays fail to detect antibodies against neuronal calcium channels in amyotrophic lateral sclerosis serum. Ann. Neurol. **40:** 695–700.

55. PROTTI, D. A., R. REISIN, T. A. MACKINLEY & O. D. UCHITEL. 1996. Calcium channel blockers and transmitter release at the normal human neuromuscular junction. Neurology **46:** 1391–1396.

56. PROTTI, D. A. & O. D. UCHITEL. 1993. Transmitter release and presynaptic calcium currents blocked by the spider toxin ω-Aga IVA. Neuroreport **5:** 333–336.

57. TORRI-TARELLI, F., M. PASSAFARO, F. CLEMENTI & E. SHER. 1991. Presynaptic localization of ω-conotoxin-sensitive calcium channels at the frog neuromuscular junction. Brain Res. **547:** 331–334.

58. ROSSONI, G., G. BERTI, L. LA MAESTRA & F. CLEMENTI. 1994. ω-Conotoxin GVIA binds to and blocks rat neuromuscular junction. Neurosci. Lett. **176:** 185–188.

59. SHER, E. & F. CLEMENTI. 1991. ω-Conotoxin-sensitive voltage operated calcium channels in vertebrate cells. Neuroscience **42:** 301–307.
60. DE LUCA, A., C. G. LI, M. J. RAND, J. J. REID, P. THAINA & H. K. WONG-DUSTING. 1990. Effects of ω-conotoxin GVIA on autonomic neuroeffector transmission in various tissues. Br. J. Pharmacol. **101:** 437–447.
61. LOGIN, I. S., Y. I. KIM, A. M. JUDD, B. L. SPANGELO & R. M. MACLEOD. 1987. Immunoglobulins of Lambert-Eaton myasthenic syndrome inhibit rat pituitary hormone release. Ann. Neurol. **22:** 610–614.
62. RICHMOND, J. E., A. CODIGNOLA, I. M. COOKE & E. SHER. 1996. Calcium- and barium-dependent exocytosis from the rat insulinoma cell line RINm5F assayed using membrane capacitance measurements and serotonin release. Pflügers Arch. **432:** 258–269.

Antigenic Sites of the Voltage-gated Calcium Channel in Lambert-Eaton Myasthenic Syndrome[a]

MASAHARU TAKAMORI, KAZUO IWASA, AND KIYONOBU KOMAI

Department of Neurology
Kanazawa University School of Medicine
Kanazawa 920, Japan

INTRODUCTION

Lambert-Eaton myasthenic syndrome (LEMS) is an autoimmune disease of neuromuscular transmission, in which antibodies directed against voltage-gated calcium channels (VGCCs) in the motor nerves play a central role in causing a deficient quantal release of acetylcholine.[1,2] Multiple VGCC types have been generally classified as L, N, P/Q, R, and T according to their electrophysiological and pharmacological properties.[3–5] In the present study, we focused attention on the P/Q-type VGCC, against which a majority of LEMS patients carry the specific antibody.[6–8] In search of antigenic sites in the molecular structure of the P/Q-type VGCC, we synthesized peptides corresponding to the extracellular region (S5–S6 linker) of each of the four domains that form the α1A subunit of the VGCC[9] and tested their antigenicity for the detection of LEMS antibodies and also for the induction of a LEMS model in Lewis rats.

METHODS

Synthesis of Peptides

The three peptides, MGKFHTTCFEEGTDDIQGESPAPCGTEEPARTCPNGTR-CQPYWEGPNNGI (N-terminus of the domain I S5–S6 linker region), GGQFN-FDEGTPPTNFDTFPAA (N-terminus of the domain II S5–S6 linker region), and KGKFFHCTDESKEFEKDCRGKYLLYEKNEVK (N-terminus of the domain III S5–S6 linker region), were synthesized by reference to a sequential residue map of the α1A subunit of the rabbit-brain calcium channel;[9] the fourth peptide, GNIGID<u>V</u>EDEDSDEDEF, was synthesized with reference to the sequence expressed in human small cell lung carcinoma,[10] which is different by only a single

[a]This work was supported by a grant-in-aid for general scientific research (No. 07457154) from the Ministry of Education, Science, and Culture of Japan; by grants from the National Center for Nervous, Mental, and Muscular Disorders; and by grants from the Neuroimmunological Disease Research Committee, the Ministry of Health and Welfare of Japan.

residue (underlined) from the N-terminus of the domain IV S5–S6 linker region of the α1A subunit of rabbit- and rat-brain calcium channels.[9,11] All four peptides were purified by reverse-phase HPLC and their synthesis was confirmed by mass spectroscopy. The antigen to immunize Lewis rats for possible induction of an animal model was the synthetic peptide, domain II S5–S6 linker region, the N-terminus of which was linked to a cysteine residue. The carrier protein, keyhole limpet hemocyanine (KLH, 5 mg/1 mg of peptide), was linked to m-maleimidobenzoyl-N-hydroxysuccinimide (MBS, 15 mg/mL of 0.05 M phosphate buffer), forming an MBS/KLH conjugate. After column purification, the MBS/KLH conjugate was cross-linked to the Cys-containing synthetic peptide.

Assay of Antipeptide Antibodies

Five μg of each of three peptides (domains I, II, and IV) and 25 μg of the peptide referring to domain III, which contains many lysine residues, were labeled with iodine (^{125}I) using Bolton-Hunter reagent (0.5 mCi). After incubation of the serum sample (1 μL) at 4 °C overnight with ^{125}I-peptide (100,000 cpm), anti-IgG antiserum (25 μL) was added and the reaction mixture was incubated at 4 °C overnight. The reaction mixture was then washed three times with saline (each by centrifugation at 3000 rpm for 10 minutes), and the radioactivity in the precipitates was counted with a gamma-counter and expressed as pmoles of ^{125}I-peptide precipitated per liter of serum.

Assay of Anti-P/Q-type Calcium Channel Antibodies

Human cerebellar tissue obtained at autopsy was homogenized in ice-cold incubation buffer and then centrifuged at 10,000g for 20 minutes. Pellets resuspended in an incubation buffer containing 2% digitonin were incubated at 4 °C for an hour and then centrifuged at 100,000g for 30 minutes. The supernatant was incubated with 25 nmol ^{125}I-ω-conotoxin MVIIC (2000 Ci/mmol) for 2 hours to form the toxin-labeled calcium channel complex. The serum (2 μL for humans; 5 μL for rats) was incubated with this complex at 4 °C overnight and precipitated with 50 μL of anti-IgG antiserum for the measurement of "binding" antibody activity (i.e., antibodies bound to the sites other than the toxin-binding site). Pellets were washed twice with ice-cold 0.1 M Tris-HC1 and 0.1 M NaCl buffer (pH 7.4) containing 0.5% Triton X-100 and centrifuged at 3000 rpm for 10 minutes. Pellet radioactivities were counted with a gamma-counter and results were expressed as pmoles of ^{125}I-ω-conotoxin MVIIC-binding sites precipitated per liter of serum. For the assay of "blocking" antibody activity (i.e., antibody bound to the toxin-binding site), the supernatant was first incubated with the test (A) or control (B) serum (2 μL) for 2 hours and then with ^{125}I-ω-conotoxin MVIIC for 2 hours, followed by 1-hour incubation with the LEMS serum that was positive for "binding" antibody and finally by precipitation with 50 μL of anti-IgG antiserum. The "blocking" activity was expressed as (B − A)/B × 100%.

Patients

Serum samples were obtained from 30 LEMS patients (16 with small cell lung carcinoma, SCLC; 1 with poorly differentiated cell lung carcinoma; 1 with stomach adenocarcinoma) whose diagnosis was made on the basis of standard clinical and electrophysiological criteria,[12] as well as from 20 disease controls (10 with SCLC without LEMS; 10 with myasthenia gravis) and 15 healthy controls.

Animals

Ten female Lewis rats, 8–10 weeks of age, were injected intradermally at multiple sites with 100 μg of the synthetic peptide (domain II S5–S6 linker peptide) conjugated with KLH and emulsified with complete Freund's adjuvant in a 200-μL volume. Injections were carried out on days 0, 7, 14, and 21, and the rats were killed 28–35 days after the initial inoculation. Ten control rats were injected with adjuvant alone and killed, following the same schedule as for the test rats.

Electrophysiological Study

The anesthetized rats were decapitated and a segment of diaphragm with its phrenic nerve was mounted in a chamber containing bathing fluid oxygenated with 95% oxygen plus 5% CO_2 at 37 °C. Normal bathing fluid contained (mM) NaCl (122), KCl (4.7), $NaHCO_3$ (15.5), $MgCl_2$ (1.2), KH_2PO_4 (1.2), $CaCl_2$ (2.6), and D-glucose (11). *d*-Tubocurarine chloride was added to inhibit muscle contraction for the study of end plate potential (EPP) evoked by nerve stimulation. Miniature end plate potential (MEPP) and EPP were recorded with a conventional intracellular microelectrode; their amplitudes were corrected for nonlinearity of the end plate response to acetylcholine assuming a –15-mV acetylcholine equilibrium potential and to a resting membrane potential of –75 mV. The acetylcholine quantal content of EPP was calculated by the variance method (coefficient of variation of the EPP amplitude distribution) using 50 EPPs after the first 10 in the train at 1-Hz repetitive nerve stimulation. This method of calculation assumes that quantal release is Poisson in nature.[13]

Statistical Analysis

Antibody titers were estimated as positive when values were more than 2.5 SD above the mean values of the 15 healthy volunteers or 10 control rats. The correlation of antipeptide antibodies and anti-P/Q-type VGCC (ω-conotoxin MVIIC–labeled cerebellar extract) antibodies in LEMS patients was estimated by Pearson's correlation coefficient (r). In the electrophysiological study of the animal experiment, differences in the means of MEPP amplitude and frequency, resting membrane potential, and EPP quantal content between the control (100 end plates, 10 end plates in each of 10 rats) and each (10 end plates) of the test rats were analyzed by one-way analysis of variance and Duncan's test for multiple comparisons.

RESULTS AND DISCUSSION

Antibodies to P/Q-type VGCC in Humans

The $\alpha 1$ subunit of the VGCC has a central role in channel functions, and multiple isoforms of this principal $\alpha 1$ subunit have been identified and designated as class A through E.[3-5] Among these isoforms, the $\alpha 1$ subunit of class A ($\alpha 1A$) is highly expressed in the cerebellum[9,11] and is specifically sensitive to ω-conotoxin MVIICl[4] and ω-agatoxin IVA.[15] Its functional properties resemble those of the VGCC known as P-type and Q-type.[16,17] We therefore referred to the $\alpha 1A$ subunit as the $\alpha 1$ subunit of P/Q-type VGCC. Recent reports have suggested that the calcium influx into the mammalian motor nerve terminal elicited by nerve stimulation occurs through this P/Q-type VGCC.[18-20] Also, an immunohistochemical study demonstrated that the presynaptic terminal in the neuromuscular junction can be highly labeled with the antipeptide antibody specific for the $\alpha 1$ subunit of P/Q-type VGCC.[21] Basing our choice of the P/Q-type VGCC on these reports, we studied human serum samples by the use of immunoprecipitation assays for which ω-conotoxin MVIIC–labeled cerebellar extract was used as an antigen. The resulting frequency (80%) of anti-P/Q-type VGCC antibodies in our 30 LEMS patients was as high as those reported previously[6-8] (TABLE 1). Seventeen of 24 LEMS patients positive for the antibody had carcinomas, including 15 patients with SCLC (TABLE 1); 2 SCLC patients were without LEMS, but were positive for the antibody (TABLE 2).

Antipeptide Antibodies in Humans

The $\alpha 1$ subunit of the VGCC, which is responsible for voltage-gating, ion conductance, and sensitivity to pharmacologic agents, possesses four repeated domains (I–IV), each containing six α-helical transmembrane segments (S1–S6).[3,5,9,11,22] The loop between segments S5 and S6 in each domain is implicated in the formation of the ion conduction pore and adjacent regions of the voltage-gated ion channel and is exposed extracellularly,[3,5,9,11,22] suggesting that the S5–S6 linker regions have a potential accessibility to circulating antibodies. In view of this molecular anatomy, we synthesized peptides that correspond to the S5–S6 linker segment of each of the four domains forming the $\alpha 1$ subunit of P/Q-type VGCC and used them as antigens to detect antibodies in 30 LEMS sera and 35 non-LEMS sera. Among the 30 LEMS sera, 6 samples (20%), 5 of whom had SCLC, were positive for antibodies to the domain II S5–S6 linker peptide, and 9 samples (30%), 6 of whom had SCLC, were positive for antibodies to the domain IV S5–S6 linker peptide (TABLE 1).[23] Only 2 of 15 antipeptide-positive sera were positive for both antibodies. Titers of antibodies to domain II, as well as those for antibodies to domain IV, correlated with those of anti-P/Q-type VGCCs, which were defined as the ability to immunoprecipitate ^{125}I-ω-conotoxin MVIIC–labeled cerebellar extract ($r = 0.39$, $p < 0.05$ for the anti-domain II; $r = 0.63$,

TABLE 1. Antibodies to P/Q-type Voltage-gated Calcium Channel (VGCC) and Synthetic Peptides Corresponding to the α1A Subunit of VGCC in Patients with Lambert-Eaton Myasthenic Syndrome

Patient No.	Age (Years)	Sex	Cancer Detected[a]	Anti-P/Q-type VGCC Antibodies (pmol/L)	Anti-Domain I S5–S6 Linker (pmol/L)	Anti-Domain II S5–S6 Linker (pmol/L)	Anti-Domain III S5–S6 Linker (pmol/L)	Anti-Domain IV S5–S6 Linker (pmol/L)
1	63	F	none	10.1	3.4	11.6	18.5	13.9
2	38	F	none	12.6	5.0	10.1	27.6	16.4
3	45	M	none	12.2	4.3	11.4	20.8	15.7
4	58	F	none	13.6	4.4	12.4	24.9	18.2
5	69	M	SCLC	53.5[b]	4.2	10.0	26.4	15.4
6	51	F	none	72.8[b]	5.5	13.0	24.0	15.7
7	64	M	PDCC	30.7[b]	4.9	12.4	25.1	16.6
8	71	M	SCLC	16.7[b]	5.7	12.4	27.6	15.6
9	72	F	none	18.5[b]	5.1	11.7	23.7	17.2
10	54	F	none	17.6[b]	5.3	17.0[b]	28.9	17.7
11	53	F	none	24.7[b]	6.5	11.4	26.9	22.4[b]
12	80	M	SCLC	164.0[b]	5.4	13.7[b]	25.9	20.1[b]
13	71	M	SCLC	94.9[b]	4.8	12.6	22.1	15.5
14	68	M	SCLC	36.8[b]	5.7	16.0[b]	23.5	17.6
15	64	F	SCLC	351.2[b]	6.6	20.4[b]	28.7	23.1[b]
16	52	F	SCLC	219.8[b]	4.0	12.7	28.8	20.8[b]
17	66	M	SCLC	36.8[b]	5.2	12.8	27.0	19.9[b]
18	60	M	SCLC	11.4	4.9	10.9	19.7	13.8
19	60	M	SCLC	34.2[b]	4.7	12.9	24.6	18.8[b]
20	63	M	SCLC	19.3[b]	4.9	9.9	25.3	17.0
21	69	M	SCLC	200.1[b]	4.5	12.7	30.1	21.4[b]
22	75	M	none	104.6[b]	4.2	11.6	30.6	19.2[b]
23	51	M	none	40.5[b]	4.1	11.2	20.8	21.3[b]
24	63	M	SC	24.2[b]	5.0	11.4	23.1	16.2
25	37	M	SCLC	20.6[b]	6.3	19.7[b]	26.8	15.6
26	69	M	SCLC	15.4[b]	5.3	19.0[b]	29.1	17.1
27	74	F	SCLC	35.2[b]	4.0	11.2	26.6	15.8
28	52	F	SCLC	38.9[b]	6.3	9.6	26.9	15.5
29	43	F	none	63.1[b]	5.5	12.1	23.5	15.7
30	61	F	none	12.5	3.8	9.1	22.7	15.3
15 controls (mean + 2.5 SD)				13.8	6.9	13.1	31.4	18.5

[a]SCLC = small cell lung carcinoma; PDCC = poorly differentiated cell lung carcinoma; SC = stomach adenocarcinoma.

[b]Significant elevation of antibody titers (more than 2.5 SD above the mean values of 15 healthy controls).

$p = 0.0001$ for the anti-domain IV).[23] Although Barry *et al.*[10] reported the expression of an acidic stretch in the domain IV S5–S6 linker region in human SCLC, our study found antibodies not only to this segment, but also to a sequence derived from the domain II S5–S6 linker in 5 LEMS patients with SCLC (TABLE 1) and also in 1 patient with SCLC without LEMS (TABLE 2).

Animal Model Induced by Immunization with Synthetic Peptide

Selective permeation of Ca^{2+} through voltage-gated Ca^{2+} channels is the primary feature of the $\alpha 1$ subunit. The loop, known as the SS1–SS2 region, in the S5–S6 link-

TABLE 2. Antibodies to P/Q-type Voltage-gated Calcium Channel (VGCC) and Synthetic Peptides Corresponding to the $\alpha 1A$ Subunit of VGCC in Patients with Small Cell Lung Carcinoma and Myasthenia Gravis

Patient No.	Age (Years)	Sex	Anti-P/ Q-type VGCC Antibodies (pmol/L)	Antipeptide Antibodies			
				Anti-Domain I S5–S6 Linker (pmol/L)	Anti-Domain II S5–S6 Linker (pmol/L)	Anti-Domain III S5–S6 Linker (pmol/L)	Anti-Domain IV S5–S6 Linker (pmol/L)
Small cell lung carcinoma							
1	67	M	5.8	4.0	6.3	27.8	14.1
2	77	M	10.9	3.8	7.5	19.6	14.4
3	69	M	7.2	5.2	9.1	22.5	14.9
4	72	F	20.8[a]	3.8	8.3	25.2	14.0
5	69	M	12.4	4.8	9.9	27.7	17.7
6	65	M	25.3[a]	4.8	15.5[a]	25.4	13.9
7	74	M	12.3	6.0	9.5	23.4	12.0
8	72	F	2.0	4.6	6.9	21.5	15.8
9	70	M	4.9	3.3	8.6	24.5	13.2
10	56	M	2.7	3.4	7.8	21.0	12.7
Myasthenia gravis							
1	23	F	6.5	4.7	4.6	24.6	15.4
2	52	F	4.1	4.9	8.5	21.0	15.2
3	14	F	8.9	5.1	6.8	28.7	16.1
4	35	F	8.3	6.2	7.9	27.4	16.3
5	56	F	2.0	6.0	7.6	23.1	14.1
6	56	M	3.0	3.6	5.2	21.7	10.6
7	61	F	4.5	4.2	7.8	31.1	14.1
8	28	F	11.3	4.4	10.9	22.4	15.6
9	34	F	3.8	4.5	12.9	28.1	16.8
10	66	F	4.4	3.9	10.6	27.3	15.5
15 controls (mean + 2.5 SD)			13.8	6.9	13.1	31.4	18.5

[a]Significant elevation of antibody titers (more than 2.5 SD above the mean values of 15 healthy controls).

er in each of the four domains of the α1 subunit folds in and then out of the membrane, thereby creating a lining in the voltage-gated Ca^{2+} selective pore of the channel.[24] Several researchers have shown that the SS2 regions of all four domains that contain Glu residues are important determinants of ion selectivity in the Ca^{2+} channel.[5,25–27] The drug- or toxin-binding sites are in close proximity to the pore lining on the α1 subunit, as suggested by the study with chimeric Ca^{2+} channels. Namely, amino-acid substitutions that replaced a portion of the ω-conotoxin GVIA–sensitive channel (N-type) with a corresponding portion of the ω-conotoxin MVIIC–sensitive channel (P/Q-type) served to markedly alter sensitivity to the toxin, thereby allocating the toxin receptor function to the extracellular loop of the S5–S6 linker in each of the four domains.[28] In view of these molecular determinants of Ca^{2+} channel function and the results from our study on human LEMS sera, the domain II S5–S6 linker was selected to immunize Lewis rats for possible induction of an animal model of LEMS. The domain IV S5–S6 linker was not available for this study because its N-terminus was not linkable with Cys as is necessary for the conjugation with KLH. The serum samples from 10 rats sacrificed after repeated immunizations showed high titers of antipeptide antibodies that reacted with sites other than the toxin-binding site of the ω-conotoxin MVIIC–labeled cerebellar extract (TABLE 3). The "blocking" activity of antibodies bound to the toxin-binding site of the channel was not detected (TABLE 3). The present study's failure to detect "blocking antibody" may suggest that the sensitivity of our assay method was too low for detection of antibodies to domain II, which may have lower toxin-binding activity than domain III.[28] Alternatively, our assumption concerning the toxin-binding site of the channel was based on the result from the study on the N-type VGCC;[28] the ω-conotoxin MVIIC–binding site in the P/Q-type may not be exactly the same as the ω-conotoxin GVIA–binding site in the N-type VGCC.

The electrophysiological study showed that the reduction in the mean quantum

TABLE 3. Antibody Assay in Rats Immunized with Domain II S5–S6 Linker Peptide

Rat No.	Antipeptide Antibodies (pmol/L)	Anti-P/Q-type VGCC Antibodies[a]	
		Binding Antibodies (pmol/L)	Blocking Antibodies (%)
control (10 rats)	1.9[b]	11.0[b]	10[b]
1	2252.1	12.0	0
2	2198.6	12.1	3
3	2261.5	11.5	0
4	2353.9	12.7	0
5	3150.7	21.8	0
6	2569.5	24.4	0
7	2680.8	16.7	0
8	3901.0	23.9	6
9	1892.1	20.2	0
10	3029.9	22.9	0

[a]VGCC: voltage-gated calcium channel (ω-conotoxin MVIIC–sensitive channel).
[b]Mean + 2.5 SD.

TABLE 4. Microelectrode Study in Rats Immunized with Domain II S5–S6 Linker Peptide[a]

Rat No. (n = 10 for each)	MEPP		Resting Membrane Potential (mV)	Quantal Content of EPP at 1 Hz (Quanta)	dTC (μg/mL)
	Amplitude (mV)	Frequency (per second)			
1	0.73 ± 0.035	2.9 ± 1.36	74 ± 5.0	136 ± 54.5	1.9
2	0.71 ± 0.020	3.4 ± 1.16	74 ± 5.1	106 ± 43.3[b]	1.6
3	0.75 ± 0.104	2.9 ± 0.29	75 ± 4.1	108 ± 24.8	1.8
4	0.71 ± 0.058	3.1 ± 0.58	75 ± 3.1	138 ± 58.9	1.9
5	0.69 ± 0.120	3.2 ± 0.75	75 ± 2.0	120 ± 44.9	1.9
6	0.74 ± 0.104	3.2 ± 0.89	74 ± 5.2	104 ± 38.5[b]	1.6
7	0.67 ± 0.096	3.4 ± 0.74	76 ± 4.9	103 ± 50.5[b]	1.6
8	0.75 ± 0.079	3.0 ± 0.91	75 ± 4.4	121 ± 27.3	1.9
9	0.69 ± 0.089	3.1 ± 0.81	76 ± 4.8	102 ± 56.7[b]	1.5
10	0.74 ± 0.022	2.9 ± 0.82	75 ± 2.9	114 ± 46.5	1.8
control (n = 100, 10 in each of 10 rats)	0.72 ± 0.104	3.2 ± 0.47	75 ± 5.3	153 ± 36.1	1.9–2.3

[a]Values in the microelectrode study are the means ± standard deviations. Terms—dTC: *d*-tubocurarine chloride concentration used to inhibit muscle contraction; MEPP: miniature end plate potential; EPP: end plate potential.

[b]Significantly different from control as estimated by one-way analysis of variance and Duncan's test for multiple comparisons.

content of EPPs at 1 Hz was significant in 4 of 10 peptide-immunized rats versus controls (TABLE 4). The repetitive nerve stimulation at a tetanic rate (50 Hz) caused early facilitation followed by less marked depression of EPP amplitudes in those end plates at which the EPP quantum content at 1 Hz ranged from 28 to 45 (FIGURE 1). These findings are similar to those both from LEMS patients and from mice treated with LEMS IgG.[1,29,30] Our experiments were all carried out in the presence of *d*-tubocurarine, which has a presynaptic action affecting acetylcholine quantal release.[31] This effect is independent of concentration over the range of 1.3 to 4.8 μg/mL;[32] any presynaptic effect at this range of tubocurarine concentration can be expected to be the same for all muscles.[30] Therefore, the tubocurarine concentration used in the present study (1.5–2.3 μg/mL) was out of the range of presynaptic modification and does not affect our conclusion.

Further studies investigating the remaining parts of the α1 subunit, as well as the search for T cell epitopes in the molecular structure, may open new avenues in the study of Lambert-Eaton myasthenic syndrome.

CONCLUSIONS

To search for antigenic sites in the molecular structure of P/Q-type VGCC, we synthesized four peptides corresponding to the extracellular region (S5–S6 linker) of each of four domains that form the α1A subunit of the VGCC and tested their anti-control

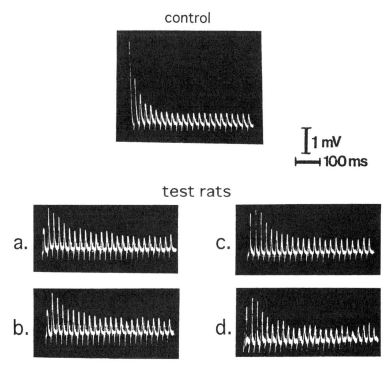

$\displaystyle \text{I}$1 mV

⊢——⊣100 ms

test rats

a.

c.

b.

d.

FIGURE 1. End plate potentials (EPPs) elicited with the repetitive nerve stimulation, recorded from the control and the test rats immunized with the domain II S5–S6 linker peptide corresponding to the α1A subunit of the voltage-gated calcium channel. The 50-Hz train of EPPs showed marked depression of amplitude in the control and early facilitation followed by less marked depression in the test rats (a–d).

genicity for the detection of LEMS antibodies and also for the induction of a rat model of LEMS. Among the sera of 30 LEMS patients, 6 (20%) were positive for anti-domain II and 9 (30%) were positive for anti-domain IV. Titers for antibodies to domain II, as well as those for antibodies to domain IV, correlated with those for antibodies to ω-conotoxin MVIIC–labeled cerebellar extract (P/Q-type VGCC). Lewis rats were immunized with the peptide (domain II S5–S6 linker) conjugated with KLH. The study of rats at sacrifice showed such characteristic LEMS features as presence of antibodies to P/Q-type VGCC and reduced EPP quantum content. Our observations suggest two potential epitopes of LEMS antibodies.

REFERENCES

1. LAMBERT, E. H. & D. ELMQVIST. 1971. Quantal components of end-plate potentials in the myasthenic syndrome. Ann. N.Y. Acad. Sci. **183:** 183–199.

2. VINCENT, A., B. LANG & J. NEWSOM-DAVIS. 1989. Autoimmunity to the voltage-gated calcium channel underlies the Lambert-Eaton myasthenic syndrome, a paraneoplastic disorder. Trends Neurosci. **12:** 496–502.

3. SNUTCH, T. P. & P. B. REINER. 1992. Ca^{2+} channels: diversity of form and function. Curr. Opin. Neurobiol. **2:** 247–253.

4. DUNLAP, K., J. I. LUEBKE & T. J. TURNER. 1995. Exocytotic Ca^{2+} channels in mammalian central neurons. Trends Neurosci. **18:** 89–98.

5. VARADI, G., Y. MORI, G. MIKALA & A. SCHWARTZ. 1995. Molecular determinants of Ca^{2+} channel function and drug action. Trends Pharmacol. Sci. **16:** 43–49.

6. LENNON, V. A., T. J. KRYZER, G. E. GRIESMANN, P. E. O'SUILLEABHAIN, A. J. WINDEBANK, A. WOPPMANN, G. P. MILJANICH & E. H. LAMBERT. 1995. Calcium-channel antibodies in the Lambert-Eaton syndrome and other paraneoplastic syndromes. N. Engl. J. Med. **332:** 1467–1474.

7. MOTOMURA, M., I. JOHNSTON, B. LANG, A. VINCENT & J. NEWSOM-DAVIS. 1995. An improved diagnostic assay for Lambert-Eaton myasthenic syndrome. J. Neurol. Neurosurg. Psychiatry **58:** 85–87.

8. TAKAMORI, M., M. TAKAHASHI, Y. YASUKAWA, K. IWASA, Y. NEMOTO, A. SUENAGA, S. NAGATAKI & T. NAKAMURA. 1995. Antibodies to recombinant synaptotagmin and calcium channel subtypes in Lambert-Eaton myasthenic syndrome. J. Neurol. Sci. **133:** 95–101.

9. MORI, Y., T. FRIEDRICH, M-S. KIM, A. MIKAMI, J. NAKAI, P. RUTH, E. BOSSE, F. HOFMANN, V. FLOCKERZI, T. FURUICHI, K. MIKOSHIBA, K. IMOTO, T. TANABE & S. NUMA. 1991. Primary structure and function expression from complementary DNA of a brain calcium. Nature **350:** 398–402.

10. BARRY, E. L. R., M. P. VIGLIONE, Y. I. KIM & S. C. FROEHNER. 1995. Expression and antibody inhibition of P-type calcium channels in human small-cell lung carcinoma cells. J. Neurosci. **15:** 274–283.

11. STARR, T. V. B., W. PRYSTAY & T. P. SNUTCH. 1991. Primary structure of a calcium channel that is highly expressed in the rat cerebellum. Proc. Natl. Acad. Sci. U.S.A. **88:** 5621–5625.

12. O'NEILL, J. H., N. M. F. MURRAY & J. NEWSOM-DAVIS. 1988. The Lambert-Eaton myasthenic syndrome: a review of 50 cases. Brain **111:** 577–596.

13. LAMBERT, E. H. & V. A. LENNON. 1988. Selected IgG rapidly induces Lambert-Eaton myasthenic syndrome in mice: complement independence and EMG abnormalities. Muscle Nerve **11:** 1133–1145.

14. HILLYARD, D. R., V. D. MONJE, I. M. MINTZ, B. P. BEAN, L. NADASDI, J. RAMACHANDRAN, G. MILJANICH, A. AZIMI-ZOONOOZ, J. M. MCINTOSH, L. J. CRUZ, J. S. IMPERIAL & B. M. OLIVERA. 1992. A new conus peptide ligand for mammalian presynaptic Ca^{2+} channels. Neuron **9:** 69–77.

15. LLINÁS, R., M. SUGIMORI, J-W. LIN & B. CHERKSEY. 1989. Blocking and isolation of a calcium channel from neurons in mammals and cephalopods utilizing a toxin fraction (FTX) from funnel-web spider poison. Proc. Natl. Acad. Sci. U.S.A. **86:** 1689–1693.

16. STEA, A., W. J. TOMLINSON, T. W. SOONG, E. BOURINET, S. J. DUBEL, S. R. VINCENT & T. P. SNUTCH. 1994. Localization and functional properties of a rat brain α1A calcium channel reflect similarities to neuronal Q- and P-type channels. Proc. Natl. Acad. Sci. U.S.A. **91:** 10576–10580.

17. RANDALL, A. & R. W. TSIEN. 1995. Pharmacological dissection of multiple types of Ca^{2+} channel currents in rat cerebellar granule neurons. J. Neurosci. **15:** 2995–3012.

18. UCHITEL, O. D., D. A. PROTTI, V. SANCHEZ, B. D. CHERKSEY, M. SUGIMORI & R. LLINÁS. 1992. P-type voltage-dependent calcium channel mediates presynaptic calcium influx and transmitter release in mammalian synapses.

19. PROTTI, D. A., R. REISIN, T. A. MACKINLEY & O. D. UCHITEL. 1996. Calcium channel

blockers and transmitter release at the normal human neuromuscular junction. Neurology **46**: 1391–1396.

20. SUGIURA, Y., A. WOPPMANN, G. P. MILJANICH & C-P. KO. 1995. A novel ω-conopeptide for the presynaptic localization of calcium channels at the mammalian neuromuscular junction. J. Neurocytol. **24**: 15–27.

21. OUSLEY, A. H. & S. C. FROEHNER. 1994. An anti-peptide antibody specific for the class A calcium channel α1 subunit labels mammalian neuromuscular junction. Proc. Natl. Acad. Sci. U.S.A. **91**: 12263–12267.

22. HOFMANN, F., M. BIEL & V. FLOCKERZI. 1994. Molecular basis for Ca^{2+} channel diversity. Annu. Rev. Neurosci. **17**: 399–418.

23. TAKAMORI, M., K. IWASA & K. KOMAI. 1997. Antibodies to synthetic peptides of the α1A subunit of the voltage-gated calcium channel in Lambert-Eaton myasthenic syndrome. Neurology **48**: 1261–1265.

24. GUY, H. R. & F. CONTI. 1990. Pursuing the structure and function of voltage-gated channels. Trends Neurosci. **13**: 201–206.

25. KIM, M-S., T. MORII, L-X. SUN, K. IMOTO & Y. MORI. 1993. Structural determinants of ion selectivity in brain calcium channel. FEBS Lett. **318**: 145–148.

26. TANG, S., G. MIKALA, A. BAHINSKI, A. YATANI, G. VARADI & A. SCHWARTZ. 1993. Molecular localization of ion selectivity sites within the pore of a human L-type cardiac calcium channel. J. Biol. Chem. **268**: 13026–13029.

27. YANG, J., P. T. ELLINOR, W. A. SATHER, J-F. ZHANG & R. W. TSIEN. 1993. Molecular determinants of Ca^{2+} selectivity and ion permeation in L-type Ca^{2+} channels. Nature **366**: 158–161.

28. ELLINOR, P. T., J-F. ZHANG, W. A. HORNE & R. W. TSIEN. 1994. Structural determinants of the blockade of N-type calcium channels by a peptide neurotoxin. Nature **372**: 272–275.

29. CULL-CANDY, S. G., R. MILEDI, A. TRAUTMANN & O. D. UCHITEL. 1980. On the release of transmitter at normal, myasthenia gravis, and myasthenic syndrome affected human endplates. J. Physiol. (Lond.) **299**: 621–638.

30. LANG, B., J. NEWSOM-DAVIS, C. PRIOR & D. WRAY. 1983. Antibodies to motor nerve terminals: an electrophysiological study of a human myasthenic syndrome transferred to mouse. J. Physiol. (Lond.) **344**: 335–345.

31. BOWMAN, W. C., C. PRIOR & I. G. MARSHALL. 1990. Presynaptic receptors in the neuromuscular junction. Ann. N.Y. Acad. Sci. **604**: 69–81.

32. AUERBACH, A. & W. BETZ. 1971. Does curare affect transmitter release? J. Physiol. (Lond.) **213**: 691–705.

Role of L-type and N-type Voltage-dependent Calcium Channels (VDCCs) on Spontaneous Acetylcholine Release at the Mammalian Neuromuscular Junction

ADRIANA LOSAVIO AND SALOMÓN MUCHNIK

Instituto de Investigaciones Medicas Alfredo Lanari
Universidad de Buenos Aires
(1427) Buenos Aires, Argentina

INTRODUCTION

Spontaneous and evoked quantal release of acetylcholine (ACh) at the mammalian neuromuscular junction are governed by dissimilar mechanisms, although both release modalities seem to require the entry of calcium ions into the presynaptic terminal through voltage-dependent calcium channels (VDCCs).[1–3]

Several types of VDCCs have been recognized in nerve cells, named L, N, P, Q, R, and T, distinguished on the basis of their electrical and pharmacological properties.[4–7] Available data indicate that multiple types of VDCCs may coexist at a given individual synapse and that they may interact to induce secretion.[8–12] The aim of our work was, first, to identify which VDCCs are involved in spontaneous ACh release in the mammalian neuromuscular junction and to evaluate the degree of synergism on the control of the secretion at individual release sites; second, to determine the influence of extracellular and intracellular calcium ion concentration on spontaneous transmitter release; and third, to study the kinetics of exocytosis related to spontaneous ACh secretion in isotonic and hypertonic saline media.

Miniature end plate potential (MEPP) frequency was recorded intracellularly from Wistar rat diaphragm muscles at the end plate region of the muscle fiber with glass microelectrodes filled with 3 M KCl (resistance, 5–10 MΩ). In the next section, n expresses the number of fibers.

RESULTS

We first studied the effect of ω-agatoxin-IVA (ω-AGA-IVA), a P/Q-type VDCC blocker, upon spontaneous ACh release. One hundred nanomolar ω-AGA-IVA is known to abolish presynaptic calcium ion currents and ACh-evoked release whether by electrical stimulation or induced by potassium ion depolarization.[13–15] As shown in FIGURE 1, panels B and C, MEPP frequency remained unaltered after the addition of ω-AGA-IVA (mean $\pm$ SD: control, 1.9 ± 0.6, $n = 38$; ω-AGA-IVA, 2.0 ± 0.5, $n = 42$), suggesting that P/Q-type VDCCs are not involved in spontaneous ACh release at the mammalian neuromuscular junction.

We then studied the effect of nifedipine on spontaneous ACh release. L-type VD-CCs are sensitive to 1,4-dihydropyridine compounds, some of which act as blockers like nifedipine.[16-18] FIGURE 1, panel A, shows that 5 μM nifedipine reduced MEPP frequency by roughly 53% (control, 3.6 ± 1.8, $n = 34$; nifedipine, 1.7 ± 0.9, $n = 32$; $p < 0.005$), indicating that nifedipine-blockable channels play a major role in resting spontaneous ACh release (see FIGURE 1, panel C).

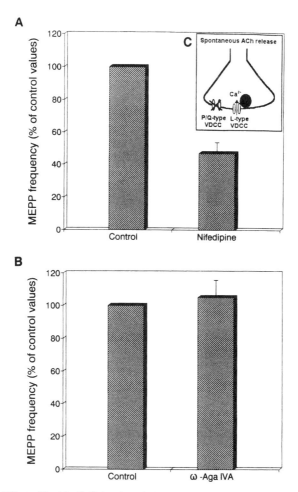

FIGURE 1. Effect of 5 μM nifedipine (panel A) and 100 nM ω-AGA-IVA (panel B) on MEPP frequency. Values are expressed as percentages of control solutions. Error bars indicate SEM. Methods for this and all subsequent figures are as follows: Isolated rat phrenic nerve diaphragm preparations were bathed in oxygenated (100% O_2) Krebs solution, at room temperature. Krebs solution contained (mM) NaCl (135), KCl (5), $CaCl_2$ (2), $MgCl_2$ (1), glucose (11), and HEPES (5), pH 7.3–7.4. Inset C: Schematic drawing of a nerve terminal showing L-type VDCC involvement and lack of participation of P/Q-type VDCC on spontaneous transmitter release.

We then evaluated the effect of the same nifedipine concentration on nerve terminals depolarized by increasing external potassium concentration to 10 and 15 mM (FIGURE 2, panel A). Nifedipine appeared to exert a selective inhibitory effect on spontaneous ACh release only in basal conditions (5 mM K$^+$), without interfering with the calcium ion current associated with nerve terminal depolarization (10 and 15 mM K$^+$). As shown in FIGURE 2, panel B, potassium ion–induced ACh release was associated with calcium ion influx through P/Q-type VDCCs, but not through L-type channels.

In order to determine whether L-type VDCCs were the only channels involved in spontaneous secretion in mammals, MEPP frequency was recorded in 0-Ca^{2+}/1 mM EGTA solution. As shown in FIGURE 3, panel A, MEPP frequency in 0-Ca^{2+}/EGTA, expressed as a percentage of that observed in the presence of normal Ringer's solution, was significantly lower than values observed after addition of nifedipine ($p <$ 0.01), indicating that more than one type of VDCC is involved (nifedipine, 47 ± 12%, $n = 32$; 0-Ca^{2+}/EGTA solutions, 33.5 ± 3.8%, $n = 60$).

Therefore, we investigated the involvement of N-type VDCCs on spontaneous release. As shown in FIGURE 3, panel B, the application of 5 μM ω-conotoxin-GVIA (ω-CgTx-GVIA), a specific blocker of N-type VDCCs,[20–22] reduced MEPP frequency to 71.5 ± 9.1% ($n = 42$). This finding suggests that N-type VDCCs also play a role

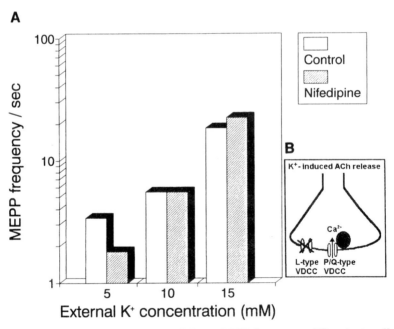

FIGURE 2. Panel A: Effect of 5 μM nifedipine on MEPP frequency at different extracellular potassium concentrations. Error bars indicate SEM. For further details, see reference 19. Panel B: Schematic drawing showing P/Q-type VDCC involvement and lack of participation of L-type VDCC on K$^+$-induced acetylcholine release.

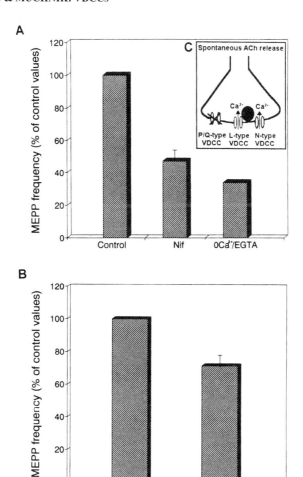

FIGURE 3. Panel A: Effect of 0-Ca²⁺/1 mM EGTA solution compared with 5 μM nifedipine on MEPP frequency. Panel B: Effect of 5 μM ω-CgTx-GVIA on MEPP frequency. Error bars indicate SEM. Inset C: Schematic drawing showing involvement of L- and N-type VDCCs, but not P/Q-type VDCCs, on spontaneous secretion.

in the modulation of spontaneous neurotransmitter release (FIGURE 3, panel C). In order to glean further data on the functional interaction between L- and N-type VDCCs on secretion control at individual release sites, the two blockers were evaluated in succession. As shown in FIGURE 4, panel A, nifedipine initially reduced MEPP frequency to 54.3% of control values, while ω-CgTx-GVIA induced a further reduction to 41.8%. In FIGURE 4, panel B, on switching blockers, ω-CgTx-GVIA initially reduced MEPP frequency to 71.5%, while nifedipine induced a further reduction to

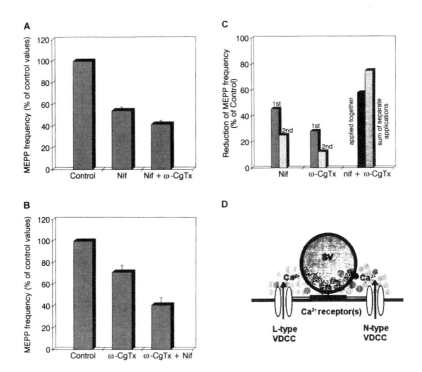

FIGURE 4. Panel A: Effect of nifedipine and of ω-CgTx-GVIA plus nifedipine on MEPP frequency. Panel B: Effect of ω-CgTx-GVIA and of nifedipine plus ω-CgTx-GVIA on MEPP frequency. Panel C: Summary of the mean reduction in MEPP frequency as shown in panels A and B. Panel D: Schematic drawing showing overlapping L- and N-type VDCC domains.

41.1%. FIGURE 4, panel C, depicts the effect of the two blockers, nifedipine and ω-CgTx-GVIA, added in succession. To simplify comparisons, the reduction in MEPP frequency is expressed as a percentage of the control value. When nifedipine was applied first, it reduced MEPP frequency by 45.7%, but only by 25.3% when applied after ω-CgTx-GVIA. An initial addition of ω-CgTx-GVIA reduced MEPP frequency by 28.5%, but only by 12.0% when added after nifedipine. Strikingly, the arithmetic sum of the individual effects of nifedipine and ω-CgTx-GVIA is 75.0%, which is quite different from the 58.0% reduction in MEPP frequency induced by simultaneous application. This result is incompatible with an additive blockade and suggests that both VDCC types act synergistically to control spontaneous release at individual release sites, with probable overlapping of their domains. It may therefore be speculated that calcium receptors triggering spontaneous release bind calcium within the L- and N-type VDCC domains so that nearby vesicles can promptly fuse (FIGURE 4, panel D).

    We then studied the kinetics of exocytosis of spontaneous ACh release through the effect of BAPTA-AM and EGTA-AM, two membrane-permeant calcium chelators. It is known that the slowly binding calcium buffer, EGTA, fails to block evoked neuro-transmitter release, whereas the rapidly binding homologue, BAPTA, efficiently blocks release.[23–26] However, data are scanty on the kinetics of spontaneous transmitter release. As shown in FIGURE 5, nerve terminals loaded with BAPTA-AM (hatched bars) displayed a reduction in MEPP frequency to $49.2 \pm 3.6\%$ ($n = 40$) and to $16.7 \pm 3.2\%$ ($n = 58$) when recordings were performed in muscles exposed to normal Ringer's solution (2 mM Ca^{2+}) and to 0-Ca^{2+} Ringer's solution, respectively. The reduction in MEPP frequency induced by EGTA-AM in both media (stitched bars; normal Ringer's solution, $75.1 \pm 19.1\%$, $n = 40$; 0-Ca^{2+} solution, $30.7 \pm 5.0\%$, $n = 40$) proved to be significantly lower than that induced by BAPTA-AM ($p < 0.018$ and $p < 0.0005$). Control values obtained in normal Ringer's solution before BAPTA-AM or EGTA-AM loading are expressed as 100% (white bars). Such results suggest that spontaneous secretion seems to follow a rapid kinetic pattern. Even though BAPTA-AM exerts a more potent effect on spontaneous release than EGTA-AM, such inhibitory action is more evident for exocytosis associated with evoked release since EGTA-AM fails to block such secretion.

In order to study osmotic response dependence on extracellular calcium ion con-

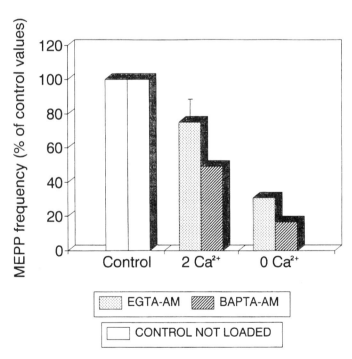

FIGURE 5. Effect of BAPTA-AM and EGTA-AM on spontaneous acetylcholine release. MEPP frequency was recorded in normal (2 mM Ca^{2+}) and in 0-Ca^{2+} Ringer's solutions after loading nerve terminals with the respective chelator. Results in control Ringer's solution before chelator loading (white bars) are expressed as 100%. Error bars indicate SEM.

centration, MEPP frequency was evaluated in 0-Ca^{2+}/EGTA solution to preclude calcium influx. As shown in FIGURE 6, panel A, a single experiment disclosed that, by increasing tonicity, MEPP frequency was raised both in control Ringer's solution and in Ringer's solution without calcium ions, but containing 1 mM EGTA. Although the magnitude of the hypertonic response in control solution was higher than in calcium-free EGTA solution (ratio of areas in control and 0-Ca^{2+}/EGTA, 4.8 ± 0.3; $n = 4$), similar ratios of peak osmotic response and mean isotonic MEPP frequencies were observed in control and experimental solutions (control, 8.0 ± 1.9; 0-Ca^{2+}/EGTA, 9.1 ± 3.5; $n = 4$). Such findings indicate that hyperosmotic response is independent of either extracellular calcium ion concentration or calcium influx through any VDCC (panel D). To investigate further the role of free calcium ion concentration within

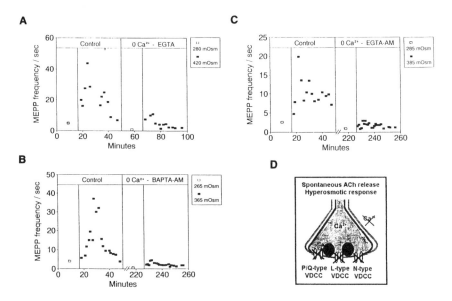

FIGURE 6. Panel A: Effect of 0-Ca^{2+}/EGTA solution on MEPP frequency when a single preparation was exposed to isotonic and hypertonic solutions. Open squares indicate the mean values from ten end plates after exposing the diaphragm to an isotonic solution and filled squares indicate the time course of osmotic response where each point represents the mean MEPP frequencies recorded from a single end plate. Panels B and C: Effect of BAPTA-AM and EGTA-AM on MEPP frequency when preparations were exposed to isotonic and hypertonic solutions. Symbols indicate MEPP frequency as described in panel A. Neurotransmitter release in BAPTA-AM and in EGTA-AM was recorded in Ca^{2+}-free Ringer's solutions after incubating the diaphragm for two hours in 0-Ca^{2+} solution containing the chelator (broken horizontal axis). Control MEPP frequency in isotonic and hypertonic solutions before chelator loading was recorded in normal Ringer's solution (2 mM Ca^{2+}). In panels A, B, and C, solutions were made hypertonic by adding sucrose to saline.[27] Panel D: Shadowed area in the schematic drawing indicates the decrease in nerve terminal volume after exposure to hypertonic solution, concomitantly with an increase in relative $[Ca^{2+}]_i$. Crosses show the lack of $[Ca^{2+}]_e$ or VDCC involvement.

nerve terminals during hypertonic response, presynaptic terminals were then loaded with BAPTA-AM or EGTA-AM. Panels B and C of FIGURE 6 depict the drastic reduction in MEPP frequency produced by BAPTA-AM and EGTA-AM, as demonstrated not only by the markedly decreased response, but also by the lower ratio between peak hyperosmotic response and mean isotonic MEPP frequency compared with values in control Ringer's solution before chelator treatment (ratio of peak osmotic response and mean isotonic MEPP frequency: BAPTA-AM, 5.6 ± 2.4; control, 9.1 ± 0.8, $n = 4$, $p < 0.01$; EGTA-AM, 4.0 ± 1.4; control, 7.6 ± 0.8, $n = 4$, $p < 0.002$). Results suggest that the presence of intracellular calcium ions within terminals is an essential requirement for hyperosmotic response. Remarkably enough, both BAPTA-AM and EGTA-AM exerted a similar effect on MEPP frequency response to hypertonicity, which contrasts with the greater potency of BAPTA-AM compared to EGTA-AM on spontaneous transmitter release observed in isotonic conditions. In this regard, such a lack of significant differences suggests that, in hypertonic conditions, calcium receptors are able to sense increased bulk intracellular calcium ion concentration, thereby inducing the observed increase in neurotransmitter release.

CONCLUSIONS

First, in the mammalian neuromuscular junction, spontaneous release is related to calcium entering the nerve terminals through at least two different channels: L-type VDCCs (blocked by nifedipine) and N-type VDCCs (blocked by ω-CgTx-GVIA). MEPP frequency is reduced mainly by nifedipine.

Second, nifedipine fails to affect the high potassium-evoked increase in MEPP frequency. On the other hand, it has been shown that ω-AGA-IVA (a P/Q-type VDCC blocker), known to inhibit presynaptic calcium ion current and acetylcholine release induced by either electrical or potassium ion depolarization in the mammalian neuromuscular junction, is not involved in spontaneous secretion, suggesting that different channels are involved in spontaneous and evoked ACh release.

Third, the combined application of nifedipine and ω-CgTx-GVIA reduces MEPP frequency to values lower than the arithmetic sum of individual drug effects, suggesting that both VDCC types have overlapping domains and act synergistically to control spontaneous release at individual release sites.

Fourth, the finding that MEPP frequency falls more sharply upon loading nerve terminals with a rapid chelator (BAPTA-AM) than with similar concentration of a slow one (EGTA-AM) indicates that spontaneous secretion seems to follow a rapid kinetic pattern. Although BAPTA-AM has a greater potency compared to EGTA-AM on spontaneous secretion, this effect is more readily discernible on evoked neurotransmitter release.

Fifth and last, neurotransmitter release in hypertonic conditions is independent of extracellular calcium ion concentration, but instead depends on intracellular values since both BAPTA-AM and EGTA-AM drastically reduce MEPP frequency. The finding that both chelators behave similarly suggests that, in hypertonic conditions, calcium receptors are able to sense increased bulk intracellular calcium ion concentration.

REFERENCES

1. HUBBARD, J. I., S. F. JONES & E. M. LANDAU. 1968. On the mechanism by which calcium and magnesium affect the spontaneous release of transmitter from mammalian motor nerve terminals. J. Physiol. (Lond.) **194:** 355–380.

2. KATZ, B. 1969. The Release of Neural Transmitter Substances. Thomas. Springfield, Illinois.

3. UCHITEL, O. D., D. A. PROTTI, V. SANCHEZ, D. CHERKSEY, M. SUGIMORI & R. LLINÁS. 1992. P-type voltage-dependent calcium channel mediates presynaptic calcium influx and transmitter release in mammalian synapses. Proc. Natl. Acad. Sci. U.S.A. **89:** 3330–3333.

4. BEAN, B. P. 1993. Classes of calcium channels in vertebrate cells. Annu. Rev. Physiol. **5:** 367–381.

5. McCLESKEY, E. W. 1994. Calcium channels: cellular roles and molecular mechanisms. Curr. Opin. Neurobiol. **4:** 304–312.

6. TSIEN, R. W., P. T. ELLINOR & W. A. HORNE. 1991. Molecular diversity of voltage-dependent Ca^{2+} channels. Trends Pharmacol. Sci. **12:** 347–354.

7. BIRNBAUMER, L., K. P. CAMPBELL, W. A. CATTERALL et al. 1994. The naming of voltage-gated calcium channels. Neuron **13:** 505–506.

8. DUNLAP, K., J. I. LUEBKE & T. J. TURNER. 1995. Exocytotic Ca^{2+} channels in mammalian central neurons. Trends Neurosci. **18:** 89–98.

9. LEMOS, J. R. & M. C. NOWYCKY. 1989. Two types of calcium channels coexist in peptide-releasing vertebrate nerve terminals. Neuron **2:** 1419–1426.

10. REGEHR, W. & I. M. MINTZ. 1994. Participation of multiple calcium channel types in transmission at single climbing fiber to Purkinje cell synapses. Neuron **12:** 605–613.

11. TAKAHASHI, T. & A. MOMIYAMA. 1993. Different types of calcium channels mediate central synaptic transmission. Nature (Lond.) **366:** 156–158.

12. MINTZ, I. M., B. L. SABATINI & W. REGEHR. 1995. Calcium control of transmitter release at a cerebellar synapse. Neuron **15:** 675–688.

13. MINTZ, I. M., V. J. VENEMA, K. M. SWIDEREK et al. 1992. P-type calcium channels blocked by the spider toxin ω-Aga-IVA. Nature (Lond.) **355:** 827–829.

14. MINTZ, I. M., M. E. ADAMS & B. P. BEAN. 1992. P-type calcium channels in rat central and peripheral neurons. Neuron **9:** 85–95.

15. PROTTI, D. A. & O. D. UCHITEL. 1993. Transmitter release and presynaptic Ca^{2+} currents blocked by the spider toxin ω-Aga-IVA. Neuroreport **5:** 333–336.

16. FOX, A. P., M. C. NOWYCKY & R. W. TSIEN. 1987. Kinetic and pharmacological properties distinguishing three types of calcium currents in chick sensory neurons. J. Physiol. (Lond.) **394:** 149–172.

17. NILIUS, B., P. HESS, J. B. LANSMAN & R. W. TSIEN. 1985. A novel type of cardiac calcium channel in ventricular cells. Nature (Lond.) **316:** 443–446.

18. NOWYCKY, M. C., A. P. FOX & R. W. TSIEN. 1985. Three types of neuronal calcium channel with different calcium agonist sensitivity. Nature (Lond.) **316:** 440–443.

19. MUCHNIK, S., B. A. KOTSIAS & E. E. ARRIZURIETA DE MUCHNIK. 1975. In vivo and in vitro miniature end-plate potentials at various external K concentrations. Am. J. Physiol. **228:** 1733–1737.

20. SANO, K., K. ENOMOTO & T. MAENO. 1987. Effects of synthetic ω-conotoxin, a new type Ca^{2+} antagonist, on frog and mouse neuromuscular transmission. Eur. J. Pharmacol. **141:** 235–241.

21. GRINNELL, A. D. & P. A. PAWSON. 1989. Dependence of spontaneous release at frog junctions on synaptic strength, external calcium, and terminal length. J. Physiol. (Lond.) **418:** 397–410.

22. FUJITA, Y., M. MYNLIEFF, R. T. DIRKSEN *et al.* 1993. Primary structure and functional expression of the ω-conotoxin-sensitive N-type calcium channel from rabbit brain. Neuron **10:** 585–598.

23. ADLER, E. M., G. J. AGUSTINE, S. N. DUFFY & M. P. CHARLTON. 1991. Alien intracellular calcium chelators attenuate neurotransmitter release at the squid giant synapse. J. Neurosci. **11:** 1496–1507.

24. NEHER, E. 1986. Concentration profiles of intracellular calcium in the presence of a diffusible chelator. Exp. Brain Res. **14:** 80–96.

25. STERN, M. D. 1992. Buffering of calcium in the vicinity of a channel pore. Cell Calcium **13:** 183–192.

26. SCHWEIZER, F. E., H. BETZ & G. J. AGUSTINE. 1995. From vesicle docking to endocytosis: intermediate reactions of exocytosis. Neuron **14:** 689–696.

27. MUCHNIK, S. & R. A. VENOSA. 1969. Role of sodium ions in the response of the frequency of miniature end-plate potentials to osmotic changes in the neuromuscular junction. Nature (Lond.) **222:** 169–171.

Activation of Opioid Receptors Inhibits Neuronal-like Calcium Channels, Distal Steps of Secretion, and Cell Proliferation in Human Small Cell Lung Carcinoma Cells[a]

AGNESE CODIGNOLA,[b,c] CRISTINA MISSALE,[d] PIERFRANCO SPANO,[d]
FRANCESCO CLEMENTI,[b] EMILIO CARBONE,[e]
AND EMANUELE SHER[b,f]

[b]CNR Cellular and Molecular Pharmacology Center
20129 Milan, Italy

[d]Institute of Pharmacology and Experimental Therapeutics
25124 Brescia, Italy

[e]Department of Neuroscience
University of Torino
10125 Torino, Italy

INTRODUCTION

Small cell lung carcinoma (SCLC) cells express neuronal-like voltage-operated calcium channels (VOCCs)[1] and release mitogenic hormones, such as serotonin (5HT).[1] We have previously shown that GLC8 human SCLC cells express only δ opioid receptors and that the selective δ agonist, [D-Pen^2,Pen^5]-enkephalin (DPDPE), potently inhibits VOCCs.[2] This modulation is dose- and voltage-dependent, pertussis toxin (PTX)–sensitive, and cAMP-independent, and mainly affects N-type VOCCs; furthermore, it is blocked by the nonselective antagonist, naloxone, while neither μ (DAMGO) nor κ (U50488) agonists have any effect.[2] With the same potency and selectivity, DPDPE also antagonizes the Ca^{2+}-dependent release of [^{3}H]-5HT. However, DPDPE inhibits not only the depolarization-induced release, but also the Ca^{2+}-dependent secretion induced by thapsigargin or ionomycin.[2] This strongly suggests that, besides inhibiting VOCCs, opioids also exert a direct depressive action on the secretory apparatus. This latter effect is also PTX-sensitive, but contrary to VOCC modulation it can be reversed by elevations of cAMP level.[2] Opioid antimitogenic effects on SCLC have been described.[3] Here, we characterize this opioid effect on cell proliferation both "unstimulated" and stimulated by different means, such as cell depolarization, intracellular Ca^{2+} mobilization, cAMP elevation, or receptor activation.

[a]This work was supported by Telethon-Italy (Grant No. 858 to E. Sher).
[c]A. Codignola is a recipient of a fellowship from the Italian Association for Cancer Research (AIRC).
[f]To whom all correspondence should be addressed. Present address: Lilly Research Centre, Erl Wood Manor, Windlesham, Surrey GU20 6PH, United Kingdom.

METHODS

Human SCLC GLC8 cells, kindly provided by G. Gaudino (University of Torino, Italy), were grown in RPMI 1640 medium supplemented with 10% fetal calf serum in a humidified atmosphere of 10% CO_2 in air at 37 °C. *In vitro* SCLC cell proliferation was assessed using a standard [^{3}H]-thymidine incorporation assay.

RESULTS AND DISCUSSION

In the last few years, different opioid receptor subtypes, as well as controversial opioid effects on cell proliferation, have been described in human SCLC lines.[3,4] We have recently demonstrated that only δ opioid receptor mRNA is expressed in human GLC8 cells. Consequently, activation of δ opioid receptors leads to inhibition of both VOCCs and [^{3}H]-5HT release.[2] We now show that activation of δ opioid receptors causes inhibition of both basal and stimulated *in vitro* cell proliferation, while neither μ nor κ is involved. As shown in FIGURE 1A, basal SCLC cell proliferation is dose-dependently inhibited by DPDPE, but not by the selective μ agonist DAMGO nor by the κ agonist U50488, and this block is abolished by the nonselective antagonist, naloxone (1 μM). As demonstrated for inhibition of both VOCCs and [^{3}H]-5HT release, also in this case DPDPE effects are mediated by a PTX-sensitive G protein: simultaneous incubation with PTX (0.1 ng/mL) reduced the inhibition obtained with 1 μM DPDPE from 63.5 ± 3.5% to 3 ± 3%. PTX alone does not have any effect on basal cell proliferation.

δ opioid receptors undergo desensitization and downregulation when chronically stimulated. In parallel, a compensatory increase in adenyl cyclase activity could be observed, suggesting a cellular adaptation to prolonged δ activation. On the other hand, δ opioid receptor activation effects on cell proliferation are usually detected after several days of treatment. We then measured the time-dependence of DPDPE effects on cell proliferation: FIGURE 1B shows that the inhibition of "unstimulated" proliferation is achieved after 5 days of treatment, with different doses of the drug.

DPDPE action is effective also on "stimulated" SCLC cell proliferation, as shown in FIGURE 2. Depolarization evoked by KC1 dose-dependently stimulates cell proliferation (38.2 ± 9.7% with 10 mM, 82 ± 12% with 20 mM, 143.5 ± 8.5% with 40 mM, and 144.7 ± 11% with 60 mM KC1): DPDPE at 1 μM reduces the response to maximal (60 mM) KC1 to 53 ± 7% (63.37% of inhibition). Internal Ca^{2+} mobilization by means of the Ca^{2+}/ATPase inhibitor, thapsigargin (1 μM), also leads to a stimulation of cell proliferation (85 ± 2.5% increase over basal): DPDPE (1 μM) reduces this increase to 50.5 ± 2.5%.

Recently, we demonstrated the dose-dependent mitogenic effect of exogenous 5HT on SCLC cell proliferation.[5] At 1 μM, 5HT stimulates SCLC proliferation by 111 ± 12%, while in the presence of DPDPE (1 μM) this effect is only 36 ± 4.2%.

Finally, elevation of intracellular cAMP with 10 mM $N^6,2'$-O-dibutyryladenosine $3',5'$-cyclic monophosphate (Bt$_2$cAMP) causes a dose-dependent stimulation of SCLC cell proliferation (0% with 10 μM, 16 ± 1% with 100 μM, 43 ± 6.1% with 1 mM, and 63.4 ± 4.2% with 10 mM), which is counteracted by the simultaneous administration of 1 μM DPDPE (33.6 ± 5.3% of increase).

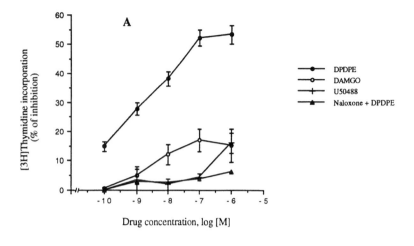

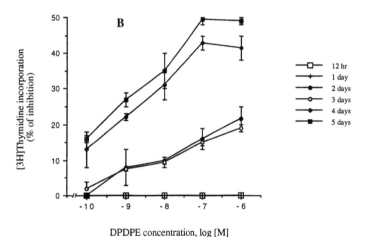

FIGURE 1. Opioid receptor effects on basal SCLC proliferation. (A) Pharmacological char-acterization indicates that only the δ selective agonist DPDPE inhibits SCLC cell proliferation, while neither the selective μ agonist DAMGO nor the κ agonist U50488 has any effect. This action is totally blocked by the nonselective antagonist naloxone at 1 μM, which, alone, does not exhibit antiproliferative activity (not shown). DPDPE effect is dose-dependent and reaches its maximum (53.3 ± 3.1% of inhibition) at 1 μM, the concentration therefore used for further characterization. (B) Time course of DPDPE effects on unstimulated cell proliferation. The maximal inhibition (49 ± 1%) is achieved after 5 days of treatment, with different doses of DPDPE; no effect is detectable before 2 days of exposure.

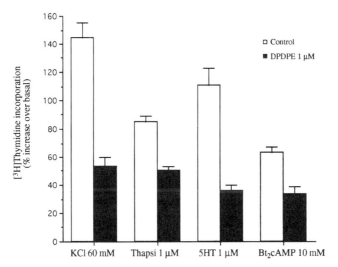

FIGURE 2. DPDPE effects on stimulated SCLC proliferation. DPDPE exerts its action not only on basal SCLC cell proliferation, but also on proliferation stimulated by different agents. Depolarization with KCl (60 mM) causes an increase in cell proliferation of 144.7 ± 11%, reduced to 53 ± 7% in the presence of 1 μM DPDPE. Also, intracellular Ca^{2+} mobilization by means of thapsigargin (1 μM) stimulates cell proliferation by 85 ± 2.5%, and this stimulation is decreased to 50.5 ± 2.5% when 1 μM DPDPE is added simultaneously (41.6% of inhibition). Serotonin (1 μM) administration as well as an increase in the intracellular cAMP levels with Bt_2cAMP (10 mM) result in stimulation of cell proliferation (111 ± 4.2% and 63.4 ± 5.3%, respectively). Both these effects are reduced by 1 μM DPDPE to 36 ± 4.2% (67.5% of inhibition) and 33.6 ± 5.3% (47% of inhibition), respectively. Each point in the curves represents the average ± SE of 3–5 experiments performed in quadruplicate in human SCLC GLC8 cells.

These data, together with those recently reported,[2] help in elucidating the complex mechanisms of opioid action in SCLC (reduction both in Ca^{2+} influx and in released hormones, and inhibition of cell proliferation) and indicate that the antimitogenic action is specific and potentially useful in exploring new therapeutic strategies.

All the data presented here have been confirmed in another human SCLC cell line (NCI-N592, not shown).

REFERENCES

1. CODIGNOLA, A., P. TARRONI, F. CLEMENTI, A. POLLO, M. LOVALLO, E. CARBONE & E. SHER. 1993. Calcium channel subtypes controlling serotonin release from a human small-cell lung carcinoma cell line. J. Biol. Chem. **268:** 26240–26247.
2. SHER, E., P. CESARE, A. CODIGNOLA, F. CLEMENTI, P. TARRONI, A. POLLO, V. MAGNELLI & E. CARBONE. 1996. Activation of δ-opioid receptors inhibits neuronal-like calcium channels and distal steps of Ca^{2+}-dependent secretion in human small-cell lung carcinoma cells. J. Neurosci. **16**(11): 3672–3684.

3. MANECKJEE, R. & J. D. MINNA. 1990. Opioid and nicotine receptors affect growth regulation of human lung cancer cell lines. Proc. Natl. Acad. Sci. U.S.A. **87:** 3294–3298.
4. ROTH, K. A. & J. D. BARCHAS. 1985. Small-cell carcinoma cell lines contain opioid peptides and receptors. Cancer Res. **45:** 760–773.
5. CATTANEO, M. G., A. CODIGNOLA, L. M. VICENTINI, F. CLEMENTI & E. SHER. 1993. Nicotine stimulates a serotonergic autocrine loop in human small cell lung carcinoma. Cancer Res. **53:** 5566–5568.

Downregulation of Nicotinic Acetylcholine Receptors by Nerve Growth Factor in Human Small Cell Lung Carcinoma Cell Lines[a]

AGNESE CODIGNOLA,[b,c] CRISTINA MISSALE,[d] PIERFRANCO SPANO,[d] FRANCESCO CLEMENTI,[b] AND EMANUELE SHER[b,e]

[b]CNR Cellular and Molecular Pharmacology Center
20129 Milan, Italy

[d]Institute of Pharmacology and Experimental Therapeutics
25124 Brescia, Italy

INTRODUCTION

Proliferation of small cell lung carcinoma (SCLC) is controlled by autocrine loops sustained by the secretion of different neurohormones and growth factors such as bombesin, insulinlike growth factor 1, bradykinin, neurotensin, cholecystokinin, and vasopressin.[1] A mitogenic autocrine loop mediated by serotonin (5HT) and modulated by neuronal-type nicotinic receptors (nAChRs) has been recently shown in SCLC.[2–5] Endogenously produced 5HT has in fact a remarkable effect on SCLC proliferation, and nicotine indirectly increases SCLC cell proliferation by specifically stimulating 5HT secretion.[2]

Nerve growth factor (NGF) is a neurotrophic protein involved in survival, growth, and differentiation of peripheral neurons of the sympathetic nervous system. NGF effects are mediated by the interaction with specific membrane receptors, composed of two different proteins: a 140-kDa tyrosine kinase, $trkA$ (gp140^{trkA}), and a 75-kDa glycoprotein (gp75^{NGFR}). The presence of the two receptors in SCLC cells has been previously reported.[6] However, the specific role exerted by NGF in the tumoral progression mechanisms has not been investigated in detail.

Here, we show that, in two human SCLC cell lines (GLC8 and NCI-N592), chronic NGF treatment remarkably inhibits both "basal" and nicotine-stimulated *in vitro* SCLC cell proliferation, while 5HT-stimulated SCLC cell proliferation is not affected by NGF. In parallel, nicotine-evoked [^{3}H]5HT release is totally abolished after NGF treatment, while KC1-stimulated secretion remains normal. These data suggest that NGF exerts its antimitogenic effects on SCLC cell proliferation at least partially by modulating the expression and/or function of the nAChRs present in these cells.

[a]This work was supported by Telethon-Italy (Grant No. 858 to E. Sher) and by the Italian Association for Cancer Research (AIRC) (grant to C. Missale).
[c]Recipient of a fellowship from AIRC.
[e]Address all correspondence to E. Sher at Lilly Research Centre, Erl Wood Manor, Windlesham, Surrey GU20 6PH, United Kingdom.

METHODS

Human SCLC GLC8 cells, kindly provided by G. Gaudino (University of Turin, Italy), and human NCI-N592 were grown in RPMI 1640 medium supplemented with 10% fetal calf serum, in a humidified atmosphere of 10% CO_2 in air at 37 °C. Cells were treated with human recombinant NGF 2.5S dissolved in RPMI 1640 for 15 days, and the medium was changed every 4 days.

In vitro SCLC cell proliferation was assessed using a standard [^{3}H]thymidine incorporation assay. [^{3}H]5HT release was performed as previously described.[2]

RESULTS AND DISCUSSION

Recently, we have studied the expression and the physiological role of nAChRs in human SCLC cell lines.[2–5] Furthermore, we have demonstrated the mitogenic effect of both exogenous nicotine and 5HT. NGF receptors are expressed in SCLC cells[6] and we recently found that their expression increases after NGF treatment, as well as the production of endogenous NGF (manuscript in preparation). An antiproliferative effect of NGF has been demonstrated in several neuronal and neuroendocrine cells. Here, we investigated whether NGF could influence the proliferative response of SCLC cells to both nicotine and 5HT.

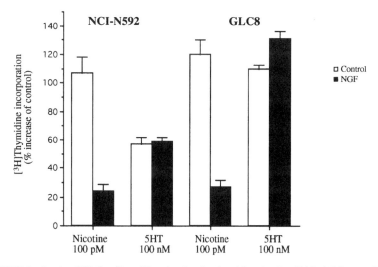

FIGURE 1. *In vitro* SCLC cell proliferation is stimulated by nicotine (100 pM) in two different human SCLC cell lines, NCI-N592 and GLC8 (107 ± 11% and 120 ± 10% over basal, respectively). NGF administration (50 ng/mL, 15 days) abolishes this stimulation (24 ± 5% and 27 ± 4.9% over basal, respectively). Also, 5HT (100 mM) is able to stimulate [^{3}H]thymidine incorporation by 57 ± 5% over basal in NCI-N592 and by 110 ± 3% over basal in GLC8 cells. In this case, NGF (50 ng/mL, 15 days) treatment does not have any inhibitory effect, with the stimulation being 59 ± 3% over basal in NCI-N592 and 131 ± 4.8% over basal in GLC8 cells.

As shown in FIGURE 1, 100 pM nicotine stimulates [³H]thymidine incorporation by 107 ± 11% in NCI-N592 cells and by 120 ± 10% in GLC8 cells. This mitogenic effect is probably due to the stimulation of secretion of different hormones, including 5HT. After chronic NGF administration (50 ng/mL, 15 days), this stimulation is strongly reduced (24 ± 5% and 27 ± 4.8% increase over "basal" proliferation in NCI-N592 and GLC8 cells, respectively). Exogenous 5HT (100 nM) also induces SCLC cell proliferation, causing an increase of 57 ± 5% in NCI-N592 and of 110 ± 3% in GLC8 cells. Moreover, NGF treatment did not influence the stimulatory action of 5HT (59 ± 3% increase in NCI-N592 and 131 ± 4.8 in GLC8 cells). This suggests that NGF action could be selective for the nicotinic receptors present in SCLC cells.

To confirm this idea, we studied the modulation exerted by NGF treatment on [³H]5HT release (FIGURE 2). Nicotine (100 nM) stimulates [³H]5HT release in both NCI-N592 and GLC8 SCLC cells (18 ± 2% and 23 ± 2% increase over basal, respectively). After NGF administration (50 ng/mL, 15 days), the response to nicotine is abolished (2.6 ± 1.8% and 2 ± 2% increase in NCI-N592 and GLC8, respectively). Also, in this case, the modulatory NGF effect is specific since the release of [³H]5HT stimulated by depolarization with KC1 (50 mM) is not affected (20.6 ± 1.8% in control versus 19 ± 1% in NGF-treated NCI-N592 cells, and 22 ± 3% in control versus 21 ± 2% in NGF-treated GLC8 cells).

These data indicate that NGF treatment could inhibit the expression, the assembly, or the function of neuronal nAChR in SCLC cells; however, transducing steps down-

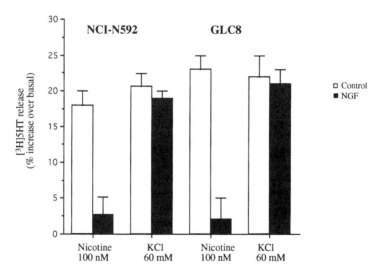

FIGURE 2. [³H]5HT release from both NCI-N592 and GLC8 human SCLC cells is stimulated by nicotine (100 nM) (18 ± 2% and 23 ± 2% increase over basal, respectively). After NGF administration (50 ng/mL, 15 days), neither NCI-N592 nor GLC8 cells respond anymore to 100 nM nicotine (2.6 ± 2% and 2 ± 2% increase over basal, respectively). On the contrary, [³H]5HT release evoked by depolarization with KC1 (50 mM) is not affected by NGF treatment (20.6 ± 1.8% in control versus 19 ± 1% in NGF-treated NCI-N592 cells, and 22 ± 3% in control versus 21 ± 2% in NGF-treated GLC8 cells).

stream of nAChRs activation could also be selectively modulated: the mechanisms underlying these NGF effects are still under investigation.

ACKNOWLEDGMENTS

We thank Genentech (San Francisco, California) for providing the human recombinant NGF (collaboration program no. 120912).

REFERENCES

1. CARNEY, D. N. 1992. Biology of small-cell lung cancer. Lancet **339:** 843–846.
2. CATTANEO, M. G., A. CODIGNOLA, L. M. VICENTINI, F. CLEMENTI & E. SHER. 1993. Nicotine stimulates a serotonergic autocrine loop in human small cell lung carcinoma. Cancer Res. **53:** 5566–5568.
3. CODIGNOLA, A., P. TARRONI, M. G. CATTANEO, L. M. VICENTINI, F. CLEMENTI & E. SHER. 1994. Serotonin release and cell proliferation are under the control of α-bungarotoxin-sensitive nicotinic receptors in small-cell lung carcinoma cell lines. FEBS Lett. **342:** 286–290.
4. CODIGNOLA, A., J. M. McINTOSH, M. G. CATTANEO, L. M. VICENTINI, F. CLEMENTI & E. SHER. 1996. α-Conotoxin Imperialis I inhibits nicotine-evoked hormone release and cell proliferation in human neuroendocrine carcinoma cells. Neurosci. Lett. **206:** 53–56.
5. TARRONI, P., F. RUBBOLI, B. CHINI, R. ZWAART, M. OORTGIESEN, E. SHER & F. CLEMENTI. 1992. Neuronal-type nicotinic receptors in human neuroblastoma and small-cell lung carcinoma cell lines. FEBS Lett. **312:** 66–70.
6. OELMANN, E., L. SRETER, I. SHULLER, H. SERVE, M. KOENINGSMANN, B. WIEDENMANN, D. OBERBERG, B. REUFI, E. THIEL & W. E. BERDEL. 1995. Nerve growth factor stimulates clonal growth of human lung cancer cell lines and a human glioblastoma cell line expressing high-affinity nerve growth factor binding sites involving tyrosine kinase signaling. Cancer Res. **55:** 2212–2219.

A Small Cell Lung Carcinoma Line and Subclone Expressing Nicotinic Acetylcholine Receptors of Muscle and Neuronal Types[a]

MICHELE A. SCIAMANNA,[b] GUY E. GRIESMANN,
AND VANDA A. LENNON[c]

*Departments of Immunology, Neurology, and
Laboratory Medicine and Pathology
Mayo Clinic
Rochester, Minnesota 55905*

INTRODUCTION

We have established in culture a cell line (SCC-37) derived from a metastatic small cell lung carcinoma (SCLC) of a patient who had myasthenia gravis (MG).[1,2] Unlike other SCLC lines,[3,4] SCC-37 expresses nicotinic (n) acetylcholine receptors (AChRs) of muscle type. Here, we summarize evidence that another α-bungarotoxin (α-BTx)–sensitive nAChR, with properties attributable to neuronal α_7 subunits, is coexpressed with muscle-type nAChR in SCC-37 cells and in a subclone, SCC-A9.

METHODS

Human cell lines used as controls were TE-671, a rhabdomyosarcoma expressing muscle-type nAChR,[5] and IMR-32, a peripheral neuroblastoma expressing neuronal-type nAChRs, including the α-BTx-sensitive α_7 subtype.[6] Cells were grown to confluency on a 24-well plate. Agonist-initiated ion influx (based on methods of Sine[5]) and ^{125}I-α-BTx binding assays (4.2 nM for 90 minutes) were performed at 37 °C. Cells were then washed and lifted, and β and γ emissions were counted. The antigenicity of α-BTx receptors was assayed by immunoprecipitation with rat IgG MAbs that distinguish α_1 from α_7 nAChRs.

RESULTS

The agonist carbachol stimulated influx of $^{22}Na^+$ in the parental cell line SCC-37, but not in the subclone SCC-A9 (FIGURE 1A). This response was inhibited by α-BTx

[a]The laboratory work was supported by grants from the National Cancer Institute (No. CA-37343) and the Admadjaja Thymoma Research Program.
[b]Recipient of a Sosin Fellowship from the National Myasthenia Gravis Foundation.
[c]To whom all correspondence should be addressed.

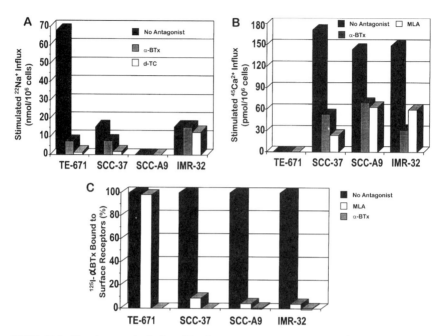

FIGURE 1. The pharmacological profile of agonist-stimulated Na^+ and Ca^{2+} influx, and of α-BTx binding to surface receptors, was determined by preincubating human tumor cell lines with an antagonist, namely, 0.1 μM α-BTx (90 min), 1 mM d-tubocurarine (dTC), or 10 μM methyllycaconitine (MLA) (each 15 min). (A) Carbachol (1 mM) stimulates $^{22}Na^+$ influx. (B) Cytisine (1 mM) stimulates $^{45}Ca^{2+}$ influx. (C) Binding of ^{125}I-α-BTx to receptors on living cells. Nonspecific binding was subtracted (determined in the presence of a stoichiometric excess of carbachol, 0.1 M).

and by dTC. Na^+ influx in IMR-32 was via non-α-BTx-sensitive nAChRs.[6] The agonist cytisine induced influx of $^{45}Ca^{2+}$ in both SCC-37 and SCC-A9, and in IMR-32. This response was inhibited by α-BTx and by MLA, a specific antagonist of α-BTx-sensitive neuronal nAChRs[7] (FIGURE 1B). Cytisine did not induce measurable $^{45}Ca^{2+}$ influx in the muscle line, TE-671. The pharmacological profiles of cytisine-initiated Ca^{2+} influx responses in SCC-37, SCC-A9, and IMR-32 are all consistent with activation of a neuronal-type nAChR containing α_7 subunits. Surface receptors for ^{125}I-α-BTx on both SCC-37 and SCC-A9 cells were blocked by α-BTx and MLA (FIGURE 1C). The results of ion influx and α-BTx binding assays imply that the SCC-37 cell line expresses functional nAChRs of both muscle and neuronal (α_7) types in its plasma membrane, while the subclone SCC-A9 expresses in its plasma membrane only neuronal-type nAChR (α_7). Receptors extracted from whole SCC-37 and SCC-A9 cells exhibited both α_1 and α_7 immunoreactivities (TABLE 1).

TABLE 1. Antigenicity of Combined Surface and Cytoplasmic Receptors[a]

		Antigenicity of Total Cell α-BTx Receptors	
Cell Line	Cell Type	α_1-Positive (MAb 35)	α_7-Positive (MAb P27)
TE-671	muscle	+	−
SCC-37	neuroendocrine	+	+
SCC-A9	neuroendocrine	+	+
IMR-32	neuron	−	+

[a]Whole cell lysates prepared in Triton X-100 buffers were clarified and complexed with ^{125}I-α-BTx (1 nM). Antigenicity of combined surface and cytoplasmic receptors was determined by immunoprecipitation. Specific binding was determined by subtracting cpm precipitated with irrelevant control rat Igs. MAb 35 distinguishes muscle-type α-BTx receptors from neuronal-type α-BTx receptors;[14] MAb P27 has converse immunoreactivity, binding selectively to α-BTx receptors derived from the neuroblastoma IMR-32, but not the skeletal muscle line TE-671. We produced the hybridoma secreting MAb P27 from the lymph node of a rat hyperimmunized with a synthetic peptide corresponding to human α_7 subunit residues 403–430.[15]

DISCUSSION

Several different types of AChR have been described in SCLC lines. These include neuronal nAChRs (both classical[8,9] and α-BTx-sensitive[4,10]) and muscarinic AChRs of M_3 subtype.[11,12] SCC-37 is unique among SCLC lines by expressing muscle-type nAChR. The original patient's development of autoimmune MG is attributed to an antibody response initiated by an immunogenic mutant form of this tumor protein.[1,2] Coexpression of both muscle and neuronal nAChRs has been reported previously in developing chick muscle cells.[13] In a highly malignant neoplasm like SCLC, these receptors would provide a mechanism for regulating Na^+ and Ca^{2+} influx, perhaps through activation by an extracellular matrix–associated agonist. Signaling via nicotinic and muscarinic AChRs in SCLC might regulate tumor growth by facilitating or inhibiting the opening of high voltage–activated Ca^{2+} channels involved in the autocrine release of growth factors.[4,11] Thus, the study of ion channels and related molecules expressed in tumors derived from patients with paraneoplastic myasthenic syndromes is pertinent to the molecular mechanisms of tumor growth as well as to the initiation of autoimmunity.

REFERENCES

1. GRIESMANN, G. E. *et al.* 1994. Muscle-type nicotinic acetylcholine receptors (AChR) expressed aberrantly in small cell lung carcinoma (SCLC) of a patient with myasthenia gravis. Muscle Nerve (Suppl.) **1:** S185.
2. GREISMANN, G. E. *et al.* 1996. Mutated autoantigen predicted by alternative RNA splicing in the P5 exon of nicotinic acetylcholine receptor (AChR) α_1 subunit expressed in a small cell lung carcinoma cell line. Mol. Biol. Cell (Suppl.) **7:** 254a.
3. CUNNINGHAM, J. M. *et al.* 1985. Acetylcholine receptors in small cell carcinomas. J. Neurochem. **45:** 159–167.

4. CODIGNOLA, A. *et al.* 1993. Calcium channel subtypes controlling serotonin release from human small cell lung carcinoma cell lines. J. Biol. Chem. **268:** 26240–26247.

5. SINE, S. M. 1988. Functional properties of human skeletal muscle acetylcholine receptors expressed by the TE671 cell line. J. Biol. Chem. **263:** 18052–18062.

6. LUKAS, R. J. 1993. Expression of ganglia-type nicotinic acetylcholine receptors and nicotinic ligand binding sites by cells of the IMR-32 human neuroblastoma clonal line. J. Pharmacol. Exp. Ther. **265:** 294–302.

7. ALKONDON, M. *et al.* 1992. Blockade of nicotinic currents in hippocampal neurons defines methyllycaconitine as a potent and specific receptor antagonist. Mol. Pharmacol. **41:** 802–808.

8. MANECKJEE, R. & J. D. MINNA. 1990. Opioid and nicotine receptors affect growth regulation of human lung cancer cell lines. Proc. Natl. Acad. Sci. U.S.A. **87:** 3294–3298.

9. TARRONI, P. *et al.* 1992. Neuronal-type nicotinic receptors in human neuroblastoma and small-cell lung carcinoma cell lines. FEBS Lett. **312:** 66–70.

10. CODIGNOLA, A. *et al.* 1994. Serotonin release and cell proliferation are under the control of α-bungarotoxin-sensitive nicotinic receptors in small-cell lung carcinoma cell lines. FEBS Lett. **342:** 286–290.

11. WILLIAMS, C. L. & V. A. LENNON. 1990. Activation of M_3 muscarinic acetylcholine receptors inhibits voltage-dependent calcium influx in small cell lung carcinoma. J. Biol. Chem. **265:** 1443–1447.

12. WILLIAMS, C. L. & V. A. LENNON. 1991. Activation of muscarinic acetylcholine receptors inhibits cell cycle progression of small cell lung carcinoma. Mol. Biol. Cell **2:** 373–382.

13. CORRIVEAU, R. A. *et al.* 1995. Expression of neuronal acetylcholine receptor genes in vertebrate skeletal muscle during development. J. Neurosci. **15:** 1372–1383.

14. LINDSTROM, J. *et al.* 1989. Molecular studies of neuronal nicotinic acetylcholine receptor family. Mol. Neurobiol. **1:** 281–337.

15. PENG, X. *et al.* 1994. Human α_7 acetylcholine receptor: cloning of the α_7 subunit from the SH-SY5Y cell line and determination of pharmacological properties of native receptors and functional α_7 homomers expressed in *Xenopus* oocytes. Mol. Pharmacol. **45:** 546–554.

Neuromuscular Blockade by Immunoglobulin G from Patients with Miller Fisher Syndrome[a]

BRIGITTE BUCHWALD,[b] JOSEF DUDEL,[c] AND KLAUS V. TOYKA[b]

[b]Department of Neurology
University of Würzburg
97080 Würzburg, Germany

[c]Institute of Physiology
Technical University of Munich
Munich, Germany

INTRODUCTION

Miller Fisher syndrome (MFS) is an acute and usually self-limiting neuropathic disorder characterized by ophthalmoplegia, ataxia, and areflexia, sometimes associated with facial and bulbar weakness.[1] It is thought to represent a variant of the Guillain-Barré syndrome, with which its shares clinical and neurophysiological features. The pathogenesis unique to MFS is still unknown. Recently, a neuromuscular blocking factor has been described in the serum of patients with MFS.[2] It has been postulated that this factor may be related to immunoglobulin G (IgG) autoantibodies directed at the ganglioside GQ1b. These ganglioside antibodies are found in acute phase sera of more than 90% of MFS patients.[3] We investigated the effect of MFS serum and immunoglobulin on neuromuscular transmission[4] and addressed the questions of which serum component mediates the observed blockade and what is the physiological mechanism of the transmission failure.

MATERIALS AND METHODS

Serum Fractions

Plasma from two patients with clinical signs of typical MFS was investigated. Serum antibodies to GQ1b were determined by ELISA and dot-blot assay. Patient 1 had mild generalized muscle weakness and complete extraocular muscle paralysis. Patient 2 had complete extraocular muscle paralysis and no generalized muscle weakness, but severe ataxia. Both patients rapidly recovered after plasma exchange treatment. By ELISA (enzyme-linked immunosorbent assay),[5] serum IgG antibodies to ganglioside GQ1b were detectable (serum titer, 200) in patient 1 (subsequently referred to as GQ1b positive), whereas in patient 2 these antibodies could not be detected (GQ1b negative). The serum of patient 2 was also negative for a panel of other

[a]This work was supported in part by Gemeinützige Hertie Stiftung, by University funds (Klinische Forschungsgruppe für Multiple Sklerose und Neuroimmunologie), and by the Sonderforschungsbereich 391 of the Deutsche Forschungsgemeinschaft.

gangliosides by dot-blot assay.[5] Both patients had no antibodies to acetylcholine receptor detectable by radioimmunoassay (modified Lindstrom assay).[6]

Plasma was obtained at therapeutic plasmapheresis. After removing fibrinogen, plasma samples were applied to a gel filtration column stocked with Sepharyl S-300 (Pharmacia, Freiburg, Germany). Fractions containing IgG were further purified by affinity chromatography using Gammabind G Sepharose (Pharmacia). IgM was prepared with Con A Sepharose affinity chromatography (Pharmacia). Purity of all fractions was assayed by SDS-PAGE.[7] All materials were diluted with the assay buffer (see below) during the final chromatographic step. Purified IgG showed bands identical to a standard IgG fraction. There was no IgG in the IgM preparation, nor IgM in the IgG preparation, as confirmed by nephelometry and SDS-PAGE.

The preparation of Fab fragments was carried out as described by Porter with some modifications:[8] IgG was digested by mercuripapain (Serva) and purified by chromatography on DEAE-Sephadex A 50 (Pharmacia). Control IgG was prepared from a commercial polyclonal IgG preparation (VenimmunR, Behringwerke, Marburg, Germany).

Nerve-Muscle Preparation

Adult mice (Balb/c, 12 to 16 weeks old) were killed by cervical dislocation, and the diaphragm with its phrenic nerve was dissected out. Hemidiaphragms were pinned down in a bath chamber and superfused with oxygenated (95% O_2, 5% CO_2) Bretag solution[9] containing (in mM) the following: NaCl (108), KCl (3.5), $CaCl_2$ (1.5), $MgSO_4$ (0.7), $NaHCO_3$ (26), NaH_2PO_4 (1.7), Na-gluconate (9.7), glucose (5.5), and saccharose (7.6), pH 7.4. Temperature was held at 20 °C by a thermostat.

Electrophysiology

End plate currents were recorded through a perfused macropatch-clamp electrode (FIGURE 1). The electrode had an approximately 10-μm-wide opening and contained a current clamp recording input as well as a stimulation electrode through which current pulses were applied to depolarize the nerve terminal in a graded manner by shifting the extracellular field potential. In addition to the two silver–silver chloride wires, each electrode was equipped with a fine tube that enabled perfusion of the tip of the electrode with pressurized solution, exchanging the volume at the tip of the electrode several hundred times per second. The standard solution for electrode perfusion was a buffer containing 162 mM NaCl, 5.3 mM KCl, 2 mM $CaCl_2$, 0.67 mM NaH_2PO_4, 15 mM HEPES (N-2-hydroxyethylpiperazine-N'-2-ethanesulfonic acid), and 5.6 mM glucose, pH 7.4. In order to prevent local excitation, 2×10^{-7} M tetrodotoxin (TTX) (Sigma) was added to the perfusate of the electrode. For direct application to the nerve terminal, the IgG was added to the perfusate of the electrode while recording from a given synaptic site.

For the measurements of quantal release, the effects of $N = 2^8$ to 2^{12} pulses were evaluated. An automatic discriminator determined whether any release occurred dur-

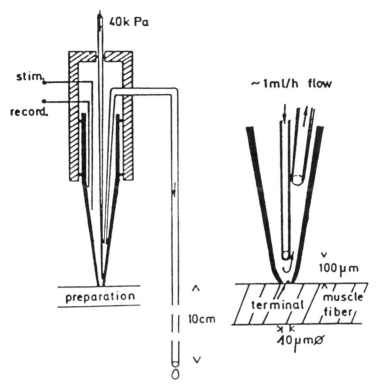

FIGURE 1. Schematic drawing of the perfused macropatch-clamp electrode. The glass electrode (dark black) contains two silver wires for stimulation and recording, and tubes for inflow and outflow of solution. A higher magnification of the tip of the electrode shows the approximately 10-μm-wide opening and the position of the polyethylene tubes. Reprinted with permission from reference 11.

ing a time window of 4 ms after each pulse and counted the rate of failures (N_0). Since control quantal excitatory postsynaptic currents (qEPSCs) were at least 10 times larger than the noise level, the discriminator worked reliably even when qEPSCs were reduced in amplitude. The average quantal release m was calculated from the proportion of failures, N_0/N, using the Poisson formula, $m = \ln(N/N_0)$.[10]

RESULTS AND DISCUSSION

In the first part of the study, we investigated a highly purified Ig fraction from plasma filtrate of a patient with typical MFS containing antibodies to the ganglioside GQ1b. Under control conditions, quantal content remained stable over about 3 hours at a given nerve terminal. As depicted in FIGURE 2, the addition of the MFS-Ig, at a concentration similar to human serum (5.93 g/L IgG, 0.015 g/L IgA, 0.71 g/L IgM, and 0.07 g/L albumin), decreased quantal content m by 20-fold within 2 minutes. Returning to control solution (washout), m came back to the baseline level within 15 minutes. This completely reversible blockade could be observed repeatedly at the same nerve terminal.

To find out which Ig fraction was responsible for the observed depression of release, purified IgM and IgG solutions from the same MFS patient were applied separately at the same concentration as before. During application of the MFS-IgM, quantal release remained at the same level ($m = 1.0134 \pm 0.19$, mean $\pm$ SD relative to the control normalized at 1). After application of the MFS-IgG, quantal content was nearly completely blocked ($m = 0.0012 \pm 0.0007$) within 2 minutes. This fast and fully reversible blockade of neuromuscular transmission could also be observed after application of monovalent Fab fragments ($m = 0.076 \pm 0.026$) from the same patient at equimolar concentrations. Application of MFS-IgG from patient 2 without any detectable ganglioside antibodies also depressed evoked quantal release ($m = 0.011 \pm 0.003$). Application of control IgG from healthy donors ($m = 1.01 \pm 0.13$) or from patients with other neurological diseases such as spasmodic torticollis did not cause any blocking effect (FIGURE 3).

Due to the procedure of its preparation, the applied MFS-IgG did not contain

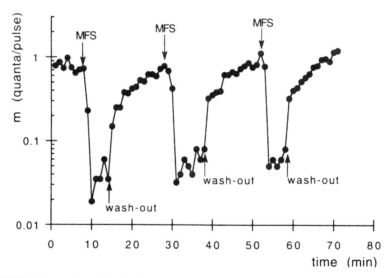

FIGURE 2. Depression of evoked quantal release by MFS plasma filtrate. Quantal content m (quanta/pulse, logarithmic ordinate scale) versus time in minutes (abscissa). Each point of the curve was determined from the results of at least 256 stimuli; quantal content was calculated using the Poisson formula. Plasma filtrate of an MFS patient (MFS) and control solution (washout) were applied. The arrows represent the time points of solution change in the electrode. Reprinted with permission from reference 4.

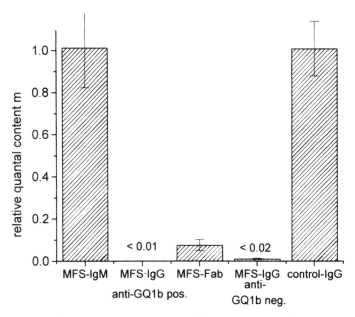

FIGURE 3. Reduction in quantal content m by different immunoglobulin preparations. The ordinate shows the quantal content m relative to the control normalized at 1 for each experiment; values are given as the mean ± SD. The abscissa shows the results for the highly purified IgM, IgG, and monovalent Fab fragments from patient 1 (anti-GQ1b positive), for the IgG of patient 2 (anti-GQ1b negative), and for the IgG preparation of healthy donors (control IgG).

complement factors or cytokines. The contamination with small peptides that theoretically could be missed by SDS-PAGE analysis was excluded by excessive dialysis using a 12-kDa cutoff tube. Efficacy of Fab fragments in our assay confirms the antibody nature of the observed blockade and demonstrates that receptor cross-linking is not likely to be an essential mechanism. Therefore, an antibody-antigen interaction is suggested as the basis for the observed blockade. In contrast to the generally held view that GQ1b is the crucial antigen, we found that the IgG fraction of an anti-GQ1b negative patient was as effective as the anti-GQ1b positive IgG fraction in blocking evoked quantal release (FIGURE 3).

In a further step, we examined the mechanism of the observed blockade in more detail. Further experiments were carried out to investigate the site of action of the MFS-IgG at the nerve terminal. The blockade by MFS-IgG could be overcome by stronger depolarization of the nerve terminal. FIGURE 4 plots quantal release m versus the depolarizing current. In the presence of MFS-IgG, the threshold depolarization for release, that is, the current needed to evoke any quantal release, was markedly increased. In general, the curve of quantal content versus depolarizing current was similar to that for controls, but obviously shifted to the right. This shift to the right resembles findings at the crayfish and frog neuromuscular junction, where lowering of the extracellular calcium concentration or prevention of calcium influx is known to

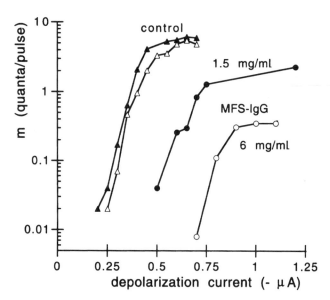

FIGURE 4. Depolarization dependence of the blockade. Quantal content m (ordinate, logarithmic scale) at different depolarization currents (1-ms pulse duration, abscissa). Filled triangles: controls at the beginning of the experiment; open triangles: repeated control after washout. After application of the MFS-IgG, the curve is shifted to larger depolarization currents. Open circles: MFS-IgG at 6 mg/mL; filled circles: MFS-IgG at 1.5 mg/mL. Each point of the curve was determined from the results of at least 256 stimuli, using up to 1028 stimuli at low release rates.

cause similar effects.[11,12]

We therefore studied the influence of the extracellular calcium concentration. MFS-IgG at two different calcium concentrations was applied at the same nerve terminal. At standard calcium concentration (2 mmol), the MFS-IgG caused the expected steep depression of release. After washout of MFS-IgG, the elevated calcium concentration (10 mmol) was applied. As shown in TABLE 1, the reduction in quantal content m by MFS-IgG could be significantly lessened by the additional calcium. Furthermore, the shift of the curve of quantal content versus depolarizing current could also be diminished by increasing the extracellular calcium concentration (not shown).

Taken together, these findings indicate that MFS-IgG may interfere with presynaptic calcium influx, possibly by blocking calcium channels. Alternatively, MFS-IgG may reduce the sensitivity of the release machinery to the intracellular calcium.

In a further step, we investigated whether the time course of release measured in distribution of the delays of quanta after the depolarizing pulse was affected by the MFS-IgG. Under control conditions, most events appeared within 4 ms after the stimulus and, after that period, only very few quanta were released (rate of late releas-

TABLE 1. Extent of Depression of Release at Different Calcium Concentrations

	Relative Quantal Content m (mean $\pm$ SD, $N = 5$) after Application of the MFS-IgG	
	At 2 mmol Calcium	At 10 mmol Calcium
Patient 1: anti-GQ1b positive	0.0029 ± 0.002	0.084 ± 0.009
Patient 2: anti-GQ1b negative	0.136 ± 0.026	0.415 ± 0.054

es under control conditions: 1.34 ± 0.13 quanta/pulse s^{-1}). After application of the MFS-IgG, these early evoked releases were nearly completely blocked, whereas the rate of late releases was rather doubled (2.21 ± 0.04 quanta/pulse s^{-1}). From the present data, it cannot be distinguished whether the occurrence of delayed releases is strictly stimulus-associated or not. Since we did not find an increase in spontaneous releases after application of MFS-IgG, we favor the possibility that, in MFS-IgG-treated end plates, the stimulus elicits a delayed asynchronous discharge of quanta. This dispersion of impulse-evoked release reminded us of the action of botulinum toxin, which is known to interfere with proteins of the exocytotic apparatus.[13] In contrast to botulinum toxin, these changes in time course by MFS-IgG were fully reversible after washout (0.78 ± 0.09 quanta/pulse s^{-1}).

We have investigated whether MFS-IgG has a postsynaptic action in addition to its obvious presynaptic effect. In the presence of MFS-IgG, the amplitude of single quanta was significantly reduced. Original recordings of qEPSCs in the control, during MFS-IgG, and after washout with all data recorded from the same nerve terminal are shown in FIGURE 5. With control solution, the average qEPSC amplitude was greater than 1 nA (1176.2 pA ± 26.2, mean $\pm$ SEM, $N = 322$). Plotted in a histogram, the distribution was Gaussian and even the smallest events were well above the noise level of the recording system. In contrast, after application of MFS-IgG, the amplitude histogram of the qEPSC was skewed with the smallest qEPSCs disappearing in the background noise. The apparent mean amplitudes were 2 times smaller (551.4 pA ± 17.3, $N = 248$) at MFS-IgG-treated end plates than at normal ones. After washout, mean amplitudes recovered fully (1341.4 pA ± 26.6, $N = 238$), indicating that the reduction in amplitude is not due to technical malfunction of the preparation or of the recording system, but rather represents an additional postsynaptic action of MFS-IgG.

Postsynaptically, the effects of MFS-IgG could be explained by a lowering of the acetylcholine receptor (AChR) channel conductance, by a decrease in the mean channel open time, or by the prevention of channel opening. The decay of qEPSC during application of control solution was 2.1 ± 0.01 ($N = 405$), which was not significantly different from decay during application of MFS-IgG ($\tau = 2.0 \pm 0.02$, $N = 210$). Therefore, we did not find that MFS-IgG induced changes in channel gating. The most-likely explanation is that MFS-IgG reduces the probability of the opening of postsynaptic channels or blocks the AChR reaction of some channels completely.

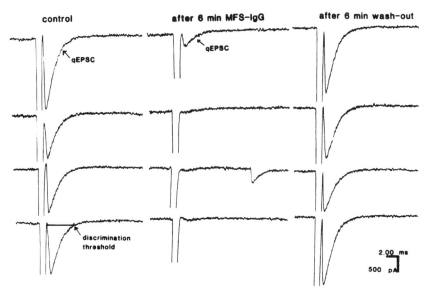

FIGURE 5. Reduction in amplitude of single quanta by the MFS-IgG. Original recordings through the perfused macropatch-clamp electrode. The partially compensated artifact is followed by quantal release (qEPSC) or failure. Currents surpassing the discrimination threshold were counted as release (at least one EPSC). In the left-hand and right-hand panels, the electrode was perfused with control solution; in the middle panels, the purified IgG fraction from patient 1 was applied. Note the reduction in amplitude of single quanta, the changes in time course, and the increase in delay time after the stimulus artifact (trace no. 3 of the middle panels). Reprinted with permission from reference 4.

CONCLUDING REMARKS

Our findings are in keeping with the hypothesis that MFS is an antibody-mediated disease of the motor nerve terminal.

In this respect, MFS resembles two other antibody-mediated disorders of the neuromuscular junction, namely, myasthenia gravis (MG) and Lambert-Eaton myasthenic syndrome (LEMS). In MG, antibodies of the IgG class and Fab fragments have been shown by passive transfer to mice to impair neuromuscular transmission[14,15] by an alteration of the postsynaptic receptor. In LEMS, IgG antibodies interfere with evoked release; LEMS IgG acts on presynaptic voltage-dependent Ca^{2+} channels to cause their loss of function by downregulation.[16–18] In contrast to MFS, the action of antibodies in MG and LEMS is more delayed. Effects that developed in the range of hours have been described for MG, LEMS, and MFS, whereas reversibility of the effects has not been examined. This very fast and fully reversible action of these antibodies of the IgG class directed to an undetermined antigen observed here in MFS is rather unique compared to the more delayed actions of antibodies in other disorders. Because of the time course and the reversibility of the reaction, it is unlikely that, in MFS, antibody binding leads to downregulation of the receptor or to morphological alterations of the nerve terminal; instead, it acts in a more direct receptor-blocking manner. Some hitherto unexplained pathophysiological features such as the rapid recovery of muscle strength after therapeutic plasmapheresis,[19,20] which occurs faster than remyelination, or sprouting at the neuromuscular junction could be possibly explained by the presence of humoral factors like IgG that interfere with presynaptic and postsynaptic ion channels as shown in this study.

FIGURE 6 summarizes the steps involved in neuromuscular transmission and some possible sites of action of MFS antibodies. The MFS-IgG does not seem to markedly affect action potentials in nerve terminals because the MFS-IgG still produces its main action in the absence of action potentials (in solutions containing TTX). Na channels would therefore not likely represent a major target of the MFS-IgG. Evidence for the action of MFS-IgG on presynaptic calcium inflow was obtained from studies of the quantal content versus depolarizing current dependence curves. The likely action of MFS-IgG on calcium inflow was supported by the finding that the increase of the extracellular calcium concentration obviously decreases the extent of depression of release and the shift of the quantal content versus depolarizing current curve by MFS-IgG. A further possible explanation is an interaction of MFS-IgG with processes occurring within the nerve terminal, such as changes of calcium sensitivity of the release machinery or interference with proteins of the exocytotic apparatus as

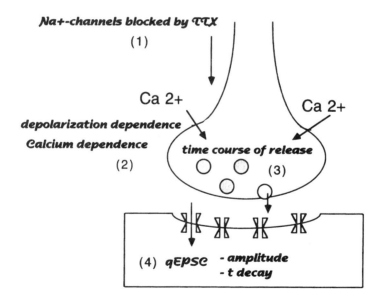

FIGURE 6. Schematic diagram of the neuromuscular junction. The general mode of synaptic transmission with the possible sites of action of the MFS-IgG and the proposed experiment to study each respective step is shown: (1) action potential; (2) Ca^{2+} influx through voltage-dependent Ca^{2+} channels; (3) intracellular processes—Ca^{2+} binding and cooperativity, vesicle fusion, and exocytosis; (4) postsynaptic site—reaction with the AChR and opening of its postsynaptic ion channels.

indicated by changes in the time course of quantal release. In addition to the striking presynaptic effect, MFS-IgG prevents the activation of postsynaptic channels, as indicated by a reduction in the amplitude of qEPSC.

Studies are currently under way to identify the putative ligand at the presynaptic and postsynaptic level possibly involved in the pathogenesis of MFS. We recently observed a similar activity of serum from a mother with Guillain-Barré syndrome and from her neonate infant with a transient paralytic syndrome, thus pointing to a more general relevance of neuromuscular blocking activity in immune-mediated neuropathies.[21]

ACKNOWLEDGMENTS

We thank A. Weishaupt for the preparation of the purified immunoglobulin fraction, J. Zielasek for performing the ganglioside antibody assays, and R. Hohlfeld for providing plasma samples from patient 2. For an extended account of the experiments described here, see references 4 and 22.

REFERENCES

1. FISHER, M. 1956. An unusual variant of acute idiopathic polyneuritis (syndrome of ophthalmoplegia, ataxia, and areflexia). N. Engl. J. Med. **255:** 57–65.
2. ROBERTS, M., H. WILLISON, A. VINCENT & J. NEWSOM-DAVIS. 1994. Serum factor in Miller-Fisher variant of Guillain-Barré syndrome and neurotransmitter release. Lancet **343:** 454–455.
3. YUKI, N., S. SATO, S. TSUJI, T. OHSAWA & T. MIYATAKE. 1993. Frequent presence of anti-GQ1b antibody in Fisher's syndrome. Neurology **43:** 414–417.
4. BUCHWALD, B., A. WEISHAUPT, K. V. TOYKA & J. DUDEL. 1995. Immunoglobulin G from patient with Miller-Fisher syndrome rapidly and reversibly depresses evoked quantal release at the neuromuscular junction of mice. Neurosci. Lett. **201:** 163–166.
5. ENDERS, U., H. KARCH, K. V. TOYKA, M. MICHELS, J. ZIELASEK, M. PETTE, J. HEESEMANN & H-P. HARTUNG. 1993. The spectrum of immune responses to *Campylobacter jejuni* and glycoconjugates in Guillain-Barré syndrome and in other neuroimmunological disorders. Ann. Neurol. **34:** 136–144.
6. BESINGER, U., K. V. TOYKA, M. HÖMBERG, K. HEININGER, R. HOHLFELD & A. FATEH-MOGHADAM. 1983. Myasthenia gravis: long-term correlation of binding and bungarotoxin blocking against acetylcholine receptors with changes in disease severity. Neurology **33**(10): 1316–1321.
7. LÄMMLI, U. K. 1970. Cleavage of structural proteins during the assembly of the head of bacteriophage T_4. Nature **227:** 680–685.
8. TOYKA, K. V., B. LÖWENADLER, K. HEININGER, U. A. BESINGER, K. L. BIRNBERGER, A. FATEH-MOGHADAM & E. HEILBRONN. 1980. Passively transferred myasthenia gravis: protection of mouse endplates by Fab fragments from human myasthenic IgG. J. Neurol. Neurosurg. Psychiatry **43:** 836–840.
9. BRETAG, A. H. 1969. Synthetic interstitial fluid for isolated mammalian tissue. Life Sci. **8:** 319–329.
10. DEL CASTILLO, J. & B. KATZ. 1954. Quantal components of the end-plate potential. J. Physiol. **124:** 560–573.

11. DUDEL, J. 1989. Calcium dependence of quantal release triggered by graded depolarization pulses to nerve terminals on crayfish and frog muscle. Pflügers Arch. **415:** 289–298.

12. DUDEL, J. 1992. Contribution of Ca^{2+} inflow to quantal, phasic transmitter release from nerve terminals of frog muscle. Pflügers Arch. **422:** 129–142.

13. VAN DER KLOOT, W. & J. MOLGÓ. 1994. Quantal acetylcholine release at the vertebrate neuromuscular junction. Physiol. Rev. **74**(4): 899–901.

14. TOYKA, K. V., D. B. DRACHMAN, D. E. GRIFFIN, A. PESTRONK, J. A. WINKELSTEIN, K. H. FISCHBECK & I. KAO. 1977. Myasthenia gravis: study of humoral immune mechanisms by passive transfer to mice. N. Engl. J. Med. **296:** 125–131.

15. STERZ, R., R. HOHLFELD, K. RAJKI, M. KAUL, K. HEININGER, K. PEPER & K. V. TOYKA. 1986. Effector mechanisms in myasthenia gravis: endplate function after passive transfer of IgG, Fab, and F(ab')2 hybrid molecules. Muscle Nerve **9:** 305–312.

16. LANG, B., J. NEWSOM-DAVIS, C. PRIOR & D. WRAY. 1983. Antibodies to motor nerve terminals: an electrophysiological study of a human myasthenic syndrome transferred to mouse. J. Physiol. **344:** 335–345.

17. LANG, B., J. NEWSOM-DAVIS, C. PEERS, C. PRIOR & D. W. WRAY. 1987. The effect of myasthenic syndrome antibody on presynaptic calcium channels in the mouse. J. Physiol. **390:** 257–270.

18. FUKUOKA, T., A. G. ENGEL, B. LANG, J. NEWSOM-DAVIS, C. PRIOR & D. W. WRAY. 1987. Lambert-Eaton myasthenic syndrome: I. Early morphological effects of IgG on the presynaptic membrane active zones. Ann. Neurol. **22:** 193–199.

19. YUKI, N. 1996. Acute paresis of extraocular muscles associated with IgG anti-GQ1b antibody. Ann. Neurol. **39:** 668–672.

20. WROBEL, C. J. & D. WATSON. 1992. Plasmapheresis in chronic demyelinating polyneuropathy. N. Engl. J. Med. **326:** 1089–1090.

21. LUIJCKX, G. J., J. VLES, M. DE BAETS, B. BUCHWALD & J. TROOST. 1997. Guillain-Barré syndrome in mother and newborn child. Lancet **349:** 27.

22. BUCHWALD, B., A. WEISHAUPT, K. V. TOYKA & J. DUDEL. 1998. Pre- and postsynaptic blockade of neuromuscular transmission by Miller-Fisher syndrome IgG at mouse motor nerve terminals. Eur. J. Neurosci. **10:** 101–110.

An Autoimmune Animal Model of the Lambert-Eaton Syndrome[a]

YONG I. KIM,[b] ERIC H. MIDDLEKAUFF,[b] MICHAEL P. VIGLIONE,[b]
JUN-ICHI OKUTSU,[c] YASUSHI SATOH,[c] NAOHIDE HIRASHIMA,[c]
AND YUTAKA KIRINO[c]

[b]Departments of Biomedical Engineering and Neurology
University of Virginia School of Medicine
Charlottesville, Virginia 22908

[c]School of Pharmaceutical Sciences
University of Tokyo
Bunkyo-ku, Tokyo 113, Japan

INTRODUCTION

Paraneoplastic neurological syndromes (PNS) are a collective group of disorders caused by immune responses against particular tumor antigens.[1] The most frequently encountered form of neoplasm in PNS is small-cell lung cancer, and one of the best defined PNS is the Lambert-Eaton myasthenic syndrome (LES). In LES, the autoantibodies pathologically compromise presynaptic function of the neuromuscular junction (NMJ) by impairing evoked quantal release of acetylcholine (ACh). The evidence implicating voltage-dependent calcium channels (VDCCs) as a primary target of these antibodies stemmed from diverse experimental studies. In patch-clamp assessment of the ion channel function, LES IgG was directly shown to inhibit the function of endogenous Ca^{2+} channels expressed in several cell types.[2,3] With no alteration in single-channel kinetics, the autoantibodies downregulate the number of functional VDCCs, presumably by cross-linking of the channels and antigenic modulation.[4]

Despite overwhelming evidence for an autoimmune pathogenesis, no animal model of LES by active immunization has been developed. Success in such a research effort will constitute ultimate verification of voltage-gated Ca^{2+} channels as a novel autoimmune triggering factor and as the putative autoantigen in the syndrome. The autoimmune animal model of LES will be a major advance in understanding this Ca^{2+} channel disorder and can be used to define and manipulate many immunological, morphological, and electrophysiological aspects of the disease. It may even provide new therapeutic approaches for the treatment of LES and related paraneoplastic disorders. Thus, the objective of our present work has been to develop and characterize

[a]This study was supported by research grants from the National Institutes of Health (No. NS-18607) (to Y. I. Kim), the Muscular Dystrophy Association (to Y. I. Kim), the Sankyo Foundation of Life Science (to Y. Kirino), and the Ministry of Education, Science, Sports, and Culture, Japan (Grants-in-Aid for Scientific Research, Nos. 06404076 and 08457591) (to Y. Kirino).

an active immunization model of the disorder—experimental autoimmune Lambert-Eaton syndrome.

In the study of experimental autoimmune myasthenia gravis, acetylcholine receptor (AChR) proteins isolated from postsynaptic membranes of *Torpedo* electric organ have served as a highly valuable antigen.[5] In a variety of animals immunized with this *Torpedo* preparation, clinical features of myasthenia gravis (MG) were consistently reproduced and the induction of pathologically active anti-AChR antibodies was ascertained. In an attempt to produce a similar autoimmune model, we have immunized mice and rats with synaptosomes isolated from the electric organ of Japanese electric ray, *Narke japonica*. These synaptosomes consist of pure cholinergic nerve terminals and are free from postsynaptic membranes. Their presynaptic mechanisms governing ACh transmitter release are similar to those demonstrated in the skeletal neuromuscular junction. Our recent pharmacological studies also revealed that these synaptosomes possess P/Q-, N-, and L-type Ca^{2+} channels.[6] This composition of the channels is similar to that found in H-146 small-cell lung cancer cells, the presumptive source of immunogen(s) in LES.[7] Furthermore, we have ascertained the cross-reactivity of LES antibodies with these synaptosomal VDCCs. Of the three channel types, the autoantibodies caused a pronounced downregulation of the P/Q-type Ca^{2+} channels. These characteristics provide a rationale for the use of the electric ray synaptosomes to induce autoimmunity to Ca^{2+} channels.

MATERIALS AND METHODS

Preparation of Electric Organ Synaptosomes and Animal Immunization

Synaptosomes, prepared from the electric organs of electric ray, *Narke japonica*, captured off the coast of Nagasaki and Fukuoka Prefectures, Japan, were used as autoantigens. Detailed protocols used for preparing the synaptosomes have been published.[8]

In the first series of studies, Swiss-Webster mice and Lewis rats were subcutaneously injected with 50 μg of synaptosome proteins mixed with Freund's complete adjuvant and were given three subsequent boost injections (50 μg) during a three-month period. Mice used in the second series of experiments were immunized with 100 μg of synaptosomes followed by one boost injection (100 μg) after three weeks. Control animals received the same volume of adjuvants free of synaptosomes.

Electrophysiological Studies of the Neuromuscular Junction

Development of LES was assessed in isolated phrenic nerve–diaphragm muscle preparations by standard intracellular recording of spontaneously occurring miniature end plate potentials (MEPPs) and neurally evoked end plate potentials (EPPs). All NMJ parameters were analyzed by a computer-aided data acquisition and analysis system.[9] To determine the quantal content (*m*) of EPPs, muscles were exposed to low $[Ca^{2+}]_o$/high $[Mg^{2+}]_o$ solution. Quantal content at each junction was computed by three different methods: (1) m_d by direct method, (2) m_i by indirect variance method, and (3) m_f by failure method. Although the accuracy of m_i and m_f is limited by the sampling error of the variance and by the assumption that the transmitter release follows a Poisson process, these estimates were used to check the consistency of the measurements.

RESULTS

Quantal Content of the Nerve-evoked EPPs

Among the first group of animals subjected to three boost injections, three out of four synaptosome-immunized mice exhibited a prejunctional deficiency, characterized by a reduction in the amplitude of evoked EPPs with relatively no change in MEPP parameters (FIGURE 1A). In comparison with that found in the control mice, m in these three animals fell significantly ($p < 0.05$), with the percent reduction ranging from 40% to 42% (TABLE 1). Similarly, quantal content from two out of three immunized rats was lower than the control; m was reduced by 26% and 37% from the control. In the second series of studies in which eight mice received a single boost injection, we found that m in five synaptosome-immunized mice was distinctively smaller than the control (TABLE 1). The quantal content reduction observed in these mice varied from 26% to 43%. Three synaptosome-immunized animals, however, did not show any evidence of presynaptic impairment. Thus, approximately 60% of animals immunized with synaptosomes exhibited significant reduction in m.

Spontaneous MEPPs in Normal Ringer's Solution and High $[K^+]_o$

In contrast to a marked decline in EPP quantal content, spontaneous MEPPs measured in normal Ringer's solution appear to be relatively unaffected by immunization (TABLE 1). As measured in normal Ringer's solution, the rate of spontaneous quantal discharge did not appear to be altered in the immunized animals (FIGURE 1B). When the diaphragm muscles were exposed to high $[K^+]_o$ (17.5 mM), MEPP frequency increased sharply. In some motor end plates of the immunized mice, there was a clear trend that the K^+-induced increase in MEPP frequency was smaller than the control (FIGURE 1B). This phenomenon is consistent with the inhibition of presynaptic VDCCs and supports the development of prejunctional deficiency resembling human LES.

In three synaptosome-immunized mice, there was a moderate, but statistically significant increase (17%, $p < 0.05$) in MEPP amplitude. Although the physiological basis of this increase is unexplained at this time, the small sample size might have influenced the outcome. The mean MEPP amplitude in the synaptosome-immunized rats, however, remained unchanged from the control. Likewise, no significant change in the resting membrane potentials (RMPs) was observed.

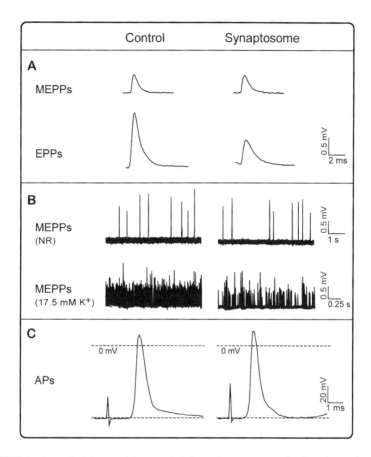

FIGURE 1. Synaptic biopotentials recorded from the neuromuscular junctions of **control** mice and those immunized with electric ray **synaptosome.** Recordings in panels **A** and **B** were obtained from the mouse phrenic nerve–diaphragm muscles, and those in panel **C** were from the rat soleus muscle fibers. **(A)** Spontaneous MEPPs and nerve-evoked EPPs recorded from the neuromuscular junctions exposed to 1.4 mM $[Ca^{2+}]_o$/10 mM $[Mg^{2+}]_o$. The biopotentials depicted in each row represent ensemble signal-averaged waveforms of 15 consecutive MEPPs and 40 EPPs evoked at 2 Hz. **(B)** Spontaneous MEPPs recorded in normal Ringer's solution (5 mM $[K^+]_o$, upper traces) and in high-potassium solution (17.5 mM $[K^+]_o$, lower traces). **(C)** Indirectly elicited muscle fiber action potentials recorded in normal Ringer's solution.

Muscle Fiber Action Potentials

It is relevant to note that the reduction in *m* could also arise from a specific modification in nerve fiber action potentials (APs), which transiently depolarize the motor nerve terminals during the depolarization-secretion coupling process. To explore this possibility, we recorded indirectly elicited muscle fiber APs from the extrajunctional

TABLE 1. Presynaptic and Postsynaptic Parameters of Neuromuscular Transmission in Animals Immunized with *Narke japonica* Electric Organ Synaptosomes[a]

Parameter	Animal	Control	Synaptosome
EPP quantal content at 2 Hz[b] [1.6 mM Ca^{2+}/10 mM Mg^{2+}]	Mouse[d] [diaphragm]	3.68 ± 0.27 (19)	2.21 ± 0.25 (19)[f]
EPP quantal content at 2 Hz [1.2 mM Ca^{2+}/10 mM Mg^{2+}]	Mouse[d] [diaphragm]	1.77 ± 0.20 (17) 1.39 ± 0.12 (21)	1.69 ± 0.15 (28) 0.91 ± 0.08 (20)[f] 0.90 ± 0.08 (16)[f]
EPP quantal content at 2 Hz [1.4 mM Ca^{2+}/10 mM Mg^{2+}]	Mouse[e] [diaphragm]	2.31 ± 0.33 (13) 1.72 ± 0.20 (15) 2.09 ± 0.42 (13) 2.39 ± 0.21 (15) 2.02 ± 0.20 (15) 2.30 ± 0.23 (16)	1.93 ± 0.24 (15) 1.61 ± 0.16 (14)[f] 1.24 ± 0.19 (15)[f] 1.48 ± 0.17 (17)[f] 1.58 ± 0.21 (14)[f] 1.48 ± 0.18 (15)[f] 2.00 ± 0.23 (15) 2.53 ± 0.50 (18)
EPP quantal content at 2 Hz [0.8 mM Ca^{2+}/4 mM Mg^{2+}]	Rat[d] [soleus]	9.32 ± 0.69 (15) 9.59 ± 0.63 (14) 9.09 ± 0.51 (17)	11.43 ± 0.86 (16) 6.87 ± 0.54 (19)[f] 5.87 ± 0.58 (20)[f]
MEPP amplitude (mV)[c] MEPP frequency (Hz) RMP (mV)	Mouse[e] [diaphragm]	0.87 ± 0.05 (43) 1.40 ± 0.07 (39) −74.2 ± 1.2 (43)	1.02 ± 0.06 (41)[f] 1.34 ± 0.09 (41) −75.4 ± 1.4 (41)
MEPP amplitude (mV) MEPP frequency (Hz) RMP (mV)	Rat[d] [soleus]	0.34 ± 0.01 (35) 1.93 ± 0.19 (35) −78.7 ± 1.5 (35)	0.36 ± 0.02 (31) 1.71 ± 0.19 (31) −78.4 ± 1.9 (31)
AP amplitude (mV)[c] AP duration (ms) Maximum dV/dt (mV/ms) Minimum dV/dt (mV/ms) RMP (mV) Overshoot (mV)	Rat[d] [soleus]	85.8 ± 1.0 (25) 1.03 ± 0.04 (25) 313.8 ± 14.4 (23) −90.8 ± 3.9 (24) −75.4 ± 1.2 (25) 10.2 ± 1.6 (25)	86.2 ± 1.4 (25) 1.18 ± 0.02 (24)[f] 259.6 ± 12.2 (24)[f] −92.0 ± 4.4 (25) −75.8 ± 0.9 (25) 10.3 ± 1.7 (25)

[a]Data are shown as mean ± SEM; numbers in parentheses indicate the number of fibers studied.

[b]EPP quantal content was measured using solutions containing low $[Ca^{2+}]_o$/high $[Mg^{2+}]_o$ as indicated.

[c]MEPPs and muscle fiber APs were measured in normal Ringer's solution.

[d]Animals received three monthly boost injections after the initial immunization.

[e]Animals received a single boost injection at three weeks after the initial immunization.

[f]$p < 0.05$ by Student's t test compared to the control mean.

region of the fibers (FIGURE 1C). Although no systematic studies were made, our preliminary results suggest no evidence implicating an explicit change in the overall waveform and size of the APs (TABLE 1). We found the two AP parameters (½ maximal duration and maximum rate of rise, dV/dt) measured from the rat soleus fibers to differ significantly from the control, but such alterations appeared to be inconsistent. The diaphragm muscle fibers of the immunized mice exhibited effects opposite to this (data not shown). In general, peak-to-peak amplitude, RMPs, overshoot, and maximum rate of fall ($-dV/dt$) of the APs were not significantly different from the corresponding control values.

DISCUSSION

To summarize, this study demonstrates that active immunization of mice and rats with *Narke japonica* electric ray synaptosomes containing P/Q-type Ca^{2+} channels causes a reduction in EPP quantal content, a primary defect of neuromuscular transmission associated with the pathophysiology of LES. The data based on MEPPs suggest that immunization with the synaptosomes does not significantly modify postjunctional sensitivity to ACh. In view of the nearly identical ion channel mechanisms underlying the prejunctionally and postjunctionally produced APs, normal muscle fiber APs in the immunized animals may be interpreted as indicating that their motor nerve terminals encounter normal AP-evoked depolarization. It is unlikely that the reduction in EPP quantal content is a result of varied membrane excitability in the production and propagation of the neuronal APs.

The immunologically induced presynaptic abnormality was observed in about 60% of the animals inoculated with the synaptosomes. The degree of presynaptic inhibition in general was not as severe as that seen in animals with passively transferred LES or in patients with LES. However, these results provide preliminary evidence for an autoimmune animal model of LES, which may be used to characterize the precise antigen-antibody interaction responsible for the autoimmune response.

REFERENCES

1. LANG, B. & A. VINCENT. 1996. Autoimmunity to ion-channels and other proteins in paraneoplastic disorders. Curr. Opin. Immunol. **8:** 865–871.
2. KIM, Y. I. & E. NEHER. 1988. IgG from patients with Lambert-Eaton syndrome blocks voltage-dependent calcium channels. Science **239:** 405–408.
3. GRASSI, C., V. MAGNELLI, V. CARABELLI, E. SHER & E. CARBONE. 1994. Inhibition of low- and high-threshold Ca^{2+} channels of human neuroblastoma IMR32 cells by Lambert-Eaton myasthenic syndrome (LEMS) IgGs. Neurosci. Lett. **181:** 50–56.
4. PEERS, C., I. JOHNSTON, B. LANG & D. WRAY. 1993. Cross-linking of presynaptic calcium channels: a mechanism of action for Lambert-Eaton myasthenic syndrome antibodies at the mouse neuromuscular junction. Neurosci. Lett. **153:** 45–48.
5. LINDSTROM, J. 1979. Autoimmune response to acetylcholine receptors in myasthenia gravis and its animal model. *In* Advances in Immunology. Vol. 27, p. 1–50. Academic Press. New York.
6. SATOH, Y., N. HIRASHIMA, H. TOKUMARU, M. P. TAKAHASHI, J. KANG, M. P. VIGLIONE, Y. I. KIM & Y. KIRINO. 1998. Lambert-Eaton syndrome antibodies inhibit acetylcholine release and P/Q-type Ca^{2+} channels in electric ray nerve endings. J. Physiol. (Lond.) In press.
7. VIGLIONE, M. P., T. J. O'SHAUGHNESSY & Y. I. KIM. 1995. Inhibition of calcium currents and exocytosis by Lambert-Eaton syndrome antibodies in human lung cancer cells. J. Physiol. (Lond.) **488:** 303–317.

8. O'HORI, T., C-Y. WANG, H. TOKUMARU, L-C. CHEN, K. HATANAKA, N. HIRASHIMA & Y. KIRINO. 1993. Action of binding of omega-conotoxin on the putative calcium channel of synaptosomal plasma membrane from electric organ of Japanese electric ray, *Narke japonica*. Neuroscience **54:** 1043–1050.
9. O'SHAUGHNESSY, T. J. & Y. I. KIM. 1995. A computer program for the study of synaptic transmission at the neuromuscular junction. Comput. Methods Programs Biomed. **46:** 79–90.

Specificity of the Lambert-Eaton Syndrome Antibodies

Downregulation of P/Q-type Calcium Channels in Bovine Adrenal Chromaffin Cells[a]

YONG I. KIM, TAICK S. NAM,[b] SUNG H. KIM,[c]
MICHAEL P. VIGLIONE, AND JUN KIM[d]

Departments of Biomedical Engineering and Neurology
University of Virginia School of Medicine
Charlottesville, Virginia 22908

INTRODUCTION

The development of paraneoplastic neurological disorders, such as the Lambert-Eaton syndrome (LES), is thought to be triggered by the presence of a tumor, particularly small-cell lung cancer (SCLC).[1] As the antibodies from LES patients pathologically target calcium channels at the neuromuscular junction (NMJ), it is reasonable to hypothesize that the putative autoantigen in this disorder may share common antigenic features with the prejunctional Ca^{2+} channels. Several lines of evidence indeed support the view that the SCLC tumor cells possess the putative immunogen for LES, namely, the P/Q-type calcium channels. These include the following: (1) ω-agatoxin IVA (ω-AgTX IVA)–sensitive, P/Q-type Ca^{2+} channels mediate cholinergic transmitter release at the human NMJ;[2] (2) P/Q-type Ca^{2+} channels sensitive to ω-AgTX IVA are also expressed in SCLC cells;[3,4] (3) autoantibodies from patients with LES immunoprecipitate the same Ca^{2+} channel subtype;[5] and (4) LES IgG primarily downregulates P/Q-type Ca^{2+} channels in SCLC cells.[3]

In studying the pathogenic action of LES IgG on voltage-dependent Ca^{2+} channels (VDCCs), bovine adrenal chromaffin (BAC) cells have been a valuable preparation.[6] These adrenal medullary cells express a high density of Ca^{2+} channels and other voltage-gated ion channels. The depolarization-excitation coupling system in these cells have increasingly served as a valid, effective model of a presynaptic nerve terminal. In the present experiments, we utilized BAC cells with the aim of determining (1) the presence of ω-AgTX IVA–sensitive, P/Q-type Ca^{2+} channels; (2) specificity of LES autoantibodies for P/Q-type VDCCs; (3) action of LES IgG on Ca^{2+}-dependent potassium channels; and (4) dependency of LES IgG action on temperature.

[a]This work was supported by National Institutes of Health Grant No. NS-18607 and a research grant from the Muscular Dystrophy Association.

[b]Present address: Department of Physiology, Yonsei University, Seoul, Korea.

[c]Present address: Department of Electronic Engineering, City University of Seoul, Seoul, Korea.

[d]Present address: Department of Physiology, Seoul National University, Seoul, Korea.

MATERIALS AND METHODS

Cell Culture

Bovine adrenal medullary chromaffin cells were isolated and maintained in culture for patch-clamp experiments as previously described.[6] Cells were kept at 37 °C in suspension in flasks containing Medium 199 supplemented with 10% heat-inactivated fetal bovine serum and were continuously aerated with 5% CO_2 and 95% air. Most of the experiments were performed on cells in culture for 1–3 days.

Solutions

All patch-clamp measurements of whole-cell calcium (I_{Ca}), potassium (I_K), and calcium-activated potassium ($I_{K(Ca)}$) currents were done using an external bath solution consisting of (in mM) NaCl 140, KCl 2.8, $CaCl_2$ 2, $MgCl_2$ 2, and HEPES (NaOH) 10. To measure I_{Ca}, we used the internal or pipette solution containing (in mM) CsCl 120, TEACl 20, EGTA (NaOH) 11, $CaCl_2$ 1, $MgCl_2$ 2, and HEPES (NaOH) 10. For the patch-clamp recordings of I_K and $I_{K(Ca)}$, the internal solution had the following composition (in mM): KCl 129, EGTA (KOH) 11, $CaCl_2$ 1, $MgCl_2$ 2, and HEPES (KOH) 10, pH 7.2. The synthetic toxin ω-AgTX IVA (Peptide International, Louisville, Kentucky) was dissolved in the external recording solution and frozen as aliquots at –20 °C.

Incubation of BAC Cells with Control and LES Antibodies

Preparation of control and LES patients' serological samples and the procedures for incubating the cells with plasma, serum, or IgG have been reported.[3,6] Plasmas or sera were obtained from three patients who were clinically and electromyographically diagnosed as having LES. The disorders of patients 2 and 3 were associated with SCLC, while patient 1 had no evidence of neoplasm. Unless otherwise noted, a 24-hour incubation period was used for all experiments.

Patch-Clamp Experiments and Data Analysis

All patch-clamp measurements were conducted at room temperatures (23 to 25 °C). The data acquisition and analysis method was the same as previously described.[3,6] Briefly, whole-cell currents were recorded at 1 minute after establishing the whole-cell configuration using a List EPC-7 patch-clamp amplifier. To directly compare currents between cells having different cell sizes, the whole-cell current in each cell was normalized by dividing it with cell membrane capacitance (C_m). Where appropriate, results are presented as the mean ± SEM and the number of cells (n) tested. Differences between means were evaluated by Student's t test, assuming $p <$ 0.05 as the limit of statistical significance.

RESULTS

BAC Cells Express ω-AgTX-sensitive, P/Q-type Ca²⁺ Channels

In vitro application of ω-agatoxin IVA to BAC cells caused dose-dependent inhibition of whole-cell Ca^{2+} currents (FIGURE 1A). The toxin produced similar inhibitory effects on the depolarization-induced increases in C_m (data not shown). Thus, BAC cells, like SCLC tumor cells, undergo exocytosis, which is mediated by P/Q-type Ca^{2+} channels. When fitted by a second-order linear regression, the dose-response curve (with ω-AgTX IVA concentrations of 3, 10, 40, and 100 nM) gave rise to a half-inhibition concentration (IC_{50}) of 6.5 nM (FIGURE 1A).

Downregulation of P/Q-type Ca²⁺ Channels by LES Antibodies

If LES IgG preferentially reacts with one subtype of VDCCs, the extent of I_{Ca} inhibition by an antagonist specific to that channel type is expected to diminish in cells pretreated with LES IgG. To test whether LES antibodies specifically interfere with the function of P/Q-type VDCCs, we examined the efficacy of ω-AgTX IVA after the BAC cells were exposed to LES antibodies.

In control serum–treated (2 mg/mL IgG, 24-h incubation) cells, ω-AgTX IVA, applied at a saturating concentration of 100 nM, caused a reduction in I_{Ca} of 45 ± 3.0% ($n = 24$ cells, $p < 0.001$) as compared to the control (FIGURE 1B). Upon incubation with serum (2 mg/mL IgG) from LES patient 1, I_{Ca} was reduced by 47 ± 4.3% ($n = 33$, $p < 0.001$). When 100 nM ω-AgTX IVA was applied to these LES cells, however, I_{Ca} fell by only an additional 7% ($p > 0.05$), far below that found with the control cells (45%). The overall reduction found under this condition was 51 ± 3.7% ($n = 26$) relative to the control I_{Ca}. Thus, in LES serum–treated cells, the toxin was 84% less effective in blocking the current. All effects observed with the toxin and sera were without alteration in the I-V relationships (FIGURE 1B).

In BAC cells incubated with antibodies from another LES patient, we consistently found the same trend. Incubation with IgG (2–3 mg/mL) of patient 2 resulted in a decrease of I_{Ca} by 48 ± 5.1% ($n = 24$) as compared to the currents recorded from control IgG (2–3 mg/mL)–treated cells. In the presence of ω-AgTX IVA (100 nM), I_{Ca} in these LES cells declined further, but the effect was markedly compromised. LES IgG and the toxin in combination produced a 57 ± 3.8% ($n = 16$) inhibition of Ca^{2+} currents relative to those measured from the cells incubated with control IgG. Hence, ω-AgTX IVA caused an additional 17% decrease ($p > 0.05$) in LES cells, indicating that the efficacy of the toxin was 75% lower than that demonstrated using the control IgG–incubated cells.

Action of LES IgG on K⁺ and Ca²⁺-activated K⁺ Channels

Among the three types of K^+ channels found in BAC cells, BK type is Ca^{2+}-activated with the largest unitary conductance.[7] Since the current flowing through these K^+ channels is directly dependent upon the activity of VDCCs, one would expect a

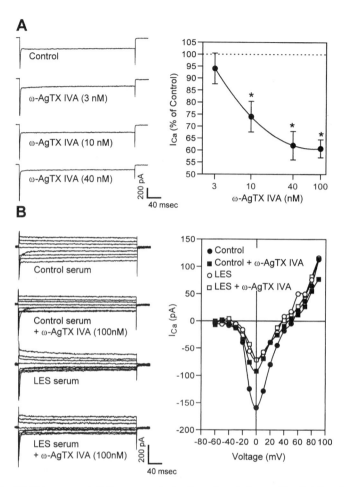

FIGURE 1. (A) Voltage-gated Ca^{2+} currents in bovine adrenal chromaffin (BAC) cells are blocked by ω-AgTX IVA *(left panel)*. The current traces shown were acquired with step-depolarization to 0 mV from a holding potential of –80 mV. The effects of the toxin are dose-dependent, saturating at 100 nM with an IC_{50} of 6.5 nM *(right panel)*. An asterisk indicates a significant difference from control (normal untreated cells) by Student's *t* test ($p < 0.05$). **(B)** I_{Ca} recorded from BAC cells that were incubated with control and LES sera (2 mg/mL IgG, patient 1) for 24 h, and the effects of 100 nM ω-AgTX IVA applied to these serum-treated cells *(left panel)*. Note that the toxin applied to LES cells is not as effective as shown in the control cells. Plotted in the *right panel* are I-V relationships for the same cells depicted in the *left panel*.

secondary inhibitory effect of LES antibodies on these channels. In the present study, we explored whether LES IgG also modifies Ca^{2+}-dependent K^+ channel currents, $I_{K(Ca)}$.

Cells were incubated for 24 hours with plasma (1 mg/mL IgG) from LES patient 3 and healthy control subjects. Whole-cell K^+ currents were recorded from cells held at –80 mV and depolarized to –30 to +120 mV (exposed to 2 mM Ca^{2+} buffer). Peak $I_{K(Ca)}$ was analyzed by the graphical method[7] from I-V curves (FIGURE 2A). In 15 LES plasma–treated cells, $I_{K(Ca)}$ was markedly smaller, 55 ± 13 pA/pF ($p < 0.001$), a reduction of 86% from the currents found in the control plasma–treated cells, 394 ± 42 pA/pF ($n = 22$) (FIGURE 2B). Unexpectedly, I_K elicited at high membrane voltages

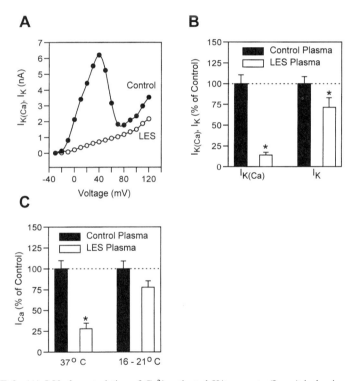

FIGURE 2. (A) I-V characteristics of Ca^{2+}-activated K^+ currents ($I_{K(Ca)}$) in bovine adrenal chromaffin cells incubated in the presence of control or LES plasma (1 mg/mL IgG, patient 3). The I-V curve for the control cell exhibits the characteristic hump that peaks at +40 mV, which is used to estimate $I_{K(Ca)}$.[7] Note that the Ca^{2+}-activated K^+ current is virtually absent in this particular LES plasma–treated cell. **(B)** Inhibition of $I_{K(Ca)}$ and voltage-dependent K^+ (I_K) currents by LES plasma (1 mg/mL IgG, patient 3). Data show the mean $\pm$ SEM of the current amplitudes measured from 15 LES and 22 control cells. An asterisk indicates a significant difference from control by Student's t test ($p < 0.05$). **(C)** Efficacy of LES antibodies in downregulating Ca^{2+} channels is diminished at low temperatures. I_{Ca} measured from BAC cells incubated (16 h) with control and LES plasma (1 mg/mL IgG, patient 3) at 37 °C was compared with data obtained upon similar incubation at 16–21 °C. An asterisk indicates a significant difference from control by Student's t test ($p < 0.05$).

also noticeably declined. In LES cells, I_K appearing at +120 mV was 332 ± 54 pA/pF; and in control cells, 465 ± 40 pA/pF. This reduction (29%) was statistically significant ($p < 0.05$) (FIGURE 2B). Although the clinical implication of this finding is yet to be determined, these results provide evidence for a distinctive inhibition of Ca^{2+}-activated K^+ channel currents in LES patients.

Action of LES IgG on I_{Ca} at Low Temperatures

The antigenic modulation produced by autoantibodies from patients with myasthenia gravis (MG) is critically dependent upon temperature. This dependency is well demonstrated by practically no loss of AChRs when temperature was lowered from 37 °C to 10 °C.[8] Despite a markedly increased rate of myasthenic IgG binding to the receptors, the antigenic modulatory effect was found to be consistently absent.

In an attempt to demonstrate similar antigenic modulation of Ca^{2+} channels, we tested the ability of LES IgG in inhibiting the function of VDCCs at low temperatures. Cells were incubated in LES or control plasma (1 mg/mL IgG) at 37 °C and I_{Ca} was measured with 2 mM $[Ca^{2+}]_o$. After 16-h exposure to plasma, LES cells displayed an I_{Ca} that fell by $72 \pm 6.6\%$ ($n = 31$, $p < 0.001$) relative to the control (FIGURE 2C). When identical incubations were performed at 16–21 °C, LES plasma was found to be significantly ineffective at reducing I_{Ca}. The autoantibodies caused a decrement of only $22 \pm 7.7\%$ ($n = 24$, $p > 0.05$) as compared to control cells incubated at the same low temperatures.

DISCUSSION

The present experiments provide evidence that the pathogenic LES antibodies, applied to bovine adrenal chromaffin cells, predominantly downregulate ω-AgTX IVA–sensitive, P/Q-type Ca^{2+} channels. This finding is consistent with the two recent studies in which similar Ca^{2+} channel specificity was revealed: (1) 95% of patients with LES possess antibodies that immunoprecipitate P/Q-type Ca^{2+} channels labeled with $[^{125}I]$-ω-conotoxin MVIIC;[5] and (2) LES antibodies produce functional inhibition of P-type Ca^{2+} channels in small-cell lung cancer cells.[3] Although the heterogeneity of Ca^{2+} channel specificities among different LES patients is a likely possibility, these findings support the concept that the principal target of LES autoantibodies is a P/Q-type Ca^{2+} channel and that the downregulation of this channel type plays a critical role in the clinical manifestation of this disorder.

Pathological consequences of the inhibitory effects of LES antibodies on $I_{K(Ca)}$ are not clear at this time. Calcium-activated K^+ channels are found in a wide variety of excitable and nonexcitable cells,[9] including motoneurons. These channels may be important in synaptic transmitter release by regulating action potential (AP) repolarization and thereby its duration, a factor impacting the influx of presynaptic Ca^{2+} current. Reduction in $I_{K(Ca)}$ is expected to prolong AP duration, causing augmentation of presynaptic Ca^{2+} entry. Despite the lack of evidence implicating SK or BK channels in the motor nerve terminal function, such an outcome is intriguing as it would tend to counteract the primary presynaptic deficiency in LES patients. In view of the complex role of calcium-activated K^+ channels in controlling membrane excitability, repetitive AP firing, and neurotransmitter release, it is uncertain how precisely the dysfunction of these channels would be manifested as clinically relevant characteristics. Nevertheless, a marked 86% inhibition of $I_{K(Ca)}$, as observed with antibodies from LES patient 3, is likely to induce alteration in the integrated functions of as yet undefined cell types and synapses. It is also noteworthy that LES antibodies suppress the function of voltage-dependent K^+ channels in BAC cells. Although the inhibition of I_K was minor compared to that found with $I_{K(Ca)}$, the effect was statistically significant. This particular finding is corroborated by a previous study in which similar inhibition of I_K was demonstrated in DRG neurons upon exposure to LES serum.[10] The immunological basis and specificity of action of LES IgG involved in the execution of this effect are currently unknown.

Finally, significant impediment of LES IgG action ensued at low temperatures, a phenomenon consistent with the antigenic modulatory effects of the pathogenic antibodies. Such temperature dependency conforms to the finding that monovalent Fab fragments of LES IgG are incapable of downregulating the channels[11] and upholds *antigenic modulation* as a mechanism to explain the loss of VDCCs.

REFERENCES

1. LANG, B. & A. VINCENT. 1996. Autoimmunity to ion-channels and other proteins in paraneoplastic disorders. Curr. Opin. Immunol. **8:** 865–871.
2. PROTTI, D. A., R. REISIN, T. A. MACKINLEY & O. D. UCHITEL. 1996. Calcium channel blockers and transmitter release at the normal human neuromuscular junction. Neurology **46:** 1391–1396.
3. VIGLIONE, M. P., T. J. O'SHAUGHNESSY & Y. I. KIM. 1995. Inhibition of calcium currents and exocytosis by Lambert-Eaton syndrome antibodies in human lung cancer cells. J. Physiol. (Lond.) **488:** 303–317.
4. MERINEY, S. D., S. C. HULSIZER, V. A. LENNON & A. D. GRINNELL. 1996. Lambert-Eaton syndrome immunoglobulins react with multiple types of calcium channels in small-cell lung carcinoma. Ann. Neurol. **40:** 739–749.
5. LENNON, V. A., T. J. KRYZER, M. S. GRIESMANN, P. E. O'SUILLEABHAIN, A. J. WINDEBANK, A. WOPPMANN, G. P. MILJANICH & E. H. LAMBERT. 1995. Calcium-channel antibodies in the Lambert-Eaton syndrome and other paraneoplastic syndromes. N. Engl. J. Med. **332:** 1467–1474.
6. KIM, Y. I. & E. NEHER. 1988. IgG from patients with Lambert-Eaton syndrome blocks voltage-dependent calcium channels. Science **239:** 405–408.
7. MARTY, A. & E. NEHER. 1985. Potassium channels in cultured bovine adrenal chromaffin cells. J. Physiol. (Lond.) **367:** 117–141.
8. KAO, I. & D. B. DRACHMAN. 1977. Myasthenic immunoglobulin accelerates acetylcholine receptor degradation. Science **196:** 527–529.
9. SAH, P. 1996. Ca^{2+}-activated K^+ currents in neurones: types, physiological roles, and modulation. Trends Neurosci. **19:** 150–154.
10. GARCIA, K. D., M. MYNLIEFF, D. B. SANDERS, K. G. BEAM & J. P. WALROND. 1996. Lambert-Eaton sera reduce low-voltage and high-voltage activated Ca^{2+} currents in murine dorsal root ganglion neurons. Proc. Natl. Acad. Sci. U.S.A. **93:** 9264–9269.
11. PEERS, C., I. JOHNSTON, B. LANG & D. WRAY. 1993. Cross-linking of presynaptic calcium channels: a mechanism of action for Lambert-Eaton myasthenic syndrome antibodies at the mouse neuromuscular junction. Neurosci. Lett. **153:** 45–48.

Neuronal Staining Patterns in Sera from Patients with Lambert-Eaton Myasthenic Syndrome[a]

AGATA POLIZZI, BETHAN LANG, ELIZABETH AMYES,
JOHN NEWSOM-DAVIS, AND ANGELA VINCENT

Neurosciences Group
Institute of Molecular Medicine
John Radcliffe Hospital
Oxford OX3 9DS, United Kingdom

The Lambert-Eaton myasthenic syndrome is due to antibodies to voltage-gated calcium channels (VGCCs) and recent evidence suggests that the P/Q-type VGCCs are the main pathogenic target (see Lang *et al.* in this volume). These VGCCs are found at the neuromuscular junction and also in the central nervous system (CNS), particularly in the cerebellum where they are expressed on Purkinje cells and in the granular layer.[1] However, there have been no reports of immunostaining of cerebellum with LEMS sera. LEMS is a paraneoplastic syndrome because about 60% of patients have an associated small cell lung cancer (SCLC). SCLC can also be associated with subacute sensory neuronopathy, brain stem encephalomyelitis, or limbic encephalitis, and in these cases serum antibodies to neuronal nuclei (ANNA-1 or anti-Hu) are frequently present. For a recent brief review, see reference 2.

Although LEMS is characterized by muscle weakness, in some patients cerebellar symptoms are present (Newsom-Davis, unpublished observations). Paraneoplastic cerebellar ataxia is usually associated with antibodies to the cytoplasm of Purkinje cells (APCA-1 or anti-Yo). However, some cases of paraneoplastic cerebellar ataxia

TABLE 1. LEMS Patients and Results of Indirect Immunohistochemistry on Sections of Rat Cerebellum and Brain Stem[a]

Patient	Sex	Anti-P/Q-type VGCC (pM)[b]	Tumor	Cerebellar Signs	Staining Pattern	Western Blotting Hu	Western Blotting Yo
1	F	68	SCLC	+	nuclei in brain stem	+	n.d.
2	M	1200	none	+	nuclei in brain stem	n.d.	n.d.
3	F	349	SCLC	none	nuclei/cytoplasm	–	n.d.
4	F	1348	none	none	nuclei/cytoplasm	–	n.d.
5	M	290	none	none	Purkinje cell cytoplasm	–	–

[a]In addition, 5 further patients with SCLC, 1 with breast cancer, and 9 without tumors were negative for antineuronal antibodies by immunohistochemistry. n.d. = not determined.
[b]Control values < 30 pM.

[a]This work was supported by the Medical Research Council of Great Britain.

684

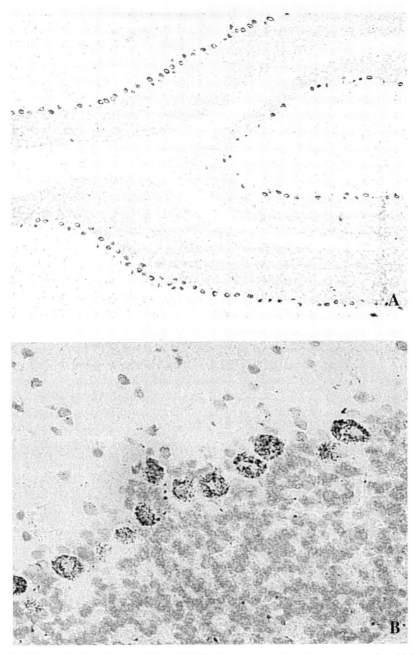

FIGURE 1. Binding of serum (diluted 1:100) from patient #5 to the cytoplasm of Purkinje cells on frozen sections of unfixed adult rat cerebellum, demonstrated by indirect immunohistochemistry. A coarse granular cytoplasmic staining can be seen: (A) ×30; (B) ×150.

with or without associated LEMS have raised anti-VGCC antibodies rather than anti-Yo antibodies.[3] Taken together, these findings suggest that serum antibodies from LEMS patients might bind detectably to CNS neurons. We tested sera from 20 patients by standard immunohistochemistry on frozen sections of adult rat brain and by Western blotting of recombinant Hu and Yo antigen. Eighteen out of the 20 were positive for anti-P/Q-type VGCC antibodies. Seven patients had small cell lung carcinoma (SCLC) and 1 had breast cancer. Two developed cerebellar symptoms during follow-up.

The results are summarized in TABLE 1. Only 5 of the 20 LEMS sera showed binding to neuronal antigens. One (#1) of the 2 sera from patients with cerebellar symptoms had antineuronal nuclear antibodies binding to the periventricular gray matter of the brain stem, and this serum was positive for binding to Hu on Western blots; the other (#2) showed nuclear staining in the brain stem and in the diencephalon, but has not been tested on Western blots. Two sera (#3 and #4), including 1 with SCLC, stained neuronal nuclei and cytoplasm mainly along the lateral aspects of the brain stem. A further patient (#5), who had neither a tumor nor cerebellar signs, exhibited a distinct pattern of coarse granular cytoplasmic staining of the Purkinje cells (FIGURE 1); this serum was negative for binding to recombinant Yo.

This preliminary study demonstrates that some sera from LEMS patients recognize CNS antigens. A possible target would be the P/Q-type VGCCs found on Purkinje cells and in the granular layer of the cerebellum, but none of the staining patterns that we saw are consistent with binding to membrane-expressed VGCCs. Rather, our data suggest possible involvement of other neuronal antigens. Although these antibodies might be relevant for the pathogenesis of central symptoms in a minority of LEMS patients, a clear correlation between cerebellar symptoms, the presence of SCLC, and different staining patterns was not found (see TABLE 1).

REFERENCES

1. VOLSEN, S. G. et al. 1995. The expression of neuronal voltage-dependent calcium channels in human cerebellum. Mol. Brain Res. **34:** 271–282.
2. LANG, B. & A. VINCENT. 1996. Autoimmunity to ion-channels and other proteins in paraneoplastic disorders. Curr. Opin. Immunol. **8:** 865–871.
3. MASON, W. P. et al. 1997. Small-cell lung cancer, paraneoplastic cerebellar degeneration, and the Lambert-Eaton myasthenic syndrome. Brain **120:** 1279–1300.

Differential Effect of Lambert-Eaton Myasthenic Syndrome Immunoglobulin on Cloned Neuronal Voltage-gated Calcium Channels[a]

ASHWIN PINTO,[b] FRASER MOSS,[c] BETHAN LANG,[b] JOHN BOOT,[c]
PAUL BRUST,[d] MARK WILLIAMS,[d] KENNETH STAUDERMAN,[d]
MICHAEL HARPOLD,[d] AND JOHN NEWSOM-DAVIS[b]

[b]Neurosciences Group
Institute of Molecular Medicine
John Radcliffe Hospital
University of Oxford
Oxford OX3 9DS, United Kingdom

[c]Lilly Research Center Limited
Windlesham, Surrey GU20 6PH, United Kingdom

[d]SIBIA Neurosciences Incorporated
La Jolla, California 92037-4641

INTRODUCTION

Lambert-Eaton myasthenic syndrome (LEMS) is an autoimmune disorder in which antibodies to presynaptic calcium channels at the neuromuscular junction lead to muscle weakness. Around 60% of patients with LEMS have an associated small cell lung carcinoma (SCLC), which is known to express voltage-gated calcium channels (VGCCs). Immunoglobulin (IgG) from patients with LEMS causes inhibition of calcium flux in an SCLC cell line.[1] This inhibition has been shown to correlate with disease severity.[1]

Neuronal VGCCs can be classified into P-, Q-, N-, L-, and R-type according to their electrophysiological and pharmacological properties. Around 92% of LEMS patients have antibodies that immunoprecipitate P/Q-type (^{125}I-ω-CTx-MVIIC labeled) VGCCs and around 30% have antibodies to N-type (^{125}I-ω-CTx-GVIA labeled) VGCCs.[2] In addition, antibodies from LEMS patients have been shown to abolish the component of neurotransmitter release subserved by both P-type and Q-type VGCCs in sympathetic and parasympathetic neurons of mice injected with LEMS IgG.[3]

Neuronal VGCCs consist of an α_1 subunit with β and $\alpha_2\delta$ subunits. Several of the human genes encoding the different types of VGCC have now been cloned and sequenced, including the α_{1A}, α_{1B}, α_{1D}, α_{1E}, β_{1-4}, and $\alpha_2\delta$ subunits. Human embryonic

[a]This work was supported by funds from the Wellcome Trust (to A. Pinto), the Sir Jules Thorne Charitable Trust (to B. Lang), and the Medical Research Council (United Kingdom) (to J. Newsom-Davis and B. Lang).

kidney (HEK) cell lines transfected with different VGCC subunits have been generated. In this study, we describe the action of different toxins, drugs, and LEMS IgG on calcium flux in transfected HEK cell lines.

MATERIALS AND METHODS

Four transfected cell lines were studied: 10-13 (α_{1A-2}, $\alpha_2\delta$, β_{4a}), G1A1 (α_{1B-1}, $\alpha_2\delta$, β_{1b}), 5D12-20 (α_{1D}, $\alpha_2\delta$, β_{3a}), and E52-3 (α_{1E-3}, $\alpha_2\delta$, β_{1b}). Transfected cells were cultured in Dulbecco's modified Eagle's medium. Cells were transferred from trilayer flasks into 96-well plates precoated with poly-*l*-lysine and incubated overnight at 37 °C. The cells were then washed extensively with Tyrode solution and incubated with the fluorescent calcium-sensitive dye fluo-3AM (20 μM) for one hour at room temperature. Cells were depolarized by exposure to either 70 mM KCl (10-13, G1A1, 5D12-20) or 40 mM KCl (E52-3) and the fluorescence (F) was measured in real time using the Labsystems Fluoroskan II. For each well, maximum fluorescence (F_{max}) and minimum fluorescence (F_{min}) were measured following sequential exposure to NP40 and then EDTA. Intracellular calcium concentration could then be estimated from the fluorescence intensity values using the equation, $[Ca^{2+}]$ (nM) = $[(F - F_{min})/(F_{max} - F)]K_d$, where K_d is the dissociation constant for Ca^{2+} binding (400 nM).[4] Calcium flux can then be calculated by subtracting the basal intracellular calcium concentration from the peak calcium concentration.

IgG was prepared from patients by the ethacridine lactate–ammonium sulfate method. IgG at a concentration of 4 mg/mL was added to each well and the plates were incubated overnight at 37 °C. Calcium flux was measured with the fluorescent dye fluo-3AM as described above. Calcium flux in cells exposed to IgG was compared to flux in cells cultured in medium alone run on the same plate.

RESULTS

TABLE 1 shows the IC_{50} values of different toxins and drugs on the transfected cell lines. Results are expressed as the mean ± SEM of between three or four experiments, each of six replicates.

A total of four LEMS patients were studied. All four patients had antibodies to

TABLE 1. IC_{50} Values for Transfected HEK Cell Lines

	ω-Aga-IVA	ω-CTx-MVIIC	ω-CTx-GVIA	Nicardipine
10-13 α_{1A-2}, $\alpha_2\delta$, β_{4a}	106 ± 20 nM	202 ± 12 nM	<20% reduction (1 μM)	<20% reduction (3 μM)
G1A1 α_{1B-1}, $\alpha_2\delta$, β_{1b}	<20% reduction (1 μM)	4.2 ± 2.6 nM	1.4 ± 0.3 nM	<20% reduction (3 μM)
E52-3 α_{1E-3}, $\alpha_2\delta$, β_{1b}	<20% reduction (1 μM)	<20% reduction (1 μM)	<20% reduction (1 μM)	28% reduction

P/Q-type (^{125}I-ω-CTx-MVIIC labeled) VGCCs and two out of the four LEMS patients had antibodies to N-type (^{125}I-ω-CTx-GVIA labeled) VGCCs on radioimmunoassay. IgG from all four LEMS patients caused a highly significant reduction in K$^+$-stimulated calcium flux in the α_{1A} (10-13) cell line (mean reduction 75%, $p <$ 0.01) as compared to either healthy or disease control IgG (see FIGURE 1A). However, LEMS IgG caused no inhibition of calcium flux in the α_{1B} (G1A1) cell line (FIGURE

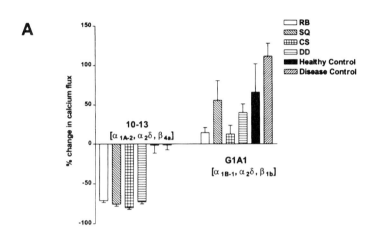

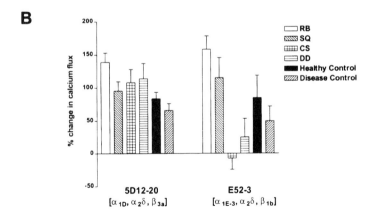

FIGURE 1. Differential effect of LEMS IgG on K$^+$-stimulated calcium flux in transfected HEK cell lines. Results are expressed as the % change in calcium flux as compared to the flux in cells grown in medium alone from a representative experiment of six replicates. (A) LEMS IgG (RB, SQ, CS, and DD) causes a significant reduction in calcium flux in the 10-13 cell line, but not in the G1A1 line. (B) LEMS IgG causes no inhibition of calcium flux in the 5D12-20 and E52-3 cell lines.

1A). We also saw no significant inhibition with either LEMS or control IgG in the α_{1D} (5D12-20) and α_{1E} (E52-3) cell lines (see FIGURE 1B). More recent experiments have established that there is no significant difference between the calcium flux of LEMS or control IgG-treated cells in the α_{1B}, α_{1D}, and α_{1E} cell lines (data not shown).

DISCUSSION

Calcium flux in the α_{1A} (10-13) cell line is inhibited most potently by ω-Aga-IVA and ω-CTx-MVIIC, but is relatively insensitive to ω-CTx-GVIA or nicardipine. This pharmacological sensitivity is consistent with a P/Q-type VGCC. Similarly, the pharmacological sensitivity of the α_{1B} (G1A1) and α_{1E} (E52-3) cell lines is consistent with N-type and R-type VGCCs, respectively.

LEMS IgG caused a highly significant reduction in calcium flux in the α_{1A} (10-13) cell line as compared to control IgG. However, incubation with LEMS IgG caused no reduction of calcium flux in the α_{1B}, α_{1D}, and α_{1E} cell lines. The results of these experiments indicate that antibodies to the P/Q-type calcium channel are the principal factor underlying the impaired neurotransmission characteristic of LEMS.

REFERENCES

1. LANG, B., A. VINCENT, N. M. MURRAY & J. NEWSOM-DAVIS. 1989. Lambert-Eaton myasthenic syndrome: immunoglobulin G inhibition of Ca^{2+} flux in tumor cells correlates with disease severity. Ann. Neurol. **25:** 265–271.
2. MOTOMURA, M., B. LANG, I. JOHNSTON, J. PALACE, A. VINCENT & J. NEWSOM-DAVIS. 1997. Incidence of serum anti-P/Q-type and anti-N-type calcium channel autoantibodies in the Lambert-Eaton myasthenic syndrome. J. Neurol. Sci. **147:** 35–42.
3. WATERMAN, S. A., B. LANG & J. NEWSOM-DAVIS. 1997. Effect of Lambert-Eaton myasthenic syndrome antibodies on autonomic neurons in the mouse. Ann. Neurol. In press.
4. KAO, J. P., A. T. HAROOTUNIAN & R. Y. TSIEN. 1989. Photochemically generated cytosolic calcium pulses and their detection by fluo-3. J. Biol. Chem. **264:** 8179–8184.

Lambert-Eaton Myasthenic Syndrome

Antigenicity of Recombinant Human P/Q-type Calcium Channel α₁ Subunit Putative Ion Pore Region (Domain IV, S5–S6)[a]

JOHN L. BLACK,[b] GUY E. GRIESMANN,[c] JEAN ERICKSON,[c]
THOMAS J. KRYZER,[c] GEOFFREY T. LAMKE,[c,d]
AND VANDA A. LENNON[c]

[b]*Departments of Psychiatry and Psychology*
[c]*Departments of Immunology, Neurology, and
Laboratory Medicine and Pathology
Mayo Clinic
Rochester, Minnesota 55905*

INTRODUCTION

IgG autoantibodies are the pathogenic agents that impair acetylcholine release in the paraneoplastic neuromuscular disorder, Lambert-Eaton myasthenic syndrome (LES). Immunoprecipitation assays implicate presynaptic P/Q-type Ca^{2+} channels as the primary target of these autoantibodies.[1] Small cell lung carcinomas (SCLC) express voltage-gated Ca^{2+} channels of L-, N-, and P/Q-subtypes.[1–3] A neuronal P/Q-channel-related tumor protein is thought to incite production of the autoantibodies responsible for LES. The principal subunit in each high voltage–activated Ca^{2+} channel is a class-specific α_1 (e.g., P/Q, α_{1A}; N, α_{1B}; L, α_{1D}). Each α_1 has four homologous domains (I–IV) with six transmembrane segments (S1–S6), and each domain contributes to the channel's voltage-sensing, ion-translocating, and ligand-binding activity. Barry *et al.*[4] generated affinity-purified rabbit antibodies using a synthetic peptide corresponding to a portion of the P/Q channel's α_1 subunit (α_{1A}, domain IV S5–S6). When applied to SCLC cells (NCI-H146), those antibodies bound to the cell surfaces (visualized by immunofluorescence) and inhibited Ca^{2+} currents (measured by whole-cell patch-clamp). We report here our experience with antibodies raised in rats against a fusion protein corresponding to a larger segment of the P/Q channel's domain IV S5–S6 region. These antibodies bound to solubilized native P/Q-type channels and bound to permeabilized, but not intact H146 SCLC cells. Immunoglobulins in LES patients' sera did not bind to this engineered segment of the P/Q-type Ca^{2+} channel.

[a]This study was supported by NCI Grant No. CA-37343 and an unrestricted educational grant from Solvay Pharmaceuticals.
[d]G. T. Lamke was awarded a Viets Scholarship from the National Myasthenia Gravis Foundation and a Summer Undergraduate Research Fellowship from Abbott Laboratories.

METHODS

Using a DNA probe specific for the human α_{1A} sequence reported by Oguro-Okano et al.,[2] we screened a Lambda Zap® II custom cDNA library (Stratagene), prepared from RNA of the SCLC line SCC-9. An isolated positive plasmid was cloned. Its DNA sequence (3758 bp) corresponded to the C-terminal region of the human P/Q-type Ca^{2+} channel's α_{1A} subunit,[2,5,6] beginning at the domain III–IV link. A subregion encompassing the putative "cation pore" (domain IV S5–S6) was ligated into the pET25 B$^+$ (Novagen) protein expression vector to produce the recombinant protein 1A-D4S56 (TABLE 1, legend). After purification on Ni-agarose, its homo-

TABLE 1. Immunoprecipitation of Fusion Protein and Native P/Q-type Ca^{2+} Channels

Source of Antibodies	^{125}I-1A-D4S56 Fusion Protein (%)	^{125}I-ω-Conopeptide MVIIC Receptors (pmol/L)
Rat Sera		
1A-D4S56 hyperimmune pool[a]	100[b]	570
A1 (25-mer)–specific Ig[a]	73	0
adjuvant control	1	0
Human Subjects' Sera		
healthy #1	2	0
#2	2	0
#3	1	0
#4	2	0
#5	2	0
autoimmune cerebellar ataxia #1	2	0
LES patient #1	2	1080
#2	2	1890
#3	1	31,700
#4	1	200
#5	1	810
#6	1	1230

[a]The full-length fusion protein, 1A-D4S56, includes a cleavable pel B leader, a herpes simplex tag, and a hexahistidine tag. Amino-acid sequences for the domain IV S5–S6 products used as immunogen and for affinity purification of peptide-specific antibodies are as follows:

fusion protein 1A-D4S56: IGIDVEDEDSDEDEFQITEHNNFRTFFQALMLLFRSATGEAW-HNIMLSCLSGKPCDKNSGILTRECGNEFA;

synthetic peptide A1: GNIGIDVEDEDSDEDEFQITEHNNY.

The sequence of this region of the human α_{1A} subunit, derived from an SCLC, was reported by Oguro-Okano et al. in 1992.[2] The underlined sequence indicates the antigenic peptide used in the study of Barry et al.[4] It is 93% homologous to the rat brain α_{1A} sequence.

[b]Percent of 9200 cpm precipitated (1A-D4S56 immune sera as 100%). IgG purified by adsorption to the A1 peptide bound exclusively to the α_{1A} sequence of interest, that is, 1A-D4S56, but not to unrelated fusion proteins made with the pET25 B$^+$ plasmid (not shown).

geneity was assessed by electrophoresis in 10% SDS-PAGE and its identity was confirmed by partial amino-acid sequencing.

Female Lewis rats were injected on four occasions with 33–100 μg of 1A-D4S56 protein emulsified in complete Freund's adjuvant *(id)* and *B. pertussis* vaccine *(sc)* as supplementary adjuvant. Control rats received adjuvants only. Rats were weighed, examined for neurologic signs, bled weekly over a period of 20 weeks, and fed an iron and vitamin supplement weekly. Sera from immunized rats and from LES patients and control subjects were tested by immunoprecipitation with ^{125}I-labeled fusion protein 1A-D4S56 and with ^{125}I-labeled ω-conopeptide MVIIC complexed to P/Q-type Ca^{2+} channels (i.e., high-affinity receptors) solubilized in digitonin from rat or human cerebrocortical membranes.[1] High titered rat sera were pooled and antibodies were purified from an aliquot by adsorption to an agarose-conjugated 25-mer synthetic peptide (A1) that included the 13-residue segment of α_{1A} domain IV S5–S6 used by Barry *et al.*[4] (TABLE 1, legend). Both pools of rat antibodies were tested by indirect immunofluorescence on NCI-H146 SCLC cells, using viable cells in suspension and cells fixed with acetone after cytospinning.

RESULTS

Rats immunized with the recombinant protein 1A-D4S56 produced high titers of antibodies against both the recombinant protein (TABLE 1) and the synthetic peptide A1 (ELISA data not shown). No abnormality of grooming, nutrition, equilibrium, sensation, muscle tone, or strength was observed clinically. Autoantibodies that bound to solubilized native P/Q-type Ca^{2+} channels were produced transiently, but titers in individual rats were not sustained for sufficiently long intervals to warrant performance of microelectrophysiological tests of neuromuscular transmission. In contrast to the rat antibodies, serum IgG from patients with LES did not immunoprecipitate the ^{125}I-labeled recombinant protein (TABLE 1). In indirect immunofluorescence studies (FIGURE 1), the rat antibodies did not bind detectably to intact NCI-H146 cells, but immunoreactivity was revealed when the membranes were delipidated with acetone. Antibodies that were purified by adsorption to peptide A1, the antigenic 25-mer (TABLE 1), bound to the ^{125}I-labeled fusion protein 1A-D4S56, but did not bind to living or permeabilized SCLC cells, or to native P/Q-type Ca^{2+} channels complexed with ^{125}I-ω-conopeptide MVIIC.

DISCUSSION

Antibodies produced by immunizing rats with a putative ion pore region of the P/Q-type Ca^{2+} channel (α_{1A} subunit, domain IV, S5–S6 loop) bound to native channels solubilized from cerebrocortical membranes (i.e., high-affinity receptors for ^{125}I-ω-conopeptide MVIIC), but they did not bind detectably to the plasma membrane of living small cell carcinoma cells (NCI-H146 line), and no rat exhibited gross neurologic impairment. The immunoreactivity detected in delipidated NCI-H146 cells may represent intramembranous epitopes of the channel's α_{1A} subunit or

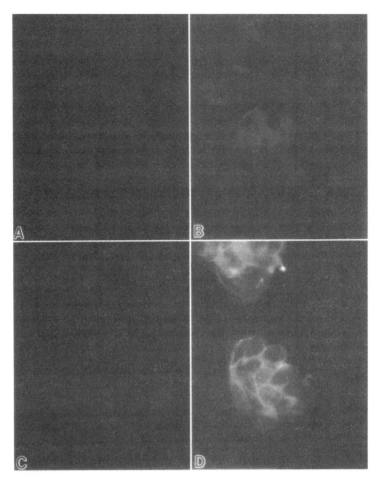

FIGURE 1. SCLC cells of the NCI-H146 line were obtained from the American Type Culture Collection, Rockville, Maryland, and were cultured in RPMI medium supplemented with 10% calf bovine serum. Living cells (A and C) or cells fixed and delipidated by momentary immersion in acetone (B and D) were incubated with one of two pools of sera, diluted 1:200, from adjuvant-immune rats (A and B) or from rats hyperimmunized with the fusion protein 1A-D4S56 (C and D). The latter serum pool bound per liter 570 pmol of ^{125}I-ω-conopeptide MVIIC complexed to high-affinity receptors solubilized from human brain synaptic membranes (TABLE 1). After washing three times, fluorescein-conjugated affinity-purified goat anti-rat IgG and IgM were added (Southern Biotechnology Associates, Birmingham, Alabama) and washing was repeated. The cells were visualized by fluorescence microscopy and photographed (Olympus AX70 system; final magnification, ×130). Immunoreactivity was detected only in permeabilized cells exposed to the P/Q-type Ca^{2+} channel–reactive antibodies (D, peripheral membrane or cytoplasmic staining of individual cells in two clusters). Antibodies purified by affinity adsorption to the 25-mer peptide A1 (TABLE 1) did not bind detectably to living or permeabilized cells.

α_{1A} in the cytoplasmic compartment. Our results contrast with the finding by Barry *et al.*[4] that rabbit antibodies produced against a peptide sequence that was included in our immunogen, and which we used to affinity-purify our rat antibodies (TABLE 1, legend), bound to the extracellular face of viable NCI-H146 cells and impaired ion conductance through P/Q-type Ca^{2+} channels. Because LES patients' sera did not immunoprecipitate the fusion protein, we conclude that, if this region of the α_{1A} subunit is a target for pathogenic autoantibodies, the epitopes that stimulate human B lymphocytes must be highly dependent on the native conformation of the P/Q-type Ca^{2+} channel.

ACKNOWLEDGMENTS

We thank Terry Snutch (University of British Columbia, Vancouver, British Columbia) for preparing RNA from which the Lambda Zap® II cDNA library was constructed and for providing the α_{1A} cDNA probe. We also thank Jim Thoreson, Cheryl Bernard, Ann Schmeichel, and Evelyn Posthumus for excellent technical assistance.

REFERENCES

1. LENNON, V. A. *et al.* 1995. Calcium-channel antibodies in Lambert-Eaton myasthenic syndrome and other paraneoplastic syndromes. N. Engl. J. Med. **332:** 1467–1474.
2. OGURO-OKANO, M. *et al.* 1992. Molecular diversity of neuronal-type calcium channels identified in small cell lung carcinoma. Mayo Clin. Proc. **67:** 1150–1159.
3. MERINEY, S. D. *et al.* 1996. Lambert-Eaton myasthenic syndrome immunoglobulins react with multiple types of calcium channels in small cell lung carcinoma. Ann. Neurol. **40:** 739–749.
4. BARRY, E. L. *et al.* 1995. Expression and antibody inhibition of P-type calcium channels in the human small-cell lung carcinoma cells. J. Neurosci. **15:** 274–283.
5. OPHOFF, R. *et al.* 1996. Familial hemiplegic migraine and episodic ataxia type 2 are caused by mutations in the Ca^{2+} channel gene CACNL1A4. Cell **87:** 543–552.
6. ZHUCHENKO, O. *et al.* 1997. Autosomal dominant cerebellar ataxia (SCA6) associated with small polyglutamine expansions in the α_{1A}-voltage-dependent calcium channel. Nat. Genet. **15:** 62–69.

Electrodiagnosis of Disorders of Neuromuscular Transmission

RICARDO A. MASELLI

Department of Neurology
University of California, Davis
Davis, California 95616

INTRODUCTION

The two most common electrodiagnostic tests to study neuromuscular transmission are repetitive stimulation and the analysis of "jitter" with single-fiber electromyography (SFEMG). Electrodiagnostic studies can be performed alone or in combination with pharmacologic testing. The most common pharmacologic study is the edrophonium or Tensilon test. Single-fiber electromyography can be done with voluntary activation or with electrical stimulation of fine motor nerve branches, a technique referred to as stimulated single-fiber electromyography (SSFEMG). Ideally, an electrodiagnostic test should be highly sensitive, specific for junctional diseases, and able to discriminate the different forms of failure of junctional transmission. Unfortunately, neither repetitive stimulation nor SFEMG meets these ideal standards. Repetitive nerve stimulation is relatively specific for disorders of neuromuscular transmission and can often discriminate some forms of presynaptic and postsynaptic failure; however, it has a limited sensitivity. Certainly, a normal repetitive stimulation study cannot exclude an underlying failure of neuromuscular transmission. In contrast, SFEMG jitter analysis is an extremely sensitive test, but unfortunately not very specific for disorders of neuromuscular transmission because other neuromuscular diseases can show jitter abnormalities as well. Stimulated SFEMG is also very sensitive, but technical factors can potentially complicate the interpretation of the test. Stimulated SFEMG is particularly useful in children and uncooperative patients. Another clear advantage of SSFEMG is the control of the interdischarge frequency, which can be of help in discriminating postsynaptic from some forms of presynaptic failure.

FUNDAMENTS OF THE TESTS

Repetitive Stimulation

The test of repetitive stimulation is based on the universal principle that synapses with high quantal content show a decline of synaptic potential amplitudes during repetitive stimulation. The neuromuscular junction is a synapse with very high quantal content and consequently shows a decrement of end plate potential (EPP) amplitudes during repetitive stimulation.[1] FIGURE 1 displays examples of EPPs recorded *in vitro* with intracellular microelectrodes from a patient without neuromuscular disease. The muscle fiber was partially depolarized; hence, it could not fire action potentials due to inactivation of sodium channels. In spite of the obvious decrement of EPP amplitudes, all EPPs fall above an arbitrarily set threshold level to fire action potentials. Therefore, with an appropriate resting membrane potential, all EPPs elicited in this fiber would have fired action potentials and there would have been no significant decrement of the electrical field generated by this fiber during stimulation. The compound muscle action potential (CMAP) recorded with surface electrodes is contributed by the field generated by thousands of muscle fibers, which in normal circumstances behave similarly as the fiber shown in this example. The result is no decrement of CMAP amplitudes even when there is underlying EPP decrement at the majority of the muscle end plates. In the bottom of the same figure, there are EPPs from a myasthenic patient recorded under similar conditions as in the previous example. Notice that the slope of decline is similar in both examples; however, in the myasthenic case, because the starting EPP amplitude is very small, subsequent EPPs fail to reach the threshold level and fail to generate action potentials. In the *in vivo* situation, this would have been reflected in a gradual decline in the percentage of fibers that contribute to the amplitude of the CMAPs as the train of stimulation progresses. Certainly, the decrement of the CMAP amplitudes is not due to a decline in

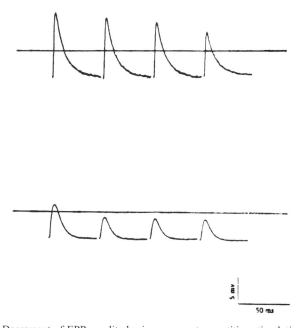

FIGURE 1. Decrement of EPP amplitudes in response to repetitive stimulation at 1 Hz: On the top, the EPPs recorded from a control muscle biopsy showed decrement of EPP amplitudes. All EPP amplitudes exceed an arbitrarily set threshold level to fire action potentials. On the bottom, the recording obtained from the muscle biopsy of a myasthenic patient is displayed. Notice that the slope of the decrement is similar in both cases. However, since the amplitude of the first EPP recorded from the myasthenic muscle is small, subsequent EPPs elicited by the train of stimulation failed to reach the threshold level to fire action potentials.

the amplitudes of muscle fiber action potentials, but rather due to a reduction in the percentage of muscle fibers that generate action potentials and contribute that way to the amplitude of the CMAP.

The reason for the decline of the EPP amplitudes during a train of stimuli is a transient depletion of vesicles in the nerve terminal. Synaptic vesicles are organized in at least two well-defined pools: one is the reserve pool or quantal store and the other is the pool of vesicles available for immediate release.[2,3] In electrophysiologic terms, the pool for immediate release is often referred to as n and presumably is formed by vesicles that are positioned at the active zones ready to be released.[4] The reserve pool is referred to as N. Repetitive stimulation empties docking sites of the available pool and forces mobilization of vesicles from the reserve pool and local recycling of vesicles. When the replenishment of vesicles equals the release, no further decrement of EPP amplitudes occurs. The percentage of vesicles that are released from the releasable pool n with each stimulation depends on the probability of release p, which in turn relies on calcium entry into the nerve terminal. The quantal content of the EPP, which is often referred to as m, depends on n and p according to the formula, $m = n \times p$. With long trains of low frequency stimulation, usually no further decline of EPP amplitudes is seen after the first ten stimuli and the EPP amplitudes are distributed normally (FIGURE 2). In the myasthenic case, the EPP amplitudes are also distributed normally, but naturally shifted to the lower amplitude end. In contrast, in a patient with a presynaptic disorder such as the Lambert-Eaton syndrome (LES), the EPP amplitudes vary in a stepwise or quantal manner and are arranged following a Poisson distribution.[5] Experimentally, a postsynaptic pattern of failure can be reproduced by treating a muscle preparation with curare or alpha-bungarotoxin. A presynaptic pattern can be mimicked by magnesium, which decreases the probability of release by antagonizing the effect of calcium. Using microelectrode studies in unblocked preparations, it is relatively simple to differentiate a postsynaptic from a presynaptic pattern of failure of neuromuscular transmission. Unfortunately, electrodiagnostic techniques cannot discriminate with accuracy presynaptic from postsynaptic defects and microelectrode studies are often needed to characterize the nature of the underlying problem.

An important consideration for the interpretation of the electrodiagnostic test is that, during repetitive nerve stimulation, two processes occur simultaneously. On the one hand there is a transient depletion of vesicles that results in transient depression, but on the other hand there is entry of calcium into the nerve terminal that results in facilitation.[6,7] FIGURE 3 shows an example of repetitive stimulation at 50 Hz in a patient with LES. In this case, repetitive stimulation at fast rates induced a decrement-increment response. The initial decrement is most likely due to depletion of vesicles and the ensuing increment probably results from calcium accumulation in the nerve terminal, which produces facilitation of synaptic vesicle release. The right upper corner of the figure shows that the decrement persists even after calcium facilitation, thus indicating that the two mechanisms are independent from each other. Fortunately, calcium facilitation does not occur at low frequencies of stimulation, but vesicle depletion does. Therefore, low frequencies of nerve stimulation are preferred for eliciting decrement without contamination of calcium-dependent facilitation. Of course, this strategy does not apply to presynaptic conditions such as botulism and LES where calcium facilitation is an important finding for the diagnosis.

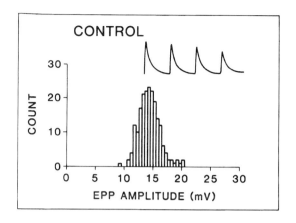

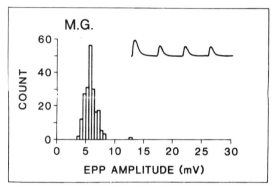

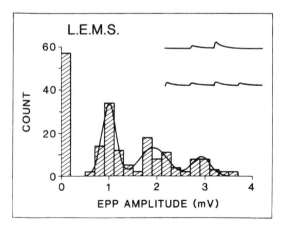

FIGURE 2. Distribution of EPP amplitudes: The amplitudes of EPPs recorded from the control and myasthenic end plates from FIGURE 1 are distributed normally (top and middle). In contrast, in a presynaptic condition such as ALS (bottom), the EPP amplitudes are distributed in multiple Gaussian curves or Poisson distributions.

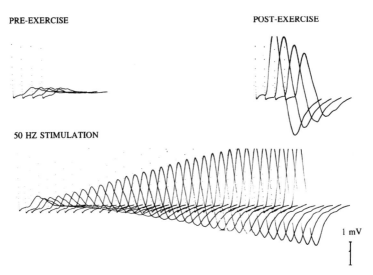

PRE-EXERCISE   POST-EXERCISE

50 HZ STIMULATION

1 mV

FIGURE 3. Repetitive stimulation in Lambert-Eaton syndrome: Repetitive stimulation at 2 Hz (top) showed decrement before (left) and after (right) exercise. Fifty-Hz stimulation (bottom) resulted in an initial decrement, which was followed by a striking incremental response.

Single-Fiber EMG

The principle of SFEMG is another general phenomenon of synaptic transmission. This principle is the natural variability of onsets of action potentials with respect to the synaptic potentials that trigger them. At normal neuromuscular junctions, the dispersion of action potential onsets with respect to the EPPs is minimal, but increases dramatically when there is a decrease of the EPP amplitudes for whatever reason (presynaptic or postsynaptic). This concept is illustrated in FIGURE 4, which shows the intracellular recording performed *in vitro* in a patient intoxicated with botulism during electrical stimulation. At the beginning of the stimulation (top), the EPPs are large and there is minimal dispersion of action potential onsets. As the stimulation continues, depletion of vesicles occurs, the EPP amplitudes diminish, and there is dispersion of action potential onsets (middle). Further stimulation (bottom) results in more pronounced decreases of EPP amplitudes and in more temporal dispersion of action potential onsets, along with impulse blocking (failure of the EPP to trigger an action potential). Clinically, intramuscular nerves are stimulated with a needle electrode and muscle action potentials are recorded with an SFEMG needle placed away from the stimulating needle. EPPs cannot be seen with this method of extracellular electrode recording. However, since only with rare exceptions EPPs are time-locked to the stimulus artifact, the jitter is calculated by estimating the interdischarge variability of the muscle action potential onset with respect to the stimulus artifact. For voluntarily activated SFEMG jitter analysis, it is necessary to record from a motor unit potential formed by at least two distinctive action potentials that fire synchronously by virtue of belonging to the same motor unit. One of the muscle fiber pairs is used to trigger the sweep in the computer monitor and the other one displays

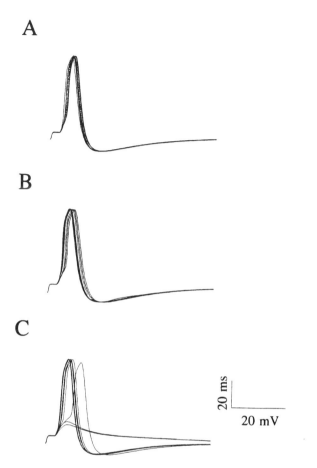

FIGURE 4. Single-fiber EMG: *In vitro* recording of action potentials and EPPs in the muscle biopsy of a patient intoxicated with botulism. Mild dispersion of EPP onsets (A) became more pronounced as the continued stimulation at 1 Hz depleted the synaptic vesicles (B). In addition, EPPs failed to reach the threshold point to trigger action potentials (C).

the jitter variability. It should be noted that in this situation the jitter represents the algebraic summation of the jitter of both fibers with respect to their corresponding EPPs, which are time-locked with each other and with the action potential impulse in the motor neuron axon.[8]

The SFEMG jitter is not only increased when the EPP amplitudes are low, but it is also increased when the end plate region is depolarized. There are two reasons for this phenomenon. First, since the amplitudes of the underlying end plate currents (EPCs) are linearly dependent on the resting membrane potential (RMP) of the muscle fiber,[9] low RMPs are associated with diminished EPC amplitudes. By Ohm's law, at constant resistance, low-amplitude EPCs result in decreased EPP amplitudes. Second, depolarization of the end plate region inactivates sodium channels that surround the end plate.[10] As a result of that, the threshold level is increased.

PATTERNS OF NEUROMUSCULAR TRANSMISSION FAILURE

From a physiologic perspective, impaired neuromuscular transmission can be classified according to the level of failure. Five levels of failure have been identified. It should be noted that pure levels of failure are hypothetical concepts because, in practice, multiple mechanisms operate simultaneously.

PREJUNCTIONAL LEVEL

This level of failure results from a nonconductive state of the motor neuron axons and motor nerve branches proximal to the nerve terminal (FIGURE 5). This type of failure is characteristic of immature motor axon branches with incomplete myelinization.[11] This is usually seen in newborns or premature babies and at early stages of reinnervation. The two classical examples of this mechanism are the failure of neuromuscular transmission observed with fast rates of stimulation in newborns and that in patients with neurogenic conditions such as amyotrophic lateral sclerosis (ALS). Clinically, a decremental response to fast rates of stimulation in a newborn child may be a normal finding. Similarly, a decremental response to fast rates of stimulation in an ALS patient may not necessarily imply an additional process at the neuromuscular junction.

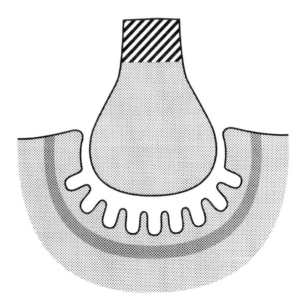

FIGURE 5. Prejunctional failure.

Repetitive Stimulation

Prejunctional level of failure is characterized by a strictly frequency-dependent and often dramatic decrement. When the number of motor neurons is reduced such as in patients with ALS, often a steplike decrement occurs.[12] This suggests that each of the steps represents a failure of a motor neuron activation due to blockade of impulse conduction in the motor neuron axons.

SFEMG

The most distinctive characteristic of SFEMG is the presence of neurogenic or concomitant blocking (simultaneous blockade of two or more fibers).[8] As with repetitive stimulation, concomitant blocking is also more pronounced with fast rates of stimulation.

Microelectrode Studies

The *in vitro* studies show failure of the electrical stimulus to generate EPPs.[13] This can easily be confused with random failures of action potentials to release quanta in presynaptic disorders. However, prejunctional failures occur in association with higher levels of EPP quantal content, and failures increase with higher rates of stimulation. In contrast, presynaptic failures diminish with higher rates of stimulation. Another finding suggestive of prejunctional failure is a paradoxical lower EPP quantal content calculated by the indirect method (variance method) in comparison with that calculated by the direct method (EPP/MEPP amplitudes).

PRESYNAPTIC LEVEL

Deficit of neurotransmitter release from the nerve terminals can result from multiple and complex mechanisms. The most common mechanisms are a low probability of release, a decreased pool of readily available vesicles, and a diminished reserve pool of vesicles (FIGURE 6).

Repetitive Stimulation

In a proportion of cases, presynaptic failure is associated with incremental responses to fast rates of repetitive nerve stimulation; however, this occurs only when the release probability p is low due to an impairment of calcium entry into the nerve terminal. The typical example of this is LES (FIGURE 3). Low probability of release is also present at immature nerve terminals during early stages of reinnervation. This may explain the occasional finding of incremental responses in early stages of ALS.[12,13] Incremental responses can also be seen when the pool of readily available vesicles or factor n is diminished. An example of this is botulism, where there is

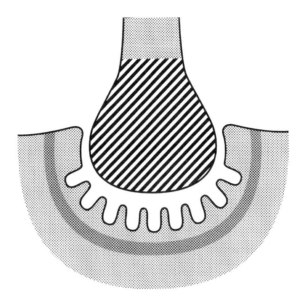

FIGURE 6. Presynaptic failure.

blockade of vesicle docking to the presynaptic membrane.[14] However, in this situation, incremental responses are not consistent and when present are rather modest.[15] In other forms of presynaptic failure, which represent the largest proportion of cases, there is a diminished reserve pool of synaptic vesicles N and repetitive stimulation results in decremental responses. This mechanism has been demonstrated with microelectrode recordings in congenital end plate acetylcholinesterase deficiency (CEAD)[16] and slow-channel myasthenic syndrome (SCMS).[17] Structurally, a diminished reserve pool is associated with small-diameter, but mature nerve terminals. Other mechanisms of presynaptic failure have been postulated, especially in congenital myasthenic syndromes. These include a putative deficiency of synthesis and packing of neurotransmitter in familial infantile myasthenia[18] and a congenital paucity of synaptic vesicles with diminished quantal content.[19] Repetitive nerve stimulation in these rare congenital myasthenic syndromes shows no abnormalities or decrement.

SFEMG

In presynaptic disorders with decreased probability of release, such as LES, the jitter is high (sometimes exceptionally high), but it becomes less pronounced as the discharge frequency increases.[20] This phenomenon can also be encountered in botulism. However, due to the patchy distribution of nerve terminal involvement in this disease, the influence of the discharge frequency on jitter is less predictable than in LES.[21] In presynaptic failure due to diminished N, the jitter increases with increment of the discharge frequency.

Microelectrode Studies

When the failure results purely from a low probability of release, MEPP amplitudes are normal, EPP quantal content is low, and EPP amplitudes are arranged following Poisson's distribution. In other forms of presynaptic failure, presumably as a result of a decrease of the quantal size, there is some degree of reduction of MEPP amplitudes as well. This is particularly true in human botulism type A[14] and in denervation atrophy.[13]

POSTSYNAPTIC LEVEL

This is the most common and most complex level of failure (FIGURE 7). From a physiologic standpoint, it is convenient to follow the classification proposed by Engel,[22] who divides postsynaptic disorders into those with or without kinetic abnormalities of the AChR ion channel. Postsynaptic disorders without kinetic changes of the ion channel are most common and are best exemplified by myasthenia gravis. The classical examples of postsynaptic failure with kinetic changes are some forms of congenital myasthenic syndromes (CMSs) associated with mutations of the AChR subunit genes. The best characterized of these disorders is the SCMS. However, kinetic changes of the ion channel can also result from pharmacologic[23] and even antibody interaction with the AChR.[24]

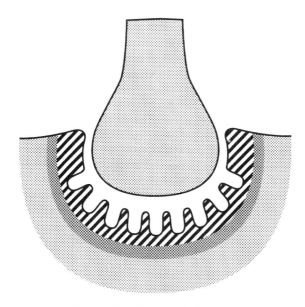

FIGURE 7. Postsynaptic failure.

Repetitive Stimulation

Slow rates of stimulation result in decrement. The decrement is usually partially corrected by exercise or fast rates of stimulation due to the calcium facilitation mechanism. In SCMS and CEAD, a single stimulation of the nerve results in repetitive CMAP (RCMAP). This is due to EPPs remaining above the threshold level longer than the refractory period of the muscle fiber, enough to fire additional action potentials. However, if the presynaptic and postsynaptic failures associated with these conditions are severe, even the first EPP is small and is unable to fire more than one action potential. Therefore, absence of RCMAP does not rule out SCMS or CEAD. In this situation, the application of a recently described end plate electromyography with Fast Fourier Transform (FFT) analysis of electromyographic end plate noise may be useful.[25]

SFEMG

This shows increased jitter and impulse blocking. Increasing the frequency of activation commonly accentuates jitter because at the usual frequency of muscle firing during voluntary SFEMG the calcium facilitation mechanism is already partially activated.

Microelectrode Studies

Typically, MEPPs are very small or undetectable, whereas the EPP quantal content is normal. Furthermore, EPP amplitudes are distributed normally. In postsynaptic disorders without kinetic changes of the AChR ion channel, voltage-clamp experiments show normal time constants of miniature end plate currents (MEPCs) and EPCs.[26] In contrast, changes of EPC and MEPC time constant decays are observed in postsynaptic conditions associated with kinetic changes of the AChR ion channel. The abnormalities of the AChR ion channel kinetics can be further characterized using FFT analysis of iontophoretic-induced end plate noise or patch clamp.

PERIJUNCTIONAL LEVEL

Perijunctional failure results from an impaired generation of action potentials in the muscle membrane adjacent to the end plate (FIGURE 8). This could be due to either a transient inactivation or a diminished density of sodium channels surrounding the end plate. The classical example of transient inactivation of perijunctional sodium channels is the failure of neuromuscular transmission associated with organophosphate intoxication (OPI).[10] An example of diminished density of sodium channels around the end plate is myasthenia gravis.[27]

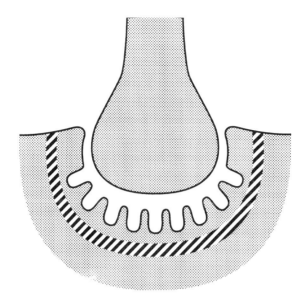

FIGURE 8. Perijunctional failure.

Repetitive Stimulation

At early stages of OPI, a single nerve stimulation results in RCMAP. This is due to the acute inactivation of the AChE. Repetitive nerve stimulation results in the classical sharp-decline-rise (SDR) response, which indicates an underlying depolarization with transient inactivation of perijunctional sodium channels.[28] The response is frequency-dependent, being more pronounced with higher frequencies of stimulation. Sharp-decline-rise responses can also be seen in other conditions—for instance, in neuromyotonia.[29] Furthermore, OPI is not always associated with SDR, particularly in late stages of the intoxication when failure of neuromuscular transmission is dominated by desensitization of the ion channel (postsynaptic failure).[23] In this situation, repetitive stimulation shows a decremental response that is also frequency-dependent.

SFEMG

There is no experience with SFEMG in perijunctional failure. Theoretically, it could be speculated that it may show frequency-dependent increments of jitter and impulse blocking.

Microelectrode Studies

Animal models of OPI have shown that the RCMAP in response to a single nerve stimulation results from inactivation of the AChE and prolongation of EPP decays.[10] In OPI, as in CEAD and in SCMS, EPPs remain above the threshold level longer than the refractory period of the muscle fiber, so they can fire additional action potentials. Sharp-decline-rise response results from a "staircase summation" of prolonged EPPs. Because the first stimulus of the train elicits multiple EPPs that summate upon each other, the depolarization and the inactivation of perijunctional sodium channels are maximal after the first stimulus.[30] This explains why the decline is maximal between the first and second CMAP of the train. The subsequent rise is due to a progressive repolarization of the perijunctional area and recovery from inactivation of sodium channels. Sharp-decline-rise is not commonly seen in CEAD and SCMS. A possible explanation for that is the intense presynaptic defect associated with CEAD and the postsynaptic defect associated with SCMS preventing the abrupt depolarization that occurs in OPI at the beginning of the stimulation train. However, the fact that these conditions usually clinically worsen with the administration of anticholinesterase medication suggests that depolarization block indeed occurs.

POSTJUNCTIONAL LEVEL

Postjunctional failure results from abnormal generation and propagation of action potentials in the muscle membrane (FIGURE 9). The most frequent causes are congen-

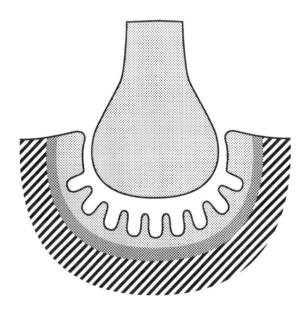

FIGURE 9. Postjunctional failure.

ital disorders involving voltage-gated channels of the muscle membrane. The classical example is myotonia congenita.

Repetitive Stimulation

As in the prejunctional level, there is a strictly frequency-dependent and often dramatic decrement. The decrement is more prominent with higher frequencies of stimulation.[31]

SFEMG

A distinctive SFEMG feature of postjunctional failure is the decrement of the amplitude of the single action potential itself.[32] This is often associated with changes in the configuration and propagation of the action potential.

Microelectrode Studies

Studies of neuromuscular transmission in disorders of muscle membrane ion channels are not available. A recent patch-clamp study in paramyotonia congenita showed marked prolongation of whole-cell-recorded sodium current decays with significant steady-state openings of sodium channels.[33]

COMBINED FAILURE

As stated earlier, combined failures are more common than failures involving a selective level. For instance, the characteristic postsynaptic defect of myasthenia gravis is often associated with presynaptic and perijunctional failure due to diminished release of neurotransmitter and decreased density of perijunctional sodium channels. In OPI, the initial perijunctional depolarization block is followed by desensitization of the AChR, leading to postsynaptic failure. A prejunctional failure due to stimulus-induced antidromic backfiring has also been postulated in OPI.[34] In CEAD, there is evidence for both presynaptic and perijunctional failure. More complex mechanisms have been postulated in recently described CMSs due to mutations of the AChR subunit genes.[35,36] The combined use of repetitive stimulation and single-fiber and end plate electromyography may provide an initial characterization of the defect of neurotransmission. However, an in-depth analysis of the underlying process requires *in vitro* microelectrode and molecular studies.

REFERENCES

1. ELMQVIST, D. & E. H. LAMBERT. 1965. A quantitative study of end-plate potentials in isolated human muscle. J. Physiol. **178:** 505–529.

2. DEL CASTILLO, J. & B. KATZ. 1954. Quantal components of the end-plate potential. J. Physiol. **124:** 560–573.
3. STEVENS, C. F. 1993. Quantal release of neurotransmitter and long-term potentiation. Neuron **10:** 55–63.
4. CECCARELLI, B. & W. P. HURLBUT. 1980. Vesicle hypothesis of the release of quanta of acetylcholine. Physiol. Rev. **60:** 396–441.
5. BOYD, I. A. & A. R. MARTIN. 1956. The end-plate potential in mammalian muscle. J. Physiol. **132:** 74–91.
6. MASELLI, R. A. 1994. Pathophysiology of myasthenia gravis and Lambert-Eaton syndrome. Neurol. Clin. North Am. **12:** 285–303.
7. STOCKBRIDGE, N. & J. W. MOORE. 1984. Dynamics of intracellular stimulation and its possible relationship to phasic transmitter release and calcium facilitation at the frog neuromuscular junction. J. Neurosci. **4:** 803–811.
8. STÅLBERG, E. & J. V. TRONTELJ. 1994. Single-Fiber Electromyography: Studies in Healthy and Diseased Muscle. Second edition. Raven Press. New York.
9. MASELLI, R. A., D. J. NELSON & D. P. RICHMAN. 1989. Effects of a monoclonal anti-acetylcholine receptor antibody on the avian end-plate. J. Physiol. **411:** 271–283.
10. MASELLI, R. A. & B. C. SOLIVEN. 1991. Analysis of the organophosphate-induced electromyographic response to repetitive nerve stimulation: paradoxical response to edrophonium and D-tubocurarine. Muscle Nerve **14:** 1182–1188.
11. DENNIS, M. J. & R. MILEDI. 1974. Non-transmitting neuromuscular junctions during an early stage of end-stage reinnervation. J. Physiol. **239:** 553–570.
12. NORRIS, F. H. 1975. Adult spinal neuron disease progressive muscular atrophy (Aran's disease) in relation to amyotrophic lateral sclerosis. *In* Handbook of Clinical Neurology: System Disorders and Atrophies. Vol. 22, p. 1–56. Elsevier. Amsterdam/New York.
13. MASELLI, R. A., R. L. WOLLMANN, C. LEUNG, B. DISTAD, S. PALOMBI, D. P. RICHMAN, E. F. SALAZAR-GRUESO & R. P. ROOS. 1993. Neuromuscular transmission in amyotrophic lateral sclerosis. Muscle Nerve **16:** 1193–1203.
14. MASELLI, R. A., W. ELLIS, R. N. MANDLER, F. SHEIKH, G. SENTON, S. KNOX, H. SALARI-NAMIN, M. AGIUS, R. L. WOLLMANN & D. P. RICHMAN. 1997. Cluster of wound botulism in California: clinical, electrophysiologic, and pathologic study. Muscle Nerve **20:** 1284–1295.
15. CHERINGTON, M. 1982. Electrophysiologic methods as an aid in diagnosis of botulism: a review. Muscle Nerve **5:** S28–S29.
16. ENGEL, A. G., E. H. LAMBERT & M. R. GOMEZ. 1977. A new myasthenic syndrome with end-plate acetylcholinesterase deficiency, small nerve terminals, and reduced acetylcholine release. Ann. Neurol. **1:** 315–330.
17. ENGEL, A. G., E. H. LAMBERT, D. M. MULDER, C. F. TORRES, K. SAHASHI, T. E. BERTORINI & J. N. WHITAKER. 1993. A newly recognized congenital myasthenic syndrome attributed to a prolonged open time of the acetylcholine receptor. Muscle Nerve **16:** 1284–1292.
18. MORA, M., E. H. LAMBERT & A. G. ENGEL. 1987. Synaptic vesicle abnormality in familial infantile myasthenia. Neurology **37:** 206–214.
19. WALLS, T. J., A. G. ENGEL, A. S. NAGEL, C. M. HARPER & V. F. TRASTEK. 1993. Congenital myasthenic syndrome associated with paucity of synaptic vesicles and reduced quantal release. Ann. N.Y. Acad. Sci. **681:** 461–468.
20. TRONTELJ, J. V. & E. STÅLBERG. 1991. Single motor end-plates in myasthenia gravis and LEMS at different firing rates. Muscle Nerve **14:** 226–232.
21. MANDLER, R. N. & R. A. MASELLI. 1996. Single fiber EMG in wound botulism. Muscle Nerve **19:** 1171–1173.
22. ENGEL, A. G. 1994. Congenital myasthenic syndromes. Neurol. Clin. **12:** 401–437.
23. MASELLI, R. A. & C. LEUNG. 1993. Analysis of anticholinesterase-induced neuromuscular transmission failure. Muscle Nerve **16:** 548–553.

24. Tamamizu, S., D. H. Butler, J. A. Lasalde & M. G. McNamee. 1996. Effects of antibody binding on structural transitions of the nicotinic acetylcholine receptor. Biochemistry 35(36): 11773–11781.

25. Maselli, R. A. 1997. End-plate electromyography: use of spectral analysis of end-plate noise. Muscle Nerve 20: 52–58.

26. Maselli, R. A., D. P. Richman & R. L. Wollmann. 1991. Inflammation at the neuromuscular junction in myasthenia gravis. Neurology 41: 1497–1504.

27. Ruff, R. L. 1998. Electrophysiology of postsynaptic activation. This volume.

28. Maselli, R. A., J. H. Jacobsen & J. P. Spire. 1986. Edrophonium: an aid in the diagnosis of acute organophosphate poisoning. Ann. Neurol. 19: 508–510.

29. Lo Monaco, M., M. Milone, L. Padua, M. R. Neri, B. Gregori, E. M. Valente, F. Odoardi & P. Tonali. 1997. Decrement-increment phenomenon in two patients with neuromyotonia. This conference.

30. Besser, R., I. Wessler & L. Gutmann. 1992. Analysis of the organophosphate-induced electromyographic response to repetitive nerve stimulation: two types of end-plate depolarization account for the two most common patterns of decrement. Muscle Nerve 15: 1369–1371.

31. Brown, J. C. 1974. Muscle weakness after rest in myotonic disorders: an electrophysiologic study. J. Neurol. Neurosurg. Psychiatry 37: 1336–1342.

32. Trontelj, J. V., M. Mihelin & E. Stålberg. 1986. Extracellularly recorded single muscle fiber responses to electrical stimulation in myotonia congenita. Electroencephalogr. Clin. Neurophysiol. 66: S106.

33. Lerche, H., N. Mitrovic, V. Dubowitz & F. Lehmann-Horn. 1996. Paramyotonia congenita: the R1448P Na^+ channel mutation in adult human skeletal tissue. Ann. Neurol. 39: 599–608.

34. Besser, R., L. Gutmann, U. Dillmann, L. S. Weilemann & H. C. Hopf. 1989. End-plate dysfunction in acute organophosphate intoxication. Neurology 39: 561–567.

35. Ohno, K., P. A. Quiram, M. Milone, H. L. Wang, M. C. Harper, J. N. Pruitt II, J. M. Brengman, L. Pao, K. H. Fischbeck, T. O. Crawford et al. 1997. Congenital myasthenic syndromes due to heteroallelic nonsense/missense mutations in the acetylcholine receptor epsilon subunit gene: identification and functional characterization of six new mutations. Hum. Mol. Genet. 6: 753–766.

36. Milone, M., H. L. Wang, K. Ohno, T. Fukudome, J. N. Pruitt, N. Bren, S. M. Sine & A. G. Engel. 1997. Slow-channel myasthenic syndrome caused by enhanced activation, desensitization, and agonist binding affinity attributable to mutation in the M2 domain of the acetylcholine receptor alpha subunit. J. Neurosci. 17: 5651–5665.

Mechanisms of Fatigue in Normal Young and Old Mice

MURALI PAGALA, TATSUJI NAMBA, AND DAVID GROB

Neuromuscular Research Lab
Maimonides Medical Center
and
SUNY Health Sciences Center
Brooklyn, New York 11219

INTRODUCTION

Aging is associated with a steady decline in essentially every physiological process in the body after the age of sexual maturity. Diminution in skeletal muscle function is one of the most debilitating consequences of old age. Significant reductions in muscle strength and in speed of muscle contraction and relaxation have been reported to occur in human subjects after 70 years[1] and in aged rats.[2] Endurance of the muscles during electrically evoked contractions was found to be unchanged,[3] increased,[4] or decreased[5] in the elderly compared to the young. In isolated soleus and laternal omohyoideus muscles of aged rats, no change was observed in fatigability following direct muscle stimulation.[6] However, increased fatigue or reduced endurance is a consistent complaint in old age. Hence, the present study was undertaken to evaluate the role played by impairment in both central and peripheral physiological processes in the development of fatigue in old age. This has been accomplished by monitoring the time course of fatigue in isolated skeletal muscles and on spontaneous motor activity and endurance of young and old mice.

MATERIALS AND METHODS

These studies were carried out using C57BL/6J male mice of 3 to 6 months (young) and 34 to 37 months (old) of age, obtained from Charles River Laboratories. To evaluate peripheral fatigue, the extensor digitorum longus (EDL) and soleus muscles were isolated from young and old anesthetized mice and mounted in an *in vitro* multimuscle chamber,[7] containing 30 mL of oxygenated physiological solution at 20 °C. Fatigue was induced by simultaneously stimulating all four muscles with square wave pulses of 7 to 10 V and 0.3 ms at 30 Hz for 0.5 s every 2.5 s until the original tension of the slowest fatiguing muscle declined by about 50%. Isometric tension response of each muscle was monitored through a separate force transducer and recorded with a Nicolet 4 channel digital oscilloscope, using a 10-ms sampling interval for 10 min at each channel. Spontaneous motor activity of the young and old mice was monitored using Columbus Instruments Opto-varimax-mini Model "B" activity meters interfaced to a microcomputer. Endurance of the young and old mice was monitored using the Columbus Instruments Treadmill CT-2 controller with a four-lane exercise unit. Swimming endurance of the mice was evaluated using a new monitor,[8] which consisted of a thermostatic water bath partially filled with distilled water at 30 °C. A rubber bulb dipped in the water bath, and attached at the other end to a force transducer, registered the force of water waves caused by swimming of the mouse. It was recorded using the Nicolet digital oscilloscope with a sampling interval of 10 ms for 30 min.

RESULTS

Time Course of Fatigue in Isolated Muscles

In 5 mice, the extrapolated mean time for a 50% drop in original tetanic tension was 109 s in young EDL and 129 s in old EDL muscle, while it was 482 s in young soleus and 1134 s in old soleus muscle (FIGURE 1). These results indicate that peripheral fatigue is not affected in fast-twitch EDL muscles, but is significantly reduced in slow-twitch soleus muscles of aged mice.

Spontaneous Motor Activity of Young and Old Mice

In 8 young mice, there were 9700 movements over a period of 24 h, and about 5300 of these were static stereotypic movements and 4400 were true ambulatory movements. In 8 old mice, there were 4267 movements, of which 3670 were stereotypic and only 597 were true ambulatory. These movements were significantly less

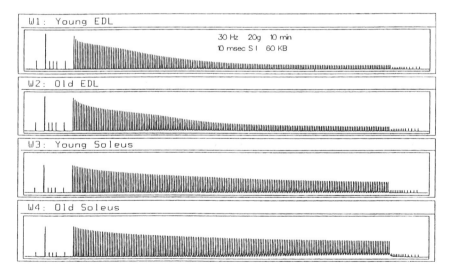

FIGURE 1. Tension decline during fatigue of EDL and soleus muscles from young and old mice.

than in the young mice. These results indicate that old mice are spontaneously less active than young mice.

Treadmill Endurance of Young and Old Mice

Young mice could run at belt inclinations of up to 10° and at belt speeds of up to 30 meters/min. At an inclination of 0° and belt speed of 10 meters/min, 8 young mice ran for 35 to 45 min, taking 0 to 3 rest periods of 10-s duration each. Old mice could not run when the inclination of the belt was set at 5°. At an inclination of 0° and belt speed of 10 meters/min, 8 old mice ran for 10 to 30 min, taking 8 to 21 rest periods of 10-s duration each. These results show that old mice have reduced endurance on a treadmill, indicating that they get exhausted or fatigued faster than young mice.

Swimming Endurance of Young and Old Mice

The swimming patterns of a young and an old mouse are shown in FIGURE 2. Five of the 6 young mice swam for 30 min, while 1 young mouse could swim for only 20 min. The mean swimming time before exhaustion was 28.3 min. For young mice, the mean value of the integrated swimming force was 366 g · s by 10 min, 696 g · s by 20

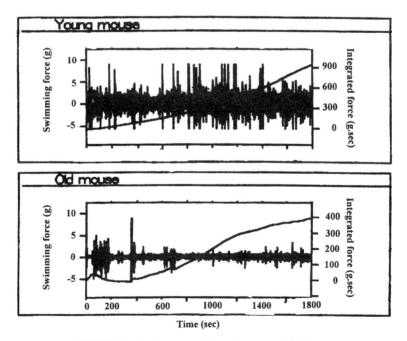

FIGURE 2. Swimming activity of young and old mice.

min, and 1002 g · s by 30 min. Two of the 6 old mice swam for 30 min, 1 for 20 min, another for 18 min, another for 13 min, and another for 10 min. The mean swimming time was 20.2 min. For old mice, the mean value of the integrated swimming force was 279 g · s by 10 min, 353 g · s by 20 min, and 401 g · s by 30 min. These studies show that the old mice have reduced swimming endurance.

CONCLUSIONS

These results indicate that, in old age, development of muscle weakness and fatigue involves considerable impairment in central neuronal and extramuscular processes, in addition to impairment in peripheral neuronal, neuromuscular, and muscular processes.

REFERENCES

1. CAMPBELL, M. J., A. J. McCOMAS & F. PETITO. 1973. Physiological changes in aging muscles. J. Neurol. Neurosurg. Psychiatry **36:** 174–182.
2. LARSSON, L. & L. EDSTROM. 1986. Effects of age on enzyme-histochemical fiber spectra and contractile properties of fast- and slow-twitch skeletal muscles in the rat. J. Neurol. Sci. **76:** 69–89.
3. CUPIDO, C. M., A. L. HICKS & J. MARTIN. 1992. Neuromuscular fatigue during repetitive stimulation in elderly and young adults. Eur. J. Appl. Physiol. **65:** 567–572.
4. DAVIES, C. T. M., M. J. WHITE & K. YOUNG. 1983. Electrically evoked and voluntary maximal isometric tension in relation to dynamic muscle performance in elderly male subjects, aged 69 years. Eur. J. Appl. Physiol. Occup. Physiol. **51:** 37–43.
5. NARICI, M. V., M. BORDINI & P. CERETELLI. 1991. Effect of aging on human adductor pollicis muscle function. J. Appl. Physiol. **71:** 1277–1281.
6. McCARTER, R. & J. McGEE. 1987. Influence of nutrition and aging on the composition and function of rat skeletal muscle. J. Gerontol. **42:** 432–441.
7. PAGALA, M. 1995. An *in vitro* multi-muscle tension recording chamber. FASEB J. **9:** abstract 5471.
8. PAGALA, M. 1995. Mouse swimming-force monitor. Unpublished.

Repetitive Nerve Stimulation in Studies of Respiratory Involvement in Myasthenia Gravis

U. ZIFKO,[a] C. B. BOLTON,[b] AND M. W. NICOLLE[b,c]

[a]Department of Neurology and Psychiatry
Kaiser Franz Josef Hospital
Vienna, Austria

[b]Neuromuscular Group
Department of Clinical Neurological Sciences
University of Western Ontario
London Health Sciences Center
London, Ontario, Canada N6A 5A5

INTRODUCTION

The recognition of respiratory difficulties in myasthenia gravis (MG) is important. Moreover, the clinical diagnosis of MG or of the Lambert-Eaton myasthenic syndrome (LEMS) can be difficult if respiratory compromise occurs without weakness elsewhere.[1,2] To appropriately manage MG or LEMS patients, it is important to be able to differentiate between the potential causes of dyspnea. These include impaired neuromuscular transmission at the diaphragm, the effects of coexistent cardiac or pulmonary diseases, or the effects of previous thoracic surgery. We have been disappointed in the ability of pulmonary function tests to discriminate between these possibilities and have further developed the technique of repetitive nerve stimulation (RNS) of the phrenic nerves as a means of assessing neuromuscular transmission at the diaphragm.[3] In this report, we describe the results in patients with MG and LEMS.

METHODS

Subjects

Control—Ten healthy volunteers were studied (7 male, 3 female), aged 25 to 57 (mean age 41). *MG/LEMS*—The patients followed in our clinic ($n = \approx 150$) are routinely asked about respiratory symptoms. Thirty-two patients were studied (5 MG without subjective respiratory complaints; 2 LEMS and 25 MG with respiratory complaints).

[c]To whom all correspondence should be addressed.

Pulmonary Function Tests

Standard pulmonary function tests (PFTs) were done on MG patients, usually on the same day as electrophysiological testing.

Electrophysiology

Three-Hz RNS was performed on one or more peripheral nerves (facial, accessory, median) using standard techniques. During the same session, phrenic nerve stimulation was performed.[3–5] The right phrenic nerve was stimulated percutaneously in the supraclavicular fossa with single square-wave pulses (0.1-ms duration). Recordings were made from the ipsilateral diaphragm with surface electrodes at 5 cm superior to the xiphoid process (G1) and at the costal margin 16 cm from the G1 electrode (G2). Supramaximal stimuli were used (150% of the stimulus intensity producing a maximal response). Accurate placement of the stimulator over the phrenic nerve just above the clavicle, avoidance of stimulation of the brachial plexus, and steady application of the stimulator were all important technical maneuvers. To minimize the effects of changes in diaphragm position, all stimuli were instituted at functional residual capacity (the end of a quiet expiration) and subjects were asked to hold their breath during stimulation. Measurements included negative peak diaphragm CMAP amplitude (NP amplitude), negative peak CMAP area (NP area), and CMAP duration (from the negative peak onset to the return to baseline). The values from the first CMAP were compared to either the fifth or sixth CMAP. Each train consisted of six stimuli at 3 Hz. At least three trains were performed for each individual at rest, and average values were calculated. Individual studies were scrutinized manually and discarded if artifacts (movement, ECG, etc.) were judged to have affected the results. The percent increment/decrement was calculated by computer (Advantage Medical, Clark Davis Medical Systems, London, Ontario). Normal values were calculated as the mean ± 2 SD.

RESULTS

Healthy Subjects

After phrenic nerve RNS, the change in the NP area was –2.1% (±4.2). Therefore, a decrement of >11% (mean controls + 2 SD) was taken as abnormal in subsequent studies.[3] The NP area measurement was more consistent between subjects than either NP amplitude or duration. Pseudofacilitation of the M wave was seen, with an increased NP amplitude (+12.1% ± 8.3) and a decreased duration (–8.7% ± 9.6). Thus, the NP area was judged to be a better measurement of neuromuscular transmission at the diaphragm.[3] Reproducibility between the results of two studies performed 4–6 weeks apart was excellent, with a variation in the mean decrement of the NP area of only 5.7% ± 2.8.

TABLE 1. Repetitive Stimulation of Phrenic and Nonphrenic Nerves in MG and LEMS Patients[a]

Group	n	PFTs Abnormal	RNS Nonphrenic[b]	RNS Phrenic
LEMS with dyspnea	2	2	2/2	2/2
MG, no dyspnea	5	4/4	1/4	2/5
MG with dyspnea[c]	25	17/20	15/23[d]	15/23[d]

[a]PFTs = pulmonary function tests. RNS = repetitive nerve stimulation.
[b]Nonphrenic nerves included facial, accessory, or median.
[c]Detailed results of MG with dyspnea are as follows:

Phrenic

	+	−
Nonphrenic +	12	3
−	3	5

[d]Two patients who had RNS of phrenic nerves, but not nonphrenic nerves, on the same day were not included.

MG and LEMS Patients

Twenty-seven of 32 patients had dyspnea (see TABLE 1). The majority of these had at least one other potential cause of dyspnea (e.g., asthma, CHF, COPD, etc.). PFTs were frequently abnormal, even in nondyspneic patients. The most common abnormalities were decreased maximal inspiratory or expiratory pressures. The significance of this was often uncertain, owing to suboptimal effort or to a poor seal around the mouthpiece secondary to facial weakness.

In 2 of the 5 nondyspneic MG patients, a decrement with phrenic RNS was seen (TABLE 1). In most dyspneic patients (17/23; 74%), the results of phrenic RNS correlated with nonphrenic RNS (decrement or not; see footnote c of TABLE 1). In 17 of 25 (68%) dyspneic MG/LEMS patients, a decrement of >11% with phrenic RNS was seen (FIGURE 1). In 3 of these, a decrement was only seen with RNS of the phrenic nerves (see footnote c of TABLE 1). In 6 patients studied with needle EMG, decreased diaphragm CMAP amplitudes and/or positive sharp waves and fibrillation potentials were occasionally seen, and these changes also disappeared with clinical improvement (not shown).

CONCLUSIONS

Dyspnea is a common complaint in MG and LEMS patients and often more than one possible cause for this is apparent clinically. Pulmonary function tests may not allow the differentiation between effort-related changes, artifactual results secondary to facial weakness, the effects of coexistent diseases, or weakness as a result of disordered neuromuscular transmission. The technique of repetitive stimulation of the

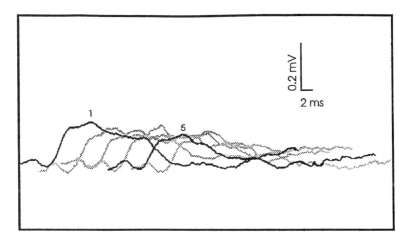

FIGURE 1. Repetitive stimulation of the phrenic nerves in a patient with LEMS produced a 26% decrement (1st to 5th) in the NP area.

phrenic nerves may be helpful in the differentiation of which of many possible causes of dyspnea are important in a given patient and it is a promising tool for the management of MG patients with respiratory symptoms.

REFERENCES

1. NICOLLE, M. W. *et al.* 1996. Lambert-Eaton myasthenic syndrome presenting with severe respiratory failure. Muscle Nerve **19:** 1328–1333.
2. MAHER, J. *et al.* 1997. Diagnostic difficulties in myasthenia gravis. Muscle Nerve. In press.
3. ZIFKO, U. *et al.* 1997. Repetitive phrenic nerve stimulation study in normal subjects. J. Clin. Neurophysiol. In press.
4. MIER, A. *et al.* 1990. Repetitive stimulation of the phrenic nerves in myasthenia gravis. Thorax **47:** 640–644.
5. CHEN, R. *et al.* 1995. Phrenic nerve conduction study in normal subjects. Muscle Nerve **18:** 330–335.

Plasma Exchange and Intravenous Immunoglobulin in Autoimmune Myasthenia Gravis[a]

PHILIPPE GAJDOS,[b] SYLVIE CHEVRET,[c] BERNARD CLAIR,[b]
CHRISTINE TRANCHANT,[d] AND CLAUDE CHASTANG[c]

[b]Service de Réanimation Médicale
Hôpital Raymond Poincaré
92380 Garches, France

[c]Département de Biostatistique et Informatique Médicale
Hôpital Saint Louis
Paris, France

[d]Service de Neurologie
Hospices Civils
Strasbourg, France

Plasma exchange (PE) was used in the treatment of myasthenia gravis (MG) as early as 1979. The effect of PE on MG has been documented through many open retrospective or prospective studies. In a review, Seybold[1] has summarized the results observed in three open studies and has reported a beneficial effect in 73% of the patients.

Dau reported an improvement in 44 out of 60 patients treated by weekly PE and immunosuppressive drugs.[2] Perlo[3] has treated 17 MG patients with 3–5 exchanges given over a period of 1–2 weeks. Results were graded as good or excellent for 11 and as fair for 7. Fornasari[4] has reported a series of 33 patients with MG who underwent a total of 49 cycles of PE. Patients were evaluated with a functional scale. An improvement was obtained for 20 patients (61%).

Antozzi[5] with a protocol of 2 PE at 1 day apart observed a positive outcome in 70% of 70 patients. However, PE has not been subject to clinical controlled trials and many questions are unanswered. First, the comparison of these studies is difficult. Some studies include chronic MG as well as patients with crisis or more or less acute forms of the disease, while others include only acute MG. The end point is different from one study to another, with some using a quantitative score, while others use a more subjective functional scale. The associated treatments, namely, steroids and/or immunosuppressive therapy, are not standardized in many studies and it may be difficult to dissociate their effects from those of PE. Anyway, given the number of confounding factors involved in the evaluation of treatment of MG, the lack of a placebo-treated control group in all these studies makes the objective assessment of PE

[a]This work was supported by the Delegation à la Recherche Clinique (Contract No. 912304, Assistance Publique, Hôpitaux de Paris), the Association Française contre les Myopathies, and the Laboratoire Français du Fractionnement et des Biotechnologies (LFB).

benefits difficult. Second, the schedule of PE is different from one study to another. Most authors use 3 to 5 sessions for 5 to 15 days,[3,6] but Antozzi[5] has obtained good results with only 2 PE every other day. Exchanged volumes range from 1 to 4 liters per session.

Nevertheless, based on all these studies and on a large clinical experience, there is a consensus to consider PE as the standard treatment for myasthenic crisis or in MG with acute deterioration.[7]

The efficacy of high-dose intravenous infusion of immunoglobulin (IVIg) was first shown in idiopathic thrombocytopenic purpura at the daily dose of 0.4 g/kg/day for 5 days.[8] Thereafter, IVIg has been widely used in other autoimmune diseases[9] and in MG as early as 1984.[10,11] The effect of IVIg has been documented by several reports. A recent review[12] summarizes the results observed in seven open studies of at least 10 patients. In a total of 119 treated patients, 90 (76%) improved. Arsura[13] has treated 12 patients with IVIg at a daily dose of 0.4 g/kg for 5 days. Eleven patients improved, beginning within 5 days after the start of treatment, with sustained improvement lasting up to 12 weeks. In a series of 21 patients treated with the same protocol, reported by us,[14] a significant increase of muscular score was observed at 10 days after the first infusion of IVIg and was maintained for up to 25 days. In this series, the success rate, defined as a gain of at least 20 points in the muscular score, was obtained in 50% of the patients. Such success was observed only in the acute forms and never in the chronic forms of the disease. Cosi[15] treated 37 patients. A one-degree improvement of a global functional scale was recorded at 12 days after the beginning of the treatment in 70% of the patients and persisted for up to 60 days in 59%. A two-degree improvement was observed in 54%. The percentage of improvement did not significantly differ between patients with a chronic form and patients with an acute phase of MG. In these different studies, side effects were limited. Arsura[16] reported a transient decrease in strength before improvement in 4 out of 9 patients; this observation was reported also by Evoli,[17] but not by other authors.

Concerning the course of AChR Ab titers after IVIg, decreased concentrations have been shown in some series, while in others AChR Ab remained unchanged.[9,16] In our initial pilot study,[14] the mean AChR Ab titer decreased by one-third at day 15 to reach baseline value on day 25.

Finally, as for PE, one must be cautious in interpreting these results of IVIg treatment. Indeed, the comparison of the different series is hazardous. Some include only acute forms of the disease, while in other studies patients have a more or less progressive or chronic stable MG. Clinical evaluation was performed according to a muscular score in some studies, while others relied on various subjective functional classifications.

There is also some questions with the IVIg dosage used. All the series used a daily dose of 0.4 g/kg/day for 5 days. This schedule is based on the first reports of IVIg therapy for idiopathic thrombocytopenic purpura. However, the optimal regimen in term of clinical benefits has not yet been determined. Other schedules have been successfully proposed for idiopathic thrombocytopenic purpura including a single dose of 0.8 g/kg[18] or a daily dose of 0.5 g/kg for 2 days.[19] Considering the drawback of IVIg and the high costs, lower doses of IVIg in MG need to be evaluated. Finally, all these studies are retrospective or open prospective and the effect of IVIg has never been compared with placebo or other treatments.

These considerations have led, in France, to a clinical trial. As it is a large consensus on the efficacy of PE in myasthenic crisis, a placebo-controlled study appeared, irrelevant on an ethical point of view. Therefore, the mean objective was to randomly assess the efficacy and tolerance of IVIg in acute MG as compared to PE. Second, we experimented and compared two different schedules of IVIg, namely, a daily dose of 0.4 g/kg for 3 or 5 days. The results of this multicenter trial have been recently published[20] and will be briefly reported here.

From December 1991 to April 1995, 87 patients with exacerbations of MG were included. Exacerbation was defined by at least one of the following: difficulty in swallowing, acute respiratory failure, or major functional disability responsible for the discontinuation of physical activity. Patients were randomized to receive either PE or IVIg. Forty-one patients received 3 PE, of 1.5 volume each, performed every other day. Forty-six received IVIg (0.4 g/kg/day, with 23 being further allocated to a 3-day schedule and 23 to a 5-day schedule).

Immunosuppressive treatment with steroids or other drugs was carried out during the 2 weeks of the trial as before inclusion without any change in dosage. The main end point was the absolute variation of a myasthenic muscular score between randomization and day 15. Other end points were the time to the occurrence of treatment response (defined as an increase of at least 20 points in the myasthenic muscular score), variation of anti-AChR Ab titers, and adverse effects.

The myasthenic muscular score variation at day 15 was similar in both groups: the mean variation of score was 16.6 (95% confidence interval 11.6–21.6) in the PE group and 15.6 (95% confidence interval 10.9–20.3) in the IVIg group ($p = 0.65$, Wilcoxon test). In the IVIg group, a similar efficacy was observed in both IVIg schedules: mean variation of 18.9 (95% confidence interval 13.1–24.7) in the 3-day group and 12.4 (95% confidence interval 5–19.8) in the 5-day group ($p = 0.14$, Wilcoxon test). The median score variation over time is given in FIGURE 1.

FIGURE 2 displays the estimated time to reach a 20-point gain in score value within the first 15 days. Such a 20-point gain was observed for 48 out of the 87 patients included. The median response time was 9 days in the PE group and greater than 15 days in the IVIg group, with an estimated relative risk of 0.67 (95% confidence interval 0.38–1.18; $p = 0.14$, log rank test). It is noteworthy that this gain in score value could be of short duration: on day 15, only 36 of these 48 patients still had an increased score value of 20 points (18 in the PE group and 18 in the IVIg group).

Among the patients with baseline detectable AChR Ab, 62% exhibited on day 15 a decrease in concentration as compared to that measured at randomization. The mean variation in AChR Ab titer was similar in both groups: –13.8% (95% confidence interval –40.8% to +13.2%) in the PE group and –16.8% (95% confidence interval –24.9% to +58.5%) in the IVIg group ($p = 0.36$, Wilcoxon test). However, the meanings of these data are not clear. Indeed, we do not know anything about the variations of the antibody titers between randomization and day 15.

Adverse events were observed in 8 patients in the PE group and, in 2 of these patients, the PE were discontinued. In the IVIg group, one side effect was observed (TABLE 1).

Improvement rates observed in this trial are in agreement with previously published noncontrolled studies of PE or IVIg efficacy. No difference in outcome was observed in the two compared treatments, that is, 3 PE and IVIg at 0.4 g/kg daily for

median score variation   **A**

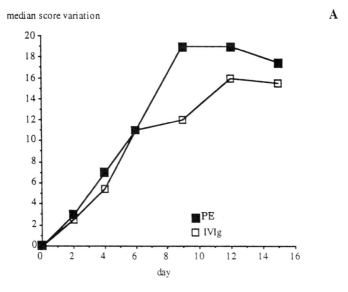

median score variation   **B**

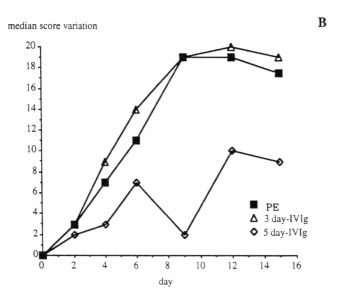

FIGURE 1. Evolution of the myasthenic muscular score from randomization in the three randomized groups, according to the first (A) or second (B) randomization. (From reference 20.)

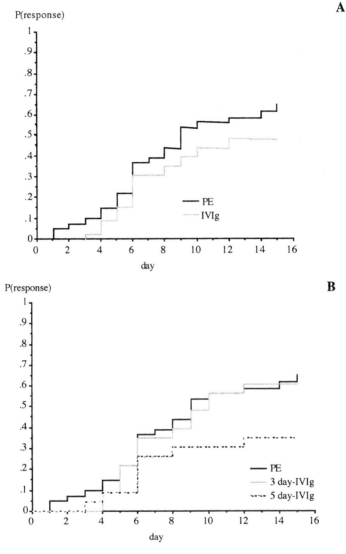

FIGURE 2. Time to reach a 20-point variation from randomization in the myasthenic muscular score value, according to the first (A) or second (B) randomization. (From reference 20.)

3 or 5 days. Five days of infusion of IVIg did not appear better than a 3-day schedule. However, given the number of patients included in each IVIg group, the power of the study does not allow a final conclusion on this point. The more-important number of side effects in the PE group and their severity for 2 patients are also in agreement with the literature. However, one must keep in mind that some severe effects, al-

TABLE 1. Adverse Events Observed in Each Randomized Group[a]

Adverse Event	Plasma Exchange ($n = 41$)	IVIg ($n = 46$)
Hemolysis	1	0
Bleeding disorders	2	0
Catheter-related venous thrombosis	1	0
Fever ($\geq 38\ °C$)	2	0
Chills	2	0
Headaches	0	1
Nausea, vomiting	1	0
Systolic blood pressure < 80 mmHg	2	0
Tachycardia	1	0
Other	2	0
Patients with at least one event	8 (20%)	1 (2%)

[a]From reference 20.

though rare, have been reported with IVIg, such as renal failure or aseptic meningitis, and there is a potential risk of transmission of blood-borne pathogens.

In conclusion, the results of this clinical trial of PE and IVIg in exacerbation of myasthenia gravis did not show any marked difference in the efficacy of both treatments and exhibited a very limited risk of IVIg. This latter treatment appears to be a therapeutic alternative for the acute phase of MG especially when PE are contraindicated or when vascular access is difficult.

However, this is the first controlled trial comparing PE and IVIg. As for all new therapy, the results have to be confirmed by another controlled trial. Furthermore, the small sample size of each IVIg arm does not allow a conclusion concerning the optimal dosage of IVIg.

Finally, many questions were not addressed by this trial. For example:

(1) How long is the effect of IVIg?
(2) Is IVIg effective in more chronic forms of MG?
(3) Is there any role for IVIg as a steroid-sparing agent?
(4) What is the mechanism of action of IVIg in MG?

REFERENCES

1. SEYBOLD, M. E. 1987. Plasmapheresis in myasthenia gravis. Ann. N.Y. Acad. Sci. **505:** 584–587.
2. DAU, P. C. 1981. Response to plasmapheresis and immunosuppressive drug therapy in sixty myasthenia gravis patients. Ann. N.Y. Acad. Sci. **377:** 700–708.
3. PERLO, V. P., B. T. SHAHANI, C. E. HUGGINS, J. HUNT, K. KOSINSKI & F. POTTS. 1981. Effect of plasmapheresis in myasthenia gravis. Ann. N.Y. Acad. Sci. **377:** 709–724.
4. FORNASARI, P. M., G. RIVA, G. PICCOLO, V. COSI & M. LOMBARDI. 1985. Short and long term clinical effects of plasma exchange in 33 cases of myasthenia gravis. Int. J. Artif. Organs **8:** 159–162.

5. ANTOZZI, C., M. GEMMA, B. REGI, E. BERTA, P. CANFALANIERI, D. PELUCHETTI, R. MANTEGAZZA, F. BAGGI, M. MARCONI, F. FIACCHINO & F. CORNELIO. 1985. A short plasma exchange protocol is effective in severe myasthenia gravis. J. Neurol. **238:** 103–107.

6. LEWIS, R. A., J. F. SELWA & R. P. LISAK. 1995. Myasthenia gravis: immunological mechanisms and immunotherapy. Ann. Neurol. **37**(S1): S51–S62.

7. BERGAMINI, E. L., D. COCITO, U. L. DURELLI & G. QUATTROCOLO. 1983. Opinions about plasma exchange and associated treatments in the therapy of myasthenia gravis. Muscle Nerve **6:** 457–458.

8. IMBACH, P., S. BARUNDUN, U. D'APUZZO, G. BAUMGARTNER, A. HIRT, A. MORICE, E. ROSSI, M. SCHONI, M. VEST & H. D. WAGNER. 1981. High dose intravenous gamma globulin for idiopathic thrombocytopenic purpura in childhood. Lancet **1:** 1228–1231.

9. DWYERS, J. M. 1992. Manipulating the immune system with immune globulin. N. Engl. J. Med. **326:** 107–116.

10. GAJDOS, PH., H. D. OUTIN, D. ELKHARRAT, D. BRUNEL, P. DE ROHAN-CHABOT, J. C. RAPHAEL, M. GOULON, C. GOULON-GOEAU & E. MOREL. 1984. High dose intravenous gamma globulin for myasthenia gravis. Lancet **1:** 406–407.

11. FATEH-MOGHADAM, A., M. WICK, U. BESINGER & R. G. GEURSEN. 1984. High dose intravenous gamma globulin for myasthenia gravis. Lancet **1:** 848–849.

12. VAN DER MECHÉ, F. G. A. & P. A. VAN DORN. 1997. The current place of high-dose immunoglobulins on the treatment of neuromuscular disorders. Muscle Nerve **20:** 136–147.

13. ARSURA, E., A. BICK, N. G. BRUNNER, T. NAMBA & D. GROB. 1986. High dose intravenous immunoglobulin in the management of myasthenia gravis. Arch. Intern. Med. **146:** 1365–1368.

14. GAJDOS, PH., H. D. OUTIN, E. MOREL, J. C. RAPHAEL & M. GOULON. 1987. High-dose intravenous gamma globulin for myasthenia gravis: an alternative to plasma exchange. Ann. N.Y. Acad. Sci. **505:** 842–844.

15. COSI, V., M. LOMBARDI, G. PICCOLO & A. ERBETTA. 1991. Treatment of myasthenia gravis with high dose intravenous immunoglobulin. Acta Neurol. Scand. **84:** 81–84.

16. ARSURA, E. 1989. Experience with intravenous immunoglobulin in myasthenia gravis. Clin. Immunol. Immunopathol. **53:** S170–S179.

17. EVOLI, A., M. T. PALMISONI, E. BARTACCIONI, L. PADUA & P. TONALI. 1993. High dose intravenous immunoglobulin in myasthenia gravis. Ital. J. Neurol. **14:** 233–237.

18. BLANCHETTE, V., P. IMBACH, M. ANDREW, M. ADAMS, J. MCMILLON, E. WANG, R. MILNER, K. ALI, D. BARNARD, M. BERNSTEIN, K. W. CHAN, D. ESSELTINC, B. DE VEBER, S. ISRAELS, N. KOBRINSKY & B. LUKE. 1994. Randomized trial of intravenous immunoblobulin G, intravenous anti-D, and oral prednisone in childhood acute immune thrombocytopenic purpura. Lancet **1:** 703–707.

19. GODEAU, B., S. LESAGE, M. DIVINE, V. WIRQUIN, J. P. FARCET & P. BIERLING. 1993. Treatment of adult chronic autoimmune thrombocytopenic purpura with repeated high dose intravenous immunoglobulin. Blood **82:** 1415–1421.

20. GAJDOS, PH., S. CHEVRET, B. CLAIR, C. TRANCHANT & C. CHASTANG. 1997. Clinical trial of plasma exchange and high dose intravenous immunoglobulin in myasthenia gravis. Ann. Neurol. **41:** 789–796.

Polyclonal Immunoglobulins Induce Apoptosis in a Small Proportion of Peripheral Lymphocytes *in Vitro*

FELIX BISCHOF AND ARTHUR MELMS

Department of Neurology
University of Tübingen
72076 Tübingen, Germany

INTRODUCTION

Intravenous application of high-dose polyclonal immunoglobulin G (IgG) preparations results in dramatic clinical improvement in a wide range of disorders associated with circulating antibodies against self antigens, including myasthenia gravis.[1,2] The mechanisms of action of this expensive therapy remain obscure. Several *in vitro* effects of IVIG have been demonstrated[3–7] that do not sufficiently explain the acute and long-term effects of IVIG treatment *in vivo*. We therefore investigated whether the inhibition of lymphocytes by immunoglobulins is due to induction of apoptosis.

METHODS

Cells

PBMCs were isolated from healthy volunteers by density gradient centrifugation (Lymphoprep, Nycomed) and were cultured in RPMI1640 containing 10% heat-inactivated fetal calf serum, 100 U/mL penicillin, and 100 μg/mL streptomycin. A commercially available immunoglobulin preparation (Polyglobin N, Bayer, Germany) was extensively dialyzed against culture medium and diluted to a final concentration of 25 mg/mL.

Cell Staining with Propidium Iodide

Cells were cultured in culture medium alone, in the presence of 1 mg/mL dexamethasone (Fortecortin, Merck, Germany), or in 25 mg/mL immunoglobulin for 24 and 48 h and stained with anti-CD19-FITC (Sigma, Germany). Propidium iodide was added to a final concentration of 10 μg/mL and FACS analysis was performed within 15 minutes.

In Situ *DNA End-Labeling (TUNEL) and FACS Analysis*

PBMCs were cultured as described above for 60 h at 37 °C, stained with anti-CD19-FITC, washed twice, and fixed for 30 min in 4% paraformaldehyde. Fluorescein staining of DNA strand breaks was performed using the "*In Situ* Cell Death Detection Kit, Fluorescein" (Boehringer, Mannheim, Germany) according to the instructions of the manufacturer, and two-color FACS analysis was performed.

RESULTS

After incubation for 24 h, 0.7% of control cells, 50% of dexamethasone-incubated cells, and 2.5% of the immunoglobulin-incubated cells were positive for propidium iodide uptake, indicating disturbances of membrane integrity as a measure of apoptosis. After 48 h, 0.1% of control cells, 85% of dexamethasone-incubated cells, and 1.2% of the immunoglobulin-incubated cells showed propidium iodide uptake (FIGURE 1).

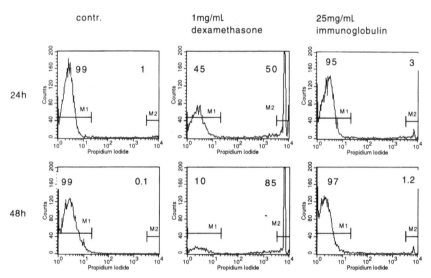

FIGURE 1. Peripheral lymphocytes show disturbances of membrane integrity after incubation with 25 mg/mL of polyclonal immunoglobulin preparations. Cells were incubated with medium alone, 1 mg/mL dexamethasone, or 25 mg/mL immunoglobulins and were stained with anti-CD19-FITC and propidium iodide. After 24 h, 1.3% of control cells, 55% of dexamethasone-incubated cells, and 4.6% of the immunoglobulin-incubated cells were positive for propidium iodide uptake. After 48 h, 0.9% of control cells, 89% of dexamethasone-incubated cells, and 3.4% of the immunoglobulin-incubated cells showed propidium iodide uptake. Thus, immunoglobulin-incubated cells showed disturbances of membrane integrity in a higher proportion than control cells.

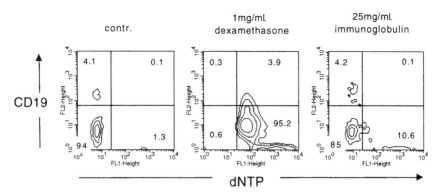

FIGURE 2. Control cells, dexamethasone-incubated cells, and immunoglobulin-incubated cells were stained for CD19 PE, and *in situ* DNA end-labeling with FITC-labeled dNTP and FACS analysis were performed: 1.6% of control cells, 99% of dexamethasone-incubated cells, and 11% of the cells incubated with immunoglobulin were TUNEL-positive.

Thus, the proportion of cells that show disturbances of membrane integrity is higher in the immunoglobulin-incubated cells than in cells incubated in medium alone. The effect is only moderate in contrast to the effect of dexamethasone, which is a known inductor of apoptosis in these cells. Staining for CD19 and two-color FACs analysis showed that T cells and B cells were equally affected (data not shown).

Similar results were obtained by *in situ* end-labeling of DNA strand breaks by the TUNEL reaction, which serves as a measure of late apoptosis (FIGURE 2). Here, 11% of the cells incubated with immunoglobulin, 1.6% of the control cells, and 99% of the dexamethasone-incubated cells were TUNEL-positive after 60 h. Most of the immunoglobulin-incubated TUNEL-positive cells were CD19−.

DISCUSSION

We found disturbances of membrane integrity and TUNEL-positive cells in peripheral lymphocytes after incubation with immunoglobulins. The concentration of immunoglobulin in our experiments is efficient *in vivo* and has been shown to inhibit proliferation of lymphocytes *in vitro*. To confirm that the immunoglobulins were responsible for the measured effect, the preparation was extensively dialyzed against medium. Our results indicate that immunoglobulins have the potential to induce apoptosis in peripheral lymphocytes, although in this system the effect was only moderate as compared to the effect of dexamethasone. Thus, immune modulation by intravenous immunoglobulins on various levels of the immune response may result in induction of apoptosis in a proportion of peripheral lymphocytes *in vivo*.

REFERENCES

1. IMBACH, P., S. BARANDUN, V. D'APUZZO *et al.* 1981. High-dose intravenous gamma globulin for idiopathic thrombocytopenic purpura in childhood. Lancet **1:** 1228–1231.
2. COOK, L., J. F. HOWARD, JR. & J. D. FOLDS. 1988. Immediate effects of intravenous IgG administration on peripheral blood B and T cells and polymorphonuclear cells in patients with myasthenia gravis. J. Clin. Immunol. **8:** 23–31.
3. MCGUIRE, W. A., H. H. YANG, E. BRUNO *et al.* 1987. Treatment of antibody-mediated pure red-cell aplasia with high-dose intravenous gamma globulin. N. Engl. J. Med. **317:** 1004–1008.
4. JUNGI, T. W., M. SANTER, P. G. LERCH *et al.* 1986. Effect of various treatments of gamma-globulin (IgG) for achieving intravenous tolerance on the capacity to interact with human monocyte Fc receptors: a comparative study. Vox Sang. **51:** 18–26.
5. KURLANDER, R. J. 1980. Reversible and irreversible loss of Fc receptor function of human monocytes as a consequence of interaction with immunoglobulin G. J. Clin. Invest. **66:** 773–781.
6. KONDO, N., T. OZAWA, K. MUSHIAKE *et al.* 1991. Suppression of immunoglobulin production of lymphocytes by intravenous immunoglobulin. J. Clin. Immunol. **11:** 152–158.
7. VAN SCHAIK, I. N., I. LUNDKVIST, M. VERMEULEN *et al.* 1992. Polyvalent immunoglobulin for intravenous use interferes with cell proliferation *in vitro*. J. Clin. Immunol. **12:** 325–334.

Thymectomy in Childhood Myasthenia Gravis

MARJORIE E. SEYBOLD

Department of Neurology
Veterans Administration San Diego Health Care System
San Diego, California 92161
and
Department of Neurosciences
University of California, San Diego
La Jolla, California 92093

INTRODUCTION

Thymectomy is a well-accepted treatment for young adults with autoimmune myasthenia gravis (MG). This acceptance has occurred despite the absence of controlled studies or a definite explanation for its effectiveness.

Logic supports the use of thymectomy. At least 80% of MG patients have thymic abnormality, either hyperplasia or thymoma.[1] Myoid cells within the thymus display acetylcholine receptor (AChR), the antigen targeted in MG.[2] This thymic AChR may serve as an antigenic stimulus in the disease. The thymus in patients with MG also contains autoreactive T cells,[3,4] although whether these cells originate in the thymus or migrate there secondarily is not clear.[1] Hyperplastic thymus tissue, taken from MG patients at surgery, can produce AChR-antibodies (AChR-ab) *in vitro*,[5] testifying to the role of the thymus as a source of antibody production. Whether one (or more) of these factors initiates or sustains MG is not known, but their existence suggests that removal of the gland may be helpful in treatment of the disease.

Support for thymectomy also comes from a matched retrospective study that found that the incidence of remission of MG symptoms improved following thymectomy[6] and from numerous unmatched series. Favorable personal experience by physicians dealing with MG on a frequent basis has also encouraged the use of thymectomy.[7] Positive outcome appears most likely when thymectomy is done within a year after the onset of symptoms.[8,9] Prethymectomy disease severity and AChR-ab are less clearly linked to outcome, and thymic pathology found at the time of surgery is not definitely related to outcome.[10]

In the absence of a large controlled study of thymectomy (which is unlikely to ever occur) or of a cure for MG, it is doubtful that thymectomy for young adult MG patients will be further challenged. However, there remain several MG patient groups in which thymectomy continues to be questioned: older adults, patients with detectable AChR-ab (seronegative MG), patients with only ocular symptoms (ocular MG), and children.

The controversy regarding thymectomy in children will be explored here. Issues investigated are the incidence of postthymectomy and spontaneous remission, risk of postthymectomy immune deficiency, risk of postthymectomy neoplasm, uncertainty of the diagnosis of MG in seronegative children, and adverse effects of alternative immunosuppressive therapies.

METHODS AND STUDIES INCLUDED

An attempt was made to examine the pertinent literature from 1966 to the present, using a computer search based on keywords such as child, infant, thymectomy, immune deficiency, steroids, azathioprine, and myasthenia gravis in various combinations. When possible, full articles were reviewed. In some cases only abstracts were available and occasionally articles could not be obtained at all. Surely, some articles were missed and I would appreciate being informed by the reader if pertinent articles have been omitted.

Large single-center studies were sought in an attempt to determine remission frequency, occurrence of infection or neoplasm after thymectomy, and AChR-ab sensitivity in identification of MG. Consideration was given to studies of nonwhite children for information suggesting different patterns of disease in these groups. Individual case reports of children with MG were also examined for reports of immune impairment following thymectomy. Studies of immunologic status in children who underwent thymus removal during cardiac surgery and descriptions of immunosuppression in children and young adults with disorders other than MG were also utilized.

Studies involving children were not uniform, and ages and groupings varied among the reports. The upper age limit for inclusion was generally 15 to 19 years. Some authors divided the children by prepuberty and postpuberty ages or into prepuberty, peripuberty, and postpuberty groups. Other authors separated the children into early (i.e., less than 2 years) and late onset. The disparity in groupings made it difficult to combine the data in any logical way. Some series were excluded (e.g., references 11 and 12) because only children that had failed to improve on steroids received thymectomy. Others were excluded from the remission section if children below an arbitrary age were not considered for thymectomy,[13,14] although data within these papers were used in other parts of the discussion. For purposes of the study of results and remissions, only reports without age or thymectomy limitations, involving more than 20 children, and containing extractable information on remissions were used.

Most authors separated or removed children with neonatal MG (i.e., born to a mother with MG) or congenital MG (i.e., presumed or proven to have a developmental disorder of neuromuscular transmission) from those presumed to have autoimmune MG. However, separation of the latter two disorders was not always clear as the clinical course may be similar for developmental and autoimmune MG patients. AChR-ab, when detected, is a reliable indicator of autoimmune MG. However, some studies were done prior to the availability of AChR-ab studied.[10] After AChR-ab tests became commercially available, not all children were studied. Even when studied, some children were initially seronegative, but became seropositive later in the course of their disease, sometimes after multiple tests. Thus, the incidence of AChR-ab detection, and therefore its sensitivity, varies with the frequency of determination in the individual as well as with severity (AChR-ab is generally lower and less often detectable in patients with only ocular findings). This problem will be further discussed below.

RESULTS

Incidence of Postthymectomy versus Spontaneous Remission

Five studies from North America[8–10,15,16] were used (TABLE 1). (Data from the Mayo Clinic by Rodriguez et al.[8] included some of the same patients reported earlier by Seybold et al.[10] so that the two studies, although analyzing the data differently, are not entirely distinct.)

The early study of Millichap and Dodge[15] described 35 children with onset of MG between ages 2 and 16, of whom 21 underwent thymectomy. The medically treated group, followed for an average of 9.7 years, had a 14% incidence of remission. Surgically treated patients, followed for an average of 3.4 years after thymectomy, had a 28% remission rate. For those operated within the first 2 years after onset of MG, the remission rate was 50%.

The data from Rodriguez et al.[8] indicate a spontaneous remission rate of 8% over 3 years as compared with 38% in the 3 years postthymectomy. After follow-up of 15

TABLE 1. Spontaneous and Thymectomy-related Remissions in Children with Myasthenia Gravis

Reference	Age (Years)	Number	Spontaneous Remissions	Postthymectomy Remissions	Follow-up Duration (Years)[a]
15	2–16	35	14.3% (n = 14)	28.5% (n = 21)	9.7 MT 3.4 ST
10	2–16	95	27.7% (n = 47)	37.5% (n = 48)	19.3 MT 12.7 ST
	prepuberty		30%[b] (n = 20)	28.5% (n = 7)	
8	1–16	149	30.1% (n = 149)	52.9%[c] (n = 85)	15 MT + ST 15 ST
	≤11	41	45% (n = 41)	31% (n = 16)	
16	1.5–16	24		67%[d] (n = 24)	10.1 ST
9	1–19	115	15% (n = 20)	16%[e] (n = 51)	1–39

[a]MT = medical treatment; ST = surgical treatment.
[b]Two patients in remission had received thymic irradiation.
[c,d,e]Remission of 67%, 67%, and 58%, respectively, in patients with thymectomy within 1 year of onset of MG.

years or more in the two Mayo Clinic studies,[8,10] the incidence of spontaneous remission was 28–30%. Patients treated with thymectomy in those series experienced a 38–53% remission rate over approximately the same time period.

Andrews et al.,[9] analyzing data from Duke and the University of North Carolina, found a remission rate of 15% in nonoperated white patients ($n = 12$) and of 16% in operated patients ($n = 51$). However, when evaluated separately, the remission rate of patients operated within the first year after the onset of their disease was 58% ($n = 12$). African-American patients followed by the same group had no spontaneous remissions ($n = 12$), 7% remissions if operated at all ($n = 30$), and 15% remission rate if operated within the first year after the development of symptoms ($n = 13$).

The Adams series from Toronto[16] contained only operated patients, generally operated within the first year of their disease. They reported a remission rate of 67% ($n = 24$) with a mean duration of follow-up of 10.1 years.

Asian patients were reported by Wong et al. from Hong Kong.[12] Most of their 101 patients had ocular MG (71%). They reported a 43% spontaneous remission rate ($n = 56$), while operated patients, all of whom had generalized MG, had a remission rate of only 17% ($n = 12$). These data cannot be fairly compared with the series included above as only children with moderately severe generalized MG who had failed medical treatment were operated. Japanese patients are also reported to frequently have only ocular findings (75–90% of children under 12 years) and to have a 55–60% rate of combined spontaneous improvement and remission.[17] Remission alone appears from their data to be only about 10% of this combined total. This study was not included in the tables as thymectomy was apparently not performed in these patients.

Several problems become apparent in the analysis of these data. Puberty is differently defined among the various studies, so comparisons across groups are essentially impossible except for the preadult group as a whole. Response to thymectomy appears to relate to duration of symptoms, again making comparisons difficult unless this information is explicitly given. Also, racial background may influence the natural course of MG, making cross-racial comparisons suspect.

Despite these problems, the patients treated with thymectomy in the Millichap series[15] and Mayo series,[8,10] the patients in the Andrews report[9] who were operated within the first year of onset of symptoms, and the Adams patients,[16] when compared with the nonthymectomized patients in these series, all experienced a higher likelihood of remission (TABLE 2). The degree of benefit from the thymectomy relative to spontaneous remission is hard to estimate. If the Mayo figures are used and thymectomy is accepted to be the determining factor (not necessarily a valid assumption), a 10–23% improvement in remission rate, 15 years postthymectomy, is suggested. If only those patients operated within the first 2 years after onset of MG are included, the remission rate is 57% as compared with 25% of those operated later and 20% for those without thymectomy (TABLE 3).

Risk of Postthymectomy Immune Deficiency

Two sources of information were examined: children without MG who received thymectomy in association with cardiac surgery and children with MG who under-

TABLE 2. Incidence of Remissions with Early, Late, and No Thymectomy in Childhood MG[a]

Reference	Treatment	No.	Remission
15	TX ≤ 24 mo	10	50%
	TX > 24 mo	11	9%
	no TX	14	14%
10	TX ≤ 24 mo	29	44.8%
	TX > 24 mo	19	26%
	no TX	54	24%
8	TX < 12 mo	31	67%
	TX > 12 mo	54	44%
16	TX ≤ 24 mo	24	67%
9	TX ≤ 12 mo	12	58%
	TX > 12 mo	39	3%
	no TX	20	15%

[a]TX = thymectomy.

went thymectomy.

Brearley et al.[18] reported that cardiac surgery–thymectomy patients operated within the first 3 months of life showed a deficiency in absolute T cell numbers, but no abnormality in B cell numbers or in responsiveness to phytohemagglutinin (PHA) or concanavalin A (ConA). Follow-up was 9 months to 3 years after thymectomy. No important clinical consequences were appreciated in these patients. Four patients reported by Rubinstein et al.[19] operated for suspected thymic malignancy at ages 3.5 to 9.5 months showed reduced response to oral polio vaccination and skin tests for delayed hypersensitivity. They had no clinical abnormalities from 5 to 14 years after operation.

Ramos et al.[20] compared 13 children with thymectomy during the first year of life and 10 children operated at ages 1.5 to 4 years. Follow-up was 4.8 years in the younger group and 8.3 years for the older children. T cell subsets were decreased and natural killer cells (NK) increased in those children operated before the age of 1 year, but no abnormality was detected in those operated later. Reszke et al.[21] also reported

TABLE 3. Summary of Remissions[a]

Treatment	Remission/Total	% Remission
early TX[b]	61/106	57%
late TX	31/123	25%
no TX	18/88	20%

[a]TX = thymectomy.
[b]TX ≤ 2 years after onset of MG.

no immunologic abnormality (T cell count, PHA reactivity, humoral immunity, NBT test, or complement C3c and C4) in 6 patients thymectomized between ages 2 months and 15 years and followed for 6 to 12 years after surgery. These patients also had no history of increased number of infections. In the retrospective thymectomy report by Rodriguez et al.,[8] long-term survival was slightly better for patients who were operated upon (median follow-up, 14–17 years). No difference in autoimmune disease was apparent between operated and nonoperated patients. Infection incidence was not mentioned.

Risk of Postthymectomy Neoplasm

In the studies by Rodriguez et al.[8] and Seybold et al.,[10] no difference in the frequency of neoplasm in the operated and nonoperated patients was present.

Uncertainty of the Diagnosis of MG in Seronegative Children

Children with MG appear less likely than adults to have detectable AChR-ab.[11,22] In the study by Andrews et al.,[22] seronegativity was particularly prevalent in patients with onset in the prepuberty period (<9.3 years for males, <8.9 years for females). In this group, only 56% (5/9) of patients with generalized MG were AChR-ab positive and, of those, 2 converted to positive at or after puberty. Peripuberty (ages 9.3–16.5 for males, 8.9–15.3 for females) had a 89% positive AChR-ab rate (16/18) and all 18 postpuberty patients had detectable AChR-ab. Snead et al.[11] found 58% of children with generalized MG to have AChR-ab (mean age, 7.7 years); 40% of patients with ocular MG were AChR-ab positive. Assays in the Andrews study[22] used human AChR as antigen; those in the Snead study[11] used rat AChR, which is less sensitive.

Seronegativity was more common among children with mild MG.[22] Forty-three percent of patients (3/7) in remission or with only ocular findings were seronegative. Only 13% (5/39) of patients with generalized MG were seronegative.[22]

The problem of differentiating congenital MG from seronegative autoimmune MG is addressed by Andrews et al.[22] They used a positive response to plasmapheresis or immunosuppression, lack of family history or consanguinity, lack of beneficial response to anticholinesterase medications, and absence of characteristic clinical or electrophysiologic features of congenital MG to help in the separation of the two disorders. In three seronegative patients (3/11), they were unable to comfortably distinguish between autoimmune and congenital MG. These patients had onset of symptoms at ages 1.7, 6.7, and 9 years.

Adverse Effects of Alternative Immunosuppressive Therapies

The potential adverse effects of steroid medications[23] and other immunosuppressant drugs such as azathioprine[24,25] are well known. Of particular concern in children are the impact of steroids on growth, the potential teratogenic effects on future offspring, and the enhanced incidence of neoplasm in patients treated with azathioprine.

Data from MG patients are scant. Most information comes from studies of children treated with steroids and/or azathioprine for disorders other than MG.

Studies in asthmatic children aged 6 to 10 years found that those treated with less than 3 mg/m^2/day of prednisone grew normally, while those treated with ≥4 mg/m^2/day grew less than half of that expected for their age.[26] Children with nephrotic syndrome treated with steroids for less than 3 months experienced no growth change, 3/14 treated for less than 6 months had a decreased growth velocity, and all had returned to normal at 5 to 10 years later. Of children treated for longer than 6 months, 12/16 had a failure in growth velocity and 4 of these failed to return to the normal rate at 5 to 10 years after steroids were stopped.[27] Morris[28] found a similar timetable for asthmatic children. Alternate-day steroids appear to have less adverse effect on growth[28] and fewer other side effects.[29]

In a comprehensive review of immunosuppressive drugs, Roubenoff et al.[30] failed to find convincing evidence of physical deformity in children born to mothers receiving azathioprine. They did describe an increased incidence of prematurity and low weight for gestational age; however, many of the series that they examined involved women with renal transplants, a confounding factor. A warning was included regarding possible infantile immune suppression in women receiving azathioprine and steroids, with mention of 5 cases of congenital athymia, lymphopenia, and immune deficiency being reported.[30] The exact role of each drug, and of maternal immunosuppression, in these cases could not be determined.

A recent report on cancer risk in multiple sclerosis patients treated with azathioprine indicated no increased risk during the first 10 years of treatment, but a possible increased risk thereafter.[31] In a large group of patients with rheumatoid arthritis ($n = 202$) treated with high doses of azathioprine (median, 300 mg/day) and followed for 10 years or more, there was a very small increased risk of lymphoma (one extra case of lymphoproliferative disease in 1000 patient-years of treatment).[32]

DISCUSSION

Available data support the view that thymectomy in white children with MG improves the possibility of remission, perhaps by 12–22% or more, especially if done within the first 2 years after onset of symptoms.[8–10,16] Thymectomy done after the second year may not improve greatly upon the natural spontaneous remission rate in children (TABLE 3). African-American patients, in one report, also benefit from early thymectomy, but the number of patients studied is small.[9] For Chinese and Japanese children with MG, the role of thymectomy is not at all clear as they appear to more frequently have ocular MG, and spontaneous improvements and remissions appear to be common.[12,17]

Postthymectomy immunologic and clinical follow-up studies do not indicate any consistent or clinically apparent loss of immune protection in children thymectomized after the first year of life.[20,21] This compares favorably with immunologic studies of young adults with MG after thymectomy who have shown no significant alterations in humoral immunity,[33] CD4 T cells,[34] B cells or T cells, and T cell subsets,[35] and modest and seemingly unimportant changes in proliferative activity.[36]

Thymectomy in children with MG also does not appear to lead to any enhanced risk of cancer.[8] This is comparable to studies in adults with MG, including the early reports of Vessey and Doll[37] and of Papatestas *et al.*[38] and the recent report in 288 nonthymoma patients by Masaoka *et al.*[39] Masaoka *et al.* found no enhancement of malignancy postthymectomy; in fact, the incidence of malignancy was lower than expected for their operated patients.[39]

The problem of recognition of autoimmune MG in prepubertal children is an important one. Most children who develop MG during or after puberty will have detectable AChR-ab,[22] and AChR-ab may be detected in children as early as the first and second year of life.[40,41] However, prepubertal children often have no detectable AChR-ab and, for these children, the possibility that they suffer from a form of congenital MG remains a consideration for the clinicians caring for them. Response to plasmapheresis or other immunosuppressive measures, as used by Andrews *et al.*,[22] or sophisticated electrophysiologic and electron-microscopic studies, as done at a few centers, are alternative diagnostic measures in difficult cases. The distinction is important as thymectomy for patients with congenital MG, a developmental disorder, would have no therapeutic benefit.

Immunosuppressant therapy with steroids and/or azathioprine is an alternative to thymectomy in children with MG. Studies in children with disorders other than MG suggest that daily steroid therapy for longer than 6 months leads to growth retardation in some children.[27,28] Alternate-day therapy appears to have less adverse effect on growth,[28] but the exact extent to which it, too, could lead to growth retardation is not known.

The use of azathioprine in young women of child-bearing age is very rarely associated with birth defects.[30] The risk of the development of lymphoproliferative disease in patients treated with azathioprine for less than 10 years also does not appear to be increased.[31,32] An extremely small increase in risk may exist for those treated for more than 10 years. Studies involving patients treated for 20 or more years are not yet available.

CONCLUSIONS

Thymectomy appears to enhance the opportunity for remission in white children with MG, especially (and perhaps only) when done within the first 2 years after the onset of symptoms. Data for African-American patients are very limited, but a benefit is suggested in these patients as well. The benefit of thymectomy in young Chinese patients is less clear, in large part because of the higher frequency of ocular MG and spontaneous remission in these patients. No adverse immunologic or neoplastic effects are evident in children operated after the age of 1 year.

Prepubertal children are more likely to be seronegative for AChR-ab than older children or adults. Certainty regarding their diagnosis is therefore often more difficult and response to other immunosuppressant measures, such as plasmapheresis, is often used in an attempt to confirm the autoimmune nature of their disease.

Daily steroid treatment for more than 6 months can lead to growth retardation in some children. Azathioprine has a low teratogenic effect in the women studied thus far (most of the reports were of patients with disorders other than MG). Azathioprine is not associated with an increased risk of neoplasia in patients treated for less than

10 years, but the risk for patients treated for longer periods may be slightly elevated and longer studies are needed. These risks must be weighed when selecting an immunosuppressant approach in children.

REFERENCES

1. HOHLFELD, R. & H. WEKERLE. 1994. The thymus in myasthenia gravis. Neurol. Clin. **12:** 331–341.
2. KAO, I. & D. B. DRACHMAN. 1977. Thymic muscle cells bear acetylcholine receptors: possible relation to myasthenia gravis. Science **195:** 74–75.
3. MELMS, A., B. C. SCHALKE, T. KIRCHNER, H. K. MULLER-HERMELINK, E. ALBERT & H. WEKERLE. 1988. Thymus in myasthenia gravis: isolation of T-lymphocyte lines specific for the nicotinic acetylcholine receptor from thymuses of myasthenic patients. J. Clin. Invest. **81:** 902–908.
4. SOMMER, N., N. WILLCOX, G. C. HARCOURT & J. NEWSOM-DAVIS. 1990. Myasthenic thymus and thymoma are selectively enriched in acetylcholine receptor–reactive T cells. Ann. Neurol. **28:** 312–319.
5. VINCENT, A., G. K. SCADDING, H. C. THOMAS & J. NEWSOM-DAVIS. 1978. *In-vitro* synthesis of anti-acetylcholine-receptor antibody by thymic lymphocytes in myasthenia gravis. Lancet **1:** 305–307.
6. BUCKINGHAM, J. M., F. M. HOWARD, JR., P. E. BERNATZ, W. S. PAYNE, E. G. HARRISON, JR., P. C. O'BRIEN & L. H. WEILAND. 1976. The value of thymectomy in myasthenia gravis: a computer-assisted matched stucy. Ann. Surg. **184:** 453–458.
7. LANSKA, D. J. 1990. Indications for thymectomy in myasthenia gravis. Neurology **40:** 1828–1829.
8. RODRIGUEZ, M., M. R. GOMEZ, F. M. HOWARD, JR. & W. F. TAYLOR. 1983. Myasthenia gravis in children: long-term follow-up. Ann. Neurol. **13:** 504–510.
9. ANDREWS, P. I., J. M. MASSEY, J. F. HOWARD, JR. & D. B. SANDERS. 1994. Race, sex, and puberty influence onset, severity, and outcome in juvenile myasthenia gravis. Neurology **44:** 1208–1214.
10. SEYBOLD, M. E., F. M. HOWARD, JR., D. D. DUANE, W. S. PAYNE & E. G. HARRISON, JR. 1971. Thymectomy in juvenile myasthenia gravis. Arch. Neurol. **25:** 385–392.
11. SNEAD, O. C., J. W. BENTON, D. DWYER, B. J. MORLEY, G. E. KEMP, R. J. BRADLEY & S. J. OH. 1980. Juvenile myasthenia gravis. Neurology **30:** 732–739.
12. WONG, V., B. R. HAWKINS & Y. L. YU. 1992. Myasthenia gravis in Hong Kong Chinese. 2. Paediatric disease. Acta Neurol. Scand. **86:** 68–72.
13. SZOBOR, A., A. MATTYUS & J. MOLNAR. 1988. Myasthenia gravis in childhood and adolescence: report on 209 patients and review of the literature. Acta Paediatr. Hung. **29:** 299–312.
14. BATOCCHI, A. P., A. EVOLI, M. T. PALMISANI, M. LO MONACO, M. BARTOCCIONI & P. TONALI. 1990. Early-onset myasthenia gravis: clinical characteristics and response to therapy. Eur. J. Pediatr. **150:** 66–68.
15. MILLICHAP, J. G. & P. R. DODGE. 1960. Diagnosis and treatment of myasthenia gravis in infancy, childhood, and adolescence. Neurology **10:** 1007–1014.
16. ADAMS, C., D. THEODORESCU, E. G. MURPHY & B. SHANDLING. 1990. Thymectomy in juvenile myasthenia gravis. J. Child. Neurol. **5:** 215–218.
17. FUKUYAMA, Y., Y. HIRAYAMA & M. OSAWA. 1981. Epidemiological and clinical features of childhood myasthenia gravis in Japan. *In* Myasthenia Gravis—Pathogenesis and Treatment, pp. 19–27. University of Tokyo Press. Tokyo.
18. BREARLEY, S., T. A. GENTLE, M. I. BAYNHAM, K. D. ROBERTS, L. D. ABRAMS & R. A.

THOMPSON. 1987. Immunodeficiency following neonatal thymectomy in man. Clin. Exp. Immunol. **70:** 322–327.

19. RUBINSTEIN, A., B. PELET & V. SCHWEIZER. 1976. Immunological decay in thymectomized infants. Helv. Paediatr. Acta **30:** 425–433.

20. RAMOS, S. B., A. B. GARCIA, S. R. VIANA, J. C. VOLTARELLI & R. P. FALCAO. 1996. Phenotypic and functional evaluation of natural killer cells in thymectomized children. Clin. Immunol. Immunopathol. **81:** 277–281.

21. RESZKE, S., E. SMOGORZEWSKA, G. BORYSEWICZ, J. TRACZYK, A. BIELOWICZ-HILGIER & H. SIWINSKA-GOLEBIOWSKA. 1990. Evaluation of immune response after thymectomy. Probl. Med. Wieku Rozwojowego **16:** 75–80.

22. ANDREWS, P. I., J. M. MASSEY & D. B. SANDERS. 1993. Acetylcholine receptor antibodies in juvenile myasthenia gravis. Neurology **43:** 977–982.

23. RIMSZA, M. E. 1978. Complications of corticosteroid therapy. Am. J. Dis. Child. **132:** 806–810.

24. KISSEL, J. T., R. J. LEVY, J. R. MENDELL & R. C. GRIGGS. 1986. Azathioprine toxicity in neuromuscular disease. Neurology **36:** 35–39.

25. MERTENS, H. G., G. HERTEL, P. REUTHER & K. RICKER. 1981. Effect of immunosuppressive drugs (azathioprine). Ann. N.Y. Acad. Sci. **377:** 691–699.

26. KERREBIJN, K. F. & J. P. M. DEKROON. 1968. Effect on height of corticosteroid therapy in asthmatic children. Arch. Dis. Child. **43:** 556–561.

27. LAM, C. N. & G. C. ARNEIL. 1968. Long-term dwarfing effects of corticosteroid treatment for childhood nephrosis. Arch. Dis. Child. **43:** 589–594.

28. MORRIS, H. G. 1975. Growth and skeletal maturation in asthmatic children: effect of corticosteroid treatment. Pediatr. Res. **9:** 579–583.

29. SOYKA, L. F. 1967. Treatment of the nephrotic syndrome in childhood: use of an alternate-day prednisone regimen. Am. J. Dis. Child. **113:** 693–701.

30. ROUBENOFF, R., J. HOYT, M. PETRI, M. C. HOCHBERG & D. B. HELLMANN. 1988. Effects of anti-inflammatory and immunosuppressive drugs on pregnancy and fertility. Semin. Arthritis Rheum. **18:** 88–110.

31. CONFAVREUX, C., P. SADDIER, J. GRIMAUD, T. MOREAU, P. ADELEINE & G. AIMARD. 1996. Risk of cancer from azathioprine therapy in multiple sclerosis: a case-control study. Neurology **46:** 1607–1612.

32. SILMAN, A. J., J. PETRIE, B. HAZLEMAN & S. J. EVANS. 1988. Lymphoproliferative cancer and other malignancy in patients with rheumatoid arthritis treated with azathioprine: a 20-year follow-up study. Ann. Rheum. Dis. **47:** 988–992.

33. SCADDING, G. K., A. D. WEBSTER, M. ROSS, H. C. THOMAS & C. W. HAVARD. 1979. Humoral immunity before and after thymectomy in myasthenia gravis. Neurology **29:** 502–506.

34. MELMS, A., G. MALCHEREK, U. GERN, N. SOMMER, R. WEISSERT, H. WIETHOLTER & H. J. BUHRING. 1993. Thymectomy and azathioprine have no effect on the phenotype of CD4 T lymphocyte subsets in myasthenia gravis. J. Neurol. Neurosurg. Psychiatry **56:** 46–51.

35. HAYNES, B. F., E. A. HARDEN, C. W. OLANOW, G. S. EISENBARTH, A. S. WECHSLER, L. L. HENSLEY & A. D. ROSES. 1983. Effect of thymectomy on peripheral lymphocyte subsets in myasthenia gravis: selective effect on T-cells in patients with thymic atrophy. J. Immunol. **131:** 773–777.

36. VAN DE GRIEND, R. J., M. CARRENO, R. VAN DOORN, C. J. LEUPERS, A. VAN DEN ENDE, P. WIJERMANS, H. J. OOSTERHUIS & A. ASTALDI. 1982. Changes in human T lymphocytes after thymectomy and during senescence. J. Clin. Immunol. **2:** 289–295.

37. VESSEY, M. P. & R. DOLL. 1972. Thymectomy and cancer—a follow-up study. Br. J. Cancer **26:** 53–58.

38. PAPATESTAS, A. E., K. E. OSSERMAN & A. E. KARK. 1971. The relationship between thymus

and oncogenesis: a study of the incidence of nonthymic malignancy in myasthenia gravis. Br. J. Cancer **25:** 635–645.

39. MASAOKA, A., Y. YAMAKAWA, H. NIWA, I. FUKAI, Y. SAITO, S. TOKUDOME, K. NAKAHARA & Y. FUJII. 1994. Thymectomy and malignancy. Eur. J. Cardiothorac. Surg. **8:** 251–253.

40. SEYBOLD, M. E. & J. M. LINDSTROM. 1981. Myasthenia gravis in infancy. Neurology **31:** 476–480.

41. LEFVERT, A. K., K. BERGSTRÖM, G. MATELL, P. O. OSTERMAN & R. PIRSKANEN. 1978. Determination of acetylcholine receptor antibody in myasthenia gravis: clinical usefulness and pathogenetic implications. J. Neurol. Neurosurg. Psychiatry **41:** 394–403.

Risk of Cancer in Patients with Myasthenia Gravis

A. EVOLI, A. P. BATOCCHI, P. TONALI,
AND M. MARCIANO[a]

Institute of Neurology
Catholic University
00168 Rome, Italy

INTRODUCTION

To assess the risk of cancer in myasthenia gravis (MG) related to the presence of thymoma and immunosuppressive therapy, we performed a case-control study comparing patients with and without extrathymic tumors for exposure to these factors.

METHODS

Population

We reviewed the records of patients with confirmed diagnosis of MG who had been followed for at least 1 year from the disease onset. Our series consists of 643 patients, 284 males and 359 females; the age at MG onset ranged from 2 to 83 years.

A thymoma was present in 149 patients (23%). All these cases underwent surgery and those with invasive thymoma were generally submitted to mediastinal radiotherapy after surgery. In unthymectomized patients, thymoma was ruled out by mediastinal CT scan.

Immunosuppressive therapy was performed in 393 patients with corticosteroids (CS) and/or azathioprine (Aza); only treatments longer than 6 months were considered. CS were used in 305 cases. According to the schedule previously described,[1] patients were given prednisone on a high daily dose (1 mg/kg-bw) at the start of treatment. This dosage was maintained until obvious improvement of MG was observed (3–4 weeks in most cases), after which it was changed to an equivalent alternate-day (a.d.) administration. Prednisone was then reduced slowly to a maintenance a.d. dose (10–25 mg in most cases) or, when possible, to complete withdrawal. Aza was administered to 88 patients, generally in association with CS. The starting dose was 2–3 mg/kg-bw/day and it was maintained for at least 1 year; then, Aza was gradually reduced to a maintenance dose of 1–1.5 mg/kg-bw/day.

---

[a]Statistical doctor.

Cases

Our cases were all those patients included in the study who developed an extrathymic cancer after the onset of MG before February 1997. A total of 18 cases were found. Follow-up was considered as the time interval between the onset of MG and the diagnosis of malignancy.

Controls

Each patient with cancer (case) was matched to cancer-free MG patients (controls) by gender, age at MG onset (±2 years), and follow-up duration (equal or longer). For each control, follow-up was the time interval between the onset of MG and the diagnosis of malignancy in the matched case. To avoid selection, all eligible controls for each case were considered. We found a total of 105 controls.

Statistical Analysis

The relative risk of cancer was evaluated in relation to both presence of thymoma and exposure to immunosuppressive therapy by conditional logistic regression adjusted for age. We also considered different durations of immunosuppressive therapy (<5 years, 5–10 years, >10 years).

RESULTS

Eighteen patients developed an extrathymic cancer after the onset of MG. Cancers consisted of adenocarcinomas of the prostate (3), colon (3), breast (3), lung (2), thyroid (2), bladder (2), kidney (1), and uterine corpus (1), and metastatic adenocarcinoma of unknown origin (1).

Cases were 12 males and 6 females (M/F = 2); age at onset of MG ranged from 30 to 75 years (mean 54.9 ± 12 years); follow-up duration varied from 2 to 28 years (mean 9.7 ± 7.4 years).

The 105 controls were 77 males and 28 females (M/F = 2.75); age at onset of MG ranged from 28 to 77 years (mean 56 ± 12.5 years); follow-up duration varied from 3 to 28 years (mean 12.4 ± 6.9 years).

MG was associated with thymoma in 9/18 (50%) cases and in 27/105 (25.7%) controls. Thymoma was invasive in 4/9 cases and in 13/27 controls; these patients also received radiotherapy.

Immunosuppressive therapy was performed in 15/18 (83.3%) cases and in 82/105 (78.1%) controls. In particular, CS were employed in 11/18 (61.1%) cases and in 64/105 (60.9%) controls; CS and AZA were administered to 4/18 (22.2%) cases and to 18/105 (17.1%) controls.

The presence of thymoma significantly increased the risk of extrathymic malignancy (odds ratio [OR] = 1.73; 95% confidence interval [CI] = 1.01–2.96; $p < 0.05$), while exposure to immunosuppressive therapy did not. These data are shown in

TABLE 1. When different duration of immunosuppressive therapy was considered, only patients treated for more than 10 years had an increased, although not significant, risk of developing cancer. These findings are shown in TABLE 2.

DISCUSSION

In patients with MG, both immunosuppressive therapy and presence of thymoma might increase the risk of cancer.

It has long been reported that prolonged immunosuppression may favor the development of malignancy,[2–5] cancer types most frequently observed being lymphoid malignancies, squamous cell skin carcinoma, and vulvar and perineal carcinoma.[3–5] On the other hand, the occurrence of extrathymic tumors has been reported to be higher in thymomatous than in nonthymomatous MG patients.[6–9] In those reports, different cancer types have been described with a prevalence of tumors of the hematopoietic organs.[8]

In order to evaluate the risk of cancer related to these factors, we performed a case-control study; this approach should prevent bias such as differences between cases and controls in age, sex, association with MG, and duration of disease.[4]

The types of cancer in our patients are those commonly observed in the general population. On the contrary, we did not find lymphomas or other tumors usually reported in immunosuppressed patients.

TABLE 1. Cancer Risk in Relation to Thymoma and Immunosuppressive Therapy in Cases and Controls

	Cases ($N = 18$)	Controls ($N = 105$)	OR[a]	95% CI[b]	p
Thymoma	9/18 (50%)	27/105 (25.7%)	1.73	1.01–2.96	<0.05
Immunosuppressive therapy	15/18 (83.3%)	82/105 (78.1%)	1.40	0.45–4.36	0.59

[a]OR: Odds ratio.
[b]95% CI: 95% confidence interval of OR.

TABLE 2. Cancer Risk in Relation to Duration of Immunosuppressive Therapy in Cases and Controls

	Cases ($N = 18$)	Controls ($N = 105$)	OR[a]	95% CI[b]	p
Never treated	3 (16.6%)	23 (21.9%)	—	—	—
Duration of treatment:					
0.5–5 years	5 (27.7%)	31 (29.5%)	0.54	0.17–1.75	0.31
5–10 years	4 (22.2%)	34 (32.4%)	1.03	0.35–2.72	0.96
>10 years	6[c] (33.3%)	17[c] (16.2%)	2.20	0.91–5.72	0.13

[a]OR: Odds ratio.
[b]95% CI: 95% confidence interval of OR.
[c]Thymoma cases in these groups were 4/6 (66.6%) and 9/17 (52.9%), respectively.

The risk induced by immunosuppressive therapy appears to be low as only treatment longer than 10 years shows an increased, although not significant, association with cancer. Unfortunately, we were not able to distinguish between CS and Aza due to the small number of cancer patients treated with Aza. However, our results are in agreement with previous studies.[4,10] We do not have sufficient data on long-term effects of other immunosuppressants such as cyclophosphamide and cyclosporine, which have been reported as being associated with an increased incidence of cancer.[3,11]

Our results show that the risk of developing extrathymic malignancies is significantly higher in thymomatous than in nonthymomatous MG patients, thus confirming previous reports. The association with thymoma appears to act as an independent risk factor, suggesting the need for tumor surveillance in these patients.

REFERENCES

1. EVOLI, A. *et al.* 1992. Long-term results of corticosteroid therapy in patients with myasthenia gravis. Eur. Neurol. **32:** 37–43.
2. OOSTERHUIS, H. J. G. H. 1984. Myasthenia Gravis. Churchill Livingstone. Edinburgh.
3. PENN, I. 1990. Cancer complicating organ transplantation. N. Engl. J. Med. **323:** 1767–1769.
4. CONFAVREUX, C. *et al.* 1996. Risk of cancer from azathioprine therapy in multiple sclerosis: a case-control study. Neurology **46:** 1607–1612.
5. DEEG, H. J. *et al.* 1996. Malignancies after marrow transplantation for aplastic anemia and Fanconi anemia: a joint Seattle and Paris analysis of results in 700 patients. Blood **87:** 386–392.
6. PAPATESTAS, A. E. *et al.* 1971. The relationship between thymus and oncogenesis: a study of incidence of non-thymic malignancy in myasthenia gravis. Br. J. Cancer **25:** 635–645.
7. GOULON, M. *et al.* 1980. Myasthenia gravis and associated diseases. Int. J. Neurol. **14:** 61–72.
8. MONDEN, Y. *et al.* 1991. Extrathymic malignancy in patients with myasthenia gravis. Eur. J. Cancer **27:** 745–747.
9. MASAOKA, A. *et al.* 1994. Thymectomy and malignancy. Eur. J. Cardiothorac. Surg. **8:** 251–253.
10. ELLISON, G. W. *et al.* 1989. A placebo-controlled, randomized, double-masked, variable dosage, clinical trial of azathioprine with and without prednisolone in multiple sclerosis. Neurology **39:** 1018–1026.
11. DRACHMAN, D. B. 1996. Immunotherapy in neuromuscular disorders: current and future strategies. Muscle Nerve **19:** 1239–1251.

Remission of Myasthenia Gravis in Association with Unresectable, Invasive Thymoma

LISSETTE JIMENEZ

359 De Diego Avenue
Santurce, Puerto Rico 00909

INTRODUCTION

Most patients with myasthenia have a favorable outcome with current therapeutic methods.[1] Yet, at age over 40, a short history of severe disease and thymoma is associated with a less favorable prognosis.[2]

Histologically, most thymomas have a benign appearance. They are staged based on the extent of disease and invasiveness.[3] Invasive thymomas, present in 4–6% of myasthenics,[4,5] show, among the thymomas, the shortest survival.[6]

There is no consensus regarding therapy for unresectable tumors. High-dose steroids,[5] radiation,[7] and combination therapies[4] have been advocated. This case illustrates the indolent course of myasthenia gravis in a patient with an invasive, unresectable thymoma treated with combination therapy.

CASE REPORT

A 57-year-old woman complained of ptosis. The examination showed horizontal gaze nystagmus and mild fatigable weakness of facial, neck, and shoulder muscles. The symptoms improved with intravenous edrophonium and pyridostigmine, 60 mg qid. Repetitive nerve stimulation showed no significant decrement. Antiacetylcholine receptor and antistriated muscle antibodies were elevated. The complete blood counts, chemistries, liver enzymes, protein electrophoresis, and thyroid function tests were normal. The CT of the chest showed a large anterior mediastinal mass. The patient developed myasthenic crisis. She received five plasma-exchange treatments over the course of a week with marked symptomatic improvement. A median sternotomy was performed, but no tumor excision was made because of tumor size and massive invasion of the pleura, lung, aorta, and pericardium. The tumor histology was epithelial, according to the traditional classification.[3] She received three courses of cisplatin, doxorubicin, and cyclophosphamide.[8] She had increasing weakness that resolved with prednisone 80 mg qid, pyridostigmine 60 mg qid, and one Timespan 180 mg qhs. Chemotherapy was followed by radiation therapy. As she was asymptomatic, a slow taper of her medications was started. One year later, she developed back pain, but no weakness. An MRI showed T8 and T9 compression fractures and metastasis, without cord compression. She received no further therapy. A repeat scan at one year later showed early similar changes in T4, T5, and thoracic cord atrophy. The patient is presently on pyridostigmine 60 mg qid and prednisone 10 mg qod. Over three years after her diagnosis, she is asymptomatic and able to maintain her

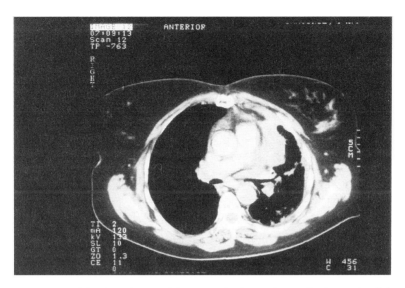

FIGURE 1. CT of the chest shows nodular masses in the anterior mediastinum. They join and become confluent below the aortic arch and extend down to the left paracardial location. The masses are adjacent to the pleura in the left hemithorax, lateral wall, extending to the upper lower segment.

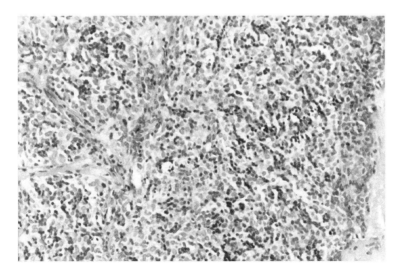

FIGURE 2. Tumor pathology: epithelial thymoma.

full-time job and active lifestyle on the previously mentioned medications. (See FIG-URES 1 and 2.)

DISCUSSION

This patient presented with acute fulminating myasthenia gravis. The severity of her symptoms, a large tumor unamenable to resection, invading adjacent thoracic structures, and epithelial histology, heralded a poor prognosis.[6,7,9]

The benign course of myasthenia gravis in this patient is unusual in various ways. First, those patients with invasive thymomas that had good outcome were shown to have tumor shrinkage with resection, high doses of steroids, or combination therapy.[4-7] This patient's tumor failed to reduce in size and showed progression, involving the spine. Second, contrary to what was expected,[7] tumor progression was not associated with disease deterioration. Third, in spite of the above, she remained asymptomatic throughout and in the two subsequent years after tapering off her medication. This case illustrates that remission can be seen in myasthenic patients in spite of invasive, unresectable thymoma.

REFERENCES

1. DRACHMAN, D. B. 1994. Medical progress: myasthenia gravis. N. Engl. J. Med. **330**(25): 1798–1810.
2. MANTEGAZZA, R. *et al.* 1990. A multicenter follow-up study of 1152 patients with myasthenia gravis in Italy. J. Neurol. **237**: 339.
3. MORGENTHALER, T. I. *et al.* 1993. Symposium on intrathoracic neoplasms: thymoma. Mayo Clin. Proc. **68**: 1110–1123.
4. WAKATA, N. *et al.* 1993. Myasthenia gravis and invasive thymoma: a 20-year experience. Eur. Neurol. **33**: 115–120.
5. GOLDMAN, A. J. *et al.* 1975. Myasthenia gravis and invasive thymoma: a 20-year experience. Neurology **25**: 1021–1025.
6. MAGGI, G. 1986. Thymomas: a review of 169 cases, with particular reference to results of surgical treatment. Cancer **58**(3): 765–776.
7. PALMISANI, M. T. *et al.* 1994. Myasthenia gravis associated with thymoma: clinical characteristics and long-term outcome. Eur. Neurol. **34**(2): 78–82.
8. LOEHRER, P. J. *et al.* 1990. Chemotherapy for advanced thymoma: preliminary results of an intergroup study. Ann. Intern. Med. **113**: 520–524.
9. MASAOKA, A. *et al.* 1981. Follow-up study of thymomas with special reference to their clinical stages. Cancer **48**: 2485–2492.

Video-assisted Thoracoscopic Extended Thymectomy (VATET) in Myasthenia Gravis

Two-Year Follow-up in 101 Patients and Comparison with the Transsternal Approach

R. MANTEGAZZA,[a] P. CONFALONIERI,[a] C. ANTOZZI,[a] L. NOVELLINO,[b]
M. T. FERRÒ,[c] M. PORTA,[c] G. PEZZUOLI,[b] AND F. CORNELIO[a]

[a]Department of Neuromuscular Diseases
"C. Besta" National Neurological Institute
20133 Milan, Italy

[b]Division of Surgery
[c]Division of Neurology
Policlinico S. Marco
Zingonia, Bergamo, Italy

INTRODUCTION

Thymectomy is a landmark therapeutical procedure in myasthenia gravis (MG): the aim of surgery is to eradicate the site for autoantigen (muscle nicotinic acetylcholine receptor, AChR) sensibilization and self-sustainment of the autoimmune reaction. Thymectomy efficacy correlates with the amount of thymic tissue removed, its precocity from diagnosis, the young age of patients, and the absence of thymoma.[1,2] Extended thymectomy (ETT) removes the thymus and the fat tissue (which may contain ectopic functional thymic tissue) from the thyroid gland to the diaphragm muscle in the space comprised between the two phrenic nerves.[2] ETT, usually obtained by median sternotomy, is a major surgery whose indication may be limited in patients affected by severe forms of MG and in cases where surgical morbidity may have detrimental effect on the patients' condition. As a peak of MG onset is usually observed in females around the age of 20–30 years, ETT might be a negative factor for the compliance of therapy.

We present our experience with video-assisted thoracoscopic surgery (no need of sternotomy) of mediastinal masses. Our approach, denominated VATET, is similar to that employed by others (reviewed in reference 2) with the substantial difference of a bilateral exploration of the mediastinum. VATET achieves a higher removal of thymic tissue than ETT, improves clinical care, minimizes side effects, and shortens hospitalization of MG patients undergoing thymectomy.

METHODS

One hundred four consecutive myasthenic patients seen as outpatients or inpatients were considered and proposed for thymectomy between February 1994 and

January 1997. Diagnosis was established according to clinical, pharmacological, and electrophysiological criteria; anti-AChR antibody titer was performed as described.[1] A clinicobiological protocol inclusive of prethymectomy and postthymectomy evaluations of clinical stage, immunological, histological, and radiological data (described in references 3 and 4) was adopted for patients' follow-up: 2, 6, 12, and 24 months. Patients affected by MG respiratory symptoms were excluded from the surgery proposal. Preoperative mediastinic evaluation was performed either by computerized tomography (CT) with contrast medium or by nuclear magnetic resonance (NMR) scan. The main clinical features of patients submitted to VATET are illustrated in TABLE 1.

The surgical approach employed for VATET is that described in reference 5. Briefly, after a transverse cervical incision and a revision of the perithyroid space, the sternum is drawn upward by a lifter and surgery continues by video-assisted thoracoscopy; three trocars are introduced in both pleural cavities, while a double lumen tube allows separate ventilation of the contralateral lung; the thymus and fat tissue are completely isolated on thoracoscopy and removed from the thorax through the cervical incision. Recovered tissue is then fractionated in three portions (thymus gland, pericardic fat, perithyroid fat) and weighed separately immediately after removal; tissue weight is expressed as grams of corresponding wet tissue. Thymic specimens are fixed in 10% formalin or frozen in liquid nitrogen for histopathological evaluation. Hyperplasia was defined by the presence of lymphoid follicles, usually not seen in normal adult thymus, and thymic involution was defined by the degree of fatty replacement of thymic tissue; thymoma was classified according to Müller-Hermelink criteria.[6]

To evaluate the efficacy of VATET, the following endpoints were considered: the presence of true remissions (no symptoms and no drugs); the frequency of asymptomatic patients with or without therapy; changes in the clinical status according to defined outcomes and the amount of thymic and mediastinic fat tissue removed.

TABLE 1. Clinical Features of MG Patients Proposed for VATET

MG Population	Sex	Age at Thymectomy (Years)	Age at Onset	Disease Duration (Months)	Anti-AChR Ab (% Positive Patients)	Therapy[a]
Whole MG population (n = 104)	F 76 M 28	32.6 ± 12.6	<40 years (80) >40 years (24)	43.4 ± 54.2	85.2%	Antichol. 47 (45.2%) Immunos. 55 (52.8%)[b]
MG, no thymoma (n = 82)	F 66 M 16	29.2 ± 9.3	<40 years (74) >40 years (8)	47.8 ± 55.9	81%	Antichol. 40 (48.8%) Immunos. 55 (67.1%)
MG with thymoma (n = 22)	F 11 M 11	45.1 ± 15.3	<40 years (6) >40 years (16)	26.6 ± 44.3	100%	Antichol. 7 (31.8%) Immunos. 15 (68.2%)

[a]Terms: Antichol. = anticholinesterase inhibitors; Immunos. = immunosuppressive drugs.
[b]Two patients were already in remission by the time of thymectomy.

TABLE 2. Comparison of MG Patients Thymectomized by VATET versus ETT: Follow-up at 1 and 2 Years

(a) Clinical Outcome

Clinical Status	VATET (1 Year)	ETT (1 Year)	VATET (2 Years)	ETT (2 Years)
Remission	11 (17.4%)	4 (6.2%)	8 (26.7%)	11 (18.6%)
Pharmacological remission	29 (46%)	8 (12.5%)	13 (43.3%)	8 (13.6%)
Symptomatics	23 (36.6%)	52 (81.3%)	9 (30%)	40 (67.8%)
Total	63 (100%)	64 (100%)	30 (100%)	59 (100%)

(b) Total Thymic Tissue Removed

Histological Diagnosis	VATET (Grams)	ETT (Grams)	VATET vs. ETT (*t* Test)
All cases	55.6 ± 38.2	35.5 ± 23.5	$p = 0.001$
No thymoma	43.6 ± 21.5	26.3 ± 23.5	$p = 0.0001$
Thymoma	60.9 ± 39.7	64.9 ± 47.9	$p = 0.7798$

RESULTS

One hundred one patients out of 104 were successfully operated by VATET; 3 patients could not complete surgery by VATET and were operated by ETT because of cardiomegaly, infiltrating thymoma, and pleuropulmonary adhesions. Analysis of both populations, VATET and ETT, of myasthenics who underwent therapeutic thymectomy revealed the following results:

(a) The number of true remissions (absence of symptoms and drug-free patients) in VATET-treated patients was 11 (17.4%) and 8 (26.7%) at 1 and 2 years of follow-up, respectively (see TABLE 2a); the number of asymptomatic patients in the VATET group was 40 (63.5%) at 1 year and 21 (70%) at 2 years of follow-up versus 12 (18.8%) and 19 (32.2%), respectively, of the ETT surgical group. Comparison of remission, pharmacological remission, and symptomatic patient frequency revealed a significant increase of remission and of pharmacological remission frequencies in VATET versus ETT at both 1- and 2-year follow-up. Statistics comparison was performed by Contingency Table Analysis: $\chi^2 = 26.393$ (df 2), G Statistic 27.559 with a $p = 0.0001$ at 1-year follow-up; $\chi^2 = 13.232$ (df 2), G Statistic 13.244 with a $p = 0.0013$ at 2-year follow-up.

(b) Analysis of the outcome of the thymectomized patients showed a positive outcome (remission, pharmacological remission, and improved patients) in 53 patients of the VATET group versus 45 of the ETT group, but the statistical comparison between the two groups at 1 and 2 years of follow-up did not reveal any significant difference.

(c) The total thymic tissue (including nonneoplastic and neoplastic diagnosis) removed by VATET compared to ETT was 55.6 ± 38.2 grams versus 35.5 ± 23.5 grams. If thymoma cases were subtracted, the following weights were obtained in the same groups: 43.6 ± 21.5 grams versus 26.3 ± 23.5 grams. If thymomas only were considered, the following results were obtained: 60.9 ± 39.7 grams versus 64.9 ± 47.9. The statistical analysis, performed by t test, revealed a significant difference in the comparison of the whole sample ($p = 0.001$) and of the nonthymomatous patients ($p = 0.0001$) (see TABLE 2b).

REFERENCES

1. BEGHI, E., C. ANTOZZI, A. P. BATOCCHI et al. 1991. Prognosis of myasthenia gravis: a multi-center follow-up study of 844 patients. J. Neurol. Sci. **106:** 213–220.
2. JARETZKI, A., III. 1997. Thymectomy for myasthenia gravis: analysis of the controversies regarding technique and results. Neurology **48**(S5): 52–63.
3. CONFALONIERI, P. 1997. In Epithelial Tumors in the Thymus: Pathology, Biology, Treatment. Plenum. New York. In press.
4. MANTEGAZZA, R., C. ANTOZZI, D. PELUCCHETTI, A. SGHIRLANZONI & F. CORNELIO. 1988. Azathioprine as a single drug or in combination with steroids in the treatment of myasthenia gravis. J. Neurol. **235:** 449–453.
5. NOVELLINO, L., M. LONGONI, L. SPINELLI et al. 1994. Extended thymectomy without sternotomy, performed by cervicotomy and thoracoscopic technique in the treatment of myasthenia gravis. Int. Surg. **79:** 378–381.
6. MARINO, M. & H. K. MÜLLER-HERMELINK. 1985. Thymoma and thymic carcinoma: relation of thymoma epithelial cells to the cortical and medullary differentiation of thymus. Virchows Arch. A Pathol. Anat. Histopathol. **407:** 119–149.

A Treatment Algorithm for Autoimmune Myasthenia in Adults

JOHN KEESEY

Department of Neurology
UCLA School of Medicine
Los Angeles, California 90095

Matters concerned with conduct and questions of what is good for us have no fixity, any more than matters of health. The general account being of this nature, the account of particular cases is yet more lacking in exactness; for they do not fall under any science or precept, but the agents themselves in each case consider what is appropriate to the occasion, as happens also in the art of medicine and navigation.
—Aristotle, *Nicomachean Ethics II 2, 1104a7*

A clinical algorithm is a method of structuring clinical decisions into a sequential set of presumably logical steps. Such clinical pathways for myasthenia gravis (MG) consist of assertions of "accepted" behavior based upon clinical experience[1-4] since none of the interventions suggested for MG meet modern standards for "evidence-based" outcome analysis, that is, prospective, double-blind, randomized clinical trials on defined populations sufficiently large for statistical analysis.[5] Until such information is available, clinical algorithms for MG should be regarded as advisory only; they are not meant to substitute for clinical judgment in the care of individual patients. An overview (FIGURE 1) of the presently proposed algorithm begins with confirmation of the diagnosis of MG.

STEP 1: CONFIRM THE DIAGNOSIS OF AUTOIMMUNE MYASTHENIA (FIGURE 2)

MG is characterized clinically by fluctuating asymmetrical weakness and fatigue of extraocular, oropharyngeal, neck, and/or limb skeletal muscles, with normal sensation and reflexes. Once MG is suspected clinically, the diagnosis should be confirmed by at least one of three methods: (a) immunological, (b) electrophysiological, or (c) pharmacological.

Immunological Confirmation

Although there are several serological tests available,[6] measurement of the acetylcholine receptor (AChR) binding antibody in the serum is the most specific; a positive AChR binding antibody test provides near-certainty of the diagnosis.[7]

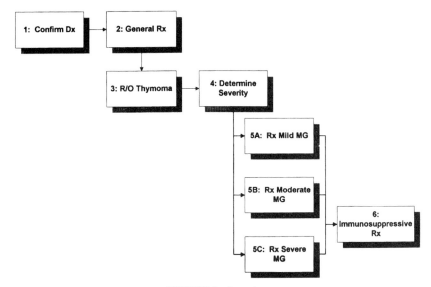

FIGURE 1. Overview.

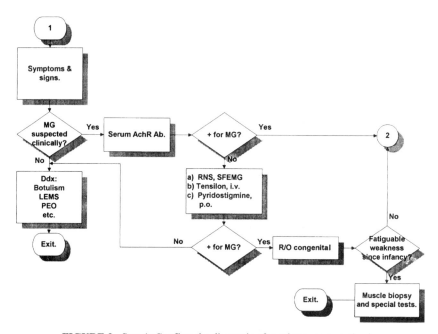

FIGURE 2. Step 1: Confirm the diagnosis of autoimmune myasthenia.

AChR modulating or blocking antibodies add very little to the usual diagnostic confirmation of MG, although they may help when a patient presents a diagnostic challenge.

Electrophysiological Confirmation

Only when the binding antibody test is negative, in about 15% of all patients with myasthenia, is it necessary to resort to one of the other less-specific methods of confirmation.[8] Of the two electrophysiological tests available, namely, repetitive nerve stimulation (RNS) and single-fiber electromyography (SFEMG), SFEMG in experienced hands is the more sensitive for detecting neuromuscular dysfunction from any cause, but it is not specific for MG and it is still not generally available. RNS usually requires testing of two or more (warm) nerve-muscle combinations to confirm the diagnosis.

Pharmacological Confirmation

The most rapid (and sometimes dramatic) pharmacological test involves the intravenous injection of 2 to 5 mg of edrophonium chloride or "Tensilon". A positive test requires a *measurable* change in some measurable sign such as ptosis, gaze paresis, grip strength, or respiratory function. This is compared to a previous placebo injection of saline or atropine, the latter to block the muscarinic effects of this short-acting anticholinesterase.

Because of vagal bradycardia, particularly in elderly patients, some hospitals now require that the Tensilon test be done in an emergency room with electrocardiographic monitoring. When this is not appropriate, it is often safer and more convenient for the patient to take a small amount of the longer-acting oral anticholinesterase pyridostigmine bromide or "Mestinon." The response can be assessed an hour or two later by the physician or by the patient over several days at home. The medication is taken after meals to minimize muscarinic stimulation of the gut.

Differential Diagnosis

If all these attempts to confirm the suspected diagnosis of myasthenia are negative or equivocal, clinical myasthenia is still not ruled out, but other conditions with fluctuating weakness should be considered in the differential diagnosis. Conditions that have been mistaken for myasthenia include Lambert-Eaton myasthenic syndrome (LEMS), botulism, progressive external ophthalmoplegia (PEO), oculopharyngeal muscular dystrophy, mitochondrial myopathies, polymyositis, progressive muscular atrophy, benign essential blepharospasm, Parkinson's disease, and even sleep apnea. Most patients suspected of having myasthenia will undergo routine electrodiagnostic testing—needle electromyography and nerve conduction studies—to exclude many of these possibilities.

Congenital Myasthenic Syndromes

The congenital myasthenic syndromes are one group of myasthenic disorders that are not autoimmune. These rare conditions usually begin in infancy, although some patients reach near-adulthood before the diagnosis is made. Some of these syndromes respond positively to anticholinesterases and have myasthenic responses on electrophysiological testing, but none of them has elevated serum titers of AChR antibodies. Since they do not respond to autoimmune therapies, they should be considered and excluded from the algorithm at this point, although many of the general therapeutic measures recommended in the next step are also of benefit to some patients with congenital myasthenia.

STEP 2: GENERAL TREATMENT MEASURES, INCLUDING MESTINON (FIGURE 3)

General Treatment Measures

General measures that can be very effective in coping with MG include education of the patient to pace activities, to get plenty of rest, and to eat a well-balanced diet

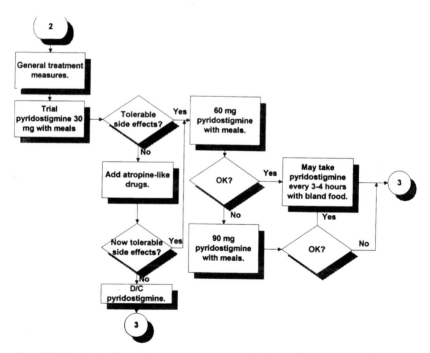

FIGURE 3. Step 2: General treatment measures, including anticholinesterase therapy.

containing foods high in potassium. Exacerbations of weakness caused by infections, fever, heat, cold, pain, overexertion, or emotional stress should be minimized. Patients should be assessed for treatable autoimmune diseases by obtaining blood levels of thyroid-stimulating hormone (TSH) and cobalamin (vitamin B_{12}). Correction of either too much or too little thyroid hormone sometimes can make myasthenic symptoms disappear. Sometimes, discontinuation of a drug known to exacerbate MG, such as beta-blocker eyedrops or cholesterol-lowering agents, may help to relieve the symptoms of MG. On occasion, blockade of menstrual periods by long-acting progesterone or even by hysterectomy has eliminated recurrent myasthenic crises.

Mestinon

Every MG patient deserves a trial of anticholinesterase medication for symptomatic relief since it is the safest and most rapidly acting medication available. To begin with, small doses should be taken after meals to minimize muscarinic side effects of abdominal cramps and diarrhea. There is no fixed dose; however, if half a tablet (30 mg) of Mestinon is well tolerated after 2 to 3 days, then the patient can try 60 mg three times a day after meals for a few more days. Not all weakness will respond equally. Because MG is naturally such a fluctuating condition, the patient should be educated to make only one change at a time and to make it gradually. If the symptoms are only partially relieved by 60 mg, the patient can then try 90 mg in a similar manner. The maximum safe individual dose is two tablets (120 mg) each time, but if possible this should be kept in reserve for potential myasthenic exacerbations. On the other hand, if Mestinon is of no real benefit after a reasonable trial, it should be discontinued altogether since it only treats the symptoms of the disease.

Shortening the Interval between Doses

Once the optimal individual dose of Mestinon is determined (and different amounts may be needed at different times of the day, depending upon the individual), then the doses can be moved as close together as every 3 hours. In most patients, the effect of Mestinon usually peaks between 1 to 2 hours after ingestion and the medication wears off in 3 or more hours. A sustained-release Mestinon Timespan, which releases 60 mg immediately and the remaining 120 mg over 6–8 hours, is available for nighttime use. Mestinon syrup, 60 mg/5 mL, is available for patients who have trouble swallowing pills.

Anticholinesterase Toxicity

It is wise to keep the daily dose of anticholinesterase medication as low as possible to minimize cholinergic toxicity. Oral atropine-like drugs such as pro-banthine (15 mg) or oral hyoscyamine sulfate (0.125 mg) can be used to counteract muscarinic side effects, but their use thickens secretions and may cover up warning signs of too much medication.

Anticholinergic medication usually does not relieve the patient's symptoms completely; however, even if it does, one should try to rule out the presence of a thymoma in every patient.

STEP 3: LOOK FOR THE PRESENCE OF A
THYMOMA (FIGURE 4)

Almost all MG patients with a thymoma have elevated titers of antistriated-muscle antibodies in their sera, but so do about one-third of MG patients without a thymoma.[9] Although the absence of an elevated serum titer of antistriated-muscle antibodies therefore argues against the presents of a thymoma,[10] in practice imaging of the anterior mediastinum is always required, either by computed tomography (CT) or by magnetic resonance imaging (MRI).[10] The sensitivity of these techniques is about equal, although CT provides better thymic definition in a much shorter scanning time, while MRI may be better for assessing possible invasion of vascular structures if an invasive thymoma is suspected.[11] Chest radiographs, even with obliques, miss many thymomas.[10,11]

Surgical Treatment

If a thymoma is detected by imaging and the patient is a suitable surgical candidate, the thymoma should be removed along with any remaining thymus on the theo-

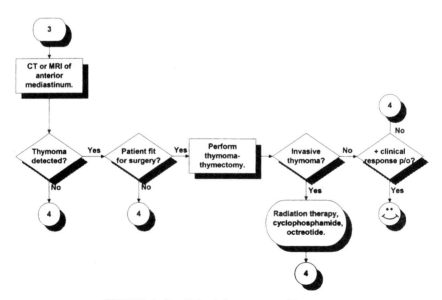

FIGURE 4. Step 3: Look for presence of thymoma.

ry that these tissues are contributing to the pathogenesis of the disease. Although usually benign and encapsulated, thymomas can be invasive, as determined by the surgeon at the time of operation. If the thymoma is found to be invasive, the patient should be considered for radiation therapy, cyclophosphamide,[12] and/or the recently described octreotide.[13]

Occasionally, patients go into remission after removal of a thymoma (and residual thymus), but usually further therapy is required to bring the MG under control, depending upon its severity.

STEP 4: DETERMINE THE SEVERITY OF THE DISEASE (Figure 5)

There have been several classification schemes for this heterogeneous and highly variable disease; however, for the purposes of this algorithm, the continuum of MG severity is divided into three groups: mild or ocular myasthenia; moderate generalized myasthenia; and severe generalized myasthenia gravis. Therapy for MG should be tailored to the severity of the disease.

Severe Generalized Myasthenia Gravis

Some available therapies for MG are so invasive, risky, and/or expensive that they should be reserved for only the most serious ("gravis") cases. These patients usually have predominantly oropharyngeal muscle weakness and have difficulty swallowing and/or breathing. These are the patients who are most at risk for developing "crisis". Crisis is defined as acute respiratory insufficiency, but it may also include the inabil-

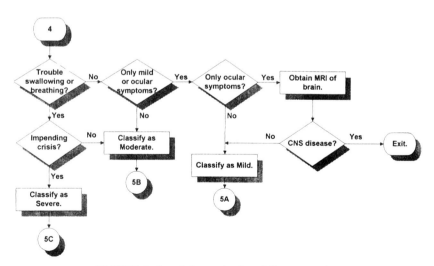

FIGURE 5. Step 4: Determination of disease severity.

ity to swallow medications or saliva. Treatments for these patients are discussed in step 5C.

Mild or Ocular Myasthenia

For those patients with only mild or ocular symptoms, on the other hand, conservative treatments with a favorable risk/benefit ratio should be preferred (step 5A). Patients with only ocular symptoms have been discovered on occasion to have central nervous system causes for their symptoms, either instead of MG or in addition to MG,[14] and thus an MRI of the brain should be considered for patients with purely ocular symptoms if there is any doubt, especially if they are negative for AChR binding antibody.

Moderate Generalized Myasthenia

The conditions of most patients will lie somewhere in between these two extremes. They are classified here as moderate generalized myasthenia and they are eligible for a somewhat different choice of therapies, discussed in step 5B. It is important to remember that MG is a fluctuating and variable condition and that the severity of an individual's condition can change from one category to another, usually for the worse and sometimes rather rapidly.

STEP 5A: TREATMENT OF MILD OR OCULAR MYASTHENIA (Figure 6)

Often, patients with mild involvement are content to treat their symptoms with Mestinon and do not consider it worthwhile to embark upon more risky or expensive treatments such as steroids, thymectomy, or immunosuppression.

Low-Dose Steroids

However, what one patient thinks is mild, another patient may find incapacitating. Double vision for a dental hygienist or ptosis for an actor is serious. This latter type of patient may wish to consider "low-dose" prednisone therapy as an outpatient, beginning at 10–20 mg on alternate days to minimize any steroid adverse effects. Patients should be informed about the potential adverse effects of prednisone. Relative contraindications to steroid therapy include severe obesity, diabetes mellitus, uncontrolled hypertension, ulcer disease, osteoporosis, and ongoing infections. In particular, tuberculosis should be ruled out before beginning steroid therapy.

To mimic the body's natural circadian rhythms of adrenal corticosteroid output, synthetic prednisone is taken once a day, early in the morning (6 A.M.) on an empty stomach. If after 2 weeks at a low dose (10–20 mg q.o.d.) the response is not satisfactory, the dose of prednisone can be increased by 10 mg every fifth dose until symptoms begin to improve or until 60 mg q.o.d. is reached. This or the lesser effective

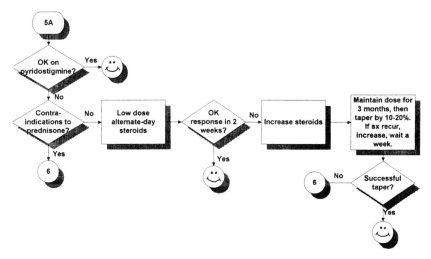

FIGURE 6. Step 5A: Treatment of mild or ocular myasthenia.

dose is maintained for at least 3 months with the goal of eliminating the patient's myasthenic symptoms completely. If this occurs, very slow tapering of prednisone may be considered, by less than 20% of the previous dose every month. If symptoms recur, the prednisone dose should be increased by 10–20 mg every week until the patient is again free of symptoms.[8]

Other Treatments

Some physicians, especially in Europe,[2] regard azathioprine as preferable to prednisone, even for mild myasthenia; however, in this present algorithm, azathioprine is considered for mild or ocular symptoms only if prednisone is contraindicated, has been unsuccessful in relieving symptoms, or is difficult to taper.

On occasion, even thymectomy has been considered in young healthy patients with only ocular symptoms. Since approximately 85% of myasthenics who present with purely ocular symptoms will become generalized within 2 years,[15] early thymectomy might prevent or minimize this occurrence. However, thymectomy is generally reserved for patients with moderate generalized myasthenia.

STEP 5B: TREATMENT OF MODERATE GENERALIZED MYASTHENIA (Figure 7)

Thymectomy

Thymectomy is recommended for those relatively healthy patients whose myasthenic symptoms interfere with their lives enough for them to consider undergoing major thoracic surgery. While it is expensive and invasive, thymectomy is the only

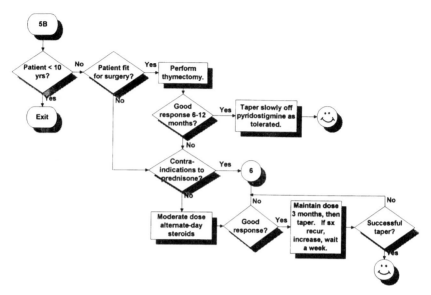

FIGURE 7. Step 5B: Treatment of moderate generalized myasthenia.

treatment available that offers a chance of an eventual drug-free remission. This chance seems to be better earlier in the disease than later. The potential benefit of thymectomy also decreases as the adult patient gets older and as the thymus naturally involutes with time. Furthermore, the risks of surgery increase with age. The age at which the risks outweigh the potential benefits must be individualized for every patient. (See the accompanying papers by Andrews and by Seybold for whether there is a lower age-limit for thymectomy.)

Steroids also cause involution of the thymus as well as inhibition of wound healing, so ideally their use before thymectomy is avoided. Nonetheless, some patients require the rapid improvement (within months) that careful prednisone treatment offers before they undergo thymectomy.

Likewise, after thymectomy, most (but not all) patients will be willing to wait up to a year to assess any improvement from the surgery before contemplating additional treatments. With improvement, the patient should gradually taper off Mestinon as tolerated, either by decreasing the dose by half a tablet (30 mg) or by prolonging the interval between doses, depending upon how soon symptoms recur each time. Improvement from thymectomy can continue for 5 to even 20 years after surgery.[16]

Moderate-Dose Steroids

If the response to thymectomy is not promising after a year and there are no contraindications, "moderate-dose" alternate-day prednisone therapy may be begun, starting at low doses of 10–20 mg every other day to minimize the chances of deterioration of symptoms, a unique initial response of some myasthenic patients to moderate amounts of prednisone. The dose is gradually increased by 10 mg every 3 weeks (10 doses) until symptoms begin to improve or until 100 mg q.o.d. is reached. The effective dose is maintained for at least 3 months. The goal is to eliminate the patient's symptoms completely. Some patients discover that Mestinon is no longer necessary once they are asymptomatic on prednisone; thus, Mestinon can be discontinued gradually at this point.

Once the patient has been asymptomatic on prednisone for at least 3 months, a very slow tapering of the prednisone every 4 weeks by less than 20% of the previous daily dose can be attempted. Eventually, the patient may experience temporary worsening for a week or so after decreasing a dose, and this may be a warning that the pace of tapering should be slowed or even halted for a while. Once symptoms recur during a taper, it is often difficult to eliminate them again by returning to the previous dose; thus, relatively large prednisone increases of 10–20 mg may be required to restore the previous condition.

Other Treatments

If there are contraindications to prednisone or the patient is unable to taper off prednisone, immunosuppressive agents such as azathioprine should be considered. Courses of pooled immunoglobulins intravenously (IVIG) every 3–4 weeks can also help patients tolerate steroid-tapering.

Patients with severe myasthenia teetering on the brink of crisis should be stabilized and improved to a "moderate" (or at least a "chronic severe") level of severity before thymectomy is performed.

STEP 5C: TREATMENT OF SEVERE GENERALIZED MYASTHENIA (Figure 8)

Expensive short-term treatment modalities such as plasma exchange (plasmapheresis) and intravenous immunoglobulin (IVIG) are justified if a patient is in immediate danger of requiring treatment in an intensive care unit (ICU) for respiratory insufficiency and/or inability to swallow medications. Although some patients respond to one and not the other of these modalities, it makes at least theoretical sense to try treatments of plasma exchange first, if venous access is available. Five treatments, either daily or every other day, are recommended as the initial plasma exchange regimen. If a good response does not occur before the end of the course of plasma exchanges, IVIG is then administered, usually as 400 mg IVIG per kg body weight per day for 5 days, or as 1 g/kg/day for 2 days.

If neither of these temporary treatments produces improvement in the patient's condition and the vital capacity is around 30 mL/kg (the threshold below which hypercarbia frequently occurs), it will probably be necessary to support the patient's ventilation by endotracheal intubation and mechanical ventilation while a precipitating cause of the crisis is investigated. One of the most-common reasons for deterioration in patients with severe MG is intercurrent pulmonary infection, often caused by

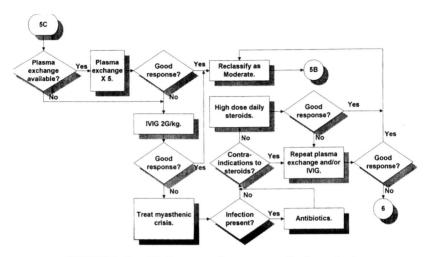

FIGURE 8. Step 5C: Treatment of severe generalized myasthenia.

aspiration because of severe dysphagia. The myasthenia will not improve until after the infection is eradicated. Another course of plasma exchange and/or IVIG treatments can be tried after intubation to facilitate eventual extubation of the patient.

High-Dose Steroids

Once the patient is intubated, it is safe to begin "high-dose" daily prednisone because now the patient's ventilation can be supported mechanically during any initial worsening that may occur. Sixty to 100 mg is given daily until several days of improvement have occurred. Eighty-five percent of patients improve within 21 days and 100% of responders improve within 2 months.[17]

When it is safe to do so, the daily dose of prednisone is slowly decreased by 10 mg each week to 50 mg daily, before converting to alternate-day maintenance by "seesawing" the dose up 5 mg and down 5 mg every 4 days (i.e., 45 mg one day, 55 mg the next for 4 days; then 40 mg alternating with 60 mg for 4 days; 35 mg with 65 mg for 4 days; and so on) until the patient is on 100 mg q.o.d. After several months on high-dose alternate-day therapy, very slow tapering can be considered if the patient is asymptomatic (see step 5B).

In refractory cases of severe myasthenia gravis, immunosuppressive medication may be required as well.

STEP 6: IMMUNOSUPPRESSIVE THERAPY (FIGURE 9)

As stated above, some physicians prefer to initiate MG therapy with azathioprine as well as prednisone.[2] In this algorithm, however, therapies are added only one at a

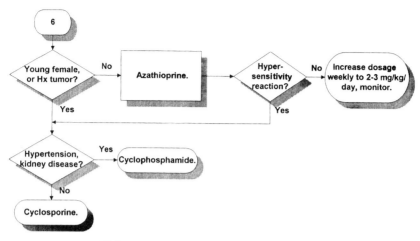

FIGURE 9. Step 6: Immunosuppressive therapy.

time, with enough time allowed to assess the positive (or negative) response of the patient to each therapy before adding a further regimen.

MG patients with moderate generalized autoimmune myasthenia are considered for immunosuppressive therapy if they (a) have not responded to thymectomy, (b) are too old for surgery, (c) have relative contraindications or toxic reactions to steroids, or (d) are unable to taper off steroids.

Azathioprine

The first choice of immunosuppressive drug for MG is usually azathioprine, unless the patient is a young woman who wishes to have children or is a patient with a history of previous cancer. These two relative contraindications reflect azathioprine's potential to cause skeletal teratogenicity and possibly increased malignancy. If these do not apply, baseline blood values for complete blood count, liver function tests, and amylase (or lipase) are obtained before starting azathioprine at one tablet (50 mg) a day, taken at bedtime to minimize nausea. Blood is monitored every week while beginning or increasing the dose of azathioprine because of the drug's adverse effects of dose-related bone marrow depression and liver dysfunction. Occasional patients develop an early hypersensitivity reaction to azathioprine consisting of myalgias, fever, abdominal pain, and flu-like symptoms, in which case the drug must be discontinued.

If blood tests are stable and the patient tolerates the medication, it is increased by 25–50 mg weekly, taken at bedtime, until a dose of 2–3 mg/kg/day is reached. This dose is required for eventual effectiveness of azathioprine in MG,[18] but the response is extraordinarily gradual and slow, beginning 3 to 6 months after starting the medication, with a maximum response at 12–36 months.[18] A dose of 150 mg/day costs $1000 per year.[8]

The dose of azathioprine is decreased if amylase or liver function tests increase greater than two times the normal values or if the white blood count drops below 2800/cm³. Lymphopenia is less worrisome than neutropenia. Azathioprine causes a macrocytosis of red blood cells with increased mean corpuscular volume, which has been suggested[19] as a way of monitoring dosage (and compliance). If azathioprine is discontinued, there is a 50% relapse rate and thus patients rarely come off this drug completely unless some other intervention such as thymectomy has been effective.

Cyclosporine

If azathioprine is toxic, contraindicated, or ineffective, the next immunosuppressive medication that may be tried is cyclosporine. Cyclosporine is nephrotoxic, so the presence of hypertension and kidney disease are relative contraindications. Cyclosporine is the only therapeutic modality used in MG that has been the subject of a preliminary randomized controlled trial.[20] The dose chosen was 5 mg/kg/day in two divided doses. Serum creatinine was followed to assess renal toxicity, which was the limiting adverse effect. Hypertension was reversible, but headache, nausea, and hirsutism were also reported.[20] Response was more rapid than that for azathioprine, averaging 2 weeks to onset of any response and 6 months for maximal response. Cyclosporine is the most expensive of the immunosuppressives, at $4300 per year for 250 mg/day.[8]

Cyclophosphamide

Cyclophosphamide is the third and usually last immunosuppressive therapy tried, but it occasionally produces dramatic improvement in refractory myasthenic patients. It has been administered as 3–5 mg/kg/day orally in divided doses, or as 200 mg intravenously once a week. The advice of a hematologist or oncologist is usually sought for the presently preferred dose and route of administration. Serious adverse effects are expected,[21] including alopecia (75%), leukopenia (35%), cystitis (8%), anorexia (17%), nausea, and vomiting (25%).

Unfortunately, some MG patients exist for whom all these treatments have been tried and the patient still has severe disease. The physician faced with this problem must consider extraordinary measures, such as rethymectomy,[22] high-dose methylprednisolone,[23] or perhaps even methotrexate (untried in myasthenia). More effective and more specific therapies are needed for these patients, whose hope lies in the future of presently experimental therapies.

CONCLUSIONS

Algorithms, decision trees, and practice guidelines are often resisted because they seem to commit physicians to a certainty that they know is unrealistic, especially when confronted by a disease as heterogeneous and variable as MG. This algorithm, however, may serve a useful purpose if it emphasizes those aspects of diagnosis, thymoma detection, general therapeutic measures, and anticholinesterase treatment that are common to all patients. It may also be of benefit if it makes clear that treatment must be appropriate to the severity of the present and potential disease for each individual patient, and that it must be tailored to the wishes of the informed patient. Structuring one reasonable approach based on clinical experience may help clarify where, in a treatment algorithm, different clinical decisions might be equally appropriate. It may also help frame those questions that need to be answered in the future by evidence-based outcome analysis.

ACKNOWLEDGMENTS

Lola W. Hackett, Coordinator of the Clinical Effectiveness Initiative of the UCLA Medical Center, provided excellent advice and assistance in creating these algorithms.

REFERENCES

1. NEWSOM-DAVIS, J. 1981. Myasthenia gravis: immune mechanisms and implications. Clin. Exp. Neurol. **18:** 14–26.
2. TOYKA, K. V. 1990. Myasthenia gravis. *In* Current Therapy in Neurologic Disease. Volume 3, pp. 385–391. B. C. Decker. Philadelphia.
3. GARCIA, C. A. 1993. Myasthenic disorders. *In* Decision Making in Adult Neurology. Second edition, pp. 238–241. Mosby–Year Book. St. Louis.
4. MENDELL, J. 1994. Neuromuscular junction disorders: a guide to diagnosis and treatment. Adv. Neuroimmunol. **1:** 9–16.
5. JABLECKI, C. K., M. T. ANDARY, M. DI BENEDETTO *et al.* 1996. American Association of Electrodiagnostic Medicine guidelines for outcome studies in electrodiagnostic medicine. Muscle Nerve **19:** 1626–1635.
6. LENNON, V. A. 1994. Serological diagnosis of myasthenia gravis and the Lambert-Eaton myasthenic syndrome. *In* Handbook of Myasthenia Gravis and Myasthenic Syndromes, pp. 149–164. Dekker. New York.
7. PHILLIPS, L. H. & P. A. MELNICK. 1990. Diagnosis of myasthenia gravis in the 1990s. Semin. Neurol. **10:** 62–69.
8. SEYBOLD, M. E. 1995. Myasthenia gravis: diagnostic and therapeutic perspectives in the 1990s. Neurologist **1:** 345–360.
9. LANSKA, D. J. 1991. Diagnosis of thymoma in myasthenics using anti-striated muscle antibodies: predictive value and gain in diagnostic certainty. Neurology **41:** 520–524.
10. KEESEY, J. C., M. BEIN, J. MINK *et al.* 1980. Detection of thymoma in myasthenia gravis. Neurology **30:** 233–239.
11. BATRA, P., C. HERRMANN & D. MULDER. 1987. Mediastinal imaging in myasthenia gravis: correlation of chest radiography, CT, MR, and surgical findings. Am. J. Radiol. **148:** 515–519.
12. GOLDMAN, A. J., C. HERRMANN, J. C. KEESEY *et al.* 1975. Myasthenia gravis and invasive thymoma: a 20-year experience. Neurology **25:** 1021–1025.
13. PALMIERI, G., S. LASTORIA, A. COLAO *et al.* 1997. Successful treatment of a patient with a

thymoma and pure red-cell aplasia with octreotide and prednisone. N. Engl. J. Med. **336:** 263–265.

14. MOORTHY, G., M. M. BEHRENS, D. B. DRACHMAN *et al.* 1989. Ocular pseudo-myasthenia or ocular myasthenia "plus": a warning to clinicians. Neurology **39:** 1150–1154.

15. SIMPSON, J. F., M. R. WESTERBERG & K. R. MAGEE. 1966. Myasthenia gravis, an analysis of 295 cases. Acta Neurol. Scand. **42**(suppl. 23): 27.

16. MASAOKA, A., Y. YAMAKAWA, H. NIWA *et al.* 1996. Extended thymectomy for myasthenia gravis patients: a 20-year review. Ann. Thorac. Surg. **62:** 853–859.

17. PASCUZZI, R. M., H. B. COSLETT & T. R. JOHNS. 1984. Long-term corticosteroid treatment of myasthenia gravis: report of 116 patients. Ann. Neurol. **15:** 291–298.

18. MERTENS, H. G., G. HERTEL, P. REUTHER & K. RICKER. 1981. Effect of immunosuppressive drugs (azathioprine). Ann. N.Y. Acad. Sci. **377:** 691–699.

19. WITTE, A. S., D. R. CORNBLATH, N. J. SCHATZ & R. P. LISAK. 1986. Monitoring azathioprine therapy in myasthenia gravis. Neurology **36:** 1533–1534.

20. TINDALL, R. S. A., J. A. ROLLINS, J. T. PHILLIPS *et al.* 1987. Preliminary results of a double-blind, randomized, placebo-controlled trial of cyclosporine in myasthenia gravis. N. Engl. J. Med. **316:** 719–724.

21. PEREZ, M. C., W. L. BUOT, C. MERCADO-DANGUILAN *et al.* 1981. Stable remissions in myasthenia gravis. Neurology **31:** 32–37.

22. MILLER, R. G., A. FILLER-KATZ, D. KIPROV & R. ROAN. 1991. Repeat thymectomy in chronic refractory myasthenia gravis. Neurology **41:** 923–924.

23. ARSURA, E., N. G. BRUNNER, T. NAMBA & D. GROB. 1985. High-dose intravenous methylprednisolone in myasthenia gravis. Arch. Neurol. **42:** 1149–1153.

Reliability Testing of the Quantitative Myasthenia Gravis Score[a]

RICHARD J. BAROHN, DONALD McINTIRE, LAURA HERBELIN,
GIL I. WOLFE, SHARON NATIONS, AND WILSON W. BRYAN

Department of Neurology
University of Texas Southwestern Medical School
Dallas, Texas 75235-8897

INTRODUCTION

Besinger *et al.*[1] introduced a clinical scoring system to assess the degree of disease severity in myasthenia gravis (MG) patients. Their system consisted of 8 items, each graded 0 to 3, with 3 being the most severe. They found that the acetylcholine receptor antibody (AChR-Ab) correlated with the severity of the MG score. Tindall *et al.*[2,3] expanded the scale to 13 items and utilized it to serve as the primary efficacy measurement in two studies that determined that cyclosporine was an effective therapy for MG. In their 1992 study,[3] there was a mean decrease in the quantitative myasthenia gravis score (QMG) scale of 3.5 units in the treated group versus a mean change of 0 in the placebo group. Based on Tindall *et al.*'s standard deviation of 4.03, we estimated that a placebo-controlled study to determine the effectiveness of an investigational drug in MG would require a sample size of 22 patients in each arm to provide for sufficient power (0.80) in detecting a difference of 3.5 units of change for a significance level of 0.05.

Interrater reliability testing results for the QMG were not published. Interrater reliability determinations can determine the reliability of QMG with the subject effect removed. We performed interrater reliability testing using a modified QMG in order to determine the reliability of the scale and the number of patients needed to perform a randomized clinical trial. Three parameters in the prior scale that could not be easily quantified (facial muscles, chewing, swallowing) were modified (TABLE 1).

METHODS

Thirteen objective parameters were measured on a 0 to 3 point scale (total score range 0–39). Nine subjects, five with MG and four normals, were independently examined by seven clinical evaluators (CEs). Five CEs examined five subjects and three CEs examined four subjects. All MG patients had positive serum AChR-Ab titers. The reliability of the QMG was estimated as the pooled standard deviation estimate using an analysis of variance.

[a]This work was supported by grants from the Muscular Dystrophy Association and by FDA Orphan Products Development Grant No. F-D-R-001362-01-1.

TABLE 1. Quantitative MG Scale[a]

Test Items Weakness	None	Mild	Moderate	Severe
Double vision on lateral gaze **right** or **left** (circle one)	61	11–60	1–10	spontaneous
Ptosis (upward gaze)	61	11–60	1–10	spontaneous
Facial muscles	normal lid	complete, weak, some resistance	complete, without resistance	incomplete
Swallowing 4 oz. water (½ cup)	normal	Minimal coughing or throat clearing	severe coughing/ choking or nasal regurgitation	cannot swallow (test not attempted)
Speech following counting aloud from 1 to 50 (onset of dysarthria)	none at #50	dysarthria at #30–49	dysarthria at #10–29	dysarthria at #9
Right arm outstretched (90° sitting)	240	90–239	10–89	0–9
Left arm outstretched (90° sitting)	240	90–239	10–89	0–9
Vital capacity (% predicted)	≥80%	65–79%	50–64%	<50%
Right hand grip (kg)				
male	≥45	15–44	5–14	0–4
female	≥30	10–29	5–9	0–4
Left hand grip (kg)				
male	≥35	15–34	5–14	0–4
female	≥25	10–24	5–9	0–4
Head lifted (45° supine)	120	30–119	1–29	0
Right leg outstretched (45° supine)	100	31–99	1–30	0
Left leg outstretched (45° supine)	100	31–99	1–30	0

[a]Total QMG score range 0–39.

RESULTS

Summary statistics for the nine subjects are compiled in TABLE 2.

The pooled standard deviation or the interrater reliability is a weighted average of the standard deviations given in TABLE 2. This value, expressed as a standard deviation, is 1.342. Consequently, at the 95% confidence level (1.96 SD), QMG scores do not differ from the observed values by more than ± 2.63 units (1.96SD × 1.342).

TABLE 2. Summary Statistics for the Nine Subjects

Subject	Sample Size (Clinical Evaluations)	QMG Score Mean	QMG Score Standard Deviation	Clinical Symptoms/Signs
(1) MG	5	6.2	0.45	34 M, ptosis, intermittent diplopia
(2) MG	5	13.4	1.67	63 F, ptosis, moderate proximal weakness, dyspnea, occasional dysphagia
(3) MG	5	3.6	2.07	55 M, asymptomatic, persistent facial weakness and slight ptosis
(4) MG	2	2.5	2.12	59 M, asymptomatic, slight proximal weakness
(5) MG	2	5.5	3.00	64 F, intermittent ptosis and dyspnea, minimal proximal weakness
(6) Normal	5	1.4	0.89	
(7) Normal	4	0.5	1.00	
(8) Normal	2	0.5	0.71	
(9) Normal	2	⌐.5	0.71	

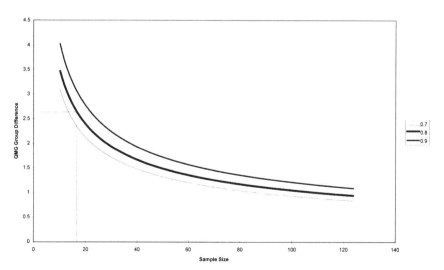

FIGURE 1. QMG group difference for two-sample Student's *t* test.

CONCLUSIONS

If QMG is to be used as a primary efficacy measurement in clinical trials, a treatment must produce more than 2.6 units of change to be of clinical significance. QMG score changes of up to 2.6 units are expected to occur due to variability of repeated observations. With this variability estimate for a placebo-controlled trial, a sample size of 34 patients (17 in each group) is necessary for a power of 0.80 to detect a difference in QMG of 2.6 units (FIGURE 1).

As the standard deviation reported by Tindall et al.[3] is 4.03 and the measured interrater reliability is 1.34, the greater part of the QMG variation is due to differences in the subjects. The implication is that the majority of QMG variation is due to subject variability.

REFERENCES

1. BESINGER, U. A., K. V. TOYKA, M. HOMBERG et al. 1983. Myasthenia gravis: long-term correlation of binding and bungarotoxin blocking antibodies against acetylcholine receptors with changes in disease severity. Neurology 33: 1316–1321.
2. TINDALL, R. S. A., J. A. ROLLINS, J. T. PHILLIPS et al. 1987. Preliminary results of a double-blind, randomized, placebo-controlled trial of cyclosporine in myasthenia gravis. N. Engl. J. Med. 316: 719–724.
3. TINDALL, R. S. A., J. T. PHILLIPS, J. A. ROLLINS et al. 1993. A clinical therapeutic trial of cyclosporine in myasthenia gravis. Ann. N.Y. Acad. Sci. 681: 539–551.

Oral Functions of Patients with Myasthenia Gravis

F. G. WEIJNEN,[a] A. VAN DER BILT,[a] J. H. J. WOKKE,[b]
M. W. M. WASSENBERG,[a] AND I. OUDENAARDE[a]

[a]Department of Oral-Maxillofacial Surgery, Prosthodontics,
and Special Dental Care
[b]Department of Neurology
Universiteit Utrecht
3508 TA Utrecht, the Netherlands

INTRODUCTION

Myasthenia gravis (MG) patients with bulbar involvement may suffer from difficulties in swallowing and chewing, changed facial expression, and dysarthria. The aim of our research is to quantify these oral dysfunctions by a series of standardized measurements.

METHODS

A group of 20 bulbar MG patients has been compared with a group of 20 healthy controls, matched for age, gender, and dental status. The series of standardized measurements were aimed at chewing problems (maximal bite force and surface EMG registrations of the masticatory muscles, combined with chewing efficiency), impaired facial expression (lip-length and snout indices), and swallowing problems (maximal tongue force measurements and examination of the swallowing process). All measurements were performed at the same time of day for each subject and were alternated with a pause of 10 minutes to avoid the influence of earlier measurements. In addition, all patients were asked to stop taking anticholinesterase drugs a few hours before the measurements took place. Differences between patients and controls were tested on significance with the Wilcoxon matched-pairs signed-rank test.

CHEWING PROBLEMS

First, the maximal voluntary contraction of the jaw-closing muscles was determined by asking the subjects to clench as hard as possible on a bite force transducer,[1] while surface EMG recordings were made of the masseter and temporal muscles. In addition, the maximal activity of the jaw-opening muscles was measured while subjects tried to open their mouth as hard as possible while the investigator applied an opposing force with her hand, positioned under their chin. Significantly lower values were found in bulbar MG patients for maximal bite force ($p = 0.0009$) and maximal

EMG activity of the jaw-closing ($p = 0.003$) and jaw-opening muscles ($p = 0.013$). A summary of the results is given in TABLE 1.

Second, the chewing efficiency was evaluated by measuring the degree of comminution of test food after 15 chewing strokes.[2] The consistency of this test food is comparable to cheese. The results indicate that chewing efficiency is impaired in the patient group. Mean particle size after 15 chewing strokes is larger than in the control group ($p = 0.0004$).

IMPAIRED FACIAL EXPRESSION

Smiling is a very important part of facial expression and is known to be impaired in part of the MG patients (the so-called "flattened smile"). The ability to smile (and the ability to pout the lips) can be quantified with the use of indices that are based on intercommissural distance measurements and that express the degree to which the mouth can be lengthened (lip-length index) or shortened (snout index).[3] The lip-length index (LL index) represents the function of the buccinator, risorius, and (part of the) zygomaticus major muscles. The snout index (S index) expresses the function of the orbicularis oris muscle. The results show that the lip-length and snout indices are significantly lower in bulbar MG patients ($p = 0.0008$ and 0.008, respectively). This means that these patients are significantly less able to smile and to pout their lips.

SWALLOWING PROBLEMS

The force of the tongue, which plays an important role in the swallowing process, was measured with the use of a tongue force transducer.[4] Measurements of maximal tongue force were performed while the subject pushed the tongue in upward and sideward direction against a lever. The results, which are depicted in FIGURE 1, indicate that maximal tongue force in the patient group is significantly lower in all directions ($p = 0.0004$–0.013). Besides these low tongue force levels, the swallowing

TABLE 1. Overview of the Results of the Series of Standardized Measurements

Measurement	Control Group	Bulbar MG Group	p Value
maximal bite force	517 N ± 52	295 N ± 45	0.0009
max. EMG (jaw-closing muscles)	939 μV ± 145	620 μV ± 130	0.003
max. EMG (jaw-opening muscles)	192 μV ± 24	148 μV ± 25	0.013
chewing efficiency[a]	3.2 mm ± 0.3	5.5 mm ± 0.5	0.0004
lip-length index	39.0% ± 2.3	25.7% ± 2.5	0.0008
snout index	34.0% ± 1.7	25.1% ± 2.6	0.008
maximal upward tongue force	8.3 N ± 0.8	5.5 N ± 0.5	0.013
swallowing duration	2.2 s ± 0.1	2.9 s ± 0.3	0.03
number of swallows	1.1 ± 0.01	1.3 ± 0.1	0.03

[a]Mean particle size after 15 chewing strokes (initial particle size = 8.0 mm).

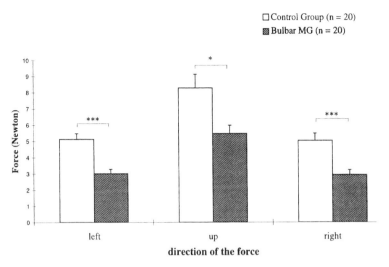

FIGURE 1. Maximal tongue force measurements (in upward and sideward direction) in the control and patient groups.

process may also be affected by weakness of submental and swallowing muscle complexes. Therefore, we examined the surface EMG of these muscles, combined with chin and larynx movement registrations, while the subject swallowed. The time and the number of swallows needed to swallow 10 mL of water were compared for both groups. The bulbar MG patients swallowed slower ($p = 0.03$) and needed more swallows to ingest 10 mL of water ($p = 0.03$). The role of the tongue was evaluated further by calculating the Spearman correlation coefficient of maximal tongue force and the duration of the swallowing process. A significant correlation was found ($p = 0.03$), which indicates that patients with lower maximal tongue force tend to swallow slower.

SUMMARY

With the use of the methods developed to quantify oral dysfunctions in bulbar MG patients, our results indicate that we can distinguish the patients from their matched controls. These results can add to our knowledge of myasthenia gravis and these methods may improve diagnosis and therapy evaluation in individual patients. In addition, these methods may be used in future pharmacological research.

REFERENCES

1. SLAGTER, A. P., F. BOSMAN, H. W. VAN DER GLAS & A. VAN DER BILT. 1993. Human jaw-elevator muscle activity and food comminution in the dentate and edentulous state. Arch. Oral Biol. **38:** 195–205.

2. OLTHOFF, L. W., A. VAN DER BILT, F. BOSMAN & H. H. KLEIZEN. 1984. Distribution of particle sizes in food comminuted by human mastication. Arch. Oral Biol. **29:** 899–903.
3. JANSEN, C., F. G. I. JENNEKENS, J. H. J. WOKKE, G. J. LEPPINK & H. J. A. WIJNNE. 1990. Lip-length and snout indices: methods for quantitative assessment of peri-oral facial muscle strength. J. Neurol. Sci. **97:** 133–142.
4. ROBINOVITCH, S. N., C. HERSHLER & D. P. ROMILLY. 1991. A tongue force measurement system for the assessment of oral-phase swallowing disorders. Arch. Phys. Med. Rehabil. **72:** 38–42.

Late-Onset Myasthenia Gravis

Follow-up of 113 Patients Diagnosed after Age 60

GERHARD SLESAK,[a] ARTHUR MELMS,[a,b] FRIEDERIKE GERNETH,[c]
NORBERT SOMMER,[a] ROBERT WEISSERT,[a] AND
JOHANNES DICHGANS[a]

[a]Department of Neurology
Eberhard-Karls-University Tübingen
72076 Tübingen, Germany

[c]Institute of Medical Information Processing
72070 Tübingen, Germany

INTRODUCTION

There is not much known about the benefits of modern treatment in patients with very late onset of myasthenia gravis (MG). In general, therapy with anticholinesterase agents, corticosteroids, and other immunosuppressive drugs, mainly azathioprine (Aza), is effective as in the treatment of young-onset cases. However, there is a broad consensus to not perform thymectomies after age 60, except for a suspected thymic tumor.[1] The main objective of our study was to evaluate the benefit of specific treatment applied in elderly MG patients.

MATERIALS/METHODS

We identified 113 patients diagnosed after age 60 between 1978 and 1996. The diagnosis was based on a typical medical history and distribution of myasthenic weakness, positive anti-AChR antibody titers (>0.4 nM/L), pathological decrement (>10%) after repetitive nerve stimulation, and positive Tensilon test. In cases with ocular MG, but without anti-AChR antibodies and electrophysiological abnormalities, typical clinical signs, positive Tensilon test, and treatment response to Mestinon were accepted for diagnosis.[2]

A last follow-up questionnaire was sent to general practitioners with a 94% feedback. The data were processed using the MYA-DATA program, developed by the Institute of Medical Information Processing, University of Tübingen, Germany. The JMP program was used for statistical analysis.

We defined standardized time points (months after diagnosis) for follow-up (range, median): 0 years (0–4; 0 months), 1 year (5–20; 12 months), 3 years (29–44; 36 months), and 5 years (53–68; 60 months).

The signs (FIGURE 1) were classified as follows: complete remission (no signs af-

---

[b]To whom all correspondence should be addressed.

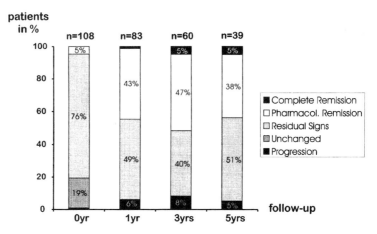

FIGURE 1. Course of signs after diagnosis in elderly patients.

ter exertion, minor complaints, no specific treatment), pharmacological remission (no signs after exertion, minor complaints, specific treatment), residual signs (good improvement after specific treatment, minor signs, no restrictions in daily life), unchanged (no satisfactory improvement with specific treatment nor progression), and progression (aggravating signs and increasing severity in spite of specific treatment).

Pharmacological remission (PR) and residual signs (RS) were classified as successful treatment. In this subgroup (PR/RS, FIGURE 2), patients took the following medication: (1) anticholinesterase agents only (AChE-Inhib. only), (2) steroids only (Steroids), (3) Aza and occasionally other immunosuppressants (Immunosuppressives), and (4) steroids and Aza (Steroids + Immunosupp.). A number of patients in groups 2–4 were also taking AChE inhibition.

RESULTS AND DISCUSSION

One hundred thirteen MG patients (30% of our total number since 1978) were diagnosed after age 60 (median age: 70 years; maximum: 87 years). The median follow-up period was 4.5 years, with a range up to 16 years. Females and males were equally represented. Over time, 33 patients died; in 6 cases, there was evidence for MG progression. One fatality was due to invasive thymoma. Age at death ranged from 65 to 77 years (median: 72 years) if patients died from MG-associated complications, as compared to 61 to 95 years (median: 77 years) if they died from unrelated causes. Thymectomy was performed in 15 patients (13%). Thymoma was found in 10, thymic carcinoma in 1, and hyperplasia and atrophic thymus in 2 cases, respectively.

At diagnosis, 40 patients (35%) had purely ocular signs and only 4 of them (10%) developed generalized MG subsequently. Other studies,[2,3] including all age groups, reported generalization of ocular MG in 31–49%. In the natural course of MG, with-

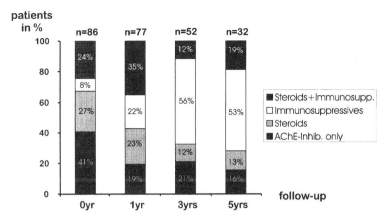

FIGURE 2. Course of treatment in the elderly with good impact (pharmacological remission and residual signs).

out steroids or other immunosuppressive treatment, this proportion was even higher (69%).[4] In our survey, 19 patients with generalized signs at diagnosis reported pure ocular symptoms at the very beginning. We estimate that about 23 of 59 cases (39%) with primary ocular symptoms developed generalized MG. Complete remission at follow-up after 0 years (1/3/5 years) was rarely observed (1–5%). However, most patients were in PR/RS (87–93%) receiving specific therapy. Only 5–8% were progressive in spite of therapy. After successful treatment (PR/RS), steroids were tapered and the majority were taking Aza only (8% at 0 years and 53% at 5 years follow-up, Figure 2). The considerable side effects of steroids,[5] especially in elderly people (diabetes, osteoporosis, cataract, glaucoma, etc.), argue in favor of that strategy.

The proportion of patients with cholinesterase inhibition only decreased from 41% (0 years) to 16% (5 years). We assume that patients on AChE inhibition only had a more benign course and hence were often lost for follow-up.

On 5 years follow-up, 23 patients (72%) of PR/RS were still taking immunosuppressive drugs (Aza, only in one case: low-dose cyclophosphamide). Hence, the optimal duration of immunosuppression after sustained remission is not known and requires further investigation.[6] Discontinuation may be tried after stable disease for several years or if there are severe side effects. This study documents that MG of very late onset has a favorable prognosis, but myasthenic weakness still contributes to the mortality in elderly patients.

REFERENCES

1. LANSKA, D. J. 1990. Indications for thymectomy in myasthenia gravis. Neurology **40:** 1828–1829.
2. SOMMER, N. *et al.* 1997. Ocular myasthenia gravis: response to long-term immunosuppressive treatment. J. Neurol. Neurosurg. Psychiatry **62:** 156–162.

3. BEVER, C. T. *et al.* 1983. Prognosis of ocular myasthenia gravis. Ann. Neurol. **14:** 516–519.
4. OOSTERHUIS, H. J. G. H. 1989. The natural course of myasthenia gravis: a long-term follow-up study. J. Neurol. Neurosurg. Psychiatry **52:** 1121–1127.
5. EVOLI, A. *et al.* 1992. Long-term results of corticosteroid therapy in patients with myasthenia gravis. Eur. Neurol. **32:** 37–43.
6. HOHLFELD, R. *et al.* 1985. Myasthenia gravis: reactivation of clinical disease and of autoimmune factors after discontinuation of long-term azathioprine. Ann. Neurol. **17:** 238–242.

Thymoma Recurrences in Myasthenia Gravis Patients

A. EVOLI,[a] A. P. BATOCCHI,[a] M. M. LINO,[a] P. TONALI,[a] L. LAURIOLA,[b]
AND G. B. DOGLIETTO[c]

[a]Institute of Neurology
[b]Institute of Pathology
[c]Institute of Surgery
Catholic University
00168 Rome, Italy

INTRODUCTION

The prognosis of thymoma appears to depend mainly on the tumor invasiveness and on the radicality of surgical resection.[1,2] These factors could determine, apart from the short-term outcome, the chance of tumor relapse. The role of adjuvant therapies such as radiotherapy and chemotherapy in the treatment plan of thymoma is not yet codified. With respect to tumor recurrences, it is well known that they can occur late after thymectomy and are generally intrathoracic.[3–5] However, there are only a few reports about their surveillance and treatment and on their possible influence on MG outcome.

We report our experience of diagnosis and treatment of thymoma recurrences in MG patients.

PATIENTS AND METHODS

Our series consists of myasthenic patients who had undergone thymectomy for thymoma during the last 24 years and with at last 2 years of follow-up from the time of the first operation.

They were 143 patients, 73 males and 70 females, with age at thymectomy ranging from 15 to 72 years.

Surgical approach was by posterolateral thoracotomy in 5 cases; median sternotomy followed by extended thymectomy was performed in all the other patients. Extended thymectomy included complete resection of the thymoma together with the thymic gland and perithymic fat tissue; when necessary, it was associated with resection of pleura, pericardium, lung, phrenic nerve, and pleural implants.

Tumor extent at surgery was evaluated retrospectively according to Masaoka staging:[6] 70 patients had a capsulated thymoma (state I) and 73 had an invasive neoplasm (stages II, III, and IVa).

Mediastinal irradiation at doses of 40–50 Gy was performed postoperatively in most cases with invasive thymoma; no patients received chemotherapy at the time of the first operation. Postoperative follow-up was performed with mediastinal CT scan every 1–2 years. In patients who complained of thymoma relapse, histologies of both the first tumor and recurrence were reviewed according to Marino and Müller-Hermelink classification.[7]

Patients with multiple recurrences received chemotherapy based on a combination of prednisolone, doxorubicin, cyclophosphamide, and cisplatin.[8]

RESULTS

Thirteen patients out of 143 (9%) complained of 14 thymoma recurrences (in one case, the tumor relapsed twice). All of them had an invasive thymoma.

They were 5 females and 8 males, with age at thymectomy ranging from 27 to 48 years. At that time, 3 patients had no signs of MG; 1 patient had purely ocular myasthenia and 9 had generalized disease. MG patients were treated with anticholinesterases associated, in most cases, with corticosteroids.

Five patients had a thymoma with invasion through the capsule or into mediastinal pleura (stage II); 5 had a tumor infiltrating the surrounding tissues (stage III); 3 had an intrathoracic disseminated thymoma (stage IVa). Postoperative radiotherapy was performed in 9/13 cases.

According to Marino and Müller-Hermelink classification,[7] 8 patients had a cortical thymoma often with small foci of epidermoid differentiation and 5 had a well-differentiated thymic carcinoma (WDTC).

Thymoma relapses were only intrathoracic. Their histology was the same as at the first operation. In patients who did not undergo further surgery, histological diagnosis was made by needle biopsy.

Five cases had 1 or 2 recurrences confined to the anterior mediastinum; in the others, multiple nodules were present on the pleura or on the pleura and pericardium, with lung infiltration in 1 case.

Four patients with 1–2 mediastinal masses underwent complete surgical resection associated with radiotherapy when it had not been performed at the time of the first operation. One of these cases complained of 2 recurrences; she underwent surgery twice and was submitted to radiotherapy after the last operation. All these patients are alive and tumor-free at the last CT scan. Their follow-up ranges between 1 and 8 years (mean 6.5 years).

Six patients with multiple nodules were treated with subtotal surgery associated with chemotherapy (3 cases) or with chemotherapy alone (3 cases). All of them are alive and tumor-free at the last CT scan. Their follow-up ranges from 2 to 5 years (mean 3 years).

One case treated with radiotherapy only died after 4 years. Two patients with multiple pleural nodules refused any treatment: 1 of them died after 2 years and the other is still alive after 7 years.

Immunosuppressive therapy for MG was performed in most cases.

The time interval between thymectomy and the radiological detection of recurrence ranged from 2 to 16 years. It is shown in FIGURE 1.

When recurrences were detected, 7 out of 10 MG patients showed a mild deterioration and 3 had no change in disease severity. In the 3 patients without MG at the first operation, the onset of MG was as follows: when recurrence was detected (2 years after the first operation) in the first patient; 1 year before recurrence detection

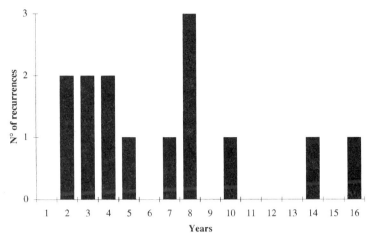

FIGURE 1. Interval between thymectomy and radiological detection of thymoma recurrences.

(3 years after thymectomy) in the second patient; at the time of the second recurrence detection (10 years after thymectomy) in the third patient.

DISCUSSION

The origins of thymoma recurrences are likely to be either tumor remnants due to incomplete surgical resection or pleural seedings possibly undetected at the first operation or due to surgical manipulation.[3,4] As a consequence, the extent of the first tumor and the radicality of surgical exeresis appear to be the strongest predicting factors.[9] It has also been reported that the histology has an independent prognostic value and that types related to cortical cells often show an aggressive behavior.[10]

Our data are in accordance with these reports. In our series, only invasive thymomas were complicated by relapses and all recurrences were from cortical thymomas or WDTC.

With respect to surgical approach, in accordance with other authors[11] we consider extended thymectomy as the technique of choice to ensure adequate exposure.

As far as adjuvant therapies are concerned, postoperative radiotherapy is generally recommended for invasive thymomas, while the role of chemotherapy is less defined. We perform radiotherapy in thymomas from stage II onwards, but so far we have little experience with preoperative or postoperative chemotherapy.

The treatment of recurrences is not yet codified. In our experience, reoperation with radical exeresis, when feasible, proved both effective and safe; in patients with multiple nodules, chemotherapy alone or associated with surgery gave good results.

As thymoma relapses can occur many years after thymectomy, surveillance should be quite prolonged. Moreover, as recurrences of stage I tumors have been occasionally reported,[9,12] postoperative follow-up should perhaps include also patients with encapsulated thymomas.

REFERENCES

1. URGESI, A. *et al.* 1992. Aggressive treatment of intrathoracic recurrences of thymoma. Radiother. Oncol. **24:** 221–225.
2. WILKINS, E. W., JR. *et al.* 1991. Role of staging in prognosis and management of thymoma. Ann. Thorac. Surg. **51:** 888–892.
3. OHMI, M. & M. OHUCHI. 1990. Recurrent thymoma in patients with myasthenia gravis. Ann. Thorac. Surg. **50:** 243–247.
4. KIRSCHNER, P. A. 1990. Reoperation for thymoma; report of 23 cases. Ann. Thorac. Surg. **49:** 550–555.
5. MAGGI, G. *et al.* 1991. Thymoma: results of 241 operated cases. Ann. Thorac. Surg. **51:** 152–156.
6. MASAOKA, A. *et al.* 1981. Follow-up study of thymomas with special reference to their clinical stages. Cancer **48:** 2485–2492.
7. MARINO, M. *et al.* 1985. Thymoma and thymic carcinoma: relation of thymoma epithelial cells to the cortical and medullary differentiation of the thymus. Virchows Arch. Pathol. Anat. **407:** 119–149.
8. HU, E. *et al.* 1986. Chemotherapy of malignant thymoma. Cancer **57:** 1101–1104.
9. REGNARD, J-F. *et al.* 1996. Prognostic factors and long-term results after thymoma resection: a series of 307 patients. J. Thorac. Cardiovasc. Surg. **112:** 376–384.
10. MARTINEZ, L. Q. *et al.* 1994. Thymoma: histologic subclassification is an independent prognostic factor. Cancer **74:** 606–617.
11. MASAOKA, A. *et al.* 1996. Extended thymectomy for myasthenia gravis patients: a 20-year review. Ann. Thorac. Surg. **62:** 853–859.
12. MASUNAGA, A. *et al.* 1995. A case of encapsulated noninvasive thymoma (stage I) with myasthenia gravis showing metastasis after a 2-year dormancy. Surg. Today **25:** 369–372.

Calcium Channel and β-Receptor Antagonists and Agonists in MG[a]

GEORG MATELL,[b] SAPKO BJELAK,[b] IRIS JONKERS,[c]
RITVA PIRSKANEN,[b] JORINE VAN VLIET,[c] AND
CHRISTER SWERUP[d]

Myasthenia Gravis Center
Karolinska Institute
S-171 77 Stockholm, Sweden

INTRODUCTION AND AIM

Certain membrane-acting drugs increase the symptoms of MG.[1,2] Calcium channel blockers and β-adrenoreceptor blockers (β-blockers) are considered as contraindicated.[3–5] These drugs may be lifesaving in common cardiovascular diseases. Some case reports concerning these drugs in MG have been published,[6–10] but our studies[11] are to our knowledge the first controlled systematic ones on human MG. We aimed at (i) determining the effects of intravenous (iv)[11] as well as oral β- and calcium channel–blocker drugs on MG both clinically and neurophysiologically and (ii) developing methods for the prediction of the individual responses of these drugs. In this short paper, we summarize the results of two studies.

MATERIALS, METHODS, AND PROTOCOL

Selection criteria for these two single, blind, placebo-controlled, crossover studies were stable, moderately severe disease (in order to allow for both worsening and improvement), and absence of contraindications for the test drugs. Two series of experiments were performed with 10 patients in each. Five patients participated in both studies. In the first study, acute effects were studied following iv injections of the test drugs. Long-term effects were studied during oral treatment using iv injection protocol for evaluation. *Muscle function test* (MFT): Peak expiratory flow (PEF), repetitive handgrip strength with a sphygmomanometer, and eye tests (diplopia or ptosis) were tested. The test results were given as a percentage of the normal. *Repetitive nerve stimulation* (RNS): Supramaximal stimulations at a frequency of 3 Hz on both

[a]This study was supported by a grant from the Paul Ferb Memorial Fund and was performed at Söder Hospital in Stockholm.
[b]Present address: Department of Neurology, Karolinska Hospital, S-171 76 Stockholm, Sweden.
[c]Present address: Faculty of Medicine, University of Leiden, the Netherlands.
[d]Present address: Department of Neurophysiology, Huddinge Hospital, S-141 86 Huddinge, Sweden.

a proximal (deltoid) and a distal (abductor digiti minimi, ADM) muscle were performed. RNS was made on the contralateral side to the muscle function tests. The decrement of the muscle action potential (AP) was calculated as the percentage decline in amplitude (baseline-to-peak) between the first and the fourth compound muscle APs. *Statistical analysis* was performed using the Wilcoxon matched-pair test. *P* values of <0.05 were considered as significant.

Drugs given intravenously: Propranolol (Inderal® 0.1 mg/kg, 1 mg/min), terbutaline (Bricanyl® 0.01 mg/kg, 0.1 mg/min), verapamil (Isoptin® 0.1 mg/kg, 1 mg/min), and calcium glubionate (Calcium-Sandoz® 1 mg/kg, 9 mg/min). *Oral drugs:* Propranolol capsules, 0.8 mg/kg, three times daily during two weeks; washout period: placebo capsules given three times daily for one week; verapamil capsules, 1.2 mg/kg, three times daily during two weeks. Drug capsules were prepared by the pharmacy of the hospital to be identical in shape and color.

Procedure: In the first study,[11] the patients were examined at two different days with a similar sequence of actions: MFT + RNS + edrophonium + MFT + RNS. After a 30-min rest, test drug was injected + MFT + RNS + edrophonium + MFT + RNS + antidote + MFT + RNS. In the second study (FIGURE 1), these examinations were performed repeatedly during oral treatment for fortnight periods. The study was approved by the ethical committee of the Karolinska Institute.

RESULTS

All patients had abnormal results in MFT and RNS before the drugs. Neither propranolol nor verapamil injections caused significant decrements in RNS or worsening of muscle strength in MFT. Oral treatment during two weeks did not cause any significant alterations in MFT or RNS decrement either (FIGURE 2). Terbutaline improved the RNS a little, but calcium improved the RNS nearly as much as edrophonium. The effects of iv injections of edrophonium and agonist were similar after injection or oral treatment with the two test drugs. Subjectively, a few patients reported increased and some reported decreased fatigability after the drugs.

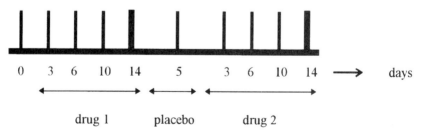

FIGURE 1. Schedule according to which the patients were investigated. Day 0: investigation before entering the experiment, baseline investigation. (❙): control investigation with MFT and RNS. (❚): injection with natural antidotes followed by MFT and RNS.

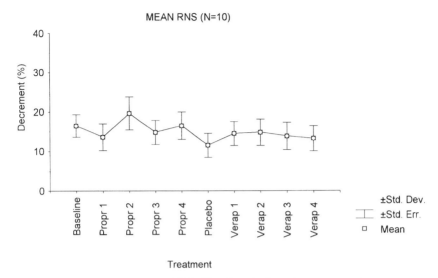

FIGURE 2. Mean RNS in 10 patients in the oral treatment study.

CONCLUSIONS

Propranolol or verapamil may be given to moderately severe MG patients without severe worsening. Emergency use of β- or calcium-blockers may thus be tried in MG. Any undesirable effect of these drugs may be immediately reversed by giving its antagonist iv. Calcium injection has nearly the same reversing effect as edrophonium on a myasthenic decrement.

REFERENCES

1. ADAMS, S. L., J. MATHEWS & L. C. GRAMMAR. 1984. Drugs that may exacerbate myasthenia gravis. Ann. Emerg. Med. **13:** 532–538.
2. ARGOV, Z. & F. L. MASTAGLIA. 1979. Disorders of neuromuscular transmission caused by drugs. N. Engl. J. Med. **301:** 409–413.
3. BARAR, F. S. K. & B. R. MADAN. 1973. Effect of some beta adrenoceptor blocking agents on skeletal neuromuscular transmission and motor coordination. Indian J. Med. Res. **1:** 1054–1061.
4. CHANG, C. C., S-O. LIN, S. J. HONG & L. C. CHIOU. 1988. Neuromuscular block by verapamil and diltiazem and inhibition of acetylcholine release. Brain Res. **454:** 332–339.
5. CONFAVREUX, C., N. CHARLES & G. AIMARD. 1990. Fulminant myasthenia gravis soon after initiation of acebutolol therapy. Eur. Neurol. **30:** 279–281.
6. KÓMÁR, J. & M. SZALAY SZÉL. 1987. Myasthenische Episode nach Einnahme grosser Mengen Betablocker. Fortschr. Neurol. Psychiatr. **55:** 201–202.
7. LEE, S. C. & S. T. HO. 1987. Acute effects of verapamil on neuromuscular transmission in

patients with myasthenia gravis. Proc. Natl. Sci. Counc. Repub. China Part B **11:** 307–312.

8. NOGUÉS, M. A. & A. RIVERO. 1993. Arterial hypertension, nifedipine, and myasthenia gravis. Muscle Nerve **16:** 797.

9. SHAIVITZ, S. A. 1979. Timolol and myasthenia gravis. JAMA **242:** 1611–1612.

10. SWASH, M. & D. A. INGRAM. 1992. Adverse effect of verapamil in myasthenia gravis. Muscle Nerve **15:** 396–398.

11. JONKERS, I., C. SWERUP, R. PIRSKANEN, S. BJELAK & G. MATELL. 1996. Acute effects of intravenous injection of beta-adrenoreceptor and calcium channel antagonists. Muscle Nerve **19:** 959–965.

A Treatment Algorithm for Autoimmune Myasthenia Gravis in Childhood

P. IAN ANDREWS

School of Pediatrics
University of New South Wales
and
Sydney Children's Hospital
Randwick 2031, Australia

INTRODUCTION

Three forms of myasthenia gravis (MG) occur in childhood. Autoimmune MG, sometimes known as juvenile myasthenia gravis (JMG), is the subject of this report. Congenital myasthenia gravis (CMG), or genetic MG, is a heterogeneous group of inherited disorders associated with dysfunction of various components of the neuro-muscular junction (NMJ), without evidence of an immune-mediated process.[1] Transient neonatal MG is a distinctive disorder of infants of mothers with autoimmune MG, in which circulating maternal autoantibodies cross the placenta to inhibit function of the acetylcholine receptor (AChR) in the fetus and during the first weeks after birth.

Autoimmune MG is an antibody-mediated process, with crucial roles for the cell-mediated immune system and complement, directed against the AChR in skeletal muscle.[2,3] This process results in reduced numbers and function of AChRs, which parallels disease severity.[2] Despite advances in our understanding of the disease, factors involved in initiation and persistence of the process remain largely unknown.

There is no evidence to suggest that the pathogenic mechanisms underlying autoimmune MG differ significantly between children and adults. There is little reported difference in the clinical manifestations of autoimmune MG among children and adults. Like other systems, however, the immune system undergoes considerable change and maturation throughout childhood. Age and sex hormones influence the incidence of JMG,[4–8] and different HLA antigens are linked to autoimmune MG in Japanese patients with onset before age 6 compared to patients with later onset.[9] It is conceivable, therefore, that maturation of the immune system influences the natural history and response to therapy of JMG. Thus, therapeutic strategies might vary with the age of the child. In addition, long-term consequences of therapies for autoimmune MG may differently affect the developing child and the already-developed adult.

In North America, onset of autoimmune MG before age 20 accounts for about 10–15% of all patients with myasthenia, with an annual incidence of 1.1 per million total population.[10] In other populations, however, the relative age distribution, incidence, and prevalence vary considerably. For instance, among Chinese, 43% of patients manifest disease before age 20;[11] a similar high proportion with early-onset disease is reported in Japan;[12] and the incidence and prevalence of JMG in North

Carolina among prepubertal black children are approximately threefold higher than among prepubertal white children.[8,13] These demographic differences may represent differences in genetic predisposition and/or environmental trigger factors. Might these putative genetic or environmental differences also modify the pathogenic process and response to therapy?

This paper will outline current therapeutic strategies for children and adolescents with autoimmune MG and will focus upon specific issues posed by pediatric myasthenic patients. It is based upon review of the English-language literature and 115 patients with onset of autoimmune MG before age 20.[8]

THE DEVELOPING IMMUNE SYSTEM

The human neonate is relatively immunologically incompetent compared to the adult.[14] Maturation of humoral, cell-mediated, and nonspecific arms of the immune system proceeds through childhood. Total immunoglobulin levels are low during infancy and reach adult levels by 2 years for IgM, 4–6 years for IgG, and puberty for IgA;[15] moreover, during and after puberty, females have higher levels of IgG, IgG1, IgM, and IgA than males.[16] Female sex hormones also increase the number of antibody-producing cells, the rapidity and duration of antibody response,[16] and the avidity of antibody binding.[17] The thymus achieves its greatest relative weight by the end of fetal life and exhibits reasonable functional maturity.[18] Absolute thymic weight increases until puberty, after which the thymus progressively involutes.[18] Release of T cells from the thymus is maximal in young animals and roughly correlates with thymic size.[14] Sex hormones are involves with thymic involution and have other important effects on cell-mediated immunity. In general, female sex hormones enhance immune responsiveness and male sex hormones have mixed effects, often inhibitory in nature.[16,19] Levels of many cytokines are lower in young children that in adolescents or adults,[20] and cytokine production and macrophage function may also be influenced by sex hormones.[19]

DIAGNOSIS

Fluctuating and fatigable weakness are the hallmarks of the disease and most frequently affect the extraocular, bulbar, and limb muscles.[5,21,22] Most patients have reached maximum disease severity within 2 years of onset. A transient response to edrophonium, significant decremental response to repetitive nerve stimulation, excessive "jitter" with single-fiber EMG, and response to therapy provide a total clinical picture that is the basis of diagnosis. Spontaneous remissions may accumulate over many years.

The most important differential diagnosis in childhood is CMG. Other potential diagnoses include cranial nerve palsies, Guillain-Barré syndrome, myopathies, botulism, Lambert-Eaton syndrome, venoms, toxins, drug effects, and hysteria. An accurate diagnosis is essential for management, both to offer potentially effective immunotherapies to children with JMG and to avoid ineffective therapy in children with other disorders.

If AChR antibody (Ab) levels are elevated, the diagnosis of autoimmune MG is certain. AChR Ab levels, however, are not elevated in all patients (seronegative). Indeed, the highest proportion of seronegative patients is among the youngest patients: 36–50% of prepubertal patients are seronegative, compared to 25–32% of peripubertal patients and 0–9% of postpubertal adolescent patients.[4,8,23] It is in these youngest patients that discrimination between seronegative JMG and CMG is most important and most problematic. TABLE 1 outlines some features that facilitate differentiation between JMG and CMG. Even so, inability to report symptoms, frequent daytime sleeps, and imprecise examination make distinction between CMG and JMG very difficult in young children. Repeated AChR Ab measurements over years may identify a conversion from seronegative to seropositive, supporting a diagnosis of JMG. Where clinically indicated (e.g., severe weakness), a therapeutic response to plasma exchange (PEX), or more feasibly intravenous immunoglobulin (IVIG), may provide benefit to patients with JMG, may support a diagnosis of JMG, and may exclude a diagnosis of CMG.

OVERVIEW OF CURRENT THERAPEUTIC STRATEGIES

Therapeutic strategies for autoimmune MG in adults are the foundation of treatment of children and adolescents with autoimmune MG. These strategies have been excellently reviewed recently[23] and during this conference. Four categories of treatment are currently employed: (1) anticholinesterase medications, which enhance transmission at the NMJ; (2) short-term immunomodulation (plasma exchange and intravenous immunoglobulin infusion); (3) thymectomy; and (4) long-term immunosuppression. The introduction of these therapies and improved respiratory support have dramatically improved the prognosis for children and adolescents with autoimmune MG. Prior to the 1940s and 1950s, approximately one-third of patients died, one-third deteriorated or remained unchanged, and one-third improved.[2,24,25] In contrast, the Mayo Clinic[22] reported no deaths in pediatric patients after 1972; and none of our 115 pediatric patients, followed for 1–44 years after disease onset, died due to

TABLE 1. Clinical Features[a]

Clinical Feature	Autoimmune MG	Congenital MG
Age at onset	after 12 months	usually from birth
Weakness	fluctuating	relatively stable
Spontaneous remission	sometimes	no
AChR Ab level	normal or elevated	normal
Pyridostigmine	often effective	variable effect
Immunotherapy	often effective	not effective
Thymectomy	often effective	not effective
Family history	no	often positive
Distinctive features	no	some syndromes

[a]Clinical features that help distinguish between CMG and JMG. "Distinctive features" refers to both clinical and electrographic features (see references 1 and 4).

the disease.[8] The decision to offer any treatment implies that the expected benefits outweigh the expected risks and that the family understands the concepts involved.

CHOLINESTERASE INHIBITORS

Pyridostigmine, a long-acting cholinesterase inhibitor, is often the first therapy. The initial dose is on the order of 1 mg/kg/dose every 4–6 hours. Comparison of peak strength and activity at one hour after a dose and immediately before the next dose facilitates individualized tailoring of the dosage schedule. This drug, however, does not influence the underlying autoimmune process and it infrequently controls all symptoms. Response may diminish with time, although a "drug holiday" may reestablish efficacy. The main side effects are nausea, vomiting, abdominal pain, diarrhea, sweating, and (potentially) cholinergic crisis (i.e., exacerbated weakness due to excess cholinesterase inhibition).

SHORT-TERM IMMUNOMODULATION

Plasma Exchange (PEX)

PEX removes antibodies and other proteins from the circulation. It produces improvement in symptoms and signs within days. The beneficial effect lasts about 4 to 10 weeks. Response roughly parallels the reduction in AChR Ab titer in seropositive patients,[2] and is seen equally in seronegative patients.[2–4] Although PEX is usually a short-term therapy, repeated PEX may be helpful in some patients who fail to respond to other therapies. Selective PEX using a specially designed immunoadsorbent may bind and remove AChR Abs without removing so many other normal plasma constituents.[26] This technique may lend itself to longer-term therapy, but is not available in most centers.

PEX is effective in pediatric patients.[4,6,7,27] It has a specific role in the preoperative period, when preparatory PEX reduces perioperative morbidity; in acute care of very weak patients; and at initiation of immunosuppressive therapy, to provide rapid control until the drugs take effect. PEX usually requires insertion of a double-lumen central venous catheter under general anesthesia in children younger than 7 years. Thereafter, PEX is often possible via peripheral intravenous cannulae. Our regime includes five or six single-volume exchanges, over 8 to 10 days, with not more than 2 consecutive days of PEX. We replace volume with albumin and saline, and monitor fluid balance, calcium, magnesium, and electrolytes.

Intravenous Immunoglobulin (IVIG)

Following successful use of IVIG therapy for Kawasaki's disease,[28] IVIG has been usefully applied to the treatment of several autoimmune diseases, including MG.[29–31] No studies have specifically addressed pediatric patients, although children and adolescents have been part of other series and have shown good response. Approximately 70% of patients improve with IVIG, typically within 5 days of initiating treatment.[2,3,29–31] The standard dose is 2 g/kg, given as slow infusions of 400 mg/kg daily over 5 days. Based on data from Kawasaki's disease, suggesting that infusion of the dose over a shorter period is equally or more beneficial and cheaper,[32,33] we have given 1 g/kg daily on 2 consecutive days without significant complications. Indications for IVIG are similar to those for PEX, that is, prior to thymectomy to reduce perioperative morbidity, for severe weakness to produce rapid improvement until immunosuppressive therapy takes effect, and in selected patients for long-term treatment. Ease of administration makes this an attractive acute therapy for young patients. However, improvement tends to be less than with PEX, and patients have failed to respond to IVIG, but have responded to PEX.[34] Improvement lasts 3 to 6 weeks and up to 17 weeks in patients already on long-term immunosuppression.[30,31] The main side effects in children are headache and aseptic meningitis, especially in migraineurs; transient flu-like illnesses; and hyperactivity; in addition, note that congestive cardiac failure, deep venous thrombosis, and acute renal failure are reported in adults, who usually have other risk factors.[35] It is also expensive. Patients with IgA deficiency may develop antibodies to IgA in the infusion, with subsequent anaphylaxis; therefore, IgA levels should be checked prior to infusion. Hepatitis C has been reported following some IVIG preparations.[36]

THYMECTOMY

Interpretation of the effect of thymectomy in MG must be cautious, due to the absence of controlled series and the selection bias that determines whether a patient will have early, late, or no thymectomy. Included among patients who remit after early thymectomy are some who may have remitted spontaneously, whereas patients treated with delayed thymectomy are those who have failed to remit spontaneously. In addition, different management strategies, assessment criteria, and duration of follow-up hinder interpretation of reported data.

Several studies have addressed thymectomy for children and adolescents with generalized and/or bulbar weakness[5,7,8,21,22,27,37–42] and have reached a broad consensus that thymectomy is generally effective, producing complete remission in 11–75% and improvement in 57–95%. These pediatric series suggest that early thymectomy (within the first 12 months of onset of symptoms) is more effective than delayed thymectomy. Although controversial, adults and children with purely ocular weakness have undergone thymectomy, with comparable success to that in patients with more severe disease.[39,43,44] Controversy exists regarding the preferred surgical approach, but complete excision of the thymus is crucial. Other potential benefits of thymectomy include likely reduction of doses and of side effects of steroids and other immunosuppressants, and identification and treatment of the very rare pediatric patients with thymoma.

Thymectomy, performed in experienced centers, is relatively safe. Preoperative preparation with cholinesterase inhibitors, PEX, IVIG, or corticosteroids optimizes the patients' strength and respiratory function and limits complications. Neonatal thymectomy in mice enhances autoimmune disease propensity and results in relative immune incompetence.[14] This has prompted some authors to advise against thymectomy in prepubertal patients.[2,6,8] T cell depletion, which follows neonatal thymectomy, however, varies among species—humans have a relatively mature thymus before birth, whereas mice have a very immature thymus at birth.[14,45] Pediatric series have not identified deleterious clinical consequences of thymectomy for MG even in the youngest patients, although follow-up has often been limited.[8,21,22,25,38–41] In addition, thymectomy (which may be incomplete) during open-heart surgery in infants before 3 months of age has not produced clinical consequences, despite lower numbers of total, helper, and suppressor T cells.[46] Some studies have reported a decreased incidence of cancer after thymectomy for MG.[47,48] Rodriguez et al.[22] reported that long-term cancer risk in JMG was identical whether or not thymectomy was performed.

Thymectomy in Prepubertal Patients

The incidence of autoimmune MG in prepubertal patients is low, diagnosis and differentiation from CMG can be difficult, and some clinicians are reluctant to offer thymectomy to young patients. Therefore, data regarding the natural history and response to various therapies in this group are limited.

We observed that remission, especially spontaneous remission, was relatively common among white patients with prepubertal onset (i.e., before 8.9 years in girls and before 9.3 years in boys[49]). Conversely, spontaneous remission among black patients with prepubertal disease onset and among black or white patients with peripubertal (i.e., 8.9–15.3 years in girls and 9.3–16.5 years in boys[49]) or postpubertal disease onset was infrequent.[8] In addition, the proportion of white patients with prepubertal disease onset, who had persistence of active disease for more than 10 years, was significantly less than the proportion with persistent disease for more than 10 years among black patients with prepubertal, peripubertal, and postpubertal onset and white patients with peripubertal and postpubertal onset.[8] Review of the literature detailing patients with JMG beginning prepubertally[5–7,21,24,27,37–42] similarly shows more frequent remissions among prepubertal patients than among older children, especially spontaneous remissions (i.e., without thymectomy); see TABLES 2 and 3. The Mayo Clinic[22] reported that 45% of the children with onset before 11 years (i.e., mostly prepubertal) achieved spontaneous remission 15 years later, whereas only 22% of the adolescents aged 12–16 years at disease onset achieved spontaneous remission 15 years later. Among children with onset before 11 years, thymectomy did not influence the remission rate.[22] Taken together, these data suggest that, among patients with prepubertal onset, remission is relatively common and that thymectomy may make little difference to the rate of remission.

Early Thymectomy in Peripubertal Patients

We have observed an excellent response to thymectomy among peripubertal white patients operated upon within 1 year of disease onset.[8] Also, the only remissions among black patients occurred in peripubertal patients treated with thymectomy

TABLE 2. Remissions and Persistent Active Disease[a]

| Pubertal Stage at Disease Onset | White Patients | | Black Patients | | Literature |
	Remissions	Persistent Disease > 10 Years	Remissions	Persistent Disease > 10 Years	Remissions
Prepubertal	4/9 (44%)	1/9 (11%)	0/11 (0%)	5/11 (45%)	16/39 (41%)
Peripubertal	6/41 (15%)	22/41 (54%)	2/17 (12%)	6/17 (35%)	37/112 (33%)
Postpubertal	1/21 (5%)	9/21 (43%)	0/14 (0%)	4/14 (29%)	19/62 (31%)

[a]The proportion of patients in remission (i.e., normal examination without treatment for at least 3 months), and the proportion of patients with ongoing active disease for more than 10 years after disease onset, stratified according to age and pubertal status at disease onset and race, from a previously reported group of 115 patients with onset of autoimmune MG before age 20.[8] Note significantly more remissions among white patients with prepubertal onset than among older white patients or among black patients. Also note that a significantly smaller proportion of white patients with prepubertal disease onset have active disease persisting for more than 10 years than among black patients or older white patients. Remissions among English-language literature series detailing age at disease onset are included for comparison.[5–7,21,24,27,37–42] Many of these series, however, only described patients treated by thymectomy and are potentially biased towards more remissions, especially among older patients who are more commonly treated by thymectomy.

TABLE 3. Outcome: Pubertal Stage and Thymectomy[a]

| Response to Treatment | Prepubertal | | | Peripubertal | | | Postpubertal | | |
	T < 1	T > 1	No T	T < 1	T > 1	No T	T < 1	T > 1	No T
Remission	3	6	7	23	10	2	6	7	1
	27%	30%	35%	61%	14%	6%	32%	18%	8%
Improved	7	8	7	11	37	18	10	23	8
	64%	40%	35%	29%	54%	50%	53%	58%	62%
No change or worse	1	6	6	4	22	16	3	10	4
	9%	30%	30%	11%	32%	44%	16%	25%	31%

[a]Outcome data for patients with JMG described in pediatric series that detailed age at disease onset, whether or not thymectomy was performed, and time between disease onset and thymectomy.[5–8,21,27,37,39,41,42] "Remission" includes patients with normal examination without medications. "Improved" includes patients with normal examination while taking medications or those with improved clinical status. "No change or worse" includes patients with little change or worsening of weakness or death. As described in the text, caution must be applied to interpretation of these data. Note the lack of influence of thymectomy upon the likelihood of remission in patients with prepubertal disease onset, the high proportion of remissions among peripubertal patients treated with thymectomy within 1 year of disease onset, as well as the trend to the same in older patients. Since most pediatric series limit their populations to less than 16 or 18 years of age at disease onset, the postpubertal group has a disproportionate contribution from our series.[8] Terms—T < 1: thymectomy within 12 months (1 year) of disease onset; T > 1: thymectomy more than 12 months (1 year) after disease onset; No T: thymectomy not performed.

within 1 year of disease onset.[8] As shown in TABLE 3, meta-analysis of the pediatric literature[5–8,21,27,37,39,41,42] suggests that peripubertal patients treated with early thymectomy have significantly more remissions than other patients treated with early thymectomy or patients treated by late thymectomy or without thymectomy. Olanow *et al.* also observed a better response among adolescents than adults treated with early thymectomy.[50] Hence, it seems appropriate to consider early thymectomy for all peripubertal patients with bulbar or generalized weakness.

CORTICOSTEROIDS

Long-Term Oral Prednisolone

Corticosteroids suppress multiple facets of the humoral, cell-mediated, and nonspecific arms of the immune system.[2,3] Although no controlled trials have been performed, retrospective review of predominantly adult patients with ocular, bulbar, or generalized weakness suggests that long-term oral corticosteroids are beneficial in about 80% of patients.[51,52] Pediatric series identified significant improvement in only 10–61% of patients treated with corticosteroids.[7,53] Corticosteroid treatment does not influence the likelihood of remission following thymectomy.[54]

Corticosteroids supplement treatment with cholinesterase inhibitors in patients whose symptoms are not adequately controlled. Some initiate treatment with a high dose (1–2 mg/kg/day of oral prednisolone, to a maximum of 60–80 mg/day). Following this schedule, a small proportion of patients (8%) will develop severe weakness in the first 3 weeks.[51] This approach requires hospitalization for initiation of therapy. Some minimize the initial exacerbation of weakness by starting with a small dose and titrating according to the patient's response. Improvement usually begins within 4 weeks and maximal effect by 3 to 9 months.[2,3,51] Preparatory PEX or IVIG will likely avoid or limit the initial weakness induced by high-dose corticosteroids and will allow for the slow onset of therapeutic benefit. Long-term treatment utilizes the lowest effective dose, given on alternate days (where possible) to minimize side effects.

The side effects of chronic corticosteroid therapy are many and potentially serious. Among a predominantly adult population, two-thirds experienced significant side effects.[51] For the growing child and adolescent, even more long-term risks are associated with corticosteroid therapy. Growth may be retarded in children with as little as 4 mg/m^2/day of oral prednisolone (an 8-year-old child has a surface area of about 1 m^2), which is reduced by an alternate-day schedule.[55] Steroid-induced growth retardation is related to duration of treatment and cumulative dose and is maximal in peripubertal boys.[56] In addition, childhood and adolescence are crucial periods for bone mineralization and development that determine the adult risk of osteoporosis. Corticosteroid therapy leads to loss of trabecular and cortical bone, which predisposes to later osteoporosis:[57] for example, a cumulative dose of 17.1 g ± 10.8 g of prednisolone significantly adversely affected bone density. This equates to a dose of 10 mg ± 6 mg on alternate days for 9.4 years, which is well possible in the treatment of JMG.

High-Dose Intravenous Methylprednisolone (Pulse MP)

Pulse MP is used in many autoimmune disorders to provide therapeutic benefit and to limit side effects of chronic immunosuppressive therapies. Reported use in children and adolescents with autoimmune MG is limited. Sustained improvements lasting months, following variable regimes of pulse MP, have been reported in some patients with ocular and more severe disease.[53,58–60]

Side effects are uncommon, but can be serious. Sudden death,[61] atrial fibrillation,[62] muscarinic effects of cholinesterase inhibitors, peptic bleeding, and transient psychosis[58] have been reported. One teenager with autoimmune generalized MG, who deteriorated after initiation of oral steroids, developed severe, acute, myopathic weakness after pulse MP.[63]

We have used pulse methylprednisolone cautiously in a dose of 1 g/(1.73 m^2)/day (given sixth-hourly, by slow intravenous infusion) for 5 days, with beneficial effect and no significant side effects in children with ocular MG and other neuroimmunologic disorders. We monitor fluid balance, electrolytes, blood pressure, hematuria, and glycosuria. We also monitor the electrocardiogram during infusions and provide short-term cover with ranitidine.

OTHER IMMUNOSUPPRESSIVE THERAPIES

Azathioprine

Azathioprine is metabolized to the cytotoxic compound, 6-mercaptopurine, which inhibits DNA and RNA synthesis and interferes with T cell function.[2,3,64] It is easy to use and has been given to adults and children with MG and to children with other autoimmune disorders to limit disease severity, corticosteroid dose, and side effects. The usual dose is approximately 2 mg/kg/day, initiated with weekly increments of 0.5 mg/kg/day. Onset of the therapeutic response is slow, with maximal benefit often delayed for 3 to 12 months.[2,3,64] Improvement is seen in 30–91% of patients in predominantly adult series,[3] with comparable benefit in one pediatric series.[53] It is usually well tolerated. The main side effects include an idiosyncratic flu-like response in 10% and some patients rapidly develop dramatic elevations of liver enzymes, which may be treated by drug withdrawal and cautious retrial.[3] Leukopenia, pancytopenia, and immunosuppression can be problematic, but respond to dose reduction. Teratogenesis is a serious potential side effect with specific relevance to young women with MG. Late development of malignancy following prolonged usage is also of concern.[65]

Cyclosporin A

Cyclosporin A is a fungal metabolite that reversibly inhibits T helper function and T cell–dependent antibody responses, and allows activation of T suppressor functions.[66] In adult MG series, this drug has improved strength in 40%, lowered AChR

Ab levels, and facilitated reduction of corticosteroid doses.[2,3,66] Improvement was apparent within the first 2 months. A standard dose is 5 mg/kg/day given in two oral doses. The main side effects are nephrotoxicity, hypertension, and headache and it is expensive.[2,3,66]

Cyclophosphamide

Cyclophosphamide is an alkylating agent that inhibits B cell proliferation and immunoglobulin synthesis.[3] It has been used with good effect in small series of MG patients, including children.[53,67,68] Most conclude that cyclophosphamide produces more significant and more rapid improvement than azathioprine, but its side effects are more severe, with particular issues of immunosuppression, sterility, teratogenesis, and potential late induction of malignancy.[3,68]

AN ALGORITHM FOR TREATMENT

Treatment needs to be individualized for each patient and family. Increasingly, we aim for cure, complete resolution of signs and symptoms, or sufficient improvement to enable a full and active lifestyle. After making the diagnosis, treatment begins with education of the family. As suggested in FIGURE 1, initial medical treatment is with cholinesterase inhibitors, titrated to the most effective dose with the least side effects. Most patients, however, will continue to exhibit signs and symptoms. Further therapy then requires a balance of potential risks and benefits.

With purely ocular weakness, low-dose, alternate-day steroids, perhaps initiated with 2 to 4 weeks of prednisolone at 1–2 mg/kg/day, may resolve symptoms. Chronic side effects may emerge and steroid-sparing alternatives such as pulse methylprednisolone or azathioprine are the next choices. Thymectomy is usually not performed for purely ocular disease, but discussion with the patient and family regarding progress, side effects of drugs, and risks and benefits of thymectomy, especially in the child about to enter or in early puberty, may make thymectomy a consideration.

With bulbar or generalized weakness, thymectomy is appropriate for those not adequately controlled by cholinesterase inhibitors, especially more severely affected patients and peripubertal patients. PEX and IVIG are effective transient therapies in severe cases, and in patients with moderate or severe weakness, performed approximately 2 weeks prior to initiation of steroids or thymectomy. If thymectomy is likely, it seems appropriate, especially in peripubertal patients, to offer thymectomy in the first year after disease onset. Initiation of steroids before or after thymectomy needs to be individualized, with subsequent titration to the lowest, effective, alternate-day schedule. Failure of combined cholinesterase inhibitors, thymectomy, and chronic low-dose, alternate-day steroids, or emergence of chronic steroid side effects, prompts therapeutic trials with steroid-sparing alternatives. A suggested order for such therapies is as follows: azathioprine or pulse methylprednisolone (with or without IVIG) in either order; then cyclosporin A; then cyclophosphamide, modified by the patient's age, response to treatment and disruption of lifestyle, side effects, desire

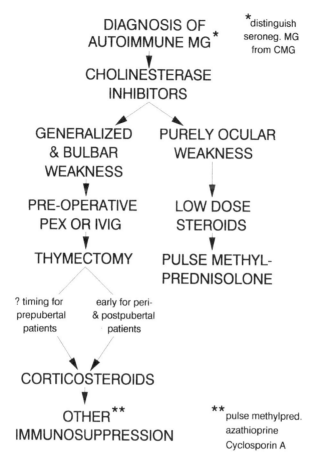

FIGURE 1. An algorithm for treatment of autoimmune MG in childhood and adolescence (see text).

or chance of pregnancy, and family preferences after education regarding risks and benefits.

What therapy should we offer prepubertal patients with generalized or bulbar weakness? At least among white patients, the limited available data suggest that there is a considerable chance of spontaneous remission, which is comparable to the remission rate after thymectomy. A specific effort to retrospectively and prospectively collect data on these patients may help plan their management. Perhaps, a randomized (necessarily multicenter) trial of thymectomy, considering race, puberty, and timing of thymectomy, is warranted. Currently, we offer early thymectomy in patients with moderate or severe disease, despite the above uncertainties, and find it useful in reducing disease severity.

There is a great need for effective, disease-specific, low-toxicity immunomodulation. Developing therapies, such as oral or mucosal tolerization, and further progress in our understanding of disease pathogenesis, and factors that initiate and maintain the disease process, will facilitate continued advances in the diagnosis and management of autoimmune MG.

REFERENCES

1. ENGEL, A. G. 1984. Myasthenia gravis and myasthenic syndromes. Ann. Neurol. **16:** 519–534.
2. DRACHMAN, D. B. 1994. Myasthenia gravis. N. Engl. J. Med. **330:** 1797–1810.
3. LEWIS, R. A. *et al.* 1995. Myasthenia gravis: immunological mechanisms and immunotherapy. Ann. Neurol. **37**(suppl. 1): S51–S62.
4. ANDREWS, P. I. *et al.* 1993. Acetylcholine receptor antibodies in juvenile myasthenia gravis. Neurology **43:** 977–982.
5. MILLICHAP, J. G. & P. R. DODGE. 1960. Diagnosis and treatment of myasthenia gravis in infancy, childhood, and adolescence: a study of 51 patients. Neurology **10:** 1007–1014.
6. SNEAD, O. C., III *et al.* 1980. Juvenile myasthenia gravis. Neurology **30:** 732–739.
7. BATOCCHI, A. P. *et al.* 1990. Early-onset myasthenia gravis: clinical characteristics and response to therapy. Eur. J. Pediatr. **150:** 66–68.
8. ANDREWS, P. J. *et al.* 1994. Race, sex, and puberty influence onset, severity, and outcome in juvenile myasthenia gravis. Neurology **44:** 1208–1214.
9. MATSUKI, K. *et al.* 1990. HLA antigens in Japanese patients with myasthenia gravis. J. Clin. Invest. **86:** 392–399.
10. PHILLIPS, L. H., II *et al.* 1992. The epidemiology of myasthenia gravis in central and western Virginia. Neurology **42:** 1888–1893.
11. CHIU, H-C. *et al.* 1987. Myasthenia gravis: population differences in disease expression and acetylcholine receptor antibody titers between Chinese and Caucasians. Neurology **37:** 1854–1857.
12. UONO, M. 1980. Clinical statistics of myasthenia gravis in Japan. Int. J. Neurol. **14:** 87–99.
13. DEPARTMENT OF HUMAN RESOURCES, DIVISION OF HEALTH SERVICES, OFFICE OF MANAGEMENT, NORTH CAROLINA VITAL STATISTICS. 1980. 1979, Vol. 1: births, deaths, population, marriages, divorces.
14. SPRENT, J. 1993. T lymphocytes and the thymus. *In* Fundamental Immunology. Third edition, pp. 75–109. Raven Press. New York.
15. LAWTON, A. R. & M. D. COOPER. 1989. Ontogeny of immunity. *In* Immunologic Disorders in Infants and Children. Third edition, pp. 1–14. Saunders. Philadelphia.
16. GROSSMAN, C. J. 1984. Regulation of the immune system by sex steroids. Endocr. Rev. **5:** 435–455.
17. FURUKAWA, F. *et al.* 1988. Estradiol enhances binding to cultured human keratinocytes of antibodies specific for SS-A/RO and SS-B/LA: another possible mechanism for estradiol influence of lupus erythematosus. J. Immunol. **141:** 1480–1488.
18. VON GAUDECKER, B. 1991. Functional history of the human thymus. Anat. Embryol. **183:** 1–15.
19. PAAVONEN, T. 1994. Hormonal regulation of immune responses. Ann. Med. **26:** 255–258.
20. ELSASSER-BEILE, U. *et al.* 1995. Comparison of cytokine production in blood cell cultures of healthy children and adults. Pediatr. Asthma Allergy Immunol. **6**(3): 170–174.
21. SEYBOLD, M. E. *et al.* 1971. Thymectomy in juvenile myasthenia gravis. Arch. Neurol. **25:** 385–392.

22. RODRIGUEZ, M. *et al.* 1983. Myasthenia gravis in children: long-term follow-up. Ann. Neurol. **13:** 504–510.
23. VINCENT, A. *et al.* 1993. Seronegative myasthenia gravis: evidence for plasma factor(s) interfering with acetylcholine receptor function. Ann. N.Y. Acad. Sci. **681:** 529–538.
24. KEYNES, G. 1954. Surgery of the thymus gland: second (and third) thoughts. Lancet **1:** 1197–1202.
25. SIMPSON, J. A. 1958. An evaluation of thymectomy in myasthenia gravis. Brain **81:** 112–114.
26. SHIBUYA, N. *et al.* 1994. Immunoadsorption therapy for myasthenia gravis. J. Neurol. Neurosurg. Psychiatry **57:** 578–581.
27. ADAMS, C. *et al.* 1990. Thymectomy in juvenile myasthenia gravis. J. Child Neurol. **5:** 215–218.
28. FURUSHO, K. *et al.* 1984. High-dose intravenous gamma globulin for Kawasaki disease. Lancet **2:** 1055–1058.
29. GAJDOS, P. 1994. Intravenous immune globulin in myasthenia gravis. Clin. Exp. Immunol. **97**(suppl.): 49–51.
30. EVOLI, A. *et al.* 1993. High-dose intravenous immunoglobulin in myasthenia gravis. Ital. J. Neurol. Sci. **14:** 233–237.
31. EDAN, G. & F. LANDGRAF. 1994. Experience with intravenous immunoglobulin in myasthenia gravis. J. Neurol. Neurosurg. Psychiatry **57**(suppl.): 55–56.
32. KLASSEN, T. P. *et al.* 1993. Economic evaluation of intravenous immune globulin therapy for Kawasaki syndrome. J. Pediatr. **122:** 538–542.
33. NEWBURGER, J. W. *et al.* 1986. The treatment of Kawasaki syndrome with intravenous gamma globulin. N. Engl. J. Med. **315:** 341–347.
34. STRICKER, R. B. *et al.* 1993. Myasthenia crisis: response to plasmapheresis following failure of intravenous gamma globulin. Arch. Neurol. **50:** 837–840.
35. BRANNAGAN, T. H., III *et al.* 1996. Complications of intravenous immune globulin treatment in neurologic disease. Neurology **47:** 674–677.
36. FASANO, M. B. 1995. Risks and benefits of intravenous immunoglobulin treatment in children. Curr. Opin. Pediatr. **7:** 688–694.
37. BUNDEY, S. 1972. A genetic study of infantile and juvenile myasthenia gravis. J. Neurol. Neurosurg. Psychiatry **35:** 41–51.
38. CAMPBELL, J. R. *et al.* 1983. Surgical treatment of myasthenia gravis in childhood. J. Pediatr. Surg. **18:** 857–861.
39. HANSSON, O. *et al.* 1972. Thymectomy in juvenile myasthenia gravis. Neuropaediatrie **3:** 429–463.
40. RYNIEWICZ, B. & B. BADURSKA. 1977. Follow-up study of myasthenic children after thymectomy. J. Neurol. **217:** 133–138.
41. SARNAT, H. B. *et al.* 1977. Effective treatment of infantile myasthenia gravis by combined prednisone and thymectomy. Neurology **27:** 550–553.
42. YOUSSEF, S. 1983. Thymectomy for myasthenia gravis in children. J. Pediatr. Surg. **18:** 537–541.
43. MASAOKA, A. *et al.* 1996. Extended thymectomy for myasthenia gravis patients: a 20-year review. Ann. Thorac. Surg. **62:** 853–859.
44. NAKAMURA, H. *et al.* 1996. Delayed remission after thymectomy for myasthenia gravis of the purely ocular type. J. Thorac. Cardiovasc. Surg. **112:** 371–375.
45. MILLER, J. & D. OSOBA. 1967. Current concepts of the immunological function of the thymus. Physiol. Rev. **47:** 437–520.
46. BREARLEY, S. *et al.* 1987. Immunodeficiency following neonatal thymectomy in man. Clin. Exp. Immunol. **70:** 322–327.

47. PAPATESTAS, A. E. *et al.* 1972. Ketosteroid excretion, myasthenia gravis, and breast cancer. Lancet **1:** 691–692.
48. VESSEY, M. P. & R. DOLL. 1972. Thymectomy and cancer—a follow-up study. Br. J. Cancer **26:** 53–58.
49. TANNER, J. M. & P. S. W. DAVIES. 1985. Clinical longitudinal standards for height and height velocity for North American children. J. Pediatr. **107:** 317–329.
50. OLANOW, C. W. *et al.* 1987. Thymectomy as primary therapy in myasthenia gravis. Ann. N.Y. Acad. Sci. **505:** 595–606.
51. PASCUZZI, R. M. *et al.* 1984. Long-term corticosteroid treatment of myasthenia gravis: report of 116 patients. Ann. Neurol. **15:** 291–298.
52. KUPERSMITH, M. J. *et al.* 1996. Beneficial effects of corticosteroids on ocular myasthenia gravis. Arch. Neurol. **53:** 802–804.
53. BADURSKA, B. *et al.* 1992. Immunosuppressive treatment for juvenile myasthenia gravis. Eur. J. Pediatr. **151:** 215–217.
54. LINDBERG, C. *et al.* 1992. Remission rate after thymectomy in myasthenia gravis when the bias of immunosuppressive therapy is eliminated. Acta Neurol. Scand. **86:** 323–328.
55. KERRIBIJN, K. F. & J. P. M. DE KROON. 1968. Effect on height of corticosteroid therapy in asthmatic children. Arch. Dis. Child. **43:** 556–561.
56. REES, L. *et al.* 1988. Growth and endocrine function in steroid sensitive nephrotic syndrome. Arch. Dis. Child. **63:** 484–490.
57. LETTGEN, B. *et al.* 1994. Influence of steroid medication on bone mineral density in children with nephrotic syndrome. Pediatr. Nephrol. **8:** 667–670.
58. ARSURA, E. *et al.* 1985. High-dose intravenous methylprednisolone in myasthenia gravis. Arch. Neurol. **42:** 1149–1153.
59. SAKANO, T. *et al.* 1989. Treatment for refractory myasthenia gravis. Arch. Dis. Child. **64:** 1191–1193.
60. TANAKA, J. *et al.* 1994. Intermittent methylprednisolone pulse therapy for myasthenia gravis in childhood. Brain Dev. **26:** 14–19.
61. BOCANEGRA, T. S. *et al.* 1981. Sudden death after methylprednisolone pulse therapy. Ann. Intern. Med. **95:** 122.
62. MCLUCKIE, A. E. & R. W. SAVAGE. 1993. Atrial fibrillation following pulse methylprednisolone therapy in an adult. Chest **104:** 622–623.
63. PANEGYRES, P. K. *et al.* 1993. Acute myopathy associated with large parenteral dose of corticosteroid in myasthenia gravis. J. Neurol. Neurosurg. Psychiatry **56:** 702–704.
64. COSI, V. *et al.* 1992. Azathioprine as a single immunosuppressive drug in the treatment of myasthenia gravis. Acta Neurol. **15:** 123–131.
65. CONFAVREUX, C. *et al.* 1996. Risk of cancer from azathioprine therapy in multiple sclerosis: a case-control study. Neurology **46:** 1607–1612.
66. TINDALL, R. S. A. *et al.* 1993. A clinical therapeutic trial of cyclosporine in myasthenia gravis. Ann. N.Y. Acad. Sci. **681:** 539–551.
67. PEREZ, M. C. *et al.* 1981. Stable remissions in myasthenia gravis. Neurology **31:** 32–37.
68. NAIKAN, E. *et al.* 1986. Immunosuppressive drug therapy in myasthenia gravis. Arch. Neurol. **43:** 155–156.

Plasma Treatment in Diseases
of the Neuromuscular Junction

F. CORNELIO, C. ANTOZZI, P. CONFALONIERI, F. BAGGI,
AND R. MANTEGAZZA

Department of Neuromuscular Disorders
Istituto Nazionale Neurologico "C. Besta"
20133 Milan, Italy

Acquired autoimmune diseases of the neuromuscular junction share a common pathogenesis mediated by autoantibodies to different components of the motor end plate. The clinical features of myasthenia gravis (MG) and Lambert-Eaton myasthenic syndrome (LEMS) are due to antibodies to postsynaptic acetylcholine receptors (AChR) and presynaptic voltage-gated calcium channels, respectively.[1,2] Recently, pathogenic autoantibodies to potassium channels have been demonstrated in acquired neuromyotonia.[3]

Treatment of autoimmune diseases of the neuromuscular junction relies upon immunosuppression.[4] The neurological impairment observed in these disorders is frequently severe, requiring long-term administration of corticosteroids and immunosuppressive drugs. Apart from the pharmacological inhibition of the autoimmune process, a significant improvement can be obtained by removing circulating pathogenic factors via therapeutic plasma exchange (PE). PE is easily applicable, the main indication being the necessity for a rapid and massive reduction of specific autoantibodies, and its efficacy has been clearly demonstrated.[5] The clinical response of autoimmune disorders of the neuromuscular junction to pharmacological therapy is not easily predictable and the percentage of treatment failures is not negligible.[4,6] Moreover, the incidence of side effects (particularly from long-term corticosteroid treatment) cannot be overlooked. The periodic removal of pathogenic autoantibodies might be of considerable help in patients with a poor response to pharmacological treatment, frequent clinical relapses, or major contraindications to high-dose immunosuppression. However, the complete lack of PE selectivity limits the amount of plasma that can be exchanged due to inevitable protein loss. Because of this drawback, PE cannot be easily considered for patients requiring repeated treatments over extended periods. In such patients, a more-selective approach able to remove pathogenic autoantibodies, but obviating the need for replacement fluids, would be preferable.

The selective removal of pathogenic autoantibodies is still not available for disorders of the neuromuscular junction. However, semiselective techniques have been proposed in recent years with encouraging results.[7–10] Among these, staphylococcal protein A, a membrane protein of the bacterial cell wall, has unique properties:[10] (a) it has a high affinity for human immunoglobulins (particularly IgG, subclass 1, 2, and 4) that are efficiently removed from plasma; (b) it is stable to changes in temperature and to exposure to low pH; (c) it can be covalently linked to a support matrix without loss of binding properties or leakage; and (d) it can be easily regenerated.

Because of these features, protein A is suitable as a chromatographic reagent for extensive reuse, without loss in its binding capacity.

We report our experience with prolonged treatment with protein A immunoadsorption in six patients with treatment-resistant MG and in one patient with LEMS.

PATIENTS AND METHODS

The main clinical features of MG patients are summarized in TABLE 1. All patients were affected with severe forms of the disease unresponsive to high-dose prednisone (associated with other immunosuppressive drugs in patients 1, 2, 3, and 6). Patients 1 and 2 did not improve with plasma exchange, while patients 3 to 6 needed repeated sessions to avoid bulbar muscle impairment. Anti-AChR Ab were detectable in all patients but one (patient 4).

The LEMS patient was a 50-year-old woman, operated on for ovarian adenocarcinoma at the age of 43. One year after surgery, the patient complained of generalized weakness of proximal muscles (particularly those of the lower limbs), abnormal fatigability on exertion, dry mouth, decreased lacrimation, nasal voice, and difficulty in chewing and swallowing. Deep tendon reflexes were absent. Neurophysiological studies showed a CMAP markedly reduced in amplitude (0.6 mV); a decremental response was found at low rates of stimulation together with an abnormal increment at high rates. The patient was treated elsewhere with a course of several plasma exchanges, and courses of intravenous immunoglobulins (IVIG), without significant improvement. Anti-voltage-gated calcium channel antibodies were undetectable. The disease showed a progressive course, with the patient being wheel-chair-bound when admitted at our institution two years from the onset. The patient was first treated with

TABLE 1. Clinical Features of MG Patients[a]

| | Patient No. | | | | | |
	1	2	3	4	5	6
Sex	F	F	F	F	F	M
Age (years)	20	23	20	54	36	35
Disease duration (years)	3	2	3	17	18	6
Thymectomy	yes	yes	yes	yes	yes	yes
Ongoing treatment	P + A	P + A	P + CyA	P	P	P + CF
Response to PE	no	no	yes	yes	yes	yes
Response to IVIG	nd	no	no	nd	nd	nd
Frequent relapses	no	no	yes	yes	yes	yes
Anti-AChR Ab (pmol/mL)	15.5	13.7	89.7	negl	144	5.4
Pretreatment Osserman classification	2B	2A	2B	2B	2B	2B
Number of PAI sessions performed	12	8	50	19	8	4

[a]PE: plasma exchange; IVIG: intravenous immunoglobulins; PAI: protein A immunoadsorption; CyA: cyclosporin A; CF: cyclophosphamide; P: prednisone; A: azathioprine; nd: not done; negl: negligible.

prednisone and azathioprine with progressive improvement, being again able to walk autonomously. Prednisone was slowly tapered up to 10 mg every other day, and she experienced fatigability; because of osteoporosis and increased intraocular pressure, prednisone was not increased and the patient was submitted to immunoadsorption.

Indications to Protein A Immunoadsorption

The main inclusion criteria for immunoadsorption with protein A in MG patients were the severity of the disease and prolonged unresponsiveness to long-term immunosuppression. Moreover, the following additional criteria were taken into consideration: (1) frequent clinical relapses; (2) unresponsiveness to plasma exchange; (3) need for frequent plasma exchanges to avoid bulbar impairment; and (4) contraindications to high-dose corticosteroids due to side effects. The LEMS patient was considered for immunoadsorption due to the severity of the disease and steroid side effects.

Clinical Evaluation

The clinical evaluation was performed with our MG score system, as reported.[11] The patient with LEMS was also evaluated with the MRC manual muscle test.

Immunoadsorption Procedure

The patient's plasma was obtained by continuous flow centrifugation and then passed on-line to the immunoadsorption monitor at a flow rate of 20–35 mL/min. ACD-A was used as anticoagulant. The immunoadsorption monitor operated two columns containing protein A covalently linked to agarose. Plasma was passed through one column, while the second was washed with pH 7.0 buffer solution followed by elution of immunoglobulins with sodium citrate, pH 2.2. Each immunoadsorption cycle lasted ten minutes. After ten minutes, the columns were switched automatically. The alternate regeneration of each column allows the immunoadsorption of unlimited amounts of plasma. At the end of the procedure, both columns were eluted, extensively washed, and stored with 0.1% Merthiolate solution at 3 °C until the next procedure.

Treatment Protocol

The first immunoadsorption course consisted of three sessions on alternate days; the following courses (one or two sessions according to pretreatment IgG levels) were performed every four to six weeks (or earlier in case of severe clinical relapse). About 1.5–2 plasma volumes calculated on body weight and patient's hematocrit were processed during each procedure.

Biochemical and Immunological Monitoring

The following hematological and immunological parameters were monitored before and after each immunoadsorption procedure: blood cell count; serum electrolytes; fibrinogen; blood coagulation; serum IgG, IgM, and IgA; and antiacetylcholine receptor antibodies.

RESULTS

Clinical Efficacy

All MG patients improved significantly after immunoadsorption. The improvement in bulbar muscle impairment was always time-related to immunoadsorption, being evident within 24 hours from the procedure. An example of the efficacy of protein A immunoadsorption in patient 2 is shown in FIGURE 1A: the patient was affected with generalized MG with severe fatigability that did not respond to plasmapheresis and high-dose IVIG. Immunoadsorption improved significantly the patient's conditions up to disappearance of fatigability after repeated immunoadsorption cycles performed over four months. Immunoadsorption was particularly helpful in patient 3, who showed frequent clinical relapses with severe bulbar impairment, in spite of immunosuppression with full doses of prednisone and cyclosporin A. Because of her responsiveness to plasma exchange, the patient was shifted to protein A immunoadsorption that was repeated at every clinical relapse. The patient was treated repeatedly for two years before immunoadsorption could be stopped. The response to immunoadsorption in patient 3 is shown in FIGURE 1B. The procedure was comparably effective in patient 4, in whom anti-AChR antibodies were not found in several assays.

The LEMS patient was submitted to eight immunoadsorption cycles over one year, to avoid an increase of immunosuppressive drugs, because of corticosteroid side effects; the patient started to worsen when prednisone was tapered to 10 mg every other day. Therefore, the patient started immunoadsorption, showing a progressive clinical improvement that did not require an increase of prednisone dosage. A significant improvement of her proximal muscle strength, as well as in walking, was observed. The CMAP increased from 1.28 mV before immunoadsorption to 5.2 mV after one year of follow-up.

Immunoadsorption procedures were always well tolerated and no major side effects occurred; mild paresthesia due to ACD was easily controlled with calcium gluconate infusion.

Biochemical and Immunological Monitoring

The percentage reductions of the following immunological parameters were observed: anti-AChR Ab 82 ± 18%, IgG 71 ± 10%, IgM 46 ± 12%, and IgA 22 ± 12%. As expected, a progressive increase of serum immunoglobulins and anti-AChR Ab was observed during follow-up, with values reaching pretreatment levels three to

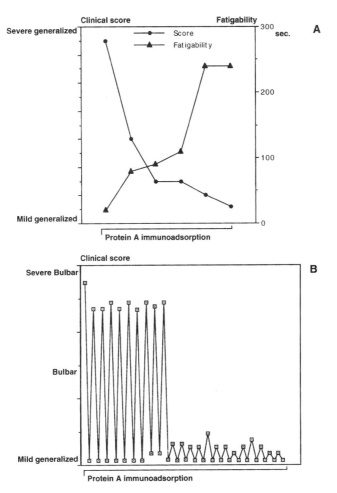

FIGURE 1. Clinical efficacy of protein A immunoadsorption in patient 2 (panel A) and patient 3 (panel B).

four weeks after immunoadsorption, a time course consistent with immunoglobulin turnover time. Albumin and fibrinogen reductions were $19 \pm 6\%$ and $20 \pm 8\%$, respectively. No significant modifications in blood coagulation parameters were noticed.

DISCUSSION

The observation of immunoglobulins as pathogenetic effectors in disorders of neuromuscular transmission is the rationale for the application of apheretic techniques for their treatment. Pharmacological protocols have been established for myasthenia gravis and Lambert-Eaton myasthenic syndrome and, recently, immuno-suppression has been proposed for acquired neuromyotonia.[1–3,12,13] The degree of neurological impairment in these disorders is usually severe and pharmacological therapy may require a long time before exerting a positive effect. Moreover, some patients respond poorly to long-term high-dose immunosuppression. In this context, the removal of pathogenic factors from plasma may be considerably helpful in modifying the natural history of the disease.

Plasmapheresis has been widely accepted as an effective and easily applicable technique and is able to remove a significant amount of plasma, and hence pathogenic immunoglobulins, in a short period of time. In MG, the response to plasma exchange can be dramatic, the main indication being severe relapses with bulbar muscle involvement. LEMS may improve with plasmapheresis, but several repeated procedures are usually necessary to obtain a significant improvement.[14,15] The efficacy of plasma exchange has been recently demonstrated in some patients with neuromyotonia.[13] All the diseases mentioned above are chronic and require prolonged immunosuppression. The percentage of treatment-resistant myasthenic patients is small, but not negligible; moreover, it is a source of neurological handicap, usually associated with severe side effects from long-standing steroid treatment.

Therapeutic plasma exchange, with the major drawback of lacking selectivity, can be problematic for patients requiring repeated treatments over extended periods. Semiselective techniques would be preferable in these situations. We investigated the use of protein A immunoadsorption, a technique able to remove IgG with high efficiency from plasma, with nonsignificant modifications of other plasma proteins. Severely compromised patients, nonresponsive to treatment and/or requiring repeated exchanges, were selected.

From a clinical standpoint, we confirm our preliminary observation of the efficacy of protein A immunoadsorption in MG.[16] We further confirm the efficacy of this approach for long-term management of treatment-resistant MG patients. Improvement was always significant and time-related with each procedure. Protein A was particularly helpful in patient 2, who recovered completely from severe fatigability, and in patients 3 and 4, who showed periodic severe relapses with bulbar involvement. It is worth noting that protein A was effective in patient 4, in whom anti-AChR antibodies were undetectable in several assays (tested also in the eluate from the columns). It is also interesting to observe that patients 1 and 2 did not respond to plasmapheresis and patients 2 and 3 did not improve with intravenous immunoglobulins. The high efficiency in IgG depletion achievable with protein A might account for this finding. The patient with LEMS, in whom antibodies to calcium channels were undetectable, benefited from immunoadsorption performed repeatedly over one year. The periodic removal of IgG was able to improve and then stabilize the clinical conditions of this patient without the need to increase immunosuppression.

From a technical standpoint, the high affinity of protein A for IgG and specific autoantibodies together with the continuous regeneration of the columns during the procedure allow the treatment of unlimited amounts of plasma without the need for replacement fluids. Because of this feature, protein A offers the opportunity to reduce IgG by more than 90% of pretreatment values in one session. The same degree of IgG removal cannot be achieved with plasma exchange with albumin alone as the replacement fluid. Immunoadsorption with tryptophan polyvinyl alcohol gel (TRY-PVA), a resin able to absorb IgG and anti-AChR antibodies, has been employed in MG patients.[7–9] Reported protocols were designed for the short-term management of MG, but data on the application of this technique for chronic apheresis are not available. Clinical improvement was significant in the majority of treated patients. However, TRY-PVA is less selective than protein A in its interaction with different plasma components; a significant reduction of fibrinogen and an activation of complement were also reported with TRY-PVA.

Modulation of specific autoantibodies has been proposed among several mechanisms to account for the efficacy of high-dose intravenous immunoglobulins in autoimmune diseases.[5] Intravenous immunoglobulins, in cases of proven efficacy, must be administered repeatedly to maintain clinical improvement. In terms of cost-effectiveness, we think that protein A immunoadsorption could be a promising alternative to immunoglobulins in the long-term management of disorders of the neuromuscular junction and deserves further investigation. Moreover, protein A immunoadsorption eliminates the risk of transmissible viral diseases.

In conclusion, we propose protein A immunoadsorption as a safe, efficient, and effective apheretic approach to long-term management of treatment-resistant patients with disorders of the neuromuscular junction. The results obtained suggest the use of protein A in other immune-mediated disorders. The selectivity of protein A could be a promising research tool in disorders of suspected, but still not confirmed, immune etiology.

REFERENCES

1. ENGEL, A. G. 1994. Acquired autoimmune myasthenia gravis. *In* Myology. Vol. 2, pp. 1769–1797. McGraw-Hill. New York.

2. ENGEL, A. G. 1994. Myasthenic syndromes. *In* Myology. Vol. 2, pp. 1798–1835. McGraw-Hill. New York.

3. SHILLITO, P., P. C. MOLENAAR, A. VINCENT, K. LEYS, W. ZHENG, R. J. VAN DEN BERG, J. J. PLOMP, G. T. H. VAN KEMPEN, G. CHAUPLANNAZ, A. R. WINTZEN, J. G. VAN DIJK & J. NEWSOM-DAVIS. 1995. Acquired neuromyotonia: evidence for autoantibodies directed against K+ channels of peripheral nerves. Ann. Neurol. **38**: 714–722.

4. DRACHMAN, D. B. 1996. Immunotherapy in neuromuscular disorders: current and future strategies. Muscle Nerve **19**: 1239–1251.

5. THORNTON, C. A. & R. GRIGGS. 1994. Plasma exchange and intravenous immunoglobulin treatment in neuromuscular disease. Ann. Neurol. **35**: 260–268.

6. CORNELIO, F., C. ANTOZZI, R. MANTEGAZZA, P. CONFALONIERI, E. BERTA, D. PELUCHETTI, A. SGHIRLANZONI & F. FIACCHINO. 1993. Immunosuppressive treatments: their efficacy on myasthenia gravis patients' outcome and on the natural course of the disease. Ann. N.Y. Acad. Sci. **681**: 594–602.

7. HEININGER, K., K. V. TOYKA, A. GACZOWSKI, H-P. HARTUNG, H. BORBERG & B. GRABENSEE. 1986. Selective removal of pathogenic factors in neurologic diseases. Plasma Ther. Transfus. Technol. **7**: 351–357.

8. SHIBUYA, N., T. SATO, M. OSAME, M. TAKEGAMI, S. DOI & S. KAWANAMI. 1994. Immunoadsorption therapy for myasthenia gravis. J. Neurol. Neurosurg. Psychiatry **57**: 578–581.

9. GROB, D., D. SIMPSON, H. MITSUMOTO, B. HOCH, F. MOKHTARIAN, A. BENDER, M. GREEN-

BERG, A. KOO & S. NAKAYAMA. 1995. Treatment of myasthenia gravis by immunoadsorption of plasma. Neurology **45:** 338–344.

10. GIORSTRUP, P. & R. WATT. 1990. Therapeutic protein A immunoadsorption: a review. Transfus. Sci. **11:** 281–302.

11. MANTEGAZZA, R., C. ANTOZZI, D. PELUCHETTI, A. SGHIRLANZONI & F. CORNELIO. 1988. Azathioprine as a single drug or in combination with steroids in the treatment of myasthenia gravis. J. Neurol. **235:** 449–453.

12. SINHA, S., J. NEWSOM-DAVIS, K. MILLS, N. BYRNE, B. LANG & A. VINCENT. 1991. Autoimmune aetiology for acquired neuromyotonia (Isaacs' syndrome). Lancet **338:** 75–77.

13. NEWSOM-DAVIS, J. & K. R. MILLS. 1993. Immunological associations of acquired neuromyotonia (Isaacs' syndrome). Brain **116:** 453–469.

14. DAU, P. C. & E. H. DENYS. 1982. Plasmapheresis and immunosuppressive drug therapy in the Eaton-Lambert syndrome. Ann. Neurol. **11:** 570–575.

15. NEWSOM-DAVIS, J. & N. M. F. MURRAY. 1984. Plasma exchange and immunosuppressive drug treatment in the Lambert-Eaton myasthenic syndrome. Neurology **34:** 480–485.

16. ANTOZZI, C., E. BERTA, P. CONFALONIERI, M. ZUFFI, F. CORNELIO, R. MANTEGAZZA & F. CORNELIO. 1994. Protein-A immunoadsorption in immunosuppression resistant myasthenia gravis. Lancet **383:** 124.

3,4-Diaminopyridine (DAP) in the Treatment of Lambert-Eaton Myasthenic Syndrome (LEMS)[a]

DONALD B. SANDERS

Department of Medicine
Division of Neurology
Duke University Medical Center
Durham, North Carolina 27710

Aminopyridines facilitate synaptic transmission by prolonging the open time of voltage-gated K^+ channels, which prolongs the duration of nerve action potentials and increases the release of transmitter at central and peripheral synapses. Unlike other aminopyridines, 3,4-diaminopyridine (DAP) has limited penetration into the brain and thus produces few CNS side effects at doses sufficient to improve neuromuscular transmission in most patients with LEMS.

DAP has been used to treat patients with LEMS for over 20 years in Europe, but has never been approved for clinical use in this country. In our experience, more than 80% of LEMS patients have significant clinical benefit from DAP; in over half of these, the improvement is marked. The optimal dose varies considerably among patients, from 5 mg tid to more than 25 mg qid, and the optimal dose and dosing schedule must be determined for each patient. In most patients, pyridostigmine enhances and prolongs the duration of action of DAP and permits use of lower doses. The effect of DAP begins about 20 minutes after an oral dose, the effect of each dose lasts about 4 hours, and the maximum effect of a given dosage may not be seen for 2 to 3 days. Patients with or without underlying cancer benefit from DAP. Side effects are minimal and usually are limited to brief perioral and digital paresthesias after doses of 10 to 15 mg or more. DAP also enhances the gastrointestinal side effects of pyridostigmine. Seizures may occur when doses greater than 100 mg/day are given. Experience with this agent consistently indicates that DAP is a safe, effective, and valuable treatment for LEMS.

TREATMENT OF LEMS

When the diagnosis of LEMS has been confirmed, an extensive search for underlying malignancy is performed since about half the patients have underlying cancer,

[a]This work was supported by Grant No. MO 1 RR-30 from the General Clinical Research Centers Program, National Center for Research Resources, NIH, and by Grant No. FD-R-001068 from the USPHS.

usually small cell lung carcinoma (SCLC). The initial treatment is aimed at any tumor that is found since the weakness may improve dramatically with effective cancer therapy[1–3] and some patients require no further treatment for LEMS. Cholinesterase inhibitors do not usually produce significant improvement in weakness in patients with LEMS, but may reduce symptoms of dry mouth in some patients. Guanidine hydrochloride, which increases the release of acetylcholine (ACh), temporarily improves strength in many patients with LEMS,[4] but the use of this agent is limited by frequent and severe side effects.[5]

When weakness is severe, plasma exchange (PLEX)[6–9] or high-dose intravenous immunoglobulin (IVIG)[10,11] may be used to induce rapid, albeit transitory, improvement. Immunosuppressants given with or following PLEX or IVIG may prolong or sustain this improvement,[6–8] but patients with LEMS rarely become functionally normal despite aggressive immunotherapy. Because of the theoretical possibility that immunosuppression may accelerate tumor growth, there is some reluctance to use such treatments in patients who have SCLC or who have a major risk of harboring an occult cancer, such as those who have had symptoms of LEMS for less than 4 years.[12]

3,4-Diaminopyridine (DAP) has been used in the treatment of disorders of neuromuscular transmission for many years in Europe, but has undergone only limited clinical testing of safety and efficacy in this country and has not been approved for clinical use by the FDA.

MECHANISM OF ACTION OF DAP

The aminopyridines increase chemical transmission at central and peripheral synapses by increasing transmitter release.[13,14] These agents improve neuromuscular transmission by facilitating the release of ACh from the motor nerve terminal. In rat diaphragm muscle, 4-aminopyridine (4-AP) and DAP enhance transmitter release during sustained nerve stimulation at high frequencies (50/s) and block facilitation, presumably by increasing the statistical probability of release to its maximum.[15] The therapeutic action of these agents is attributed primarily to their ability to increase the releasable store of ACh and its mobilization by increasing the duration of end plate potentials[15] and muscle action potentials.[15,16] Their action requires the presence of calcium.[16] These observations are compatible with the hypothesis that aminopyridines enhance calcium entry into excitable membranes by blocking voltage-sensitive potassium channels. Since they act on central as well as peripheral synapses, aminopyridines can produce convulsions. 4-AP produces marked improvement in LEMS,[17–21] but CNS side effects, especially seizures, limit its clinical use.[22,23] DAP penetrates the CSF significantly less than does 4-AP and thus has less convulsant activity. DAP has been used in Europe to treat LEMS for many years[21,24,25] and has undergone limited testing in this country.[22,23] It has also been shown to be beneficial in some patients with myasthenia gravis[23,26] and congenital myasthenic syndromes.[27] Variable results have been reported from its use in botulism.[28–30] All previous reports indicate that most LEMS patients are significantly improved by DAP.

PHARMACOKINETICS OF AMINOPYRIDINES

4-AP is eliminated with a half-time of 3.6 ± 0.9 hours after intravenous or oral administration.[31] Sixty-five percent of a dose is excreted into the urine after 6 hours and 85% after 24 hours.[31] Peak serum levels are reached 193 ± 51 minutes after oral administration.[31]

In patients with LEMS, intravenous administration of 8 to 9 mg DAP produces clinical improvement in less than 5 minutes;[32] after oral administration, maximum improvement is seen 1.5 hours after a dose[32,33] and beneficial effects last for 3 to 8 hours. The effective oral dose is approximately three times the dose given intravenously.[12] Improvement of EMG responses is seen within 10 to 20 minutes after an oral dose, becomes maximal within 30 minutes, and persists for over 3 hours after a dose. The improvement induced by DAP is lost within 24 hours after the drug is withdrawn (personal observations).

TOXICITY OF DAP

The toxicity of the aminopyridines appears to relate directly to their effect on synaptic transmission. In mice, the LD_{50} of DAP is 13 mg/kg after intravenous injection,[34] 20 mg/kg after intraperitoneal injection,[35] and 35 mg/kg after subcutaneous administration.[35] Death in mice is due to uncontrolled convulsions.

OUR EXPERIENCE WITH DAP

We have held an IND to administer DAP to patients with myasthenia gravis (MG) and LEMS since 1987. We initially treated 19 LEMS patients with DAP in a pilot study, which demonstrated significant benefit in most patients. Based on this experience, we undertook a placebo-controlled, parallel treatment protocol to demonstrate that DAP is an effective and safe treatment for patients with LEMS. This study involves an initial double-blinded, placebo-controlled phase of DAP administration and a subsequent open-label phase during which the dose of DAP is optimized for each patient, usually with pyridostigmine. Since this study is still ongoing, results of the blinded phase are not yet known and the following conclusions include observations made during the open-label phase.

PREPARATION OF ORAL DAP

Purified DAP is obtained in powdered form from Jacobus Pharmaceuticals (Princeton, New Jersey) and packaged into hard gelatin capsules with lactose by the Duke University Medical Center Hospital Pharmacy. Capsules are stored at $-20\ ^{\circ}C$ until dispensed in light-tight containers and are kept refrigerated until used.

With my colleagues, Janice Massey and James Howard, I have treated 45 LEMS patients with DAP in the past 10 years. At the time of this writing, 40 LEMS patients had taken DAP for an average of 31 months (range, 1 to 109 months): 6 patients had taken DAP continuously for more than 5 years and 13 patients for more than 3 years. Fifteen patients had SCLC and the others had no evidence of lung cancer during the time that they have been followed. Forty-seven percent of patients achieved essentially normal function while taking DAP, but usually had some persistent fatigue or weakness. Another 38% had significantly better function in activities of daily living while taking DAP. Four patients had no benefit from DAP and 3 others noted subjective improvement, but had no significant improvement in function. Thus, 85% of LEMS patients derived functionally significant improvement from DAP.

Patients notice the onset of effect less than 30 minutes after taking a dose and the benefit from single doses lasts for 2.5 to 4 hours. The optimal dose schedule and dosage are determined empirically for each patient and are based on the patient's subjective reports of strength and function as well as on a quantitative assessment of strength that is performed at each clinic visit. Many patients notice a cumulative effect of fixed doses, with the maximum response occurring 3 to 4 days after a dose change. DAP effects begin to wear off after less than 8 hours following the last dose and have cleared entirely in less than 2 days. In some studies, it has been noted that the benefit from a fixed dose of DAP becomes less with chronic administration and that patients require occasional "drug holidays" to reestablish the optimal response to DAP.[12] We have not noted this in our patients.

Patients frequently have circumoral paresthesias after taking doses of DAP higher than 10 mg. These sensations occur within several minutes after a dose and last for 5 to 10 minutes. They do not always occur after every dose and may be more marked when DAP is taken on an empty stomach or together with pyridostigmine. Only one patient found these symptoms sufficiently unpleasant to require altering the dose. Abdominal cramps and diarrhea may occur when DAP is taken with pyridostigmine and can be minimized by reducing the dosage of pyridostigmine. Some patients have had insomnia when DAP was taken less than 2 hours before bedtime.

Seizures attributable to DAP occurred in one patient who was receiving 100 mg DAP/day. An EEG was normal before beginning DAP and within 12 hours after the seizure, which did not recur when the dose was reduced. Another patient who had cancer metastatic to the brain had seizures while taking 60 mg DAP/day. A third patient who was taking 100 mg DAP/day had seizures while receiving toxic doses of theophylline; seizures did not recur on the same dose of DAP after theophylline was discontinued.

We have found no changes in blood tests of renal, hematologic, or endocrine function in any of our patients. Transient mild elevations of blood pressure have been seen in animals receiving DAP, but this has not been reported in humans and we have not seen it in any of our patients. Asthma attacks have been reported by others after DAP was taken by patients with known asthma. Lundh *et al.* reported a patient who died of a myocardial infarction a few weeks after starting DAP for LEMS,[12] possibly secondary to a sudden increase of physical activity. There is no information about the teratogenicity or mutagenicity of DAP.

CONCLUSIONS

Most LEMS patients have improvement after starting DAP, which may be dramatic and sufficient to maintain relatively normal function in some. Experience from many years of use in other countries and from preliminary studies that we and others have carried out in the United States indicates that DAP is a safe and effective treatment for LEMS. Used alone or together with immunosuppression, it can frequently make the difference between severe disability and relatively normal function in these patients.

REFERENCES

1. JENKYN, L. R., P. L. BROOKS, R. J. FORCIER, L. H. MAURER & J. OCHOA. 1980. Remission of the Lambert-Eaton syndrome and small cell anaplastic carcinoma of the lung induced by chemotherapy and radiotherapy. Cancer **46:** 1123–1127.
2. BERGLUND, S., M. ERIKSSON, F. E. VON EYBEN, C. HELLEKANT & W. MATTSSON. 1982. Remission by chemotherapy of the Eaton-Lambert myasthenic syndrome in a patient with small cell bronchogenic carcinoma. Acta Med. Scand. **212:** 429–432.
3. CHALK, C. H., N. M. MURRAY, J. NEWSOM-DAVIS, J. H. O'NEILL & S. G. SPIRO. 1990. Response of the Lambert-Eaton myasthenic syndrome to treatment of associated small-cell lung carcinoma. Neurology **40:** 1552–1556.
4. CHERINGTON, M. 1976. Guanidine and germine in Eaton-Lambert syndrome. Neurology **26:** 944–946.
5. NORRIS, F. H., J. M. EATON & C. H. MIELKE. 1974. Depression of bone marrow by guanidine. Arch. Neurol. **30:** 184–185.
6. DAU, P. C. & E. H. DENYS. 1982. Plasmapheresis and immunosuppressive drug therapy in the Eaton-Lambert syndrome. Ann. Neurol. **11:** 570–575.
7. NEWSOM-DAVIS, J. & N. M. MURRAY. 1984. Plasma exchange and immunosuppressive drug treatment in the Lambert-Eaton myasthenic syndrome. Neurology **34:** 480–485.
8. ILLA, I., M. CODINA, P. SALISACHS & J. PRADAS. 1986. Plasmapheresis and prednisone in Lambert-Eaton syndrome. Muscle Nerve **9:** 155.
9. JOST, W. H., U. MIELKE & K. SCHIMRIGK. 1991. Therapeutic approaches to Lambert-Eaton myasthenic syndrome in the intra-individual comparison. Wien. Klin. Wochenschr. **103:** 629–632.
10. BIRD, S. J. 1992. Clinical and electrophysiologic improvement in the Lambert-Eaton syndrome with intravenous immunoglobulin therapy. Neurology **42:** 1422–1423.
11. BAIN, P. G., M. MOTOMURA, J. NEWSOM-DAVIS et al. 1996. Effects of intravenous immunoglobulin on muscle weakness and calcium-channel antibodies in the Lambert-Eaton myasthenic syndrome. Neurology **47:** 678–683.
12. LUNDH, H., O. NILSSON, I. ROSEN & S. JOHANSSON. 1993. Practical aspects of 3,4-diaminopyridine treatment of the Lambert-Eaton myasthenic syndrome. Acta Neurol. Scand. **88:** 136–140.
13. THESLEFF, S. 1980. Aminopyridines and synaptic transmission. Neuroscience **5:** 1413–1419.
14. MOLGÓ, J. 1982. Effects of aminopyridines on neuromuscular transmission. Adv. Biosci. **35:** 95–116.
15. THOMSEN, R. H. & D. F. WILSON. 1983. Effects of 4-aminopyridine and 3,4-diaminopyri-

dine on transmitter release at the neuromuscular junction. J. Pharmacol. Exp. Ther. **227:** 260–265.

16. KIM, Y. I., M. M. GOLDNER & D. B. SANDERS. 1980. Facilitatory effects of 4-aminopyridine on neuromuscular transmission in disease states. Muscle Nerve **3:** 112–119.

17. LUNDH, H., O. NILSSON & I. ROSEN. 1977. 4-Aminopyridine: a new drug tested in the treatment of Eaton-Lambert syndrome. J. Neurol. Neurosurg. Psychiatry **40:** 1109–1112.

18. AGOSTON, S., T. VAN WEERDEN, P. WESTRA & A. BROEKERT. 1978. Effects of 4-aminopyridine in Eaton-Lambert syndrome. Br. J. Anaesth. **50:** 383–385.

19. SANDERS, D. B., Y. I. KIM, J. F. HOWARD & C. A. GOETSCH. 1980. Eaton-Lambert syndrome: a clinical and electrophysiological study of a patient treated with 4-aminopyridine. J. Neurol. Neurosurg. Psychiatry **43:** 978–985.

20. MURRAY, N. M. F. & J. NEWSOM-DAVIS. 1981. Treatment with oral 4-aminopyridine in disorders of neuromuscular transmission. Neurology **31:** 265–271.

21. LUNDH, H. 1982. Therapeutic applications of aminopyridines in diseases of neuromuscular transmission. Adv. Biosci. **35:** 287–296.

22. MCEVOY, K. M., A. J. WINDEBANK, J. R. DAUBE & P. A. LOW. 1989. 3,4-Diaminopyridine in the treatment of Lambert-Eaton myasthenic syndrome. N. Engl. J. Med. **321:** 1567–1571.

23. SANDERS, D. B., J. F. HOWARD, JR. & J. M. MASSEY. 1993. 3,4-Diaminopyridine in Lambert-Eaton myasthenic syndrome and myasthenia gravis. Ann. N.Y. Acad. Sci. **681:** 588–590.

24. NEWSOM-DAVIS, J. 1986. Treatment of neuromuscular junction disorders: current status and new frontiers. Muscle Nerve **9**(suppl.): 14.

25. LUNDH, H., O. NILSSON & I. ROSEN. 1984. Treatment of Lambert-Eaton syndrome: 3,4-diaminopyridine and pyridostigmine. Neurology **34:** 1324–1330.

26. LUNDH, H., O. NILSSON & I. ROSEN. 1985. Improvement in neuromuscular transmission in myasthenia gravis by 3,4-diaminopyridine. Eur. Arch. Psychiatry Neurol. Sci. **234:** 374–377.

27. PALACE, J., C. M. WILES & J. NEWSOM-DAVIS. 1991. 3,4-Diaminopyridine in the treatment of congenital (hereditary) myasthenia. J. Neurol. Neurosurg. Psychiatry **54:** 1069–1072.

28. SIEGEL, L. S. & J. I. PRICE. 1987. Ineffectiveness of 3,4-diaminopyridine as a therapy for type C botulism. Toxicon **25:** 1015–1018.

29. DAVIS, L. E., J. K. JOHNSON, J. M. BICKNELL, H. LEVY & K. M. MCEVOY. 1992. Human type A botulism and treatment with 3,4-diaminopyridine. Electromyogr. Clin. Neurophysiol. **32:** 379–383.

30. HOWARD, J. F., A. S. WEISS, M. K. DONOVAN, W. P. CHESHIRE & T. G. BRAUN. 1992. 3,4-Diaminopyridine effects on compound muscle action amplitudes in a patient with botulism. Muscle Nerve **15:** 1202–1203.

31. UGES, D. R. A., Y. J. SOHN, B. GREIJDANUS, A. H. J. SCAF & S. AGOSTON. 1982. 4-Aminopyridine kinetics. Clin. Pharmacol. Ther. **31:** 587–593.

32. LUNDH, H., O. NILSSON & I. ROSEN. 1983. Novel drug of choice in Eaton-Lambert syndrome. J. Neurol. Neurosurg. Psychiatry **46:** 684–687.

33. MURRAY, N. M. F., J. NEWSOM-DAVIS, Y. KARNI & C. M. WILES. 1984. Oral 3,4-diaminopyridine in the treatment of the Lambert-Eaton myasthenic syndrome (LEMS) [abstract]. J. Neurol. Neurosurg. Psychiatry **47:** 1052–1053.

34. LECHAT, P., M. DEYSSON, M. LEMEIGNAN & M. ADOLPHE. 1968. Toxicité aiguë composee de quelques aminopyridines in vivo (souris) et in vitro (cultures cellulaires). Ann. Pharm. Fr. **26:** 345–349.

35. VOHRA, M. M. & S. N. PRADHAN. 1964. Pharmacology of 3,4-diaminopyridine. Arch. Int. Pharmacodyn. Ther. **150:** 413–424.

A Treatment Algorithm for Lambert-Eaton Myasthenic Syndrome

JOHN NEWSOM-DAVIS

Neurosciences Group
Institute of Molecular Medicine
John Radcliffe Hospital
University of Oxford
Headington, Oxford OX3 9DU, United Kingdom

The Lambert-Eaton myasthenic syndrome (LEMS) is an antibody-mediated autoimmune disease characterized by muscle weakness, depressed tendon reflexes, posttetanic potentiation, and autonomic dysfunction that can include dry mouth, constipation, and erectile impotence in males.[1] About 60% of patients have a small cell lung cancer that may not become radiologically evident for at least 2 years after the onset of the neurological syndrome, and sometimes for as long as 5 years.[2] In the remainder, who are typically nonsmokers, no clear neoplastic association has been established, although lymphoma may occur at slightly increased frequency.[3]

Voltage-gated calcium channels (VGCCs) of the P/Q subtype appear to be the primary targets for the IgG autoantibodies.[4,5] At the neuromuscular junction, the autoantibodies downregulate motor nerve terminal VGCCs, reducing the number of acetylcholine quanta released by each nerve impulse. Anti-P/Q-type VGCC antibodies also interfere with postganglionic sympathetic and parasympathetic function,[6] which is likely to account for the autonomic symptoms.

LEMS is diagnosed by the presence of serum anti-P/Q-type VGCC antibodies, detected in over 90% of patients by radioimmunoassay using ^{125}I-ω-conotoxin MVIIC.[4,5] In addition, patients show a characteristic reduction in the CMAP amplitude and a striking enhancement following voluntary activation.[7] Some patients who are "seronegative" for anti-P/Q-type VGCC antibodies may nevertheless have an antibody-mediated disorder since they appear to respond to immunological treatment.

An algorithm for the treatment of LEMS is proposed in FIGURE 1. 3,4-Diaminopyridine (3,4-DAP) will virtually always produce symptomatic improvement. Its benefits, and relative lack of serious side effects at recommended dosage, have been well documented.[8,9] It acts by blocking voltage-gated potassium channels, thereby prolonging the action potential at motor nerve terminals and lengthening the open time of the VGCCs.[10] The consequent increased influx of Ca^{2+} results in a greater quantal release of transmitter, compensating for the reduced number of functional VGCCs. A starting dose (in adults) of 10 mg given four or five times daily can be increased to a maximum daily dose of 80–100 mg if necessary. Most patients experience perioral and distal parasthesias about an hour after drug ingestion. Overdosage results in central excitation and seizures. Seizures have very occasionally been reported at recommended dosage. When 3,4-DAP is unavailable, guanidine should be considered.[11] Although this medication is unquestionably effective, side effects can be serious, in-

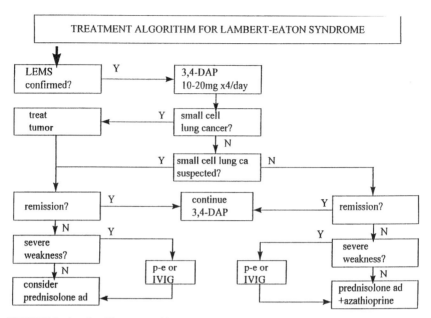

FIGURE 1. An algorithm to provide an outline guide to therapy in the Lambert-Eaton myasthenic syndrome.

cluding bone marrow suppression, renal failure, atrial fibrillation, and dermatitis. Patients can also have some of the central excitatory effects of 3,4-DAP.

Some LEMS patients find that the addition of pyridostigmine (30–60 mg given five times daily) to 3,4-DAP treatment is beneficial.

PATIENTS WITH SMALL CELL LUNG CANCER (SC-LEMS)

In patients with small cell lung cancer (SCLC), treatment of the tumor will be implemented in its own right, but an added benefit is the improvement that this is likely to induce in the neurological disorder. Chalk et al.[12] showed that 7 of 11 SC-LEMS cases surviving specific tumor therapy by more than 2 months subsequently showed progressive improvement in their neurological symptoms. This was confirmed by the parallel recovery in the CMAP amplitudes, which in all patients studied had returned to the normal range within 6–12 months of starting therapy. The specific tumor therapy included chemotherapy, surgical resection, and local radiotherapy. The longest surviving patient underwent right lower lobectomy and local radiotherapy over 12 years ago and remains free of tumor recurrence and features of LEMS. The explanation for this unexpectedly long survival probably lies with the evidence that LEMS IgG blocks K^+-stimulated Ca^{2+} influx into SCLC cell lines,[13,14] suggesting that tumor VGCCs provoke the anti-VGCC antibody response. Treatment of the tumor, especially its surgical removal, would presumably reduce—or even eliminate—antigenic driving of the autoantibody response. Histological examination of the tumor in SCLC cases reveals a far greater degree of macrophage infiltration than in SCLC tumors from non-LEMS patients, implicating the tumor as the initial site of antibody production in SC-LEMS cases.[15]

If treatment of the tumor has resulted in remission, no further action other than continuing 3,4-DAP need be taken (FIGURE 1). When remission does not develop, however, further immunotherapy should be considered. Prednisolone may induce improvement and would not be contraindicated by the continued presence of tumor. It can be prescribed in doses up to 1–1.5 mg/kg body weight on alternate days; the use of corticosteroids on alternate days may reduce the risk of side effects. I have tended to avoid using azathioprine in this group because of its likely slowness in exerting an effect, typically 15 months or more.

Respiratory and bulbar muscle weakness can occasionally be life-threatening in LEMS patients. In patients with such severe weakness, plasma exchange (plasmapheresis) can produce a short-term benefit when given as a 5-day course.[16] The improvement in muscle strength develops after a longer time interval (about 10 days) than is the case in myasthenia gravis, where the response is typically evident within 2 days.[17] This observation might suggest a slower turnover rate for VGCCs as compared with acetylcholine receptors. The improvement attributable to plasma exchange will only last for a few weeks, so additional corticosteroid treatment will be needed.

We[18] have shown that intravenous immunoglobulin treatment is beneficial in the short term in LEMS patients without evidence of cancer (NC-LEMS), as discussed below; there is no a priori reason why such therapy should not also be effective in SC-LEMS patients.

PATIENTS IN WHOM SMALL CELL LUNG CANCER IS SUSPECTED

These patients will be cigarette smokers in whom no tumor can be detected. They will need to be rescanned at regular intervals even after 5 years because of the rare reports of SCLC becoming apparent after this interval. The long survival of such patients, in the presence of cancer that is typically highly malignant, implies that the anti-VGCC antibodies may be playing a role in controlling tumor growth or, alternatively, that the small cell cancers that provoke LEMS may be more highly differentiated (and slower growing) than is usually the case with these tumors.

PATIENTS WITHOUT SMALL CELL LUNG CANCER (NC-LEMS)

This group will principally comprise nonsmokers, or smokers with an LEMS history of <10 years. If 3,4-DAP medication has satisfactorily controlled symptoms, no further treatment will be needed other than its continuation (FIGURE 1). In the remainder who require further treatment, plasma exchange can be undertaken as immediate treatment if weakness is severe.[16] Alternatively, intravenous immunoglobulin (IVIG) could be considered, which has been reported to be beneficial in individual case reports.[19,20] In our recently completed double-blind crossover trial of IVIG infusion (1 g/kg body weight given on 2 consecutive days; total dose of 2 g/kg body weight) in 9 patients,[18] there was a significant increase in strength measures on the active preparation as compared with placebo (albumin). Each arm of the trial lasted 8 weeks, and the interval between the first and second limbs of the trial for the first 4 patients was 14–18 weeks, but in the remainder the crossover was immediate. Statistically significant improvement in strength measures was evident. This was first observed at 2 weeks, was at its best at 2–4 weeks, and was declining by 8 weeks. Anti-P/Q-type VGCC antibodies were measured throughout both arms of the trial. A clear-cut and significant reduction in mean titer was seen at 2–6 weeks (but not at 1 week) in the active arm of the trial, the time course being inversely related to the improvement in muscle strength. No change in titer was seen during the placebo arm.

How the IVIG was able to depress anti-P/Q-type VGCC antibody levels is not clear. The effect did not seem to be a direct anti-idiotypic neutralization of anti-VGCC antibodies since it was not observed at 1 week, although it was well developed by 2 weeks. Moreover, we were unable to demonstrate *in vitro* inhibition by the IVIG preparation of anti-VGCC antibody binding in the radioimmunoassay.[18]

In practical terms, IVIG treatment as used in the trial can be expected usefully to increase muscle strength for 6–8 weeks. We do not have objective evidence either for or against the repeated use as long-term therapy, although uncontrolled observations in a few patients do not suggest any cumulative benefit.

In those with significant symptoms despite 3,4-DAP, long-term treatment with prednisolone and/or azathioprine should be considered (FIGURE 1). Clinical improvement was inversely related to the anti-P/Q-type antibody response in a longitudinal study of a patient with NC-LEMS treated with prednisolone.[21] The effectiveness of combined prednisolone and azathioprine therapy in LEMS has been demonstrated in a retrospective study,[16] but has not been subjected to a prospective randomized controlled trial. However, such a trial in a related disorder (myasthenia gravis) clearly demonstrated that combined treatment with prednisolone and azathioprine was more effective than treatment with prednisolone alone.[22]

When remission has been obtained in LEMS patients receiving prednisolone plus azathioprine therapy, the dose for prednisolone should be tapered to the minimum required to maintain remission. It is not usually possibly to fully withdraw medication without symptoms returning. Patients receiving azathioprine require full blood count and liver function tests weekly for 8 weeks and then monthly for 3 months thereafter. In non-SC patients who are unable to tolerate azathioprine, oral cyclosporine or methotrexate therapy can be considered.

CONCLUSIONS

All patients with LEMS, whether a tumor is present or not, will benefit from 3,4-DAP. When this medication is not available, guanidine can be considered as an alternative, but the risk of side effects is much greater. Subsequent therapy will depend on whether or not the patient has an SCLC. Specific tumor therapy will often improve muscle strength, which is reflected in recovery in the CMAP amplitude. Severely weak patients in either group will benefit from plasma exchange or IVIG. Prednisolone treatment should be considered in patients with SC-LEMS who are unresponsive to 3,4-DAP and specific tumor therapy. Prednisolone combined with azathioprine is appropriate long-term treatment in NC-LEMS patients who are not adequately controlled by 3,4-DAP alone.

REFERENCES

1. LANG, B. & J. NEWSOM-DAVIS. 1995. Immunotherapy of the Lambert-Eaton myasthenic syndrome. Springer Semin. Immunopathol. **17:** 3–15.
2. O'NEILL, J. H., N. M. MURRAY & J. NEWSOM-DAVIS. 1988. The Lambert-Eaton myasthenic syndrome: a review of 50 cases. Brain **11:** 577–597.
3. ARGOV, Z., Y. SHAPIRA & I. WIRGUIN. 1994. Lambert-Eaton myasthenic syndrome (LEMS) in lymphoproliferative disorders (LPD). J. Neurol. **241:** S36,
4. MOTOMURA, M., I. JOHNSTON, B. LANG, A. VINCENT & J. NEWSOM-DAVIS. 1995. An improved diagnostic assay for Lambert-Eaton myasthenic syndrome. J. Neurol. Neurosurg. Psychiatry **58:** 85–87.
5. LENNON, V. A., T. J. KRYZER, G. E. GRIESMANN, P. E. O'SUILLEABHAIN, A. J. WINDEBANK, A. WOPPMAN, G. P. MILJANICH & E. H. LAMBERT. 1995. Calcium-channel antibodies in the Lambert-Eaton syndrome and other paraneoplastic syndromes. N. Engl. J. Med. **332:** 1467–1474.
6. WATERMAN, S. A., B. LANG & J. NEWSOM-DAVIS. 1997. Effect of Lambert-Eaton myasthenic syndrome antibodies on autonomic neurons in the mouse. Ann. Neurol. **42:** 147–156.
7. LAMBERT, E. H., E. D. ROOKE, L. M. EATON & C. H. HODGSON. 1961. Myasthenic syndrome occasionally associated with bronchial neoplasm: neurophysiologic studies. *In* Myasthenia Gravis, pp. 362–410. Thomas. Springfield, Illinois.
8. LUNDH, H., O. NILSSON & J. ROSEN. 1977. 4-Aminopyridine—a new drug tested in the treatment of Eaton-Lambert syndrome. J. Neurol. Neurosurg. Psychiatry **40:** 1109–1112.
9. MCEVOY, K. M., A. J. WINDEBANK, J. R. DAUBE & P. A. LOW. 1989. 3,4-Diaminopyridine in the treatment of Lambert-Eaton myasthenic syndrome. N. Engl. J. Med. **321:** 1567–1571.
10. MOLGO, J., H. LUNDH & S. THESLEFF. 1980. Potency of 3,4-diaminopyridine and 4-aminopyridine on mammalian neuromuscular transmission and the effect of pH changes. Eur. J. Pharmacol. **61:** 25–34.
11. OH, S. J. & K. W. KIM. 1973. Guanidine hydrochloride in the Eaton-Lambert syndrome: electrophysiologic improvement. Neurology **23:** 1084–1090.
12. CHALK, C. H., N. M. MURRAY, J. NEWSOM-DAVIS, J. H. O'NEILL & S. G. SPIRO. 1990. Response of the Lambert-Eaton myasthenic syndrome to treatment of associated small-cell lung carcinoma. Neurology **40:** 1552–1556.
13. ROBERTS, A., S. PERERA, B. LANG, A. VINCENT & J. NEWSOM-DAVIS. 1985. Paraneoplastic myasthenic syndrome IgG inhibits $^{45}Ca^{2+}$ flux in a human small cell carcinoma line. Nature **317:** 737–739.
14. DE AIZPURUA, H. J., E. H. LAMBERT, G. E. GRIESMANN, B. O. OLIVERA & V. A. LENNON. 1988. Antagonism of voltage-gated calcium channels in small cell carcinomas of patients with and without Lambert-Eaton myasthenic syndrome by autoantibodies, ω-conotoxin, and adenosine. Cancer Res. **48:** 4719–4724.
15. MORRIS, C. S., M. M. ESIRI, A. MARX & J. NEWSOM-DAVIS. 1992. Immunocytochemical

characteristics of small cell lung carcinoma associated with the Lambert-Eaton myasthenic syndrome. Am. J. Pathol. **140:** 839–845.

16. NEWSOM-DAVIS, J. & N. M. MURRAY. 1984. Plasma exchange and immunosuppressive drug treatment in the Lambert-Eaton myasthenic syndrome. Neurology **34:** 480–485.

17. NEWSOM-DAVIS, J., A. J. PINCHING, A. VINCENT & S. G. WILSON. 1978. Function of circulating antibody to acetylcholine receptor in myasthenia gravis: investigation by plasma exchange. Neurology **28:** 266–272.

18. BAIN, P. G., M. MOTOMURA, J. NEWSOM-DAVIS, S. A. MISBAH, H. M. CHAPEL, M. L. LEE, A. VINCENT & B. LANG. 1996. Effects of intravenous immunoglobulin on muscle weakness and calcium-channel autoantibodies in the Lambert-Eaton myasthenic syndrome. Neurology **47:** 678–683.

19. BIRD, S. J. 1992. Clinical and electrophysiologic improvement in Lambert-Eaton syndrome with intravenous immunoglobulin therapy. Neurology **42:** 1422–1423.

20. TAKANO, H., M. TANAKA, R. KOIKE, H. NAGAI, M. ARAKAWA & S. TSUJI. 1994. Effect of intravenous immunoglobulin in Lambert-Eaton myasthenic syndrome with small cell lung cancer: correlation with the titer of anti-voltage-gated calcium channel antibody. Muscle Nerve **17:** 1073–1075.

21. MOTOMURA, M., B. LANG, I. JOHNSTON, J. PALACE, A. VINCENT & J. NEWSOM-DAVIS. 1997. The incidence of serum anti-P/Q-type and anti-N-type calcium channel autoantibodies in the Lambert-Eaton myasthenic syndrome. J. Neurol. Sci. **147:** 35–42.

22. PALACE, J., J. NEWSOM-DAVIS, B. LECKY & MYASTHENIA STUDY GROUP. 1996. A multicenter, randomized, double-blind trial of prednisolone plus azathioprine versus prednisolone plus placebo in myasthenia gravis. Neurology **46:** A332.

Lambert-Eaton Myasthenic Syndrome (LEMS)

Clinical and Electrodiagnostic Features and Response to Therapy in 59 Patients

RICHARD W. TIM, JANICE M. MASSEY, AND
DONALD B. SANDERS

Duke University Medical Center
Durham, North Carolina 27710

INTRODUCTION

The Lambert-Eaton myasthenic syndrome (LEMS) is a rare autoimmune presynaptic disorder of neuromuscular transmission, which has an association with bronchial neoplasms.[1] We reviewed the records of 59 patients with LEMS seen at Duke University Medical Center since 1986 and present our clinical experience.

RESULTS

There were 25 males and 34 females. The age of symptom onset ranged from 8 to 84 years; the mean was 56 years. The diagnosis of LEMS was based upon a combination of symptoms and signs including proximal muscle weakness, hyporeflexia or areflexia, autonomic dysfunction (dry mouth, dry eyes, or orthostatic hypotension), and abnormalities in repetitive nerve stimulation studies. Twenty-four patients were diagnosed with small cell carcinoma of the lung (SCLC). In 18, the diagnosis of LEMS was made from 1 week to 20 months (mean, 4.1 months) before the diagnosis of SCLC. Of the 6 patients in whom SCLC was diagnosed before LEMS, 2 had symptoms of LEMS for 2 and 7 months, respectively, before lung cancer was diagnosed.

Fifty-one patients had tests for antibodies to the acetylcholine receptor (AChRAbs), which gave normal results in 49. Binding AChRAbs were elevated in an 8-year-old female (0.04 nmol/L, reference range ≤ 0.02) and in a 50-year-old male (0.12 nmol/L). Both patients had markedly elevated levels of antibodies to the voltage-gated calcium channel (VGCC). Antibodies to the VGCC were elevated in 14 of 20 patients in whom measurements were done (4 of 5 with SCLC).

The responses to therapy for LEMS were graded as follows (see FIGURE 1):

marked—the patient noted very little weakness or fatigue in daily activities;
moderate—significant improvement in activities of daily living (e.g., from being nonambulatory to ambulatory);
mild—a sense of improved strength, but no changes in functional status.

Patients

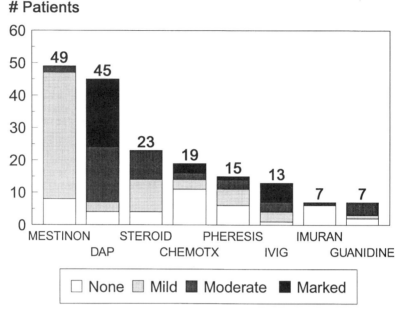

FIGURE 1. The graded responses to therapies in 59 LEMS patients. Terms: DAP = 3,4-di-aminopyridine, Steroid = prednisone, Chemotx = chemotherapy for small cell lung cancer, Pheresis = plasmapheresis, IVIG = intravenous immunoglobulin.

Mestinon (pyridostigmine bromide) was used in 49 patients and produced mild improvement in strength in 80% and no benefit in 16%. Many patients reported that Mestinon improved their dry mouth. No patient had marked improvement with Mestinon alone.

Forty-five patients were treated with 3,4-diaminopyridine (DAP), usually in combination with Mestinon: improvement was marked in 47%, moderate in 38%, and mild in 7%. When Mestinon was given to patients taking DAP, they often reported increased strength, which had not been noted with Mestinon alone, or prolongation of the effect of DAP. Three patients had seizures while on DAP. One was taking 100 mg per day and her seizures did not recur when the dose was reduced. Another patient had SCLC metastatic to brain when the seizures began, and the third had toxic blood levels of theophylline.

Twenty-three patients were treated with high-dose daily prednisone: 84% of these had mild to moderate improvement in strength, which did not persist when the steroid dose was reduced. Of the 15 patients treated with plasmapheresis, 1 had marked, but transient improvement in strength; 5 had mild benefit; and 6 (40%) had no benefit. In the 13 patients treated with intravenous immunoglobulin (IVIG), 46% had marked improvement and 23% had moderate improvement. Responses to IVIG were not sustained. In the 19 patients undergoing chemotherapy for SCLC, 16% had marked improvement in strength and 58% had no improvement. Seven patients had been treated with guanidine. Four reported moderate benefit, which did not persist as therapy continued.

In 51 patients, repetitive nerve stimulation (RNS) studies were performed in the abductor pollicis brevis (APB), abductor digiti quinti (ADQ), and extensor digitorum brevis (EDB) muscles. There was an abnormal decrement to 3-Hz RNS in both hand muscles in 98% of the patients. Baseline compound muscle action potential (CMAP) amplitude was low in the ADQ in 94% and low in the APB in 96%. In 1 patient, the CMAP amplitudes were within control range in all three muscles. CMAP amplitude potentiation after 10–15 seconds of maximum voluntary contraction (MVC) was 100% or greater in the ADQ in 78% of the patients and in at least one of the three tested muscles in 88%. Potentiation was greater than or equal to 100% in all three muscles in only 39% of the patients. The largest post-MVC potentiation was seen in the ADQ in 51% of the patients. RNS was performed in the trapezius muscle in 29 patients. There was an abnormal decrement to 3-Hz RNS in 90%, and a 100% or greater post-MVC potentiation in 24%. Potentiation was never greater in the trapezius than in the other tested muscles (see FIGURE 2).

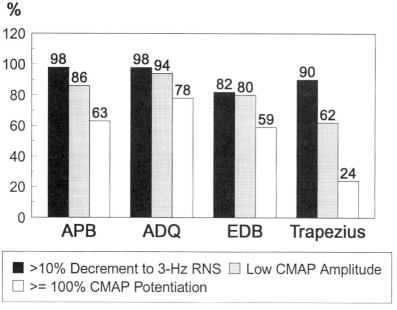

FIGURE 2. Prevalence of electrophysiologic abnormalities in 51 LEMS patients. Testing consisted of measuring the baseline compound motor action potential (CMAP) amplitude, the decrement in the CMAP amplitude to a 3-Hz train of supramaximal stimuli delivered to the appropriate nerve, and the CMAP amplitude potentiation after 10–15 seconds of maximum voluntary activity. All 51 were tested in the APB, ADQ, and EDB muscles; 29 were also tested in the trapezius. Terms: APB = abductor pollicis brevis, ADQ = abductor digiti quinti (hand), EDB = extensor digitorum brevis.

DISCUSSION

Many of these patients were referred to us for inclusion in a treatment trial of DAP. Patients with advanced, unresponsive, or poorly responsive SCLC or patients who had a good response to other treatment modalities were not likely to be referred to us. This certainly could have affected our analysis of the response to treatment, and our experience should not be used to directly compare one treatment modality to another.

CMAP amplitude potentiation of 100% or greater is an arbitrary criterion frequently used in diagnosing LEMS. Twelve percent of our LEMS patients did not meet this criterion in any of the three muscles tested, and only 39% met it in all three muscles. The diagnosis of LEMS should be based upon clinical criteria in conjunction with CMAP potentiation and VGCC antibody measurements.

REFERENCE

1. LAMBERT, E. H., L. M. EATON & E. D. ROOKE. 1956. Defect of neuromuscular conduction associated with malignant neoplasms. Am. J. Physiol. **187:** 612–613.

Wide Spectrum of Symptomatic Treatment in Lambert-Eaton Myasthenic Syndrome

SHIN J. OH, DAE S. KIM, KEE H. KWON, ANNA TSENG,
HOLLY MUSSELL, AND GWEN C. CLAUSSEN

Department of Neurology
University of Alabama at Birmingham
Veterans Affairs Hospital
Birmingham, Alabama 35294

The best drug for symptomatic treatment of Lambert-Eaton myasthenic syndrome (LEMS) is considered to be 3,4-diaminopyridine (DAP).[1,2] Unfortunately, this drug is not commonly available in many parts of the world, including the United States. Thus, an alternative choice of medications becomes necessary for symptomatic relief in this disorder. We report here our experience with pyridostigmine, guanidine, and 3,4-DAP in LEMS.

PATIENTS AND METHODS

The diagnosis of LEMS was based on clinical features (easy fatigability, proximal leg weakness, and diminished or absent muscle stretch reflexes), together with the classic triad of findings on the repetitive nerve stimulation (RNS) test—low compound muscle action potential amplitude, abnormal decremental response (>7%) at 2–5 Hz stimulation rate, and abnormal incremental response (>100%) at 50 Hz stimulation rate. Severity of disease was graded according to the strength of pelvic girdle muscles: 0 (asymptomatic), 5 MRC scale; I (mild), 4; II (moderate), 3; III (severe), 0–2. When the clinical severity was improved by one grade, symptomatic treatment was defined as satisfactory.

Among 31 patients with LEMS, 14 patients (6 males and 8 females, ranging in age from 28 to 75 years) were selected for this study because all had symptomatic treatment with various drugs for more than 3 months. Seven of the 14 patients were known to have cancer—small cell lung cancer (SCLC) in 6 and thyroid medullary cancer in 1.

Anticancer treatment was provided to all patients with cancer. In noncancer patients, symptomatic treatment with drugs alone was offered first. If this was not effective, immunotherapy was added. Pyridostigmine was tried as the first drug in all cases. If the result was not satisfactory, low-dose guanidine was added. If guanidine and pyridostigmine were not helpful, 3,4-DAP was used as an experimental drug during the past 2 years.

RESULTS

Pyridostigmine alone was tried to maximum benefit in 6 patients, including 2 who could not take guanidine because of adverse side reactions (TABLE 1). Of 3 patients

TABLE 1. Clinical Features and Treatment Effects of Pyridostigmine, Guanidine, and 3,4-Diaminopyridine[a]

Case No.	Sex/Age	Associated Tumor	Duration of Therapy (months)	Guanidine Dose (mg/day)	Pyridostigmine Dose (mg/day)	3,4-DAP Dose (mg/day)	Side Reactions	Clinical Improvement[b]	Concomitant Treatment	Immunotherapy, Cancer Treatment	Final Treatment
Guanidine and Pyridostigmine											
1	F/46	(−)	20	187.5–375	180		none	II–0	none	none	remission
2	F/26	(−)	10 (7 + 3)	1875[c] 375	480–1200		fainting spell GI upset[e]	II–I	none	thymectomy PE	PS, IVIG
3	F/53	SCLC	55	375–1500[f] (625–750)	240–600		nausea, vomiting	II–0	none	surgery, chemotherapy	G, PS
4	M/58	thyroid cancer	48	750–2500 (1000)[f]	none[d]		tingling fingers, insomnia, diarrhea	I–0	none	surgery	G
5	M/70	(−)	5	375	240		nausea, epigastric pain[e]	I–0	prednisone, 7.5 mg/day	prednisone	PS, prednisone
6	M/75	(−)	12	375–500	180–240		abdominal pain[e]	II–I	none	none	3,4-DAP
7	F/59	(−)	57	500–750	240–420		none	II–0	ATP, 100 mg/day	IVIG	G & ATP
8	F/36	(−)	102	500	240–360		none	II–0	none	PE	G
9	M/53	SCLC	36	625	360		tingling sensation	II–0	none	radiation	G, PS
10	F/72	SCLC	7	400	360		none	III–II	prednisone, 20 mg/day	PE, IVIG, chemotherapy	G, PS, prednisone

Pyridostigmine

2[h]	F/26	(–)	120	none	480–1200	II–I	none	thymectomy, PE	PS, IVIG
5[h]	M/70	(–)	36	none	240	I–0	prednisone, 7.5 mg/day	prednisone	PS, prednisone, died from LEMS
11	F/69	(–)	5	epigastric pain	240[g]	III–II	prednisone, 60 mg/day	PE, IVIG	PE, IVIG
12	M/56	SCLC	24	none	360	I–0	none	chemotherapy	PS
13	F/57	SCLC	18	none	180	I–0	prednisone, 10 mg/day	PE, chemotherapy	PS, prednisone, died from SCLC
14	M/64	SCLC	11	none	420	I–0	none	chemotherapy	PS

3,4-Diaminopyridine

6[h]	M/75	(–)	12	tingling sensation	35	1–0	none	none	3,4-DAP

[a] Abbreviations: PE, plasma exchange; IVIG, intravenous immunoglobulin; ATP, azathioprine; DAP, diaminopyridine; G, guanidine; PS, pyridostigmine.
[b] Clinical improvement was graded according to the change in the iliopsoas muscle power in MRC grade.
[c] Initial high dose (1875 mg/day) produced frequent fainting and had to be discontinued. Low dose (375 mg/day) was tried 10 years later and again was discontinued due to GI trouble.
[d] Pyridostigmine produced severe abdominal cramping pain and could not be used in this case.
[e] Guanidine was discontinued due to the side reactions.
[f] At the beginning, more than 1000 mg was given. This was soon followed by 1000 mg or less.
[g] Initially, guanidine (500 mg/day) was given together with pyridostigmine. Inadvertently, guanidine was discontinued. Pyridostigmine was given alone. This had to be discontinued due to side reactions.
[h] These are cases in which other medications were tried.

with mild (I) severity of LEMS and SCLC, this drug induced satisfactory symptomatic improvement in 2 cases and in the third when accompanied by prednisone. In
all 3 patients, SCLC was controlled with chemotherapy. In 1 patient (case 11), pyridostigmine alone was given along with a high dose of prednisone, but this combination had to be discontinued because of GI side reactions. Shortly thereafter, this patient developed adult respiratory syndrome and died. In this case, another drug was
given in place of guanidine inadvertently by the local internist. Of 2 patients (cases 2
and 5) who could not take guanidine, satisfactory improvement was noted with intermittent IVIG in 1 and with prednisone in the other.

Pyridostigmine and low-dose guanidine (1000 mg/day) were tried in 10 patients
(TABLE 1).[3] In all cases, pyridostigmine was given first to maximum benefit and then
guanidine was added between pyridostigmine doses. All patients improved at least to
the point that they did not require assistance in their usual activities, and 6 experienced improvement in strength to near-normal levels. None of these patients developed any serious bone marrow suppression or renal dysfunction during an average
34-month follow-up period. Because of side reactions, 2 patients stopped guanidine
and preferred pyridostigmine alone: 1 became symptom-free with prednisone. In 1
patient, 3,4-DAP was tried because of side reactions to guanidine and pyridostigmine. In 3, guanidine alone was enough to sustain an improved state. In 1 patient, remission was induced after 20 months of treatment. Most of the tested patients
showed electrophysiological improvement after treatment. All RNS test parameters
improved in all 5 tested cases. Among these, the compound muscle action potential
(CMAP) amplitude showed the most definite change, demonstrating a 96–900% improvement. Although responses to low and high rates of stimulation also showed improvement, the degree of change was not as dramatic as that of the initial CMAP. The
SFEMG was performed in 3 cases: 2 showed a definite improvement in all parameters, but the third showed no essential change after treatment despite clear evidence
of clinical improvement.

In 1 patient (case 6) who could not take pyridostigmine, guanidine, or prednisone
because of side reactions, 3,4-DAP was tried as an experimental drug in a random
double-blind test comparing this drug with a placebo. In this case, unequivocal benefit was documented with 3,4-DAP. Subsequently, with 35 mg of 3,4-DAP daily, satisfactory clinical improvement was achieved, together with improvement on SFEMG
and RNS tests and no serious side reactions.

DISCUSSION

Our study clearly showed that satisfactory symptomatic treatment can be achieved
in almost all LEMS patients with various options of pyridostigmine, guanidine, and
3,4-DAP. Although anticholinesterase is reported to have only a limited effect in
LEMS,[4] our study showed that, in some mild LEMS cases, pyridostigmine alone is
enough to induce a satisfactory symptomatic treatment when LEMS is stable with
immunotherapy or anticancer therapy. Our study also showed that combination therapy with pyridostigmine and low-dose guanidine (<1000 mg/day) is a relatively safe
and effective therapy for symptomatic treatment of LEMS, confirming the previous
findings[5,6] of a strong synergistic effect of pyridostigmine on guanidine based on the

clinical and electrophysiological improvement in a patient with LEMS. We were able to avoid serious side reactions of bone marrow suppression in early stages of treatment and renal insufficiency in later stages of treatment associated with guanidine by using a dose of less than 1000 mg/day, yet still achieving a significant clinical and electrophysiological improvement by combining liberal doses of pyridostigmine. Thus, we conclude that pyridostigmine alone or in combination with low-dose guanidine can be used as an alternative symptomatic treatment for LEMS when 3,4-DAP is not readily available. In a single patient who could not take pyridostigmine or guanidine, we confirmed the effectiveness of 3,4-DAP.

REFERENCES

1. NILSSON, L. H. & R. I. JOHANSSON. 1993. Practical aspect of 3,4-diaminopyridine treatment of the Lambert-Eaton myasthenic syndrome. Acta Neurol. Scand. **88:** 136–140.
2. MCEVOY, K. M., A. J. WINDERBANK, J. R. DAUBE & P. A. LOW. 1989. 3,4-Diaminopyridine in the treatment of Lambert-Eaton myasthenic syndrome. N. Engl. J. Med. **321:** 1567–1571.
3. OH, S. J., D. S. KIM, T. C. HEAD & G. C. CLAUSSEN. 1997. Low-dose guanidine and pyridostigmine: relatively safe and effective long-term symptomatic therapy in Lambert-Eaton myasthenic syndrome. Muscle Nerve **20:** 1146–1152.
4. LAMBERT, E. H. 1966. Defects of neuromuscular transmission in syndromes other than myasthenia gravis. Ann. N.Y. Acad. Sci. **135:** 367–384.
5. OH, S. J. & K. W. KIM. 1973. Guanidine hydrochloride in the Eaton-Lambert syndrome. Neurology **23:** 1084–1090.
6. HENRIKSSON, K. G., O. NILSSON, I. ROSEN & H. H. SCHILLER. 1977. Clinical, neurophysiological, and morphological findings in Eaton-Lambert syndrome. Acta Neurol. Scand. **56:** 117–140.

Index of Contributors